Histocompatibility Testing 1984

Report on the Ninth International Histocompatibility Workshop and Conference
Held in Munich, West Germany, May 6–11, 1984
and in Vienna, Austria, May 13–15, 1984

Edited by
E.D. Albert M.P. Baur W.R. Mayr

Coeditors* and Organizing Committee
E.D. Albert, Munich M.P. Baur, Düsseldorf J. Bertrams*, Essen
S. Goldmann*, Ulm H. Grosse-Wilde*, Essen W.R. Mayr, Vienna
G. Opelz*, Heidelberg C. Rittner*, Bonn D.J. Schendel*, Munich
S. Scholz*, Munich R. Wank*, Munich

With 226 Figures and 432 Tables

Springer-Verlag
Berlin Heidelberg New York Tokyo

Professor Dr. Ekkehard D. Albert
Labor für Immungenetik, Kinderpoliklinik der Universität
Pettenkoferstraße 8a, 8000 München 2
Bundesrepublik Deutschland

Priv.-Doz. Dr. Max P. Baur
Diabetes Forschungsinstitut an der Universität, Biometrische Abteilung
Auf'm Hennekamp 65, 4000 Düsseldorf 1
Bundesrepublik Deutschland

Professor Dr. Wolfgang R. Mayr
Institut für Blutgruppenserologie der Universität
Spitalgasse 4, 1090 Wien
Österreich

Library of Congress Cataloging in Publication Data. International Histocompatibility Workshop and Conference (9th: 1984: Munich, Germany and Vienna, Austria) Histocompatibility testing 1984. 1. Histocompatibility testing–Congresses. I. Albert, E. D. (Ekkehard D.) II. Baur, M. P. (Max Peter), 1948– . III. Mayr, W. R. (Wolfgang Richard), 1944– . IV. Title.
QR184.3.I56 1984 616.07'9 84-26847
ISBN-13:978-3-642-69772-2 e-ISBN13:978-3-642-69770-8
DOI: 10.1007/978-3-642-69770-8

Softcover reprint of the hardcover 1st edition 1984

Offsetprinting and Binding: K. Triltsch, Würzburg/Germany

2123/3140-5 4 3 2 1 0

Acknowledgements

We would like to express our sincere gratitude to all the co-workers who have contributed so much to the production of this book. In the first place we thank our secretaries Ms. Petra Heinle (Munich) and Ms. Barbara Quernhorst (Düsseldorf) for their untiring help in organizing the conference, in taking on menial tasks like typing hundreds of tables, and in providing moral support when difficult decisions had to be made.
We gratefully acknowledge the enormous efforts of Ms. A. McNicholas, Ms. E. Keller, and Dr. S. Scholz in changing the entire book to the new nomenclature, in looking up endless numbers of addresses and references, and in proof-reading and correcting all contributions. Last but not least, we admire the friendly and efficient attitude of Ms. B. Montenbruck, Mr. D. Roseveare, and Mr. H. Schwaninger at Springer-Verlag, who had to put up with all our wishes for last-minute changes. It is due to the great spirit of the entire team that we can honestly say that – in spite of all the hard work – we enjoyed the "ordeal" from beginning to end.

Autumn, 1984 The Editors

Committee

Chairmen:	E.D. Albert, Munich, West Germany W.R. Mayr, Vienna, Austria
President:	P.I. Terasaki, Los Angeles, USA
Past Presidents:	D.B. Amos, Durham, USA J.J. van Rood, Leiden, The Netherlands R. Ceppellini, Turin, Italy J. Dausset, Paris, France F. Kissmeyer-Nielsen, Aarhus, Denmark W.F. Bodmer, London, UK
Councillors:	M. Aizawa, Sapporo, Japan F. Bach, Minneapolis, USA H. Bashir, Sydney, Australia J.R. Batchelor, London, UK J.G. Bodmer, London, UK C.B. Carpenter, Boston, USA L. Degos, Paris, France B. Dupont, New York, USA C.P. Engelfriet, Amsterdam, The Netherlands P. Ivanyi, Amsterdam, The Netherlands Z. Layrisse, Caracas, Venezuela P.J. Morris, Oxford, UK R. Payne, Stanford, USA A. Piazza, Turin, Italy P. Rubinstein, New York, USA A. Svejgaard, Copenhagen, Denmark E. Thorsby, Oslo, Norway R. Tosi, Rome, Italy K. Tsuji, Isehara, Japan R.L. Walford, Los Angeles, USA E.J. Yunis, Boston, USA

Staff of the Host Laboratory (Munich):

Adriane Andreas
Angelika Albert
Michael Albert
Sabine Albert
Helga Bechmann-Holzner
Helga Fuchs
Elke Glitscher
Peter Haas
Petra Heinle
John Herminghaus
Erika Höfner
Elisabeth Keller
Rudolf Kreutinger
Daphne Langgassner
Erdmute Lipper
Ann McNicholas
Otto Richter
Beate Schiessl
Siegfried Scholz
Barbara Siegmund
Gabi Sierp
Reinhard Stier
Sabine Wallis
Rosi Wastlhuber
Helmut Zander
Martin Zietz
Ingeborg Zöbisch

Supported by:

Deutsche Forschungsgemeinschaft (DFG)
Bonn Al 92/13-1, Al 92/13-2
Deutscher Akademischer Austauschdienst (DAAD)
Bonn
World Health Organization (WHO)
Geneva

The following companies have supported the workshop:

Amersham Buchler	Braunschweig, West Germany
Austria Tabakwerke AG	Vienna, Austria
Behring-Werke	Marburg, West Germany
Biotest	Frankfurt, West Germany
Bio-Chrom	Berlin, West Germany
Cooper Biomedical Inc.	Malvern, USA
Fresenius	Oberursel, West Germany
Gödecke	Freiburg, West Germany
Greiner & Söhne	Nürtingen, West Germany
Heraeus Christ	München, West Germany
Hoffmann-La Roche & Co AG	Basel, Switzerland
Knut H. Escher GmbH	Duisburg, West Germany
Leitz Austria	Vienna, Austria
Leitz	Köln, West Germany
LKB-Instruments	Gräfelfing, West Germany
Dr. Molter	Heidelberg, West Germany
Novo Industrie GmbH	Vienna, Austria
Ortho-Diagnostiks	Heidelberg, West Germany
Pharmig	Vienna, Austria
Pel-freez	Brown Deer, USA
Rank Xerox	Düsseldorf, West Germany
Dr. C. Reissigl	Innsbruck, Austria
Robbins Scientific	Mountain View, USA
Schwab & Co. GmbH	Vienna, Austria
Siemens	Düsseldorf, West Germany
Dipl.-Ing. Z. Szabo GmbH	Vienna, Austria
Tecnomara	Fernwald, West Germany
Wiener Gebietskrankenkasse für Arbeiter und Angestellte	Vienna, Austria

The financial fund of the Thirteenth Annual HLA-Meeting (Hannover)

Table of Contents

Introductory Remarks

E. D. Albert, M. P. Baur, and W. R. Mayr

Aims of the Ninth Workshop

The Ninth International Histocompatibility Workshop started at a time when the technology for testing B cell alloantigens and information on ten DR alleles and several supertypic specificities had already been well established through the Eighth International Histocompatibility Workshop and spread among the HLA laboratories of the world. The nature and the genetic organization of the supertypic specificities were very much in dispute. A number of antigens belonging to new loci were postulated, and these claims were supported by biochemical evidence for the existence of several different classes of DR-like antigens. However, it was not clear exactly which allotypic specificities reside on which molecules, because most of the biochemical data were obtained using monoclonal antibodies directed at monomorphic determinants. Monoclonal antibodies defining polymorphic HLA determinants were just beginning to appear. It was therefore a logical consequence that one of the major aims of the Ninth Workshop was the utilization of the great potential of monoclonal antibodies for further dissection of the HLA polymorphisms by direct serological testing, as well as by biochemical analysis of molecules precipitated by the same polymorphic monoclonal antibodies. One of the major questions to be resolved was the organization of the HLA-D region. Which loci exist in the D region? Which antigenic specificities are governed by which loci? What is the precise relationship between serologically defined antigens and the HLA-Dw antigens? One of the keys to the understanding of the serology of the D region was to be the definition of the elusive specificity DRw6. At the same time, it was hoped that in the definition of HLA antigens by cellular reagents, the standard procedure of typing with homozygous typing cells (HTCs) could be complemented by proliferating and cytotoxic T cell clones.

In 1980 the first HLA genes were cloned, and since then a great deal of information about the genes in the HLA region has been obtained with recombinant DNA technology. Although it was too late to accommodate the DNA research in the workshop, activities in both fields were coordinated, particularly by W. Bodmer and J. Dausset and their groups.

One further aim of the Workshop was to include a significant amount of testing for the HLA-linked complement polymorphisms. Particular emphasis was to be placed on the highly polymorphic C4 A, B-system. Aside from the analysis of possible functional interaction with other HLA gene products, for example in determining disease susceptibility, the C4 polymorphism would provide a powerful marker for the fine mapping of the HLA-B, D region.

In the field of the clinical application of HLA research, the aim was to analyze the relationship between HLA and a number of diseases in cases where a specific question could be answered best by international cooperation, for example the question of whether the rare cases of B27-negative ankylosing spondylitis exhibit an association with another HLA allele. (We know today that the answer is: no.) For the specific aims of the various disease studies, we refer to the joint reports in this volume.

During the Eighth Workshop, a transplant study had provided at best only inconclusive evidence for the beneficial effect of HLA matching in kidney transplantation. Therefore the organizers of this workshop felt – with the very reluctant approval of some of the protagonists of HLA matching – that the Workshop owed it to the community to make another attempt at solving this very important question in a convincing way.

Organization of the Workshop

In order to distribute the organizational workload, the regional concept of the Seventh Workshop in Oxford was again applied. A network of 21 regions was established, each with one regional representative through whom information from the central organizers was distributed to the participating laboratories.

The collection of workshop reagents and later of the data was organized by the regions, who then sent the materials to the center in Munich. This system helped a great deal to limit the burden of the

Histocompatibility Testing 1984
Edited by E. D. Albert et al.

central organizers, and we would like to express our sincere gratitude for this help, as we are aware that it involved a great amount of work, time, and expense. The regional organization of the workshop had, however, the disadvantage of a sometimes slow flow of information, due to the rapidly deteriorating postal services in many parts of the world.

In June 1982 a total of over 3000 reagents (sera and monoclonal antibodies) were collected and distributed to councillor laboratories for prescreening, ensuring that each reagent was tested by at least five laboratories. Based on the results of the prescreening, the final workshop reagents were selected using certain principles. First, it was the aim to include at least four to five reagents which would define a given specificity in a reliable way, in other words with reagents which would present only a very small percentage of false-negative reactions with this specificity.

Second, an attempt was made to include sera which appeared to be splitting a given specificity which would be suspected if a large number of false-negative reactions were observed for the "unsplit" specificity. Such sera, however, had to fulfill the criterion of strong reactivity.

Third, we included a number of broadly reactive sera with the hope of providing reagents which in their tail contained reactivity with so far unknown specificities. In cases where a specificity could not be defined by a number of operationally monospecific sera, an attempt was made to include duo- and oligospecific antisera of different combinations of specificities in order to obtain a clear definition of such antigens.

In the selection of antisera for the DR antigens, an attempt was made to provide a clear definition of already well-established DR antigens and to include a large number of antisera which showed some degree of relationship with the elusive specificity DRw6. Such sera were included even if the strength of reactivity was less than satisfactory. For the definition of supertypic specificities of the DR and DQ series, it was the aim to select antisera showing all possible different types of broad reactivity patterns.

It was the overall strategy of serum selection to include a relatively large number of sera in order to reflect the complexities, particularly of the HLA-D region specificities. In addition, it should be mentioned that the organizers had expected that a certain percentage of antisera selected after the prescreening might not arrive for the production of the final reagent set. Therefore the number of antisera requested for the final set exceeded the planned size of the final set by about 15%. The compliance of the HLA community was, however, so good that approximately 97% of the antisera requested did indeed arrive in Munich. At this stage it was then felt that all sera that had arrived in Munich should indeed be used. For this reason the final reagent set became considerably larger than had been anticipated.

A number of known and hidden controls were included in the reagent set. The workshop numbers and the specificities of controls are given in Table 1.

Due to the fact that practically all laboratories submitting antisera kept to the given deadlines (a very rewarding experience for the organizers), it was possible to distribute the reagents to the regions in the early part of February 1983.

Selection of Cells To Be Tested

Following the experience from many previous workshops that the definition of new antigens was most convincing when their segregation in families could be shown, especially in the splitting of already established antigens, it was most helpful if it

Table 1. The controls used in the Ninth Workshop Serum Set

Card no.	Workshop no.	Specificity given	Identity and true specificity	
17	9w805	HU	Neg. control	
	9w806	New ABC	Neg. control	
21	9w798	Control moab	SEA-35.1	Anti-T cell (anti-TP50)
	9w799	Control moab	SEA-B1	Anti-Pan-B
22	9w643	DRw9	9w643	Anti-DR7
	9w800	Control moab	SEA 7.2	Anti-Ia monomorphic
	9w802	Control	9w537	Anti-DR2
23	9w801	Control moab	SEA-20.2	Anti-monocyte
24	9w803	DR5+w8	9w522	Anti-DR1+
	9w804	DR7 split	Bach-Chartier	Anti-B12
	9w540	DR4+7	9w540	Anti-DR2

could be shown that a particular split segregated with a number of different haplotypes. For this reason it was decided to ask for the typing of families and to select the families in such a way that they were as informative as possible, either by inclusion of a large number of children or by inclusion of several generations. Also, the disease studies were to be done on the level of family studies. The typing of family members, particularly of HLA-identical siblings, provided a set of built-in controls who yielded additional genetic information. In the disease studies, the genotyping of patients provided the opportunity to investigate the question of associations with particular haplotypic combinations and analyze the orientation of disease susceptibility genes within the HLA region. For example, it could be deduced in the study of juvenile chronic arthritis that the increase of HLA-A2 is independent, and not due to linkage disequilibrium with either DR5 or DRw8.

The choice of families as the sole target of investigation was also of benefit for the inclusion of data on the complement polymorphisms, particularly of the alleles of the C4 system, where it is mandatory to validate the phenotyping of single individuals by genotype analysis of the family. Due to the unexpectedly high frequency of gene duplications in this region, and due to the variable degree of detectability of null alleles at C4 A and C4 B, even family studies did not always allow unequivocal deduction of the C4 A,B genotypes of the families, so additional techniques such as typing for α and β chains (see joint report by C. Rittner and G. Mauff, C4 Polymorphism, this volume) had to be included.

Also in the analysis of the relationship between serologically and cellular defined alleles of the HLA region, the family structure allows the observation of joint segregations, which yields more information than a mere association on the population level.

In the selection of cells to be tested it was a second major aim of the workshop to include as many different populations as possible. It has been the experience of many workshops that the comparison of reaction patterns in ethnically different populations allows clearer definition of specificities. Furthermore, the qualitative differences of different race groups in the linkage disequilibria displayed by the HLA region has been instrumental in sorting out complexities, for example those of the HLA-D region. The fact that HLA-DR5, which in the Caucasian population is almost always associated with DQw3, has been found on the same haplotype with the DQw1 in Negroid populations has greatly helped to sort out the genetic organization of the broad and narrow specificities of the HLA-D region. With such situations in mind, the participating laboratories, particularly those in North America, Latin America, and Southeast Asia, were encouraged to include families of various ethnic backgrounds, so as to ensure that rare specificities and rare haplotypic combinations would be represented in the workshop master file.

Nomenclature for Factors of the HLA System 1984

This Article Will Also Be Published in The WHO Bulletin, vol. 63:2, April 1985

The HLA nomenclature committee met under the auspices of the WHO after the 9th International Histocompatibility Testing Workshop to consider revisions and additions to the nomenclature of factors identified by serological and cellular typing following the principles established successively in previous reports [1–6]. The nomenclature for the variants of the complement components controlled by genes of the HLA region was not considered as it was assumed that this was the responsibility of those with a special interest in complement, see e.g. [7]. Special attention was given to establishing a revised system of nomenclature for the products (sometimes called class II) of what can now be called the HLA-D region, based on the recent advances in our understanding of the biochemistry and genetics of these products.

The decision to upgrade a specificity, namely to drop its "w" designation, took into account the correlation in the overall workshop data between the local laboratory assignment of a specificity and that arrived at by the central computer analysis. A correlation coefficient of around 0.95 or higher together with general availability of appropriate antisera was taken as a sufficient indication of adequate clarity of definition of a specificity to drop the "w" designation. This criterion was applied equally to broader and narrower specificities even though, in some cases, the splits of the broader specificity were not so well defined. This is, for example, still the case for HLA-B5 with its splits B51 and Bw52. The retention of a "w" in the designation remains an indication that the specificity, though clearly identified, may not always be easily defined.

HLA-A, B and C Specificities

As before, the HLA-A and -B specificities are numbered jointly with non-overlapping numbers. The "w" designation is retained for all HLA-C specificities to avoid confusion with the nomenclature for complement components.

Newly upgraded HLA-A and -B specificities are listed in table 1. In addition to Cw1, Cw2, Cw3, Cw4 and Cw5, Cw6 approaches the clarity of definition that would be required for dropping the "w" designation. Cw5 remains, however, slightly more difficult to define than Cw1, Cw2, Cw3 or Cw4.

New provisional designations for HLA-A and HLA-B specificities are listed in tables 2 and 3 respectively. Aw66 (previously LN) is effectively another split of A10 and cannot so far be defined serologically in the presence of A26. Aw69 (previously A2/28) is a split of A28 that is most clearly defined by monoclonal antibodies with reactivity

Table 1. New designations for HLA-A and HLA-B specificities upgraded to full HLA status

New	Previous equivalents
A23	Aw23
A24	Aw24
A30	Aw30
A31	Aw31
A32	Aw32
B16	Bw16
B21	Bw21
B35	Bw35
B38	Bw38
B39	Bw39
B44	Bw44
B45	Bw45
B49	Bw49
B51	Bw51

Table 2. New provisional designations of HLA-A specificities

New	Previous equivalents
Aw66	LN
Aw68	A28 and negative to A2/28
Aw69	A2/28

Table 3. New provisional designations for HLA-B specificities

Bw64	B14.1, (8w63)
Bw65	B14.2, (8w62)
Bw67	SN-2, Te90, (8w57), Te75
Bw70	Bu + SV, K5, Da(6), (8w59)
Bw71	Bu
Bw72	SV
Bw73	KA, IEH

Histocompatibility Testing 1984
Edited by E. D. Albert et al.

only against A2 and Aw69, and cannot so far be defined serologically in the presence of A2. This is the first example of an officially recognised specificity identified by a monoclonal antibody. Given the potential exquisite specificity of monoclonal antibodies, criteria for designation of new specificities identified by them need careful consideration. Aw69 has been designated because at least two monoclonal antibodies agree in defining a new specificity that is clearly distinct from any previously identified specificity. Aw68 is defined as the split of A28 that is complementary to Aw69. Since Bw71 (previously Bu) cannot be identified serologically other than by lack of reactivity to sera containing antibodies against Bw72 (previously SV), it was also necessary to designate the broad specificity Bw70 [previously Bu+SV, K5 or Da(6)].
Other suggested HLA-A or -B specificities discussed, but not yet considered to be sufficiently well defined to merit official provisional designation, included 9.3, Th (a possible further split of Aw19 in negroid populations), 19bac, 33.1, 33.2, St16 (a possible further split of B39), 15.3 and Te74 (another B15 split sometimes referred to as 8w66, an informal designation that should be avoided to prevent any possible confusion with Aw66). Special attention clearly needs to be given to clarification of the many possible further splits of B15 seen especially in oriental populations.
Individual workshop sera suggested a new specificity that may fill part of the HLA-C blank, and a split of Cw3. Other sera suggested splits of Cw7. However none of these suggestions were considered to be sufficiently well founded to merit an official provisional designation. The combination of Cw1 and Cw3 seen in association with haplotypes containing Bw46, was not given a separate designation as it is not yet clear whether this is simply a reflection of gene duplication (in whole or in part) or truly represents a novel serological specificity.

The HLA-D Region

Biochemical and molecular genetical analyses of the products and genes associated with the HLA-Dw and HLA-DR(w) specificities have led to a considerable advance in our understanding of the HLA-D region and its products. It is now clear that there are at least three well defined subsets of products, which until now have been informally designated DR, DC (MB or DS) and SB. Each product consists of a non-covalently associated combination of an α- and a β-chain. The α and β chains are substantially different from each other, and there is evidence for at least six α chain genes and seven β chain genes all in the HLA region. These genes, for the most part, appear to be arranged in subsets corresponding to the three subsets of products, where α and β chain genes within a subset are significantly more similar to each other than they are to the genes of one of the other subsets. While presently available knowledge concerning the genes of the HLA-D region is not yet adequate to give them each an official designation, it was decided that the division into three subsets of products is sufficiently well established to merit an official designation and that this could be done without prejudicing future decisions on nomenclature for the specificities and genes of the HLA-D region. The chosen designations are HLA-DR, HLA-DQ (previously DC etc.) and HLA-DP (previously SB). Current evidence suggests one α and two or three β chain genes for HLA-DR, and two α and two β chains each for HLA-DQ and HLA-DP. It is anticipated that when eventually gene names are officially designated they will consist of HLA-DR, HLA-DQ, HLA-DP, followed by a combination of numbers and letters (A for an α-chain gene and B for a β-chain gene) that uniquely defines each gene. The HLA-D region is the counterpart of the I-region of the mouse H-2 system, whose determinants are sometimes called Ia, with I-A corresponding to DQ, and I-E to DR.
The serologically defined specificities of the HLA-D region can be associated predominantly with either the HLA-DR or HLA-DQ sets of products, while the different HLA-DP products are so far only defined using the primed lymphocyte, or PLT test. Certain monomorphic monoclonal antibodies can however clearly distinguish between these three sets of products.
The HLA-Dw specificities defined by the mixed lymphocyte culture or MLC test cannot yet be clearly associated with one or other of the three subsets of products, though it seems likely that they mostly involve HLA-DR. Where new specificities are clearly identified as being associated predominantly with one or other of the subsets of HLA-D products we have followed previous practice in assigning to them the designation HLA-DR, HLA-DQ or HLA-DP (followed by "w" to indicate the designation is provisional) and appropriate numbers, usually in sequence. The designation HLA-Dw, with no further indication of subdivisions, is retained for the MLC defined specificities.

HLA-DR Specificities

The previously defined HLA-DR1, DR2, DR3, DR4, DR5, DRw6, DR7, DRw8, DRw9 and

DRw10 specificities are all clearly associated with the HLA-DR products. They therefore retain their previous designations, since it was decided that none of DRw6, DRw8, DRw9 or DRw10 deserved to be upgraded to full HLA-status. Amongst HLA-DR specificities with full HLA status, DR5 remains the most difficult to define.

New provisional designations for HLA-DR specificities are given in table 4. DRw11 (previously LB5) and DRw12 (previously LB5 x 8 etc.) are splits of DR5, while DRw13 (previously 6.6, 6.1, 6Z) and DRw14 (previously 6.3, 6.9, 6X, 901) are splits of DRw6.

DRw52 (previously MT2) and DRw53 (previously MT3) were originally identified in the 7th and 8th Workshops as apparently crossreacting specificities involving DR3, DR5, DRw6 and DRw8 for DRw52, and DR4, DR7 and DRw9 for DRw53. Following the 8th Workshop it was suggested that these two specificities might be on molecules from a different locus (sometimes also referred to as BR) to that controlling the then designated HLA-DR specificities, or possibly on molecules from both the then assumed HLA-DR locus and another locus, and this remains true. But it is now clear that all such molecules must be members of the HLA-DR subset. High numbers were chosen for these two broad, operationally supertypic, specificities to separate them clearly from the other narrower HLA-DR specificities. DRw6, in particular, seems operationally to be completely included in DRw52 (previously MT2).

Other suggested HLA-DR specificities discussed, but not yet considered sufficiently well defined to merit official provisional designation, included 4.1, 4.2, 4.3 and DR2 splits.

HLA-DQ Specificities

New provisional HLA-DQ specificities are listed in table 5. As in the case of DRw52 (previously MT2) and DRw53 (previously MT3), DQw1 (previously DC1, MB1, MT1, LB-E12), DQw2 (previously MB2, DC3, Te24, LB-E17) and DQw3 (previously MB3, MT4, DC4, TB21) were originally identified in the 7th and 8th Workshops as apparently crossreacting specificities including DR1, DR2, DRw6 and DRw10 for DQw1, DR3 and DR7 for DQw2 and DR4 and DR5 for DQw3. These also were suggested at the time of the 8th Workshop to be on different locus products from the HLA-DR specificities. Subsequent studies, in this case, have clearly associated these specificities with the HLA-DQ (previously DC etc.) products. TA10 and LB-E13 were discussed as possible HLA-DQ specificities, apparently splitting DQw3, but it was felt that their

Table 4. New provisional designations for HLA-DR specificities

New	Previous equivalents
DRw11	LB5
DRw12	LB5 × 8, DR5 short, FT23
DRw13	6.6, 6.1, 6Z
DRw14	6.9, 6.3, 6X, 901
DRw52	MT2
DRw53	MT3

Table 5. New provisional designations for HLA-DQ specificities

New	Previous equivalents
DQw1	DC1, MB1, MT1, LB-E12
DQw2	MB2, DC3, Te24, LB-E17
DQw3	MB3, MT4, DC4, TB21

Table 6. New provisional designations for HLA-DP specificities

New	Previous equivalents
DPw1	SB1, PL3A
DPw2	SB2
DPw3	SB3
DPw4	SB4, PL3B
DPw5	SB5
DPw6	SB6

Table 7. New provisional designations for HLA-Dw specificities

New	Previous equivalents
Dw13	DB3
Dw14	LD40
Dw15	DYT, YT
Dw16	DB8, B8
Dw17	7A, (Dw7A)
Dw18	6A, (Dw6A)
Dw19	6B, (Dw6B)

Table 8. Dw and DR relationships

Dw specificities	Associated DR specificities
Dw1	DR1
Dw2, Dw12	DR2
Dw3	DR3
Dw4, Dw10, Dw13, Dw14, Dw15	DR4
Dw5	DRw11 (5)
Dw6, Dw18, Dw19	DRw13 (w6)
Dw9, Dw16	DRw14 (w6)
Dw7, Dw11, Dw17	DR7
Dw8	DRw8

Table 9. Complete listing of recognised HLA specificities

HLA						
A	B	C	D	DR	DQ	DP
A1	B5	Cw1	Dw1	DR1	DQw1	DPw1
A2	B7	Cw2	Dw2	DR2	DQw2	DPw2
A3	B8	Cw3	Dw3	DR3	DQw3	DPw3
A9	B12	Cw4	Dw4	DR4		DPw4
A10	B13	Cw5	Dw5	DR5		DPw5
A11	B14	Cw6	Dw6	DRw6		DPw6
Aw19	B15	Cw7	Dw7	DR7		
A23(9)	B16	Cw8	Dw8	DRw8		
A24(9)	B17		Dw9	DRw9		
A25(10)	B18		Dw10	DRw10		
A26(10)	B21		Dw11(w7)	DRw11(5)		
A28	Bw22		Dw12	DRw12(5)		
A29(w19)	B27		Dw13	DRw13(w6)		
A30(w19)	B35		Dw14	DRw14(w6)		
A31(w19)	B37		Dw15			
A32(w19)	B38(16)		Dw16	DRw52		
Aw33(w19)	B39(16)		Dw17(w7)	DRw53		
Aw34(10)	B40		Dw18(w6)			
Aw36	Bw41		Dw19(w6)			
Aw43	Bw42					
Aw66(10)	B44(12)					
Aw68(28)	B45(12)					
Aw69(28)	Bw46					
	Bw47					
	Bw48					
	B49(21)					
	Bw50(21)					
	B51(5)					
	Bw52(5)					
	Bw53					
	Bw54(w22)					
	Bw55(w22)					
	Bw56(w22)					
	Bw57(17)					
	Bw58(17)					
	Bw59					
	Bw60(40)					
	Bw61(40)					
	Bw62(15)					
	Bw63(15)					
	Bw64(14)					
	Bw65(14)					
	Bw67					
	Bw70					
	Bw71(w70)					
	Bw72(w70)					
	Bw73					
	Bw4					
	Bw6					

The listing of broad specificities in parenthesis after a narrow specificity, e.g. HLA-A23(9) is optional. The following is a listing of these specificities which arose as clear-cut splits of other specificities.

Original broad specificities	Splits
A9	A23, A24
A10	A25, A26, Aw34, Aw66
Aw19	A29, A30, A31, A32, Aw33
A28	Aw68, Aw69
B5	B51, Bw52
B12	B44, B45
B14	Bw64, Bw65
B15	Bw62, Bw63
B16	B38, B39
B17	Bw57, Bw58
B21	B49, Bw50
Bw22	Bw54, Bw55, Bw56
B40	Bw60, Bw61
Bw70	Bw71, Bw72
DR5	DRw11, DRw12
DRw6	DRw13, DRw14
Dw6	Dw18, Dw19
Dw7	Dw11, Dw17

The following are the generally agreed inclusions of HLA-B specificities into Bw4 and Bw6.

Bw4: B5, B13, B17, B27, B37, B38(16), B44(12), Bw47, B49(21), B51(5), Bw52(5), Bw53, Bw57(17), Bw58(17), Bw59, Bw63(15).

Bw6: B7, B8, B14, B18, Bw22, B35, B39(16), B40, Bw41, Bw42, B45(12), Bw46, Bw48, Bw50(21), Bw54(w22), Bw55(w22), Bw56(w22), Bw60(40), Bw61(40), Bw62(15), Bw64(14), Bw65(14), Bw67, Bw70, Bw71(w70), Bw72(w70), Bw73.

The following specificities are generally agreed to be associated with DRw52 and DRw53:

DRw52: DR3, DR5, DRw6, DRw8, DRw11(5), DRw12(5), DRw13(w6), DRw14(w6)

DRw53: DR4, DR7, DRw9

relationship with HLA-DQ products required some further independent confirmation, and so they were not assigned official provisional designations.
The fact that DQw1 (previously DC1 etc.) and DRw6 are on different sets of products clearly indicates that DQw1 does not contribute to the definition of DRw6. The strong population associations between these and other analogous combinations of specificities can now be seen clearly to be due to strong linkage disequilibrium between alleles at very closely linked loci coding for DR and DQ products.

HLA-DP Specificities

New provisional HLA-DP specificities as defined by PLT typing are listed in table 6.

HLA-Dw Specificities

HLA-Dw1, Dw2 and Dw3 now approach the clarity of definition by MLC typing that would justify dropping their "w" designation. However, in order to distinguish the MLC identified specificities from those clearly assigned to one of the HLA-D region products it was decided, at least for the time being, to use the prefix Dw for all the MLC identified specificities however well defined they are.
New provisional designations for HLA-Dw specificities are listed in table 7. Dw13 (previously DB3), Dw14 (previously LD40), Dw15 (previously DYT, found predominantly in oriental populations) together with Dw4 and Dw10 are all associated with the serological specificity DR4. Dw2 and Dw12 have similarly previously been associated with DR2. Dw17 (previously 7A) is the complementary split of Dw7 to Dw11, while Dw18 (previously 6A) and Dw19 (previously 6B) are splits of Dw6, which is in turn associated with the serological specificity DRw13, one of the splits of DRw6. The other split of DRw6, DRw14 is associated with Dw9 and Dw16. These multiple relationships between Dw and DR specificities, further confounded by patterns of association with DQ specificities that are probably due to linkage disequilibrium between alleles at DR and DQ loci, emphasise again that it is no longer possible to maintain any relationship between the numbering of Dw and DR specificities. A list of the known relationships between officially designated Dw and DR specificities is given in table 8.

Other specificities not officially designated included DB6 (originally defined by the cell Herluf), DB9, and a split of Dw8, informally called 8.2, which appears to occur especially in Eskimo and American-Indian populations. These specificities, probably for technical reasons, were not well defined in the final workshop analysis.
A complete listing of the recognised HLA specificities is given in table 9. Further background to the basis for the decisions reported here can be found in Histocompatibility Testing 1984 [8].

Acknowledgements. The contributions of Drs. Max Baur, Hans-Grosse Wilde and Ieke Schreuder who acted as coopted members of the committee producing this report are gratefully acknowledged.

References

1. Bulletin of the World Health Organization (1968) 39:483
2. WHO terminology report, Histocompatibility Testing 1970, p 49, Terasaki PI ed, Munksgaard, Copenhagen 1970
3. Bulletin of the World Health Organization (1972) 47:659
4. Bulletin of the World Health Organization (1975) 52:261
5. Bulletin of the World Health Organization (1978) 56:461
6. Histocompatibility Testing 1980, Terasaki PI ed, UCLA Tissue Typing Laboratory, Los Angeles, Calif. p 18–20, 1980
7. Statement on the Nomenclature of Human C4 Allotypes. Mauff G, Alper CA, Awdeh Z, Batchelor JR, Bertrams J, Bruun-Petersen G, Dawkins RL, Demant P, Edwards J, Grosse-Wilde H, Hauptmann G, Klouda P, Lamm L, Mollenhauer E, Nerl C, Olaisen B, O'Neill G, Rittner C, Roos MH, Skanes V, Teisberg P, Wells L. Immunobiology, vol. 164, pp 184–191 (1983)
8. Histocompatibility Testing 1984, Albert ED, Baur MP, Mayr WR eds, Springer Verlag, Heidelberg 1984

List of members involved in preparing this report with affiliations:

Bodmer WF, Imperial Cancer Research Fund, London England (Rapporteur)
Albert E, Kinderpoliklinik der Universität München, München, Germany
Bodmer JG, Imperial Cancer Research Fund, London, England
Dausset J, Institut de Recherches sur les Maladies du Sang, Hôpital St. Louis, Paris, France
Kissmeyer-Nielsen F, The University Hospital, Aarhus, Denmark
Mayr W, Institut für Blutgruppenserologie, Universität Wien, Wien, Austria
Payne R, Stanford University School of Medicine, Stanford, California, United States
Rood JJ van, University of Leiden, Leiden, The Netherlands (Chairman)
Trnka Z, Basel Institute for Immunology, Basel, Switzerland
Walford RL, UCLA School of Medicine, University of California, Los Angeles, California, United States

Joint Reports

The HLA System, 1984 *

W. F. Bodmer

Imperial Cancer Research Fund, P.O. Box No. 123, Lincoln's Inn Fields, London WC2A 3PX, U.K.

The HLA region, though only about one thousandth of the total human genome, continues to challenge us with its complexity and diversity. This summary is intended to give a kaleidoscopic view of the system, biased inevitably by my own prejudices, following the four successive meetings – on molecular genetics in Strasbourg; on biochemical analysis, followed by the Histocompatibility Testing Workshop itself, in Munich; and finally, the conference in Vienna.

The HLA Map

The conventional map of the HLA system, developed gradually from family data, puts the complement genes between the HLA-D region and the *ABC* loci. The order *DP* (*SB*), *DQ* (*DC* or *MB*) and *DR* seems most probable, and for *DQ* and *DR* best matches the mouse sequence, but recombination data have not established the order of C4 and C2, or unequivocally placed the gene (or genes) for 21 hydroxylase (21OH) in the HLA region. Not to be forgotten are the human equivalents of the mouse *QA* and *TL* loci, especially as they presumably occupy a large part of the HLA region, based on the analogy with the mouse.

The workshop data and molecular analysis have now, however, considerably refined this picture. A genetic map based on recombination fractions places *A* somewhat further from *C* than *C* is from *B*, because the estimated *A* to *C* recombination fraction is at least three to four times that from *C* to *B*. Similarly, the recombination fraction from *DP* to *DQ* is thought to be substantially bigger than that from *DP* to *DR* based both on family data and on a relative lack of linkage disequilibrium between *DQ* and *DR* alleles. However, in molecular terms, the distances involving the higher recombination fractions are probably no larger than the rest. It seems most likely rather that they are associated with recombination "hot spots", entirely analogous to the one described in some detail in the mouse I region by Steinmetz and Hood. Thus virtually all the recombinants within the I region have occurred in one particular section encompassing a few hundred base pairs. At the nucleotide level recombination may be distributed very unevenly. It should be remembered that per meiosis recombination only occurs on average about one in every hundred million base pairs, and so there may be enormous differences, perhaps up to ten or even one hundred fold, between recombination frequencies in sequences where it is more likely to occur than in other sequences. Over long distances such heterogeneity averages out, so that recombination fractions may give reasonable estimates of physical distance. Over short distances, however, the particular distribution of recombination hot spots can considerably distort the relationship between recombination fractions and physical distance, depending on whether a hot spot happens to lie in the region being studied or not. Genes that are quite close together in nucleotide pair terms, but separated by recombination hot spots, will be much more loosely linked than expected and as a result will give rise to much less linkage disequilibrium than expected. That is no doubt why *DP* can easily be separated from *DQ* and *DR*, and also probably why there was originally little difficulty in separating the *A* and *B* loci, the prediction being that each of these intervals includes a recombination hot spot.

Four *BC* recombinants have been reported in this workshop, at least one of which (reported by Du Toit) seems very clear cut, and these are consistent with the order ...*B–C–A*... A family reported by Erna Möller in addition supports the HLA-D region order ...*DQ–DR–B*... For further mapping information, however, we must turn to the molecular data which have, of course, revolutionised our knowledge of the region. Perhaps, strikingly, at this level the complement region is now the best characterised, based on the work of the Oxford and Boston groups together with the work on 21OH by White and colleagues. The best estimate of the overall order now appears to be

...*DR*...C2–Bf–C4B–21OH–C4A–21OH'...*B*...

all the genes from C2 to the second 21OH gene being connected by overlapping genomic clones. This

*This is an edited version of the final summary talk given at the conference in Vienna

Histocompatibility Testing 1984
Edited by E. D. Albert et al.

order is consistent with mouse data from Steinmetz and others and also with data on deletions involving 21OH and C4A in association with certain *B* alleles and 21OH deficiency. The molecular geneticists still have to link up C4A and 21OH′ with *B*, and C2 with the HLA-D region. The C4 allelic variation has been confirmed at the molecular level to be in the C4d fragment, and it is interesting to note that restriction fragment polymorphism does not easily pick up this variation. In addition, C4 deletions have been identified in association with 21OH deletions, as well as C4 duplications. Molecular variation associated with complement and 21OH deficiency diseases can now be analyzed following the same approaches used for the classical studies of the haemoglobinopathies.
C4 is somewhat analogous to C3, the third complement component, which maps not in the HLA region but to chromosome 19. This suggests that C4 was transposed into the HLA region after the evolutionary establishment of HLA class I and class II products and complement, leading to an association between C4 and HLA that was selectively advantageous. Perhaps when that happened, C4 brought 21OH with it simply as a bystander, because it was the neighbouring gene and no counteracting disadvantage followed from its transposition. In that case one should look for enzymes similar to 21OH, which is a P450 mixed-function oxidase, next to, for example, C3 on chromosome 19. Such a finding would be a striking confirmation of this predicted evolutionary history of the relationship between the C4 genes and the HLA region.

Class I Genes and Products

Detailed knowledge of the class I region at the molecular level has on the whole progressed less far. It is more complicated, there are more genes and they are more similar to each other than are, for example, most of the D region genes. There are some complete DNA sequences, for example from the groups of Jordan, Weissman and others, and there are now indications of differences that are locus specific as well as allele specific. Variations in gene number have been found associated with particular HLA-A and B determinants, but it is not known whether all of these genes are expressed. Some of the genes are extraordinarily similar to each other, suggesting comparatively recent duplication and, perhaps, a more fluid situation for the evolution of the class I than the other genes. Work in the mouse by Steinmetz and Hood, Flavell and others shows that the vast majority of class I genes (25 to 30) are in the QA and TL regions, with only five or six in *K*, *D* and *L*, the equivalents of *A*, *B* and *C*. In the mouse, H-2K is out of line with the human sequence (lying on the centromeric side of the I region), and it is interesting that Flavell's group has suggested that DNA segments can be transposed from the H-2L, QA region to the K region because of similarities between sequences found in these two parts of the H-2 region. This supports the suggestion I made a few years ago, namely that in the mouse K was transposed to its present position from the L, QA neighbourhood. A key question is clearly: what are the functions of all these QA and TL genes? The human equivalents of QA are beginning to be defined serologically, and there are monoclonal antibodies to some TL-like human products. Molecular data from mutants also clearly indicates that in man, as in the mouse, there is going to be a comparable set of genes in this region within the HLA system, of which, however, only about half may be expressed. The QA and TL determinants are called differentiation antigens, but this is only a description of their restricted tissue distribution and says little or nothing about their function. The challenge for the future is to unravel the function of these genes together with their molecular organisation, coupled, of course, with a more detailed clarification of the molecular organisation of the *HLA-A*, *B* and *C* loci.

The HLA-D Region

Our view of the HLA-D region, one of the most frequently shown pictures in the Workshop (Fig. 1), has been enormously clarified by a combination of work at the molecular level, conventional serology, work with monoclonal antibodies and biochemical analysis. The region codes for three main sets of molecules, DP, DQ and DR. There is, intriguingly, a further set, indicated by a new α gene different from any of the DP, DQ or DR α genes, which we have called DZ and which appears to be the same as that described independently by Inoko and Tsuji. This suggests that there may not be many, if any, more genes to be found in this particular HLA subfamily. The structure of the DP subregion is established in complete detail from the work of Trowsdale, Mach, Peterson and Strominger and their colleagues and shows that there are two β and two α genes, though there may, in addition, be limited polymorphism for the number of these genes. There are, similarly, two pairs of β and α genes in the DQ subregion, corresponding to DX and DC, but these are not yet linked together at the molecular level. In the DR subregion there are probably three β genes, one of which is a pseudo-gene, but there is only one DR α gene and this does not vary very much. The only highly poly-

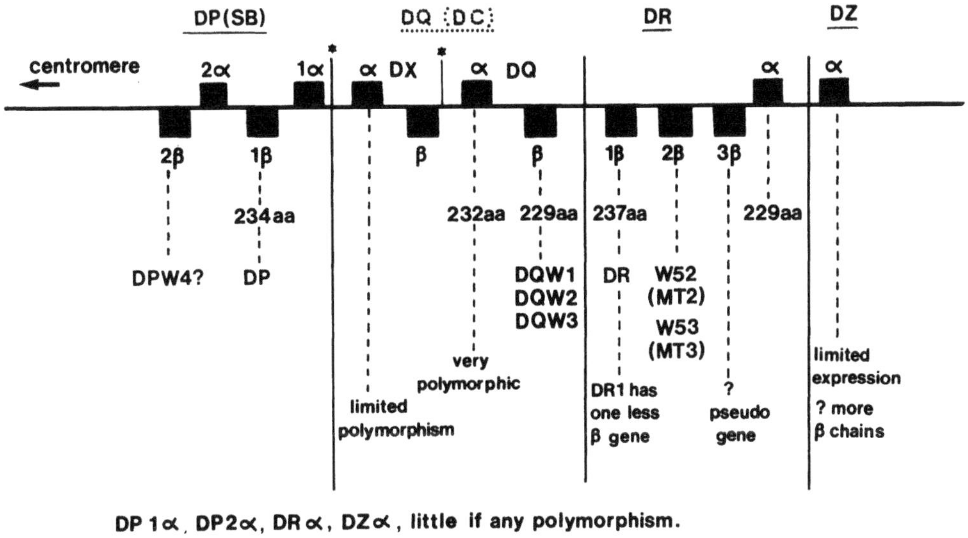

Fig. 1. Schematic map of the HLA-D region based on the general consensus from the work of many different laboratories. The numbers in front of α or β, such as in *2α* and *1α*, simply identify different genes. The order of DX and DQ (DC) within the DQ region is that suggested by the lack of linkage disequilibrium between DXα variations and DC and DR variations. *234aa* etc. indicate the number of amino acids predicted by the nucleotide sequence. The position of DZα is not clearly defined, though it is somewhere between the DP region and *HLA-B*

morphic α gene appears to be the DQ subregion DC α gene. Though all the β genes are polymorphic there are clearly differences in the extent of their variation. One of the DR β genes is most probably associated with the original DR determinants and the other with DRw52 and 53 (formerly MT2 and MT3). DQw1, 2 and 3 (formerly the MB or DC determinants) go with one of the DQ β genes, probably DC β. The picture of the HLA-D region is perhaps nearly complete, though there are still gaps to be filled in to join up its different parts.

Recombination hot spots and their effects on linkage disequilibrium contribute to the interpretation of the HLA-D region. Many of the problems involved in sorting out its complexity are because of the very close linkage, and therefore close linkage disequilibrium, between the DQ and DR α and β genes. Linkage disequilibrium between alleles at very closely linked loci is almost entirely a function of that closeness. Thus, alleles at such closely linked loci will stay together in a population for very long periods of time. Only when the recombination fraction increases beyond 0.5% – 1% do these associations get dissipated, leading to a disappearance of linkage disequilibrium. When determinants that are closely associated because of linkage disequilibrium also cross-react, even when they are controlled by different loci, then the serological data may be very hard to interpret in terms of the contributions of the various loci, and this interpretation has been a major aim of this workshop. As already mentioned, there is probably a recombination hot spot between DP and DQ, which could mean that the physical distance between DP and DQ is likely to be comparable to that between DQ and DR. There is a possible second hot spot in the DQ region because, as Spielman has shown with some of our probes working in London and Philadelphia, the DX α variation is not stronlgy associated with DC or DR and probably also not with DP. These two recombination hot spots would thus explain the pattern of association among serological HLA-D determinants, namely very strong between DQ and DR, and quite weak between these and DP. One very interesting family described from Leiden, involving the mixed lymphocyte culture (MLC) type called locally LBQ1, can be interpreted as a recombinant between two of the β chain genes in the DR region.

Other HLA Functions?

Apart from class I and class II products and complement factors and 21OH, what else might there be in the HLA region? Are there other functions controlled by HLA still to be found? A special type of transposable sequence, sometimes called a retroposon, has been found by Trowsdale and his colleagues in our laboratory in London in the course of a search for expressed sequences other than those we now know about. It was found by screening cosmids with cDNA probes made from message from T lymphocytes and other cells, but probably has no functional significance. Clearly, given genomic clones that cover the whole of the HLA region, they should be screened with mRNA or cDNA probes from a variety of tissue sources, including perhaps especially liver because of its multiplicity of related products, to determine whether any other HLA region functions can be identified. It was interesting, in this context, that Meo in Strasbourg mentioned that they had found an activity in the liver coded for by mouse C4-containing clones which now is most likely to be 21OH or something very similar to it. McDevitt's group have also described the so-called low-molecular-weight proteins. Personally, I do not expect to find many, if any, more novel gene products in the HLA region. The average observed ratio of coding to non-coding DNA suggests that there may already be enough products to fill the HLA region as we now know it.

HLA Serology

The core of the workshop activity is still the serology. The whole HLA system started from the serology. Its discovery was based on a relatively few sera, some quite unreproducible techniques that gave rise to many incorrect apparent recombinants, and some simple statistics. These initial problems led to the need for serum exchanges, and so for workshops in order to establish an agreed definition of specificities. There followed, over the past 20 years, the truly remarkable phenomenon of international co-operation in science, giving rise to the international histocompatibility testing workshops, which as far as I am aware are a unique occurrence, at least in the biomedical field. The workshops are not only scientific gatherings, but also constructive and enjoyable social gatherings, in which by coming together we stimulate each other and so stimulate scientific collaboration on HLA on a world-wide basis. This workshop was undoubtedly every bit as effective as its eight predecessors.

The A, B, C serology report suggests that we may be reaching the limit of antigen splitting, except perhaps for B15. It is reassuring to see that previously suggested antigens, however tentative they were initially, seem to remain and so have stood the test of time. The fact that none have disappeared, at least in recent workshops, shows the value of a somewhat conservative approach to the formal designation of the existence of an antigen by the WHO Nomenclature Committee. Now, clearly, we must hope that molecular studies will throw further light on the sometimes complex serology. What, for example, are the old BW4 (4a) and BW6 (4b) really? Are they, as suggested many years ago, in some sense the oldest of the differences between the B locus alleles, seen also in other species? Thus, alloantisera from one species tested on the determinants of another species most readily reflect the BW4, BW6 difference. Most of the C locus blank has been filled in, but we still do not know whether there are any true blanks, namely absence of expression of any C locus product.

The D region serology has progressed extraordinarily well. Schreuder and her colleagues have done a remarkable job in sorting out DRw6. The serology, helped by the biochemistry and the molecular genetics, appears to have sorted out DQw1, 2 and 3 (formerly DC or MB1, MB2, MB3 etc.), TA10 and DRw52, 53 (formerly MT2 and MT3). Thus the nature of these serological specificities, nearly all of which were already seen quite clearly in the first workshop in Oxford, where the DR types were defined, has been substantially clarified. Some DR splits, namely of DR5 and DRw6, are convincing and have now been officially recognised in the updated WHO nomenclature.

Cellular Typing

I have little or no direct experience of the cellular techniques, but have always admired the heroic efforts of the relatively small band of cellular typers. The homozygous typing cells (HTCs) have provided a valuable guide to the discovery of new serological determinants and to the analysis of the HLA-D region. However, it is becoming increasingly clear that the old notion of a distinction between types defined by cellular techniques and those defined by serology is now becoming very blurred. There is no reason why those parts of the HLA-D molecules that are important for stimulation in cell culture cannot be identified by appropriate antibodies, especially, of course, monoclonal antibodies. As described by Julia Bodmer and her colleagues in the D region monoclonal antibodies report, serology can, for example, now distinguish between some of the components of DR4 defined by HTCs, and also between the new Dw6 splits Dw18 (6A) and Dw19 (6B). The HTCs are surely mixed reagents just like conventional alloantisera, but with perhaps greater biases towards particular products. They may, for example, detect mainly DR (including DRw52 and 53) because the MLC response is dominated by the numerically more frequent helper T cells. Thus perhaps DQ, as has been suggested before, is more involved in suppression than help and so does not contribute to the same extent as DR to MLC stimulation. Undoubtedly, DP may also be involved in stimulation, and so the MLC response is just like a mixed serological reaction.

Degos suggested that some of the differences between HTCs associated with the same DR specificity, such as the DR2-associated Dw2 and DB9, were due simply to differently associated DQ determinants. In this case DQw1 is associated with Dw2 and TA10 with DB9, so that the suggestion is that it is the DQ difference that causes the MLC difference between these two HTCs. However, strong linkage disequilibrium between DQ and DR genes suggests an alternative explanation consistent with the notion that MLC stimulation is mainly due to DR differences. Thus, within the DR2 haplotypes there are likely to be differences in the DRβ genes that have not yet been recognised either serologically or biochemically, and which will be expected to be in strong linkage disequilibrium with DQ variations such as DQw1 and TA10. It is therefore likely to be such associated DR variations, and not the known DQ differences, that distinguish HTCs such as Dw2 and DB9.

The other major cellular technique, primed lymphocyte typing (PLT), in which primed cells are used to stimulate in a secondary test, now, of course, often carried out using clones, has most importantly identified the DP (formerly SB) determinants. This is the first workshop in which DP has been clearly defined by the cellular techniques. It is perhaps ironic that the conventional serology can hardly even detect the DP products, though there are good monoclonal antibodies for them, and yet within the HLA-D region it is the DP subregion that is most completely characterised at the molecular level. That may well be due to a mixture of chance, in picking up good DP genomic clones, and the fact that DP is probably expressed at a relatively low level. Cellular techniques, using clones, are going to become increasingly important. The T cell clones are obviously cellular equivalents of monoclonal antibodies, and in addition to D region specificities are also defining interesting subdivisions of class I determinants such as A2 and B44.

Monoclonal Antibodies

Another first in this workshop was a substantial contribution from monoclonal antibodies. It is quite clear that the monoclonal antibodies can already reveal a great deal of the serological specificity within the HLA region, including nearly all the DQ and DR determinants with their new splits, provided they are treated with care and attention. Being abundantly available, they can easily be used by all serologists and should not require complicated special techniques for their handling. They will surely become more and more important in the future. There are already some very good monoclonal antibodies for HLA-A and B locus specificities, and the challenge is to make more of them and to fill in the gaps. Some new specificities have been defined by monoclonal antibodies, especially the various determinants associated with A2 and A28, and one in particular has been given an official WHO designation, namely Aw69 (formerly A2/28), and so as a result has the complementary split of A28, namely Aw68 (A28 and not Aw69). Monoclonal antibodies have also clearly identified HLA-A and B inter-locus cross-reactions. The old observation of an association between antibodies to A9 and BW4 in alloantisera is now reflected by monoclonal antibodies with just that combination specificity. It should be remembered that the clarity with which it was possible originally to define the *HLA-A* and *B* loci in man, as compared to the difficulty in the mouse in separating H-2K from D, was largely due to differences between the species in inter-locus cross-reaction. Thus, there is much less cross-reaction between *HLA-A* and *B* locus determinants than between H-2K and D. It is to be expected that cross-combinations identified by monoclonal antibodies will eventually be found in alloantisera, which are, after all, nothing but mixtures of monoclonal antibodies. The specificity of an alloantiserum is determined effectively as the lowest common denominator of its constituent individual antibodies. It must, however, be borne in mind that the mouse may see us a little differently than we see ourselves.

The greatest contribution so far of the monoclonal antibodies has surely been to the resolution of the D region serology and biochemistry, including the definition of the DRw6-associated determinants, and the sorting out of the three sets of products DP, DQ and DR. They have also identified inter-allele and inter-locus cross-reaction. One of their particular contributions has, of course, been to the analysis of the biochemistry of the HLA-D region products. Collaboration in work on the biochemistry of the class II products was another first for this workshop. This was based, as described in the joint report, on an exchange of antibodies, an exchange of cell lines and an attempt to use a common analytical technique, namely a standardised two-dimensional gel immunoprecipitation analysis. Though many problems of the technique were revealed, there were many areas of considerable common ground. The collaboration showed how, even in such a complicated area, working together with a variety of approaches, namely two-dimensional gels and immunoprecipitation, radio-immunoassays, peptide and amino acid sequence analyses, can really contribute to understanding the nature of the class II molecules. An important outcome was simply the further clarification of the definition of the set of HLA-D region products. Another contribution was to the understanding of the polymorphic differences, including the fact that DQw1 and other similar determinants are supertypic specificities. Variation within the DR4-associated MLC types, differences between Dw2 and Dw12 and polymorphism for the DQ (DC) α chain were either established or confirmed biochemically and fitted together with the amino acid and nucleotide sequence data. The biochemical analyses further emphasised the extraordinarily strong linkage disequilibrium between the alleles of the DQ α, β and DR β chain genes, which contributes to the difficulty in using the conventional alloserology to resolve the different gene products.

Molecular Genetics and Transfection

Molecular genetics can be very effectively combined with serological and cellular techniques through the use of the technique of transfection. Thus, a well-defined particular cloned gene can now be inserted into an alien cell, where it can be expressed, and so studied, against an effectively neutral background. In this way one can study the specificity and function of a single gene product, avoiding mixtures and problems of linkage disequilibrium. Interesting work along these lines has been done, for example, by the French group for the *A* locus specificities, in Stanford for B17 and by Mach and others for HLA-DR. Transfectant cell lines promise to be unique reagents for studying gene expression and for making monoclonal antibodies and cloned T cell lines of defined specificity. Using the techniques of in vitro mutagenesis followed by transfection, the expression of cloned genes altered in defined positions can be studied. How, for example, are the expression of serological determinants and other functions affected by switching around different parts of the molecule or by changing, deleting or inserting sequences in defined regions? These techniques will define the functionally important parts of the molecules and so provide the basis for understanding how variations influence immune response and disease susceptibility.

There will be puzzles created by these novel approaches using interspecific combinations of genes and cells. It has, for example, been observed by several groups that cytotoxic T cells (CTLs) mostly do not effectively attack their specific human determinants against a mouse cellular background. Similarly Mach and Thorsby and their colleagues have found that human class II products on a mouse L cell background do not stimulate as expected in an MLC. In both situations there appears to be something missing that a human cell can provide but a mouse cell cannot, some other determinant perhaps. Using mouse L cell transfectants for human class II products for antigen presentation may circumvent these problems. Thus in our laboratory Austin and Trowsdale have obtained L cell transfectants expressing a DP product on their surface which is derived from the '1β' gene (see Fig. 1) and either, or both, DPα genes. Using either FACS analysis or an ELISA assay, the transfectants react with monoclonal antibodies such as TÜ39, SG171 and B7/21(FA) known to react with DP products, while they are negative with monomorphic DR and DQ antibodies such as L203 and TÜ22. The reaction with B7/21(FA) (from Trowbridge and Bach) is especially significant, as the joint biochemical analysis showed that this antibody is, so far, unique in reacting exclusively with one subset of products, namely DP. Clearly the transfectants, once characterised, will be very useful for the definition of serological specificities.

In collaboration with J. Lamb in London, it has been shown, using DP-restricted T cell clones specific for flu virus neuraminidase, that these transfectants can present specific antigen. This contrasts with the reported inability of CTLs to recognise human determinants against a mouse background. Perhaps in the latter case the equivalent of the antigen added for studying antigen presentation is lacking. Thus the CTLs may be recognising a monomorphic cell surface determinant in association with the class I products, so that on human cells they are specific for the class I polymorphism. The lack of CTL recognition on the mouse cell is then, presumably, because this lacks the relevant monomorphic human cell surface determinant recognised by CTLs. Perhaps this could be provided, and mapped to a chromosome, using appropriate human-mouse somatic cell hybrids as targets. Transfectants may be encouraged to stimulate in an MLC by, for example, adding IL2 or using them to restimulate. These approaches should help to provide functional assays for transfectants and so enable these very powerful tools to be used for a broad range of functional studies.

Variations in Expression

Studies with transfectants to some extent are analogous to the use of mutants, pioneered by Pious, and Kavathos and De Mars, which have made substantial contributions to the characterisation of monoclonal antibodies and gene clones. These mutants, however, can also provide interesting examples of variations in the control of expression of HLA region products.

There are now many interesting examples of natural variation in expression of HLA-D region products. At first it was thought that class II products were present on B cells and most monocytes and macrophages, but not on other cells. Perhaps the first indication that the situation was more complicated came from Hirschberg and Thorsby, who showed that endothelial cells could stimulate in an MLC and, subsequently, that some melanomas were found to express HLA-D products. Now class II products are appearing unexpectedly on a wide range of tissues, for example, sometimes on epithelial cells and even on fibroblasts. Differential expression of DQ as compared to DR has been found on some leukaemic cells. Increased expression can often be induced by, for example, the phorbol esther TPA or by gamma interferon, provided in pure form using recombinant DNA techniques. What is the significance of such induction of expression of HLA-D products, especially by gamma interferon, which may reflect a natural mechanism for controlling expression? Is it, for example, an adaptation to emergency presentation of antigen in the absence of macrophages? Does it then help the immune response to focus on viruses attacking different tissues? But then, as in other aspects of enhanced protective immune response, is there a price to pay, as suggested by Bottazzo and colleagues, because triggering D region expression in certain tissues, such as the thyroid epithelium, may sometimes enhance the possibility of auto-immune attack and so contribute to the development of auto-immune disease?

The "bare lymphocyte" syndrome and related deficiences are fascinating examples of in vivo mutants. They were first described as combined immunodeficiencies associated with a reduction in HLA class I expression, and then later with reduced or absent class II expression. It now appears that there is probably a variety of related mutants controlling expression of one or more HLA products. The mutations are not in the HLA region, because affected individuals within a family are not necessarily HLA identical. Molecular and cellular studies should help elucidate the nature of these intriguing mutations. Somatic cell hybrids, for example made between DR-negative lymphoblastoid cell lines from these patients and Ia-positive mouse cell lines, might enable the mapping of the gene(s) controlling D region expression.

Class I determinant variation on human tumour cells was first clearly seen in the Burkitt-lymphoma-derived Daudi cell line, which was shown to lack HLA-ABC and β_2 microglobulin (β_2m) surface expression because it was a recessive mutant for β_2m production. This led to our speculation, some years ago, that the absence of surface HLA class I expression protected Daudi as a tumour from cellular immune response with respect to Epstein-Barr virus determinants. More generally, it was suggested that lack of HLA-ABC expression may tend to be selected for during tumour progression whenever a tumour needs to escape from the host's immune response to tumour-specific antigens, including especially viral determinants. Many examples of reduced expression of HLA-ABC determinants in tumours have now been found. In our own laboratory, for example, we have observed that a majority of colorectal cell lines lack HLA-ABC expression. Ferrone and his colleagues have described an intriguing correlation between lack of HLA-ABC expression and metastasis in melanomas, and Michael Feldman and others have done experiments in the mouse suggesting a role for altered class I determinant expression in relation to the potential for tumour metastasis and progression. More work is clearly needed along the lines of that described by Sanderson, Beverly and others relating, in human tissue sections, class I expression on primary and secondary tumours with clinical outcome.

These natural mutants, which arise and are selected for during tumour progression, will be interesting to study in their own right and because of what they tell us about the immune response to tumours. Thus it has, for example, been shown recently by Van der Erb and others that certain transforming adenoviruses reduce class I antigen expression in the rat, and Rigby and colleagues have described an intriguing induction of expression of H-2 TL or perhaps H-2 L or D-like determinants in transformed mouse cells. This recalls the classical observation that mouse thymocytes, which have increased expression of TL, have a correspondingly reduced expression of H-2K and D, and the same is true for human thymocytes and T-ALL. Perhaps one way to reduce H-2K, D, L, or HLA-ABC expression is to mimic thymocytes and, by mutation, switch control of expression to TL, which may not function, or functions less efficiently, as a joint target for CTLs. In most trophoblasts the *HLA-A*, *B* and *C* loci are co-ordinately switched off (most probably as a major part of the mechanism by which the foetus survives as an allograft), and that could also be a basis for mutations which mimic the natural process and switch off all these three genes together.

Transplantation

The transplantation study in this workshop was another extraordinary example of how much can be achieved by international collaboration among a considerable number of centres providing data on a very large number of transplants. It also shows the importance of the serological collaboration, since it seems that the HLA effects are seen more clearly in those transplants which have been typed using the workshop serology than in the others. This shows, incidentally, the importance of good serology for effective studies on HLA and transplantation. The role of the HLA-D region appears to be established, but further work is needed on the intriguing effects of DRw6. More work is also needed to further understanding of the role of donor-specific blood transfusion. Hopefully, the HLA associations will be more finely dissected and established by the use of monoclonal antibodies and molecular techniques.

Disease Associations

Studies on disease associations, as in previous workshops, have yielded interesting results. These include further data on the association between AIDS and Kaposi's sarcoma and DR5 and DRw52, and on juvenile rheumatoid arthritis, emphasising especially the importance of proper clinical classification and how the HLA associations can help to analyse disease heterogeneity. The clear description of the lack of any true B27-negative ankylosing sponylitis is reassuring, considering the unsuccessful effort made to find it in 1977 in the Oxford workshop. It seems clear that B27-negative ankylosing spondylitis, if it exists, is a different disease from that associated with B27. The study on leprosy was the first in a workshop on an infectious disease. The HLA association with gold-induced nephropathy surely must be taken into account in planning treatment for severe rheumatoid arthritis. Intriguing results were reported on interactions between gamma endorphins and HLA determinants by Van Rood and colleagues, and between antibodies to HLA-A and B antigens and human T-cell leukemia virus by Dean Mann and his colleagues. Among the variety of other interesting data I wish to focus on the contrasting interpretations of the HLA associations with rheumatoid arthritis (RA), Hodgkin's disease (HD) and juvenile-onset insulin-dependent diabetes mellitus (IDDM).

It is striking that, while the RA association with DR4 remains high and very convincing, the sib pair HLA distribution shows no significant distortion. This is an apparent paradox which has at least two explanations. One is that, as emphasised by Glenys Thomson, if the relevant HLA-linked disease gene is effectively dominant and has a relatively high frequency and therefore a low penetrance, there may be a minimal disturbance of the HLA distribution in affected sib pairs which could be difficult to detect. The second possible explanation arises if there is a mixture of HLA-associated and non-HLA-associated, or sporadic, forms of the disease. The sporadic forms could involve other non-HLA-linked genes as well, of course, as environmental effects. Suppose, for example, that 50% of rheumatoids are HLA-associated and 50% are not, i.e. are sporadic. Then, in the absence of any other distinguishing feature between these two forms of the disease, and especially given the likely low penetrance of the HLA-linked effect, only about a quarter of affected sib pairs will both involve HLA associations. In the face of these two likely factors, namely a low-penetrance, high-frequency, dominant HLA-linked gene, and a relatively high frequency of sporadic cases, it is perhaps not surprising that there is no distortion of the HLA distribution among sib pairs with RA. It is therefore striking that the only clue to the genetic effect of HLA on RA remains the population association. Classical family studies simply do not help, unless, at least, there is some way to distinguish the HLA-linked from the non-HLA-linked cases. And, moreover, do not use lod scores for analysis of linkage between HLA and diseases that have no simple Mendelian basis! The potential errors in the model are greater than the estimated recombination fractions, whose limits are much more tightly set by the linkage disequilibrium that gives rise to the HLA association with the disease in the population. This can only exist if the recombination fraction is very small, probably less than 0.5%.

Hodgkin's disease presents a very interesting picture, complementary to that of RA. In this case the population association is very weak, as first observed in 1967 by Amiel, and is only convincing because it has been studied so much. In families, on the other hand, as first clearly shown by De Hors et al., then by Mary Claire-King and her colleagues and now again in the workshop, the HLA distortion among sib pairs with HD is very clear and highly significant, even with comparatively small numbers. The situation is thus exactly the opposite to RA, where the association with HLA in the population is significant, but that in the family is not. The HD pattern can be accounted for, as suggested before, by a very rare gene, perhaps with a frequency of only one in a thousand, which is such that almost all homozygotes get HD while the penetrance in heterozygotes is very low, possibly no more than 5%. On the other hand, there may be few, if any, sporadic non-HLA-linked cases, so that almost everyone with HD has this particular HLA-linked gene. The challenge is, clearly, to find that gene, which must be somewhere in the HLA region. The weak population association between

HLA and HD suggests a gene in the HLA region that is not in linkage disequilibrium with those so far studied, namely *A*, *B*, *C*, *DR* and *DQ*. What about DP or DX? Perhaps that is where the search for the HD gene in the HLA region should be concentrated.

The third contrasting example of an HLA disease association is IDDM, which has been a human geneticists' conundrum even before the discovery of its HLA association. There can be no doubt about its familial concentration and a relatively high penetrance, perhaps 25% or more, in complete contrast to both RA and HD. In a family study of 43 IDDM cases carried out by Winearls, Julia Bodmer and myself in collaboration with colleagues in Oxford, all cases were either DR3, DR4 or both. This very strong association, stronger perhaps than in most other studies, may be due to the fact that all patients were under 16 years old and ascertained, presumably at random, from a paediatric clinic. The strength of the association emphasises, in contrast to RA, that there is little or no room for sporadic, non-HLA-involved cases, at least in relatively severe IDDM. The possible effect of additional non-HLA genes is of course allowed for in the penetrance parameter, which includes both the effects of other genes and environmental factors. In our data, as previously seen by others, especially Svejgaard and Dausset and their collaborators, a high proportion of cases are DR3/DR4 heterozygotes, though we also see a relatively high proportion of DR4/DR4 homozygotes, consistent with a relatively high DR4 association. But, in addition, we found that among DR4 heterozygotes who are not DR3/DR4, 10 out of 14 were DR4/DR1, which is undoubtedly significant. This finding is consistent with some earlier suggestions of an involvement of DR1 in RA, and also in other diseases, and brings to mind the existence of monoclonal antibodies that cross-react between DR1 and DR4. In the workshop data on IDDM it was notable that after taking account of DR3 and DR4, all the other antigens were decreased in frequency except DR1, and this too suggests a positive association with DR1. The workshop also, of course, added further to the large body of data showing a marked HLA association with IDDM among affected sib pairs. The combined overall IDDM data on sib pair distributions, population incidence, incidence in relatives and the population distribution of HLA genotypes are only really compatible with a comparatively low frequency gene or genes which, in homozygotes or heterozygotes for just these genes, has a relatively high penetrance. Numerical calculations suggest a combined gene frequency of, at most, 5%–6% and a penetrance of anywhere from 30% to 70%, so that most HLA-identical sibs within an IDDM family should have a relatively high probability of eventually developing the disease. This is clearly important from the point of view of preventative approaches to dealing with children in such families. In order to accommodate the fact that about 30% or more of IDDM patients in the population are heterozygotes only for DR3 or DR4 (i.e. DR3/*X* or DR4/*X*, where *X* is not DR3 or DR4), there has to be a small chance, perhaps no more than a few per cent, that individuals with just one copy of the relevant diseased gene(s) get IDDM. This overall interpretation of the data does matter from a practical point of view, since the alternative of one or more relatively frequent genes with low penetrance would give rise to a much lower disease concordance amongst HLA identical sibs. IDDM is thus different from RA and HD in that it associates strongly with HLA both in population and family studies.

There is another interesting contrast with RA. While the DR4 haplotypes associated with RA are similar to those in the normal population, the IDDM-associated DR4 haplotypes are strongly associated with B15, CW3 and probably Dw4, and so are clearly a particular subset of those found in the population at large. This suggests that either DR4 is not the gene responsible for susceptibility, but a neighbouring gene in linkage disequilibrium with both DR4 and B15 is involved, or that there is another gene involved in addition to DR4 and that this is associated with B15. The extraordinary heterozygote effect, which applies to both DR3/DR4 and DR4/DR1, needs to be explained. Svejgaard and I have suggested independently that it could be due to heterozygous determinants formed by particular combinations of D region α and β chains, and Charron has shown formally that, as expected, such combinations are formed by α and β chains from different haplotypes. Since DRα is essentially invariant, and DP shows little or no association with DR, these combinations must involve the DQ, and most probably DC, α and β chains, both of which are known to be very polymorphic. This is because α and β chain combinations from different D region subsets are unlikely to be functionally effective. Thus, suppose that the relevant DQ α and β alleles on the DR3 haplotype are αx and βx, while those on the DR4 haplotype are αy and βy. Then for DQ, the genotype of the DR3/DR4 heterozygote would be $\alpha x\ \beta x/\alpha y\ \beta y$. Such an individual can make four types of DQ (or DC) products, namely the parental combinations ($\alpha x\ \beta x$ and $\alpha y\ \beta y$) and the hetero combinations ($\alpha x \beta y$ and $\alpha y\ \beta x$). It is these latter products which could give rise to determinants seen only, or almost only, in such heterozygotes, since linkage disequilibrium between the very closely linked DQ or DC α and β genes would ensure that the haplotypes $\alpha x\ \beta y$, or $\alpha y\ \beta x$ do not occur, or at least are very rare. Indeed, it could be argued that particular haplotypes such as $\alpha x\ \beta x$ have been selected for because the (αx βx) product forms combination determinants that were selectively advantageous. This might provide a rationale for preserving close linkage, and so strong linkage disequilibrium, between corresponding α and β chain genes and their alleles.

The hetero-determinants formed by particular combinations of α and β chains have their analogy in the fact that an antibody's idiotypic specificity generally depends on the combination of both L and H chain variable regions. Since only a minority of the DQ products in a DR3/DR4 heterozygote will involve a specific combination of chains, the combination itself must have a "dominant" effect. It could, for example, specifically enhance or suppress a particular immune response.

The DNA probes should help to confirm this predicted involvement of DQ α and β chain combinations in determining IDDM susceptibility. It is important, though, to point out that such DNA polymorphism studies should be carried out in *random* diseased individuals, because family studies do not in practice help to resolve linkage differences at such very low recombination levels. What is being sought is not so much a marker that is further increased in frequency in the diseased population (since after all 100% is the limit, as in ankylosing spondylitis and as almost reached by DR3 and DR4 combined in IDDM), but one that is substantially decreased in frequency in controls, and so has much greater specificity for the disease. A remarkable example of this was the report by Tilanus, Van Rood and colleagues, of a fragment identified by a DR β chain probe that correlated perfectly with Felty's syndrome. The next challenge is to identify the critical DNA sequence responsible for the disease susceptibility and to explain its function.

Natural Selection

The HLA and disease associations are the price we now pay for the fact that our ancestors in less hygienic times were protected, at least to some extent, from infectious diseases. One of the most important lines of evidence for natural selection is when one gene is much more variable than another. This is because, in the absence of selection (or major differences in the overall mutation rates), all genes are expected, on average, to be equally variable, since random drift in the absence of selection depends on parameters of the population structure which are the same for all genes. Thus, the extraordinary differences in level of polymorphism between different α chains, and indeed between different parts of the same gene, surely indicate that selection is at play. Data from McDevitt and others show that a major part of the class II protein polymorphism lies in the N-terminal domain, with a tendency to cluster around certain positions, and the situation is probably similar for the highly polymorphic class I products. This pattern clearly suggests that natural selection has pulled out alleles with changed amino acid sequences in functionally important regions of the molecule, presumably those which give rise to immune response differences. The high level of polymorphism for DCα in comparison to the other α genes thus suggests that the DC α gene is more likely to give rise to functionally significant immune response variation. The patterns of polymorphism seen using DNA probes and restriction enzymes seem to match quite closely the serologically determined protein variation. However, most of the restriction enzyme variation is not within the gene and so cannot be detecting the serological differences directly. These DNA polymorphisms are thus going along with the variation within the gene because of strong linkage disequilibrium. One possible explanation for their origin is that in the course of producing the mutations in the gene which give rise to the immune response differences that are selected for, variants at some distance away are also produced. Thus, the mutation mechanism may give rise to both functionally relevant and functionally irrelevant variation, but because of close linkage both are pulled together into the population and remain associated through linkage disequilibrium. It is also possible that a new selected allelic variant happens to occur in a haplotype carrying one or more pre-existing polymorphisms in a flanking region or intron. This associated variant is likely to be selectively neutral and will also be carried into the population by linkage disequilibrium. Such associated variations will be broken into clusters by recombination hot spots, as has been observed in the haemoglobin gene cluster.

Gene Conversion

Gene conversion is nowadays invoked to explain all sorts of phenomena in the HLA region. Historically, gene conversion was discovered as a departure from expected Mendelian segregation, and established in *Neurospora* by the geneticist Lindegren, and nobody at first believed him. In *Neurospora* one can classify the immediate meiotic products, so that an $A \times a$ mating (it is haploid) should always segregate exactly $2A : 2a$. However, very occasionally, one observes instead say $3A : 1a$, and this is due to gene conversion. Subsequently, with the development of molecular genetics, a number of explanations were put forward for this phenomenon. Basically they involve the transfer, by copying, of a segment of DNA from one homologous chromosome to the other. In this way the recipient chromosome has acquired the copied chromosome's sequence in place of its own. Essentially, the same mechanism can lead to transfer of sequences from one gene on a chromosome to another related gene on the *same* (rather than the homologous) chromosome. This is unequal *intra*-chromosomal gene conversion. A double unequal intra-chromosomal cross-over may also have a similar effect. In the mouse, Flavell and Nathanson and their colleagues have produced convincing evidence for gene conversion as the mechanism by which some of the H-2 mutants were produced. Thus Flavell et al. have shown, for example, that the I-A β chain mutant bm12 has probably acquired a sequence from an I-E β chain gene, and this accounts for the mutation. Unequal intra-chromosomal gene conversion, for example between DQ and DR β genes, could account for cross-reactions between the products of alleles at different loci, as revealed by monoclonal antibodies. Since such a gene conversion event would have happened on one particular haplotype, the converted and original alleles will initially be on this same haplotype. Then, if they are sufficiently close together, which is likely, they will stay together in strong linkage disequilibrium, and that explains why there can be strong linkage disequilibrium between cross-reacting determinants on different locus products. Clearly, subsequent evolution may lead to divergence between the original allele and its converted partner. The converted segment may also take on a slightly different configuration in the alien background of the gene into which it has been inserted. In either case, the serological specificities detected in the two cross-reacting products will not be expected to be precisely the same. These phenomena make it very difficult to establish unequivocally the evolutionary history of alleles, as was originally tried for the alleles of the HLA-A and B loci and is now being attempted in the HLA-D region.

Structure and Function

A major goal of HLA studies must be to understand function, especially of course in relation to transplantation and disease associations, and function must ultimately be studied through structure. The basic structure of the class I (and β2m) and class II molecules is of course already established through protein and DNA sequence analysis. They have a similar organisation, with pairs of domains near the surface, pairs of domains distal to the surface which carry most of the polymorphic determinants, and transmembrane and short intracytoplasmic segments. The membrane proximal domains are clearly similar in sequence and structure to immunoglobulin constant regions. At the DNA level there is a striking relationship between the genomic exons and the protein domains. Sequence comparisons clearly show that DR is the homologue of mouse I-E, and DQ of I-A, which differ on average by no more than about 30%. Different types of products, such as α and β genes, or class I and class II products, have only about 25%–30% of their sequences in common, and this is comparable to the relationship with immunoglobulins. It is this extent of sequence similarity, which applies especially to amino acids that are critical for structural conformation and so predicts structural similarity, which places the HLA class I and class II products and the immunoglobulins in the same superfamily of related genes. Using the known three-dimensional structure of immunoglobulins, one can begin to predict the detailed structure of parts of the HLA-D region products. These predictions, for example, indicate that the points of contact between the α and β chains are different for DR and DQ to such an extent that it seems most unlikely that combinations of, say, a DR α chain and a DQ β chain would form stable, fully functional, products. Clearly the aim must be to obtain the complete three-dimensional structure of these products using X-ray crystallographic techniques, and from this discern, for example, the nature of the external polymorphic domains and their contribution to immune response control. Recombinant DNA techniques will be needed to obtain these molecules in sufficient amounts to study their structure.

The structures of the HLA products must be studied in relation to those of the T cell receptor molecules with which they interact to carry out their function. The T cell receptor, which is the T cell's equivalent of antibody, has now been shown by the work of Davies and others to be another most important member of the immunoglobulin-related superfamily of products. T cell receptors will surely be found to be subdivided into functionally different classes, according for example to whether they work on cytotoxic, helper or suppressor T cells, and so according to their interactions with class I and class II products. Perhaps, as already mentioned, since DQ may be more related to suppression than to help and vice versa for DR, this will be reflected in their preferential associations with different classes of T receptor molecules. This distinction may also be an important clue to disease susceptibility mechanisms, so that, for example, a DQ-associated disease may be more likely to involve suppression than help as the basis of the immune response difference. Variation in the T cell receptor itself may, of course, also influence immune response and interact with HLA differences in determining disease susceptibility. These are all exciting and important questions for future investigation.

The Way Forward

The next workshop will take us forward together into the realms of molecular genetics and the challenge of using these newer techniques to understand the nature of the polymorphic variation within the HLA region in relation to its function. Monoclonal antibodies and recombinant DNA techniques will be used in conjunction with the serological and cellular tools that have formed the basis for the definition of the HLA region. The DNA typing procedures will not easily replace the serology, and one must avoid circular arguments in typing with the DNA markers instead of the serology, for sooner or later, even with very close linkage disequilibrium, the association between the two may be broken. And if we do find that little sequence in a DQ α chain that really helps to cause susceptibility to IDDM, I suspect it will eventually be typed for by means of a monoclonal antibody made to recognise just that short sequence.
Ekkehart Albert, having organised this marvellous workshop, becomes our President, and now Bo Dupont, our new organiser, is going to take us forward into the new era in which we combine molecular and biochemical with serological and cellular techniques in the Tenth International Histocompatibility Testing Workshop.

Acknowledgements. To have documented this HLA overview with references would have been a considerable and hopefully superfluous task, since the material referred to is all well documented in the rest of this volume. I clearly owe an enormous debt to all my many colleagues in the HLA field, to the many workshop participants and especially, of course, to the workshop and conference organisers, Ekkehard Albert, Wolfgang Mayr and their colleagues. I have throughout used the nomenclature established by the WHO Committee, which met and reported after the workshop conference.

HLA at the Gene Level

J. Dausset and D. Cohen

Institut de Recherches sur les Leucémies, Unit 93, Institut National de la Santé et de la Recherche Médicale,
Hôpital Saint-Louis, 2, Place du Dr. Fournier, 75010 Paris, France

After years of exciting research on the products of the HLA complex, it is now possible, using the powerful tools of moleculear biology, to reach the HLA genes themselves. A great deal has been learned recently about the organisation of this complex, including the number of genes in each class, their arrangement in exons and introns, and even their nucleotide sequences [1–3].
Numerous class I genes exist, at least 20. Each region (A, B, and C) contains a limited number of genes which may be functional or nonfunctional. However, the majority of them appear to be the human analogue of the murine Qa and Tla genes. An interesting possibility is that some genes may code for soluble antigens which could be involved in transplantation tolerance. The comparison of class I and II molecules with the immunoglobulin gene (Fig. 1) is striking and suggests the existence of a common ancestor for these genes involved in self and nonself recognition [4–12].
Class II genes code for the α and β chains of the class II molecules. There are at least seven β genes and five α genes (two DPα, two DPβ; two DQα, two DQβ; one DRα and three DRβ) (Fig. 2). Cell surface molecules which are presently well characterized include one DP molecule, one DQ molecule and two DR molecules; however, it is likely that other weakly expressed molecules will be detected later (a DP and a DQ have been postulated) [13–28].

Histocompatibility Testing 1984
Edited by E. D. Albert et al.

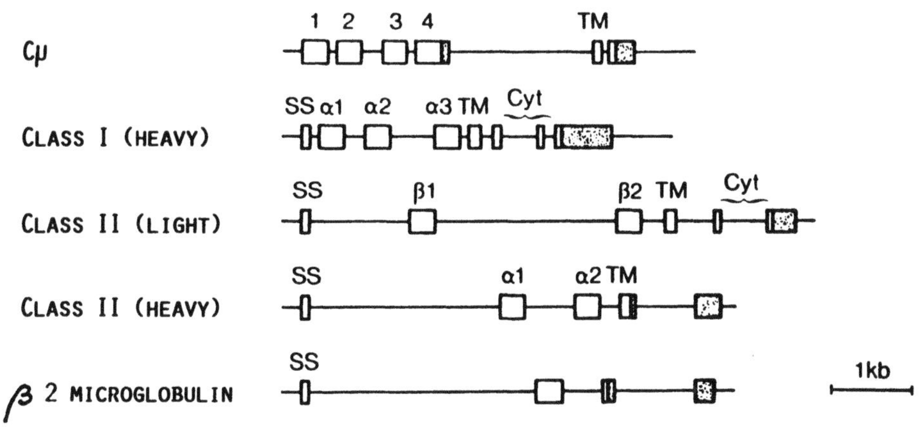

Fig. 1. Comparison of the gene organization of the $C\mu$ immunoglobulin genes with the HLA genes coding for the heavy chain of class I, for the β and α chains of class II, and for the β 2 microglobulin of class I. The exons are represented by *squares* and introns by a *line*. *SS*, signal sequence; α and β correspond to the various domains of the chains; *TM*, transmembrane; *Cyt*, intracytoplasmic. The *shaded areas* correspond to the 3′-untranslated regions

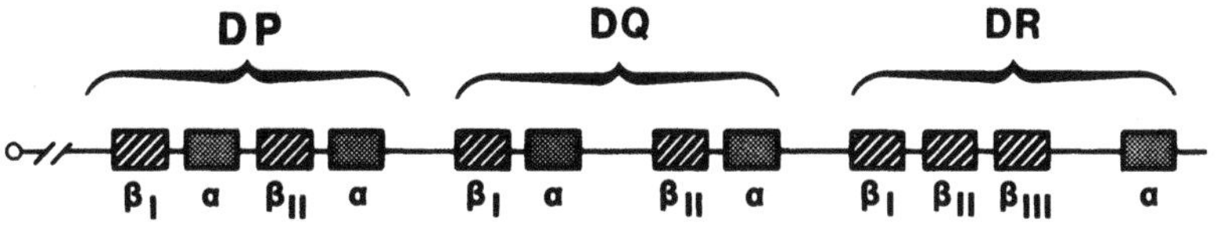

Fig. 2. Organization of the human HLA-D region (from Bernard Mach). The HLA-D region is subdivided into three subregions: DP (SB) with two α and two β genes, DQ (DC) with two α and two β genes, and DR with three β and one α gene. The DP is centromeric, but the order of the other two subregions is not known, as is the α, β organization within them. The distance between DP and the other class II subregions is about 1 centimorgan

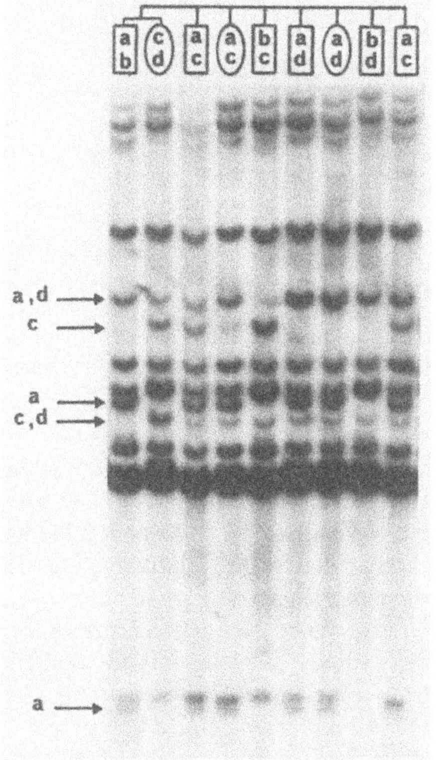

Fig. 3. Segregation in a family of *BglI* class I restriction fragments. Each lane corresponds to one individual. The two parents, with *a, b* and *c, d* HLA haplotypes, are on the *left*, the children on the *right*. Note that some bands marked *a* or *c* segregate with a corresponding haplotype. Note also that the band marked *a, d* is much more intense in children *a, d*, indicating that they are homozygous for this fragment

As for class III, the order of the genes is now well established as Bf, C2, C4A, C4B, but the position of the centromere (on one side or the other) is unknown. Bf and C2 genes are very closely associated (only a few nucleotides apart) and have a strong homology. The genes C4A and C4B are separated from the Bf, C2 complex by a larger distance. Bf possesses 18 exons. In the mouse, there are two 21-hydroxylase genes, each of which is close to each C4 gene. The same situation probably occurs in man [29, 30].

Our contribution to the unravelling of the HLA genes has included a systematic study, using the Southern blot technique, of restriction fragment length polymorphisms (RFLP or allogenotopes). We used five different enzymes to study the DNA of the parents and children of 23 families. The fragments were visualized by a class I cDNA probe (Weissman) and several class II cDNA probes: DQα (Strominger), DRβ, and DQβ (Peterson).

In most of these cases (99%) it was possible to assign the allogenotopes in a given haplotype, even when a family was not directly informative. Indeed, the homozygosity for a given gene can easily be deduced from the intensity of the band (Fig. 3). It must be emphasized that the allogenotope always segregates with the HLA haplotype, indicating that there are probably no polymorphic homologous genes outside the human MHC.

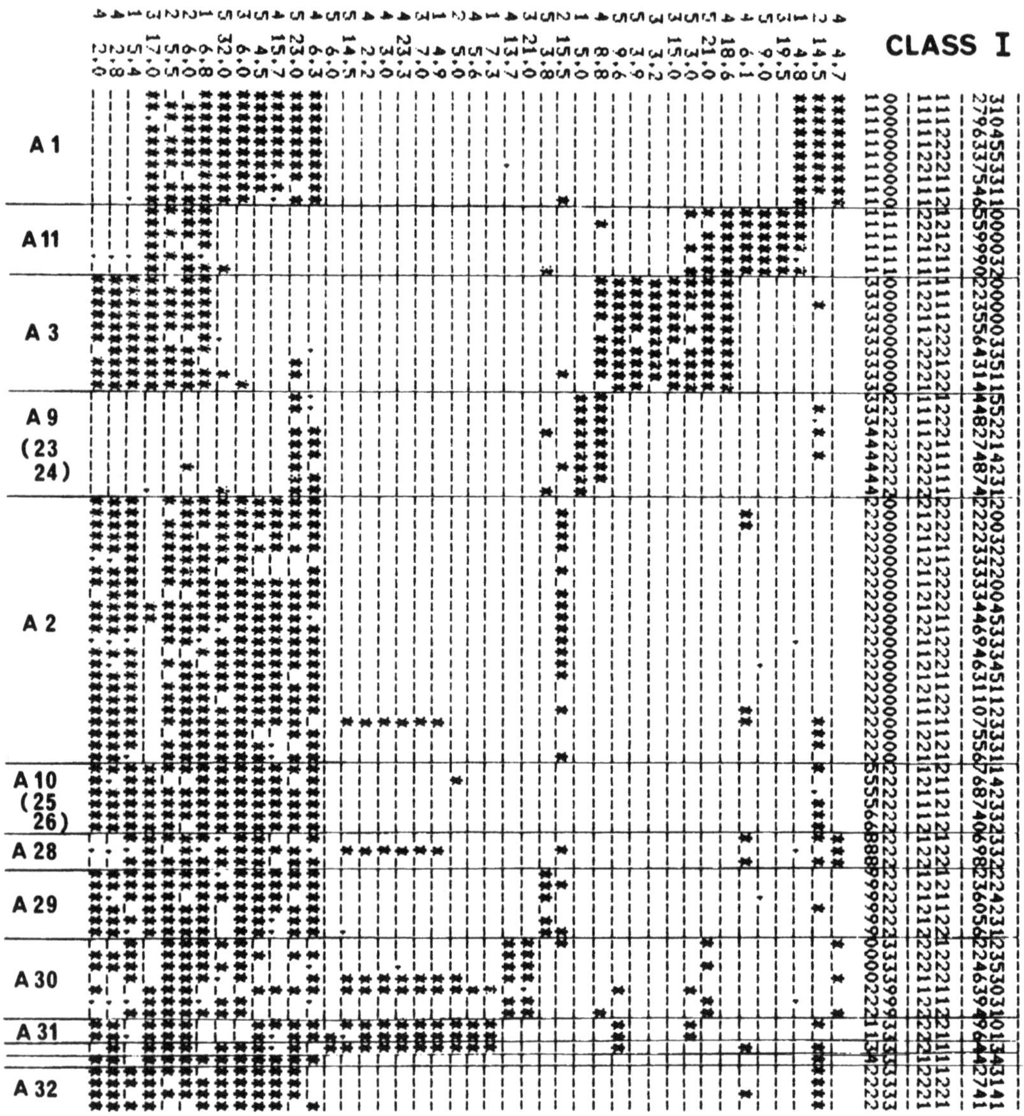

Fig. 4. Distribution among 88 haplotypes of 56 class I restriction fragments correlating with HLA-A alleles. Each *horizontal line* corresponds to a haplotype while each *vertical line* corresponds to a given fragment. The *stars* indicate the presence of a fragment. A *dot* indicates "not done" or "unreadable." The *figures* at the top of each vertical line indicate the enzymes used (*1, Hin*dIII; *2, Eco*RV; *3, Eco*RI; *4, Pvu*II; *5, Bam*HI) as well as the length in kilobases of the fragment. The haplotypes have been classified according to the HLA-A alleles that they carry (for further explanation, see text)

Class I

With five enzymes we have observed 152 different fragments of which 88 are polymorphic. Surprisingly, 63% of these polymorphisms correlated with alleles of the HLA-A locus, and only 13% and 5% with the HLA-B and C alleles respectively. This striking difference suggests that the A region is more divergent than the B and C regions. About 19% of variable bands do not correlate with any known serologically defined HLA alleles.

In Fig. 4, it can be seen that clusters of variable allogenotopes correlate positively with alleles A1, A11, A3, A9 (A23 and A24) and some of the Aw19 crossreacting group (A30, A31, Aw33). Four other clusters, found in most haplotypes, are defined by negative correlations with A1, A11, A9; A9 alone; A11, A3, A9; and A11, A3 respectively. The most striking observation is that A9 (A23 and A24) haplotypes are associated with relatively few restriction fragments, suggesting that these haplotypes carry fewer gene copies than the others. On the contrary, some Aw19 haplotypes seem to carry more class I gene copies than the others. The fact that a single A2 and a single A28 haplotype also carry the Aw19-specific cluster may indicate that they are recombinant haplotypes between genes of the HLA-A gene family.

The variation from one haplotype to another could be the result of deletion or duplication. Among the genes of the A, B, and C families, probably only one is expressed, as indicated by preliminary data

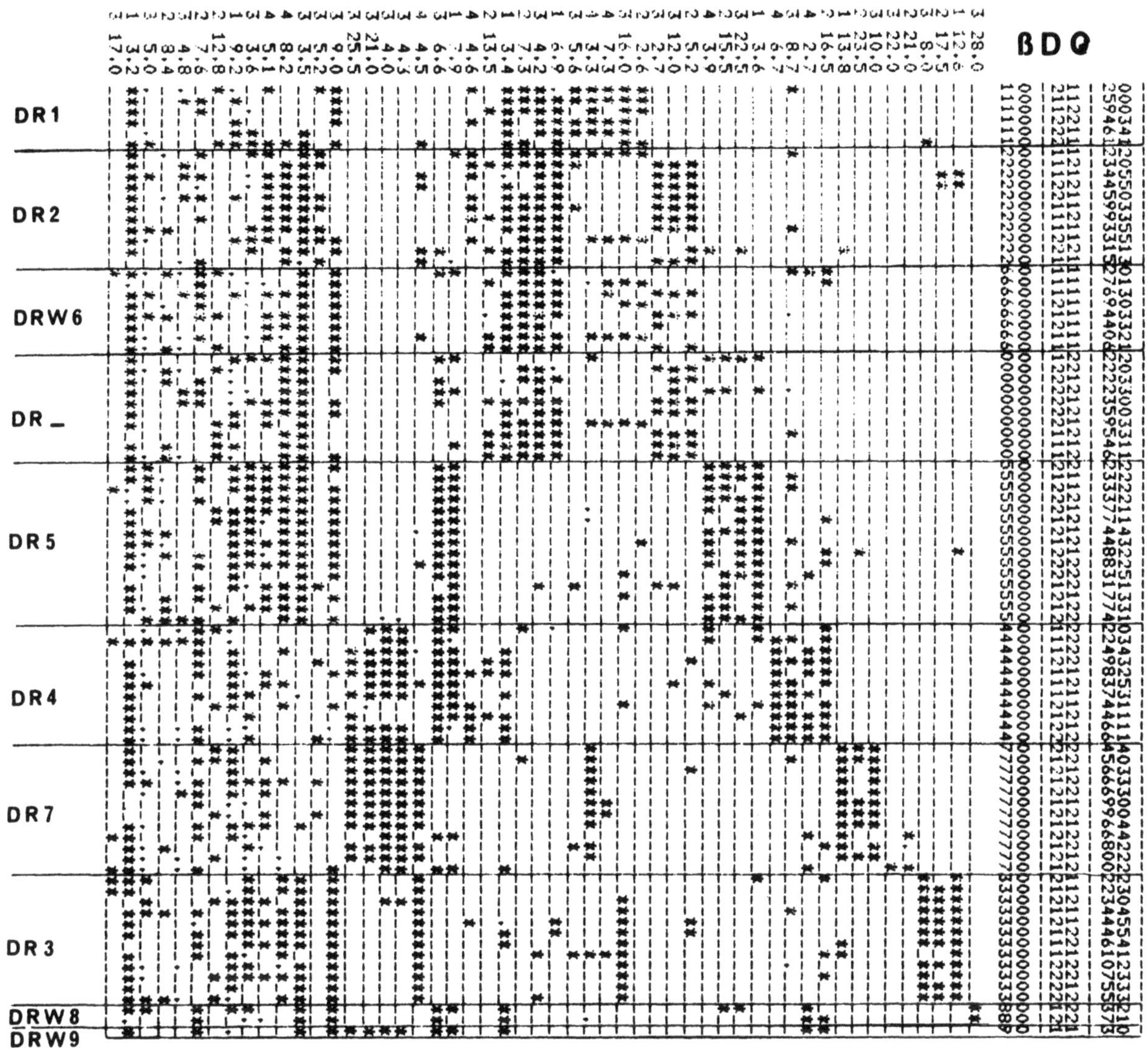

Fig. 5. Distribution among 88 haplotypes of the 52 restriction fragments observed with a DQβ probe and four enzymes. See legend, Fig. 4, for interpretation. The *figures* at the top of the *vertical lines* correspond to the enzymes used (*1, Hind*III; *2, Eco*RV; *3, Eco*RI; *4, Bam*HI). The seven fragments on the *left* of the figure do not correlate with any known specificity

on gene transfection. Already several A genes have been successfully transfected: A1 by Orr (personal communication), A2 by Barbosa et al. [12], A3 by Lemonnier et al. [11], A9 by Jordan (personal communication), A11 and A26 by Paul et al. (unpublished observation).

Correlations of allogenotopes with B and C alleles are much less numerous.

Class II

Genomic DNA from the same families was hybridized with DQβ, DRβ, and DQα probes. Using six different enzymes and a DQβ probe, 52 allogenotopes were detected. Those which have been considered as DQβ fragments are (1) those which were seen with the DQβ probe but not with the DRβ probe, and (2) those which hybridized with both probes but showed a more intense signal with the DQβ probe.

The 88 haplotypes studied have been arranged in Fig. 5 in order to show the various clusters of allogenotopes and their correlations with the DR, the DQ, and the MT (DRw52 and 53). On the right side of the figure are displayed the clusters which correlate well with the DR series: DR5, DR4, DR7, and DR3. Only one allogenotope correlated with DRw8. In the middle of the figure are the clusters correlating with the DQ series. At the top is a large cluster correlating with DQw1 (DR1, 2, w6, blank). This cluster is associated with two other subclusters, subdividing the same haplotype into two groups. Another cluster correlates with DQw2 (DR5 + 4), and only one allogenotope correlates with DQw3 (DR7 + 3). Finally, on the left of the figure, one can see clusters correlating with the MT series; two DRβ clusters correlate with MT3 (DRw53, i.e. DR4 + 7 + w9), one positively and one negatively associated with this specificity. When the distinction between the DQ and DR bands is made, the data suggests that the DQβ allogenotopes correlate mostly with DR and DQ specificities, while the DRβ allogenotopes correlate mostly with the MT (DRw52, 53) and less obviously with DR specificities.

Our interpretation is that DQβ correlates with the DR specificities by virtue of a strong linkage disequlibrium between polymorphic sequences associated with most DQβ and DRβ genes (Fig. 6). Products of the polymorphic sequence existing in the DQβ genes are not presently serologically identified. This could be due either to non- or weak immunogenicity of the corresponding epitopes or to the fact that anti-DQ antibodies are usually confused with anti-DR antibodies (as was the case for a long time between some anti-B and anti-Cw antibodies).

With a DQα probe, four variable *Hin*dIII restriction fragments were noted. These four fragments behave as alleles in the population. One correlates with DR4 + 7 (DRw53) and another with DR3 + 5 (DRw52). The other two split the DQw1 specificity but in a different way from the DQβ probes.

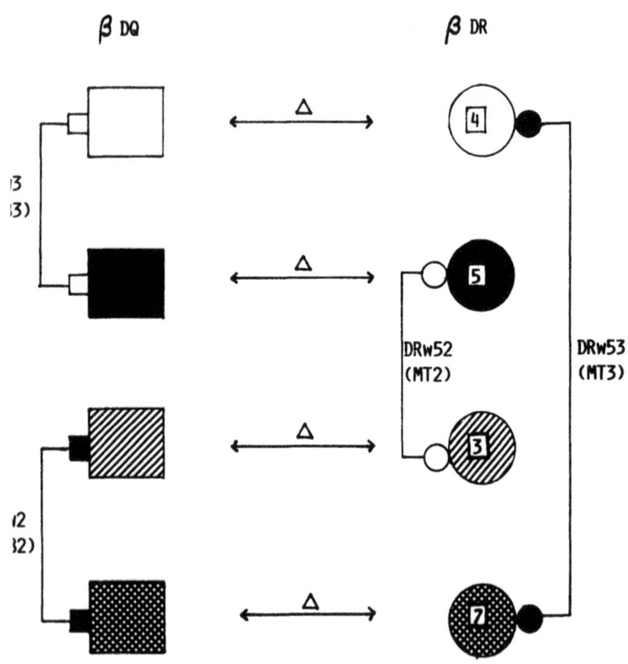

Fig. 6. The correlation observed between βDQ and βDR allogenotopes and DR, DQ, and MT (DRw52, 53) serologically determined specificities: βDQ (*squares*) and βDR (*circles*) genes carry private sequences (*white, black, shaded* and *cross-hatched*) in strong linkage disequilibrium (Δ) as well as supertypic sequences (*small connecting squares and circles*) corresponding to the DQ (MB) and DRw52 (MT2) series

If we assume that the DRw52 and 53 epitopes are borne not by the DR molecules but by the β chain of a second DR-like (BR?) molecule, it follows that the α polymorphism is in linkage disequilibrium with the allelic variation of the β chain of this DR-like molecule.

In conclusion, allogenotopes are a new tool for studying polymorphism of the HLA genes. There are good but not complete correlations with the already known cell surface polymorphism. DNA typing [31] will give information differing from that of classical HLA typing, since for the first time we have a means of studying the noncoding regions of the HLA complex, either in the introns or in flanking regions. The latter are known to be the site of regulatory mechanisms for the expression of genes. This could be of considerable importance to the understanding of HLA and disease association.

HLA and Disease Association

One of the most interesting diseases is juvenile insulin-dependent diabetes mellitus (IDDM) [32, 33]. The excess of affected HLA-identical siblings indicates that both haplotypes are involved. In Caucasians, heterozygous DR3/DR4 patients are very frequent, and DR2 patients are rare. We studied 35 patients and an equal number of DR matched controls using five restriction enzymes and a DQβ probe. Several bands were found to be significantly increased or decreased in frequency among patients compared to controls. With some bands, a significant difference in frequency was found only when the comparison was made within a given DR or DQ specificity. One band was particularly interesting. An *Eco*RI 2.2-kb fragment was absent from the seven DR2 patients studied, while present in 14 of 15 DR2 controls ($p = 0.00005$).

Two characteristic patterns of bands could be observed. The first was among DR1 patients: the absence of an *Eco*RI 8.0-kb fragment and the presence of *Bam*HI 8.2-, 4.6-, and 3.3-kb fragments ($p = 0.0006$) (Table 1). The second pattern was among the DR3/DR4 patients: the presence of *Taq*I 14.5- and 1.8-kb fragments and the absence of a *Taq*I 12.7-kb fragment. This pattern was observed in 11 of the 12 DR3/4 patients and not in the 12 DR-matched controls ($p = 0.000005$). Moreover, the *Taq*I 14.5-kb fragment is a DR fragment, while the *Taq*I 1.8-kb fragment is a DQ fragment. The relative risk for IDDM among DR3/4 individuals carrying this pattern is over 400, about 10 times higher than the risk calculated using only serologically defined markers (Table 1).

A less extensive study has been conducted in multiple sclerosis (MS). An *Eco*RI 12.8-kb DQβ frag-

Table 1. Specific Distribution of Some Class II β Allogenotopes in Diabetic Patients

					All DR		
*Eco*RI 8.0	*Bam*HI 8.2	*Bam*HI 4.6	*Bam*HI 3.3 kb		All DR	DR1	
–	+	+	+	IDDM	2/35	1/8	$p=0.0006$
				Controls	9/35	8/8	
*Taq*I 14.5	*Taq*I 12.7	*Taq*I 1.8 kb			All DR	DR3/4	
+	–	+		IDDM	11/35	11/12	$p=0.000005$
				Controls	0/35	0/12	
*Eco*RI 2.2 kb					All DR	DR2	
+				IDDM	2/35	0/7	$p=0.00005$
				Controls	7/35	14/15	

ment was found in 22 patients and 26 controls. Among the HLA-DRw6 or DR- (blank) individuals, 12 of the 16 controls and none of the seven patients carried this fragment ($p=0.001$). Interestingly enough, the *Eco*RI 2.2-kb fragment, absent in DR2 IDDM patients, is usually present in DR2 MS patients.

Conclusion

Human genetics is entering a new era, thanks to the introduction of molecular biology. The HLA complex, deeply involved in the defence of the organism, is one of the most interesting parts of the human genome. Restriction enzymes, which digest the DNA molecules both in the coding and noncoding regions, considerably increase our insight into the HLA complex. It is amazing that with only a few enzymes and four different probes (one class I, and three class II), we have already been able to detect more than 150 polymorphic markers in the HLA complex. Moreover, our results are in complete agreement with the serological and biochemical data accumulated during the past 20 years.

Important applications will quickly follow. Among the earliest will be the refinement of the known associations with disease. New polymorphic markers, more closely associated with susceptibility or resistance to diseases, will be found. It is possible that new diseases will be added to the list of those associated with HLA when associations are found with new DNA polymorphisms which have no associations with the classical HLA series. Predictive and preventive medicine will take advantage of these advances.

The ultimate goal, however, is to achieve understanding of the true pathophysiological mechanism of these diseases by the exact identification and characterization of the gene or genes responsible for the diseases, thus hopefully leading to therapeutic management.

Acknowledgements. This work was made possible by the dedication and enthusiasm of Odile Cohen, Marie-Pierre Font, Isabelle LeGall, Agnes Marcadet, Pascale Paul, Brigitte Sayagh for their work in molecular biology. We are deeply indebted to Jean-Marc Lalouel for the computer analysis. We are grateful to Drs. C. Raffoux and V. Lepage for the HLA typing, and to Professor J. Hors, Dr. I. Deschamps and Professor H. Lestradet for their contribution to the study of juvenile insulin-dependent diabetes. We also wish to thank Dr. Elizabeth Robbins and Ms. Elizabeth May for translation and typing of the paper.

References

1. Steinmetz M, Hood L (1983) Genes of the major histocompatibility complex in mouse and man. Science 222:727–733
2. Kaufman JF, Auffray C, Korman AJ, Shackelford DA, Strominger J (1984) The class II molecules of the human and murine major histocompatibility complex. Cell 36:1–13
3. Cohen D, Dausset J (1983) HLA genes polymorphism. In: Proceedings of Fifth Congress of Immunology, Kyoto, August
4. Sood AK, Pereira D, Weissman SM (1981) Isolation and partial nucleotide sequence of a cDNA clone for human histocompatibility antigen HLA-B by use of an oligodeoxynucleotide primer. Proc Natl Acad Sci USA 78:616
5. Malissen M, Malissen B, Jordan BR (1982) Exon/intron organization and complex nucleotide sequence of an HLA gene. Proc Natl Acad Sci USA 79:893–897
6. Ascanio L, Paul P, Narcadet A, Mahouy G, Fradelizi D, Cohen D, Dausset J (1982) Polymorphisme des gènes HLA (I): Mise en évidence d'une étroite corrélation entre des fragments d'ADN déterminés par l'enzyme de restriction *Bgl*I et des antigènes HLA de classe I. CR Seances Acad Sci (Paris) 295:433
7. Orr HT (1983) Use of Southern blotting to analyze the size and restriction fragment polymorphism of HLA class I DNA in the human population. Transplant Proc 15:1900–1906
8. Cann HM, Ascanio L, Paul P, Marcadet A, Dausset J, Cohen D (1983) Polymorphic restriction endonuclease fragment segregates and correlates with the gene for HLA-B8. Proc Natl Acad Sci USA 80:1665

9. Cohen D, Paul P, Font MP, Cohen O, Sayagh B, Marcadet A, Busson M, Mahouy G, Cann HM, Dausset J (1983) Analysis of HLA class I genes with restriction endonuclease fragments: implications for polymorphism of the human major histocompatibility complex. Proc Natl Acad Sci USA 80:6289
10. Jordan B (1983) Structure and expression of HLA-A gene. Proceedings of Fifth Congress of Immunology Kyoto, August
11. Lemonnier FA, Dubreuil PC, Layet C, Malissen M, Bourel D, Mercier P, Jabobsen BK, Caillol DH, Svejgaard A, Kourilsky FM, Jordan BR (1983) Transformation of MLTK⁻ cells with purified HLA class I genes. II. Serological characterization of HLA-A3 and Cw3 molecules. Immunogenetics 18:65
12. Barbosa JA, Kamarck ME, Biro PA, Weissman SM, Ruddle FH (1982) Proc Natl Acad Sci USA 79:6327–6331
13. Korman AJ, Auffray C, Schamboeck A, Strominger JL (1982) The amino acid sequence and gene organization of the heavy chain of the HLA-DR antigen: homology to immunoglobulins. Proc Natl Acad Sci USA 79:6013–6017
14. Larhammar O, Gustafsson K, Claesson L, Bill P, Wiman K, Shenning L, Sundelin J, Widmark E, Peterson PA, Rask L (1982) Alpha chain of HLA-DR transplantation antigens is a member of the same protein superfamily. Cell 30:153–161
15. Auffray C, Korman AJ, Roux-Dosseto M, Bono R, Strominger JL (1982) cDNA clone for the heavy chain of the human B cell alloantigen DC1: strong sequence homology to the HLA-DR heavy chain. Proc Natl Acad Sci USA 79:6337–6341
16. Lee JL, Trowsdale J, Travers PJ, Carey J, Grosveld F, Jenkins J, Bodmer WF (1982) Sequence of an HLA-DR chain cDNA clone and intron-exon organization of the corresponding gene. Nature 299:750–752
17. Auffray C, Ben-Nun A, Roux-Dosseto M, Germain RN, Seidman JG, Strominger JL (1983) Polymorphism and complexity of the human DC and murine Ia α chain genes. EMBO J 2:121
18. Trowsdale J, Lee J, Carey J, Grosveld F, Bodmer J, Bodmer W (1983) Sequences related to HLA-DRα chain on human chromosome 6: restriction enzyme polymorphism detected with DCα chain probes. Proc Natl Acad Sci USA 80:1972
19. Auffray C, Lillie JW, Arnot D, Grossberger D, Kappes D, Strominger JL (1984) Isotypic and allotypic variation of human class II histocompatibility antigen α-chain genes. Nature 308:327–333
20. Andersson M, Böhme J, Andersson G, Möller E, Thorsby E, Rask L, Perteson PA (1984) Genomic hybridization with class II transplantation antigen cDNA probes as a complementary technique in tissue typing. Hum Immunol (in press)
21. Wiman K, Larhammar D, Claesson L, Gustafsson K, Schenning L, Bill P, Böhma J, Denaro M, Dobberstein B, Hämmerling U, Kuist S, Servenius B, Sundelin J, Peterson PA, Rask L (1982) Isolation and identification of a cDNA clone corresponding to an HLA-DR antigen beta chain. Proc Natl Acad Sci USA 79:1703–1707
22. Wake CT, Long EO, Mach B (1982) Allelic polymorphism and complexity of the genes for HLA-DR β-chains direct analysis by DNA-DNA hybridization. Nature 300:372
23. Larhammar D, Schenning L, Gustafsson K, Wiman K, Claesson L, Rask L, Peterson PA (1982) Complete amino acid sequence of an HLA-DR antigen-like β chain as predicted from the nucleotide sequence: similarities with immunoglobulins and HLA-A, -B and -C antigens. Proc Natl Acad Sci USA 79:3687
24. Long FO, Wake CT, Gorski J, Mach B (1983) Complete sequence of an HLA-DRβ chain deduced from a cDNA clone and identification of multiple non-allelic DR chain genes. EMBO J 8:389–394
25. Larhammar D, Anderson G, Andersson M, Bill P, Böhme J, Claesson J, Denaro M, Emmoth E, Gustafsson K, Hammerling U, Heldin E, Hyldil-Nielsen JJ, Lind P, Schnning L, Servenius B, Widmark E, Rask L, Peterson PA (1983) Molecular analysis of human class II transplantation antigens and their genes. Hum Immunol 8:95–103
26. Roux-Dosseto M, Auffray C, Lillie JW, Boss JM, Cohen D, De Mars R, Mawas C, Seidman JG, Strominger JL (1983) Genetic mapping of a human class II antigen β chain cDNA clone to the SB region of the HLA. Proc Natl Acad Sci USA 80:6036
27. Owerbach D, Lernmark A, Rask L, Peterson PA, Platz P, Svejgaard A (1983) Detection of HLA-D/DR-related DNA polymorphism in HLA-D homozygous typing cells. Proc Natl Acad Sci USA 80:3758
28. Gustafsson R, Emmoth E, Widmark E, Böhme J, Peterson PA, Rask L (1984) Isolation of a cDNA clone coding for an SB β-chain. Nature 309:76–78
29. Whitehead AS, Woods DE, Fleischnick E, Chin JE, Yunis EJ, Katz AJ, Gerald PS, Alper CA, Colten HR (1984) DNA polymorphism of the C4 genes. A new marker for analysis of the major histocompatibility complex. N Engl J Med 310:88–91
30. Carroll MC, Campbell RD, Bentley DR, Porter RR (1984) A molecular map of the human major histocompatibility complex class III region linking complement genes C4, C2 and factor B. Nature 307:237–240
31. Marcadet A, Fischer A, Griscelli L, Cohen D, Dausset J (1984) HLA genotyping using DNA probes in two cases of bare lymphocyte syndrome. N Engl J Med (submitted)
32. Owerbach D, Lernmark A, Platz P, Ryder LP, Rask L, Peterson PA, Ludvigsson J (1983) HLA-D region β-chain DNA endonuclease fragments differ between HLA identical healthy and insulin-dependent diabetic individuals. Nature 303:815
33. Cohen D, Cohen O, Massart C, Lathrop M, Descamps I, Hors J, Schuller E, Dausset J (1984) HLA class IIβDC DNA restriction fragments differentiate among HLA-DR2 individuals in insulin-dependent diabetes and multiple sclerosis. Proc Natl Acad Sci USA 81:1774–1778

Biochemistry of Class II Antigens: Workshop Report

M.J. Crumpton, J.G. Bodmer, W.F. Bodmer, J.M. Heyes, J. Lindsay, and C.E. Rudd

Imperial Cancer Research Fund, P. O. Box 123, Lincoln's Inn Fields, London WC2A 3PX, U.K.

Introduction

The structure of the HLA-D region has been enormously clarified by the results of recent gene cloning studies [1–4]. These results, when combined with those of cellular responses, serology and immunoprecipitation, lead to the suggested genetic complement and arrangement shown in Fig. 1.

The D region incorporates three subregions, arranged in the order DR, DQ (DC) and DP (SB) towards the centromere. The DR subregion comprises three β genes and one α gene, whereas the DQ and DP subregions each comprise two sets of α and β genes (DQ and DX, DP1 and DP2 respectively). A further α chain gene (namely DZα) has been distinguished, although it is at present uncertain whether this gene is located to the left or right of the DR subregion. All of the β genes are polymorphic, although it is apparent that they differ in the extent of their variation. In contrast, the only highly polymorphic α gene appears to be DQα. It is currently not known whether all haplotypes possess all of these genes, whether all the genes are expressed and whether the expression of particular genes is related to the DR type.

The sizes of the respective primary gene products (i.e. the polypeptides) differ slightly. Thus, the DP1β and DQβ polypeptides are respectively three and eight amino acids shorter than the DRβ polypeptide, whereas the DQα polypeptide is three amino acids larger than the DRα polypeptide. Although the primary products of the respective α and β gene have similar sizes, these are subsequently modified by intracellular processing, especially through glycosylation [5]. In particular, the α gene products possess two *N*-linked carbohydrate moieties of about 3 kdaltons each, whereas the β chains possess one *N*-linked moiety only. The above differences in size are generally reflected in the relative mobilities of the respective polypeptides on sodium dodecylsulphate-polyacrylamide gel electrophoresis (SDS-PAGE), although the small variations in number of amino acid residues do not necessarily lead to the expected differences in mobilities (e.g. see Fig. 5).

Screening for cell surface class II antigens by serology and cellular responses has provided compelling evidence for the presence of multiple gene products. In particular, serology has not only indicated the presence of DR antigens, but also provided direct evidence for the existence of families of supertypic specificities (previously named DC, MB, MT and BR) in linkage disequilibrium with the DR subregion antigens. Current results suggest that the DC and MB families are equivalent and are coded by genes within the DQ subregion. Also,

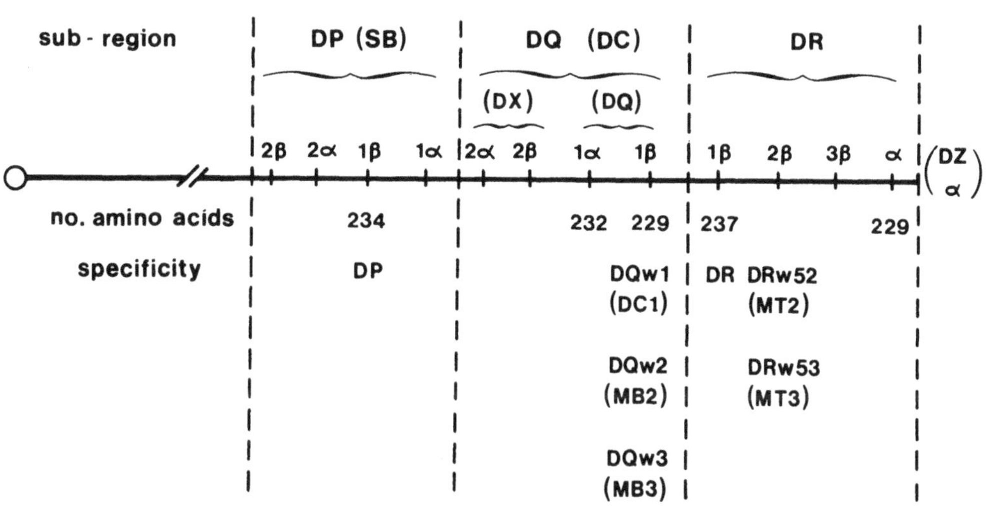

Fig. 1. A schematic map of the HLA-D region derived from the results of a large number of laboratories. The nomenclature used is that established by the WHO Committee which met after the Workshop conference. The numbers in front of α or β (e.g. "2α", "1β") identify different genes

it appears that the DRw52 and DRw53 antigens are the products of genes located within the DR subregion [6], in which the product of a β gene distinct from that responsible for the DR specificities is associated with the common, non-polymorphic DRα gene product [7].

Given the gene structure of the D region it is theoretically possible that up to six α and seven β gene products may be expressed on the surfaces of cells. Previous analyses of the expressed class II antigens have, however, failed to reveal such a large number of products. The principal and most informative analytical procedure employed has been two-dimensional non-equilibrium pH gel electrophoresis (2D-NEPHGE)/SDS-PAGE of immunoprecipitates prepared from [^{35}S]methionine biosynthetically labelled lymphoblastoid cells from homozygous consanguineous individuals, by using monoclonal antibodies against HLA-D region antigens. Figure 2a shows a representative pattern of spots revealed by such an analysis. In this experiment [^{35}S]methionine-labelled WT46 cells (DRw6, Dw6) were immunoprecipitated using the monomorphic anti-HLA-DR monoclonal antibody TAL-1B5. It can be clearly seen that this pattern includes an unresolved splotch of radioactivity in the position of the α chain (molecular weight about 33 000), suggesting that this area includes a number of polypeptides. As well, three distinct sets of β chains can be distinguished (molecular weight about 28 000), providing direct evidence for the presence in these cells of three separate class II antigens.

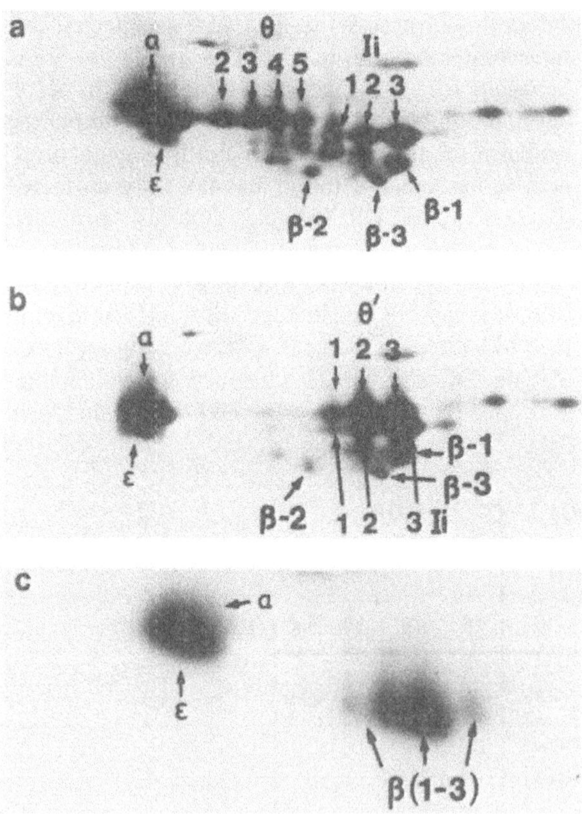

Fig. 2a–c. 2D-NEPHGE/SDS-PAGE analyses of immunoprecipitates prepared from WT46 cells (DRw6, Dw6) by using the monomorphic HLA-DR monoclonal antibody TAL-1B5. **a** Immunoprecipitate prepared from [^{35}S]methionine biosynthetically labelled cells. **b** As for **a** except that the immunoprecipitate was digested with neuraminidase prior to analysis. **c** Immunoprecipitate prepared from cells labelled at the surface by lactoperoxidase-catalysed iodination. Experimental conditions and labelling of spots is as described in [10]

The interpretation of such patterns is, however, complicated by two features. Firstly, as shown originally in the mouse [8] and more recently in humans [9, 10], the class II antigens are associated intracellularly with a family of basic invariant polypeptides (labelled θ, Ii and σ in Fig. 2a). There is thus an absolute requirement to distinguish the α and β gene products from these invariant polypeptides. The latter polypeptides are coded by a single gene, which is not located in the HLA region, and arise through various processing procedures including *N*- and *O*-glycosylation [10, 11]. Secondly, because of intracellular processing, multiple α and β spots do not necessarily represent separate gene products. For instance, maturation of *N*-linked carbohydrate is frequently associated with the differential addition of sialic acid residues, leading to multiple spots for the same gene product in the first (pH) dimension of 2D gel analyses. Under these circumstances, as is to be anticipated, digestion of immunoprecipitates with neuraminidase prior to analysis leads to a decrease in the number of spots. This is strikingly apparent in Fig. 2b for the θ invariant polypeptide, but the patterns of α and β spots are also simplified.

Since polypeptides expressed on the cell surface (compared with their intracellular precursors) have mature forms of the carbohydrate moieties, and as the invariant polypeptide(s) is apparently not expressed on the cell surface [12], analysis of cell surface class II antigens should also yield a very much simpler pattern of spots. This prediction is confirmed by Fig. 2c which shows an analysis of the immunoprecipitate prepared from WT46 cells which had been labelled at the surface by lactoperoxidase-catalysed iodination. Most importantly, this pattern again shows the presence of at least three β chains, indicating that three class II antigens are expressed on the surface of a consanguineous HLA- DRw6 cell line.

In spite of the difficulties associated with the interpretation of the 2D gel patterns, this procedure has yielded valuable data. In particular, it has previously proved possible to describe the β chain mediating the DR serological specificities, to iden-

Table 1. Binding activity (ELISA) of core antibodies with core cell lines

Antibody	Reference no.	Submitted specificity	Cell lines DR2 PGF	DR3 WT49	DR4 Leif-T	DR4 KT3	DRw6 WT46	DR7 Mann
IB5	[16]	Anti-α	•	•	•	•	•	•
L203	[17]	DR	•	•	•	•	•	•
Q2.70	[18]	DR	•	•	•	•	•	•
DA6.164	[19]	DR (except 7)	•	•	•	•	•	
III.E.3	[20]	DR		•	•	•		•
17.3.3	[21]	DR7 only						•
Tü22	[22]	DC	•	•	•	•	•	•
SDR4.1	[23]	DC1	•				•	
IV.D.12	[24]	MB3			•	•		
SG171	[25]	DR, DC	•	•	•	•	•	•
Tü39	[22]	SB, DR	•	•	•	•	•	•
MHM4	[26]	SB	•	•	•	•	•	•
B7/21	[27]	FA	•	•	•	•	•	•

A blank space indicates no detectable reaction

tify the α and β chains comprising the DQw1 (DC1) antigens, and to obtain direct evidence for polymorphism of the DCα gene and for the expression of three distinct sets of class II antigens [13–15].

Aims and Approaches

These earlier studies, although informative, failed to identify the gene products of the DP subregion and to answer unequivocally questions concerning the number of D region gene products expressed by cells. As a result, a co-operative study between a group of laboratories was organised by the authors as part of the Ninth Histocompatibility Workshop. The study was centred around 2D NEPHGE/SDS-PAGE analyses of immunoprecipitates prepared using a core set of monoclonal antibodies and homozygous cell-lines which were distributed to the participating laboratories. The specificities of the core antibodies, assigned by the donating laboratory, are recorded in Table 1 together with the results of binding experiments (as assessed by ELISA) carried out using the core cell lines. As can be seen, the latter results agreed with the assigned specificities.

The aims of the study were twofold: firstly, to identify for each cell line the β spots encoded by the DR, DQ and DP genes and to describe their positions on 2D gels; secondly, to define more exactly the specificities of the core antibodies. Laboratories were also encouraged to use the core antibodies or cell lines to explore local issues such as the specificity of a new monoclonal antibody or the application of different techniques.

Results and Conclusions

The laboratories listed in Table 2 submitted data to the Workshop. All of these laboratories except those of Giphart/van Rood, Capra and Tanigaki provided results of 2D-NEPHGE/SDS-PAGE analyses. Giphart's laboratory analysed immunoprecipitates by 1D gel electrophoresis, whereas Capra's laboratory characterised the immunoprecipitated α and β polypeptides by *N*-terminal amino acid sequence analysis using radioactive tyrosine and phenylalanine. Tanigaki's laboratory provided peptide fingerprint analyses of the precipitated α and β chains.

Table 2. Laboratories submitting data

Peptide fingerprints:	Tanigaki
Amino acid sequence:	Capra
2D-NEPHGE/SDS-PAGE:	Aizawa
	Bach
	Bodmer, J.
	Charron
	Crumpton
	Ferrone/Igarashi
	Gandini
	Nepom/Hansen
	Juji
	Katagiri
	Knowles
	Maeda
	McMichael
	Peterson
	Raghupathy/Strominger
	D'Apice/Russ
	Sasazuki
	Schwartz
	Tsuji
1D-IEF gel or 1D-SDS-PAGE	Giphart/van Rood

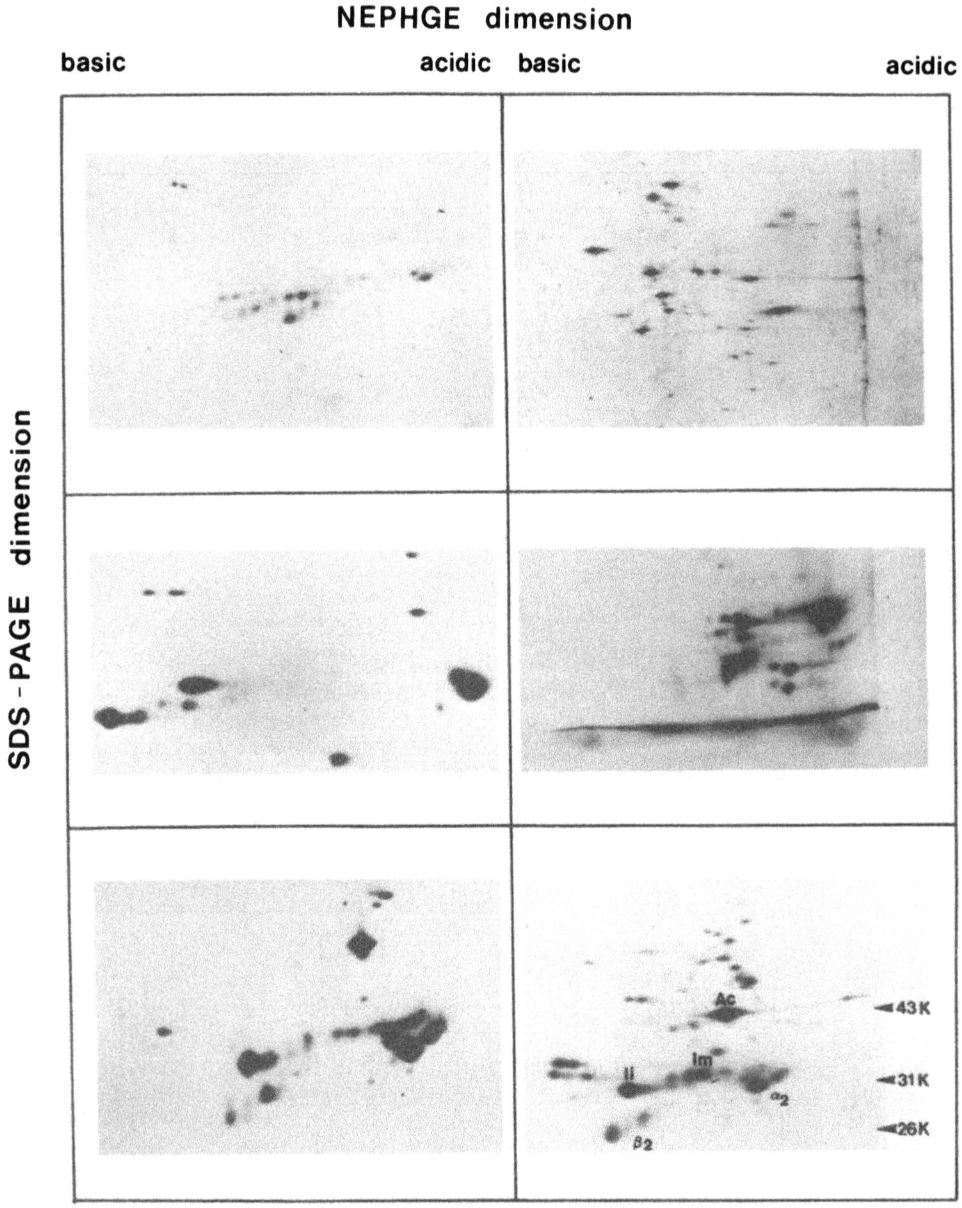

Fig. 3. Comparison of 2D gel patterns submitted by six different laboratories. In each case, immunoprecipitates prepared from [^{35}S]methionine-labelled WT46 cells by using the monoclonal antibody SDR4.1 were analysed by NEPHGE/SDS-PAGE using a supposedly standard set of experimental conditions

2D Gel Analyses

A representative selection of the 2D gel results submitted by different laboratories for the same combination of antibody and cell line is shown in Fig. 3. Obviously, the level of reproducibility achieved between the different laboratories was disappointing. The individual patterns differed considerably, not only in the degree of background and in the number of invariant polypeptides, but also in respect of the number and positions of the *β* spots. The reasons for the extensive variation in patterns have not been unequivocally established, but it appears most likely that they are primarily technical in origin. Variables that probably have a marked effect on the patterns include the period of biosynthetic labelling, variation in which can influence the number of labelled polypeptides, and the conditions used for immunoprecipitation and washing the precipitate, which can affect the precipitate's composition, especially the spectrum of more loosely associated polypeptides (i.e. background and invariant polypeptides). Variation in the separation conditions used for the gel analyses is also likely to be of crucial importance. Although the latter conditions were specified (see [10] for experimental details), variations between different laboratories were noted in the pH gradient, %

acrylamide (10%, 11%, 12.5% or 12%–15% gradient) and especially the conditions (volt h) of the first dimension (between 1600 and 3500 volt h). Of these, changes in the volt h should have a pronounced effect on the relative positions of the spots owing to the non-equilibrium nature of the first dimension.

Computer Analyses of 2D Gels

An attempt was made by Dr. Warwick Grant (ICRF Laboratories in collaboration with Image Analysis Group, Department of Physics, University College London) to analyse the various 2D gel patterns by using a computer specifically designed for image analysis. An essential requirement of such comparative analyses is the presence of a number of standard spots which allow the computer to "map" the position of each spot relative to a set of common reference points. The preliminary data are promising, but because the gel patterns did not contain a sufficiently large number of suitable reference points, this approach failed to resolve the problem of the variation between laboratories in 2D patterns.

Specificities of Core Antibodies

Although there was considerable variation in the patterns obtained by different laboratories for the same immunoprecipitate, individual laboratories derived similar conclusions from the analysis of their own data. As a result, it proved possible to reach consensus opinions with respect to the particular specificities of the core monoclonal antibodies. These conclusions are summarised in Table 3. The results, in general, confirm the assignments ascribed by the donating laboratory. However, in some cases new features were revealed. Of the antibodies studied, Tü39 gave the most extensive pattern of β spots that apparently comprised the products of the DR, DQ and DP genes. When assayed using WT46 cells, SG171 had a similar spectrum of reactivity to Tü39. This result was unexpected in view of the specificity ascribed to this antibody by the donating laboratory [25]. It appears likely, however, that antibody specificity depends upon the cell lines used to define the specificity. Indeed, SG171 has been reported to react with DR only, except with cells of DR7 type, where it reacts with both DR and DQ gene products [25]. In contrast to Tü39 and SG171, the antibodies TAL-1B5, Q2.70 and DA6.164 showed a more restricted pattern, recognising products mainly of the DR and to a lesser extent the DQ subregions. For example, Fig. 4 shows a comparison of the patterns given by Tü39 and TAL-1B5 with WT46 cells (panels *c* and *a* respectively). Figure 4 also shows that SDR4.1 gave a similar number of spots to TAL-1B5, but that different α and β chains, which represent the products of the DQ subregion, were preferentially precipitated. Antibody Tü22 behaved in a similar manner to SDR4.1, as did antibody IV.D.12, which was submitted as an anti-MB3 antibody. As a re-

Table 3. Specificities of the core monoclonal antibodies

Antibody	Specificity		
	Submitted	Concluded	
		Class II antigen[a]	Polypeptide[b]
1B5	anti-α	DR*; DQ	DRα*, DQα
L203	DR	DR*; DQ	
Q2.70	DR	DR*; DQ	
DA6.164	DR (except 7)	DR* (except 7, w9); most DQs	DR1β
111.E.3	DR3, 4, 7 (MT3?)	DR3, 4, 7	DR2β
17.3.3	DR7 only	DR7	DR1β7
Tü22	DC	DR; DQ*	
SDR4.1	DC1 (i.e. DR1, 2, w6)	DR1, 2, w6; DQw1*	DQβ
IV.D.12	MB3 (i.e. DR4, 5)	DR4; DQw3*	
SG171	DR, DC	DR; DQ; DP	DQβ
Tü39	SB, DR	DR; DQ; DP	
MHM4	SB	DP (possibly DP2)[c]	
B7/21	FA	DP	

[a] Based on 2D gel analyses
[b] Deduced from polymorphic specificity and/or results of Western blotting
[c] Based principally on the results of binding studies using the Kavathas and DeMars mutants
* Preferential reactivity

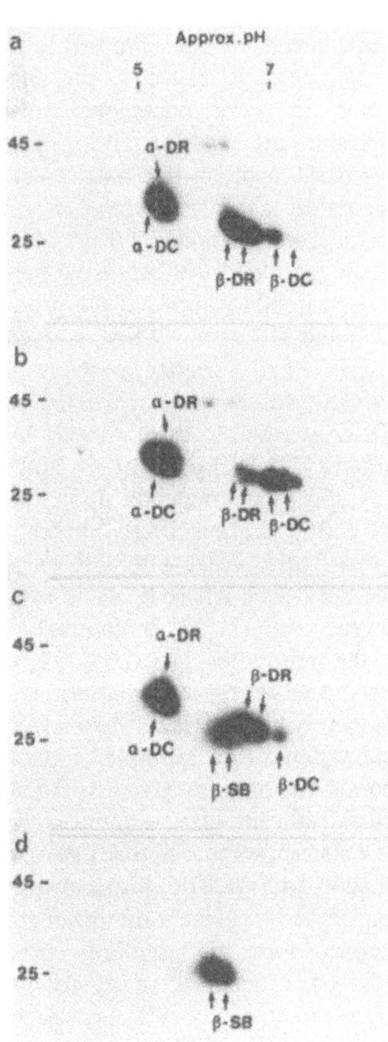

Fig. 4. 2D-NEPHGE/SDS-PAGE analyses of immunoprecipitates prepared from surface-[^{125}I]-labelled WT46 cells by using the monoclonal antibodies **a** TAL-1B5; **b** SDR4.1; **c** Tü39; **d** B7/21 (SB = DP; DC = DQ)

sult, the DQw3 (MB3) specificity must be coded by DQ subregion genes. It is notable that as judged by 2D gel patterns, the antibodies Tü22 and SDR4.1 possessed a broader specificity than that ascribed by serology (binding) (i.e. they recognised the products of DR subregion as well as DQ subregion genes). The basis of the difference between serology and immunoprecipitation is not clear, although various explanations are feasible, including in particular a difference in the effective antibody affinity in different assays and the presence of complexes of the DR and DQ antigens in detergent lysates. On the other hand, whereas Tü22 is monomorphic, recognising all DQ subregion antigens, SDR4.1 is polymorphic, recognising, by immunoprecipitation, only the DQ (and DR) subregion antigens normally expressed by HLA-DR1,2,w6 individuals. In one instance, namely a subset (Dw18) of DRw6 cells, SDR4.1 failed to precipitate recognisable class II antigens even though it reacted positively by serology [23].

Contrary to the above antibodies, B7/21 failed to recognise the products of the DR and DQ subregions that were precipitated by Tü39, SG171, TAL-1B5, Q2.70 and DA6.164, but gave a subset of β spots that coincided with the extra β spots precipitated by Tü39 and SG171. These spots are most probably coded by DP subregion genes (vide infra). Antibody B7/21 was unique amongst the core antibodies in respect of its restricted pattern of spots. This unique character is demonstrated in Fig. 4d, which shows the pattern given by an immunoprecipitate derived from surface-[^{125}I]-labelled WT46 cells. Only two β spots were detected that were distinct from those previously ascribed to the DRβ and DQβ genes. Interestingly, no α spots were detected, as reported previously [27]. Because α spots were identified in immunoprecipitates from [^{35}S]-methionine-labelled cells, the most probable explanation for their absence in Fig. 4d is that they are not labelled by lactoperoxidase-catalysed iodination. The very restricted pattern of spots precipitated by B7/21 contradicts the suggestion that the DP antigens form complexes with the DQ and/or DR antigens (see above), and also indicates that hybrids of DPβ polypeptides with DR or DQα chains do not occur.

Most laboratories failed to detect any spots in analyses of immunoprecipitates prepared using the antibody MHM4. As judged from the results of binding studies using the Kavathas and DeMars mutants and of inhibition of T cell killing (A. J. McMichael), it is possible that this antibody recognises a subset of the DP antigens, perhaps that coded by the DP2α and 2β genes (Fig. 1). Antibody III.E.3, which was submitted as an anti-DR antibody, is polymorphic, recognising HLA-DR3, 4, 7 antigens, and thus probably has a specificity related to DRw53 (MT3) [6].

Characterisation of Gene Products

Figure 5 shows the composite patterns of spots derived from the Workshop data for the WT46 and Leif-T cell lines; the genetic origin of the respective polypeptides is also indicated. Similar patterns were obtained for the other Workshop cell lines. The two β polypeptides precipitated from WT46 cells by antibody B7/21 were resistant to neuraminidase digestion and thus probably represent the products of separate genes. Similarly, as indicated in Fig. 4, the DR and DQ subregions also probably code for two β polypeptides each. Thus, it appears that the total number of β polypeptides ex-

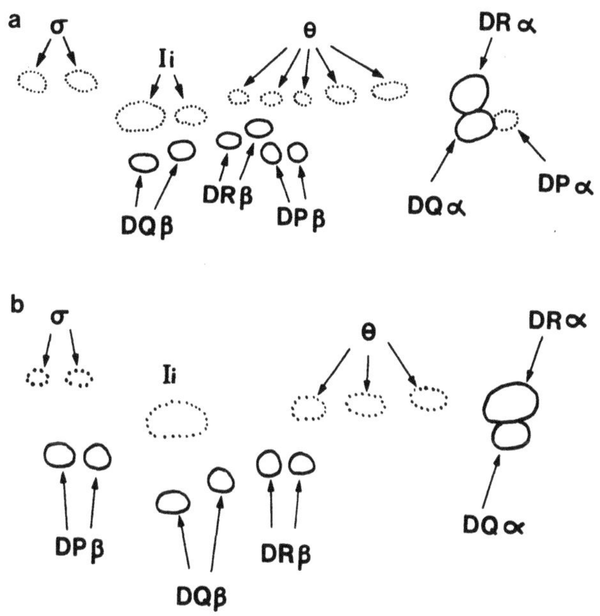

Fig. 5. Characterisation of the HLA-D region gene products expressed by **a** WT46 and **b** Leif-T cells. The 2D gel patterns and the assignment of particular polypeptides to particular genes represent the composite data of the Workshop analyses. The pattern and assignments for Leif-T cells are based primarily on results from Professor Aizawa's laboratory

pressed in WT46 and Leif-T cells (i.e. six) is close to that expected from the gene complement of the D region (Fig. 1). Independent evidence for the expression of five distinct β chains by cells of various DR serological specificities was provided by *N*-terminal amino acid sequence analyses (Capra).

Although the Workshop was primarily concerned with characterising the β spots, information was also acquired on the number and distribution of the α spots. Thus, on the basis that the DPα chain is not labelled by lactoperoxidase-catalysed iodination and that the DQα chain has a faster mobility in the second dimension (i.e. SDS-PAGE), it proved possible to delineate the portion of the α area that is occupied by the DRα chain. Such analyses provided evidence for three distinct α polypeptides, a figure which was supported by *N*-terminal amino acid sequence analyses.

The DR Subregion Codes for the MT2/MT3 (DRw52/53) Specificities

Capra reported data on the *N*-terminal amino acid sequences of the α and β polypeptides precipitated by the monoclonal antibodies L203 (Table 3), 1-LR2 [anti-DRw52 (MT2)] and 109α6 [anti-DRw53(MT3)]. The results, shown in Table 4, indicate that the polypeptides precipitated by 1-LR2 and 109α6 had the same amino acid sequences as those of the DRα and β polypeptides precipitated by L203. On the other hand, the precipitated antigens were shown by cross-depletion experiments to be distinct from the DR antigens. The most satisfying interpretation of these experiments is that the above antibodies recognise a distinct subset of DR-like antigens which comprise polypeptides coded by the DRα and DR2β genes of the DR subregion (Fig. 1). Obviously, this interpretation depends crucially upon the results of the depletion experiments. In this respect, the results of more extensive sequence analysis of the β polypeptide will be invaluable, since they should ultimately reveal differences from the DR1β polypeptide.

Future Aims

The present lack of agreement between the 2D gel patterns from different laboratories appears to rule out a previous suggestion that such patterns may provide a more informative way than serology of typing cells for HLA-D region antigens. However, more rigorous standardisation of the immunoprecipitation and separation conditions

Table 4. *N*-terminal amino acid sequences of α and β chains precipitated by the anti-DR (L203), anti-DRw52 (MT2) (I-LR2) and anti-DRw53 (MT3) (109α6) monoclonal antibodies (Data from Capra's laboratory)

Cell line	DR type	Antibody specificity	α chain position						β chain position								
			12	13	22	24	26	32	7	10	13	17	18	26	30	31	32
127	3	DR	F	Y	F	F	F	F	F	Y	–	F	F	Y	Y	F	–
127	3	DRw52	F	Y	F	F	F	F	F	Y	–	F	F	Y	Y	F	–
3105	5	DR	F	Y	F	F	F	F	F	Y	–	F	F	F	Y	F	Y
3105	5	DRw52	F	Y	F	F	F	F	F	Y	–	F	F	F	Y	F	Y
Priess	4	DR	F	Y	F	F	F	F	F	–	–	F	F	F	Y	F	Y
Priess	4	DRw53	F	Y	F	F	F	F	F	–	–	F	F	F	Y	F	Y
3163	7	DR	F	Y	F	F	F	F	F	–	Y	F	F	F	–	F	Y
3163	7	DRw53	F	Y	F	F	F	F	F	–	Y	F	F	F	–	F	Y

F, phenylalanine; Y, tyrosine

should yield more reproducible patterns. The incorporation in such patterns of an adequate number of reference points should make computer analyses of the patterns feasible, including quantitative estimation of the relative intensities of the different spots.

Up to now, the α spot(s) have been neglected relative to the β spots, primarily because the different α chains fail to separate well in NEPHGE. As suggested by the results of A. J. McMichacl's experiments in which a different mixture of ampholines (20% pH 3–10, 80% pH 5–7) was used, small changes in the pH gradient should give increased separation of the α spots. Such manipulations may permit the separate identification of the DRα, DQα, DXα, DP1α and DP2α gene products on 2D gels.

Past studies have used principally biosynthetically labelled cells as a source of antigen. There are now two reasons for concentrating on the antigens expressed at the cell surface: firstly, it is the surface molecules which mediate function; secondly, this approach should restrict (or eliminate) the multiplicity of spots for a single gene product that arise at present through sampling of the variably processed (i.e. intracellular and surface) forms.

Finally, there is clearly a need for more monoclonal antibodies of restricted specificity. Antibody B7/21 was unique amongst those studied in precipitating the product(s) of a single subregion (namely DP). Ideally, monomorphic antibodies are required that are specific for the distinct class II antigens and their constituent α and β chains, including the different DR, DQ and DP subregion products.

References

1. Auffray C, Lillie JW, Arnot C, Grossberger D, Kappes D, Strominger JL (1983) Isotopic and allotypic variation of human class II histocompatibility antigen α chain genes. Nature 308:327–333
2. Larhammar D, Hyldig-Nielsen JJ, Servenius B, Andersson G, Rask L, Peterson PA (1983) Exon-intron organization and complete nucleotide sequence of a human major histocompatibility antigen DCβ gene. Proc Natl Acad Sci USA 80:7313–7317
3. Long EO, Wake CT, Gorski J, Mach B (1983) Complete sequence of an HLA-DRβ chain decuded from a cDNA clone and identification of multiple non-allelic DRβ chain genes. EMBO J 2:389–394
4. Spielman RS, Lee J, Bodmer WF, Bodmer JG, Trowsdale J (1984) Six HLA-Dα chain genes on human chromosome 6: polymorphisms and associations of DCα-related sequences with DR types. Proc Natl Acad Sci USA 81:3461–3465
5. Kaufman JF, Auffray C, Korman AJ, Shackelford DA, Strominger J (1984) The class II molecules of the human and murine major histocompatibility complex. Cell 36:1–13
6. Hurley CK, Giles RC, Nunez G, DrMars R, Nadler L, Winchester R, Statsny P, Capra JD (1984) Molecular localization of human class II MT2 and MT3 determinants. J Exp Med 160:472–493
7. Suzuki M, Maeda H, Mukai R, Yabe T, Hamaguchi U (1983) Identification of the MT3 molecule using two-dimensional gel electrophoresis and alloantisera. Immunogenetics 18:575–583
8. Jones PP, Murphy DB, Hewgill D, McDevitt HO (1978) Detection of a common polypeptide chain in I-A and I-E sub-region immunoprecipitates. Mol Immunol 16:51–60
9. Charron DJ, McDevitt HO (1979) Analysis of HLA-D region associated molecules with monoclonal antibody. Proc Natl Acad Sci USA 79:6567–6571
10. Rudd CE, Bodmer JG, Bodmer WF, Crumpton MJ (1984) HLA-D region antigen associated invariant polypeptides as revealed by 2-D gel analysis: glycosylation and structural interrelationships. J Biol Chem (in press)
11. Strubin M, Mach B, Long EO (1984) The complete sequence of the mRNA for the HLA-DR-associated invariant chain reveals a polypeptide with an unusual transmembrane polarity. EMBO J 3:869–872
12. Owen MJ, Kissonerghis AM, Lodish HF, Crumpton MJ (1981) Biosynthesis and maturation of HLA-DR antigens in vivo. J Biol Chem 256:8987–8993
13. Shackelford DA, Mann D, van Rood JJ, Ferrara GB, Strominger JL (1981) Human B-cell alloantigens DC1, MT1 and LB12 are identical to each other but distinct from the HLA-DR antigen. Proc Natl Acad Sci USA 78:4566–4590
14. de Kretser TA, Crumpton MJ, Bodmer JG, Bodmer WF (1982) Two-dimensional gel analysis of the polypeptides precipitated by a polymorphic HLA-DR1,2,w6 monoclonal antibody: evidence for a third locus. Eur J Immunol 12:600–606
15. de Kretser TA, Crumpton MJ, Bodmer JG, Bodmer WF (1983) Biochemical analysis of the polymorphism of three HLA-D region antigens. Mol Biol Med 1:59–76
16. Adams TE, Bodmer JG, Bodmer WF (1983) Production and characterisation of monoclonal antibodies recognising the α-chain subunits of human Ia alloantigens. Immunology 50:613–624
17. Lampson LA, Levy R (1980) Two populations of Ia-like molecules on a human B cell line. J Immunol 125:293–299
18. Quaranta V, Indiveri F, Glassy MC, Ng A, Russo C, Molinaro GA, Pellegrino MA, Ferrone S (1980) Serological, functional, and immunochemical characterization of a monoclonal antibody (MoAb Q2/70) to human Ia-like antigens. Hum Immunol 3:211–223
19. van Heyningen V, Guy K, Newman R, Steel CM (1982) Human MHC class II molecules as differentiation markers. Immunogenetics 16:459–469
20. Hurley CK, Shaw S, Nadler L, Schlossman S, Capra JD (1982) Alpha and beta chains of SB and DR antigens are structurally distinct. J Exp Med 156:1557–1562
21. Ozato K, Mayer N, Sachs DH (1980) Hybridoma cell lines secreting monoclonal antibodies to mouse H-2 and Ia antigens. J Immunol 124:533–540
22. Wernet P, Ziegler A, Shaw S, Blaurock M, Pawelec G (1983) Monoclonal antibodies against Ia-like antigens inhibiting HLA-D and/or SB-directed secondary proliferative responses. Transplant Proc XV:94–98
23. Bodmer J, Heyes J, Lindsay J (1984) Study of monoclonal antibodies to the HLA-D region products DQw1 and DRw 52. This volume
24. Giles RC, Nunez G, Hurley CK, Nunez-Roldan A, Winchester R, Stastny P, Capra JD (1983) Structural analysis

of a human I-A homologue using a monoclonal antibody that recognises an MB3-like specificity. J Exp Med 157:1461–1470
25. Goyert SM, Shively JE, Silver J (1982) Biochemical characterization of a second family of human Ia molecules, HLA-DS, equivalent to murine I-A subregion molecules. J Exp Med 156:550–566
26. Makgoba MW, Hildreth JEK, McMichael AJ (1983) Identification of a human Ia antigen that is different from HLA-DR and DC antigens. Immunogenetics 17:623–635
27. Watson AJ, DeMars R, Trowbridge IS, Bach FH (1983) Detection of a novel human class II HLA antigen. Nature 304:358–361

The Central Data Analysis of the Ninth Workshop *

M. P. Baur [1], E. D. Albert [2], and W. R. Mayr [3]

1 Biometrical Department, Diabetes Research Institute, Auf'm Hennekamp 65, 4000 Düsseldorf, Federal Republic of Germany
2 Laboratory of Immunogenetics, Pettenkoferstr. 8 a, 8000 München 2, Federal Republic of Germany
3 Institute for Blood Group Serology, University of Vienna, Spitalgasse 4, 1090 Vienna, Austria

As in all previous Workshops, the aims of the Ninth International Histocompatibility Workshop (IHW) could be defined according to the following five major topics:

1. Typing techniques
   a) serology
   b) monoclonal antibodies
   c) cellular techniques
2. Disease studies
3. Transplantation
4. Frequency studies (total MHC)
5. Mapping (total MHC).

Since the limited nature of the information to be gained from typing unrelated individuals had become apparent for the study of a chromosomal region with numerous tightly linked, highly polymorphic loci, it was decided during the early phase of organization that for all topics except transplantation, only family data would be accepted for the central data analysis. Consequently, already at this stage the structure of data collection, data checking, and data analysis had to be organized according to the complexities of general pedigrees with multilocus information.

Organization of Data Collection

The coding forms (Figs. 1–8) were very similar to those used for the Eighth IHW [1], because participating laboratories were already used to these formats, which in addition already provided for a unique definition of family relationships. The compulsory card 1 for each family member contained all identification, defined relationship to other family members, gave information about the individual's age, sex, ethnic group, etc., and indicated the presence or absence of the other cards containing the following information:

Cards 2– 7	Lab assignments for genetic markers
Cards 11–24	Serology
Cards 31–33	Monoclonal antibodies
Cards 51–72	Disease information
Cards 75–93	Cellular tests

Each card had the first 13 columns reserved for the following hierarchical identification variables:

	Columns
Card number	1– 2
Region code (workshop-assigned)	3– 5
Lab code (workshop-assigned)	6– 8
Family identity (laboratory-assigned)	9–10
Individual identity (laboratory-assigned)	11–13

allowing for easy sorting, merging, or extraction of subfiles for special purposes.

The submission of data for central analysis was organized in a way similar to the procedure of the Seventh IHW [2]. In order to reduce the enormous amount of work involved in the communication and data transfer between the Biometrical Department of the Diabetes Research Institute and the 220 participating laboratories, 21 regional representatives were asked to coordinate the data collection within the group of laboratories assigned to them and to submit their regional file after formal and logical checking for central data analysis in Düsseldorf (Fig. 9).

* The central data analysis of the Ninth Workshop was supported by Deutsche Forschungsgemeinschaft Al 92/13-2

N I N T H   I N T E R N A T I O N A L   H I S T O C O M P A T I B I L I T Y   W O R K S H O P   1 9 8 4

C E N T R A L   D A T A   A N A L Y S I S   -   C O D I N G   F O R M S

CARD 01

Individual identification and data set information. This card should be submitted for each individual tested. In addition, submit card 01 for each ID assigned to nontested persons as necessary to complete pedigrees.

GENERAL INSTRUCTIONS

Photocopy these forms for the number of cells you intend to test. It is extremely important that data be entered and keypunched carefully. Please submit keypunched cards after testing about 4 families to your regional data collection center to confirm that both testing and data entry are going well. In case of doubt contact regional organizer or directly:
Max P. Baur, Diabetes Research Institute, Auf'm Hennekamp 65, D-4000 Düsseldorf, W.-Germany
Tel.: (211) 3382-258 Telex: 858 2052 diab d

Section	Field	Columns
IDENTIFICATION	Card Number	1–2 (Ø1)
	Region Code	3–4
	Typing Lab Code	5–8
	Family ID Number	9–10
	Individual ID Number	11–13
	(X)	14
PEDIGREE DATA	Father's ID Number	15–17
	Mother's ID Number	18–20
	Birth Order	21–22
	Recombinant Family (codes below)	23–24
	Selection status (codes below)	25
	(X)	26
INDIVIDUAL DATA	NAME Last / First	27–42
	Age in years (01-99)	43–44
	Sex (M or F)	45
	Ethnic group (codes below)	46–47
	Disease (codes below)	48–49
	Recombinant Indiv. (codes below)	50
	(X)	51
LOCAL DATA	HLA-A and C Card 02	52
	HLA-B Card 03	53
	HLA-DR Card 04	54
	HLA-Dw Card 05	55
	Other markers Card 06-07	56
	(X)	57
WORKSHOP DATA	ABC serology Card 11-17	58
	DR serology Card 21-24	59
	DR monoclonal Card 31-32	60
	ABC monoclonal Card 33	61
	MLC	62
	PLT	63
	CML	64
	Family included in	65
	WS disease study (codes below)	66
	Disease data cards	67
	(X)	68–80

Identification Col. 1-13

Region code: WS assigned
Lab code : WS assigned
Family ID : local 01-99
Indiv. ID : local 001-999

Name Col. 27-42

Local use only. Will be deleted from masterfile.

Recomb. Indiv. Col. 50

0 No information
1 No
2 Yes

Local data Col. 52-56
WS data Col. 58-64

Data sets submitted for this individual

0 None
1 One set

Multiple sets not allowed.

Pedigree data Col. 15-25

ID numbers: Pedigrees will be reconstructed through offspring relationships, so we need both father's and mother's IDs for each individual. These IDs are coded as "NPR" (No PaRent) for first generation individuals or for individuals marrying into the pedigree (pedigree entries). If persons necessary to completely define the pedigree were not tested in the workshop, IDs must be assigned for these persons and a Card 01 submitted for them.

Birth order: Important for identifying monozygotic twins. Number siblings in order of birth, being sure that monozygotic twins have the same number. Range 01-99.

Recombinant type in family:

00	No information	09	C/(Bf,C2,C4)	18	(Bf,C2,C4)/SB
01	Non recombinant	10	C/DR	19	(Bf,C2,C4)/GLO
02	A/C	11	C/SB	20	DR/SB
03	A/B	12	C/GLO	21	DR/GLO
04	A/(Bf,C2,C4)	13	B/(Bf,C2,C4)	22	SB/GLO
05	A/DR	14	B/DR	23	D/DR
06	A/SB	15	B/SB	24	Intra (Bf,C2,C4)
07	A/GLO	16	B/GLO	25	Other
08	C/B	17	(Bf,C2,C4)/DR	26	Multiple

Selection status:

0	No information	1	Random healthy family	2	Disease family
3	Recombinant family	4	Family selected for antigen or homozygousity	5	Other selection

Ethnic group Col. 46-47

00 No information

Negroid
01 African
02 American
03 Cape Coloured
04 Other Negroid

Mongoloid
11 Chinese
12 Japanese
13 No. Americ. Indians
14 So. Americ. Indians
15 Mexican
16 Thai
17 Malaysian
18 Indonesian
19 Austr. Aborig.
20 Maori
21 Other Mongoloid

Caucasoid
31 American
32 Amish
33 Asian Indian
34 Australian
35 Austrian
36 Canadian
37 Czech
38 Dutch
39 English
40 French
41 German
42 Hispanic
43 Hungarian
44 Italian
45 Jewish-Ashk.
46 Jewish-Non-Ashk.
47 Russian
48 Scandinavian
49 Scot
50 So. African
51 Spanish
52 Swiss
53 Yugoslav
54 Other Caucasoid

Disease codes Col. 48-49 / 65-66

00 No information
01 Healthy
02 AIDS syndrome
03 B27 neg. AS
04 Coeliac disease
05 Diabetes
06 d-pen-induced MG
07 Gold-induced nephropathy
08 Hodgkins disease
09 Juvenile chronic arthritis
10 Leprosy
11 Melanoma
12 RA without drug side effects
13 Scleroderma
14 Other disease

Disease data cards Col. 67

Disease data sets submitted for this individual

0 None
1 One set

Fig. 1

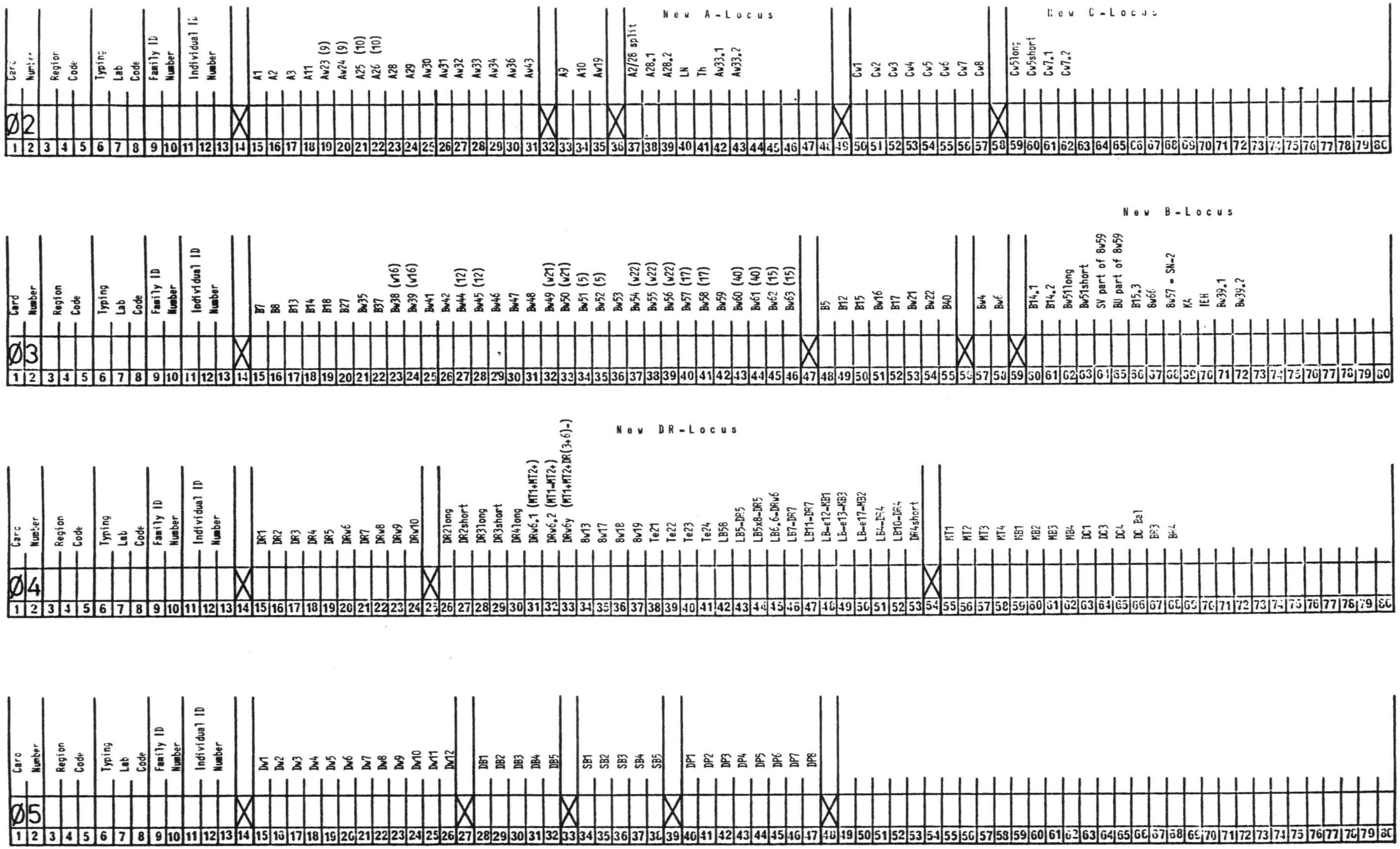

CARDS 02 - 05

HLA specificities (WHO)

New HLA specificities

Fig. 2

Score each specificity as follows:
0 Not tested
1 Negative
4 Doubtful
8 Present

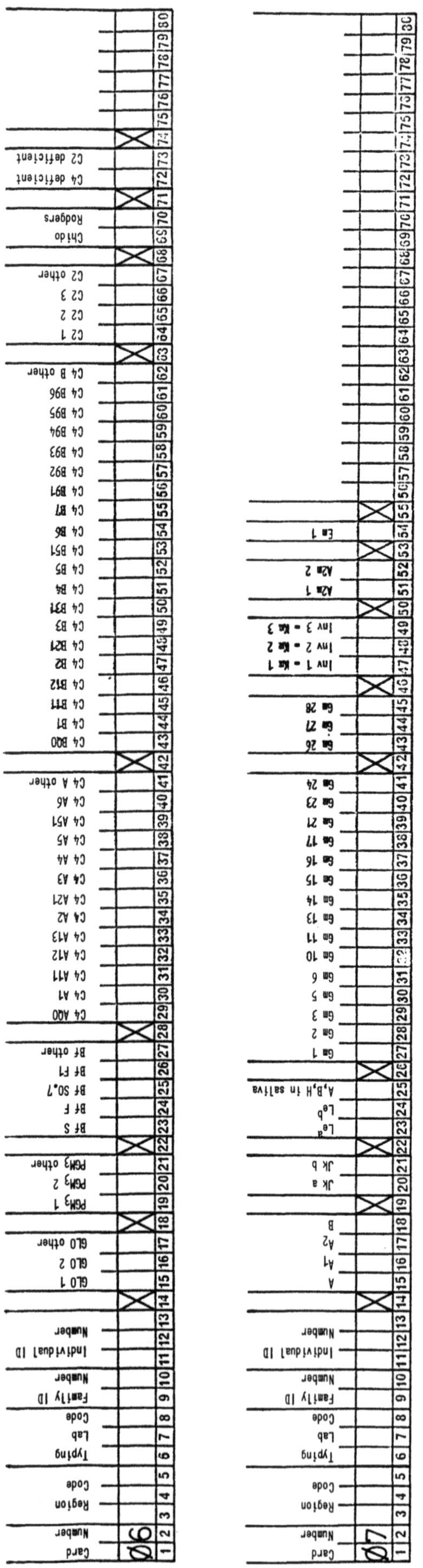

Fig. 3 CARDS 06–07 Other genetic markers
Score each specificity as follows: 0 Not tested 1 Negative 2 Doubtful 8 Present

Data Checking and Correction

Regional data was formally checked after arrival in Düsseldorf using the program FADE (J. Willems) according to a checklist similar to the one of the Seventh IHW [2], which included checking for column shifts, predefined ranges of values for variables like serum reactions, antigen coding, age, sex, etc., consistency of genetic coding, pedigree coding, submitted card set for each individual, and other formal tests. Most of the large amount of flagged formal errors were corrected in Düsseldorf and the data of complete families with no errors was added to the regional Workshop masterfile. Parallel to the formal checks all families were analyzed for consistency in segregation, using the laboratory assignments as given on cards 2–7 and the family analysis package (FAP; see M. Neugebauer et al., Analysis of Multilocus Pedigree Data by Computer, this volume) [3]. The results of FAP – haplotype interpretation for all family members plus a pedigree plot of the most likely solution (see M. Sigmund, PEDPLO, this volume) or error messages pointing out the individuals and loci with discrepant coding – were returned to the regions together with output from FADE concerning formal errors which were not straightforward to correct. In addition, the tape contained the output of a program displaying serological patterns on the family level. Participating laboratories were asked to check family interpretations by means of the output of FAP and the pedigree plot and to resubmit corrected data. Corrections were checked formally again before admission to the regional files, which at the end of March 1984 contained submitted and checked data as listed in Table 1.

Consequently, the masterfile WS9DAT of the Ninth Workshop contained 21 regional subfiles comprising:

Families	2300
Family members	14765
Disease families	866
Unrelated individuals	1223
ABC typing	13929
DR typing	13083
ABC monoclonals	12822
DR monoclonals	11346
Other markers	8562
MLCs	953
Total cards	311235

A comparison of lab codes and family names of WS9DAT with the masterfile of the 8th IHW [1] revealed an overlap of data of less than 5%. Consequently all results of this Workshop are not merely a repetition on the basis of the same retyped individuals, but on the contrary are either new findings or independent confirmation of previous results.

General instructions for the coding of cards 11 - 33 (ABC and DR serology; ABC and DR monoclonals)

Score each reaction as follows:
0 Not tested
1 Negative (0- 10% killed)
2 Doubtful negative (11- 20% killed)
4 Doubtful positive (21- 40% killed)
6 Positive (41- 80% killed)
8 Strong positive (81-100% killed)

Type of cell (col. 14):
1 PBL fresh
2 PBL frozen
3 T-Cells fresh
4 T-Cells frozen
5 B-Cells fresh
6 B-Cells frozen
7 T-line
8 B-line
9 Other line

Type of complement (col. 15):
1 Local
2 Regional
3 Other

Technique (col. 16):
1 Straw
2 SRBC rosetting
3 AET rosetting
4 Neuraminidase rosetting
5 TCF
6 Other

Columns 1-16 (cards 11, 12, 13):

Col.	1	2	3	4	5	6	7	8	9	10	11	12	13	14	15	16
Field	Card	Number	Region	Code		Typing	Lab	Code	Family ID	Number	Individual ID	Number		Type of cell	Type of complement	X

Columns 29, 42, 55 and 68 are crossed out (X).

Card 11

Col.	Specificity	Code	Col.	Specificity	Code	Col.	Specificity	Code
17	A1	01-9w001	30	A2+28	01-9w021	43	A9	01-9w038
18	A1	01-9w002	31	A28+2	01-9w023	44	A9	01-9w039
19	A1	01-9w003	32	A28+2	01-9w024	45	Aw23	01-9w041
20	A1+w36	01-9w006	33	A28+2	01-9w025	46	Aw23	01-9w042
21	A1+w36	01-9w007	34	A28+2	01-9w027	47	Aw23	01-9w043
22	A1+w36	01-9w009	35	A28+w33	01-9w029	48	Aw23	01-9w044
23	A2	01-9w011	36	A28+w33	01-9w031	49	Aw24	01-9w047
24	A2	01-9w013	37	A28+w33	01-9w032	50	Aw24	01-9w048
25	A2	01-9w014	38	A2+B17	01-9w033	51	Aw24	01-9w050
26	A2+28	01-9w017	39	A2+B17	01-9w034	52	Aw24	01-9w051
27	A2+28	01-9w018	40	A9	01-9w036	53	A3	01-9w056
28	A2+28	01-9w019	41	A9	01-9w037	54	A3	01-9w057

Col.	Specificity	Code	Col.	Specificity	Code
56	A3	01-9w059	69	A10+w34	01-9w076
57	A3	01-9w060	70	A10+w34	01-9w077
58	A3+11	01-9w061	71	A10+w34	01-9w078
59	A3+11+w19	01-9w062	72	A10+w34	01-9w079
60	A11	01-9w063	73	A10+w34	01-9w081
61	A11	01-9w065	74	A10+w34	01-9w082
62	A11	01-9w067	75	Aw34	01-9w083
63	A11	01-9w069	76	Aw34	01-9w084
64	A10	01-9w071	77	A25	01-9w085
65	A10	01-9w072	78	A25	01-9w086
66	A10	01-9w074	79	pos.control	local
67	A10	01-9w075	80	neg.control	local

Card 12

Col.	Specificity	Code	Col.	Specificity	Code	Col.	Specificity	Code
17	A25	02-9w087	30	A29	02-9w104	43	Aw30+w31	02-9w123
18	A25	02-9w090	31	A29	02-9w106	44	Aw30+w31	02-9w124
19	A25	02-9w091	32	A29	02-9w108	45	Aw30+w31	02-9w126
20	A26	02-9w093	33	Aw32	02-9w111	46	Aw30	02-9w128
21	A26	02-9w094	34	Aw32	02-9w112	47	Aw30	02-9w129
22	A26	02-9w095	35	Aw32	02-9w113	48	Aw32	02-9w130
23	A26	02-9w098	36	Aw32+25	02-9w114	49	Aw30	02-9w132
24	A26	02-9w099	37	Aw32+25	02-9w117	50	Aw30+Cw5	02-9w133
25	Aw43	02-9w100	38	Aw32+25	02-9w118	51	Aw31	02-9w134
26	Aw43	02-9w101	39	Aw30+w31	02-9w119	52	Aw31	02-9w135
27	A29	02-9w102	40	Aw30+w31	02-9w121	53	Aw31	02-9w136
28	A29	02-9w103	41	Aw30+w31	02-9w122	54	Aw31+B13	02-9w138

Col.	Specificity	Code	Col.	Specificity	Code
56	Aw31+w30	02-9w139	69	Bw51	02-9w156
57	Aw31+w33+w34	02-9w140	70	Bw51	02-9w157
58	Aw33	02-9w141	71	Bw51	02-9w158
59	Aw33	02-9w142	72	Bw51	02-9w159
60	Aw33	02-9w143	73	Bw51	02-9w160
61	Aw33+10	02-9w144	74	Bw52	02-9w161
62	Aw33	02-9w146	75	Bw52	02-9w162
63	A19+1n	02-9w147	76	Bw53	02-9w163
64	A19+1n	02-9w148	77	Bw51+w52	02-9w164
65	A19+1n	02-9w149	78	Bw51+w52	02-9w166
66	A19+1n	02-9w150	79	pos.control	local
67	A10+w33+w34+1n	02-9w151	80	neg.control	local

Card 13

Col.	Specificity	Code	Col.	Specificity	Code	Col.	Specificity	Code
17	Bw51+w52	03-9w167	30	Bw35	03-9w181	43	new ABC	03-9w201
18	Bw51+w52	03-9w169	31	Bw35	03-9w182	44	new ABC	03-9w202
19	B5+w53	03-9w170	32	Bw35	03-9w184	45	B7	03-9w203
20	B5+w35+w53	03-9w171	33	Bw35	03-9w186	46	B7	03-9w205
21	B5+w35+w53	03-9w172	34	B18	03-9w189	47	B7	03-9w207
22	B5+w49	03-9w173	35	B18	03-9w190	48	B27	03-9w209
23	B5+w49	03-9w174	36	B18	03-9w193	49	B27	03-9w210
24	B5+w49	03-9w175	37	B18	03-9w194	50	B27	03-9w211
25	B5+w49	03-9w176	38	B18	03-9w196	51	B27	03-9w215
26	B5+w35+w53+18	03-9w177	39	B18	03-9w197	52	Bw22	03-9w216
27	Bw35	03-9w179	40	B18	03-9w198	53	Bw22	03-9w217
28	Bw35	03-9w180	41	A2+B17	03-9w199	54	Bw22	03-9w218

Col.	Specificity	Code	Col.	Specificity	Code
56	Bw22	03-9w219	69	Bw56	03-9w234
57	Bw54	03-9w222	70	Bw56	03-9w235
58	Bw54	03-9w223	71	Bw42+w55	03-9w236
59	Bw54	03-9w224	72	Bw42	03-9w237
60	Bw54	03-9w225	73	Bw42	03-9w238
61	Bw55	03-9w226	74	B7+w42	03-9w239
62	Bw55	03-9w227	75	Bw22+w42	03-9w240
63	Bw55	03-9w229	76	Bw42	03-9w241
64	Bw55	03-9w230	77	B27+w42	03-9w242
65	Bw55	03-9w231	78	B27+w47	03-9w243
66	Bw55	03-9w232	79	pos.control	local
67	Bw56	03-9w233	80	neg.control	local

CARDS 11-13
ABC serology

Fig. 4

Card 14

Col.	Code	Entry
1–2	14	Card Number
3–5		Region Code
6–8		Typing Lab Code
9–10		Family ID Number
11–13		Individual ID Number
14		Type of cell
15		Type of complement
16	X	
17	04-9w245	B7+ka
18	04-9w246	B7+ka
19	04-9w247	B7+ka
20	04-9w248	B8
21	04-9w249	B8
22	04-9w250	B8
23	04-9w253	B8+w59
24	04-9w254	Bw59+5
25	04-9w255	B8+w59
26	04-9w256	Bw59
27	04-9w257	Bw59
28	04-9w258	Bw59
29	X	
30	04-9w259	Bw59+8
31	04-9w260	B14.1
32	04-9w261	B14.1
33	04-9w262	B14.2
34	04-9w263	B14.2
35	04-9w264	B14.2
36	04-9w265	B14.2
37	04-9w266	B14.2
38	04-9w267	B14
39	04-9w270	B14
40	04-9w272	B14
41	04-9w274	B14+Cw5
42	X	
43	04-9w275	B14+18
44	04-9w276	B15
45	04-9w277	Bw62
46	04-9w278	Bw62+w63
47	04-9w281	Bw62
48	04-9w282	Bw62
49	04-9w284	Bw62
50	04-9w285	Bw62
51	04-9w286	Bw62
52	04-9w289	B15+ts
53	04-9w290	Bw57+w58
54	04-9w291	B17
55	X	
56	04-9w292	B17
57	04-9w293	Bw57+w58
58	04-9w296	B17
59	04-9w298	B17
60	04-9w299	B17
61	04-9w301	B17
62	04-9w302	Bw57
63	04-9w303	Bw57
64	04-9w304	Bw57
65	04-9w305	Bw57+w58+w63
66	04-9w306	Bw57+w58
67	04-9w307	B15+w57
68	X	
69	04-9w308	B15+w57+w46+1[illegible]
70	04-9w309	B15+17
71	04-9w310	B15+w57
72	04-9w311	bu-sv
73	04-9w312	bu-sv
74	04-9w313	bu-sv
75	04-9w314	bu-sv,da[illegible]
76	04-9w315	B5+w38+w59+w[illegible]
77	04-9w316	B15+bu-sv
78	04-9w500	B14
79	local	pos.control
80	local	neg.control

Card 15

Col.	Code	Entry
1–2	15	Card Number
3–5		Region Code
6–8		Typing Lab Code
9–10		Family ID Number
11–13		Individual ID Number
14		Type of cell
15		Type of complement
16	X	
17	05-9w317	bu-sv
18	05-9w318	A1+Bw17
19	05-9w319	A2+Bw17
20	05-9w320	A2+Bw17
21	05-9w321	A2+Bw17
22	05-9w322	A2+Bw17
23	05-9w323	A9+Bw17
24	05-9w324	Bw37
25	05-9w325	Bw37
26	05-9w327	Bw37
27	05-9w329	Bw37
28	05-9w332	Bw38+w39
29	X	
30	05-9w333	Bw38+w39
31	05-9w335	Bw38+w39
32	05-9w337	Bw38
33	05-9w339	Bw38
34	05-9w340	Bw38
35	05-9w341	Bw39
36	05-9w342	Bw39
37	05-9w343	Bw39
38	05-9w344	Bw39
39	05-9w346	B13
40	05-9w348	B13
41	05-9w352	B13
42	X	
43	05-9w353	B40
44	05-9w355	B40
45	05-9w356	B40
46	05-9w357	B40
47	05-9w359	B40
48	05-9w360	Bw60
49	05-9w362	Bw60
50	05-9w363	Bw60
51	05-9w365	Bw60
52	05-9w366	Bw61
53	05-9w368	Bw60+w48
54	05-9w369	Bw60+w48
55	X	
56	05-9w370	Bw60+w48
57	05-9w372	B13+40+w47
58	05-9w373	B13+40+w47
59	05-9w374	B13+40+w47
60	05-9w376	B13+40+w47
61	05-9w377	Bw47+Aw32
62	05-9w378	B40+w41+12
63	05-9w380	Bw41
64	05-9w381	Bw41
65	05-9w384	Bw41
66	05-9w386	Bw41
67	05-9w387	B12
68	X	
69	05-9w388	B12
70	05-9w393	B12
71	05-9w394	Bw44
72	05-9w396	Bw44
73	05-9w398	Bw44
74	05-9w399	Bw44
75	05-9w400	Bw45
76	05-9w401	Bw45
77	05-9w402	Bw45
78	05-9w404	Bw21
79	local	pos.control
80	local	neg.control

Card 16

Col.	Code	Entry
1–2	16	Card Number
3–5		Region Code
6–8		Typing Lab Code
9–10		Family ID Number
11–13		Individual ID Number
14		Type of cell
15		Type of complement
16	X	
17	06-9w405	Bw21
18	06-9w407	Bw21
19	06-9w409	Bw21
20	06-9w410	Bw49
21	06-9w411	Bw49
22	06-9w413	Bw49
23	06-9w414	Bw49
24	06-9w416	Bw49
25	06-9w417	Bw50
26	06-9w418	Bw50
27	06-9w419	Bw50
28	06-9w420	Bw46+8
29	X	
30	06-9w421	Bw46
31	06-9w422	Bw46
32	06-9w423	Bw4
33	06-9w425	Bw4
34	06-9w427	Bw4
35	06-9w428	Bw4
36	06-9w430	Bw4
37	06-9w431	Bw6
38	06-9w433	Bw6
39	06-9w434	Bw6
40	06-9w436	Bw6
41	06-9w439	Bw6
42	X	
43	06-9w440	ka
44	06-9w441	new abc
45	06-9w442	new abc
46	06-9w443	sn-2
47	06-9w444	sn-2
48	06-9w445	Bw42+sn-2
49	06-9w446	Bw39+sn-2
50	06-9w447	tcn-1
51	06-9w448	Cw1
52	06-9w449	Cw1
53	06-9w450	Cw1
54	06-9w451	Cw1
55	X	
56	06-9w452	Cw1
57	06-9w453	Cw1
58	06-9w454	Cw1+
59	06-9w455	Cw2
60	06-9w456	Cw2
61	06-9w457	Cw2
62	06-9w458	Cw2
63	06-9w459	Cw2
64	06-9w460	Cw2
65	06-9w461	Cw3
66	06-9w462	Cw3
67	06-9w463	Cw3
68	X	
69	06-9w464	Cw3
70	06-9w465	Cw3
71	06-9w466	Cw3
72	06-9w467	Cw3
73	06-9w468	Cw4
74	06-9w469	Cw4
75	06-9w470	Cw4
76	06-9w471	Cw4
77	06-9w472	Cw4
78	06-9w473	Cw4
79	local	pos.control
80	local	neg.control

Card 17

Col.	Code	Entry
1–2	17	Card Number
3–5		Region Code
6–8		Typing Lab Code
9–10		Family ID Number
11–13		Individual ID Number
14		Type of cell
15		Type of complement
16	X	
17	07-9w474	Cw6
18	07-9w475	Cw6
19	07-9w476	Cw6
20	07-9w477	Cw6
21	07-9w478	Cw6
22	07-9w479	Cw4+w6
23	07-9w480	Cw4+w6
24	07-9w481	Cw4+w6
25	07-9w482	Cw4+w6
26	07-9w483	Cw5
27	07-9w484	Cw5
28	07-9w485	Cw5
29	X	
30	07-9w486	Cw5
31	07-9w487	Cw5
32	07-9w488	Cw5
33	07-9w489	Cw5+w8
34	07-9w490	Cw5+w8+B14
35	07-9w491	Cw8
36	07-9w492	Cw8+B14
37	07-9w493	Cw8
38	07-9w494	Cw7
39	07-9w495	Cw7
40	07-9w496	Cw7
41	07-9w497	Cw7
42	X	
43	07-9w498	Cw7
44	07-9w499	Cw7
45	07-9w089	st-16
46	07-9w125	Aw30+w31
47	07-9w152	Bw51
48	07-9w153	Bw51
49	07-9w244	B27+w47
50	07-9w338	bu-sv
51	07-9w350	B13
52	07-9w361	Bw60
53	07-9w805	hu
54	07-9w806	new abc
55	X	
56	local	pos.control
57	local	neg.control
58–80		

Fig. 5

CARDS 14–17

ABC serology
Codes col. 14–15 see general instructions.

General instructions

Score each reaction as follows:
- 0 Not tested
- 1 Negative (0- 10% killed)
- 2 Doubtful negative (11- 20% killed)
- 4 Doubtful positive (21- 40% killed)
- 6 Positive (41- 80% killed)
- 8 Strong positive (81-100% killed)

Type of complement (col. 15):
- 1 Local
- 2 Regional
- 3 Other

Type of cell (col. 14):
- 1 PBL fresh
- 2 PBL frozen
- 3 T-Cells fresh
- 4 T-Cells frozen
- 5 B-Cells fresh
- 6 B-Cells frozen
- 7 T-line
- 8 B-line
- 9 Other line

Card columns 1–15: Card | Number | Region | Code | Typing | Lab | Code | Family ID | Number | Individual ID | Number | Type of cell | Type of complement

Card entry: 1 8 (columns 1–2)

Column	Specificity	Serum
16	X	
17	14.1	9w260
18	14.1	9w260 1:2
19	14.1	9w261
20		RPMI
21	14.2	9w262
22	14.2	9w262 1:2
23	14.2	9w263
24	14.2	9w263 1:2
25	14.2	9w263 1:4
26	14.2	9w264
27	14.2	9w264 1:2
28	14.2	9w265
29	X	
30	14.2	9w265 1:2
31	14.2	9w265 1:4
32	14.2	9w266
33	14.2	9w266 1:2
34	14.1+14.2	9w267
35	14.1+14.2	9w268
36	14.1+14.2	9w269
37	14.1+14.2	9w270
38	14.1+14.2	9w271
39	14.1+14.2	9w272
40	14.1+14.2	9w273
41	14.1+14.2+18	9w275
42	X	
43	14.2	9w700
44	14.1+14.2	DRK Gough 752 C
45	14.1	DRK Abs. Gough
46	14.1	DRK Abs. Gough 1:4
47	14.2	BAS Dickinson
48	14.2	BAS Dickinson 1:2
49	14.2	BAS Dickinson 1:4
50	14.2	FOT Schv
51	14.2	SUF 2258
52	14.2	BOT CT 714
53	14.1+14.2	DRK Jones 375 C
54	14.2	DRK Abs. Jones (2)
55	X	
56	14.2	DRK Abs. Jones 1:4
57	14.2	DRK Abs. Jones (1)
58	pos.control	local
59	neg.control	local
60–80		

Fig. 6

Card columns 1–16 (cards 21–24):

Columns	Field
1–2	Card Number
3–4	Region Code
5–8	Typing Lab Code
9–10	Family ID Number
11–13	Individual ID Number
14	Type of cell
15	Type of complement
16	Technique

Columns 29, 42, 55 and 68 are crossed out (X) on all four cards.

Card 21

Col.	Specificity	Serum
17	DR1	10-9w502
18	DR1	10-9w504
19	DR1	10-9w505
20	DR1	10-9w507
21	DR1	10-9w508
22	DR1	10-9w509
23	DR1	10-9w510
24	DR1	10-9w511
25	DR1	10-9w512
26	DR1	10-9w514
27	DR1	10-9w515
28	DR1+w10	10-9w516
30	DR1+	10-9w518
31	DR1+	10-9w521
32	DR1+	10-9w522
33	DRw10	10-9w523
34	DRw10	10-9w524
35	DRw10	10-9w525
36	DRw10	10-9w527
37	DRw10	10-9w529
38	DR2	10-9w530
39	DR2	10-9w531
40	DR2	10-9w533
41	DR2	10-9w534
43	DR2	10-9w535
44	DR2	10-9w537
45	DR2	10-9w538
46	DR2	10-9w541
47	DR2	10-9w542
48	DR2	10-9w543
49	DR2short	10-9w545
50	DR2short	10-9w546
51	DR2short	10-9w547
52	DR2short	10-9w548
53	DR2short	10-9w549
54	DR2short	10-9w550
56	DR2short	10-9w551
57	DR2short	10-9w552
58	DR2short	10-9w553
59	DR2short	10-9w554
60	DR2short	10-9w555
61	DR3	10-9w557
62	DR3	10-9w559
63	DR3	10-9w561
64	DR3	10-9w563
65	DR3	10-9w564
66	DR3	10-9w565
67	DR3	10-9w567
69	DR3	10-9w568
70	DR3	10-9w569
71	DR3	10-9w570
72	DR3short	10-9w571
73	DR3short	10-9w572
74	DR3short	10-9w573
75	DR3short	10-9w574
76	DR4	10-9w575
77	DR4	10-9w576
78	DR4	10-9w578
79	contr.moab	10-9w798
80	contr.moab	10-9w799

Card 22

Col.	Specificity	Serum
17	DR4	11-9w580
18	DR4	11-9w581
19	DR4	11-9w582
20	DR4	11-9w584
21	DR4	11-9w585
22	DR4	11-9w587
23	DR4	11-9w589
24	DR4	11-9w590
25	DR4short	11-9w591
26	DR4short	11-9w592
27	DR4short	11-9w593
28	DR4short	11-9w594
30	DR4short	11-9w595
31	DR5	11-9w596
32	DR5	11-9w597
33	DR5	11-9w598
34	DR5	11-9w599
35	DR5	11-9w601
36	DR5	11-9w603
37	DR5	11-9w605
38	DR5	11-9w607
39	DR5	11-9w608
40	DR5short	11-9w609
41	DR5short	11-9w610
43	DR5short	11-9w611
44	DR5short	11-9w612
45	DR5short	11-9w613
46	DR5+w8	11-9w614
47	DR5+w6+w8	11-9w616
48	DRw8+5	11-9w618
49	DRw8	11-9w619
50	DRw8+	11-9w620
51	DRw8	11-9w621
52	DRw8	11-9w623
53	DRw8	11-9w624
54	DRw8	11-9w626
56	DRw8	11-9w627
57	DR7	11-9w629
58	DR7	11-9w630
59	DR7	11-9w633
60	DR7	11-9w634
61	DR7	11-9w636
62	DR7	11-9w637
63	DR7	11-9w638
64	DR7	11-9w639
65	DR7	11-9w640
66	DR7	11-9w642
67	DRw9	11-9w643
69	DRw9	11-9w644
70	DRw9	11-9w645
71	DRw9+	11-9w646
72	DRw9	11-9w647
73	DRw9	11-9w650
74	DR2+w6	11-9w652
75	DR2+w6	11-9w653
76	DR2+w6	11-9w654
77	DR2+w6	11-9w655
78	DR2+w6	11-9w656
79	contr.moab	11-9w800
80	control	11-9w802

Card 23

Col.	Specificity	Serum
17	DR2+w6	12-9w657
18	DR1+2+w6	12-9w661
19	DR1+2+w6	12-9w662
20	DR1+2+w6	12-9w663
21	DR1+2+w6	12-9w664
22	DR1+2+w6	12-9w667
23	DR1+2+w6	12-9w668
24	DR1+2+w6+w10	12-9w669
25	DR1+2+w6+w10	12-9w670
26	DR1+2+w6+w10	12-9w671
27	DR1+2+w6+w10	12-9w672
28	DR1+2+w6+w10	12-9w674
30	DR3+w6	12-9w677
31	DR3+w6	12-9w678
32	DR3+w6	12-9w679
33	DR3+w6	12-9w680
34	DR5+w6	12-9w681
35	DR5+w6	12-9w682
36	DR5+w6	12-9w683
37	DR5+w6	12-9w684
38	DR3+5+w6	12-9w685
39	DR3+5+w6	12-9w687
40	DR3+5+w6	12-9w688
41	DR3+5+w6	12-9w689
43	DR3+5+w6+w8	12-9w692
44	DR3+5+w6+w8	12-9w693
45	DR3+5+w6+w8	12-9w694
46	DR3+5+w6+w8	12-9w696
47	DR3+5+w6+w8	12-9w697
48	DR3+5+w6+w8	12-9w698
49	DR3+5+w6+w8	12-9w699
50	DRw6	12-9w700
51	DRw6	12-9w701
52	DRw6	12-9w702
53	DRw6	12-9w703
54	DRw6	12-9w704
56	DRw6	12-9w705
57	DRw6	12-9w706
58	DRw6	12-9w707
59	DRw6	12-9w708
60	DRw6	12-9w709
61	DRw6	12-9w710
62	DR3+w6	12-9w711
63	DR3+w6	12-9w712
64	DR3+w6	12-9w713
65	DR3+w6	12-9w714
66	DR3+w6	12-9w715
67	DR3+7	12-9w716
69	DR3+7	12-9w717
70	DR3+7	12-9w719
71	DR3+7+w9	12-9w720
72	DR3+7+w9	12-9w721
73	DR3+7+w9	12-9w722
74	DR3+7	12-9w723
75	DR3+7	12-9w724
76	DR3+7	12-9w726
77	DR3+7	12-9w727
78	DR4+w9	12-9w729
79	DR4+5+7	12-9w730
80	contr.moab	12-9w801

Card 24

Col.	Specificity	Serum
17	DR4+7	13-9w540
18	DR4+5+7	13-9w731
19	DR7+w9	13-9w733
20	DR4+7	13-9w734
21	DR4+7	13-9w735
22	DR4+7	13-9w736
23	DR4+7	13-9w737
24	DR4	13-9w739
25	new	13-9w740
26	DR1+7	13-9w741
27	DR4+7	13-9w743
28	DR4+5	13-9w744
30	DR4+5	13-9w745
31	DR4+5	13-9w746
32	DR4+5	13-9w747
33	DR4+5	13-9w748
34	DR4+5	13-9w750
35	DR1+4	13-9w752
36	DR4+7+5	13-9w753
37	DR4+5+w8	13-9w754
38	DR3+5+w6+w8	13-9w755
39	DR3+5+w6+w8	13-9w756
40	DR3+5+w6+w8	13-9w757
41	DR3+5+w6+w8	13-9w758
43	DR3+7	13-9w759
44	DR4+5+w8	13-9w761
45	DRw8+	13-9w763
46	new	13-9w764
47	new	13-9w765
48	new	13-9w766
49	new	13-9w767
50	new	13-9w768
51	new	13-9w769
52	new	13-9w770
53	new	13-9w771
54	new	13-9w772
56	new	13-9w773
57	new	13-9w774
58	new	13-9w775
59	new	13-9w776
60	new	13-9w777
61	new	13-9w778
62	new	13-9w779
63	new	13-9w780
64	new	13-9w781
65	new	13-9w785
66	new	13-9w786
67	new	13-9w787
69	new	13-9w788
70	new	13-9w789
71	new	13-9w790
72	new	13-9w791
73	new	13-9w792
74	new	13-9w793
75	new	13-9w794
76	new	13-9w795
77	new	13-9w796
78	DRw10	13-9w797
79	DR5+w8	13-9w803
80	DR7short	13-9w804

CARDS 21-24 **Fig. 7.**

DR serology
Codes col. 14–16 see general instructions.

Column	CARD 31	CARDS 31-32 (Card 32)	CARD 33
1–2	Card Number: 31	Card Number: 32	Card Number: 33
3–5	Region Code	Region Code	Region Code
6–8	Typing Lab Code	Typing Lab Code	Typing Lab Code
9–10	Family ID Number	Family ID Number	Family ID' Number
11–13	Individual ID Number	Individual ID Number	Individual ID Number.
14	Type of cell	Type of cell	Type of cell
15	Type of complement	Type of complement	Type of complement
16	Technique	Technique	X
17	30-9w901	31-9w959	32-9w1102
18	30-9w902	31-9w960	32-9w1103
19	30-9w903	31-9w962	32-9w1104
20	30-9w904	31-9w963	32-9w1105
21	30-9w905	31-9w964	32-9w1106
22	30-9w906	31-9w965	32-9w1107
23	30-9w907	31-9w967	32-9w1108
24	30-9w908	31-9w968	32-9w1109
25	30-9w909	31-9w969	32-9w1110
26	30-9w910	31-9w970	32-9w1111
27	30-9w911	31-9w972	32-9w1112
28	30-9w912	31-9w973	32-9w1113
29	X	X	X
30	30-9w913	31-9w974	32-9w1116
31	30-5w914	31-9w975	32-9w1117
32	30-9w915	31-9w976	32-9w1118
33	30-9w916	31-9w977	32-9w1119
34	30-9w917	31-9w978	32-9w1120
35	30-9w918	31-9w979	32-9w1121
36	30-9w919	31-9w980	32-9w1122
37	30-9w920	31-9w981	32-9w1124
38	30-9w921	31-9w982	32-9w1127
39	30-9w922	31-9w983	32-9w1128
40	30-9w923	31-9w984	32-9w1129
41	30-9w924	31-9w985	32-9w1130
42	X	X	X
43	30-9w925	31-9w986	32-9w1131
44	30-9w926	31-9w987	32-9w1132
45	30-9w927	31-9w988	32-9w1134
46	30-9w928	31-9w782	32-9w1135
47	30-9w929	31-9w783	32-9w1136
48	30-9w930	31-9w784	32-9w1137
49	30-9w931	31-9w992	32-9w1138
50	30-9w932	31-9w993	32-9w1139
51	30-9w933	31-9w994	32-9w1140
52	30-9w934	31-9w995	32-9w1141
53	30-9w935	31-9w996	32-9w1142
54	30-9w936	31-9w660	32-9w1143
55	X	X	X
56	30-9w937	pos.control – local	32-9w1146
57	30-9w938	neg.control – local	32-9w1147
58	30-9w939		32-9w1148
59	30-9w940		32-9w1150
60	30-9w941		32-9w1151
61	30-9w942		32-9w1152
62	30-9w943		32-9w1153
63	30-9w944		32-9w1154
64	30-9w945		32-9w1155
65	30-9w946		32-9w1156
66	30-9w947		32-9w1157
67	30-9w948		32-9w1158
68	X	X	X
69	30-9w949		32-9w1159
70	30-9w950		32-9w1160
71	30-9w951		32-9w1125
72	30-9w952		32-9w1126
73	30-9w953		32-9w1133
74	30-9w954		32-9w1144
75	30-9w955		pos.control – local
76	30-9w956		neg.control – local
77	30-9w957		
78	30-9w958		
79	pos.control – local		
80	neg.control – local		

CARDS 31-32
DR monoclonal
Codes col. 14-16 see general instructions

CARD 33
ABC monoclonal
Codes col. 14-15 see general instructions

Fig. 8.

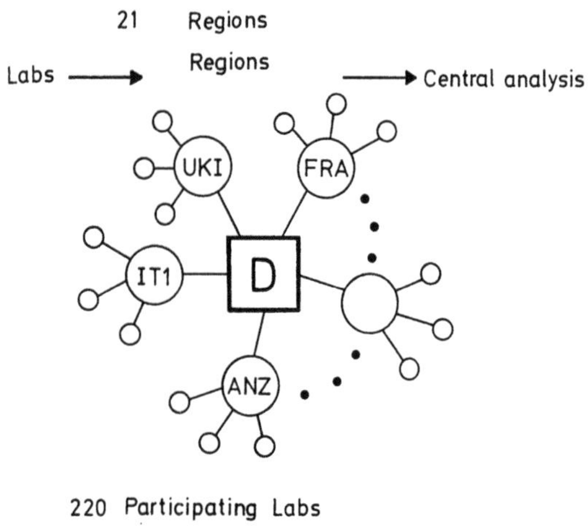

Fig. 9. Data submission for central analysis

Data Analysis

Figure 10 is a simplified flowchart of the complex and interdependent tasks involved in the attempted analyses on the basis of the available general family data. It was obvious from the beginning that a set of interfacing programs had to be developed to break up the total problem into smaller units, which could be handled separately, although dependent on the results of other units.

The analysis of typing reagents (Workshop serum set, Workshop set of homozygous typing cells) was performed in the standard way, constructing 2×2 tables for submitted serum reactions vs submitted laboratory assignments for each tested cell. A subsequent tail analysis to detect multispecificity of sera provided a list of up to four antigens besides the main specificity correlated with each serum. The characterization of sera was the basis for cell typing by computer (see H. Deppe et al., Cell Typing by Computer, this volume).

This program, which is based on ideas used in the Eighth IHW [4], assigns each cell, on the basis of submitted serum reactions and in accordance with the results of the serum analysis for each investigated locus, up to two specificities. The results of the computer assignments were compared to the original laboratory assignments and added as new cards 8–10 in analogy to the existing cards 2–5 to the card set of each individual in the masterfile WS9DAT.

Laboratory assignments as well as computer assignments for the HLA markers, and in addition the information on the class III loci, were the starting point for all further genetic analyses of this Workshop. The new situation of general family data was supposed to provide information not only about multilocus phenotypes, but also about the given genotypes of the tested individuals. Consequently the program package FAP (see M. Neugebauer et al., Analysis of Multilocus Pedigree Data by Computer, this volume) [3] was designed to derive in general predigree situations and for an arbitrary number of linked loci for each individual, paternal and maternal haplotype compatible with phenotype and family relations. FAP was used to analyze all 2300 families submitted, including problems with missing individuals, missing data, recombinant families, etc. Already at the early stage of data checking it became apparent that FAP was also an extremely important logical checking device, flagging all cases of "nonsegregation" caused by typing errors, nonpaternity, or pedigree miscoding. In the case of a nonunique solution in the haplotyping process, the program assigned each solution its conditional likelihood on the basis of involved parameters such as gene frequencies, linkage disequilibria, recombination fractions, and mendelian ratios. The solution with the highest likelihood was printed and in addition served as input to PEDPLO (see M. Sigmund, this volume), a program for the general display of multigeneration pedigree data.

In order to give the participating laboratories a feedback about our interpretation of their family data, an attempt was made to return as much information as possible in the way of outputs from FAP and plotted pedigrees from PEDPLO as early as the stage of data submission and correction. At the Workshop, the final results were given to each laboratory in a folder [8] containing for each submitted family its interpretation on the basis of laboratory assignments, its pedigree plot, the results of computer cell typing in comparison to laboratory typing, and an additional output of FAP on the basis of computer assignments.

Parallel to the results produced for the participating laboratories, the chairmen of joint analyses – disease studies, crossover registry, population study – were provided with subfiles of the masterfile containing the raw family data relevant to their study. In addition their subfile was analyzed by FAP and correct families were plotted by PEDPLO.

Finally, using all family analyses data set WS9DIPLO was created, containing the deduced multilocus diplotypes (paternal and maternal haplotypes) of each family member together with relative likelihood and all information from card 1. This data set, together with the complete results of FAP, was the basis for all joint analyses, e.g., the population study and the crossover registry.

It is obvious that the data sets compiled for the Ninth IHW contain a large amount of valuable information, extraction of which is by no means complete.

Table 1. Participating laboratories and their data in the Workshop masterfile

LAB	Code	Fam.	Mem.	Dis. Fam.	Unrel. Ind.	ABC	DR	ABC mono	DR mono	Other mark.	MLC	Total cards
REGION ANZ												
BASHIR	BSH	14	80	6	2	79	77	79	73	79	30	2231
CHEN	CHE	5	32	0	0	32	32	32	32	32	0	672
CHIEWSHILP	CHI	5	34	0	0	34	34	34	34	34	0	714
CROSS	CRS	5	29	0	0	29	29	29	29	29	0	609
CHAN SOH HA	CSH	3	34	1	0	32	32	32	32	32	0	675
DAWKINS	DAW	16	165	13	10	151	145	148	131	154	0	3182
CHANDANAYI.	DCH	6	37	0	0	37	37	37	37	37	0	777
FONG	FON	5	34	0	0	33	25	33	25	33	0	646
HAWKINS	HAW	7	40	1	0	40	40	0	0	40	0	720
HAY	HAY	8	90	2	0	83	83	83	83	82	0	1752
MEHRA	MEH	20	131	15	0	113	113	113	113	108	0	2348
ROBINSON	ROB	5	30	0	0	30	30	30	30	30	0	600
SERJEANTSON	SER	6	41	0	0	41	41	41	41	41	0	861
TAIT	TAI	9	67	2	0	63	63	63	63	63	0	1329
WOODFIELD	WOO	5	28	0	0	28	28	28	28	28	0	588
YAO	YEG	5	31	0	0	30	30	30	30	30	0	631
REGION BEN												
BOUILLENNE	BOU	1	4	1	0	3	3	3	3	3	0	64
BRUYERE	BRU	3	19	3	0	17	18	17	18	18	0	362
DUPONT	DPT	3	11	3	0	10	10	10	10	10	0	211
ENGELFRIET	ENG	18	138	6	0	126	113	126	113	43	0	2294
IVANYI	IVA	0	0	0	7	0	0	0	0	0	0	31
MUYLLE	MUY	3	15	3	0	15	15	15	6	12	0	282
REEKERS	REE	16	78	3	0	65	58	50	21	0	0	1068
VAN ROOD	ROO	16	118	9	31	143	121	116	73	99	33	5447
REGION EAE												
BARTOVA	BRT	7	72	0	0	72	68	68	10	72	0	1392
IVASKOVA	IVS	5	39	1	0	37	37	37	36	0	27	1741
KASTELAN	KAS	40	210	23	10	217	210	173	154	202	24	4560
MAYR	MYR	20	128	0	3	130	129	130	129	0	25	2701
NYULASSY	NYU	3	20	0	0	20	20	20	20	0	29	631
PETRANYI	PTR	12	83	0	1	78	77	75	71	36	47	2033
RICHTER	RIC	18	138	2	0	130	127	128	118	53	24	3309
SHABALIN	SHA	13	48	13	0	42	42	42	42	0	0	636
WALTZ	WTZ	11	90	0	0	90	90	90	90	90	0	1800
ZARETSKAYA	ZAR	6	35	6	0	29	29	29	16	0	0	525
REGION FRA												
ARNAIZ	ARN	17	91	17	0	69	63	69	63	91	31	2863
BETUEL	BET	28	184	2	4	178	170	173	162	148	29	5254
BIGNON	BIG	4	41	0	0	30	30	30	30	0	0	534
DAUSSET	DAU	22	161	3	4	148	147	143	138	118	0	5331
FAUCHET	FAU	27	192	7	1	187	185	182	178	180	0	3756
GARRIDO	GRA	5	32	0	0	32	32	31	32	0	0	575
JEANNET	JEA	10	64	1	20	64	64	64	64	0	0	1844
KREISLER	KRE	12	66	12	1	60	60	54	29	0	0	1085
LEPETIT	LEP	3	46	3	0	25	25	25	25	40	0	541
MAYER	MYE	24	175	4	0	156	136	156	126	156	0	3018
OHAYON	OHA	22	194	11	0	166	166	165	164	174	0	3421
PERRIER	PRR	8	48	3	0	42	39	42	34	0	0	733
VIVES	VIV	5	36	0	0	36	34	36	33	36	0	704
REGION GER												
ALBERT	ALB	12	91	5	15	143	143	133	134	33	0	2164
BERTRAMS	BER	39	233	32	1	105	105	104	105	211	0	2928
BRAUTBAR	BRA	6	66	0	2	42	42	41	42	42	26	1488
EWALD	EWA	6	42	5	0	33	33	33	33	33	0	680
GAZIT	GAZ	14	75	14	0	48	43	41	41	0	0	882
GOLDMANN	GOL	18	104	0	0	78	78	78	78	0	0	1493

Table 1. Continued

LAB	Code	Fam.	Mem.	Dis. Fam.	Unrel. Ind.	ABC	DR	ABC mono	DR mono	Other mark.	MLC	Total cards
GROSSE-WILDE	GSW	5	34	0	11	44	44	44	44	44	45	3037
KUEHNL	KUE	13	74	10	2	68	65	62	55	62	0	1132
MUELLER-ECKHARDT	MUE	28	249	5	46	127	130	126	129	252	0	3592
NEUMEYER	NEU	8	68	4	0	54	51	52	48	7	0	989
RITTNER	RIT	5	30	0	0	30	30	30	30	30	0	601
SCHUNTER	SCU	5	76	0	21	95	95	95	95	0	0	1730
WANK	WAN	6	47	0	5	0	0	0	0	7	60	3058
WERNET	WER	2	55	2	27	70	69	47	46	65	0	1334
WESTPHAL	WES	10	57	8	0	51	51	51	51	42	0	1074
REGION IT1												
CONTU	CON	10	66	0	0	64	64	64	64	64	0	1282
CARBONARA	CRB	20	166	7	0	160	148	160	131	159	0	3176
MENICUCCI	MCC	13	95	0	0	95	95	64	61	78	0	1767
MERCURIALI	MRC	8	37	8	0	37	37	37	37	0	0	682
MATTIUZ	MTT	16	140	13	0	130	128	130	123	130	0	2586
PURPURA	PUR	7	54	0	0	51	32	51	32	51	0	890
SALERNO	SAL	8	52	0	0	52	46	51	44	51	0	991
SAVI	SAV	10	49	10	0	48	48	48	46	0	0	861
REGION IT2												
BARBONI	BAR	6	35	4	0	31	31	31	31	31	0	652
CELADA	CEL	2	11	1	0	11	11	11	11	11	0	222
FERRARA	FER	12	112	0	3	113	113	113	113	33	30	3368
GANDINI	GAN	18	117	0	0	117	111	117	110	0	0	2062
PELLEGRIS	PEL	1	4	1	0	4	4	4	4	4	0	82
REGION JAP												
AIZAWA	AIZ	10	61	0	0	61	61	61	61	0	0	1098
JUJI	JUJ	48	279	2	0	277	277	277	276	71	0	5135
KASHIWAGI	KSH	5	30	0	34	57	57	57	57	0	49	2650
MATSUYAMA	MAT	7	39	5	1	37	32	37	32	0	0	649
MIYAJIMA	MIY	37	191	20	0	184	184	176	172	68	0	3483
NAITO	NAI	14	79	3	0	79	79	79	79	16	0	1455
OHKOCHI	OKO	7	42	0	0	42	42	41	42	0	0	755
SASAZUKI	SAS	23	102	16	7	112	105	78	67	0	27	2208
SEKIGUCHI	SEK	25	146	7	0	146	146	146	125	19	0	2665
TOKUNAGA	TOK	10	60	0	0	53	52	53	52	53	0	1061
TSUJI	TSU	55	268	47	32	278	278	278	278	204	49	6998
YOSHIDA	YOS	16	94	0	0	94	88	94	85	11	0	1666
REGION LAT												
ALVAREZ	BNO	1	6	1	0	6	5	6	6	0	0	116
FERREIRA	FRR	12	111	2	0	94	94	83	93	31	0	1873
GERBASE	GER	15	95	4	0	94	94	83	94	0	0	1801
GIRAUDO	GIR	5	43	4	0	36	32	36	33	0	0	652
GORODESKY	GOR	5	47	5	0	43	43	40	42	28	0	878
JOBIM	JOB	2	10	2	0	10	10	9	10	10	0	214
MORAES	JRM	15	136	9	0	111	111	111	111	111	0	2409
LAYRISSE	LAY	22	156	18	12	142	141	142	138	142	36	4422
MORALES	MRL	4	23	1	0	23	23	23	23	0	0	437
PRIGOSHIN	PRI	1	5	1	0	5	5	5	5	5	0	110
PEREZ	PRZ	8	48	1	0	48	44	43	38	0	0	823
ROSALES	ROS	16	102	4	0	99	94	98	89	98	0	2024
SUAREZ	SUA	4	29	0	0	26	26	26	26	26	0	539
REGION NCY												
BIAS	BIA	16	146	6	5	104	104	104	104	143	39	3302
CARPENTER	CAR	7	32	7	32	64	64	64	63	27	0	1204
FALK	FAL	9	27	9	3	25	23	24	5	0	0	409

Table 1. Continued

LAB	Code	Fam.	Mem.	Dis. Fam.	Unrel. Ind.	ABC	DR	ABC mono	DR mono	Other mark.	MLC	Total cards
FULLER	FUL	1	9	0	22	19	19	19	17	9	0	692
GOEKEN	GOE	6	36	2	22	56	54	56	55	0	0	998
KOETHE	KOE	10	60	0	0	59	0	59	0	0	0	650
MARSHALL	MAR	5	34	1	0	33	29	33	29	33	0	635
MERVART	MRV	16	103	2	36	139	139	138	139	84	0	2669
SCHACTER	SCH	3	20	1	63	82	74	81	70	12	0	1438
YAGNOW	YAG	13	86	0	0	80	79	80	79	0	0	1439
YUNIS	YUN	9	55	0	84	124	124	124	124	24	38	3473
REGION SAF												
DU TOIT	DUT	42	379	24	2	331	328	330	326	334	43	7769
HAMMOND	HAM	20	223	2	0	192	173	192	170	193	0	3739
REGION SCA												
JERSILD	JER	2	10	2	44	54	54	54	54	0	0	1088
KISSM.-NIELSEN	KIS	15	95	0	48	143	123	140	6	132	32	3359
KOSKIMIES	KOS	5	21	4	12	21	17	20	4	18	0	586
LINDBLOM	LIN	25	152	0	0	152	151	0	0	146	0	2567
LOEW	LOW	16	77	8	0	77	77	77	77	0	0	1402
MÖLLER	MOL	14	73	14	0	72	72	72	72	0	0	1368
SVEJGAARD	SVE	15	92	0	76	109	118	109	118	89	25	3922
THORSBY	TSB	28	154	21	50	192	192	192	192	34	25	4644
REGION UKI												
BATCHELOR	BAT	21	152	21	0	93	92	92	87	93	0	1996
BODMER	BOD	14	92	1	0	90	83	75	50	36	0	1735
BRADLEY	BRS	13	77	0	22	95	93	93	90	89	30	4637
EVANS	CXH	4	63	2	0	50	47	0	0	59	0	954
DEWAR	DEW	11	47	2	3	44	44	0	0	44	0	765
DICK	DIC	9	56	9	0	56	54	0	0	56	0	970
DARKE	DRK	15	83	14	79	64	63	0	0	49	0	1459
FESTENSTEIN	FES	24	138	0	10	137	90	0	5	63	98	6033
GELSTHORPE	GEL	4	35	3	0	31	31	30	13	8	0	547
HARRIS	HAR	8	50	4	1	46	46	0	0	46	0	787
JAMES	JAM	11	57	5	1	55	55	55	55	55	0	1170
JOYSEY	JOY	5	24	2	0	24	24	0	0	0	0	367
KNIGHT	KNT	28	136	28	0	113	111	113	109	114	0	2433
LAWLER	LAW	13	78	1	0	76	75	76	75	76	0	1518
MACKINTOSH	MAC	5	66	3	0	52	44	46	35	52	0	977
MIDDLETON	MID	6	39	0	0	30	26	0	0	12	0	472
MORRIS	MOR	8	55	0	0	55	55	55	53	0	0	986
WELSH	WEL	5	37	5	0	28	21	0	0	30	0	509
WOODROW	WOR	16	116	5	0	103	106	102	102	108	0	2236
REGION US1												
AMOS, KOSTYU	AMO	5	27	0	48	72	73	72	68	0	0	1329
DUQESNOY	DUQ	8	47	0	0	46	46	46	46	0	0	849
JOHN.HART.ECK.	HEJ	17	112	2	23	62	62	62	60	50	0	2577
BIEGEL, BRAHMI	IND	5	41	1	0	31	30	31	30	32	0	638
JONGH	NWO	28	197	8	29	178	106	175	103	159	0	3103
RODEY, OLDFATH.	STL	10	44	10	0	44	40	44	40	0	0	788
THOMPSON	THP	6	45	2	30	74	74	73	74	0	0	1360
WARD	WAR	4	22	0	23	39	39	39	39	0	0	708
REGION US2												
BACH, SEG.	BAC	18	125	0	5	121	116	120	102	0	31	3372
POLASKY	HFP	82	247	0	0	106	0	106	0	0	0	1307
JONASSEN, LAZDA	JON	18	54	0	0	18	18	0	0	0	0	306

Table 1. Continued

LAB	Code	Fam.	Mem.	Dis. Fam.	Unrel. Ind.	ABC	DR	ABC mono	DR mono	Other mark.	MLC	Total cards
REGION US3												
GRUMET	GRU	6	47	0	0	45	45	45	45	45	0	902
KING, THOMPSON	KAT	17	95	17	0	74	73	0	0	82	0	1404
PERKINS	PER	8	48	0	0	48	48	48	48	47	0	958
REGION US4												
BARGER	BRG	2	15	2	0	15	15	14	5	0	0	252
RADVANY	RAD	17	67	17	0	65	64	65	62	65	0	1335
SAUNDERS	SND	3	24	0	0	24	24	24	24	24	0	480
STASTNY	STA	44	220	2	0	166	166	166	166	166	32	6679
REGION US5												
WILLIAMS	ABS	11	80	0	0	79	79	79	79	0	0	1423
ALARIF	ALA	7	41	0	0	35	35	35	35	24	0	699
SUNG XING CHANG	BLT	18	109	0	0	109	0	109	0	0	0	1199
CHONG HOON LEE	CMC	11	67	0	0	67	0	67	0	0	0	737
TESTIN	FTW	12	69	0	0	69	69	69	69	0	0	1242
PARSA	ISM	7	28	7	60	84	84	84	84	0	0	1410
MITTAL	MIT	11	68	0	0	68	68	68	68	68	0	1360
SCHROEDER	MLS	4	19	4	34	53	53	53	53	19	0	1000
PAIK	PAK	22	167	22	0	81	81	81	81	0	0	1604
PEETOM	PNW	10	70	0	0	70	70	70	70	0	0	1260
REEVE	RVE	14	109	14	0	80	80	80	80	0	0	1547
SINGAL	SIN	16	75	7	23	93	93	93	92	0	0	2336
SCHWEIZER	SWE	7	42	0	0	42	42	42	42	0	0	756
TERASAKI	TER	9	66	0	0	66	0	66	0	0	0	726
REGION US6												
BLANK	BLA	13	61	13	0	61	61	61	61	0	0	1159
BRAUN	BRN	25	161	18	0	153	156	153	153	144	0	3090
TROUP	TRP	2	15	0	0	15	15	15	15	0	0	270
WALFORD	WAL	4	21	4	0	21	16	21	4	0	0	339
REGION US7												
DUPONT	DUP	13	70	9	8	72	71	67	70	54	0	1453
HANSEN	HAN	25	191	5	6	155	155	155	7	142	31	2949
REGION US8												
DECARY	DEC	10	83	0	0	63	63	63	63	64	0	1301
FOTINO	FOT	4	32	0	0	31	31	31	31	0	0	559
LEE	JLE	39	273	18	0	268	261	268	254	268	0	5386
SUCIU-FOCA	NSF	19	91	9	0	87	81	86	79	0	0	1529
RUBINSTEIN	RUB	11	75	10	0	73	73	54	0	75	0	1373

We therefore urge those who are interested in doing further analyses to contact us for transfer of the data sets:

(1) WS9DAT masterfile, (2) WS9DIPLO deduced haplotypes, and (3) disease files, as well as the available programs, (1) FAP, (2) PEDPLO, and (3) CELLTYPE, which were produced by the members of the central data analysis team (listed in alphabetical order):

Hans Deppe (Düsseldorf), Tom K. Louton (Düsseldorf), Meinhard Neugebauer (Düsseldorf), Gabi Sierp (München), Martin Sigmund (Bonn), Susanne Sigmund (Bonn), and Jürgen Willems (Düsseldorf).

In conclusion, we would like to express our belief that most of the "dubious" family situations originally submitted, such as the one presented in Fig. 11, have been corrected and that the quality of the now available masterfile has been improved as far as possible. Nevertheless, it has to be kept in mind that all the analyses of the Ninth Workshop as well as results produced in the future, depend entirely on the quality of the data submitted by the participating laboratories.

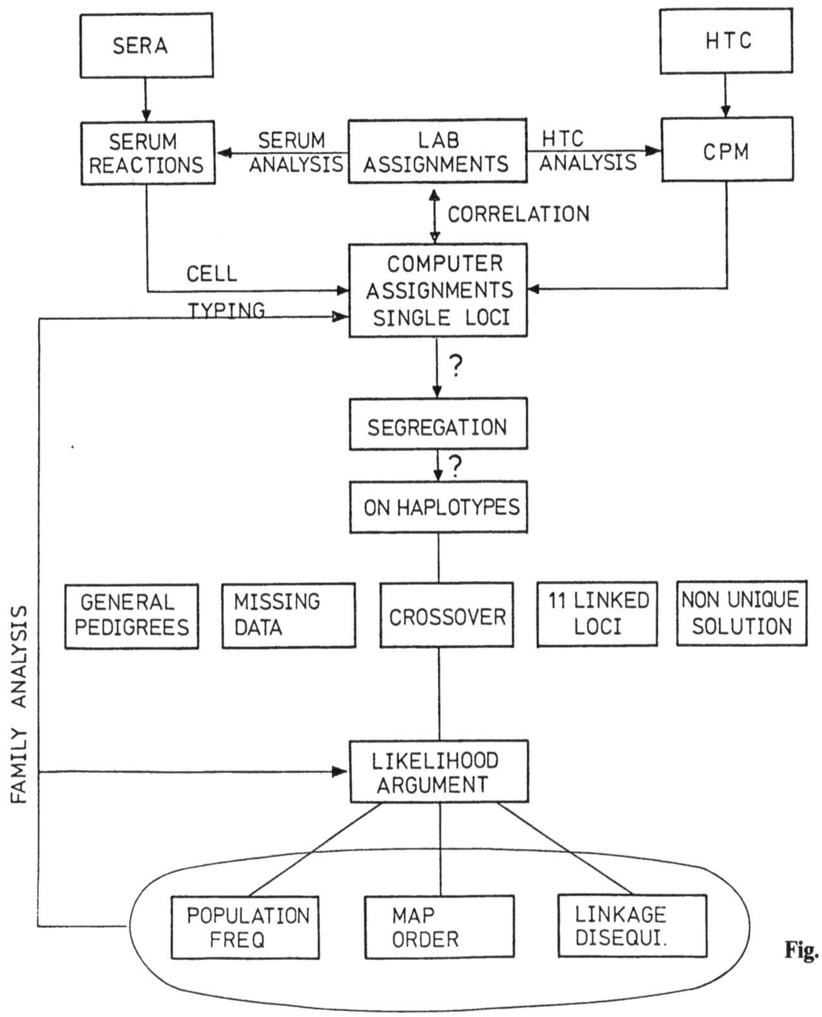

Fig. 10. Programs for family data

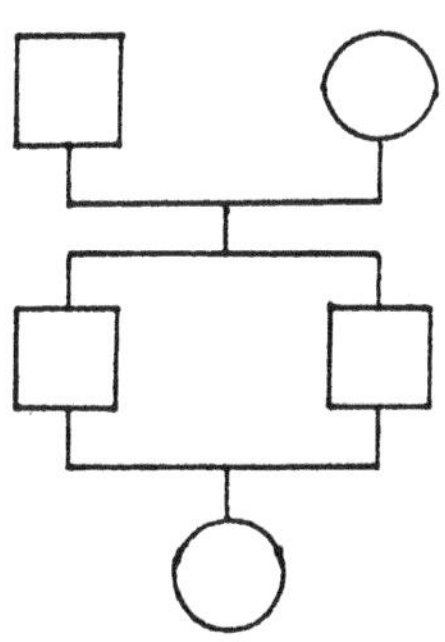

Fig. 11. Questionable family situation originally submitted and later corrected: a fertile brother-brother mating

Acknowledgments. We would like to thank Prof. G. Oberhoffer (†), Head of the Institute for Medical Statistics, University of Bonn, for his unrelenting support of our work during this and previous Workshops. Furthermore, we would like to acknowledge the total availability of the computing facilities of the Diabetes Research Institute, Düsseldorf, and the extensive access to the Central Computing Center of the University of Bonn (Director Dr. E. Jasper).

References

1. Terasaki PI (ed) (1980) Histocompatibility testing 1980. UCLA, Los Angeles
2. Bodmer WF, Batcheler JR, Bodmer JG, Festenstein H, Morris PJ (eds) (1978) Histocompatibility testing 1977. Munksgaard, Copenhagen
3. Baur MP, Neugebauer M, Sigmund M, Willems J (1984) FAP – Family analysis program. Human gene mapping 7. Cytogenet Cell Genet 37:416
4. Mickey MR, Terasaki PI (1980) The serological data of the 8th Workshop and summary analyses. In: Terasaki PI (ed) Histocompatibility testing 1980. UCLA, Los Angeles
5. Baur MP, Albert ED (1984) Central data analysis. Folder prepared for distribution at Ninth International Histocompatibility Workshop 1984

Analysis of Multilocus Pedigree Data by Computer *

M. Neugebauer, J. Willems, and M. P. Baur

Biometrical Department, Diabetes Research Institute, Auf'm Hennekamp 65, 4000 Düsseldorf 1, Federal Republic of Germany

Introduction

Pedigree analysis is a methodology used for gene mapping, risk prediction in genetic counseling, hypothesis testing in genetic epidemiology, and parameter estimation of genetic models. Therefore, mendelian likelihoods must be computed from human pedigree data with a well-defined genetic model.

The family analysis package (FAP) is a package of FORTRAN IV programs which analyzes multilocus pedigree data. The genetic model used can be freely defined, including mendelian ratios, allele frequencies, two-locus to n-locus linkage disequilibria, recombination frequencies, and penetrance values.

Given the phenotypes of n marker (HLA) and/or disease susceptibility loci for the related individuals, the program tries in a first step to uniquely assign each member of the pedigree its multi-locus diplotype, i.e., both the paternal and the maternal haplotype of length n. When a nonunique situation in the pedigree occurs, the set of diplotypes compatible with both phenotype and family relations is derived for each individual. In a subsequent step, for each compatible combination of individual diplotypes the likelihood of this explanation is calculated from the parameters of the genetic model. The diplotypic possibilities of the pedigree are printed in order of likelihood. Obviously these calculations of likelihood depend on the assumed set of genetic parameters. Conversely, it is possible to estimate these parameters by iterative application of the program to a given family sample, improving the parameter estimate(s) according to the previous cycle. In this way the program can generally be used to estimate recombination fractions, allele frequencies, multilocus haplotype frequencies, and linkage disequilibria, or to perform maximum likelihood ordering in linkage groups.

The program is able to analyze pedigrees with recombination, pedigrees with missing or partially missing phenotype data for some members, and pedigrees with inbreeding. The number of generations, pedigree members, or linked loci is limited only by computer size and time. For this purpose FAP contains five main programs:

- FAP: performs the likelihood calculations.
- FHAP: counts the haplotype frequencies from the output of FAP and gives n loci haplotype frequency tables.
- FORFREI: translates the parameter set from a formated file into a format-free file.
- WS9UM: translates the original data of the Ninth Workshop for use in FAP.
- ESTIM: estimates allele frequencies, two-way and three-way haplotype frequencies, disequilibria values, and penetrance. ESTIM creates a new input file for program FAP.

Further more, a plot-routine is available which produces pedigree plots from the results of FAP.

Description of Algorithms

In order to compute the likelihood of a complex pedigree with data of multiple loci, it is useful to minimize the calculations by formal genetic reduction. This means that the likelihood is only computed for those explanations which are compatible with the pedigree relationships.

For this analysis the following data structure is necessary:

1. Definition of the pedigree
   - pedigree identification
   - individual identification
   - father identification for each individual
   - mother identification for each individual

   (For an entry individual both father and mother identification must be missing.)
2. Phenotype data for each pedigree member
   - for each marker locus no, one, or two specificities
   - for each trait locus (disease susceptibility) only one phenotype value

   (All or part of the phenotype data of a person may be missing.)

The formal genetic analysis gives for each person a set of diplotypes which are genetically compatible with the rest of the pedigree. For each person the number of diplotypes of the set or each diplotype can be produced. The program constructs for each individual all possible diplotypes. Given the 2*n

* Supported by Deutsche Forschungsgemeinschaft Ba 660/5-1, Al 92/13-2, SFB 113 B8

Histocompatibility Testing 1984
Edited by E. D. Albert et al.

phenotype data of n marker loci, one can construct 2^n up to 3^n different diplotypes, taking in account that one haplotype is transmitted from the father, the other from the mother. The exact number of diplotypes depends on the number of loci with a recessive allele.

For disease susceptibility loci the program builds all possible genotypes ($=(n+1)*n/2$) from the available alleles of the disease locus for each person and combines these with the marker diplotype set.

For the reduction, a pedigree is divided into nuclear pedigrees, each consisting of father, mother, and children. Within such a nuclear pedigree all diplotypes are deleted which are not compatible with the inheritance from parents to children. This procedure is done iteratively for each nuclear pedigree in the way illustrated in Fig. 1.

In case of cross-over in the pedigree, the algorithm described above leads to no results (for one or more members of the pedigree all diplotypes are completely deleted). In such a pedigree the program creates the diplotype set for each person a second time and the formal genetic reduction is done with a modified algorithm.

During the reduction in a nuclear pedigree, a diplotype is deleted only if the diplotype is not compatible with all parent haplotypes that could have originated from the original haplotypes by recombination. For example, if a father has a diplotype "a b c d; e f g h" a child's diplotype "a b c h; . . . " is not deleted. If this gives no results, the program produces a phenotype data error message.

In many pedigrees the phenotype data are not available for some members, and the possible genotypes must be created from the genotypes of the typed related individuals. For individuals with completely missing phenotype data this is done in the following way: (1) The formal genetic reduction is done for the pedigree without use of the "missing individual." (2) The diplotype set for the "missing individual" is created by combination of the parental haplotypes, if the diplotype sets of both parents exists.

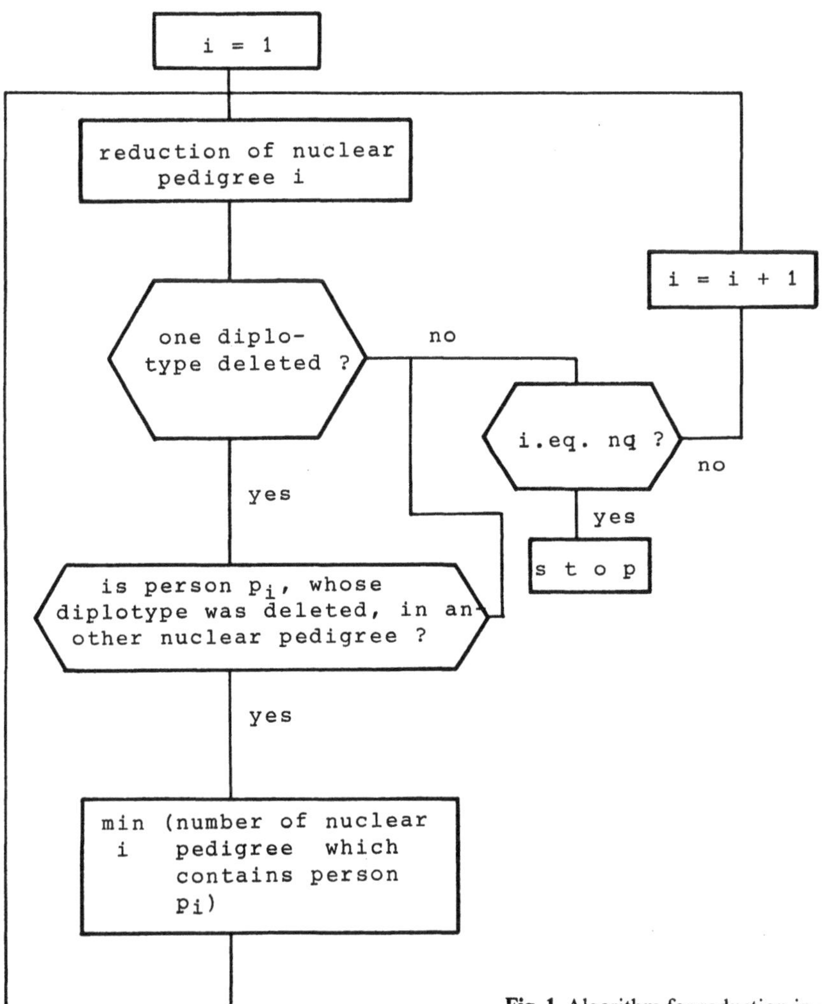

Fig. 1. Algorithm for reduction in a nuclear pedigree

If the haplotypes of the parents do not exist, the diplotype set is built up by combination of all filial haplotypes of the "missing individual." (3) The formal genetic reduction is done again. For individuals with partially missing phenotype data the program deletes all diplotypes which are not compatible with the rest of the data.

Likelihood Calculations

After the formal genetic reduction has been done, for each member of the pedigree $i=1 \ldots n_{ipi}$ a diplotype set with n_i diplotypes $(k_{i_1} \ldots k_{in_i})$ exists. From this one can give $m = n_1 \times n_2 \times \ldots \times n_i$ different possible pedigree explanations with only one diplotype per member. The summation over these m explanations gives the likelihood of the whole pedigree [1, 2]:

$$L = \sum_{k_1} \sum_{k_2} \ldots \sum_{k_{n_i}} \prod_{\text{individual with observed } i} \text{pen}(i, k_i) \times \prod_{i = \text{entry individual}} f(k_i) \times \prod \text{trans}(k_{i1}; k_{i2}, k_{i3})$$

$(k_{i1}$: child, k_{i2}: father, k_{i3}: mother)

pen(i, k_i): penetrance = probability of phenotype i under the condition of genotype k_i

$f(k_i)$: probability of diplotype k_i for the entry persons

trans: transition probability = mendelian ratios (1/2, 1/4, 1) plus recombination frequencies

The program calculates first the haplotype frequencies (diplotype frequencies) and then the likelihood of the various possibilities, prints the most likely explanations, and sums up all likelihood values.

Calculation of Haplotype Frequencies

For unassociated loci, the haplotype frequency is given by the product of the allele frequencies:

$$f(a, b, c) = f(a) * f(b) * f(c)$$

For loci with linkage disequilibria, the haplotype frequency calculation must take into account disequilibrium values. The program uses only two-loci disequilibria delta (a, b), so the frequency of a two-loci haplotype is given by:

$$f(a, b) = f(a) * f(b) + \text{delta}(a, b)$$

For a three-loci haplotype:

$$\begin{aligned} f(a, b, c) = {} & f(a) * f(b) * f(c) \\ & + f(a) * \text{delta}(b, c) \\ & + f(b) * \text{delta}(a, c) \\ & + f(c) * \text{delta}(a, b) \\ & (+ \text{delta}(a, b, c)) \end{aligned}$$

If one does not use the higher order delta values (greater than or equal to three), it is possible to compute the haplotype frequencies recursively:

$$\begin{aligned} f(a, b) &= f(a) * f(b) + \text{delta}(a, b) \\ f(a, b, c) &= f(c) * f(a, b) \\ &\quad + f(a) * \text{delta}(b, c) \\ &\quad + f(b) * \text{delta}(a, c) \\ f(a, b, c, d) &= f(d) * f(a, b, c) \\ &\quad + f(a, b) * \text{delta}(c, d) \\ &\quad + f(a, c) * \text{delta}(b, d) \\ &\quad + f(b, c) * \text{delta}(a, d) \end{aligned}$$

For an n-loci haplotype, f is given as follows:

$$f(a_1, \ldots, a_i, \ldots, a_n) = f(a_1, \ldots, a_i, \ldots, a_{n-1}) * f(a_n) + \sum_{j=1,\ldots n-1} f(a_1, \ldots, a_i, \ldots, a_{n-2})_{i \neq j;\, i \neq n} * \text{delta}(a_j, a_n)$$

Calculation of Likelihood of a Complex Pedigree

The likelihood computation for one pedigree constellation is done with the following algorithm shown in Fig. 2, where $i = 1 \ldots n_i$ persons; p = likelihood; hi · p = paternal haplotype; hi · m = maternal haplotype; θ_k = recombination frequency; n loc = number of loci.
For each explanation $j = 1 \ldots m$ a likelihood value L(j) is computed and the relative likelihood is printed:

$$L_{rel}(j) = L(j) / \sum_{k=1 \ldots m} L(k)$$

With these values, to each diplotype k of person i (D_{ik}) a relative likelihood is assigned:

$$L_{rel}(D_{ik}) = \Big(\sum_{D_{ik} \text{ in explanation } j} L(j)\Big) \quad \sum_{ks = \text{all diplotypes of ind. } i} (L(D_{iks}))$$

Program Example

Figure 3 shows the first part of the output of an example. In the first line are the region, laboratory, and family code, then come the codes for population, disease, recombinant family, and selection status. Then follow the input data for each individual, in the sequence ind id, father id, mother id,

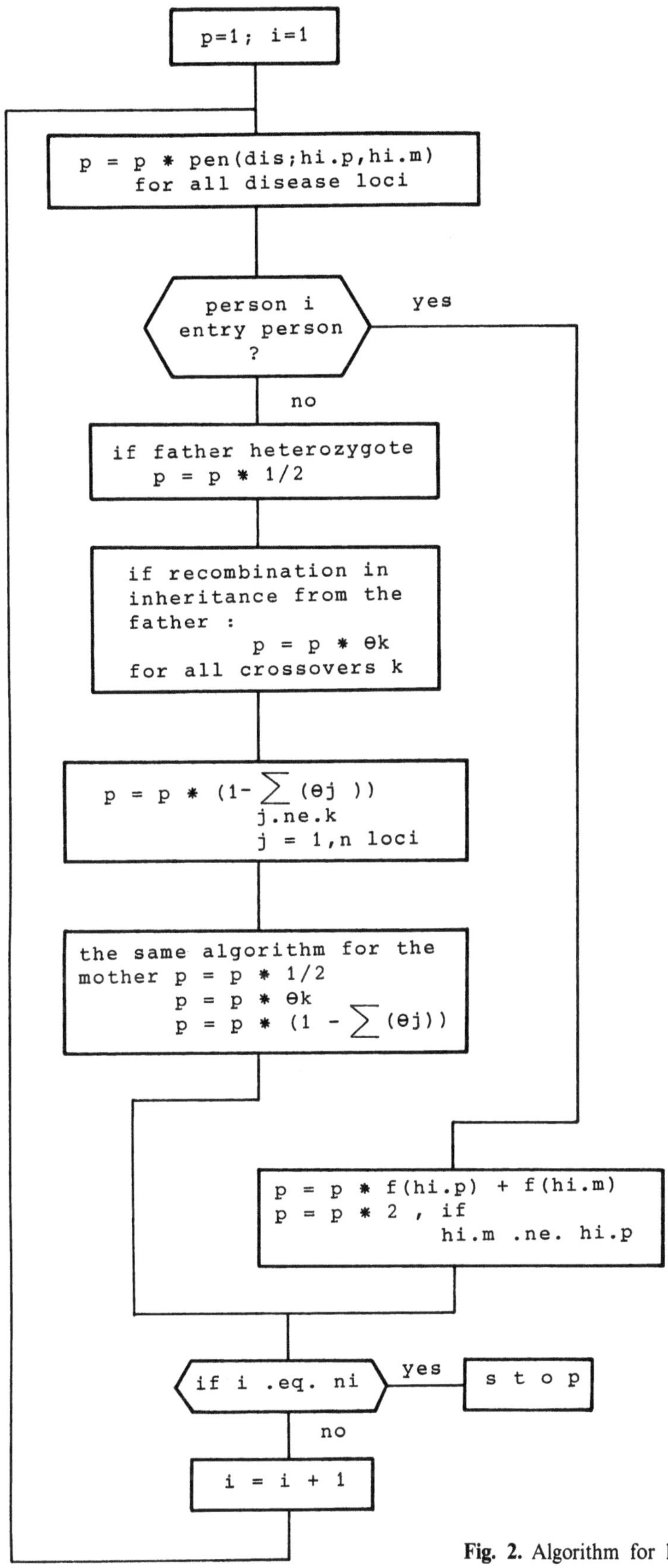

Fig. 2. Algorithm for likelihood computation of pedigree constellation

```
-----------------------------------------------------------------------------
   1 FAMILY  GER WES   1
-----------------------------------------------------------------------------

      POP : (  41) GERMAN
      DIS : (   9) JUVENILE CHRONIC ARTHRITIS
      RCF : (   1) NON RECOMBINANT
      SEL : (   2) STATUS DISEASE FAMILY

-----------------------------------------------------------------------------


 IND PAT MAT SEX POP DIS AGE RCP BRO*  PHENOTYPE                                * DIPLOTYPE *

                                   *     A   A    B   B    C   C   DR  DR   BF  BF    *    NO


   1 *** ***   1  41   1  46   1   0*    1   2   37  38    6        6        S   F    *     2

   6 *** ***   1  41   0   0   0   0*  *** ***  *** ***  *** ***  *** ***  *** ***    *    36

   7 *** ***   2  41   0   0   0   0*  *** ***  *** ***  *** ***  *** ***  *** ***    *    36

   2   6   7   2  41   1  44   1   0*    2  24    8  27    5   7    3   5    S   S    *     2

   3   6   7   1  41   9  52   1   0*    2  24    7  27    5   7    3   5    S   S    *    16

   4   1   2   1  41   1  16   1   1*    2        8  38    7        3   6    S   S    *     1

   5   1   2   1  41   9  11   1   2*    2  24   27  38    5        5   6    S   S    *     1
```

Fig. 3. Input data and number of compatible diplotypes

```
=============================================================================
NUMBER OF COMPATIBLE PEDIGREES (GE)      :          144
SUM CF THE ABS. LIKELIHOODS              :   0.7C4E-17
- LOG ( LIKELIHOOD)                      :        39.49

.............................................................................
.                                                                           .
.  REL. LIKELIHOODS OF THE COMPATIBLE PEDIGREES                             .
.                                                                           .
. PEDIGREE  LREL  0--------------------------LREL--------------------------1.
.                                                                           .
.                                                                           .
.      1   0.3575  ********************                                     .
.                                                                           .
.      2   0.3575  ********************                                     .
.                                                                           .
.      3   0.1312  *******                                                  .
.                                                                           .
.      4   0.1312  *******                                                  .
.                                                                           .
.   REST   0.0227  *                                                        .
.                                                                           .
. PEDIGREE  LREL  0--------------------------LREL--------------------------1.
.                                                                           .
.............................................................................
```

Fig. 4. Histogram of relative likelihoods of possible pedigree explanations

```
============================================================

PEDIGREE  :     1 LABS =  0.252E-17 LREL =  0.357

 IND PAT MAT SEX POP DIS AGE RCP BRO* DIPLOTYPE          *

                                   *  *    A   C   B  BF  DR

   1 *** ***   1  41   1  46   1   0* *    2   C  38   S   6
                                      *    1   6  37   F   6

   6 *** ***   1  41   0   0   0   0* *   24   5  27   S   5
                                      *  *** *** *** *** ***

   7 *** ***   2  41   0   0   0   0* *    2   7   8   S   3
                                      *    2   7   7   S   3

   2   6   7   2  41   1  44   1   0* *   24   5  27   S   5
                                      *    2   7   8   S   3

   3   6   7   1  41   9  52   1   0* *   24   5  27   S   5
                                      *    2   7   7   S   3

   4   1   2   1  41   1  16   1   1* *    2   C  38   S   6
                                      *    2   7   8   S   3

   5   1   2   1  41   9  11   1   2* *    2   C  38   S   6
                                      *   24   5  27   S   5
```

Fig. 5. Most likely pedigree explanation

sex, population code, disease, age, recombinant individual, birth order, and phenotype data. The last column contains the number of possible diplotypes after the formal genetic reduction.

Figure 4 gives the number of compatible pedigree configurations, in this case 144, and a histogram of the four most likely pedigrees.

Figure 5 shows the nongenetic input parameters, followed by the output of the diplotypes of the most likely pedigree explanation. For each pedigree member the paternal haplotype is printed first, then the maternal haplotype. This information has been plotted in Fig. 6.

Finally, the program prints the relative likelihoods of the possible diplotypes for each individual (Fig. 7). Diplotypes with relative likelihoods lower than 1/1000 are not printed.

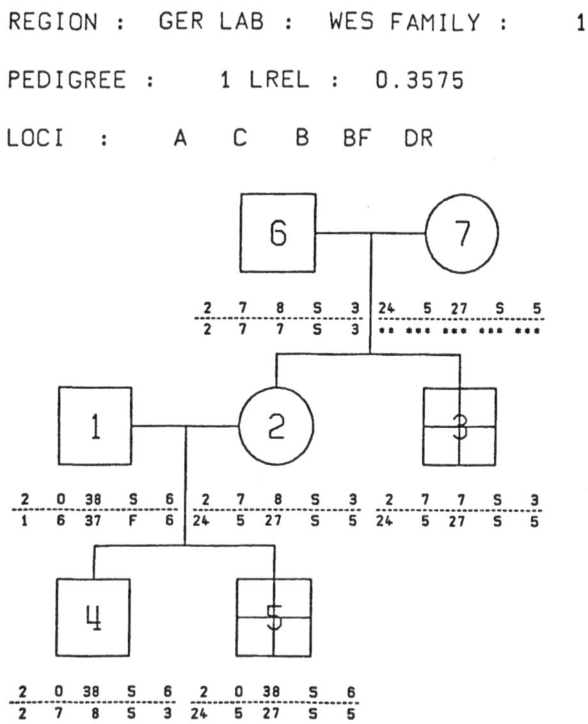

Fig. 6. Plot of most likely pedigree explanation

Conclusion

This program is a useful tool in the analysis of a wide variety of genetic problems. It has been successfully applied in the analysis of 2300 families of the Ninth Workshop data. In connection with the graphical display of families as pedigrees (PEDPLO), it served as a means to check the submitted phenotypes for logical coherence with respect to the given family structure and to present the genotypic background of the families to the submitting laboratories for comparison and/or help in the interpretation of the family data. The results of these analyses were the basis for further work in literally all disease studies. For the analysis of the diabetes families, FAP was used to compare different models for the inheritance of IDDM. The deduced haplotypes of nonrelated family members were the basis for all population analyses, and the recombinant haplotypes supplied the information for the cross-over family study.

The variety of problems for which FAP has been used, is not restricted to those involving the major histocompatibility complex; rather FAP can be

RELATIVE LIKELIHOOD OF DIPLOTYPES

PERS. :		DIPLOTYPE										LIKELIHOOD
FAM	IND	A	C	B	BF	DR	A	C	B	BF	DR	*****
1	1	2	0	38	S	6	1	6	37	F	6	0.732
1	1	2	0	38	S	6	1	6	37	F	0	0.268
1	6	2	7	8	S	3	2	7	7	S	3	0.500
1	6	24	5	27	S	5	***	***	***	***	***	0.489
1	6	24	5	27	S	5	2	7	8	S	3	0.003
1	6	24	5	27	S	5	2	7	7	S	3	0.002
1	6	24	5	27	S	5	2	7	7	S	5	0.002
1	6	24	5	27	S	5	2	5	8	S	3	0.001
1	6	24	5	27	S	5	2	7	8	S	5	0.001
1	7	2	7	8	S	3	2	7	7	S	3	0.500
1	7	24	5	27	S	5	***	***	***	***	***	0.489
1	7	24	5	27	S	5	2	7	8	S	3	0.003
1	7	24	5	27	S	5	2	7	7	S	3	0.002
1	7	24	5	27	S	5	2	7	7	S	5	0.002
1	7	24	5	27	S	5	2	5	8	S	3	0.001
1	7	24	5	27	S	5	2	7	8	S	5	0.001
1	2	24	5	27	S	5	2	7	8	S	3	0.500
1	2	2	7	8	S	3	24	5	27	S	5	0.500
1	3	24	5	27	S	5	2	7	7	S	3	0.500
1	3	2	7	7	S	3	24	5	27	S	5	0.500
1	4	2	0	38	S	6	2	7	8	S	3	1.000
1	5	2	0	38	S	6	24	5	27	S	5	1.000

Fig. 7. Relative likelihoods of diplotypes

easily applied to any multilocus analysis, if sufficient data or knowledge about underlying parameters are available.

Summary

Family analysis package (FAP) is a package of FORTRAN IV programs written for the analysis of multilocus pedigree data.
Given the phenotypes of related individuals for the up to 11 closely linked loci of the MHC (typed in the Ninth Workshop) the program derives for each individual all diplotypes (i.e., both paternal and maternal haplotypes) compatible with phenotypes and relationships. It computes for every compatible combination of diplotypes the likelihood of all possible pedigree configurations and the likelihood of each diplotype. This procedure is applicable to:

1. Analysis of a single pedigree having a genetic model with given parameters
2. Analysis of a sample of families, which estimates genetic parameters such as allele frequencies, multilocus haplotype frequencies, linkage disequilibria, and recombination fractions
3. Analysis of a sample of disease families in order to test genetic models of disease inheritance

The output of FAP has been used for the population analysis of the Ninth Workshop data and analysis of the diabetes families.

References

1. Elston RC, Stewart J (1971) A general model for the genetic analysis of pedigree data. Hum Hered 21:523 – 542
2. Lange K, Boehnke M (1983) Extensions to pedigree analysis. Hum Hered 33:291 – 301

PEDPLO: The Pedigree Plot Program *

M. Sigmund

Institute of Medical Statistics, Documentation and Data Processing, University of Bonn, Sigmund-Freud-Str. 25, 5300 Bonn, Federal Republic of Germany

Introduction

Analysis of the linkage of different loci, analysis of the association of disease and haplotype, differentiation of the MHC region, and research in histocompatibility depend widely on family analyses. For extensive analyses, as done in this workshop by the family analyses package FAP (M. Neugebauer et al., Analysis of Multilocus Pedigree Data by Computer, this volume), clear graphical presentation of inheritance becomes very important.
The pedigree plot program PEDPLO has been developed to present the results of family analyses as pedigrees. For this purpose it has been closely adapted to FAP. But this application to MHC data of human chromosome 6 is certainly only one possibility for this program, which can also present inheritance data in pedigrees of animals or historical pedigrees, due to the fact that only the individual's number, the numbers identifying the parents, and the sex of each individual are needed for the construction of the pedigree. It is especially for things such as analysis of animal breeding or plant cultivation, involving a large number of generations and numerous individuals, that the application of PEDPLO will be helpful.
During the data analysis for this workshop the family data submitted by nearly all participating laboratories were plotted by PEDPLO, resulting in approximately 2500 different pedigrees.

* This work was supported in part by Deutsche Forschungsgemeinschaft Ba 660/5-1

Description and Application of PEDPLO

Input

The pedigrees to be plotted must have the structure of disjunct pointed trees [1], i.e., the pedigree is allowed to ramify only toward the subsequent generations. This condition is satisfied, for instance, by the offspring of one or several couples. Within each pointed tree, every sort of parentage is permitted.
The input for a pedigree of n individuals consists of $2n+4$ records, the first three of which contain comments. All three comment lines will head the particular pedigree. Additionally, the first line will

 Histocompatibility Testing 1984
Edited by E. D. Albert et al.

appear as entry in the table of contents written at the end of the plot. The last input line contains a delimiter to indicate the end of the first pedigree. The input data of other pedigrees may follow. For each of the n individuals there are two input lines, structured as follows:

First line

Column

1– 4: Family number
5– 8: Individual number
10–13: Father's individual number
14–17: Mother's individual number
18–21: Sex (1 = male, 2 = female)
22–25: Disease (value greater than 1 = yes)
26–29: Birth order
33–72: First text line

Second line

Column

33–72: Second text line.

Both text lines are written below the symbol of the person concerned and may contain first and second haplotype, family name and first name, or any other information.

Limits of Program

Logical Limits. The logical limits are as follows: (1) The individuals' numbers must be unequivocal. (2) A marriage without children cannot be plotted. (A widely extended version is able to plot a childless marriage too.) (3) The parents in the first generation must have a zero entry for "father's ID" and "mother's ID." The same applies for one of a couple who him/herself is not a child of other pedigree members. Either father's and mother's ID are zero or both must be known. These limits result from the logical structure of the program and are therefore indispensable.

Size of Pedigree. The pedigree may contain up to 99 individuals in maximally 10 generations. Each individual may appear up to five times. (This may happen, for example, with someone who has children by different partners.) The size of the pedigree is subject to the dimensions of the arrays used, which can be changed easily by changing the FORTRAN IV source program. Several families can be included in one input list, and will be recognized and plotted as different families in separate pedigrees. Multiple marriages and inbreedings are accepted without problems.

Internal Procedures

The user determines the desired maximal symbol size for the person-symbols. The program then computes the maximal available size, which is dependent on the dimensions of the pedigree and the space given by the plotter hardware. If the desired size exceeds the available size, the desired size is diminished to the available size.
The size of the first and second text lines below each person-symbol is computed automatically, subject to the length of the text and the size of a person-symbol.
Persons who appear more than once in the pedigree are marked by double person-symbols. A carrier of a disease is marked by a cross within his/her person-symbol.
After plotting all pedigrees according to the input list, the program plots a table of contents with one entry for each pedigree and an explanation of the symbols for disease and multiple marriage.

Technical Data

PEDPLO is written in FORTRAN IV and developed on IBM/3081 at the RHRZ Bonn. No part of a program library is required, apart from a number of plot subroutines. These are standard plot subroutines, marked explicitly in the program, which are available at any computing center where plotting is possible. The main program and the subroutines require a total capacity of 256 Kbytes main storage.
The actual release of the program is active on CALCOMP 1670, VERSATEC 2160-A. All plots for this workshop have been produced by the VERSATEC 2160-A.

Example

Beside the heritage information in column 1-29, the input of the example (Fig. 1a) contains as text for each individual the paternal and maternal haplotype of the HLA loci A, C, B, and DR as computed by FAP.
The table of contents and the heading comment lines of the output (Fig. 1b) have been omitted. The double marriage of the individual 6 is marked by a double person-symbol. Both individual 12 and his mother, individual 8, are carriers of a disease. Below each person-symbol the diplotype is plotted by printing paternal and maternal haplotypes separated by a dotted line.
Plotting a pedigree with diplotypes is obviously only one application of PEDPLO. The output for a

genealogical tree, for example, would certainly omit the dotted line and print the name and dates of birth and death of each individual. Special forms of output can be achieved by small changes of the source program.

Acknowledgments. Special thanks are owed to the managers and operators of the RHRZ Bonn for assistance and cooperation.

Reference

1. Serre JP (1980) Trees. Springer, Berlin Heidelberg New York

```
Example/
Demonstration of multiple marriage and disease/
Order of loci: A C B DR/
 1   1  0  0  1            3  4  35  1/
                           1  4   8  3/
 1   2  0  0  2           11  4  35  1/
                          23  4  44  7/
 1   3  0  0  1           28  1  14  4/
                          29  6  44  7/
 1   4  1  2  2        1   3  4  35  1/
                          11  4  35  1/
 1   5  1  2  2        2   3  4  35  1/
                          23  4  44  7/
 1   6  1  2  1        3   1  4   8  3/
                          23  4  44  7/
 1   7  0  0  2           30  6  13  7/
                          30  5  18  0/
 1   8  0  0  2  17        2  3  51  3/
                           1  2  60  0/
 1   9  3  4  1           28  1  14  4/
                          11  4  35  1/
 1  10  6  7  1        1   1  4   8  3/
                          30  6  13  7/
 1  11  6  7  1        2  23  4  44  7/
                          30  5  18  0/
 1  12  6  8  1  17        1  4   8  3/
                           1  2  60  0/
&
```

a

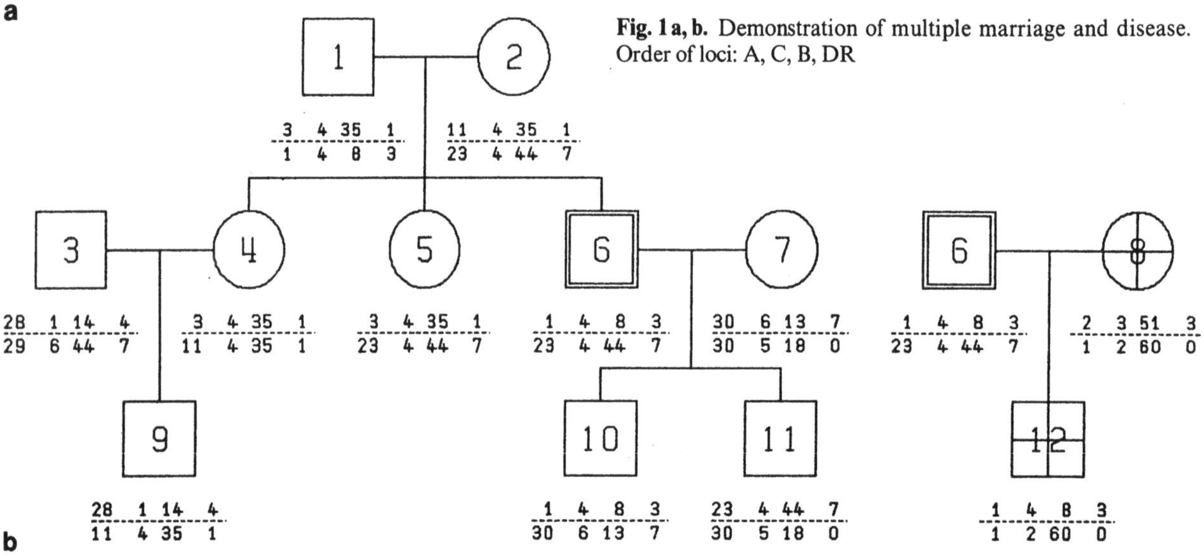

b

Fig. 1 a, b. Demonstration of multiple marriage and disease. Order of loci: A, C, B, DR

Cell Typing by Computer

H. Deppe[1], E. D. Albert[2], and M. P. Baur[1]

1 Biometrical Department, Diabetes Research Institute, Auf'm Hennekamp 65, 4000 Düsseldorf, Federal Republic of Germany
2 Laboratory for Immunogenetics, Children Polyclinic, University of Munich, Pettenkoferstraße 8a, 8000 Munich, Federal Republic of Germany

For the Ninth International Histocompatibility Workshop, a computer cell typing program was developed, as was done for the previous Workshop. Its main purpose was to assign phenotypes to all individuals submitted to the Workshop by a unified cell typing based on the reactions of all Workshop sera. In contrast to the Workshop concept that all analyses should be based on families, this cell typ-

Histocompatibility Testing 1984
Edited by E. D. Albert et al.

ing was done on an individual basis lest some serological problems be obscured.

Method of Cell Typing

The algorithm used for the computer cell typing program is basically the same as the one developed by Mickey and Terasaki [1] and used for the Eighth Workshop. After a brief summary of this method, some modifications and improvements will be described here.

Description of the Model

For a given locus and for each possible genotype, there are certain probabilities p (i) for the reaction grades of a given serum with the cell. Here, the index i indicates one of the possible reaction grades i = 1, 2, 4, 6, 8. Thus, taking the product of the p's for all sera, one has a probability for each possible outcome of all the serum reactions coded on cards 11–24 in the Workshop data set; this probability depends on the genotype of the cell. Further, using Bayes' formula, a probability can be computed for each possible genotype, which depends on the observed outcome of all serum reactions. The genotype with the highest probability will be assigned to the cell.

Triplets and New Antigens

It is clear from this description that triplets cannot be found by the computer program. Splits and new antigens are also not automatically detected; rather, information on them has to be provided in the same way as for all other antigens.

Gene Frequencies as A Priori Probabilities

For an application of Bayes' formula as described above, it is necessary to give a priori probabilities for all genotypes at the locus under consideration. Whereas in [1] these were implicitly assumed to equal each other (which means no a priori information), in this program the actual gene frequencies in the population served as a basis for computing the a priori probabilities. Different frequencies were used for the three ethnic groups: Negroid, Mongoloid, and Caucasoid. For the first run of the computer cell typing program the frequencies were taken from [2], and for later runs they stemmed from calculations based on former runs (cf. M. Baur et al., Reference Tables of Two-Locus Haplotype Frequencies for All MHC Marker Loci, this volume).

The Concept of the "Recognition Set"

Too many different probabilities would have to have been computed in the theoretical model described above. Hence, as in [1], the following simplifying assumption had to be made: the probabilities of the serum reactions are equal for all genotypes which have no antigen in common with a so-called recognition set. This recognition set includes all antigens relevant for the corresponding serum, i.e., its main specificities and all antigens (the tail) with which the serum shows some cross-reactions.

The main improvement of the present program over that in [1] is that the probabilities for the serum reactions may differ arbitrarily for the genotypes from the recognition set. In [1] it had to be assumed that a serum either types for a certain antigen or it does not. This meant that for all genotypes from the recognition set the same probabilities were applied. Further, different sera had to be grouped together, such that their characteristic distributions of the reaction grades were assumed to be equal. In contrast, this program uses different probability distributions for each serum and each relevant genotype. How this was accomplished and which practical consequences it has will now be explained.

Estimation of Probabilities for Serum Reactions

First of all, the recognition sets for each serum had to be determined. This was done on the basis of the serological analysis of the responsible Workshop group, which considered all the detailed reports on the different antigens in the Workshop (E. Albert et al., The Serological Analysis of the Data of the Ninth Histocompatibility Workshop, this volume). Probabilities for the reaction grades could then be estimated for each serum and the corresponding genotypes. This was done on a special file of unrelated random individuals from all ethnic groups. To give an example, Table 1 shows the actual counts for the different reaction grades for serum 02-9w128. The row labeled "A30" is used for all genotypes with A30, and the row labeled "A31" is used for all genotypes with A31, but without A30.

Table 1. Reaction grades for serum 02-9w128

	1	2	4	6	8	Total
A30	24	16	39	66	211	356
A31	344	3	6	3	8	364
Other	4650	13	14	3	7	4689
	5018	34	59	72	226	5409

Table 2. Probabilities p and q for serum 02-9w128

	1	2	4	6	8	Total
A30	0.067	0.045	0.110	0.185	0.593	1.000
A31	0.945	0.008	0.016	0.008	0.022	1.000
Other	0.992	0.003	0.003	0.001	0.001	1.000

Table 3. Scores for serum 02-9w128

	1	2	4	6	8
A30	−2.69	2.64	3.60	5.67	5.98
A31	−0.05	0.95	1.71	2.56	2.69

Table 2 gives the corresponding probabilities p (i) mentioned earlier. The last row shows the probabilities q (i) in case of absence of all relevant antigens. As can be seen from this table, the probability for the serum showing reaction grade 8 with a cell carrying A30 is only about 59%. Nevertheless, this serum is quite good for A30, since out of a total of 226 reactions of 8, 211 (93%) are accounted for by the presence of A30.

To abbreviate the necessary computations, the computer program uses scores derived from Table 2 by the formula log (p (i)/q (i)), as was presented in [1]. These scores are listed in Table 3. As can be seen, the scores of 1 and 8 are well separated for A30, but not for A31. This reflects the fact that this serum is a good typing reagent for A30 but shows some cross-reactions with A31.

It is clear that this method of cell typing takes into account the varying characteristics of all the different sera. As could be seen from this example, especially cross-reactions can be handled with great sensitivity.

Artificial Loci

The computer cell typing program was used for the four loci A, B, C, and DR, with each locus treated independently. In addition, some artificial loci were introduced to study the presence or absence of specific antigens. These artificial loci were for the antigens LB58 (=9wDR86), DQw1 (=MT1), DRw52 (=MT2), DRw53 (=MT3), DQw2 (=MB2), DQw3 (=MB3), and Bw4/Bw6. They were analyzed independently of the real loci. This may have led to contradictions (especially for Bw4/Bw6, where only few sera were used), but it guaranteed an unbiased analysis.

Results

All 13 961 cells for which serological data had been submitted to the Workshop were typed with the computer cell typing program. All participating laboratories received the results for the individuals they had tested.

The Printout

In the printout, not only the genotypes with the highest probabilities, but also possible solutions with a similarly high probability were listed, unless the probability of the best solution was at least 1000 times as large as those for all other genotypes. In this way, it is generally possible to find segregating solutions for a family in spite of cases in which the program yielded nonsegregating assignments for the individual family members. Here it should be noted again that in order to obtain unbiased results, the computer assignments do not consider the family structure.

Quality of Computer Cell Typing

The quality of the computer cell typing can be measured by comparing the computer and laboratory assignments for each individual antigen. This has been done in Table 4. Judging from the assigments for some well-defined antigens such as A2, A24, B8, B13, B18, and B27, all of which had a correlation coefficient of 0.99, it appears that the computer cell typing generally yielded very reliable results.

Quality of Antigen Definition

The correlation coefficients given in Table 4 can therefore be used to distinguish well-defined antigens from those in which there are still serological problems. Coefficients of less than 0.85 were obtained for the following antigens: Aw36, Aw66, Bw42, Bw46, Bw47, Bw48, Bw53, Bw59, Bw63, Bw64, Bw67, Bw71, Bw72, Bw73, Cw8, DR5, DRw6, DRw8, DRw52, DRw53, DQw1, DQw2, and DQw3. Many of these are newly defined antigens; their former names are given in Table 4.

Serum Analysis: The Quality Scores

In addition to the detailed analyses of the sera appearing elsewhere in this volume, the estimation of the scores for the cell typing program, which was

Table 4. Comparison of computer and laboratory assignments

Name of antigen	Number of cells	*r*
A1	13 733	0.98
A2	13 741	0.99
A3	13 739	0.98
A11	13 736	0.97
A23	13 287	0.96
A24	13 455	0.99
A25	13 522	0.97
A26	13 522	0.96
A28	13 736	0.96
A29	13 638	0.97
A30	13 431	0.95
A31	13 445	0.93
A32	13 502	0.98
Aw33	13 118	0.91
Aw34	12 248	0.85
Aw36	11 642	0.56
Aw43	10 909	0.86
Aw66 (LN)	4 979	0.12
9WA71 (Th)	4 028	0.34
Cw1	13 561	0.95
Cw2	13 590	0.96
Cw3	13 596	0.96
Cw4	13 614	0.97
Cw5	13 191	0.92
Cw6	13 291	0.90
Cw7	12 883	0.87
Cw8	12 343	0.80
DR1	12 866	0.94
DR2	12 865	0.94
DR3	12 865	0.93
DR4	12 863	0.92
DR5	12 854	0.83
DRw6	11 836	0.77
DR7	12 858	0.96
DRw8	12 762	0.76
DRw9	12 232	0.92
DRw10	12 346	0.86
DRw52 (MT2)	9 652	0.81
DRw53 (MT3)	8 887	0.74
9WDR86 (LB58)	2 563	0.14
DQw1 (MB1, MT1)	9 557	0.82
DQw2 (MB2)	6 143	0.73
DQw3 (MB3, MT4)	6 034	0.69

Name of antigen	Number of cells	*r*
B7	13 738	0.97
B8	13 744	0.99
B13	13 744	0.99
B18	13 747	0.99
B27	13 747	0.99
B35	13 744	0.95
B37	13 653	0.97
B38	13 340	0.97
B39	13 414	0.97
Bw41	13 450	0.89
Bw42	12 755	0.84
B44	13 681	0.98
B45	13 427	0.93
Bw46	11 905	0.81
Bw47	13 071	0.80
Bw48	12 406	0.63
B49	13 403	0.95
Bw50	13 216	0.89
B51	12 870	0.94
Bw52	12 760	0.86
Bw53	12 887	0.75
Bw54	12 335	0.90
Bw55	13 194	0.90
Bw56	13 139	0.92
Bw57	12 840	0.92
Bw58	12 645	0.92
Bw59	12 186	0.76
Bw60	13 052	0.92
Bw61	12 720	0.86
Bw62	13 179	0.93
Bw63	12 873	0.72
Bw64 (B14.1)	8 484	0.75
Bw65 (B14.2)	8 484	0.87
Bw67 (8w57)	6 485	0.69
Bw71 (BU)	7 865	0.20
Bw72 (SV)	8 217	0.32
Bw73 (KA, IEH)	6 732	0.24
9WB78 (B15.3)	4 875	0.00
9WB79 (8w66)	5 747	0.10
Bw4	13 336	0.94
Bw6	13 342	0.88

described above (Estimation of Probabilities for Serum Reactions), gave some additional information. This is the quality score (q-score), which was introduced in [1] and may serve as a simple tool for determining the quality of a serum as a typing reagent for a specific antigen. The definition of the q-score is given by the formula

$$\text{q-score} = \sum (p(i) - q(i)) * \log (p(i)/q(i))$$

where i ranges over all reaction grades i = 1, 2, 4, 6, 8. For example, it can be easily calculated from Table 2 that the q-score for serum 02-9w128 is 7.6 for A30 and 0.1 for A31. This shows that this serum is a good typing reagent for A30, but gives hardly any information at all about A31.

References

1. Mickey MR, Terasaki PI (1980) The serological data of the 8th Workshop and summary analyses. Joint report. In: Terasaki PI (ed) Histocompatibility testing 1980. UCLA, Los Angeles, p 21–136
2. Baur MP, Danilovs JA (1980) Reference tables of two and three-locus haplotype frequencies for HLA-A, B, C, DR, Bf, and GLO. Joint report. In: Terasaki PI (ed) Histocompatibility testing 1980. UCLA, Los Angeles, pp 994–1210

Unbiased Serum Analysis *

G. Sierp and E. D. Albert

Laboratory for Immunogenetics, Pettenkoferstr. 8 a, 8000 Munich 2, Federal Republic of Germany

The purpose of this analysis was an unbiased grouping of sera that test the same antigen. The only data that was used were the family relationships. That genes responsible for the serum reactions are inherited as codominant mendelian traits was the only assumption made. Only families with both parents and at least three children tested were used for input. As output, 60 groups of sera that test the same antigen were received.

Description of the Program

In the first three steps, only one family is considered in which the paternal haplotypes are called a and b and the maternal haplotypes c and d. Following the mendelian rules, children can only have the haplotype combinations ac, ad, bc and bd (recombinations are excluded). In the following, it is always assumed that the first child has ac.

In the first step, only the reactions of father (Fa), mother (Mo), and first child (C1) with all the sera are considered. Whenever a serum shows one of the following patterns, it is classified as an a-, b-, c-, or d-serum as noted on the right-hand side:

Fa	Mo	C1	
ab	cd	ac	
+	−	+	a-serum
+	−	−	b-serum
−	+	+	c-serum
−	+	−	d-serum

In the following, a serum will always be called an a-, b-, c-, or d-serum whenever it reacts with any antigen contained in the a-, b-, c-, or d-haplotype respectively.

In a second step, the haplotype combinations of the remaining children are determined. For each child, four scores according to the four sets of sera marked in the first step are computed. For each set of sera, the positive reactions of the child with the sera contained in the set are counted. By dividing this count by the total number of sera contained in this set, four scores – s_a, s_b, s_c, and s_d – are obtained. Since a child can only inherit the haplotypes a or b from the father and c or d from the mother, the maximum of s_a and s_b and the maximum of s_c and s_d give the haplotype combination of the child. If, for example, a child has scores where s_b is greater than s_a and s_c is greater than s_d, he has the haplotype combination bc. The essential idea is that if a child has the haplotype combination bc, it should react positively with all the b- and c-sera and negatively with all the a- and d-sera. Computing of scores and taking of maxima is only carried out in order to eliminate false reactions.

In a third step, the sera are classified once more. In order to do this, the haplotype combinations of the family are listed in a matrix as follows:

Fa	Mo	C1	C2	C3	C4	
ab	cd	ac	ad	bc	bd	
+	−	+	+	−	−	a-serum
+	−	−	−	+	+	b-serum
−	+	+	−	+	−	c-serum
−	+	−	+	−	+	d-serum
+	+	+	+	−	+	a + d-serum

Note that the four children happen to have the four possible haplotype combinations.

The first line shows how an a-serum must react in this family, the second line how a b-serum must react, etc.

If the first and fourth line are combined with a logical or-connection, the fifth line is obtained, which shows how an a + d-serum has to react.

A logical or-connection is defined as follows: In order to get the resulting line, the positions that code for the same person in the two input lines are considered. Whenever at least one of these positions is a plus the resulting position is a plus. Only if both positions are a minus is the resulting position then minus. All four lines can be connected with each other in this way, giving all the possible combinations: a + b, a + c, a + d, . . .

Next, each serum reaction is compared with the four lines of this haplotype matrix and its logical connections. A serum is classified according to the line with which its reaction in this family matches

* Supported by DFG Al 92/13-1 and Al 92/13-2

Histocompatibility Testing 1984
Edited by E. D. Albert et al.

without exception. For example, if a serum reacts thus:

Fa	Mo	C1	C2	C3	C4
ab	cd	ac	ad	bc	bd
+	–	–	–	+	+

it is classified as a + b-serum.

Thus, four sets of sera are obtained from each family. The three steps are repeated in 200 families, yielding 800 sets of sera.

In the next step, a 2×2 table is obtained where, for example, each entry $T_{i,j}$ stands for the number of common appearances of serum number i with serum number j in the same set of sera. Whenever $T_{i,j}$ is greater than a certain level L (the level chosen was L = 0.6) times $T_{i,i}$ (that is the total number of appearances of serum number i) sera i and j are put into the same group. Thus, for each serum, a group of sera is found that test the same antigen.

By comparing these groups and combining essentially equivalent groups, 60 final groups are obtained. Following this paragraph there is a complete listing of the groups. Not all of the antigen groups came out well. For example, B35 cannot be separated from Cw4, although there is a separate B35 group.

We are presently trying to increase the sensitivity of the program in order to distinguish the serological "fine splits."

Table 1. The 60 serum groups

Group 1	Number of sera: 8				
9W0001	A1	9W0002	A1	9W0003	A1
9W0006	A1, AW36	9W0007	A1, AW36	9W0009	A1, AW36
9W0318	A1, BW57	9W1109	A1, 11, 26, 25		
Group 2	Number of sera: 19				
9W0011	A2	9W0013	A2	9W0014	A2
9W0017	A2	9W0018	A2	9W0019	A2
9W0021	A2	9W0033	A2+B17	9W0034	A2+B17
9W0319	A2, BW57, BW58	9W1102	A2, B49	9W1103	A2, BW48
9W1104	A2, B7	9W1108	A2, 28	9W1139	A2
9W1141	A2, 28	9W1142	A2, 28	9W1151	A2, 28
9W1156	A2, 28				
Group 3	Number of sera: 4				
9W0023	A28, AW68, AW69	9W0024	A28, AW68, AW69	9W0025	A28, AW68, AW69
9W0032	A28, AW68, AW69, AW33				
Group 4	Number of sera: 9				
9W0036	A23, A24	9W0037	A24, A23	9W0038	A23, A24, AW9.3
9W0039	A23, A24, AW9.3	9W0047	A24	9W0048	A24, A23
9W0050	A24, AW9.3, A23	9W0051	A24, AW9.3, A23	9W0926	A24
Group 5	Number of sera: 3				
9W0042	A23	9W0043	A23	9W0044	A23
Group 6	Number of sera: 9				
9W0057	A3	9W0059	A3	9W0060	A3
9W0061	A3, A11	9W0062	A3, 11, W33, 31, 29, 30, W34	9W1116	A3, B7, 27
9W1131	A3	9W1146	A3	9W1152	A3
Group 7	Number of sera: 14				
9W0071	A26, A25, AW66	9W0072	A25, A26, AW43, AW66	9W0074	A26, AW43, A25, AW66
9W0075	A26, A25, AW43, AW66	9W0076	AW34, A25, A26, AW66	9W0077	A26, A25, AW43, AW66, AW34
9W0078	A26, AW34, A25, AW66	9W0079	A26, A25, AW43, AW34, AW66	9W0081	A26, A25, AW34, AW43, AW66
9W0082	A26, AW43, AW34, A25, AW66	9W0094	A26	9W0095	A26, AW43, AW66, AW34
9W0099	A26, AW43, A25	9W0147	A26, 25, 34, 66, 28, 68, 69, 43, 33, 32*		
Group 8	Number of sera: 9				
9W0071	A26, A25, AW66	9W0074	A26, AW43, A25, AW66	9W0075	A26, A25, AW43, AW66
9W0076	AW34, A25, A26, AW66	9W0079	A26, A25, AW43, AW34, AW66	9W0085	A25
9W0086	A25	9W0090	A25, AW66	9W0147	A26, 25, 34, 66, 28, 68, 69, 43, 33, 32
Group 9	Number of sera: 5				
9W0102	A29, AW43	9W0103	A29, AW43	9W0104	A29, Aw43
9W0106	A29, AW43	9W1119	A29, B51		
Group 10	Number of sera: 6				
9W0111	A32	9W0112	A32, A25	9W0114	A32, A25, AW66
9W0117	A32, A25	9W0130	A32	9W0377	B27, A32, BW47, B13
Group 11	Number of sera: 4				
9W0121	A30	9W0128	A30	9W0129	A30
9W0138	A30, B13				

* Due to lack of space "w's" are omitted

Table 1 (continued)

Group 12 Number of sera: 7

9W0133	CW5, A30	9W0483	CW5	9W0484	CW5, B44
9W0485	CW5	9W0486	CW5	9W0487	CW5
9W0488	CW5				

Group 13 Number of sera: 15

9W0156	B51	9W0157	B51	9W0160	B51
9W0164	B51, BW52	9W0166	B51, BW52	9W0167	B51, BW52
9W0169	B51, BW52	9W0170	B51, BW53	9W0173	B51, BW52, B49, BW63
9W0174	B51, BW52, B49, BW53	9W0175	B51, BW52, B49, BW63, BW53	9W0176	B51, W52, 49, W53, W63
9W0201	B51, BW52, B13	9W0253	B51, BW52, BW59	9W0153	B51

Group 14 Number of sera: 7

9W0171	B51, Bw35, BW53, CW4	9W0172	B51, BW53, B35, CW4	9W0177	BW53*, B51, BW52, Bw35*, B18
9W0199	B35, B51, BW53, BW52	9W0313	B35, 51, 52, 72, 62, 18*	9W0315	B35, 53, 51, 52, 72, 62*
9W0317	B35, 51, 52, 53, 72, 62, 18, 50*				

Group 15 Number of sera: 7

9W0179	B35	9W0180	B35, BW62	9W0181	B35, BW53, CW4
9W0468	CW4	9W0471	CW4	9W0472	CW4
9W0473	CW4				

Group 16 Number of sera: 11

9W0179	B35	9W0180	B35, BW62	9W0181	B35, BW53, CW4
9W0468	CW4	9W0469	CW4	9W0470	CW4
9W0471	CW4	9W0472	CW4	9W0473	CW4
9W0479	CW4, CW6	9W0482	CW4, CW6		

Group 17 Number of sera: 7

9W0189	B18	9W0190	B18	9W0193	B18
9W0194	B18	9W0196	B18	9W0197	B18
9W0198	B18				

Group 18 Number of sera: 5

9W0202	BW50, W56, W62, W72, 35	9W0311	BW72, BW50, BW62, B35	9W0312	BW72, 35, 15.3, 62, 50, 53, 57*
9W0315	B35, 53, 51, 52, 72, 62*	9W0338	BW50, W62, W72, B35, CW4		

Group 19 Number of sera: 7

9W0203	B7	9W0205	B7, BW73	9W0207	B7, BW73
9W0239	BW42, B7, BW55	9W0442	B7, CW7	9W1105	B7, 27, BW57, BW58, CW1
9W1111	B7, 27, 40				

Group 20 Number of sera: 6

9W0209	B27	9W0211	B27	9W0215	B27
9W0242	B27, BW47	9W0243	B27, BW47	9W0244	B27, BW47

Group 21 Number of sera: 8

9W0216	BW55, BW56, BW54, BW42	9W0217	BW55, BW56, BW54	9W0219	BW55, BW54, BW56
9W0226	BW55	9W0227	BW55	9W0229	BW55, W42, W56, W54
9W0230	BW55, BW42, BW56, W54, W67	9W0232	BW55, BW42		

Group 22 Number of sera: 5

9W0217	BW55, BW56, BW54	9W0226	BW55	9W0227	BW55
9W0231	BW55, BW42	9W0232	BW55, BW42		

Group 23 Number of sera: 10

9W0248	B8	9W0249	B8	9W0250	B8
9W0255	B8, BW59	9W0259	B8, BW59, A1	9W0420	B8, BW46
9W0574	DR3	9W1140	B8	9W1154	B8
9W1160	B8				

Group 24 Number of sera: 2

9W0256	BW59	9W0413	B49		

Group 25 Number of sera: 10

9W0262	BW65	9W0263	BW65, CW8	9W0264	BW65
9W0265	BW65, CW8, BW64	9W0266	BW65, CW8, BW64	9W0267	BW65, CW8, BW64
9W0270	BW65, BW64	9W0272	BW65, BW64	9W0500	BW65, BW64
9W0492	BW65, CW8, BW64				

Group 26 Number of sera: 9

9W0276	BW62, BW63	9W0277	BW62, BW63	9W0278	BW62, BW63
9W0281	BW62, BW63	9W0282	BW62	9W0284	BW62
9W0285	BW62	9W0286	BW62	9W0289	BW62

Group 27 Number of sera: 10

9W0290	BW57, BW58, CW6	9W0291	BW57, BW58	9W0292	BW57, BW58
9W0293	BW57, BW58	9W0296	BW57, BW58	9W0298	BW57, BW58
9W0299	BW57, BW63, BW58	9W0301	BW57, BW58, A29	9W0305	BW57, BW58, BW63
9W0306	BW57, BW58, BW63				

* Due to lack of space "w's" are omitted

Table 1 (continued)

Group 28	Number of sera: 3				
9W0302	BW57	9W0303	BW57, CW6	9W0304	BW57, BW58, CW6
Group 29	Number of sera: 2				
9W0309	BW62, W63, W57, W46	9W0310	BW62, W63, W57, W46		
Group 30	Number of sera: 3				
9W0324	B37	9W0325	B37	9W0327	B37
Group 31	Number of sera: 5				
9W0341	B39	9W0342	B39	9W0343	B39
9W0344	B39	9W0446	B39, BW64		
Group 32	Number of sera: 7				
9W0346	B13	9W0348	B13	9W0352	B13
9W0350	B13	9W1134	B13	9W1153	B13
9W1158	B13				
Group 33	Number of sera: 5				
9W0360	BW60, BW61	9W0362	BW60, BW48	9W0363	BW60
9W0365	BW60, BW48	9W0370	BW60, BW48		
Group 34	Number of sera: 8				
9W0378	B44, W57, 49	9W0388	B44, B45	9W0393	B44, B45
9W0394	B44	9W0396	B44	9W0398	B44
9W0399	B44	9W0441	BW50, B49, Bw44		
Group 35	Number of sera: 4				
9W0404	BW50, B49	9W0405	B49, BW50	9W0407	B49, BW50
9W0409	B49, BW50				
Group 36	Number of sera: 4				
9W0396	B44	9W0411	B49, A23	9W0416	B49
9W0441	BW50, B49, B44				
Group 37	Number of sera: 6				
9W0423	BW4	9W0425	BW4	9W0427	BW4, A25
9W0428	BW4, B39	9W0430	BW4, B45	9W1155	A32, BW4
Group 38	Number of sera: 6				
9W0431	BW6	9W0433	BW6	9W0434	BW6
9W0436	BW6	9W0439	BW6	9W1143	BW6
Group 39	Number of sera: 7				
9W0448	CW1	9W0449	CW1	9W0450	CW1
9W0451	CW1	9W0452	CW1	9W0453	CW1
9W0454	CW1				
Group 40	Number of sera: 5				
9W0455	CW2, B27	9W0457	CW2	9W0458	CW2
9W0459	CW2	9W0460	CW2		
Group 41	Number of sera: 7				
9W0461	CW3, BW46	9W0462	CW3, BW46	9W0463	CW3, BW46
9W0464	CW3	9W0465	CW3, BW46	9W0466	CW3
9W0467	CW3				
Group 42	Number of sera: 4				
9W0474	CW6	9W0475	CW6	9W0476	CW6
9W0477	CW6				
Group 43	Number of sera: 4				
9W0495	CW7, BW56, BW55	9W0496	CW7, B7	9W0497	CW7
9W0499	CW7, B8, B7				
Group 44	Number of sera: 15				
9W0502	DR1	9W0504	DR1, DRW10	9W0505	DR1
9W0507	DR1	9W0508	DR1	9W0509	DR1
9W0510	DR1, DRW10	9W0511	DR1, DRW10	9W0512	DR1
9W0514	DR1	9W0515	DRW10, DR1	9W0518	DR1, DRW10
9W0521	DRW10, DR1	9W0522	DR1, DRW10	9W0803	DRW10, DR1
Group 45	Number of sera: 4				
9W0523	DRW10	9W0524	DRW10	9W0527	DRW10
9W0645	DRW9, DRW10				
Group 46	Number of sera: 17				
9W0530	DR2	9W0531	DR2	9W0533	DR2, DQW1
9W0535	DR2	9W0538	DR2, DQW1	9W0541	DR2
9W0543	DR2	9W0545	DR2	9W0546	DR2
9W0547	DR2	9W0550	DR2	9W0552	DR2
9W0553	DR2	9W0554	DR2	9W0802	DQW1
9W0706	DQW1, DR2, W14	9W0540	DR2		

Table 1 (continued)

Group 47	Number of sera: 3				
9W0559	DR3	9W0568	DR3	9W0571	DR3, B8
Group 48	Number of sera: 4				
9W0559	DR3	9W0564	DR3, DRW52	9W0567	DR3
9W0568	DR3				
Group 49	Number of sera: 10				
9W0576	DR4	9W0578	DR4	9W0580	DR4
9W0581	DR4, DRW11, DQW3	9W0585	DR4, DQW3	9W0592	DR4, DQW3
9W0594	DR4	9W0595	DR4, DRW53	9W0729	DR4, DRW9 W53
9W0736	DR4, W53, W9, 7				
Group 50	Number of sera: 4				
9W0616	DRW11, W8, W12, W13, DRW52	9W0681	DRW11, 13, W52, 12	9W0709	DRW13, W52, W11
9W0757	DRW11, W8, W12, W52, W14, 3, W13				
Group 51	Number of sera: 2				
9W0626	DRW8	9W0627	DRW8		
Group 52	Number of sera: 22				
9W0629	DR7, DQW2	9W0630	DR7	9W0633	DR7, DQW2
9W0634	DR7, DQW2	9W0636	DR7, DQW2	9W0637	DR7
9W0638	DR7	9W0639	DR7, DQW2	9W0640	DR7
9W0642	DR7	9W0719	DR7, DQW2	9W0720	DR7, DQW2, DR3, W9
9W0721	DR7, DRW9, DQW2, DR3	9W0722	DR7, DQW2, DR3	9W0723	DR7, DQW2, DR3
9W0724	DR7, DRW9, DQW2, DR3, W53	9W0727	DR7, DQW2, DR3	9W0733	DR7, DQW2, DRW53
9W0734	DRW53, DR7	9W0735	DR7, W9, 4, W53, 3, DQW2	9W0743	DR7, W9, W53, 4
9W0774	DQW2, DR7, 3, W9				
Group 53	Number of sera: 22				
9W0652	DR2, DQW1, DRW14, 1, W10, W13	9W0653	DR2, DRW14, 1, W10, W13	9W0654	DR2, DQW1, DRW14, 1, W10, W13
9W0655	DQW1, DR2, W14, 1, W10, W13	9W0656	DR2, DQW1, DRW14, 1	9W0657	DR2, DQW1, DRW14, 1, W10, W13
9W0661	DQW1, DR2, W14, 1, W13	9W0667	DQW1, DR2, DR1	9W0668	DQW1, DRW14, 2, 1, W10, W13
9W0669	DQW1, DR2, 14, 1, W10, W13	9W0670	DQW1	9W0671	DQW1
9W0672	DQW1, DRW14, 1, W10	9W0674	DQW1, DR2, 14, W10, 1, W13	9W0700	DRW14, DQW1, DR1, W10, 2
9W0702	DRW14, DQW1, DR2	9W0703	DQW1, DRW14, 2, 1, W10	9W0706	DQ1, DR2, W14
9W0794	DQW1	9W0901	DQW1	9W0927	DQW1
9W0660	DQW1				
Group 54	Number of sera: 18				
9W0652	DR2, DQW1, DRW14, 1, W10, W13	9W0653	DR2, DRW14, 1, W10, W13	9W0654	DR2, DQW1, DRW14, 1, W10, W13
9W0655	DQW1, DR2, W14, 1, W10, W13	9W0656	DR2, DQW1, DRW14, 1	9W0667	DQW1, DR2, DR1
9W0668	DQW1, DRW14, 2, 1, W10, W13	9W0670	DQW1	9W0671	DQW1
9W0672	DQW1, DRW14, 1, W10	9W0674	DQW1, DR2, 14, W10, 1, W13	9W0702	DRW14, DQW1, DR2
9W0703	DQW1, DRW14, 2, 1, W10	9W0706	DQ1, DR2, W14	9W0794	DQW1
9W0901	DQW1	9W0927	DQW1	9W0660	DQW1
Group 55	Number of sera: 12				
9W0677	DR3, DRW52, W14, W11	9W0679	DR3, DRW13	9W0681	DRW11, W13, W52, W12
9W0687	DR3, DRW52, W12, W11, W14	9W0689	DR3, W12, W14, W52, W11, W13, W8	9W0696	DRW13, W12, 3, W14, W52, W11, W8
9W0697	DRW12, W11, 3, W13, W14, W8, W52	9W0709	DRW13, W52, W11	9W0713	DR3, W52, W12, W12, W13, W14
9W0715	DR3, W14, W52	9W0757	DRW11, W8, W12, W52, W14, 3, W13	9W0946	DRW52
Group 56	Number of sera: 5				
9W0679	DR3, DRW13	9W0681	DRW11, 13, W52, 12	9W0687	DR3, DRW52, W12, W11, W14
9W0713	DR3, W52, W12, W13, W14	9W0715	DR3, W14, W52		
Group 57	Number of sera: 4				
9W0581	DR4, DRW11, DQW3	9W0750	DR4, DQW3, DRW11	9W0791	DQW3, DR4, DRW11, W12
9W0908	DQW3, DR4, DR5				
Group 58	Number of sera: 5				
9W0722	DR7, DQW2, DR3	9W0759	DR3, DR7, DQW2	9W0774	DQW2, DR7, 3, W9
9W0775	DQW2, DR7	9W0792	DQW2, DR3		
Group 59	Number of sera: 8				
9W0747	DQW3, DR4, W11, W12	9W0754	DRW11, W12, TA10, DQW3, DR4	9W0779	DRW12, DQW3, DRW11
9W0786	DQW3, DRW12, W11, W9, 4	9W0789	DRW12, W11, TA10, DR3	9W0791	DQW3, DR4, DRW11, W12
9W0908	DQW3, DR4, DR5	9W0915	DQW3, DR5, DR4		
Group 60	Number of sera: 5				
9W0970	DQW3	9W0974	DRW52	9W0994	0
9W0996	0	9W0000	Pos. Contr. 32		

Selection of a Set of High-Quality Data for B Cell Antigen Analysis*

W. H. Marshall[3], G. Sierp[4], T. Barbalho[1], F. T. Christiansen[2], S. Scholz[4], and E. D. Albert[4]

1 Permanent address: HEMOPE (Centro de Hematologia e Hemoterapia de Pernambuco), Recife, Brazil
2 On sabbatical leave from the Royal Perth Hospital, Perth, Western Australia
3 On sabbatical leave from the Memorial University, St. John's, Newfoundland, Canada
4 Laboratory for Immunogenetics, Pettenkoferstr. 8a, 8000 Munich 2, Federal Republic of Germany

Introduction

In order to obtain the best definition of splits in the DR system and to facilitate analysis of the "DR" monoclonal antibodies, a file of high-quality B cell typing data was required. The aim was to select labs that had good B cell typing and, within the data of those labs, to select cells with a clear-cut separation of positive and negative scores, i.e., data in which the scores were clearly distributed between 1 and 6/8, with only a few scores of 2 or 4. Data that did not show clear bimodality were considered unsatisfactory because of the blurred distinction between positive and negative antibody reactions.

Methods

Lab Quality. The distribution of cytotoxicity scores from the pooled B cell data (regular DR and "DR" monoclonal) from each lab was calculated as percentages by computer. These were examined and plotted as histograms for easier scanning. Examples of these data are given in Table 1. It can be seen that some data sets show predominantly scores of 1 and 8, with few scores of 2, 4 or 6. These data were considered satisfactory. Other data sets show a variety of unsatisfactory patterns with flat or unimodal distributions. These data were not included in the final file.
During the data evaluations, the identity of each lab was concealed so as to avoid bias. Initial evaluation was done independently by four observers, and final conclusions were the results of a combined evaluation. Data of borderline quality were rejected in the interest of obtaining a high-quality file.

Individual Cell Quality. After initial examinations of a sample of some 60 B cells' serological results, both as raw data (Fig. 1) and as distribution of scores, two ratios with a cutoff point for each were considered appropriate for the selection of good-quality results. One ratio was the percentage of scores of 4 vs the total percentage of scores of 4, 6 and 8 (the 4-ratio). The other was the percentage of scores of 2 vs the total number of scores of 1 and 2 (the 2-ratio). In these calculations wells scored as zero were ignored, so that 100% was the number of wells with scores 1, 2, 4, 6, 8. For example, consider a cell with the following distribution of scores: 0 = 32% (of all wells on the plate), 1 = 30%, 2 = 5%, 4 = 2%, 6 = 24%, 8 = 39%. The 2-ratio would thus

* We acknowledge with gratitude the financial support from Health and Welfare Canada (Visiting Scientist Award to W.H.M.); D.F.G grant number AL 92/13-1, 13-2 (to E.D.A.) and from the Deutscher Akademischer Austauschdienst (grant as a Visiting Scientist to T.P.B.).

Table 1. Percentages of cytotoxicity scores from eight laboratories

Scores												
	Card 21						Card 24					
Lab	0	1	2	4	6	8	0	1	2	4	6	8
a	0.8	63.2	13.6	9.3	5.8	8.0	3.9	51.8	17.0	12.1	8.4	10.7
b	0.7	63.3	12.8	9.4	6.1	5.5	3.6	51.6	13.0	16.3	11.1	8.1
c	3.3	64.2	9.3	11.1	11.6	3.8	12.3	52.5	13.9	20.6	10.6	2.3
d	2.1	87.3	0.1	3.5	5.8	3.4	4.1	52.3	0.1	10.3	22.7	14.7
e	6.3	80.3	0.0	0.1	0.9	8.7	19.9	46.1	0.5	2.4	6.2	44.8
f	1.4	78.5	0.9	2.7	3.4	14.8	7.7	50.0	0.4	4.6	4.4	40.4
g	2.1	82.3	1.7	1.4	4.1	10.4	4.7	41.2	1.6	3.4	14.6	39.2
h	6.0	77.4	3.7	1.8	2.9	19.2	5.8	48.2	4.7	4.9	7.2	35.0

Histocompatibility Testing 1984
Edited by E. D. Albert et al.

Good

```
111111111111 111111148868 888886611110 618881111111 111111188618
888881888661 611146111111 110111111114 111111111111 111118888888
888888888888 111111111181 811411111111 111111111118 811111111881
681118688416 888688880116 161181600880 111118181181 188811816118
018888888118 806888111101 118811888808 811811186001 111111188181
000810818010 810881000008 080888888081 81
```

Unsatisfactory

```
686866666462 844422222212 442224222224 421222221124 121122112128
102111111021 121141111111 112121108144 620111121110 111214611164
144684466464 624111112166 662118864646 214622141248 112211112241
141111264124 444424866848 124211111121 441426611121 268414444141
444664644466 422488644644 464621888886 626444464242 412248668681
824404440444 426242442222 442111868888 82
```

Fig. 1. The cytotoxicity scores from cards 21 – 24 and 31 – 32 for two cells. The upper data is clear, the lower data much less clear

be 5/35 = 0.143, and the 4-ratio would be 2/65 = 0.03. Comparing these ratios with subjective assessments, it was found that a 4-ratio of 0.2 clearly separated the good from the bad data, whilst the 2-ratio was useful only in delineating cells judged good by subjective criteria, not in identifying poor cells. Two cutoff points were decided upon with the aim of eliminating virtually all the poor cells: thus a 4-ratio of 0.2 or a 2-ratio of 0.3 were the upper limits for a satisfactory cell.

Results

The rating of data from individual laboratories resulted in 42% being counted as satisfactory and 58% as borderline or unaccepable for this special file of B cell data.
When the computer calculated score ratios for the cells in the subfile of satisfactory lab data and eliminated unsatisfactory cells, the file was reduced from about 12 800 to about 5400 cells. Table 2 shows the technical details as coded in columns 14 – 16 on the B cell data cards. It can be seen that there are no major differences in the techniques used between the two types of laboratories (the numbers in the table do not always add up to the number of labs because sometimes a lab recorded using two techniques). Several labs used frozen B cells in their early records and later changed to fresh B cells. It seems that no simple technical differences can account for the difference in data quality between laboratories. In order to validate the selection criteria for the "good"-quality file of cells, the correlation of laboratory assignment with computer cell typing as an overall measure of serological quality was compared between the approximately 5400 selected good cells and the remaining approximately 7400 cells. As can be seen in Table 3, this correlation is far superior for every single DR antigen in the panel of good cells.

Table 2. Technical information according to acceptability (101 labs) or unsatisfactoriness (77 labs) of B cell data

	Acceptable	Unsatisfactory
Type of cells (card 14)		
1. PBIs fresh	12	7
2. PBIs frozen	6	3
3. T cells fresh		1
4. T cells frozen		
5. B cells fresh	63	54
6. B cells frozen	23	16
7. T line		
8. B line	1	
9. Other line		
Type of complement (card 15)		
1. Local	54	44
2. Regional	26	15
3. Other	23	18
Technique used (card 16)		
1. Straw	52	36
2. SRBC rosetting	5	3
3. AET rosetting	12	11
4. Neuraminidase rosetting	5	8
5. Two-color fluorescence	11	10
6. Other	18	9

Table 3. Correlation (r value) between laboratory assignment and computer cell typing as a measure of serological quality

	Good cells (n=5431)	Other cells (n=7428)
DR1	0.98	0.90
DR2	0.99	0.93
DR3	0.97	0.88
DR4	0.95	0.85
DR5	0.86	0.67
DRw6	0.83	0.64
DR7	0.99	0.93
DRw8	0.83	0.73
DRw9	0.94	0.81
DRw10	0.94	0.78
DRw52	0.84	0.73
DRw53	0.79	0.68
DQw1 (MT1)[a]	0.88	0.76
DQw1 (MB1)[a]	0.81	0.71
DQw2	0.80	0.74
DQw3	0.72	0.66

[a] The correlation for DQw1 is given twice because not all laboratories coded for MT1 *and* MB1

Discussion

We were concerned that the combination of subjective and scores ratio criteria might be biased against certain important cells or in favor of artifacts. For example, it is possible that some laboratories with low numbers of 2 and 4 may actually have that kind of data as a matter of policy, readers being told not to score 2 or 4; this would be an artifact, particularly if those wells that were really 2 and 4 were scored as 1 and 8. If this was so, then much of the less clear data could actually be from more objective and "honest" labs. On the other hand, a lab that only submitted data on good cells and rejects data on unsatisfactory cells, will be classified as a good lab for good reason. Extensive use of the score of zero *within* the scores for a single cell, instead of scoring 2 and 4, will also produce good data as judged by the score ratio, but it is questionable whether this really is good-quality data. To some extent, which we have not determined, the final B cell file contains such results.

As fully objective, automated plate reading becomes more widespread it will be interesting to see how the scores appear. In this workshop we have no information on which labs used an automated plate reader to produce their results.

One problem which this method of selection probably does very little to detect is carry-over. This could be dealt with in a future workshop by including a strong polyspecific antibody surrounded by negative control wells, but some ground rules on tray layout would be required.

A potential problem with our method of selection is that a cell with virtually no positive reactions due to lack of antigens could produce a poor ratio for this very reason (no 6 or 8). Such a cell, rare and interesting, would be lost from the file. However, in this workshop, where we are dealing with monoclonal antibodies as well as the broad-specificity B cell antisera, such cells must be very uncommon. In spite of all the above discussed possible shortcomings, our selection procedure for a high-quality panel of cells appears to be validated by the improvement seen in the correlation between laboratory assignment and computer cell typing. This correlation represents an overall measure of serologic quality, because only serologically unequivocal results can lead to computer cell typing which is in agreement with the local assignment. In addition to the serological reactions with the workshop reagents, local assignment also utilizes information on prior testing with local reagents and, more importantly, takes into account the segregation in families.

The Serological Analysis of the Data of the Ninth Histocompatibility Workshop*

E. D. Albert[1], T. Barbalho[2], M. P. Baur[3], F. T. Christiansen[4], H. Deppe[3], E. Keller[1], W. H. Marshall[5], A. McNicholas[1], T. Luton[3], C. Raffoux[6], B. Schiessl[1], S. Scholz[1], G. Sierp[1], and M. Sigmund[7]

1 Laboratory for Immunogenetics, Pettenkoferstr. 8a, 8000 Munich 2, Federal Republic of Germany
2 HEMOPE (Centro de Hematologia e Hemoterapia de Pernambuco), Recife, Brazil
3 Biometrical Department, Diabetes Research Institute, Auf'm Hennekamp 65, 4000 Düsseldorf 1, Federal Republic of Germany
4 Royal Perth Hospital, Perth, Australia
5 Memorial University, St. John's, Newfoundland, Canada
6 INSERM U93, Paris, France
7 Institute for Medical Statistics, University of Bonn, 5300 Bonn, Federal Republic of Germany

The analysis of the serological data of the workshop represents a major team effort involving interaction between biomathematicians (Baur, Deppe, Sierp, Sigmund) and serologists (the remaining authors). The final data as found in this volume are the result of an iterative input of work by the two groups in many successive cycles.

In the following we give a description of the major steps which have led to the conclusions of the antigen working groups and which were necessary for serum typing in the central and the population analysis. In a first step the serological data submitted by the participating laboratories were prepared in a way which would allow easy analysis of segregation within families. This program, prepared by G. Sierp, is based on a family listing program by Mickey used in the Fourth International Histocompatibility Workshop in 1970 [1]. After dissection of complicated pedigrees into two-generation core families, the program determines the distribution of HLA haplotypes in the family based on the sera reactions (for details see G. Sierp and E. Albert, Unbiased Serum Analysis, this volume). In a first listing, the reactions of father, mother, and all children are given for all the antisera tested in this particular family in the order in which the sera appeared on the coding sheets. This allows the user to investigate the definition of HLA antigens in the family members. In a second listing, the sera are ordered according to the segregation pattern they show in this particular family, so that the sera which mark the paternal a-haplotype segregation are listed first, then those sera which mark the paternal b-haplotype segregation followed by the sera which show the maternal c- and maternal d-haplotype segregation. Then follow the antisera which have combined reaction patterns: a + b, a + c, etc. At the end are listed the sera which show reaction patterns not in keeping with the established segregation of HLA haplotypes in this particular family. The family pattern listing was performed for all families that satisfied the family pedigree coding. A tape with the output of this program was distributed to the regions.

The second step consisted of a serum typing program written by M. Sigmund on the basis of a program described by Mickey in Histocompatibility Testing 1980 [2]. Basically, this program constructs 2x2 tables comparing the reaction pattern of one given serum with the distribution of all antigens of the HLA-A, B, C, and DR series, including the supertypic specificities. The program displays, among other things, serologically important information such as the number and percentage of false positives and false negatives, *r* values with the antigens under consideration, the average strenght of reactions with cells positive for the antigen under consideration, and the overall strength of reactions (scores of 8 as a percentage of the positive scores). The program selects the antigen with which the reaction pattern of the serum is most closely correlated (i.e., the highest *r* value) and performs a restricted analysis with cells negative for this antigen in order to determine the specificity of the extra reactions. This restricted analysis may be iterated until the number of cells to be analyzed becomes too small.

Another important feature of this program is the listing of a "remainder analysis" in which the extra reactions of the most closely associated specificities are analyzed as to those antigens which would account for the highest percentage of the extra reactions. This serum typing was performed for all antisera and monoclonal antibodies in four different population groups: Caucasians, Japanese, Chinese, and Negroes. The results were excerpted by the team of serologists, and a condensed listing was constructed which combined the result of the serum specificities in the four different populations. This list of sera specificities based on the local assignment of antigens formed the basis for the first cycle of computer cell typing. It should be stressed at this point that an attempt was made to find a set of specificities for each serum which ac-

* Supported by DFG grants Al 92-13-1 and Al 92-13-2.

 Histocompatibility Testing 1984
Edited by E. D. Albert et al.

counted for a maximum percentage of the positive reactions of this serum. This means, for example, that for an excellent anti-A1 serum which in a panel of over 3000 cells showed only 30 reactions with cells that are not A1 positive, it was observed that 25 of these 30 extra reactions were with A9-positive cells. Although this serum reacted with only a minute proportion of the A9-positive cells, A9 was added to the specificity of the serum. As was later seen in the analysis of cell typing, this addition of "tail" specificities resulted in a significant improvement of the cell typing.

The next step consisted of computer cell typing of a test panel of cells representing the major racial groups. Cell typing was performed using a program developed by H. Deppe (for details see H. Deppe et al., Cell Typing by Computer, this volume) on the basis of a cell typing program by Mickey and Terasaki [2].

This cell typing step was essential to establish a panel of cells which were uniformly typed for a set of antigenic specificities including the DQ antigens and the broad antigens DRw52 and DRw53. In addition, the computer cell typing served to eliminate a large number of miscodings in which the serological reactions indicate the presence of an antigen but the coding was wrong.

This first cycle of cell typing was then used as a basis for the second cycle of serum analysis, which was particularly important for the DR antisera and monoclonal antibodies, because the supertypic DR specificities were quite heterogeneously coded in the local assignments. This heterogeneity was eliminated by the computer cell typing. While the first-cycle serum typing information was distributed to all the groups working on antigen reports, it was the second-cycle serum typing that was available in the Munich laboratory at the time of the workshop. In order to further refine the computer typing of cells and in order to include information about new antigens and splits, several successive cycles of cell typing followed by a new estimation of convergence scores (Q-scores) based on the serum reactions with the cell-typed panel were performed. After five such cycles of iteration, the resulting scores were used for a final cell typing, which in turn provided the basis for a final typing of all sera as given in Table 1, see page 75.

Before studying the details of this table, it is important that the reader be aware of a few general points:

a) The cells used for this serum analysis represent a highly selected sample originating from all racial groups tested in the workshop so as to represent, for example, "typical" Japanese or Negro antigens or haplotypes. In addition, cells with rare antigens were selected and added to the panel. Therefore, it is impossible to use this panel for an estimate of the antigen frequencies.

b) The serum analysis includes many antigens with very weak correlations, which for practical purposes in the single laboratory are not very important. In the procedure of computer cell typing involving many thousands of cells, however, it proved to be of considerable benefit to find a set of serum specificities which accounts for a maximum number of the positive reactions of a given serum, even if this involves very weak correlations.

The table is arranged so that the first four columns give serum identification and origin. The fifth column denotes the strength, i.e., the percentage of scores of 8 among the positive reactions (scores 4, 6, and 8) of the serum. Columns 6, 7, 9, 10, and 11 give the information of the 2×2 table of antigen-vs-serum reactions. The number of "–/–" is not given, but may be calculated from column 7 minus column 9 minus column 10 minus column 11. (For serum 9w001 this is: $3919 - 580 - 116 - 10 = 3213$).

In column 8 the strength of the positive reactions in antigen-positive cells is given as the average over all positive scores. This information shows, for example, that in serum 9w007 the extra reactions with B8-positive cells are very weak (average of 5.5), while the reactions with A1-positive cells are very strong (average of 7.9).

Column 12 represents the percentage of inclusion of the antigen (given in column 6 of the same line) into the reaction pattern of the serum. For example, serum 9w001 reacts positively with 84% of the A1-positive cells. Column 13 lists the Q-scores, which were calculated by the cell typing program described by H. Deppe et al. (this volume). Since the majority of the monoclonal antibodies were not used for computer cell typing there are also no Q-scores for these reagents. In the last column is given the correlation coefficient (r) between antigen and serum reactions.

Each antiserum is analyzed in up to five cycles. In the first cycle, the antigen with the strongest correlation is selected and the 2×2 table and the other parameters are given in the first line. For example for serum 007 the strongest correlation ($r = 0.937$) is with HLA-A1. Since there is still a significant number of "extra" reactions with 74 cells, the second cycle of analysis considers only cells negative for A1. In other words, a restricted analysis is performed, the results of which are given in the second line: the reaction pattern of serum 9w007 in A1-negative cells shows the strongest correlation ($r = 0.358$) with Aw36. In the third cycle, only cells are considered wich are negative for the antigens chosen in the previous two cycles. This process of successive restricted analyses is performed up to five times until no more significant correlations are found.

In cases where one of the broad specificities (such as DQw1, DQw2, DQw3 or DRw52, DRw53) gave the strongest correlation, information on the highly associated or included antigens was given in addition. Lines with such additional information were marked by an asterisk. A particular antigen could, therefore, appear twice. Let us, for example, consider a serum with primary specificity of anti-DQw1: Since DQw1 is highly associated with DR1, DR2, DRw10, DRw13, and DRw14, information on significant correlations of these antigens is given in lines (marked with asterisks) below the first line, which contains information for DQw1. In the second cycle of analysis, where only DQw1-negative cells are considered, it may be that the serum reacted also with the rare cells which are DQw1 negative but DRw10 positive. If this reactivity amounts to a significant correlation with DRw10, this antigen will appear a second time in the listing.

In order to provide the antigen working groups with material from which to prepare the antigen reports, a "pattern analysis" program was developed by G. Sierp in which the reactivity patterns of a given set of antisera or monoclonal antibodies with cells with certain specifications, such as positive for A1 and negative for A11, were counted. This pattern program was designed to investigate the quality of definition of antigens and to provide information about possible splits (an example is shown in Table 2). In preparation of the working material for the antigen groups, the 10 best sera for each antigen were selected and the pattern program performed with this group of 10 sera. In the first step, reaction patterns with cells positive for the antigen in question and negative for any cross-reacting specificities are given (top part of Table 2). As a control, the reactivity patterns of the same antisera were also investigated in cells which were negative for the antigen under consideration (bottom part of Table 2). For a well-defined antigen it could be observed that more than 90% of the antigen-positive cells reacted with all 10 antisera defining the antigen, while among the antigen-negative cells there were rarely any patterns with positive reactivity with more than three of the 10 sera. With this pattern analysis program, "short" or "long" splits of established antigens could be found, for example the split of DR5 into DRw11 and DRw12.

If a significant number of cells positive for the antigen showed a short pattern (i.e., negative for some of the good antisera defining the antigen under consideration, as shown in Table 2) it was important to investigate whether such patterns also segregated in families, or, alternatively, were caused simply by weak and nonreproducible reactivity of some antisera. Therefore, a family pattern search program was developed by G. Sierp to search for families in which one of the parents shows a given pattern of reactivity with a given set of antisera. This program will print out the serum reaction of a given set of antisera for all family members belonging to a family in which one of the parents fulfills a given reactivity pattern with the set of sera. This family pattern programme was used in two different ways.

First, families were selected in which one of the parents was positive for the antigen under consideration and the reactivity patterns of the total set of the best antisera defining the antigen under consideration were given for all family members. From these results it could be seen how reproducible the reactivity patterns were when segregating in families.

Second, when a certain short pattern had been observed in one family it was essential to find additional families in which the same pattern segregated in order to substantiate a short split of a given antigen. Table 3 shows this for the segregation of the short DR5 pattern (= DRw12). The above-described procedure was used to assess the quality of definition of established antigens and to validate the definition of new antigens such as Aw66, Th, Bw67, Bw71, Bw72, Bw73, DRw11, DRw12, DRw13, DRw14, and TA10.

References

1. Allen F, Amos DB, Batchelor R, Bodmer W, Ceppellini R, Dausset J, Engelfriet C, Jeannet M, Kissmeyer-Nielsen F, Morris P, Payne R, Terasaki P, van Rood JJ , Walford R, Zmijewski C, Albert E, Mattiuz P, Mickey MR, Piazza A (1970) Joint report of Fourth International Histocompatibility Workshop. In: Terasaki PI (ed) Histocompatibility testing 1970. Munksgaard, Copenhagen, pp 17–47
2. Mickey MR, Terasaki PI (1980) The serological data of the 8th Workshop and summary analyses. In: Terasaki PI (ed) Histocompatibility testing 1980. UCLA Tissue Typing Laboratory, Los Angeles, pp 21–136

Table 1. Final results of the serological analysis

9wNo.:	REG	LAB.	SERUM-ID	STR	ANTIGEN	No.REAC.	AVE	+/+	MISS. +/-	EXTRA -/+	%INCL	Q-SCORE	R-VALUE
001	FRA	JEA	PGE-2232	68	A1	3919	7.2	580	116	10	84	7.0	.887
002	US4	STA	GARRET-P1734	77	A1	3929	7.5	669	33	34	96	9.5	.942
				32	A24	3203	5.7	25	855	6	3	0.11	.118
003	GER	SCN	SCN-BPL-1	88	A1	3950	7.8	699	6	33	100	11.0	.967
				15	Aw36	3244	5.0	6	23	27	21	1.3	.186
				16	DRw13	3155	4.2	9	412	15	3	0.023	.062
006	UKI	MID	MADDEN	92	A1	3900	7.9	701	3	61	100	11.0	.947
				34	Aw36	3196	7.0	29	0	32	100	7.9	.686
007	GER	SUD	SUD-HB-9436	89	A1	3937	7.9	699	4	74	100	11.0	.937
				21	Aw36	3234	6.8	17	12	57	59	3.0	.358
				10	B8	3205	5.5	11	129	46	8	1.7	.098
009	US8	LEE	TABL	83	A1	3947	7.8	690	11	86	99	9.9	.921
				31	Aw36	3246	6.2	28	1	58	97	7.7	.555
				29	A26	3217	5.8	22	331	36	7	0.24	.117
				27	Aw43	2864	4.0	3	8	33	28	2.7	.145
				36	A11	2578	5.8	10	401	12	3	0.019	.075
011	US1	SOB	SOB-313	98	A2	3947	8.0	1986	17	15	100	12.0	.984
				20	Bw57	1944	4.3	7	92	8	8	0.068	.167
				37	Cw2	1844	6.5	4	170	4	3	0.0078	.092
013	US1	AMO	SIMPSON 32482	96	A2	3941	7.9	1980	19	9	100	11.0	.986
				33	Aw69	1942	5.0	4	13	5	24	3.2	.319
014	GER	GOL	GOL-8367.4	93	A2	3882	7.8	1933	40	7	98	12.0	.976
				14	A28	1909	4.7	6	243	1	3	0.06	.131
017	SCA	SVE	COP.D-2749-79	97	A2	3919	8.0	1979	14	33	100	12.0	.976
				39	Aw69	1926	6.8	10	7	23	59	3.9	.415
				34	Bw57	1909	5.8	11	82	12	12	0.15	.220
				41	Aw68	1816	6.3	8	214	4	4	0.74	.136
018	EAE	WEG	WÖRMSDORF	96	A2	3899	8.0	1964	11	54	100	11.0	.967
				24	Aw69	1924	5.9	14	2	40	88	4.3	.470
				22	Aw68	1908	5.6	33	196	7	15	0.91	.317
019	SAF	HAM	N-628	89	A2	3845	7.7	1822	123	14	94	9.7	.930
				85	A28	1900	7.7	14	232	0	6	0.22	.223
021	IT2	FER	FE-44	83	A2	3910	7.6	1801	184	25	91	7.9	.896
				36	Aw69	1925	6.3	13	3	12	82	3.5	.646
023	SAF	DUT	CT-630	50	A28	3871	6.9	261	99	89	73	5.0	.709
				15	Aw69	3511	5.3	56	151	33	28	0.49	.390
024	IT2	FER	FE-67	76	A28	3929	7.6	348	21	44	95	10.0	.906
				13	Aw69	3560	5.1	37	171	7	18	0.55	.373
025	GER	HIL	HI-6374/80	61	A28	3873	7.9	351	5	314	99	10.0	.687
				23	Aw69	3517	6.2	151	58	163	73	2.3	.558
				14	A2	3308	5.2	157	1491	6	10	0.74	.212
027	GER	MUE	MUE-21334/II	59	A28	3939	7.9	362	6	530	99	10.0	.581
				34	Aw69	3571	6.7	170	42	360	81	2.9	.462
				26	A2	3359	5.8	341	1327	19	21	1.1	.312
029	BEN	BRX	LINDEMANS	67	A28	3904	7.6	296	69	296	82	5.9	.590
				48	Aw33	3539	6.8	184	108	112	64	3.0	.592
				41	Aw34	3247	7.3	43	9	69	41	5.0	.554
				21	Aw69	3195	4.9	25	162	44	14	0.16	.192
				29	Bw41	3008	6.0	12	76	32	14	0.034	.176
031	FRA	PAU	FRE-103	63	A28	3941	7.9	366	5	547	99	7.4	.577
				41	Aw69	3570	6.9	141	69	406	68	1.5	.360
				35	Cw8	3360	6.5	125	173	281	32	0.6	.286
				32	B8	3062	6.0	100	228	181	31	0.34	.256
				32	A2	2734	5.8	159	1282	22	12	0.22	.187
032	US4	RAD	NW-14000	55	A28	3881	7.0	268	99	144	74	5.0	.655
				38	Aw33	3514	6.4	114	169	30	41	2.4	.540
033	NCY	FUL	MGH-85.1	51	A2	3948	6.6	1395	607	171	70	2.5	.622
				58	Bw57	1946	7.3	90	9	81	91	2.5	.672
				48	Bw58	1847	6.6	67	35	14	66	1.1	.724

Table 1 (continued)

9wNo.:	REG	LAB.	SERUM-ID	STR	ANTIGEN	No.REAC.	AVE	+/+	MISS. +/-	EXTRA -/+	%INCL	Q-SCORE	R-VALUE
034	EAE	BRT	LASAKOVA	92	A2	3859	7.9	1885	75	170	97	5.1	.874
				70	Bw57	1899	7.4	85	11	85	89	1.5	.643
				63	Bw58	1803	6.9	70	28	15	72	1.0	.755
036	EAE	WEG	PEPER	87	A24	3945	7.7	958	33	148	97	8.6	.885
				86	A23	2934	7.9	122	4	26	97	9.1	.888
				30	Aw9.3	2828	6.0	2	1	24	67	3.8	.224
037	FRA	DAU	FPA-0916	67	A24	3915	7.4	879	102	166	90	6.7	.822
				17	A23	2934	5.9	62	61	104	51	2.0	.405
				8	Aw69	2785	4.8	24	271	78	9	0.13	.082
038	SAF	DUT	CT-511.3	92	A24	3901	7.9	968	17	143	99	11.0	.899
				79	A23	2916	7.8	119	3	24	98	11.0	.896
				12	Aw9.3	2794	6.0	3	0	21	100	6.3	.352
039	US5	MIT	C-6395.1	95	A24	3936	7.9	976	12	157	99	11.0	.895
				84	A23	2948	7.9	129	0	32	100	11.0	.887
				34	Aw9.3	2823	6.7	3	0	29	100	6.6	.305
041	US1	SOB	SOB-352.1	56	A24	3940	6.5	541	449	180	55	2.9	.545
				78	A23	2950	7.9	124	1	56	100	9.2	.818
				39	Bw57	2825	6.1	36	106	20	26	0.27	.420
				47	Aw69	2680	5.7	7	276	12	3	0.048	.072
042	SCA	JER	TS-105	69	A23	3946	7.4	137	8	48	95	8.7	.830
				47	A24	3801	6.2	33	941	15	4	0.1	.112
043	US1	DUQ	LOOK	61	A23	3913	7.0	129	14	15	91	7.6	.895
044	US2	BAC	MN-14121	70	A23	3918	7.6	135	8	47	95	9.1	.830
				29	A24	3775	5.8	31	927	16	4	0.14	.105
047	US8	LEE	HAMB	92	A24	3924	7.8	967	19	9	99	11.0	.981
048	US1	DUQ	KIRBY	85	A24	3945	7.7	962	25	96	98	11.0	.921
				48	A23	2958	6.5	91	35	5	73	5.5	.821
050	JAP	JUJ	MRC-37	81	A24	3948	7.6	965	28	61	98	9.5	.941
				31	A23	2955	6.1	29	97	32	24	1.2	.311
				25	Aw69	2829	5.5	12	288	20	4	0.17	.093
051	US5	STA	C 360.1	76	A24	3942	7.4	908	85	59	92	8.1	.902
				38	A23	2949	6.1	44	82	15	35	2.3	.497
056	IT2	FER	FE-136	44	A3	3931	6.4	410	259	21	62	3.6	.729
				35	Aw69	3262	5.3	8	294	13	3	0.013	.080
057	FRA	LEP	CHAMBOST	93	A3	3945	7.9	668	3	64	100	12.0	.943
				45	A24	3274	6.7	46	872	18	6	0.17	.138
				16	A11	2356	5.3	11	345	7	4	0.098	.113
059	EAE	WEG	R-181	72	A3	3947	7.7	665	10	214	99	10.0	.832
				21	A11	3272	5.9	128	318	86	29	1.4	.356
				13	Aw34	2826	5.7	12	39	74	24	0.94	.162
				10	Aw33	2775	5.1	24	227	50	10	0.3	.135
				12	A31	2524	4.4	20	186	30	10	0.38	.165
				16	TH	2318	5.0	2	5	28	29	3.1	.133
060	SAF	DUT	CT-529	94	A3	3950	8.0	672	2	35	100	12.0	.968
				25	A11	3276	5.4	28	416	7	7	0.38	.202
061	FRA	MUL	FPC-SPE	85	A3	3938	7.9	661	12	560	99	8.9	.660
				73	A11	3265	7.8	419	21	141	96	7.0	.817
				26	A29	2825	5.7	44	136	97	25	0.51	.233
				26	Aw33	2618	5.9	31	216	62	13	0.31	.157
				25	Aw34	2371	5.7	6	32	56	16	0.36	.105
062	GER	KUE	KUE-005-C	86	A3	3948	7.9	660	13	1403	99	8.1	.416
				81	A11	3275	7.8	443	4	960	100	8.0	.452
				77	Aw33	2828	7.8	238	20	722	93	5.7	.390
				71	A31	2570	7.7	194	12	528	95	5.5	.434
				65	A29	2364	7.7	155	16	373	91	5.1	.458
				56	A30	2193	7.5	143	30	230	83	4.4	.511
				*56	A25	2193	5.9	31	50	342	39	1.0	.111
				*56	A1	2193	6.2	147	374	226	29	.61	.166
				*56	Aw34	2193	7.9	31	11	342	74	3.0	.211
063	UKI	MID	BULLOCK	73	A11	3894	7.7	466	26	195	95	7.4	.788
				40	A3	3402	6.6	88	534	107	15	0.3	.171
				28	Aw33	2780	6.4	31	226	76	13	0.27	.136
				23	A1	2523	5.1	33	517	43	6	0.04	.092
				30	DR1	1969	5.6	14	200	29	7	0.11	.104
				31	B27	1759	5.4	7	77	22	9	0.007	.118
065	US5	CMC	9741 K	77	A11	3876	7.8	468	9	137	99	10.0	.852
				29	A3	3399	5.6	75	543	62	13	0.47	.194
				27	A24	2781	6.0	40	766	22	5	0.075	.118
067	EAE	WEG	R-174	75	A11	3942	8.0	494	1	225	100	11.0	.800
				23	A1	3447	5.4	118	548	107	18	0.43	.222
				24	A3	2781	6.0	58	478	49	11	0.46	.177
				20	A26	2245	5.4	29	268	20	10	0.27	.203
069	US1	DUQ	RYAN	45	A11	3919	6.4	271	216	17	56	4.4	.697

9wNo.:	REG	LAB.	SERUM-ID	STR	ANTIGEN	No.REAC.	AVE	+/+	MISS. +/-	EXTRA -/+	%INCL	Q-SCORE	R-VALUE
071	FRA	MAY	FST-01	58	A26	3901	7.0	295	82	207	79	5.6	.639
				49	A25	3524	6.9	88	17	119	84	5.5	.581
				43	A3	3419	6.8	60	565	59	10	0.24	.158
				27	Aw34	2794	6.2	9	42	50	18	0.61	.147
				24	Aw66	2743	5.7	6	22	44	22	1.6	.149
				25	Aw33	2715	5.3	12	240	32	5	0.12	.080
072	US6	BRN	CC 101.1	80	A26	3921	7.8	367	11	187	98	9.0	.778
				55	A25	3543	7.5	102	2	85	99	9.8	.722
				28	Aw66	3439	6.3	20	9	65	69	4.8	.395
				26	Aw43	3410	7.1	11	0	54	100	6.4	.408
074	JAP	JUJ	MRC-41	77	A26	3940	7.6	353	25	102	94	8.2	.834
				51	A25	3562	6.6	66	39	36	63	4.1	.627
				44	Aw43	3457	7.3	11	0	25	100	7.5	.551
				28	Aw66	3446	5.3	9	21	16	30	3.2	.323
				37	Aw34	3416	5.7	6	49	10	11	0.62	.196
075	SAF	DUT	CT-668	88	A26	3911	7.9	376	3	230	100	13.0	.758
				73	A25	3532	7.8	102	2	128	99	11.0	.646
				60	Aw66	3428	7.0	20	8	108	72	7.6	.324
				60	Aw43	3400	8.0	11	0	97	100	8.6	.315
				55	A3	3389	6.8	86	536	11	14	0.63	.312
076	FRA	KRE	FMT-810	81	A26	3939	7.6	340	41	178	90	7.8	.737
				72	A25	3558	7.6	92	12	86	89	7.8	.664
				59	Aw34	3454	7.6	51	4	35	93	7.7	.737
				25	Aw66	3399	5.9	16	14	19	54	4.1	.489
077	EAE	WEG	R-179	88	A26	3933	7.8	381	1	216	100	11.0	.773
				75	A25	3551	7.7	102	1	114	100	8.8	.672
				61	Aw34	3448	7.1	42	14	72	75	4.6	.515
				56	Aw66	3392	6.3	19	11	53	64	5.3	.401
				69	Aw43	3362	7.8	9	1	44	90	5.3	.388
078	IT2	FER	FE-116	85	A26	3903	7.9	375	5	204	99	10.0	.775
				69	A25	3523	7.4	93	6	111	94	8.7	.642
				63	Aw34	3424	7.9	56	0	55	100	10.0	.704
				30	Aw66	3368	5.7	20	9	35	69	4.6	.495
				37	Aw33	3339	6.3	24	256	11	9	0.41	.223
079	FRA	FAU	FRE-105	90	A26	3889	8.0	376	2	207	100	11.0	.776
				76	A25	3511	7.4	102	3	105	98	8.9	.680
				76	Aw34	3406	7.8	50	6	55	90	7.5	.645
				60	Aw66	3350	7.0	23	7	32	77	5.6	.561
				53	Aw43	3320	8.0	10	0	22	100	7.8	.557

9wNo.:	REG	LAB.	SERUM-ID	STR	ANTIGEN	No.REAC.	AVE	+/+	MISS. +/-	EXTRA -/+	%INCL	Q-SCORE	R-VALUE
081	UKI	DEW	DB-200	92	A26	3940	8.0	378	3	198	100	12.0	.783
				81	A25	3559	7.6	103	2	95	99	10.0	.704
				78	Aw34	3454	7.7	53	3	42	95	10.0	.721
				69	Aw66	3398	7.4	22	7	20	76	6.9	.627
				60	Aw43	3369	8.0	10	0	10	100	8.3	.706
082	SAF	HAM	N-51	76	A26	3898	7.9	345	23	319	94	5.7	.659
				56	A25	3530	6.9	87	18	232	83	4.5	.451
				53	Aw34	3425	7.5	48	7	184	88	4.7	.409
				46	Bw60	3370	6.4	103	188	81	36	0.67	.405
				46	Aw66	3079	7.2	15	9	66	63	2.8	.332
				43	Aw43	3055	8.0	9	0	57	100	5.1	.366
083	UKI	FES	NYONG	35	Aw34	3452	6.5	29	21	74	58	3.4	.392
				28	A26	3402	5.7	48	283	26	15	0.70	.277
084	FRA	FAU	FRE-127	36	Aw34	3916	6.7	41	23	134	65	3.60	.372
				31	A26	3852	6.1	75	296	59	21	0.86	.298
				23	A25	3481	6.0	13	92	46	13	0.50	.146
				26	Aw66	3376	6.0	5	25	41	17	0.64	.125
085	FRA	MAY	FST-02	87	A25	3788	7.9	102	3	17	98	9.4	.910
				47	Aw66	3683	7.0	4	25	13	14	1.1	.175
086	EAE	RIC	NR-809.2	67	A25	3892	7.4	105	6	54	95	7.5	.783
				57	Aw66	3781	5.5	4	26	50	14	0.37	.090
087	GER	GOL	GOL-12715.12	68	A25	3797	7.9	104	2	106	99	8.0	.686
				43	A26	3691	6.0	67	299	39	19	0.89	.307
				61	B51	3325	7.1	20	330	19	6	0.026	.145
090	FRA	OHA	FTO-125	52	A25	3817	6.9	90	16	37	85	7.2	.769
				37	Aw66	3711	6.0	4	26	33	14	0.88	.112
091	EAE	BRT	DOBES-140678	63	A26	3705	6.6	197	171	107	54	4.1	.548
				89	A25	3337	8.0	92	7	15	93	9.7	.891
				26	Aw66	3238	6.0	5	25	10	17	1.9	.231
093	FRA	BET	FLY-874	43	A26	3680	6.7	195	170	74	54	3.0	.588
				23	Cw7	3275	5.5	58	1121	11	5	0.023	.147
094	US8	LEE	THOM-1	61	A26	3921	7.1	330	45	40	88	8.1	.874
				22	Aw66	3546	5.4	7	22	33	25	2.1	.198
				27	A25	3517	5.2	10	94	23	10	0.38	.157
				30	A29	3413	6.5	8	174	15	5	0.19	.108

Table 1 (continued)

9wNo.:	REG	LAB.	SERUM-ID	STR	ANTIGEN	No.REAC.	AVE	+/+	MISS. +/-	EXTRA -/+	%INCL	Q-SCORE	R-VALUE
095	EAE	RIC	D-219.4	86	A26	3913	7.8	369	10	45	98	12.0	.924
				35	Aw34	3534	6.4	21	35	24	38	2.7	.410
				25	Aw66	3478	6.2	12	17	12	42	3.4	.451
				16	Aw43	3449	4.0	3	7	9	30	3.9	.272
				22	A25	3439	7.0	4	100	5	4	0.48	.124
098	SAF	DUT	CT-728	52	A26	3932	6.7	268	106	13	72	5.8	.812
				30	Aw43	3558	5.5	4	7	9	37	3.9	.332
				44	Aw66	3547	5.0	2	28	7	7	0.85	.118
099	SAF	DUT	CT-422	59	A26	3884	7.0	274	93	24	75	7.2	.813
				25	A25	3517	5.8	21	82	3	21	1.7	.416
				0	Aw43	3414	4.0	3	8	0	28	3.1	.522
100	SAF	DUT	CT-544.2	25	Aw43	3920	5.8	11	0	65	100	8.4	.377
				26	A26	3909	5.9	50	327	15	14	0.86	.296
				0	A29	3532	5.3	9	174	6	5	0.23	.162
101	SAF	DUT	CT-438	19	Aw43	3891	6.0	11	0	20	100	7.4	.594
102	IT2	FER	FE-71	80	A29	3780	7.7	183	4	20	98	9.9	.936
				30	Aw43	3593	5.0	4	6	16	40	3.9	.280
				33	Aw41	3563	6.5	4	94	11	5	0.024	.095
103	US5	ANN	B-3671.1	75	A29	3938	7.7	197	3	56	99	10.0	.869
				28	Aw43	3738	6.8	10	0	46	100	7.8	.420
				23	B8	3728	5.5	34	380	12	9	0.21	.223
				16	Aw34	3314	4.0	3	49	9	6	0.39	.114
104	FRA	KRE	FMT-125	63	A29	3939	7.9	196	3	204	99	10.0	.675
				31	A11	3740	6.2	100	390	104	21	0.81	.256
				21	Aw43	3250	7.6	10	0	94	100	6.9	.306
				14	TH	3240	6.4	5	5	89	50	2.6	.156
				13	A3	3230	4.8	44	561	45	8	0.16	.132
				17	Bw53	2625	5.4	7	45	38	14	0.27	.129
106	GER	WEI	HU-23171	83	A29	3953	7.8	198	2	33	99	11.0	.917
				18	Aw43	3753	7.0	10	0	23	100	7.3	.549
				4	DR7	3739	4.2	18	497	5	4	0.35	.147
108	FRA	MUL	FPC-101	56	A29	3845	7.7	190	2	195	99	13.0	.679
				28	A1	3653	5.8	173	488	22	27	1.6	.436
				22	Aw43	2992	5.6	5	5	17	50	4.4	.334
				17	A11	2982	5.6	9	418	8	3	0.032	.083
111	IT2	FER	FE-77	69	A32	3948	7.7	203	4	85	99	8.7	.821
				29	A25	3741	5.8	28	80	57	26	0.94	.274
				26	Bw62	3633	5.7	42	378	15	10	0.25	.245
				20	Bw57	3213	4.4	5	145	10	4	0.072	.093
112	UKI	BAT	DAVEY	61	A32	3907	7.9	207	0	337	100	10.0	.588
				40	A25	3700	7.3	103	5	234	96	6.8	.520
				25	Cw8	3592	6.1	90	233	144	28	0.41	.272
				19	A24	3269	5.5	102	799	42	12	0.24	.208
				23	A23	2368	5.4	13	97	29	12	0.36	.168
				27	Aw66	2258	5.0	4	19	25	18	0.63	.145
113	US7	HAN	SEA-1065	29	A32	3908	5.9	111	95	10	54	4.6	.692
				30	Aw69	3702	6.5	4	311	6	2	0.011	.059
114	SAF	DUT	CT-435	80	A32	3879	7.7	192	10	101	96	11.0	.776
				63	A25	3677	7.1	96	13	5	89	9.0	.912
117	IT2	FER	FE-150	72	A32	3922	7.6	205	1	86	100	12.0	.827
				40	A25	3716	6.4	79	28	7	74	5.7	.819
118	US7	HAN	SEA-1168	32	A32	3895	6.0	123	83	45	60	3.8	.644
				24	B49	3689	5.3	11	72	34	14	0.40	.166
				27	B51	3572	5.4	17	388	16	5	0.078	.122
				37	A25	3167	5.5	4	87	12	5	0.31	.094
				41	Bw57	3076	6.5	4	141	8	3	0.092	.085
119	FRA	MAY	FST-03	71	A31	3848	7.3	221	22	208	91	8.5	.658
				71	A30	3605	7.3	199	12	9	95	9.4	.947
121	FRA	BET	FLY-967	68	A30	3936	7.7	214	6	153	98	6.7	.736
				40	A31	3716	5.6	41	204	112	17	0.35	.169
				45	Cw5	3471	6.2	29	375	83	8	0.066	.081
122	US8	LEE	COLL	80	A31	3880	7.5	238	11	215	96	10.0	.684
				79	A30	3631	7.6	202	8	13	97	11.0	.948
123	US8	LEE	THOM-2	72	A30	3878	7.7	213	7	265	97	12.0	.630
				60	A31	3658	7.3	221	24	44	90	7.8	.854
				9	DR4	3407	4.4	36	910	8	4	0.081	.138
124	US3	LUG	MU-YOUNG	57	A30	3847	7.1	188	21	194	90	9.0	.641
				49	A31	3638	6.7	190	54	4	78	7.3	.866
126	UKI	BAT	TOME	75	A30	3913	7.8	218	3	205	99	12.0	.692
				58	A31	3692	6.9	198	46	7	82	7.4	.878
128	UKI	BRS	LIV-5985	66	A30	3890	7.1	188	21	14	90	8.4	.910
129	US5	KC	AMO	80	A30	3942	7.7	210	11	31	96	8.5	.904
				29	B13	3721	5.5	16	80	15	17	1.6	.283
130	GER	SUD	HB-13540/3	84	A32	3904	7.7	199	5	10	98	9.5	.962
				50	A11	3700	6.8	5	480	5	2	0.011	.057

9wNo.:	REG	LAB.	SERUM-ID	STR	ANTIGEN	No.REAC.	AVE	+/+	MISS. +/-	EXTRA -/+	%INCL	Q-SCORE	R-VALUE
132	US1	NWO	(D.)BROWN-12.361	41	A30	3375	5.9	59	140	48	30	1.6	.378
				54	A3	3176	6.5	24	559	24	5	0.10	.101
				58	A1	2593	6.8	13	494	11	3	0.037	.084
133	IT2	FER	FE-82	58	Cw5	3919	6.7	310	143	136	69	2.7	.649
				69	A30	3466	7.5	101	82	35	56	1.6	.623
				22	A1	3283	5.5	15	581	20	3	0.017	.067
				25	Aw34	2687	7.3	3	48	17	6	0.063	.083
				17	A32	2636	5.6	5	128	12	4	0.091	.090
134	US6	BRN	CC-338.3	30	A31	3907	5.6	98	150	43	40	2.8	.501
				44	A30	3659	6.6	29	118	14	14	0.56	.290
				21	Aw33	3450	4.0	5	273	9	2	0.10	.065
135	US6	BRN	CC-362.1	30	A31	3941	6.2	179	71	71	72	6.3	.697
				11	Aw33	3691	5.3	51	245	20	18	1.1	.329
				15	A30	3395	5.5	8	194	12	4	0.071	.111
136	IT2	FER	FE-78	58	A31	3944	7.2	232	20	113	93	9.1	.770
				37	A30	3692	6.2	80	135	33	38	2.6	.493
				27	Aw33	3477	5.6	27	255	6	10	0.52	.264
138	FRA	BIG	FNN-551	83	A30	3946	7.8	214	7	114	97	6.8	.781
				66	B13	3725	7.6	84	14	30	86	4.6	.789
				20	A31	3627	5.4	20	218	10	9	0.53	.222
139	US6	BRN	CC-257.1	49	A31	3902	7.0	197	52	191	80	5.7	.604
				32	A30	3653	6.4	88	121	103	43	2.3	.408
				23	A3	3443	6.3	39	594	63	7	0.080	.090
				12	Aw33	2810	5.2	18	230	45	8	0.12	.105
				11	B13	2562	6.8	5	66	40	8	0.60	.068
140	JAP	JUJ	19-50368	59	Aw33	3904	6.9	242	64	229	80	6.0	.600
				59	A31	3598	7.1	200	39	29	84	7.1	.845
				13	Aw66	3359	6.0	4	24	25	15	1.2	.133
				8	Aw69	3331	4.5	11	277	14	4	0.034	.109
141	IT2	FER	FE-123	57	Aw33	3926	7.3	280	26	147	92	7.3	.753
				26	Aw34	3620	6.7	24	34	123	42	2.2	.241
				22	A31	3562	5.4	49	187	74	21	0.81	.253
				24	A25	3326	5.6	18	88	56	17	0.58	.182
				25	A29	3220	4.8	19	162	37	11	0.38	.164
142	FRA	BET	FLY-855	53	Aw33	3931	7.1	100	205	40	33	1.5	.457
				15	Cw8	3626	5.2	20	284	20	7	0.62	.159
				15	Aw66	3322	6.0	4	24	16	15	0.56	.163

9wNo.:	REG	LAB.	SERUM-ID	STR	ANTIGEN	No.REAC.	AVE	+/+	MISS. +/-	EXTRA -/+	%INCL	Q-SCORE	R-VALUE
143	IT1	MTT	FIO-2111	51	Aw33	3929	6.9	237	69	143	78	5.4	.666
				34	Aw34	3623	7.2	36	21	107	64	3.8	.384
				22	A26	3566	5.8	53	302	54	15	0.55	.232
				16	A29	3211	5.4	17	158	37	10	0.28	.150
				16	Aw66	3036	5.0	4	26	33	4	0.95	.110
				14	A25	3000	5.1	7	88	27	8	0.35	.107
144	FRA	GRA	FGR-1059	35	Aw33	3770	6.2	132	135	147	50	2.8	.443
				31	Aw34	3503	6.9	38	20	109	66	3.9	.397
				21	A26	3445	5.7	86	239	23	27	1.5	.430
				17	Aw66	3120	5.5	4	25	19	14	0.93	.148
146	NCY	YUN	YUN-MMUL	43	Aw33	3875	6.4	174	109	49	62	4.2	.672
				34	Aw34	3592	5.8	20	34	29	38	2.0	.380
147	ANZ	ROB	LISTER	75	A26	3887	8.0	371	5	505	99	11.0	.596
				57	A25	3511	8.0	100	1	405	100	11.0	.415
				47	Aw68	3410	6.6	133	98	272	58	1.1	.381
				45	Aw34	3179	7.8	46	4	226	92	8.1	.377
				36	Aw33	3129	6.3	91	168	135	36	1.8	.324
				31	Aw66	2870	7.0	21	8	114	73	5.8	.323
				*31	A32	2870	6.0	45	136	90	25	1.2	.247
				*31	A28	2870	5.9	34	77	101	31	2.8	.246
148	JAP	JUJ	MRC-32	73	A26	3951	8.0	377	5	458	99	9.3	.622
				52	Aw33	3569	6.8	228	64	230	79	4.3	.582
				46	Aw34	3277	7.8	42	8	188	84	5.8	.375
				37	A29	3227	5.6	53	125	135	30	0.88	.247
				43	Aw66	3049	6.9	18	11	117	63	3.5	.275
				41	Aw43	3020	8.0	9	0	108	100	6.4	.272
				*41	A31	3020	5.4	34	191	83	16	0.14	.165
				*41	A25	3020	6.7	14	83	103	15	0.51	.100
				*41	A30	3020	6.6	16	160	101	10	0.14	.067
				*41	Aw69	3020	5.7	21	255	96	8	0.079	.061
				*41	Bw60	3020	6.2	21	256	96	8	0.012	.061
149	UKI	BRS	SL-6203	85	A26	3956	7.8	366	14	1161	97	5.9	.386
				83	Aw33	3576	7.5	274	19	887	94	4.7	.389
				83	A31	3283	7.5	217	15	670	94	4.7	.413
				84	A32	3051	7.9	186	4	484	98	6.2	.473
				80	A29	2861	7.7	161	8	323	96	6.0	.524
				76	A25	2692	7.9	92	1	231	99	7.4	.506
				*76	Aw34	2692	7.7	43	1	280	88	2.7	.340
				*76	B27	2692	7.4	108	46	215	71	0.97	.441

Table 1 (continued)

9wNo.:	REG	LAB.	SERUM-ID	STR	ANTIGEN	No.REAC.	AVE	+/+	MISS. +/-	EXTRA -/+	%INCL	Q-SCORE	R-VALUE
150	EAE	RIC	SU-10142	86	A26	3792	7.7	340	10	1219	98	7.1	.356
				85	Aw33	3442	7.8	260	5	959	99	7.8	.379
				84	A31	3177	7.8	203	10	756	96	6.5	.380
				81	A32	2964	8.0	185	4	571	98	7.6	.433
				76	A29	2775	7.8	164	5	407	98	7.3	.482
				70	A30	2606	7.4	164	14	243	93	5.8	.571
				*70	A25	2606	7.9	93	0	314	100	8.8	.447
				*70	Aw34	2606	7.6	43	2	364	96	7.0	.292
				*70	B13	2606	7.3	54	65	353	46	0.17	.179
				*70	Bw53	2606	7.3	25	30	382	46	0.27	.121
151	SAF	HAM	N-678	46	A26	3785	6.9	222	140	472	62	3.7	.361
				40	Aw34	3423	7.7	52	3	420	95	9.3	.299
				34	A25	3368	6.6	69	31	351	69	4.5	.299
				31	Aw33	3268	6.5	116	154	235	43	1.9	.312
				24	A31	2998	6.0	50	159	185	24	0.73	.164
				21	A3	2789	5.7	78	475	107	15	0.27	.149
				*21	TH	2789	5.0	6	4	179	60	5.0	.129
				*21	A11	2789	6.1	52	348	133	13	0.17	.105
				*21	A29	2789	5.7	23	137	162	15	0.24	.077
156	US6	BRN	CC-273.1	65	B51	3936	7.1	357	88	27	81	6.2	.848
157	US5	FTW	GREE	65	B51	3940	7.1	376	72	35	84	6.4	.861
				31	B13	3492	6.7	14	128	21	10	0.17	.183
158	US8	LEE	THOM	58	B51	3844	6.9	298	130	53	70	4.0	.743
				56	DRw12	3412	6.7	15	327	38	5	0.045	.076
159	SAF	DUT	CT-725	52	B51	3949	6.7	297	154	19	66	4.6	.766
160	US8	NSF	NSF-2032	77	B51	3560	7.6	288	72	23	80	6.4	.847
				13	Bw53	3200	4.0	3	64	20	5	0.40	.065
161	US5	MIT	C-3502	38	Bw52	3906	6.3	71	96	199	43	3.2	.297
				35	B35	3739	6.0	135	517	64	21	1.1	.315
				35	B51	3087	6.4	51	336	13	14	0.63	.295
162	JAP	TOK	JR-50-(100)-5	49	Bw52	3934	6.8	111	58	106	66	4.5	.558
				39	B51	3765	6.2	72	356	34	17	0.80	.303
163	US1	MCG	MCG-AL	62	B35	3613	7.3	509	109	1778	83	0.36	.180
				59	B51	2995	6.7	270	126	1508	69	0.052	.070
				60	Bw54	2372	6.9	93	37	1270	72	0.087	.069
164	FRA	BET	FLY-794	88	B51	3913	7.9	443	6	207	99	9.3	.794
				70	Bw52	3464	7.7	139	10	68	94	7.5	.781
				32	B18	3315	5.7	27	219	41	11	0.32	.178
				39	Bw53	3069	6.8	5	65	36	8	0.31	.077
				41	B35	3036	6.4	15	549	24	3	0.016	.058
166	US1	DUQ	(M.)Neary	69	B51	3910	7.4	418	32	174	93	7.1	.782
				49	Bw52	3460	6.8	122	31	52	80	4.6	.735
167	UKI	JOY	LEWIS	76	B51	3946	7.6	429	19	111	96	7.8	.855
				45	Bw52	3498	6.3	79	75	32	52	2.9	.589
169	NCY	MRV	9811	87	B51	3531	7.8	411	12	160	98	8.6	.812
				71	Bw52	3108	7.6	120	7	40	95	8.0	.834
				40	Bw59	2981	6.0	6	19	34	24	1.2	.181
170	US1	THP	THP-McMullin	82	B51	3941	7.8	438	12	164	98	10.0	.819
				53	Bw52	3491	7.1	117	36	47	77	5.8	.726
				25	Bw53	3338	5.8	13	60	34	18	1.1	.208
171	US6	WAL	SUTTON	87	B35	3950	7.9	641	26	536	97	8.6	.653
				78	B51	3283	7.7	400	9	136	98	9.7	.832
				52	Bw53	2874	7.7	63	3	73	96	8.0	.655
				20	Bw52	2808	5.3	24	114	49	18	0.76	.211
				22	Bw62	2670	5.8	29	312	20	8	0.17	.181
172	SAF	HAM	N-1058	93	B35	3641	8.0	576	30	483	96	7.8	.649
				86	B51	3035	7.8	376	11	107	98	9.6	.849
				59	Bw53	2648	7.8	55	1	52	99	8.7	.703
				25	Bw52	2592	6.0	21	106	31	17	0.62	.235
173	US7	HAN	SEA-1022	75	B51	3936	7.9	446	5	383	99	8.5	.687
				52	Bw52	3485	7.6	144	9	239	95	6.2	.570
				34	B49	3332	6.7	52	34	187	61	2.2	.336
				28	A28	3246	6.1	76	239	111	25	0.17	.258
				23	Bw53	2931	5.9	14	39	97	27	0.65	.161
174	US6	BRN	CCB 147.1	80	B51	3918	7.9	433	14	368	97	.680	
				64	Bw52	3471	7.8	139	11	229	93	.567	
				47	B49	3321	7.3	72	14	157	84	.494	
				35	Bw53	3235	6.7	57	15	100	80	.522	
				23	Bw63	3163	6.2	13	60	87	18	.129	
175	US1	SOB	SOB-275	82	B51	3894	7.8	434	14	339	97	12.0	.696
				72	Bw52	3446	7.8	139	5	200	97	9.7	.608
				58	B49	3302	7.7	80	6	120	94	8.8	.596
				37	Bw63	3216	6.6	40	34	80	55	3.7	.407
				28	Bw53	3142	6.4	31	34	49	48	2.6	.417
				18	Bw57	3077	5.8	24	120	25	17	0.74	.267
176	EAE	MYR	HODOSI	91	B51	3897	7.9	435	12	380	98	8.6	.676
				86	Bw52	3450	7.9	137	14	243	91	7.1	.545
				81	B49	3299	7.8	82	4	161	96	6.7	.551
				76	Bw63	3213	7.9	67	8	94	90	6.3	.598
				63	Bw53	3138	7.5	59	8	35	89	5.4	.737

9wNo.:	REG	LAB.	SERUM-ID	STR	ANTIGEN	No.REAC.	AVE	+/+	MISS. +/-	EXTRA -/+	%INCL	Q-SCORE	R-VALUE
177	NCY	CAR	BOS/CHIN	92	B35	3895	7.9	619	34	840	95	8.3	.532
				88	B51	3242	7.9	398	10	442	98	9.9	.620
				81	B18	2834	7.6	197	14	245	94	8.1	.608
				80	Bw52	2623	7.9	131	6	114	96	9.1	.696
				59	Bw53	2486	7.8	59	0	55	100	10.0	.711
				23	Bw62	2427	6.0	27	316	28	8	0.13	.153
179	US5	MIT	C-4106	66	B35	3913	7.5	620	42	263	94	7.0	.767
				35	Bw62	3251	6.2	137	270	123	44	1.3	.355
				34	Bw72	2844	5.7	27	79	99	26	5.6	.201
				35	B51	2738	6.0	50	325	49	14	0.36	.207
				34	Bw53	2363	6.1	16	43	33	28	1.0	.281
180	US4	BRG	SS-0445-79	82	B35	3944	7.9	657	11	202	99	9.3	.838
				35	Bw62	3276	6.2	134	271	68	44	1.8	.420
				32	Bw72	2871	6.0	24	83	44	23	5.6	.260
				29	Bw53	2764	5.8	16	49	28	25	1.0	.285
				28	Bw71	2699	6.0	4	6	24	40	0.97	.234
181	US6	BRN	CCB-308.1	80	B35	3859	7.7	605	52	152	93	8.1	.827
				44	Bw53	3202	7.2	61	7	91	90	7.2	.589
				27	B51	3134	5.9	68	326	23	18	0.69	.324
182	FRA	BET	FLY-806	75	B35	3926	7.4	550	107	89	84	6.3	.819
				58	Bw53	3269	7.3	54	14	35	80	6.3	.687
				34	B51	3201	5.9	26	378	9	7	0.21	.195
184	JAP	JUJ	19 20203	45	B35	3934	6.4	350	315	71	53	2.6	.612
				29	Bw53	3269	6.0	8	63	63	12	0.28	.093
				26	Bw62	3198	5.7	20	382	43	5	0.029	.083
186	SAF	DUT	CT-730	38	B35	3945	6.4	383	283	186	58	2.9	.553
				25	Bw62	3279	5.9	107	300	79	27	0.75	.336
				20	Bw72	2872	5.3	20	87	59	19	3.2	.196
189	US5	SIN	11668.1	67	B18	3944	7.8	259	6	181	98	7.2	.738
				32	B8	3679	6.1	42	373	139	11	0.022	.086
190	US1	SOB	SOB-375.2	68	B18	3871	7.4	249	15	38	95	8.0	.897
193	SCA	JER	TS-124	77	B18	3916	7.7	248	10	32	97	10.0	.917
194	SCA	SVE	D-1605/79	67	B18	3933	7.9	258	4	196	99	8.4	.727
				29	Bw65	3671	6.3	55	189	141	23	0.52	.204
				24	B8	3427	6.2	45	349	96	12	0.076	.133

9wNo.:	REG	LAB.	SERUM-ID	STR	ANTIGEN	No.REAC.	AVE	+/+	MISS. +/-	EXTRA -/+	%INCL	Q-SCORE	R-VALUE
196	IT2	FER	FE-31	81	B18	3938	7.7	260	4	24	99	11.0	.946
197	SAF	DUT	CT-718	84	B18	3927	7.8	262	4	32	99	11.0	.932
198	SAF	DUT	CT-551	83	B18	3900	7.5	243	19	16	93	8.0	.928
199	FRA	BIG	MET	88	B35	3327	7.9	500	62	536	89	5.6	.563
				82	B51	2765	7.7	313	33	223	91	5.9	.680
				73	Bw52	2419	7.5	96	20	127	83	4.6	.571
				65	Bw53	2303	8.0	46	11	81	81	4.7	.525
				45	Bw62	2246	6.2	51	246	30	18	0.33	.284
201	NCY	YUN	YUN/DEM	85	B51	3881	7.9	427	17	269	97	8.2	.773
				70	Bw52	3437	7.7	141	9	128	94	7.5	.685
				53	B13	3287	7.2	73	63	55	54	3.0	.535
				34	Bw59	3151	5.8	11	20	44	36	2.2	.257
				38	Bw53	3120	5.8	10	58	34	15	0.50	.168
202	NCY	MRV	MER-74	72	B35	3872	7.3	560	93	597	86	4.4	.550
				72	Bw62	3219	7.4	351	53	246	87	5.0	.666
				65	Bw72	2815	7.4	97	8	149	93	3.3	.583
				59	Bw56	2710	7.2	65	10	84	87	4.7	.601
				53	Bw50	2635	7.6	35	2	49	95	5.8	.621
				32	Bw71	2598	7.1	7	3	42	70	0.70	.311
203	FRA	MUL	FPC-104	71	B7	3945	7.3	546	49	21	92	7.1	.930
205	IT2	FER	FE-98	61	B7	3934	7.1	514	76	63	88	7.6	.860
				15	Bw60	3344	5.4	51	250	12	17	0.82	.348
207	EAE	RIC	E-10022	81	B7	3944	7.7	554	34	38	95	8.1	.928
				21	Bw73	3356	5.0	8	14	30	37	0.91	.270
209	US2	BAC	SCHLONECKER	76	B27	3938	7.8	203	10	52	96	8.8	.863
				15	B7	3725	4.9	38	530	14	7	0.35	.191
210	UKI	ENT	MESSENGER	90	B27	3931	7.9	207	4	17	99	11.0	.949
211	UKI	MID	STEELE	91	B27	3928	8.0	212	1	22	100	11.0	.947
215	US7	HAN	SEA-1094	92	B27	3934	8.0	210	4	14	99	13.0	.957
216	UKI	DIC	LOUGHLIN	66	Bw55	3916	7.8	137	3	149	98	11.0	.670
				44	Bw56	3776	6.8	72	20	77	79	6.7	.603
				33	Bw54	3684	6.0	48	126	29	28	1.8	.397

Table 1 (continued)

9wNo.:	REG	LAB.	SERUM-ID	STR	ANTIGEN	No.REAC.	AVE	+/+	MISS. +/-	EXTRA -/+	%INCL	Q-SCORE	R-VALUE
217	US3	PER	1317 A	71	Bw55	3946	7.9	143	0	297	100	10.0	.547
				59	Bw54	3803	6.7	155	29	142	85	5.8	.642
				64	Bw56	3619	7.6	89	5	53	95	7.7	.763
				32	Bw42	3525	6.1	14	30	39	32	1.4	.280
				30	Bw57	3481	6.3	13	154	26	8	0.26	.142
218	JAP	TOK	JR-50648	54	Bw54	3771	7.3	148	15	520	91	6.8	.407
				49	Bw55	3608	7.5	112	9	408	93	7.3	.414
				41	Bw56	3487	7.7	86	3	322	97	7.7	.428
				29	B35	3398	5.7	142	458	180	34	0.79	.224
				29	Bw59	2798	6.7	19	10	161	66	3.4	.246
				27	Bw58	2769	6.3	48	105	113	32	0.97	.264
				*27	Bw42	2769	6.1	14	21	147	40	2.2	.165
				*27	Bw53	2769	5.5	19	44	142	31	1.1	.159
				*27	Bw57	2769	5.5	29	124	132	19	0.35	.136
				*27	B7	2769	5.8	48	446	113	10	0.15	.078
219	JAP	HSE	AY-281	75	Bw54	3929	7.8	181	4	255	98	9.8	.614
				63	Bw55	3744	7.6	136	4	119	98	10.0	.707
				39	Bw56	3604	6.6	60	32	59	66	4.1	.561
				27	Bw42	3512	4.9	7	37	52	16	0.78	.125
				28	Bw57	3468	5.4	14	152	38	9	0.26	.128
222	JAP	TOK	JR-50514	82	Bw54	3951	7.8	186	0	22	100	12.0	.943
223	JAP	NIS	NS-1069	52	Bw54	3938	7.0	121	65	54	66	5.2	.655
				29	Bw55	3752	6.2	42	98	12	30	2.0	.472
224	JAP	SOW	KMU-658	64	Bw54	3906	7.3	178	7	61	97	10.0	.838
				32	Bw55	3721	6.2	43	98	18	31	1.8	.451
225	JAP	OKO	NYC-1179	54	Bw54	3875	6.9	133	47	39	74	5.7	.744
				30	Bw55	3695	6.0	29	109	10	22	1.2	.385
226	UKI	MID	FORSYTH	49	Bw55	3880	7.1	126	16	55	89	7.3	.777
				9	A25	3738	5.5	20	82	35	20	0.53	.252
227	US6	BRN	CC-283.1	55	Bw55	3904	7.1	124	19	45	87	7.9	.789
				22	Bw54	3761	5.9	29	154	16	16	0.89	.305
229	US5	RVE	V-1241	45	Bw55	3924	7.5	136	5	225	97	9.8	.583
				25	Bw56	3783	6.2	43	50	182	47	3.0	.270
				23	Bw54	3690	5.6	60	117	122	34	2.1	.300
				22	B7	3513	5.8	90	455	32	17	0.79	.305
				12	Bw42	2968	5.2	17	21	15	45	3.5	.481
230	GER	SCN	APS-55	58	Bw55	3928	7.7	140	2	195	99	11.0	.624
				36	Bw54	3786	6.3	100	82	95	55	3.8	.506
				37	Bw56	3604	6.2	53	41	42	57	4.1	.549
				35	Bw42	3510	6.5	31	12	11	73	5.7	.726

9wNo.:	REG	LAB.	SERUM-ID	STR	ANTIGEN	No.REAC.	AVE	+/+	MISS. +/-	EXTRA -/+	%INCL	Q-SCORE	R-VALUE
231	GER	MUE	MUE-25422/II	60	Bw55	3918	7.3	111	29	39	80	7.6	.757
				25	Bw42	3778	6.9	18	26	21	41	3.5	.428
232	NCY	KOE	P-3411-TH1	53	Bw55	3933	7.3	133	7	79	95	8.7	.762
				17	Bw42	3793	5.8	12	32	67	28	1.3	.191
				16	Bw56	3749	5.5	11	83	56	12	0.28	.120
				17	Bw62	3655	5.7	20	412	36	5	0.14	.092
233	FRA	BET	FLY-754	44	Bw56	3918	7.1	78	17	50	83	6.3	.699
				12	Bw55	3823	4.8	17	115	33	13	0.41	.193
234	GER	BER	1679 B	54	Bw56	3941	7.9	90	7	143	93	6.7	.585
				28	Bw63	3844	6.5	36	49	107	43	1.6	.307
				25	Aw24	3759	5.8	78	871	29	9	0.15	.188
235	NCY	MRV	11675	62	Bw56	3338	7.4	73	7	45	92	7.3	.744
				44	Bw55	3258	6.3	13	91	32	13	0.47	.173
236	US1	DUQ	FOX	51	Bw55	3843	7.6	132	8	246	95	7.6	.551
				34	Bw42	3703	7.1	41	2	205	96	9.0	.386
				28	B7	3660	6.1	136	407	69	26	1.1	.353
				18	Bw54	3117	5.4	29	141	40	18	0.74	.242
				27	Bw56	2947	5.7	18	64	22	22	1.1	.301
237	SAF	DUT	CT-679	34	Bw42	3908	7.1	30	15	71	67	5.6	.436
				21	Bw55	3863	5.6	23	117	48	17	0.88	.211
				20	B7	3723	5.2	39	520	9	7	0.36	.212
238	SAF	DUT	CT-521	34	Bw42	3948	6.3	32	14	29	70	6.1	.599
239	BEN	ENG	CLB-167	77	B7	3919	7.6	538	52	158	92	6.5	.809
				47	Bw42	3329	7.2	38	2	120	95	7.4	.468
				40	Bw55	3289	6.3	60	61	60	50	2.5	.479
				38	Bw56	3168	6.9	28	51	32	36	1.9	.394
240	US8	LEE	WILL	25	Bw55	3868	6.7	66	62	193	52	2.4	.332
				17	Bw42	3740	5.7	23	19	170	55	4.1	.239
				15	B7	3698	5.4	79	478	91	15	0.35	.193
				13	Bw54	3141	5.4	16	152	75	10	0.20	.094
				*13	B8	3141	5.2	31	359	44	8	0.19	.113
				*13	Bw41	3141	4.7	10	76	34	13	0.55	.098
241	LAT	JRM	ED 234	20	Bw41	3808	6.7	44	59	238	43	1.3	.225
				15	Bw42	3705	6.3	20	23	218	47	1.5	.177
242	US5	ABS	AZ-77	63	B27	3929	7.6	203	12	145	95	6.6	.725
				35	Bw47	3714	7.0	30	10	115	75	3.8	.383
				27	B13	3674	6.0	24	120	91	17	0.53	.157

9wNo.:	REG	LAB.	SERUM-ID	STR	ANTIGEN	No.REAC.	AVE	+/+	MISS. +/-	EXTRA -/+	%INCL	Q-SCORE	R-VALUE
243	US6	BRN	CC-182.1	65	B27	3927	7.9	212	4	304	99	6.9	.607
				43	Cw2	3710	6.3	100	146	204	41	1.7	.315
				47	Bw47	3465	7.6	31	9	173	78	3.4	.329
				40	B7	3425	5.8	78	456	95	15	0.27	.188
				52	B13	2891	6.5	24	107	71	19	0.36	.184
245	EAE	MYR	KAPPL	89	B7	3892	7.9	572	13	746	98	7.7	.568
				82	Bw60	3307	7.7	248	43	498	86	4.6	.466
				80	B27	3016	7.9	173	7	325	97	6.6	.540
				71	Bw55	2839	7.6	95	12	230	89	5.2	.481
				65	Bw48	2729	7.8	49	6	181	90	5.1	.416
				58	Bw56	2674	6.9	53	22	128	71	3.2	.432
				*58	Bw42	2674	7.9	37	2	144	95	5.8	.427
				*58	Bw73	2674	7.2	17	3	164	85	0.75	.270
				*58	Bw67	2674	7.3	6	2	175	75	3.3	.149
				*58	Cw1	2674	6.6	55	299	126	16		.136
246	EAE	RIC	N-1010	92	B7	3951	8.0	592	3	723	100	8.6	.592
				86	Bw60	3356	7.9	294	6	429	98	7.3	.583
				79	B27	3056	8.0	180	3	249	99	7.2	.613
				65	Bw48	2873	8.0	56	1	193	99	6.6	.453
				56	Bw42	2816	7.8	36	1	154	98	6.0	.431
				48	Bw55	2776	6.6	57	48	97	55	2.3	.422
				*48	Bw73	2776	7.1	19	1	154	95	0.80	.333
				*48	Bw67	2776	6.4	5	3	149	63	3.5	.134
				*48	Bw56	2776	5.8	18	61	136	23	0.45	.129
247	EAE	RIC	B-10757	89	B7	3935	8.0	584	5	599	100	8.2	.632
				81	B27	3346	7.9	192	5	407	98	6.7	.519
				74	Bw55	3149	8.0	110	5	297	96	6.3	.480
				66	Bw56	3034	7.7	74	4	223	95	5.8	.465
				57	Bw42	2956	8.0	37	1	186	98	6.5	.388
				49	Bw73	2918	7.4	17	4	169	81	0.45	.260
				*49	Bw65	2918	6.4	59	164	127	27	0.63	.236
				*49	Bw48	2918	7.2	22	34	164	40	1.4	.188
				*49	Bw67	2918	8.0	8	1	178	89		.188
248	US8	FOT	FOT-WARM	90	B8	3949	7.9	439	1	75	100	11.0	.913
				61	B7	3509	6.8	61	494	14	11	0.33	.265
249	SAF	DUT	CT-716	66	B8	3932	7.1	394	40	21	91	7.4	.920
250	US7	DUP	HINRICHS	81	B8	3904	7.6	423	14	12	81	9.8	.966
253	US3	GRU	AQ-9540	85	B51	3923	7.7	429	21	178	96	7.8	.795
				74	Bw52	3473	7.6	135	17	43	89	6.5	.812
				37	Bw59	3321	5.8	9	22	34	30	1.5	.238

9wNo.:	REG	LAB.	SERUM-ID	STR	ANTIGEN	No.REAC.	AVE	+/+	MISS. +/-	EXTRA -/+	%INCL	Q-SCORE	R-VALUE
254	JAP	TOK	50-92	36	B51	3942	6.1	120	330	102	27	1.0	.328
				31	Bw59	3492	6.5	23	10	79	70	3.8	.387
				29	Bw49	3456	5.8	13	75	65	15	0.42	.136
				27	B38	3368	6.5	11	157	54	7	0.066	.077
				22	Bw52	3200	4.5	8	137	46	6	0.16	.065
255	JAP	SAK	20616	82	B8	3863	7.9	429	8	117	99	8.6	.862
				36	Bw59	3426	7.8	30	6	87	84	5.2	.453
				18	A32	3390	5.9	15	159	72	9	0.063	.089
				16	Aw33	3114	4.9	14	250	48	6	0.10	.072
256	JAP	JUJ	1-519	50	Bw59	3947	7.2	34	6	202	85	5.5	.337
				46	B51	3907	6.6	57	386	145	13	0.30	.124
				44	B49	3464	6.7	18	69	127	21	0.83	.132
				42	B8	3377	5.9	33	382	94	8	0.10	.082
257	JAP	MNA	A-2420	38	Bw59	3928	6.2	26	14	174	65	4.0	.276
				36	B8	3888	5.8	95	336	79	23	0.72	.300
				45	B7	3457	7.3	41	511	38	8	0.21	.150
258	JAP	SAJ	35-PK-18	46	Bw59	3945	6.4	26	14	87	65	4.8	.377
				47	B8	3905	5.6	39	401	48	9	0.40	.160
				*47	B7	3905	7.3	40	550	47	7	0.17	.130
259	US4	STA	JUNGMAN	79	B8	3945	7.9	431	8	230	99	7.4	.771
				47	A1	3506	6.4	153	253	77	38	2.0	.455
				51	Bw59	3100	7.7	30	7	47	82	3.9	.555
				27	Bw65	3063	5.3	14	193	33	7	0.19	.115
260	US5	CMC	2482-K	43	Bw64	3923	6.5	65	47	34	59	4.2	.607
				41	Bw65	3811	6.8	16	241	18	7	0.24	.153
261	UKI	DEW	DB-2080	49	Bw64	3921	7.1	84	27	57	76	5.1	.661
				28	Bw65	3810	6.4	19	234	38	8	0.25	.132
262	US5	MIT	C-4170	66	Bw65	3954	7.2	250	15	25	95	8.9	.921
				36	Bw64	3684	5.7	15	88	10	15	1.0	.287
263	UKI	DEW	DB-3407	72	Bw65	3427	7.4	201	41	23	84	7.5	.853
				30	Bw64	3185	6.1	18	71	5	21	1.4	.391
264	UKI	DRK	LITCHFIELD-655-D	60	Bw65	3389	7.2	214	24	40	90	8.6	.860
				5	Bw64	3151	4.8	26	58	14	31	2.1	.439
265	GER	BRA	BRA-173-B1:2	79	Cw8	3891	7.6	310	40	34	89	7.3	.883
				*79	Bw65	3891	7.7	246	13	98	95	9.0	.810
				*79	Bw64	3891	7.2	79	24	265	77	5.9	.394
266	GER	SUD	HB-11011,1:2	75	Bw65	3916	7.7	255	11	57	96	10.0	.876
				19	Bw64	3650	5.6	47	54	10	19	3.1	.612

Table 1 (continued)

9wNo.:	REG	LAB.	SERUM-ID	STR	ANTIGEN	No.REAC.	AVE	+/+	MISS. +/-	EXTRA -/+	%INCL	Q-SCORE	R-VALUE
267	FRA	MUL	FPC-105	90	Cw8	3947	7.6	353	12	15	97	10.0	.959
				*90	Bw65	3947	7.9	264	1	104	100	14.0	.833
				*90	Bw64	3947	7.5	105	7	263	94	10.0	.496
270	NCY	YUN	YUN/SUL	82	Cw8	3943	7.9	359	7	70	99	9.0	.896
				25	Bw64	3577	6.5	4	0	60	100	9.0	.237
				24	Bw65	3573	8.0	4	0	62	100	12.0	.244
				19	B8	3569	5.4	38	350	24	10	0.33	.215
272	EAE	MYR	HEIBL	86	Cw8	3956	7.9	356	11	64	98	8.2	.897
				28	Bw65	3589	8.0	5	0	59	100	10.0	.277
				22	Bw64	3584	8.0	4	0	55	100	9.3	.258
				16	B8	3580	5.4	40	353	15	11	0.31	.247
274	US5	ABS	AZ-218	81	Cw5	3886	7.4	408	49	356	90	6.0	.639
				86	Cw8	3429	7.8	320	12	36	97	8.3	.923
				*86	Bw64	3429	7.8	100	3	256	98	4.7	.500
				*86	Bw65	3429	7.8	227	11	129	96	4.9	.761
275	IT2	FER	FE-16	76	Cw8	3930	7.7	349	16	153	96	6.5	.794
				*76	Bw65	3930	7.8	257	9	245	97	9.2	.677
				*76	Bw64	3930	7.5	106	5	396	96	9.3	.423
				48	B18	3565	6.6	128	113	25	54	3.8	.649
276	IT2	FER	FE-105	76	Bw62	3946	7.4	416	36	65	93	8.4	.878
				63	Bw63	3494	7.0	58	22	7	90	5.7	.800
277	IT1	NIE	TV-401-1	77	Bw62	3951	7.6	418	31	81	94	9.3	.867
				41	Bw63	3502	6.9	48	32	33	60	4.4	.587
				15	Bw57	3422	5.7	15	142	18	10	0.30	.193
278	GER	WEI	HU-3937	80	Bw62	3954	7.7	440	13	115	98	8.8	.860
				45	Bw63	3501	7.0	58	22	57	73	4.6	.594
				24	Bw57	3421	5.3	25	131	32	17	0.47	.245
281	JAP	JUJ	1-615	79	Bw62	3952	7.8	439	13	131	98	8.1	.846
				45	Bw63	3500	6.9	60	20	71	75	4.2	.574
				30	Bw65	3420	6.0	16	233	55	7	0.077	.085
				37	Bw54	2909	6.4	10	157	30	6		.098
282	GER	ALB	BK-947-3	89	Bw62	3952	7.8	430	23	26	95	9.0	.939
284	FRA	OHA	FTO-262	83	Bw62	3877	7.6	393	46	15	90	7.3	.920
285	FRA	MAY	FST-11	88	Bw62	3883	7.7	388	50	2	89	8.8	.932
286	BEN	ROO	vR-57467.5	85	Bw62	3940	7.6	401	51	4	89	8.4	.930
289	JAP	TOK	JR-50-903	58	Bw62	3910	6.8	314	137	12	70	5.2	.800

9wNo.:	REG	LAB.	SERUM-ID	STR	ANTIGEN	No.REAC.	AVE	+/+	MISS. +/-	EXTRA -/+	%INCL	Q-SCORE	R-VALUE
290	ANZ	BSH	BD-815	70	Bw57	3928	7.7	172	2	212	99	10.0	.646
				55	Bw58	3754	7.2	158	13	54	93	7.2	.821
				12	Cw6	3579	5.3	19	267	34	7	1.3	.126
291	NCY	MRV	5097	84	Bw57	3394	7.8	140	3	166	98	9.2	.651
				81	Bw58	3251	7.8	142	13	24	92	8.4	.879
292	LAT	GOR	GM-00025	73	Bw58	3938	8.0	176	1	327	100	8.7	.563
				60	Bw57	3761	8.0	169	0	158	100	9.1	.703
				20	A24	3592	5.4	64	873	94	7	0.022	.070
293	US5	FTV	SHOR	83	Bw57	3948	7.7	174	0	189	100	12.0	.675
				80	Bw58	3774	7.7	171	1	18	100	12.0	.946
296	US8	LEE	SWIE	87	Bw57	3928	7.8	171	1	204	100	11.0	.654
				83	Bw58	3756	7.9	168	3	36	99	10.0	.894
				36	B51	3585	6.8	15	417	21	4	0.083	.092
298	US4	STA	SPRIGGS	74	Bw57	3902	7.6	163	7	154	96	11.0	.686
				63	Bw58	3732	7.1	141	29	13	83	6.9	.866
299	EAE	WEG	R-236	58	Bw57	3921	7.2	153	17	187	90	8.5	.615
				50	Bw58	3751	6.3	118	47	69	72	5.8	.656
				68	Bw63	3586	7.2	62	12	7	84	6.7	.865
301	EAE	WEG	R-176	81	Bw57	3914	7.6	162	8	339	96	7.1	.526
				79	Bw58	3744	7.5	152	19	187	89	5.4	.609
				79	A29	3573	7.7	148	30	39	84	2.9	.801
				33	Aw43	3394	7.1	7	0	32	100	4.1	.422
302	GER	MUE	MUE-28216/2	66	Bw57	3935	7.7	167	6	78	97	10.0	.801
				23	Bw62	3762	5.8	44	400	34	10	0.23	.201
				20	Bw58	3318	5.5	11	151	23	7	0.24	.130
303	GER	GOL	8975 V	71	Bw57	3930	7.3	157	17	7	91	9.1	.926
304	NCY	YAG	KELLY	50	Bw57	3886	6.9	150	23	75	87	7.3	.748
				36	Bw58	3713	6.2	51	119	24	30	1.8	.436
305	US5	FTV	RAND	85	Bw57	3819	7.9	174	0	298	100	11.0	.582
				79	Bw58	3645	7.9	166	2	132	99	9.6	.727
				59	Bw63	3477	7.9	69	6	63	92	6.9	.685
				17	Bw62	3402	5.2	31	378	32	8	0.16	.157
306	ANZ	ROB	BATES	78	Bw57	3849	7.6	161	6	208	97	8.9	.628
				73	Bw58	3682	7.7	156	11	52	94	7.6	.829
				32	Bw63	3515	6.0	19	51	33	28	1.3	.303
				33	Bw62	3445	6.4	11	401	22	3	0.019	.065

9wNo.:	REG	LAB.	SERUM-ID	STR	ANTIGEN	No.REAC.	AVE	+/+	MISS. +/-	EXTRA -/+	%INCL	Q-SCORE	R-VALUE
307	BEN	ENG	CLB-176	82	Bw62	3908	8.0	430	4	438	100	11.0	.654
				66	Bw57	3474	7.5	164	3	274	99	8.9	.579
				56	Bw63	3307	7.9	71	0	203	100	9.4	.493
				41	Bw46	3236	7.8	72	5	131	94	6.9	.562
				16	B35	3159	5.3	61	528	70	11	0.16	.149
				15	Bw15.3	3132	6.0	3	0	123	100	0.049	.151
				*15	Bw53	3132	5.2	12	58	114	18	0.38	.101
308	GER	WES	A3624/III	92	Bw62	3913	8.0	439	4	351	100	9.9	.702
				84	Bw57	3470	7.8	156	3	195	99	8.7	.640
				79	Bw46	3311	7.7	77	3	118	97	7.8	.604
				74	Bw63	3231	7.9	71	0	47	100	8.8	.770
309	EAE	WEG	R-177	85	Bw62	3927	8.0	446	2	394	100	12.0	.684
				69	Bw57	3479	7.7	160	3	234	99	9.1	.608
				57	Bw63	3316	8.0	71	0	163	100	9.3	.537
				39	Bw46	3245	6.8	58	22	105	73	5.1	.491
				30	B13	3165	5.8	43	91	62	33	1.3	.338
				32	Bw72	3031	5.7	15	77	47	17	1.3	.178
				*32	B35	3031	5.9	30	553	32	6	0.11	.107
310	ANZ	HAY	HIGGS 180381	84	Bw62	3933	7.9	444	9	317	99	9.8	.718
				70	Bw57	3480	7.3	150	16	167	91	7.4	.632
				65	Bw63	3314	7.9	70	1	97	99	8.8	.633
				45	Bw46	3243	6.9	63	14	34	82	6.1	.722
311	UKI	BRS	6957 DUM	75	B35	3902	7.2	553	112	585	84	4.2	.540
				80	Bw62	3237	7.6	375	26	207	94	6.0	.740
				73	Bw72	2836	7.8	102	3	105	98	3.4	.677
				55	Bw50	2731	7.8	34	4	71	90	6.4	.529
				38	Bw71	2693	5.6	10	1	61	91	0.63	.353
				42	B45	2682	6.2	10	23	51	31	1.5	.210
				*42	Bw63	2682	6.7	9	64	52	13	0.31	.113
				*42	Bw57	2682	6.4	9	132	52	7	0.038	.065
312	UKI	BRS	8069 CBT	80	B35	3955	7.9	652	15	1006	98	6.8	.510
				70	Bw62	3288	7.6	389	20	617	96	5.9	.528
				61	Bw72	2879	7.7	106	1	511	100	3.4	.372
				56	Bw58	2772	7.4	104	42	407	72	2.4	.321
				51	Bw57	2626	6.8	97	46	310	68	2.4	.347
				49	Bw53	2483	7.5	50	6	260	90	4.7	.353
				*49	Bw50	2483	7.8	35	2	275	95	5.9	.306
				*49	Bw56	2483	6.6	49	25	261	67	2.3	.285
				*49	Bw71	2483	6.4	9	1	301	90	0.49	.075
				*49	Bw15.3	2483	7.0	3	0	308	100	5.8	.075
				*49	Cw1	2483	6.3	120	304	190	29	0.13	.271
				*49	Cw4	2483	7.3	55	83	255	40	1.5	.201
313	UKI	BRS	7809 CBT	86	B35	3922	8.0	652	7	1522	99	7.2	.393
				81	B51	3263	8.0	401	2	1121	100	7.0	.398
				75	Bw62	2860	7.6	354	16	767	96	5.6	.446
				69	Bw52	2490	7.9	134	2	633	99	6.1	.353
				63	B18	2354	7.5	157	35	476	82	3.4	.369
				57	Bw72	2162	7.9	99	3	377	98	4.1	.403
				*57	Bw53	2162	7.7	54	1	422	99	5.6	.297
				*57	Bw71	2162	6.9	11	0	4	100	0.51	.135
				*57	Bw15.3	2162	6.0	3	0	473	100	6.2	.070
				*57	B39	2162	6.8	87	64	389	58	1.4	.235
				*57	B38	2162	6.6	75	65	401	54	1.2	.200
				*57	Bw59	2162	6.7	22	8	454	74	1.7	.147
				*57	Cw4	2162	7.4	81	50	395	62	1.2	.244
				*57	Aw34	2162	7.4	24	13	452	65	0.25	.136
314	FRA	DAU	FPA-BERT	61	Cw7	3915	7.0	1007	331	97	76	3.4	.754
				35	B7	2577	5.7	15	87	82	15	1.1	.117
				35	B8	2475	5.4	7	65	75	10	1.5	.062
315	GER	EHR	EHR-2141/III	88	B35	3927	7.9	643	19	1145	98	6.3	.467
				84	B51	3265	7.8	385	19	760	96	5.7	.474
				81	Bw62	2861	7.6	338	31	422	92	4.9	.567
				77	Bw52	2492	7.9	132	4	290	98	5.3	.513
				68	Bw72	2356	7.5	95	9	195	92	2.4	.517
				61	Bw53	2252	7.9	53	4	142	93	6.3	.483
				*61	Bw50	2252	6.6	17	11	178	61	2.3	.208
				*61	B49	2252	7.3	30	40	165	43	1.1	.218
				*61	B18	2252	6.7	52	139	143	28	0.48	.201
				*61	Cw4	2252	7.8	47	81	148	37	1.1	.245
316	SAF	HAN	N-389	68	Bw62	3699	7.7	360	40	842	90	5.7	.428
				59	Bw35	3299	7.0	406	161	436	72	3.1	.482
				55	Bw72	2732	6.6	75	28	361	73	1.2	.307
				56	Bw63	2629	7.3	55	17	306	77	3.9	.305
				53	Bw51	2557	6.6	126	216	180	37	1.0	.301
				55	Bw53	2215	7.0	39	16	141	71	3.5	.367
				*55	Bw46	2215	7.3	40	20	140	67	2.7	.357
				*55	Bw57	2215	6.8	54	66	126	45	1.4	.323
				*55	B49	2215	6.5	17	48	163	27	0.56	.115
				*55	Bw50	2215	5.7	7	20	173	26	0.69	.072
500	US3	NES	BOWLES	72	Cw8	3935	7.4	295	63	73	83	5.0	.794
				*72	Bw65	3935	7.7	248	16	120	94	6.9	.779
				*72	Bw64	3935	6.3	58	48	310	55	2.5	.259

Table 1 (continued)

9wNo.:	REG	LAB.	SERUM-ID	STR	ANTIGEN	No.REAC.	AVE	+/+	MISS. +/-	EXTRA -/+	%INCL	Q-SCORE	R-VALUE
317	BEN	ROO	vR 26756.2	84	B35	3913	7.9	637	23	1150	97	6.3	.460
				78	B51	3253	7.9	395	11	755	98	6.4	.489
				69	Bw62	2847	7.3	285	84	470	78	3.3	.443
				67	Bw52	2478	7.8	121	12	349	91	4.9	.437
				59	B18	2345	7.1	123	70	226	64	2.1	.411
				55	Bw72	2152	6.8	74	29	152	72	2.2	.449
				*55	Bw53	2152	7.9	45	11	181	81	3.9	.372
				*55	Cw4	2152	7.6	47	84	179	36	1.1	.211
318	FRA	DAU	FPA-R-424	79	A1	3923	7.9	687	14	372	99	6.3	.746
				47	Bw57	3222	7.1	77	14	295	85	3.0	.390
				42	Bw58	3131	6.7	84	70	211	55	0.82	.351
				36	A11	2977	6.3	98	324	113	24	0.40	.256
				34	Aw36	2548	6.0	9	12	104	43	0.86	.170
				34	A24	2533	6.0	55	700	49	8	0.036	.104
319	FRA	DAU	FPA-K-1200	89	A2	3892	7.8	1892	78	200	97	4.7	.859
				75	Bw57	1922	7.7	95	2	105	98	2.5	.661
				61	Bw58	1825	7.1	89	12	16	89	1.3	.856
320	FRA	BIG	FNN-CHA	60	A2	3366	6.9	1223	478	130	72	2.6	.654
				60	Bw57	1665	7.1	68	11	62	87	1.8	.651
				56	Bw58	1586	6.7	56	37	6	61	0.90	.725
321	FRA	OHA	FTO-102	63	A2	3922	7.0	1534	457	114	78	3.2	.721
				46	Bw57	1931	6.6	63	33	51	66	0.83	.580
				45	Bw58	1835	6.6	37	65	14	37	0.24	.494
322	FRA	OHA	FTO-217	47	Bw57	3899	7.0	135	34	232	80	4.4	.514
				38	Bw58	3730	6.5	108	65	124	63	2.5	.513
				31	Aw69	3554	5.8	46	237	78	17	0.19	.205
				28	A2	3274	5.5	70	1496	8	5	0.080	.131
323	FRA	BET	FLY-723	63	A23	3936	7.9	139	4	449	98	5.0	.448
				53	Bw57	3793	6.7	131	37	318	78	3.5	.441
				52	Bw56	3625	7.8	82	11	236	89	4.1	.455
				37	Bw63	3532	7.1	57	15	179	80	3.1	.419
				28	Bw58	3460	5.6	57	95	122	38	1.3	.313
				31	Bw55	3308	5.6	36	99	86	27	0.85	.251
				*31	A24	3307	5.8	87	799	35	10	0.090	.197
324	US5	PNW	ARC-PNW-POHL	62	B37	3957	7.5	82	5	34	95	9.0	.812
				26	B18	3870	6.1	17	243	17	7	0.25	.163
325	UKI	DIC	McISAAC	59	B37	3955	7.3	84	3	29	97	9.6	.843
327	GER	SCN	SCN-AVC-37	55	B37	3914	7.8	86	0	120	100	9.2	.636
				29	B27	3828	6.1	23	191	97	11	0.16	.106
				25	Aw69	3611	5.4	19	272	78	7	0.040	.070
				24	Bw47	3475	6.0	5	33	82	14	0.42	.072
				*24	B39	3475	5.1	13	179	74	7	0.023	.066
329	UKI	GEL	TTT-10400-d	60	B37	3906	7.9	82	1	58	99	9.6	.755
				12	B8	3823	5.1	16	416	42	4	0.015	.064
332	SCA	JER	TS-43	61	B39	3910	7.9	194	8	485	97	6.5	.485
				48	B38	3708	7.8	170	2	315	99	8.2	.561
				26	A3	3536	5.7	137	469	178	23	0.30	.219
				26	Bw67	2930	7.8	9	2	169	82	1.5	.195
				23	B35	2919	5.6	60	425	109	13	0.086	.126
				29	Bw42	2441	8.0	10	27	97	28	0.57	.137
333	US4	BRG	SS-0791-82	80	B39	3918	8.0	203	2	384	100	8.7	.553
				70	B38	3713	8.0	171	0	213	100	9.5	.647
				46	Bw55	3542	6.4	51	85	162	38	1.4	.265
				46	Bw42	3406	7.4	26	17	136	61	2.8	.296
				39	Bw67	3363	8.0	8	3	128	73	2.6	.200
				35	Bw59	3352	6.2	12	22	116	36	1.3	.166
				*35	Bw41	3352	5.1	17	69	111	20	0.58	.135
				*35	B8	3352	6.0	43	357	85	11	0.21	.133
335	BEN	BRX	BOYEZ 38	87	B39	3949	7.7	196	9	180	96	9.1	.686
				86	B38	3744	7.7	175	1	5	100	11.0	.982
337	UKI	DEW	DB-1950	64	B38	3946	7.4	159	25	75	87	7.4	.754
				34	B39	3762	6.0	56	140	19	29	1.1	.446
339	GER	BRA	BRA-896	70	B38	3964	7.4	157	28	38	85	5.5	.818
				44	Bw59	3779	5.2	5	33	33	14	0.91	.123
340	NCY	KOE	SJ-142-HK-1	67	B38	3897	8.0	179	1	129	100	11.0	.747
				24	Bw59	3717	6.7	20	18	109	53	2.2	.273
				18	B51	3679	5.3	44	382	65	11	0.24	.157
				18	B49	3253	4.6	16	67	49	20	0.79	.200
				22	Bw52	3170	5.2	17	128	32	12	0.65	.181
341	JAP	TOK	JR-50-278-2	64	B39	3954	7.2	181	24	53	89	5.8	.816
				43	B38	3749	5.6	10	165	43	6	0.093	.081
342	JAP	OSA	JR-36-69	79	B39	3959	7.6	196	9	22	96	9.6	.923
				27	Bw41	3754	6.0	10	88	12	11	0.80	.206

9wNo.:	REG	LAB.	SERUM-ID	STR	ANTIGEN	No.REAC.	AVE	+/+	MISS. +/-	EXTRA -/+	%INCL	Q-SCORE	R-VALUE
343	JAP	NAI	FD-1483	81	B39	3934	7.6	188	16	23	93	8.0	.901
				43	B38	3730	5.7	6	168	17	4	0.079	.080
344	US7	DUP	MAGUILLI-800	61	B39	3948	7.5	186	16	64	93	7.6	.818
				14	B8	3746	5.4	37	392	27	9	0.16	.192
346	BEN	BRU	WOL-136	84	B13	3923	7.8	154	2	23	99	11.0	.924
348	FRA	BET	FLY-813	90	B13	3930	8.0	155	1	18	100	11.0	.941
352	ANZ	SER	BDA-FRAN	75	B13	3944	7.6	143	12	22	93	9.4	.890
353	BEN	ENG	CLB-83	79	Bw61	3928	7.6	374	42	476	90	7.7	.571
				76	Bw60	3512	7.8	292	8	184	98	10.0	.748
				49	Bw48	3212	7.7	40	9	144	82	6.7	.407
				38	B13	3163	6.2	51	87	93	37	2.0	.332
				36	B7	3025	6.3	77	447	16	15	0.69	.308
355	UKI	MOR	KEATING	84	Bw61	3947	7.8	402	12	483	98	9.8	.613
				77	Bw60	3533	8.0	289	11	194	97	9.7	.733
				46	Bw48	3233	7.6	42	6	152	88	6.9	.421
				36	B7	3185	6.0	89	441	63	17	0.53	.252
				34	B13	2655	6.1	35	99	28	27	1.3	.360
				28	Bw47	2521	6.3	7	27	21	21	1.2	.217
356	FRA	BET	FLY-1004	71	Bw60	3891	8.0	330	2	436	100	11.0	.612
				52	Bw61	3559	6.7	271	106	165	72	5.2	.626
				49	B13	3182	6.8	82	61	83	58	2.8	.510
				42	Bw48	3039	6.1	30	19	53	62	3.6	.459
				49	Bw47	2990	7.1	21	16	32	57	3.8	.466
357	JAP	TOK	JR-50-731	75	Bw61	3944	7.3	360	54	335	87	7.2	.623
				74	Bw60	3530	7.6	260	37	75	88	7.3	.807
				42	B13	3233	6.3	44	99	31	31	1.4	.407
				41	Bw47	3090	6.6	10	28	21	27	1.7	.283
359	US4	BRG	CANADY	84	Bw61	3927	7.7	383	30	463	93	8.3	.594
				82	Bw60	3514	8.0	294	5	169	99	10.0	.768
				56	Bw48	3215	7.9	44	5	125	90	6.5	.471
				41	Bw41	3166	6.0	42	54	83	44	2.6	.361
				45	B7	3070	6.7	68	453	15	14	0.45	.288
360	BEN	REE	10272	65	Bw60	3941	7.8	327	6	368	99	9.6	.642
				40	Bw41	3608	7.4	81	19	287	81	6.0	.395
				30	B7	3508	6.0	129	422	158	24	0.99	.240
				26	Bw48	2957	5.7	22	36	136	38	1.6	.205
				26	Bw61	2899	6.0	56	285	80	17	0.73	.203
				21	B13	2558	5.0	16	114	64	13	0.29	.122
				*21	B44	2558	5.8	58	635	22	9	0.25	.184

9wNo.:	REG	LAB.	SERUM-ID	STR	ANTIGEN	No.REAC.	AVE	+/+	MISS. +/-	EXTRA -/+	%INCL	Q-SCORE	R-VALUE
362	UKI	MID	FRYERS	57	Bw60	3934	6.9	282	50	43	85	7.5	.846
				25	Bw48	3602	6.3	28	33	15	46	3.0	.540
363	UKI	MID	MULHOLLAND	75	Bw60	3956	7.5	315	16	39	96	8.8	.913
				12	Bw61	3625	4.6	20	364	19	6	0.29	.138
365	US8	LEE	SZUH	81	Bw60	3946	7.9	328	5	103	99	11.0	.852
				32	Bw48	3613	6.5	34	26	69	57	3.5	.420
				28	Bw47	3553	6.2	11	28	58	11	1.2	.200
				29	B13	3514	6.0	16	131	42	11	0.31	.151
				28	Bw61	3367	5.8	18	345	24	5	0.25	.116
366	US5	CMC	11024 K	60	Bw61	3889	7.2	330	74	248	82	5.7	.640
				52	Bw60	3485	6.9	176	119	72	60	3.9	.622
				30	Bw47	3190	6.0	18	22	54	45	2.4	.324
				25	B13	3150	6.1	24	114	30	18	0.98	.259
				20	Bw41	3012	4.9	7	86	23	8	0.64	.117
368	FRA	BET	FLY-475	78	Bw61	3928	7.7	405	10	764	98	8.8	.510
				73	Bw60	3513	8.0	295	3	469	99	10.0	.570
				57	B7	3215	6.9	361	168	108	69	3.8	.675
				40	Bw48	2686	7.6	42	2	66	96	8.5	.601
				10	B13	2641	5.4	14	120	51	11	0.17	.119
369	JAP	TOK	JR-50-636	68	Bw60	3918	7.7	320	10	232	97	11.0	.722
				41	Bw61	3588	5.9	161	221	71	43	3.1	.501
				63	Bw48	3206	7.8	41	8	30	84	7.3	.690
				30	Bw41	3157	5.8	9	88	21	10	0.51	.153
370	JAP	TOK	JR-50-491	61	Bw60	3952	7.0	294	39	81	89	7.1	.816
				46	Bw48	3619	6.3	39	23	42	63	4.4	.541
				54	B13	3557	7.0	18	131	24	13	0.27	.211
372	GER	SUD	SUD-HB-7089	84	Bw61	3930	7.5	379	36	533	92	9.8	.554
				88	Bw60	3515	7.9	290	9	243	97	11.0	.696
				79	B13	3216	8.0	142	1	101	100	13.0	.749
				50	Bw47	3073	7.3	33	5	68	87	7.6	.524
				38	B27	3035	5.3	17	175	51	9	0.19	.116
				43	Bw50	2843	6.7	6	36	45	15	0.53	.115
				*43	B49	2843	6.0	8	70	43	11	0.37	.107
				*43	B44	2843	6.9	28	714	23	4	0.11	.089
373	FRA	FAU	FRE-125	91	Bw61	3872	7.9	410	4	496	100	11.0	.618
				88	Bw60	3458	8.0	280	4	216	99	10.0	.719
				74	B13	3174	7.7	135	3	81	98	10.0	.771
				54	Bw47	3036	7.4	32	5	49	87	6.0	.578
				36	Bw48	2999	6.6	25	23	24	53	3.4	.508

Table 1 (continued)

9wNo.:	REG	LAB.	SERUM-ID	STR	ANTIGEN	No.REAC.	AVE	+/+	MISS. +/-	EXTRA -/+	%INCL	Q-SCORE	R-VALUE
374	FRA	MUL	ENG	96	Bw61	3888	7.9	411	4	467	100	11.0	.632
				95	Bw60	3473	8.0	281	14	186	96	9.7	.731
				91	B13	3178	7.9	142	0	44	100	12.0	.867
				77	Bw47	3036	7.9	35	3	9	93	8.3	.854
376	JAP	OSA	JR-36-79	88	Bw61	3956	7.9	414	2	566	100	10.0	.594
				83	Bw60	3540	7.9	285	13	281	96	8.4	.659
				69	B13	3242	7.9	142	1	139	100	10.0	.692
				41	Bw47	3099	7.8	37	1	102	98	7.4	.500
				23	Bw41	3061	5.5	31	62	71	34	1.6	.296
				21	B27	2968	5.9	18	171	53	10	0.24	.122
377	BEN	REE	10903	60	B27	3934	8.0	200	16	531	93	4.8	.459
				46	A32	3718	7.5	162	25	369	87	2.9	.476
				32	B7	3531	5.9	166	370	203	31	0.78	.284
				33	B13	2995	6.4	62	77	141	45	1.3	.332
				30	Bw47	2856	6.4	23	10	118	70	2.6	.323
				29	A25	2823	5.2	25	56	93	31	0.40	.229
				*29	Bw60	2823	6.0	42	221	76	16	0.38	.189
				*29	Bw61	2823	5.9	37	313	81	11	0.13	.120
378	FRA	COR	FCO-717	70	B44	3874	7.6	784	76	396	92	5.7	.705
				39	Bw4	3014	6.2	352	1067	44	25	2.0	.326
				27	B45	1595	4.0	6	29	38	18	0.28	.132
380	GER	SCN	SCN-JCN-AGB-41	45	Bw41	3932	6.7	87	17	72	84	5.9	.666
				36	Bw42	3828	5.6	10	33	62	24	0.64	.168
				37	Bw60	3785	5.7	25	301	37	8	0.26	.146
				45	Bw47	3459	6.5	4	36	33	10	0.48	.094
381	BEN	ROO	vR-58496.7	34	Bw41	3362	6.2	67	24	41	74	4.6	.666
				19	B44	3271	5.1	20	727	21	3	0.043	.070
384	US8	CRC	L-330	40	Bw41	3918	7.0	91	13	173	88	6.7	.532
				29	Bw60	3814	6.2	101	222	72	32	1.3	.391
				18	Bw61	3491	5.3	45	330	27	12	0.43	.243
386	NCY	YUN	YUN-CUT	49	Bw41	3897	7.0	89	13	133	88	5.3	.577
				39	B13	3795	6.9	32	118	101	22	0.46	.197
				31	Bw42	3645	6.3	14	28	87	34	1.1	.201
387	NCY	YUN	YUN-BER	80	B44	3905	7.5	829	46	108	95	7.4	.890
				48	B45	3030	7.4	44	4	64	92	6.3	.603
388	EAE	ZAR	MZ-202	91	B44	3873	7.9	850	13	62	99	9.6	.946
				59	B45	3010	7.1	40	7	22	86	6.0	.736
393	US6	BRN	CCB-146.1	68	B44	3872	7.2	718	134	75	85	6.2	.840
				46	B45	3020	7.3	39	6	36	87	6.5	.665
394	NCY	YUN	YUN-BLA	85	B44	3875	7.7	832	29	31	97	8.3	.955
396	SAF	HAM	N-137	80	B44	3864	7.7	824	35	136	96	8.3	.879
				30	B27	3005	5.9	54	141	82	28	0.90	.294
				31	Bw4	2810	6.0	78	1155	4	7	2.4	.179
398	ANZ	DAW	HOULISTON 40578	87	B44	3931	7.9	872	1	172	100	9.9	.887
				35	Bw4	3058	6.0	159	1282	13	12	2.1	.222
399	US1	SOB	SOB-261	87	B44	3903	8.0	864	8	180	100	8.8	.876
				31	Bw4	3031	5.9	149	1279	31	11	2.0	.180
400	SCA	KIS	34675/79	53	B45	3871	7.4	49	2	67	97	11.0	.631
				34	B44	3820	6.1	60	795	7	8	0.38	.215
401	US1	NWO	SHERRYWARE	60	B44	3881	6.9	503	345	108	60	2.7	.633
				60	B45	3033	7.8	46	1	62	98	7.3	.639
				35	Bw50	2986	5.0	4	42	58	9	0.17	.058
402	US1	DUQ	GEBOY	46	B45	3942	7.0	48	4	45	93	6.9	.685
				26	B44	3890	6.1	32	834	13	4	0.13	.127
404	US3	PER	P.0025-A	57	B49	3916	6.9	62	24	114	73	3.8	.489
				56	Bw50	3830	7.2	30	19	84	62	3.0	.390
				50	B44	3781	6.6	29	821	55	4	0.021	.043
405	EAE	MYR	SCHERTER	75	B49	3852	7.6	82	8	79	92	6.8	.672
				67	B50	3762	7.7	38	9	41	81	5.2	.618
				46	B44	3715	5.9	21	816	20	3	0.030	.073
407	IT1	CUR	TORP 828	58	B49	3946	7.8	89	1	228	99	9.0	.511
				45	B50	3856	7.7	47	2	181	96	5.3	.433
				33	B44	3807	5.9	139	724	42	17	0.44	.289
				42	B45	2944	4.8	5	40	37	12	0.38	.102
409	SCA	KIS	7775-78	71	B49	3944	8.0	87	2	124	98	8.4	.624
				51	B50	3866	7.8	45	3	79	94	5.8	.576
				27	B44	3818	5.5	48	815	31	6	0.13	.133
410	US3	GRU	SIMPKINS	68	B49	3875	7.9	84	5	63	95	9.8	.727
				33	B52	3786	5.2	19	147	44	12	0.68	.164
				40	B51	3620	6.3	25	388	19	7	0.14	.158
411	BEN	LEU	L-254-II	59	A23	3920	7.5	119	25	362	83	3.0	.419
				51	B49	3776	7.9	74	1	288	99	6.5	.431
				40	B44	3701	6.3	181	640	107	23	0.59	.284
				29	B13	2880	5.7	37	91	70	29	0.93	.287
				28	B58	2750	5.1	17	122	53	13	0.38	.142
				*28	B51	2750	5.7	27	329	26	8	0.19	.123

9wNo.:	REG	LAB.	SERUM-ID	STR	ANTIGEN	No.REAC.	AVE	+/+	MISS. +/-	EXTRA -/+	%INCL	Q-SCORE	R-VALUE
413	IT2	FER	FE-99	56	B49	3935	7.1	71	19	19	79	5.4	.784
414	FRA	MAY	FST-08	70	Bw52	3891	7.8	138	29	248	83	6.5	.515
				60	B49	3724	7.8	88	1	160	99	9.3	.579
				41	B51	3635	6.2	101	321	59	24	1.1	.345
				35	Bw63	3213	6.6	29	47	30	39	2.0	.421
416	US5	MIT	C-5295	48	B49	3942	7.8	85	2	334	98	9.7	.424
				38	B44	3855	6.1	266	596	68	31	1.4	.423
				44	B51	2993	6.5	33	342	35	9	0.19	.166
417	US5	MIT	C-4503	32	Bw50	3941	5.4	21	28	29	43	2.0	.417
				41	B49	3892	6.9	7	83	22	8	0.36	.126
418	US5	PNW	SNYD	43	Bw50	3932	7.2	38	11	42	78	4.0	.601
				21	B45	3883	5.5	8	42	34	16	0.46	.165
				23	B49	3833	4.7	6	80	28	7	0.25	.098
419	FRA	DAU	FPA-BARO	28	Bw50	3934	6.7	42	6	219	88	5.6	.361
				23	Bw62	3886	6.0	109	334	110	25	0.72	.295
				11	Bw72	3443	5.6	26	78	84	25	1.7	.219
420	ANZ	BSH	MULLANE-BD-1169	81	B8	3947	7.7	420	16	68	97	9.5	.899
				55	Bw46	3511	6.9	55	32	13	64	4.3	.709
421	JAP	KUR	JR-02-180	50	Bw46	3941	6.9	79	9	30	90	6.3	.802
422	ANZ	CHI	S-522	63	Bw46	2868	6.7	28	37	37	44	2.8	.418
				67	B44	2803	7.6	18	612	19	3	0.028	.073
423	NCY	YUN	BH-7	83	Bw4	3933	7.6	2168	138	105	95	5.9	.873
				32	A32	1627	6.1	36	43	69	46	0.34	.360
				28	B27	1548	7.0	8	4	61	67	6.2	.266
				22	A23	1536	5.2	13	39	48	25	0.093	.202
				27	A24	1484	5.8	34	416	14	27	0.096	.161
425	NCY	SCH	CWR-NIE-2	91	Bw4	3939	7.9	2240	72	147	97	5.8	.885
				43	B13	1627	8.0	11	1	136	92	7.1	.248
				38	Bw72	1615	6.3	23	46	113	34	1.2	.190
				39	B27	1546	7.1	7	5	106	39	4.8	.173
				37	A29	1533	6.0	14	35	92	29	0.35	.155
				38	B8	1522	6.4	32	221	72	13	0.033	.103
				*38	B45	1522	6.0	6	21	66	23	0.41	.082
427	FRA	FAU	FRE-117	76	Bw4	3949	7.4	2067	250	45	90	5.7	.853
				15	A25	1632	5.8	21	10	24	68	1.0	.552
428	GER	KUE	KUE-048-M	90	Bw4	3913	7.9	2261	36	189	99	6.4	.883
				43	B39	1616	6.8	77	48	112	62	2.4	.450
				33	B13	1490	7.5	8	4	103	67	7.0	.203
				29	B35	1452	5.8	53	324	44	15	0.23	.175
				*29	Bw65	1452	6.1	21	118	76	16	0.088	.110
430	BEN	BRX	SOLNAZER 56	79	Bw4	3851	7.4	1739	522	71	77	3.5	.715
				61	B45	1590	7.7	33	2	38	95	6.5	.652
431	EAE	WEG	R-627	91	Bw6	3919	7.8	3044	164	60	95	5.8	.821
				25	B35	711	6.5	4	5	56	45	6.0	.147
433	NCY	YAG	CATO	88	Bw6	3942	7.7	3165	60	109	99	5.9	.853
				42	Bw65	717	6.4	19	6	90	76	4.6	.322
				41	B45	686	8.0	4	0	86	100	1.8	.202
				39	Cw7	682	6.1	33	96	49	26	0.28	.201
				40	B18	553	8.0	5	4	44	56	5.6	.211
				34	Bw60	544	8.0	3	1	41	75	6.6	.211
434	FRA	FAU	FRE-118	87	Bw6	3904	7.7	2998	192	147	94	3.6	.717
				76	A1	714	6.7	72	43	75	63	0.26	.455
				54	A11	599	7.2	38	9	37	81	0.59	.602
436	US1	AMO	RA	74	Bw6	3907	7.3	2623	572	11	83	5.9	.663
439	BEN	ROO	vR-480684	95	Bw6	3923	7.9	3184	26	116	100	6.4	.875
				49	Bw65	713	7.7	21	3	95	88	5.2	.360
				37	Cw1	683	6.0	33	34	56	50	0.10	.355
				30	Bw61	616	6.7	6	1	50	86	6.1	.286
				30	B35	609	4.8	5	4	45	54	5.2	.211
				*30	Bw73	604	5.3	3	2	42	60	0.28	.174
440	EAE	MYR	KERSCHNER	31	Bw46	3901	6.6	42	45	284	49	2.4	.218
				30	Cw7	3770	5.8	194	1112	78	15	0.25	.215
				*30	Bw73	3770	6.6	10	11	272	48	1.3	.117
				40	Bw54	2294	5.7	14	138	48	10	0.24	.107
441	FRA	MOP	FMO-K-430	65	B44	3935	7.2	654	213	342	76	3.8	.613
				57	B49	3068	8.0	78	2	264	98	7.3	.449
				45	Bw50	2988	8.0	46	1	218	98	5.7	.397
				34	B45	2940	6.9	34	11	184	76	3.6	.324
				29	B35	2896	6.0	85	469	99	16	0.49	.179
				31	Bw53	2342	6.1	19	47	80	29	0.61	.208
				*31	Bw62	2342	5.8	26	323	73	8	0.10	.067
				*31	Aw69	2342	5.9	18	166	81	10	0.041	.081

Table 1 (continued)

9wNo.:	REG	LAB.	SERUM-ID	STR	ANTIGEN	No.REAC.	AVE	+/+	MISS. +/-	EXTRA -/+	%INCL	Q-SCORE	R-VALUE
442	GER	REN	290113	47	Cw7	3921	6.1	600	743	178	45	1.1	.449
				38	A11	2578	6.3	85	262	93	25	0.41	.274
				40	B7	2231	6.3	24	71	69	26	1.4	.223
				36	Bw55	2136	6.5	20	62	49	25	0.26	.239
				36	A1	2045	6.3	22	258	27	8	0.23	.142
443	JAP	TOK	JR-50-322	45	Bw42	3927	7.3	25	20	335	56	2.3	.173
				42	Bw67	3882	6.9	11	0	324	100	1.8	.173
				42	Aw69	3868	6.3	78	238	246	25	0.19	.176
				41	Bw55	3555	6.6	32	99	214	25	0.50	.154
				41	B7	3514	6.6	64	452	171	13	0.11	.095
				40	B39	3385	7.1	24	149	147	14	0.27	.077
				*40	Cw7	3385	6.4	105	1027	42	10	0.076	.097
444	JAP	KUR	JR-02-62	34	B39	3953	6.3	86	120	98	42	1.7	.413
				28	Bw67	3747	6.4	5	6	93	46	2.5	.146
				26	Bw42	3736	7.1	7	38	86	16	0.41	.093
				23	Bw55	3691	4.8	12	125	74	9	0.15	.084
				25	Aw69	3552	5.6	18	266	56	7	0.059	.088
				25	Cw7	3270	5.7	36	1010	20	4	0.068	.091
445	JAP	NAI	FD-1223	50	Bw67	3941	6.0	9	2	42	82	3.2	.377
				52	Bw42	3930	7.5	13	33	29	29	0.89	.288
446	JAP	YOS	AY-483	66	B39	3931	7.6	194	11	148	95	6.6	.715
				43	Bw64	3534	6.7	63	44	85	59	3.0	.483
				37	B38	3619	5.2	29	139	56	18	0.69	.217
				48	Bw65	3451	6.3	24	214	32	11	0.28	.182
				43	Bw67	3213	6.5	4	7	28	37	3.2	.209
447	US5	CMC	11008-K	61	B38	3861	7.9	168	14	399	93	7.3	.488
				48	B37	3679	7.4	72	7	327	92	6.5	.383
				42	B44	3600	6.1	206	608	121	26	0.92	.305
				49	Bw59	2786	7.4	28	8	93	78	5.0	.412
				41	B13	2750	6.2	24	106	69	19	0.62	.186
				43	B51	2620	6.6	25	309	44	8	0.094	.116
				*43	Bw57	2620	5.7	13	112	56	11	0.19	.109
448	IT2	FER	FE-124	93	Cw1	3924	7.9	521	10	15	99	9.7	.973
449	UKI	BRS	DUN-7543	88	Cw1	3944	7.9	536	6	53	99	10.0	.940
				26	B51	3402	5.4	17	359	36	5	0.084	.084
450	JAP	TSU	I-0141	87	Cw1	3116	7.8	382	20	59	96	8.0	.893
				44	Bw55	2714	6.6	43	38	16	54	2.0	.612
451	JAP	TOK	JR-50-647	86	Cw1	3950	7.8	537	7	40	99	9.4	.952
				20	Bw57	3406	4.9	16	153	24	10	0.20	.176
452	JAP	NIS	NS-1068	70	Cw1	3939	7.2	463	76	16	86	6.8	.898
453	GER	GSW	GSW-S-632-3	88	Cw1	3887	7.9	524	9	107	99	9.8	.887
				46	B27	3354	6.7	79	54	28	60	2.2	.650
454	NCY	YAG	KUSAK	77	Cw1	3929	7.9	530	5	202	100	8.0	.820
				29	B51	3394	6.2	101	273	101	28	0.37	.313
455	NCY	YUN	YUN-SCH	72	Cw2	3913	7.4	317	39	55	90	6.3	.858
				34	B27	3557	5.8	19	78	36	20	1.8	.245
456	US8	NSF	NSF-2191	75	Cw2	3684	7.6	293	25	41	93	6.9	.889
				21	Bw42	3366	5.4	7	24	34	23	0.72	.188
				23	Bw41	3335	6.4	11	77	23	13	0.13	.188
457	US3	GRU	REIMER	74	Cw2	3936	7.4	336	14	20	96	9.2	.947
458	US1	DUQ	STEGER	74	Cw2	3952	7.4	334	26	12	93	8.8	.941
459	US5	FTW	BIRT	74	Cw2	3905	7.5	344	15	35	96	8.4	.926
				22	B7	3545	5.8	25	513	10	5	0.12	.157
460	IT1	MTT	TS-40	69	Cw2	3939	7.5	339	23	118	94	6.4	.815
				36	B51	3577	6.0	44	366	74	11	0.094	.150
				39	Bw61	3167	6.3	16	273	58	6	0.27	.067
461	SCA	SVE	COP-III0-52-76	80	Cw3	3940	7.6	1040	38	47	97	7.8	.946
				48	Bw46	2862	7.5	22	6	25	79	2.7	.602
462	US3	GRU	HOLT	68	Cw3	3942	7.2	885	192	14	83	7.0	.868
				14	Bw46	2865	6.0	3	25	11	11	0.91	.146
463	GER	NEU	GÖ-802973-C	80	Cw3	3910	7.5	1017	51	25	96	8.6	.951
				24	Bw46	2842	4.8	8	20	17	29	1.4	.296
464	EAE	RIC	FO-10324	77	Cw3	3914	7.6	994	70	191	94	7.5	.840
				38	B35	2850	6.4	150	344	41	31	0.38	.433
				24	Bw53	2356	4.8	8	58	33	13	0.29	.135
465	ANZ	HAY	ADAMS-070873	89	Cw3	3917	7.8	1059	14	89	99	11.0	.936
				44	Bw46	2844	7.8	27	1	62	31	3.2	.534
				24	Cw1	2816	6.0	29	322	33	8	0.38	.156
466	UKI	BRS	MK-6131-BWD	86	Cw3	3940	7.8	1035	41	90	97	8.6	.918
				12	Aw33	2863	5.1	18	192	78	8	0.099	.088
467	JAP	TOK	JR-50-869	81	Cw3	3929	7.6	503	569	13	47	2.7	.613

9wNo.:	REG	LAB.	SERUM-ID	STR	ANTIGEN	No.REAC.	AVE	+/+	MISS. +/-	EXTRA -/+	%INCL	Q-SCORE	R-VALUE
468	EAE	RIC	FO-10532	80	Cw4	3943	7.5	639	65	41	91	7.3	.907
				39	Cw6	3239	6.3	21	407	20	5	0.062	.127
469	EAE	MYR	FÜRLINGER	80	Cw4	3874	7.5	648	39	19	95	9.5	.948
470	BEN	BOU	54307-2.3.82	82	Cw4	3940	7.6	679	25	5	97	11.0	.974
471	US7	DUP	FIORE-557	77	Cw4	3934	7.5	667	37	10	95	9.2	.959
472	US5	MOO	McHUIE	90	Cw4	3939	7.8	700	7	21	100	10.0	.976
				28	Cw6	3232	5.0	12	413	9	3	0.048	.105
473	UKI	BRS	UK-5956-CBT	79	Cw4	3923	7.6	650	57	110	92	6.0	.861
				46	Cw6	3216	6.4	37	391	73	9	0.050	.113
474	GER	MUE	MUE-23928-II	72	Cw6	3934	7.5	464	22	126	96	7.2	.846
				38	Bw57	3448	5.7	7	9	119	44	4.0	.146
475	GER	ALB	RK-993-4	53	Cw6	3944	6.9	422	63	115	88	6.3	.801
				23	Cw4	3459	5.5	73	575	42	12	0.29	.213
476	US5	SIN	13782.2	70	Cw6	3934	7.3	449	36	158	93	5.7	.801
				51	Bw58	3449	7.1	93	39	65	71	3.7	.629
				35	Bw57	3317	7.4	13	2	52	87	6.9	.412
				25	B13	3302	7.0	21	28	31	43	3.8	.407
477	FRA	BET	FLY-956	51	Cw6	3914	6.6	355	128	36	74	5.9	.795
478	US1	DUQ	BOPPRE	46	Cw6	3939	6.7	299	188	132	62	4.4	.607
				25	Cw7	3452	5.7	124	1108	8	11	0.52	.242
479	BEN	ROO	vR-45157.9	79	Cw4	3939	7.8	696	13	561	99	8.0	.666
				63	Cw6	3230	7.5	406	21	155	96	6.6	.801
				20	Cw5	2803	5.4	55	290	100	16	0.21	.171
				24	B51	2458	5.9	36	276	64	12	0.056	.144
480	FRA	MAY	FST-14	59	Cw4	3907	7.9	697	8	925	99	6.4	.546
				31	Cw6	3202	6.4	280	143	645	67	1.4	.321
				24	Cw7	2779	5.8	329	747	316	31	0.077	.139
481	IT1	MTT	FIO-446	63	Cw4	3941	7.1	543	163	317	77	4.6	.623
				54	Cw6	3235	6.8	272	154	45	44	3.6	.708
				22	B13	2809	6.0	6	38	39	14	0.57	.121
482	BEN	ENG	CLB-105	83	Cw4	3911	7.9	689	20	215	98	11.0	.827
				41	Cw6	3202	6.3	207	218	8	49	3.6	.656
483	US7	HAN	SEA-1167	61	Cw5	3955	7.0	406	50	33	90	7.7	.896

9wNo.:	REG	LAB.	SERUM-ID	STR	ANTIGEN	No.REAC.	AVE	+/+	MISS. +/-	EXTRA -/+	%INCL	Q-SCORE	R-VALUE
484	UKI	BRS	6347-LCS	74	Cw5	3934	7.7	442	9	110	99	9.0	.870
				18	B44	3483	5.6	48	455	62	10	1.1	.150
				14	Cw6	2980	5.7	23	374	39	6	0.053	.102
485	GER	WER	HM-135	55	Cw5	3909	6.8	361	87	31	81	6.3	.845
				12	Cw8	3461	5.5	16	306	15	5	0.22	.138
486	GER	SCN	SCN-ANG-5	60	Cw5	3900	7.0	390	56	34	88	7.3	.884
487	ANZ	BSH	MANNS-BD-888	58	Cw5	3953	6.9	388	63	18	87	7.8	.896
488	US3	PER	P-0045-A	57	Cw5	3948	6.9	384	68	20	85	6.9	.886
489	EAE	MYR	CZUJAN	65	Cw8	3816	7.6	322	29	384	92	6.8	.600
				51	Cw5	3465	6.8	326	84	58	80	5.1	.799
				24	Aw43	3052	5.2	5	5	53	50	1.4	.202
				26	A11	3045	5.9	19	385	34	5	0.0022	.089
490	US8	LEE	CARM	62	Cw8	3952	7.8	359	7	308	99	9.4	.693
				26	Cw5	3586	5.8	216	204	92	52	2.4	.557
				18	Cw1	3166	5.9	32	488	60	7	0.067	.086
491	US6	BRN	CCB-239.3	47	Cw8	3879	6.4	191	168	32	54	3.0	.651
492	NCY	SCH	CWR-SEMI	58	Cw8	3954	6.8	300	65	226	83	3.8	.647
				57	Bw61	3589	7.2	82	325	144	21	0.54	.204
				*57	Bw48	3589	7.0	23	40	203	37	1.4	.166
				*57	Bw62	3589	6.7	59	375	167	14	0.15	.111
				*57	A11	3589	7.1	58	408	168	13	0.0047	.098
493	ANZ	BSH	BD-883	46	Bw65	3944	6.7	175	90	72	63	4.1	.662
				20	Bw64	3679	5.3	20	83	52	20	0.67	.214
				21	B8	3576	5.0	16	374	36	5	0.033	.077
494	JAP	TSU	I-0147	64	Cw7	3238	7.3	1059	69	186	94	5.2	.833
				20	A28	2110	5.6	51	136	135	28	0.096	.203
				*20	B49	2110	5.7	6	7	180	47	1.3	.104
495	BEN	ENG	CLB-147	59	Cw7	3916	6.8	1092	254	204	82	3.6	.739
				68	Bw55	2570	7.3	96	16	108	86	1.5	.614
				62	Bw56	2458	7.8	62	10	46	87	1.9	.693
				23	Bw42	2386	5.5	12	10	34	55	1.5	.369
496	US1	DUQ	PURNIS	55	Cw7	3860	6.8	992	335	38	45	4.6	.787
				26	B7	2533	5.9	31	66	7	32	2.6	.500
497	US6	BRN	CCB-306.1	56	Cw7	3927	6.9	1140	204	52	85	5.7	.855
				17	B18	2583	4.9	11	119	41	9	0.070	.106

Table 1 (continued)

9wNo.:	REG	LAB.	SERUM-ID	STR	ANTIGEN	No.REAC.	AVE	+/+	MISS. +/-	EXTRA -/+	%INCL	Q-SCORE	R-VALUE
498	US6	BRN	CCB-336.1	58	Cw7	3906	6.9	1026	309	39	77	5.1	.802
499	US5	TER	M-1275	57	Cw7	3955	6.9	1214	145	72	90	5.8	.878
				15	B8	2596	5.3	18	53	54	26	2.8	.231
				16	B49	2525	4.3	8	8	46	50	1.9	.264
089	US8	LEE	R-97	57	Cw7	3936	6.8	773	573	596	58	0.77	.343
				52	A11	2590	7.0	187	158	409	52	1.2	.291
				47	Cw6	2245	6.5	154	182	255	47	0.51	.300
				48	A26	1909	6.9	115	131	140	47	0.97	.377
				39	A25	1663	6.6	41	17	99	71	2.3	.426
				34	B39	1605	6.3	21	27	78	44	0.61	.274
125	US7	HAN	SEA-1171	52	A31	3919	6.6	194	58	218	77	4.6	.568
				52	A30	3667	6.9	160	52	58	76	4.4	.728
152	FRA	FAU	FRE-111	66	B51	3875	7.1	361	79	22	83	6.3	.865
				27	B13	3435	5.5	4	135	18	3	0.030	.058
153	US2	HFP	MN-THOMAS	73	B51	3924	7.3	398	47	20	90	6.6	.913
244	NCY	MRV	MER 4451	68	B27	3849	7.3	179	34	37	85	6.1	.825
				48	Bw47	3636	6.8	17	23	20	43	2.4	.436
338	FRA	DAU	FPA-BER	53	B35	3931	6.7	395	268	416	60	2.8	.434
				52	Bw62	3268	6.9	269	140	147	66	3.4	.602
				37	Bw72	2859	6.1	63	44	84	59	2.7	.480
				41	Bw50	2752	6.9	29	9	55	77	4.6	.504
				38	Bw56	2714	6.1	27	49	28	36	1.4	.404
				39	Bw71	2638	6.0	3	7	25	30	1.2	.174
350	FRA	FAU	FRE-124	85	B13	3938	7.9	150	5	25	97	9.8	.907
361	US5	ABS	AZ-99	65	Bw60	3952	7.2	275	57	34	93	6.2	.846
				32	Bw48	3620	5.9	14	47	20	23	1.1	.299
502	US3	PER	P 0059 A	74	DR1	3908	7.5	460	21	70	96	7.2	.898
504	UKI	DRK	WARNE 595 F	60	DR1	3939	7.7	488	6	411	99	8.7	.685
				30	DRw10	3445	5.9	49	14	362	78	3.2	.277
				31	DRw14	3382	5.9	186	658	176	23	0.45	.211
				30	DR2	2538	5.7	101	652	75	14	0.14	.166
505	FRA	ARN	FAR 5	71	DR1	3892	7.7	479	9	119	99	8.4	.869
				14	DRw10	3404	4.8	17	47	102	27	0.59	.174
				15	DRw14	3340	5.2	45	791	57	6	0.026	.078
507	FRA	POI	FPP-2753	65	DR1	3939	7.7	484	8	201	99	7.8	.807
				18	DQw2	3447	5.4	123	826	78	13	0.11	.188

9wNo.:	REG	LAB.	SERUM-ID	STR	ANTIGEN	No.REAC.	AVE	+/+	MISS. +/-	EXTRA -/+	%INCL	Q-SCORE	R-VALUE
508	BEN	ROO	vR 576602	52	DR1	3885	7.2	465	22	269	96	5.8	.741
				23	DQw1	3398	5.7	216	1633	53	12	0.54	.152
509	UKI	DRK	PERRY	55	DR1	3936	7.1	446	44	106	92	6.6	.836
				10	DRw10	3446	4.8	12	54	94	19	0.90	.122
510	US5	SWE	EATON 1069	65	DR1	3917	7.5	464	23	125	96	7.6	.846
				24	DRw10	3430	6.0	35	31	90	54	2.4	.396
511	US5	MOO	McSMITH	64	DR1	3938	7.4	475	14	128	98	8.9	.856
				19	DRw10	3449	6.1	26	40	102	40	1.5	.264
				15	DR2	3383	5.4	52	768	50	7	0.11	.110
512	GER	GSW	GSW-S 3713	63	DR1	3830	7.2	433	40	50	92	6.8	.892
514	IT2	FER	FE-204	49	DR1	3909	6.9	381	102	112	79	4.9	.750
				18	DR2	3426	5.6	52	773	60	7	0.057	.096
515	US1	DUQ	WEGNER	69	DR1	3818	7.5	458	22	154	96	7.8	.821
				44	DRw10	3338	7.6	64	1	90	99	7.0	.630
516	SCA	KIS	14649/81	39	DR1	3846	6.4	294	179	330	63	2.4	.467
				34	DRw10	3373	7.5	66	0	264	100	6.7	.429
				23	TA10	3239	5.8	158	1462	95	10	0.0079	.072
518	US6	BRN	CCB-921.2	62	DR1	3927	7.7	472	15	368	97	8.5	.693
				35	DRw10	3440	7.6	66	0	302	100	7.9	.404
				24	DR2	3374	5.8	204	618	98	25	0.75	.315
				18	DRw9	2552	5.3	44	203	54	18	0.67	.238
521	EAE	WEG	MR-774	61	DR1	3930	7.3	442	41	169	92	6.4	.785
				40	DRw10	3447	7.4	63	3	106	96	6.6	.586
				21	Cw4	3375	5.9	61	503	45	11	0.22	.197
522	EAE	WEG	MR-1162	62	DR1	3912	7.2	431	54	107	89	6.7	.820
				40	DRw10	3427	6.9	61	5	46	93	6.2	.720
				19	Cw4	3355	5.3	16	547	30	3	0.13	.057
523	BEN	ROO	vR-57647.2	39	DRw10	3455	7.7	58	1	304	99	7.1	.378
				29	Bw53	3396	6.7	30	30	274	50	0.90	.193
				27	DR1	3336	6.2	68	339	206	17	0.12	.115
				21	DRw14	2905	5.7	75	621	126	11	0.055	.085
524	US4	RAD	NW 14543	47	DRw10	3911	7.6	68	2	83	98	8.4	.654
525	FRA	VIV	FBA-AGUIL	48	DRw10	3937	7.4	69	2	112	98	8.7	.599
				31	DR1	3866	5.4	25	462	87	6	0.019	.051
527	US1	DUQ	MYSCEWSKI	43	DRw10	3946	7.3	67	2	53	98	8.7	.731

9wNo.:	REG	LAB.	SERUM-ID	STR	ANTIGEN	No.REAC.	AVE	+/+	MISS. +/-	EXTRA -/+	%INCL	Q-SCORE	R-VALUE
529	FRA	FAU	FRE-549	36	B8	3918	6.3	253	179	338	59	1.5	.428
				35	DRw10	3486	7.6	61	2	277	97	5.3	.399
				25	A1	3418	5.8	80	305	197	21	0.65	.165
				22	DRw11	3038	5.8	87	740	110	11	0.0045	.100
				21	B51	3013	5.5	51	330	59	14	0.063	.109
530	FRA	FAU	FRE-568	71	DR2	3925	7.5	831	32	152	97	7.4	.873
				21	DRw11	3062	5.6	63	821	89	8	0.020	.063
				*21	DRw14	3062	5.4	62	807	90	8	0.025	.063
531	BEN	ROO	vR4475.3	58	DR2	3823	7.4	810	35	445	96	5.3	.715
				26	DR1	2978	5.9	124	318	321	29	0.21	.154
				24	DRw10	2536	5.4	18	37	303	33	0.48	.090
				25	A2	2530	5.8	209	1101	111	16	0.012	.103
533	ANZ	DAW	TOOLEY R1/397	72	DR2	3924	7.6	851	14	145	99	8.7	.892
				17	DR1	3059	5.9	40	411	105	9	0.068	.081
534	US2	BAC	MN-7395	80	DR2	3869	7.7	828	15	105	99	10.0	.914
				22	DR1	3026	6.0	56	389	49	13	0.29	.207
535	ANZ	BSH	KYLE B 381	84	DR2	3888	7.8	846	8	87	100	9.5	.933
				22	DR7	3084	5.2	31	519	56	6	0.057	.078
537	EAE	RIC	MB 844	63	DR2	3904	7.6	824	34	585	97	5.8	.662
				35	DRw11	3046	6.2	332	545	253	38	0.48	.301
				30	B7	2169	6.0	47	162	206	23	0.57	.110
				29	DR1	1960	6.0	51	238	155	18	0.10	.097
				30	DRw10	1658	6.7	9	27	143	25	0.10	.082
538	JAP	MRI	AY-403	74	DR2	3907	7.8	852	13	297	99	7.3	.809
				25	DR7	3042	5.6	99	450	198	19	0.089	.131
				27	DRw10	2469	6.1	46	229	148	17	0.035	.117
				25	DRw53	2194	5.8	92	943	56	9	0.19	.081
541	FRA	BET	FLY-835	83	DR2	3900	7.7	852	7	48	100	9.8	.960
542	NCY	YUN	ZIA	76	DR2	3919	7.6	829	31	53	97	8.7	.938
543	EAE	KAS	KAS-101	62	DR2	3855	7.0	710	130	46	85	5.4	.863
545	FRA	DAU	FPA 8927	65	DR2	3877	7.2	738	109	38	88	6.4	.887
546	JAP	SEK	KS 33	45	DR2	3858	6.7	653	177	183	79	3.8	.724
				18	DRw53	3028	5.5	126	1520	57	8	0.11	.074
547	US6	BRN	CCB 986	45	DR2	3880	6.7	615	220	82	74	4.7	.760
				2	DRw52	3045	4.7	75	2305	7	4	0.13	.054

9wNo.:	REG	LAB.	SERUM-ID	STR	ANTIGEN	No.REAC.	AVE	+/+	MISS. +/-	EXTRA -/+	%INCL	Q-SCORE	R-VALUE
548	US1	DUQ	WHEELER	45	DR2	3946	6.7	565	298	102	66	3.0	.686
				12	A24	3075	5.1	60	673	40	9	0.066	.156
549	US8	LEE	DCC	50	DR2	3853	6.7	619	220	89	74	3.4	.755
				39	Bw61	3007	7.0	23	286	65	8	0.014	.091
				27	B8	2675	5.3	24	340	38	7	0.037	.113
550	NCY	MRV	9839	48	DR2	3326	6.6	529	222	38	71	3.8	.767
551	FRA	FAU	FRE-550	32	DR2	3903	6.4	507	347	473	60	1.0	.418
				22	A23	3042	5.9	41	70	430	37	0.35	.115
				21	DRw14	2938	5.7	167	666	265	21	0.016	.095
				18	A1	1927	5.6	67	325	155	18	0.0038	.088
				17	Bw57	1535	5.4	14	37	141	28	0.0098	.107
552	NCY	MRV	9887	56	DR2	3368	7.0	657	102	70	87	5.4	.852
				12	A25	2609	5.5	16	63	54	21	0.21	.192
				9	DRw14	2530	5.1	29	704	25	4	0.056	.081
553	JAP	MRI	AY 2054	54	DR2	3863	6.9	690	171	111	81	4.3	.785
				19	TA10	3000	5.3	73	1416	38	5	0.040	.063
554	UKI	BRS	BRL 6442	63	DR2	3929	7.5	808	60	333	94	5.1	.751
				28	DRw52	3061	5.8	288	2105	45	13	0.11	.070
555	US6	BRN	CCB 1000	64	DR2	3919	7.2	701	160	98	82	4.9	.804
				18	DR3	3058	5.7	30	472	68	6	0.025	.070
557	US1	AMO	IA 35	48	DR3	3738	6.9	444	76	236	86	4.2	.700
559	US6	BRN	CCB 1045.1	42	DR3	3924	6.5	345	201	29	64	4.4	.735
561	ANZ	WOO	WATSON 018887	47	DR3	3933	6.7	427	119	76	79	4.5	.786
563	FRA	FAU	FRE 570	54	DR3	3928	7.7	540	10	644	99	7.8	.598
				26	DRw52	3359	5.9	590	1755	43	26	1.8	.246
				*26	DRw8	3359	5.8	102	211	531	33	0.88	.205
				*26	DRw14	3359	6.0	267	539	366	34	1.2	.205
				*26	DRw12	3359	6.0	111	276	522	29	0.55	.091
				*26	DRw11	3359	5.9	217	703	416	24	0.50	.074
564	UKI	DRK	WILLIAMS 773 E	70	DR3	3949	7.8	546	8	212	99	9.0	.814
				18	DRw14	3375	5.3	92	715	116	12	0.32	.122
				22	DRw12	2568	5.2	36	294	80	11	0.15	.118
				27	DRw13	2238	5.6	28	376	52	7	0.061	.085
565	US8	RUB	NYBC-002	61	DR3	3886	7.1	522	28	61	95	7.9	.909

Table 1 (continued)

9wNo.:	REG	LAB.	SERUM-ID	STR	ANTIGEN	No.REAC.	AVE	+/+	MISS. +/-	EXTRA -/+	%INCL	Q-SCORE	R-VALUE
567	NCY	CAR	BOS/BUR	54	DR3	3870	6.9	473	67	99	88	6.0	.826
				26	Bw46	3330	5.8	27	54	72	34	0.48	.265
				27	DRw14	3229	5.5	31	757	39	4	0.030	.069
568	NCY	MRV	10895	48	DR3	3351	6.5	363	120	135	76	3.7	.696
				57	DRw12	2868	7.1	28	282	107	10	0.080	.071
569	SAF	HAM	N 310	55	DR3	3755	7.0	463	67	87	88	5.8	.834
				21	DRw14	3225	6.0	32	742	55	5	0.035	.050
570	US7	DUP	STILLWELL 1559	63	DR3	3904	7.5	525	24	154	96	7.8	.835
				14	DRw14	3355	5.6	62	744	92	8	0.16	.083
				9	DR7	2549	4.9	35	397	57	9	0.11	.109
				*9	DRw12	2549	4.9	22	307	70	9	0.099	.064
571	US1	DUQ	HAYWARD	34	DR3	3759	6.3	253	275	74	48	2.4	.563
				16	B8	3231	5.2	19	274	55	16	1.8	.176
572	US8	LEE	CARTLIGE	52	DR3	3891	7.5	536	14	1117	98	6.1	.451
				39	DRw52	3341	6.2	1056	1279	61	46	2.0	.484
				*39	DRw14	3341	6.5	467	337	650	59	1.4	.294
				*39	DRw11	3341	6.1	467	461	650	51	1.3	.222
				*39	DRw12	3341	6.3	192	187	925	51	1.1	.131
				29	DRw11	1006	4.7	6	12	55	34		.154
573	US1	THP	THP-EVINK	31	DR3	3869	6.0	281	247	39	54	3.0	.649
574	GER	MUE	MUE-26709	57	B8	3794	7.2	345	68	91	84	4.5	.790
				*57	DR3	3794	7.1	269	252	167	52	1.8	.502
575	US5	CMC	3504 KZ	72	DR4	3744	7.5	960	57	151	95	5.9	.865
576	US1	DUQ	EDELSTEIN	65	DR4	3898	7.4	1014	58	199	95	5.6	.844
578	GER	SCN	CWB 4	52	DR4	3814	6.9	882	157	134	85	4.2	.806
				24	DRw53	2773	6.0	59	754	74	8	1.4	.074
580	UKI	FES	LH 986	69	DR4	3885	7.7	1064	12	738	99	5.2	.652
				44	DQw3	2746	6.5	361	766	353	33	1.2	.115
				*44	DRw11	2746	6.2	267	615	447	31	0.041	.067
				41	DR1	1587	6.4	82	211	261	28	0.083	.074
581	FRA	FAU	FRE 573	58	DR4	3890	7.3	979	88	653	92	4.7	.620
				39	DRw11	2823	6.4	495	408	158	55	1.4	.515
582	FRA	VIV	F-BA-AMELI	48	DR4	3879	6.8	725	334	214	69	3.0	.633
				24	DR1	2820	6.0	60	368	154	15	0.095	.103
				21	DQw3	2326	5.7	82	911	60	9	1.0	.078
584	SAF	HAM	N 587	66	DQw3	3884	7.3	1960	223	351	90	3.0	.699
				*66	DR4	3884	7.5	1045	27	1266	98	5.8	.478
				*66	DRw11	3884	7.1	792	248	1519	77	2.3	.205
				*66	DRw12	3884	7.3	363	48	1948	89	3.5	.202
				29	DRw53	1701	6.3	212	230	139	48	1.3	.400
				*29	DRw9	1701	6.5	65	36	289	65	2.3	.271
				*29	DR4	1701	6.3	32	3	319	92		.254
				*29	DR7	1701	6.2	142	210	209	41	0.92	.249
				18	DR4	1259	6.0	15	2	124	89		.288
				16	TA10	1231	5.4	41	147	79	22	0.65	.167
585	EAE	WEG	MR 1165	61	DR4	3760	7.5	1002	28	529	98	8.1	.707
				28	DQw3	2730	5.9	452	644	77	42	2.9	.453
				*28	DRw11	2730	5.9	294	590	235	34	1.0	.243
				*28	DRw12	2730	6.0	135	160	394	46	1.1	.232
				23	DRw53	1634	6.0	44	372	33	11	1.6	.162
				*23	DRw9	1634	6.0	15	72	62	18	1.1	.140
				*23	DR7	1634	6.0	31	320	46	9	0.059	.102
587	NCY	MRV	9671	63	DR4	3509	7.2	897	73	95	93	6.2	.881
				29	DQw3	2539	5.6	64	957	31	7	1.9	.109
				*29	DRw11	2539	5.7	44	774	51	6	0.051	.059
				*29	DRw12	2539	5.8	18	261	77	7	0.034	.050
589	GER	GSW	GSW-S 346/3	66	DR4	3802	7.3	982	38	147	97	7.1	.882
				24	DRw9	2782	6.0	42	158	105	21	0.45	.196
				22	DR1	2582	5.6	45	376	60	11	0.16	.148
				23	DRw53	2161	5.7	29	517	31	6	2.1	.090
590	US7	DUP	NJ 3429-942	61	DR4	3903	7.2	958	118	106	90	5.7	.856
				17	B27	2823	5.5	19	133	86	17	0.10	.111
				18	Bw57	2671	5.2	17	113	69	14	0.095	.126
				18	Bw54	2541	5.1	7	43	62	18	1.1	.098
591	JAP	SAJ	35-P 257	45	DR4	3834	6.6	679	354	337	66	1.9	.540
				37	DQw3	2801	6.2	194	945	143	18	0.80	.127
				*37	DRw11	2801	6.2	136	766	201	16	0.043	.065
				*37	DRw12	2801	5.9	53	262	284	17	0.063	.052
592	NCY	MRV	5094	50	DR4	3555	6.8	782	202	73	80	4.7	.802
593	US8	RUB	NYBC 003	47	DR4	3912	6.8	753	320	319	71	2.4	.590
				27	DRw53	2839	6.0	144	692	175	18	0.96	.123
				*27	DRw9	2839	5.7	41	168	278	20		.075
				*27	DQw3	2003	5.8	85	665	90	12	1.0	.071
594	US8	RUB	NYBC 001	40	DR4	3894	6.5	678	382	67	64	3.3	.697
				22	DRw53	2834	5.4	34	799	33	5	1.3	.073
				*22	DRw9	2834	4.6	10	199	57	5	0.095	.045
				*22	DR7	2834	5.8	14	491	54	3	0.0002	.007

9wNo.:	REG	LAB.	SERUM-ID	STR	ANTIGEN	No.REAC.	AVE	+/+	MISS. +/-	EXTRA -/+	%INCL	Q-SCORE	R-VALUE
595	NCY	MRV	8372	60	DR4	3497	7.2	830	145	122	86	4.7	.809
				20	DRw53	2522	5.5	71	676	51	10	1.7	.141
				*20	DR7	2522	5.5	34	445	88	8	0.016	.051
				*20	DRw9	2522	5.6	10	160	112	6	0.036	.013
596	FRA	BET	FLY 802	67	DRw11	3882	7.6	1008	32	329	97	6.4	.795
				29	DRw8	2842	6.3	122	150	207	45	0.96	.338
				22	TA10	2570	5.9	108	620	99	15	2.0	.157
				17	Bw52	1839	5.1	18	66	79	22	0.13	.158
				18	Bw35	1755	5.5	24	241	55	10	0.048	.093
597	EAE	MYR	FREUNDHOFER	63	DRw11	3713	7.7	980	20	757	98	7.2	.623
				35	DRw52	2713	6.2	686	1076	71	39	1.5	.335
				*35	DRw8	2713	6.6	161	100	596	62	1.7	.246
				*35	DRw12	2713	6.3	182	161	575	54	1.4	.213
				*35	DRw14	2713	6.3	318	411	439	44	.97	.212
				22	DRw8	951	6.0	12	28	59	30		.180
598	EAE	WAL	MA 251079	70	TA10	3826	7.5	1443	353	199	81	3.8	.711
				16	DRw11	2030	6.6	10	1	189	91	7.8	.201
				14	DRw8	2019	5.2	43	150	146	23	0.53	.144
				15	DRw52	1826	5.4	120	1024	26	11	1.2	.119
				*15	DRw12	1826	5.3	6	11	140	36	3.9	.098
				*15	DRw14	1826	5.4	70	530	76	22	0.19	.095
599	NCY	FUL	DA-6	65	TA10	3927	7.3	1556	294	261	85	3.8	.716
				13	DRw11	2077	5.7	7	4	254	64	6.3	.112
601	FRA	FAU	FRE 534	72	TA10	3932	7.4	1733	119	139	94	6.2	.868
				12	DRw11	2080	6.0	7	4	132	64	5.8	.166
				10	DRw12	2069	5.6	5	11	127	32	4.2	.090
603	US5	SIN	Z 100761	55	DRw11	3874	7.2	980	55	313	95	6.9	.785
				21	DRw12	2839	5.9	179	181	134	50	1.9	.471
				14	TA10	2479	5.4	70	390	64	16	3.2	.207
				12	DRw14	2019	4.9	35	637	29	6	0.025	.082
605	US8	LEE	NOVEL	63	DRw11	2657	7.3	580	106	242	85	4.8	.684
				40	DRw52	1971	6.3	224	1025	18	18	1.0	.227
				*40	DRw12	1971	6.0	58	174	184	25	0.42	.142
				*40	DRw14	1971	6.5	104	464	138	19	0.47	.117
				*40	DRw8	1971	6.5	41	134	201	24	0.57	.106
				*40	DRw13	1971	6.4	59	253	183	24	0.26	.088
				38	DRw8	723	7.0	4	24	14	15		.152
607	US5	SWE	CARP 1074	29	TA10	3829	6.6	1276	536	43	71	4.0	.717

9wNo.:	REG	LAB.	SERUM-ID	STR	ANTIGEN	No.REAC.	AVE	+/+	MISS. +/-	EXTRA -/+	%INCL	Q-SCORE	R-VALUE
608	IT1	GAN	CO 844	68	DRw11	3935	7.6	1032	21	331	99	8.0	.805
				19	DRw52	2882	5.5	296	1582	35	16	1.1	.183
				*19	DRw12	2882	5.4	97	273	234	27	0.57	.177
				*19	DRw14	2882	5.4	152	637	179	20	0.46	.150
				*19	DRw13	2882	5.8	76	428	255	16	0.21	.052
				25	TA10	1004	6.1	25	251	10	10	2.5	.187
609	US5	SIN	15902.1	43	DRw11	3879	6.6	773	268	128	75	4.6	.732
				12	DRw8	2838	5.1	28	246	100	11	0.048	.090
				13	DRw14	2564	4.9	46	665	54	7	0.077	.082
				18	DRw13	1853	5.6	23	364	31	6	0.057	.093
610	US5	SWE	1073	66	DRw11	3853	7.5	1016	33	246	97	7.7	.835
				17	TA10	2804	5.6	116	680	130	15	2.4	.129
				16	DRw52	2008	5.2	111	1196	19	9	0.94	.112
				*16	DRw14	2008	5.3	69	602	61	11	0.14	.110
				*16	DRw8	2008	5.8	22	170	108	12	0.16	.066
				*16	DRw13	2008	4.9	39	410	91	9	0.051	.048
611	US1	ZMI	PJ-NOVE	57	DRw11	3542	7.1	796	139	175	86	6.0	.775
				27	DRw52	2607	5.7	159	1552	16	10	0.95	.142
				*27	DRw14	2607	6.1	75	658	100	11	0.37	.088
				*27	DRw8	2607	5.8	31	205	144	14	0.21	.081
				*27	DRw13	2607	5.3	50	401	125	12	0.15	.081
				*27	DRw12	2607	5.4	35	304	140	11	0.11	.056
612	NCY	BIA	SICKLER	54	DRw11	3889	6.9	903	138	99	87	5.3	.843
				16	TA10	2848	5.8	41	765	58	6	2.1	.055
613	NCY	MRV	18772	48	DRw11	3487	6.7	705	239	114	75	3.7	.736
				24	DRw10	2543	5.6	9	47	105	17	0.14	.084
614	US8	LEE	CANIS	64	DRw11	3820	7.6	1007	22	621	98	5.7	.678
				32	DRw8	2791	6.3	177	91	444	67	1.4	.343
				30	TA10	2523	6.1	268	438	176	38	2.1	.333
				23	DQw3	1817	5.7	106	401	70	21	0.75	.236
				18	A25	1307	6.0	10	14	60	42	0.47	.221
616	UKI	BOD	F 7621 A1	71	DRw52	3862	7.3	2307	557	175	81	1.7	.576
				*71	DRw11	3862	7.8	1018	15	1464	99	6.9	.432
				*71	DRw8	3862	7.6	317	12	2165	97	5.5	.204
				*71	DRw12	3862	7.3	357	49	2125	88	3.6	.169
				*71	DRw13	3862	6.8	420	100	2062	81	2.5	.136
				*71	DRw14	3862	7.3	699	225	1783	76	2.3	.133
				37	DRw8	998	6.9	38	7	137	85		.382
				33	DRw11	953	7.8	17	1	120	95		.317
				25	DRw12	935	6.0	5	1	115	84		.169
				25	DRw13	929	4.7	6	3	109	67		.163
				26	DR2	920	6.0	59	272	50	18	0.087	.139

Table 1 (continued)

9wNo.:	REG	LAB.	SERUM-ID	STR	ANTIGEN	No.REAC.	AVE	+/+	MISS. +/-	EXTRA -/+	%INCL	Q-SCORE	R-VALUE
618	JAP	SAJ	35-165	44	DRw8	3897	7.2	294	33	1015	90		.361
				38	TA10	3570	6.4	731	973	284	43		.306
				29	DRw14	1850	6.1	154	455	125	26	0.31	.201
				21	DRw13	1241	5.2	67	287	58	19	0.12	.186
				34	DRw12	887	6.4	5	4	53	23	0.78	.142
619	NCY	MRV	12560	36	DRw8	3497	6.7	221	55	260	81	3.8	.564
				22	Bw57	3214	5.6	33	114	225	23	0.083	.116
				22	TA10	3074	5.8	154	1315	73	11	0.048	.113
620	JAP	JUJ	I-1015	46	DRw8	3855	7.1	289	31	724	91	5.5	.438
				39	DRw11	3535	6.3	429	549	295	44	1.2	.358
				36	DRw12	2557	6.5	144	204	151	32	1.5	.371
621	JAP	OKO	KYO 1097	47	DRw8	3895	7.4	312	13	723	96	5.6	.474
				35	DRw12	3571	6.6	214	183	509	54	1.0	.296
				29	TA10	3174	5.9	276	1054	233	21	0.11	.109
				24	DRw14	1796	6.2	98	508	126	17	0.10	.080
623	UKI	DRK	1068 D	48	DRw8	3919	7.6	311	19	1271	95	4.5	.333
				39	DQw3	3589	6.4	1018	1028	253	50	0.32	.345
				*39	DRw11	3589	6.2	586	411	685	59	0.64	.303
				*39	DRw12	3589	6.4	214	189	1057	54	0.36	.132
				27	TA10	1543	5.8	70	134	183	35	0.36	.189
				28	Bw42	1326	7.6	11	8	166	58	0.55	.158
				25	DRw53	1310	5.6	71	319	97	19	0.013	.105
624	US4	STA	ALANIZ P16746	43	DRw8	3897	6.7	237	82	224	75	4.2	.578
				34	DQw3	3578	5.9	172	1856	52	9	0.023	.105
				*34	DR4	3578	6.2	89	919	135	9	0.085	.066
				*34	DRw14	3578	5.6	73	793	151	9	0.012	.051
				*34	DRw11	3578	5.7	82	917	142	9	0.042	.050
				*34	DRw12	3578	5.8	33	364	191	9	0.062	.030
626	US8	LEE	FOUR	39	DRw8	3908	7.1	256	68	570	80	3.6	.426
				25	TA10	3584	5.8	349	1366	221	21	0.038	.116
				17	DRw14	1676	5.8	84	481	88	15	0.061	.108
627	US1	ZMI	PJ FOUR	45	DRw8	3689	7.3	244	58	313	81	4.4	.548
				23	DQw3	3387	5.7	241	1676	72	13	0.023	.131
				*23	DRw12	3387	6.0	58	330	255	15	0.093	.071
				*23	DRw11	3387	5.7	117	826	196	13	0.058	.068
				11	DRw14	1456	5.2	39	456	33	8	0.019	.097
629	GER	NEU	GÖ 804694 B	75	DR7	3924	7.8	576	13	163	98	8.3	.849
				25	B13	3326	6.6	35	38	126	48	2.1	.301
				18	DQw2	3259	5.2	43	368	85	11	2.9	.128
				18	DRw14	2848	5.4	39	665	46	6	0.044	.086
630	GER	NEU	GÖ 810468 B	68	DR7	3938	7.3	567	25	53	96	8.7	.924
				24	DRw8	3346	5.4	14	304	39	5	0.051	.073
633	US6	BRN	CCB 979	65	DR7	3907	7.3	565	24	43	96	8.2	.934
				20	DQw2	3318	6.2	13	404	30	4	3.8	.061
				13	DQw3	2901	5.2	28	1727	2	2	0.0080	.069
634	US5	SWE	1075	54	DR7	3819	7.3	523	51	278	92	5.8	.725
				25	DRw14	3245	5.7	110	692	168	14	0.10	.105
				26	DQw3	2443	5.6	138	1429	30	9	0.036	.102
				*26	DRw11	2443	5.9	74	692	94	10	0.12	.074
				*26	DRw8	2443	5.2	26	218	142	11	0.061	.050
				*26	DR4	2443	5.5	67	753	101	9	0.025	.036
636	UKI	MID	LAVERY	73	DR7	3935	7.9	591	3	232	100	8.9	.815
				23	DQw2	3341	5.9	72	349	160	18	3.1	.152
				*23	DR3	3341	5.6	56	444	176	12	0.055	.070
				18	TA10	2920	5.4	114	1314	46	8	0.086	.108
637	US5	SWE	1078	71	DR7	3854	7.8	576	7	188	99	8.1	.836
				22	DRw14	3193	5.6	68	737	102	9	0.025	.081
638	ANZ	DAW	SIMMONS 8w977	76	DR7	3857	7.6	575	7	61	99	9.2	.935
639	US7	HAN	SEA-1126	46	DR7	3913	6.5	434	155	48	75	4.8	.786
				22	DQw2	3324	5.3	19	395	29	5	2.4	.099
				*22	DR3	3324	4.7	12	480	36	3	0.028	.035
640	IT1	GAN	CO 781	81	DR7	3939	7.6	582	13	46	98	9.5	.943
642	FRA	BET	FLY 915	70	DR7	3888	7.3	550	41	35	94	7.6	.924
643	BEN	BOU	DARAT 61278	57	DR7	3310	6.9	150	328	59	32	0.99	.423
				44	DQw2	2832	6.7	18	350	41	5	0.51	.076
644	US5	CMC	N 1943	62	DRw9	3856	7.8	262	10	191	97	7.1	.724
				24	DRw53	3584	5.6	113	1444	78	8	0.34	.075
				*24	DR7	3584	5.6	44	534	147	8	0.016	.045
				*24	DR4	3584	5.6	62	926	129	7	0.0016	.026
645	FRA	FAU	FRE 582	61	DRw9	3916	7.9	279	9	309	97	7.4	.646
				32	DRw10	3628	6.9	58	13	251	82	3.9	.370
				27	DRw53	3557	5.8	178	1383	73	12	0.36	.150
				*27	DR4	3557	6.0	119	874	132	12	0.096	.120
				*27	DR7	3557	5.8	47	531	204	9	0.038	.018
				24	DRw14	1996	5.6	38	547	35	7	0.080	.097

9wNo.:	REG	LAB.	SERUM-ID	STR	ANTIGEN	No.REAC.	AVE	+/+	MISS. +/-	EXTRA -/+	%INCL	Q-SCORE	R-VALUE
646	JAP	SAK	16821	48	DRw9	3908	7.7	275	8	693	98	6.7	.469
				34	DR7	3625	6.3	421	165	272	72	2.3	.589
				29	DRw53	3039	5.6	157	877	115	16	0.97	.157
				*29	DR4	3039	5.7	136	776	136	15	0.10	.137
647	JAP	OKU	JR-36-25 A	61	DRw9	3919	7.3	274	15	80	95	6.6	.844
650	JAP	JUJ	I-993 A	55	DRw9	3887	7.7	274	5	352	99	8.0	.621
				30	DRw53	3608	6.0	235	1336	117	15	0.49	.154
				*30	DR7	3608	6.0	98	488	254	17	0.17	.103
				*30	DR4	3608	5.9	130	868	222	14	0.041	.068
				23	DRw14	2037	5.6	51	537	66	9	0.11	.080
652	US5	CMC	2926 KZ	69	DQw1	3746	7.3	1931	281	74	88	4.7	.813
				*69	DRw14	3746	7.4	831	68	1174	93	5.4	.438
				*69	DR2	3746	7.5	766	45	1239	95	6.0	.431
				*69	DRw13	3746	6.9	374	122	1631	76	2.9	.171
				*69	DR1	3746	7.0	338	129	1667	73	2.8	.143
				*69	DRw10	3746	7.1	51	16	1954	77	2.6	.061
				31	DR2	1534	6.3	8	1	66	89		.301
				31	DRw13	1525	5.5	19	40	47	33		.275
653	BEN	ENG	EB-32	60	DQw1	3903	7.0	2008	312	128	87	4.5	.774
				*60	DR2	3903	7.5	832	30	1304	97	6.9	.447
				*60	DRw14	3903	7.0	846	83	1290	92	5.0	.408
				*60	DRw13	3903	6.8	380	140	1756	74	2.4	.145
				*60	DR1	3903	6.5	351	137	1785	72	2.3	.131
				*60	DRw10	3903	7.0	48	23	2088	68	1.7	.035
				17	DRw13	1583	5.6	17	43	111	29		.147
				17	DR2	1523	6.0	5	5	106	50		.134
654	US4	STA	CJO	68	DQw1	3876	7.3	2110	188	81	92	5.6	.859
				*68	DRw14	3876	7.3	884	36	1307	97	6.2	.445
				*68	DR2	3876	7.6	838	22	1353	98	7.3	.441
				*68	DR1	3876	7.0	397	87	1794	83	3.4	.194
				*68	DRw13	3876	7.0	399	115	1792	78	3.3	.166
				*68	DRw10	3876	7.1	53	18	2138	75	3.4	.050
				27	DR2	1578	6.7	9	1	72	90		.307
				25	DRw13	1568	4.7	14	46	58	24		.179
				29	DR1	1469	5.6	5	27	43	16		.104
655	ANZ	HAY	DUKE 060772	67	DQw1	3859	7.2	2077	224	61	91	5.4	.852
				*67	DRw14	3859	7.4	876	44	1262	96	6.6	.448
				*67	DR2	3859	7.4	803	51	1335	95	6.3	.414
				*67	DR1	3859	7.1	385	97	1753	80	3.3	.186
				*67	DRw13	3859	6.8	399	121	1739	77	3.2	.169
				*67	DRw10	3859	7.1	53	17	2085	76	3.0	.056
				19	DRw13	1558	5.0	10	46	51	18		.139

9wNo.:	REG	LAB.	SERUM-ID	STR	ANTIGEN	No.REAC.	AVE	+/+	MISS. +/-	EXTRA -/+	%INCL	Q-SCORE	R-VALUE
656	FRA	OHA	FTO 501	68	DQw1	3692	7.3	2004	204	338	91	3.4	.692
				*68	DR2	3692	7.7	794	28	1548	97	4.6	.368
				*68	DRw14	3692	7.3	817	65	1525	93	3.6	.340
				*68	DR1	3692	7.2	387	73	1955	85	2.1	.162
				*68	DRw13	3692	7.0	399	94	1943	81	1.5	.143
				*68	DRw10	3692	7.1	53	15	2289	78	0.99	.041
				34	DQw2	1484	6.0	173	395	165	31	0.079	.144
				*34	DR7	1484	5.9	111	227	227	33	0.38	.130
				33	DR2	916	6.5	4	0	161	100		.141
				34	DRw12	903	6.5	47	129	114	27	0.11	.114
802	EAE	MYR	Control	61	DR2	3794	7.5	764	79	733	91	3.8	.560
				41	DRw11	2947	6.4	365	470	368	44	0.48	.274
				37	B7	2112	6.2	64	137	304	32	0.50	.123
				37	DR1	1911	6.3	70	217	234	25	0.057	.097
657	FRA	VIV	FBA-AVILES	74	DQw1	3861	7.5	2190	107	188	96	5.4	.841
				*74	DRw14	3861	7.5	892	25	1487	98	6.0	.409
				*74	DR2	3861	7.8	832	23	1546	98	6.4	.392
				*74	DR1	3861	7.3	440	48	1938	91	3.7	.223
				*74	DRw13	3861	7.3	442	77	1936	86	3.2	.191
				*74	DRw10	3861	7.1	63	7	2315	90	3.4	.079
				21	DR1	1564	6.1	16	20	172	45		.153
				21	DRw13	1528	5.1	19	37	153	34		.140
				24	DR2	1472	6.8	5	3	148	63		.126
				*24	DR7	1472	5.5	56	281	97	17	0.28	.111
661	FRA	BET	FLY-894	77	DQw1	3924	7.6	2288	45	162	99	6.4	.891
				*77	DRw14	3924	7.7	921	11	1529	99	7.6	.419
				*77	DR2	3924	7.8	858	9	1592	99	7.5	.402
				*77	DR1	3924	7.3	473	23	1977	96	5.2	.259
				*77	DRw13	3924	7.3	476	48	1974	91	4.0	.230
				*77	DRw10	3924	7.2	66	3	2384	96	3.8	.092
				22	DRw13	1591	5.5	31	29	131	52		.272
				23	DR1	1531	5.6	18	15	113	55		.244
				24	DR2	1498	7.1	7	2	106	78		.207
662	EAE	KAS	KAS-109	76	DQw1	3869	7.5	2185	109	89	96	6.2	.894
				*76	DR2	3869	7.8	841	12	1433	99	8.0	.430
				*76	DRw14	3869	7.4	883	43	1391	96	6.6	.417
				*76	DR1	3869	7.6	473	11	1801	98	7.3	.299
				*76	DRw13	3869	7.2	417	96	1857	82	3.5	.179
				*76	DRw10	3869	7.5	59	7	2215	90	5.4	.082
				32	DR1	1575	7.0	29	6	60	83		.504
				21	DR2	1540	6.3	6	3	54	67		.249
				22	DRw13	1531	5.3	11	45	43	20		.170
				25	Bw64	1471	5.7	7	39	36	16	0.0050	.131

Table 1 (continued)

9wNo.:	REG	LAB.	SERUM-ID	STR	ANTIGEN	No.REAC.	AVE	+/+	MISS. +/-	EXTRA -/+	%INCL	Q-SCORE	R-VALUE
663	EAE	KAS	KAS-110	75	DQw1	3838	7.5	2180	93	145	96	5.6	.871
				*75	DRw14	3838	7.7	899	15	1426	99	7.5	.432
				*75	DR2	3838	7.5	786	55	1458	94	5.5	.356
				*75	DR1	3838	7.5	454	23	1871	96	5.8	.267
				*75	DRw13	3838	7.1	449	62	1876	88	4.6	.219
				*75	DRw10	3838	7.6	61	5	2264	93	4.5	.086
				26	DR1	1565	6.0	23	11	122	68		.300
				27	DRw13	1531	5.6	19	34	103	36		.195
				29	DRw9	1478	6.1	38	138	65	22	0.51	.211
				27	Bw46	1302	5.3	6	12	59	34	0.085	.154
				30	DR2	1284	4.0	4	5	55	45		.160
664	IT2	FER	FE-140	77	DQw1	3882	7.6	2259	52	152	98	6.8	.891
				*77	DRw14	3882	7.7	918	12	1493	99	7.6	.423
				*77	DR2	3882	7.6	830	27	1581	97	6.7	.381
				*77	DR1	3882	7.4	477	15	1934	97	5.8	.274
				*77	DRw13	3882	7.2	467	45	1944	92	4.8	.234
				*77	DRw10	3882	7.3	68	2	2343	98	5.8	.098
				23	DRw13	1571	5.8	33	26	119	56		.309
				22	DR1	1512	5.6	22	11	97	67		.326
				22	DRw9	1479	5.4	26	150	71	15	0.53	.122
667	NCY	YUN	YAR	70	DQw1	3873	7.3	2083	210	72	91	5.6	.854
				*70	DR2	3873	7.6	839	17	1316	99	6.9	.454
				*70	DRw14	3873	7.3	840	80	1315	92	5.1	.401
				*70	DR1	3873	7.2	412	73	1743	85	3.8	.223
				*70	DRw13	3873	7.0	385	127	1770	76	2.2	.154
				22	DR2	1580	5.3	6	4	66	60		.212
				24	Bw53	1570	6.0	5	19	61	21	0.080	.103
668	ANZ	BSH	HEMPHREYS B184	69	DQw1	3893	7.3	2170	140	68	94	6.6	.891
				*69	DRw14	3893	7.6	902	23	1336	98	7.5	.452
				*69	DR2	3893	7.3	777	79	1461	91	5.5	.357
				*69	DR1	3893	7.2	443	46	1795	91	5.2	.254
				*69	DRw13	3893	7.0	438	83	1800	85	4.7	.211
				*69	DRw10	3893	7.1	66	3	2172	96	6.1	.104
				11	DRw13	1583	5.5	16	44	52	27		.219
				11	DR1	1523	5.0	8	24	44	25		.174
669	GER	MUE	MUE 2328611	74	DQw1	3847	7.5	2255	41	162	99	6.8	.891
				*74	DRw14	3847	7.6	919	8	1498	100	8.0	.423
				*74	DR2	3847	7.6	841	11	1576	99	7.5	.396
				*74	DR1	3847	7.4	457	30	1960	94	5.3	.244
				*74	DRw13	3847	7.1	457	48	1960	91	4.7	.223
				*74	DRw10	3847	7.1	67	3	2350	96	4.6	.093
				22	DR1	1551	5.5	17	17	145	50		.194
				22	DRw13	1517	5.5	23	34	122	41		.207
				22	DR2	1460	7.0	4	5	118	45		.103
				23	DRw11	1346	5.6	63	487	46	12	0.080	.102
670	ANZ	DAW	DAW 0104873	71	DQw1	3731	7.5	2159	54	584	98	3.0	.658
				*71	DRw14	3731	7.7	884	9	1859	99	5.3	.324
				*71	DR2	3731	7.4	787	35	1956	96	2.7	.268
				*71	DR1	3731	7.3	427	29	2316	94	2.4	.170
				*71	DRw13	3731	7.2	459	40	2284	92	2.2	.164
				*71	DRw10	3731	7.4	62	2	2681	97	2.3	.070
				48	DRw9	1518	6.8	113	74	471	61	0.90	.169
				46	Bw54	1297	6.6	50	20	401	72	0.10	.184
671	ANZ	DAW	HOPKINS 30954	70	DQw1	3836	7.4	2199	86	573	97	2.9	.650
				*70	DRw14	3836	7.6	906	11	1866	99	4.1	.332
				*70	DR2	3836	7.3	789	53	1983	94	2.4	.254
				*70	DR1	3836	7.2	457	32	2315	94	2.1	.181
				*70	DRw13	3836	7.1	465	50	2307	91	1.9	.159
				*70	DRw10	3836	7.3	66	4	2706	95	2.5	.067
				48	Bw54	1547	6.5	63	32	509	67	0.064	.155
				48	DRw12	1424	6.8	111	116	381	49	0.20	.131
				*48	DRw9	1424	6.8	77	72	415	52	0.21	.123
672	BEN	BRX	DUCARME 6	73	DQw1	3899	7.5	2228	84	227	97	5.1	.835
				*73	DRw14	3899	7.7	915	10	1540	99	7.7	.415
				*73	DR2	3899	7.5	804	56	1651	94	4.7	.336
				*73	DR1	3899	7.5	452	39	2003	93	4.4	.229
				*73	DRw13	3899	7.2	458	55	1997	90	2.7	.212
				*73	DRw10	3899	7.6	64	6	2391	92	5.2	.080
				21	DRw13	1587	5.7	30	29	197	51	3.7	.205
				21	DRw8	1528	5.8	52	104	145	34	0.90	.206
				20	DR1	1372	5.3	12	20	133	38		.135
674	IT1	CUR	TORP 25	75	DQw1	3894	7.5	2239	71	138	97	6.2	.889
				*75	DRw14	3894	7.7	910	16	1467	99	7.7	.426
				*75	DR2	3894	7.6	837	23	1540	98	6.3	.396
				*75	DR1	3994	7.4	457	34	1920	94	4.6	.250
				*75	DRw13	3894	7.1	465	48	1912	91	4.8	.236
				*75	DRw10	3894	7.4	67	3	2310	96	4.9	.096
				16	DRw13	1584	5.5	34	26	104	57		.337
				17	DR1	1524	5.2	17	16	87	52		.264
				17	DR2	1491	6.0	5	4	82	56		.165
677	US5	TER	NO 467.1 Z	56	DRw52	3851	6.9	2208	658	78	78	3.1	.614
				*43	DRw14	3851	7.1	819	111	1467	89	3.1	.330
				*43	DR3	3851	7.5	523	15	1763	98	5.4	.311
				*43	DRw11	3851	6.8	809	226	1477	79	2.0	.232
				*43	DRw13	3851	6.5	381	131	1905	75	1.1	.120
				25	DQw1	985	5.8	63	451	15	13	0.031	.168
678	US6	BRN	CCB 887.2	56	DR3	3917	7.5	523	17	716	97	5.3	.561
				38	DRw52	3377	6.2	680	1678	36	29	1.7	.284

9wNo.:	REG	LAB.	SERUM-ID	STR	ANTIGEN	No.REAC.	AVE	+/+	MISS. +/-	EXTRA -/+	%INCL	Q-SCORE	R-VALUE
679	ANZ	HAY	PETT 250275	55	DRw52	3898	6.8	1743	1149	96	61		.445
				*55	DR3	3898	7.6	533	8	1306	99	6.0	.413
				*55	DRw14	3898	7.0	715	207	1124	78	2.3	.339
				*55	DRw13	3898	6.4	364	154	1475	71	1.4	.181
				*55	DRw12	3898	6.6	266	149	1573	65	1.3	.117
				30	B8	1006	6.2	13	22	83	38	1.3	.178
				27	A31	971	4.7	14	52	69	22	0.030	.122
680	FRA	JEA	FGE-2412	58	DRw52	3511	6.9	1197	1158	118	55	1.2	.380
				*58	DRw14	3511	7.2	596	215	919	74	1.7	.336
				*58	DR3	3511	7.2	408	79	1107	86	2.1	.329
				*58	DRw12	3511	6.8	197	182	1318	52	0.48	.062
				*58	DRw13	3511	6.6	252	198	1263	56	0.54	.099
				38	DQw1	956	6.2	112	371	6	24	0.18	.333
681	FRA	FAU	FRE 558	66	DRw52	3894	7.2	2075	809	74	72	2.4	.570
				*66	DRw11	3894	7.3	967	74	1182	93	5.3	.458
				*66	DRw13	3894	7.2	471	54	1678	90	3.6	.274
				*66	DRw14	3894	7.6	658	268	1491	72	2.7	.178
				18	DRw11	1010	5.7	13	5	61	73		.335
				22	DRw13	992	6.3	6	4	55	60		.226
682	ANZ	CSH	AH 3229	73	DRw52	3461	7.4	2107	472	301	82	0.75	.451
				*73	DRw11	3461	7.6	891	50	1517	95	4.6	.334
				*73	DRw13	3461	7.2	418	49	1990	90	2.9	.171
				*73	DRw12	3461	7.4	319	52	2089	86	3.0	.124
				*73	DRw14	3461	7.5	656	167	1752	80	2.3	.123
				*73	DRw8	3461	7.1	239	44	2169	85	2.2	.096
				52	DR2	882	6.9	230	79	71	75	2.4	.624
				32	DRw11	573	6.0	9	5	62	65		.249
				32	DRw8	559	6.2	11	14	51	44	2.2	.227
				31	DRw13	534	6.3	6	3	45	67		.254
				33	B38	525	7.3	6	5	39	55	0.28	.240
683	US5	CMC	2708 KZ	58	DRw52	3676	7.0	2240	481	180	83	2.0	.587
				*58	DRw14	3676	7.3	824	67	1596	93	4.0	.318
				*58	DRw11	3676	7.0	843	147	1577	86	2.7	.247
				*58	DRw12	3676	7.0	314	76	2106	81	1.7	.107
				*58	DRw13	3676	6.8	371	111	2049	77	1.1	.091
				*58	DR3	3676	7.1	386	118	2034	77	0.92	.090
				*58	DRw8	3676	6.9	236	67	2184	78	0.91	.076
				24	DQw1	955	5.8	157	338	23.	32	0.22	.341
				8	DRw8	460	5.1	7	11	16	39		.314
684	US5	TER	L 24421 Z	42	DRw52	3847	6.4	1566	1286	69	55	1.5	.425
				*42	DRw14	3847	6.8	600	317	1035	66	1.7	.259
				*42	DRw11	3847	6.3	654	387	981	63	1.5	.250
				*42	DRw13	3847	6.2	327	187	1308	64	1.0	.168
				23	TA10	995	5.9	31	251	38	11	0.35	.100
685	FRA	FAU	FRE 538	62	DRw52	3916	7.0	2310	589	40	80	4.5	.678
				*62	DRw14	3916	7.4	862	71	1488	93	4.4	.370
				*62	DR3	3916	7.8	532	9	1818	99	6.7	.313
				*62	DRw12	3916	7.2	372	46	1978	89	3.5	.205
				*62	DRw11	3916	6.8	767	279	1583	74	1.7	.164
				20	DRw14	1017	5.9	7	7	33	50		.280
687	FRA	BET	FLY 232	67	DRw52	3824	7.2	2498	352	118	88	4.2	.708
				*67	DRw11	3824	7.4	986	60	1630	95	4.9	.341
				*67	DRw14	3824	7.3	842	69	1774	93	4.1	.289
				*67	DR3	3824	7.8	533	2	2083	100	8.0	.271
				*67	DRw12	3824	7.5	372	26	2244	94	4.5	.184
				*67	DRw13	3824	6.6	370	140	2246	73	1.6	.035
				19	TA10	974	5.6	59	222	59	21	0.65	.173
				16	DRw14	693	5.1	7	5	52	59		.237
688	UKI	FES	LH 621	84	DRw52	3882	7.7	2819	62	174	98	5.8	.838
				*84	DRw11	3882	7.7	1029	18	1964	99	5.9	.306
				*84	DRw14	3882	7.8	915	7	2078	100	6.8	.294
				*84	DR3	3882	7.8	538	5	2455	100	7.0	.211
				*84	DRw13	3882	7.6	508	8	2485	99	5.3	.199
				*84	DRw12	3882	7.8	400	9	2593	98	6.2	.169
				*84	DRw8	3882	7.4	275	45	2718	86	2.1	.063
				31	DRw14	1001	7.4	13	0	161	100		.250
				27	DRw11	988	6.7	15	3	146	84		.247
				26	DRw13	970	7.0	8	2	138	80		.185
				24	DRw8	960	5.2	19	25	119	44		.180
				28	DRw12	916	7.2	5	1	114	84		.170
689	ANZ	WOO	FOWLER 032529	75	DRw52	3809	7.5	2673	139	347	96	2.8	.654
				*75	DRw14	3809	7.6	892	19	2128	98	4.1	.258
				*75	DRw11	3809	7.5	960	64	2060	94	2.7	.216
				*75	DR3	3809	7.8	522	6	2498	99	4.6	.194
				*75	DRw12	3809	7.6	392	2	2628	100	5.0	.169
				*75	DRw13	3809	7.1	454	51	2566	90	1.8	.102
				*75	DRw8	3809	7.4	274	51	2746	85	0.85	.038
				53	Cw1	997	6.9	137	114	210	55	0.020	.241
				52	DRw9	731	7.2	57	43	145	57	0.34	.261
				45	Aw34	631	7.0	10	6	135	63	0.088	.152
				43	DRw12	615	6.5	4	0	131	100		.153
692	US1	AMO	JA 350	76	DRw52	3754	7.5	2618	161	160	95	4.5	.778
				*76	DRw14	3754	7.7	857	26	1921	98	5.6	.291
				*76	DRw11	3754	7.5	962	64	1816	94	4.2	.276
				*76	DR3	3754	7.6	509	14	2269	98	5.8	.214
				*76	DRw13	3754	7.6	474	27	2304	95	4.0	.184
				*76	DRw12	3754	7.4	338	44	2440	89	2.8	.111
				*76	DRw8	3754	7.4	271	42	2507	87	2.9	.087
				26	DRw8	975	6.4	22	20	138	53		.206
				24	DRw13	933	6.6	7	2	131	78		.175
				24	A3	924	5.7	41	115	90	27	0.049	.156
				25	DRw14	768	4.9	7	4	83	64		.195

Table 1 (continued)

9wNo.:	REG	LAB.	SERUM-ID	STR	ANTIGEN	No.REAC.	AVE	+/+	MISS. +/-	EXTRA -/+	%INCL	Q-SCORE	R-VALUE
693	GER	NEU	NEU 810413 B	78	DRw52	3918	7.6	2820	85	128	98	5.8	.857
				*78	DRw11	3918	7.5	1017	39	1931	97	5.9	.296
				*78	DRw14	3918	7.7	913	17	2035	99	7.3	.296
				*78	DR3	3918	7.7	536	7	2412	99	7.9	.218
				*78	DRw13	3918	7.3	507	15	2441	98	6.0	.199
				*78	DRw12	3918	7.6	399	11	2549	98	6.4	.175
				*78	DRw8	3918	7.6	311	19	2637	95	5.7	.134
				35	DRw8	1013	7.0	35	9	93	80		.429
				24	DRw11	969	5.3	14	4	79	78		.318
				26	DRw14	951	5.5	11	3	68	79		.311
				29	DRw13	937	6.7	9	1	59	90		.331
				25	DRw12	927	6.5	4	2	55	67		.199
694	ANZ	HAY	RICE 150972	72	DRw52	3886	7.4	2701	176	88	94	5.2	.830
				*72	DRw14	3886	7.6	895	36	1894	97	6.4	.304
				*72	DRw11	3886	7.2	955	88	1834	92	4.4	.266
				*72	DR3	3886	7.8	516	3	2273	100	7.8	.241
				*72	DRw13	3886	7.1	493	27	2296	95	4.9	.201
				*72	DRw12	3886	7.5	382	30	2407	93	4.7	.160
				*72	DRw8	3886	7.3	298	25	2491	93	4.7	.137
				26	DRw8	1009	5.8	27	17	61	62		.398
				27	DRw13	965	6.0	7	3	54	70		.268
				27	DRw12	955	5.5	4	2	50	67		.210
				30	DRw14	949	6.0	5	9	45	36		.167
				33	Bw59	935	6.8	5	12	40	30	0.025	.156
696	US7	DUP	SCIARAPPA 1431	71	DRw52	3904	7.3	2710	184	100	94	5.3	.817
				*71	DRw14	3904	7.6	917	19	1893	98	6.7	.325
				*71	DRw11	3904	7.2	951	97	1859	91	4.1	.253
				*71	DR3	3904	7.5	516	21	2294	97	6.3	.214
				*71	DRw13	3904	7.3	498	25	2312	96	4.6	.204
				*71	DRw12	3904	7.5	392	19	2418	96	6.0	.179
				*71	DRw8	3904	7.1	249	75	2561	77	1.7	.033
				19	DRw14	1010	5.6	9	5	91	65		.216
				18	DRw13	996	6.0	6	4	85	60		.178
				20	DRw12	986	5.5	4	2	81	67		.162
				19	B49	980	5.2	5	9	76	36	0.040	.120
697	US7	DUP	FERNANDEZ 1366	66	DRw52	3813	7.3	2593	225	181	93	3.5	.728
				*66	DRw11	3813	7.3	956	65	1818	94	5.5	.284
				*66	DRw14	3813	7.4	855	50	1919	95	5.7	.272
				*66	DRw12	3813	7.4	385	17	2389	96	5.9	.177
				*66	DR3	3813	7.3	471	45	2303	92	4.8	.165
				*66	DRw8	3813	7.2	292	27	2482	92	4.3	.127
				*66	DRw13	3813	6.9	443	79	2331	85	3.5	.108
				23	DRw8	995	6.4	34	11	147	76		.324
				22	DQw2	950	5.9	67	185	80	27	0.044	.185
				22	DRw11	697	5.0	8	4	72	67		.229
				20	Bw42	685	5.5	4	1	68	80	0.13	.194

9wNo.:	REG	LAB.	SERUM-ID	STR	ANTIGEN	No.REAC.	AVE	+/+	MISS. +/-	EXTRA -/+	%INCL	Q-SCORE	R-VALUE
698	NCY	MRV	18660	79	DRw52	3273	7.6	2327	96	133	97	5.1	.816
				*79	DRw11	3273	7.7	865	32	1595	97	5.8	.302
				*79	DRw14	3273	7.8	743	22	1717	98	6.1	.281
				*79	DRw13	3273	7.4	435	19	2025	96	4.5	.192
				*79	DR3	3273	7.7	431	19	2029	96	5.9	.191
				*79	DRw12	3273	7.7	310	24	2150	93	4.3	.138
				*79	DRw8	3273	7.4	229	25	2231	91	3.6	.101
				20	DRw14	850	6.0	10	3	123	77		.210
				19	DRw8	837	5.4	17	15	106	54		.216
				20	DRw11	805	6.2	11	6	95	65		.224
				21	DRw13	788	6.0	5	3	90	63		.157
				21	DRw12	780	7.0	4	2	86	67		.152
699	ANZ	WOO	ZINSLEY 52496	83	DRw52	3920	7.7	2797	103	157	97	4.7	.825
				*83	DRw11	3920	7.8	1030	19	1924	99	6.2	.320
				*83	DRw14	3920	7.8	914	14	2040	99	6.9	.299
				*83	DR3	3920	7.6	522	17	2432	97	5.6	.199
				*83	DRw13	3920	7.5	501	21	2553	96	5.0	.188
				*83	DRw8	3920	7.7	319	7	2635	98	6.0	.157
				*83	DRw12	3920	7.5	377	41	2577	91	3.9	.119
				46	DRw8	1020	7.4	41	3	116	94		.458
				37	DRw14	976	6.6	13	1	103	93		.302
				35	DRw11	962	7.3	14	3	89	83		.311
				30	DRw13	945	6.3	7	3	82	70		.215
700	GER	LEN	HBKC 17378	62	DQw1	3878	7.2	2060	244	280	90	2.9	.719
				*62	DRw14	3878	7.5	913	13	1427	99	6.9	.438
				*62	DR2	3878	7.1	685	160	1655	82	2.4	.224
				*62	DR1	3878	7.2	433	54	1907	89	3.2	.221
				*62	DRw13	3878	6.8	430	88	1910	84	2.2	.182
				*62	DRw10	3878	7.2	65	5	2275	93	3.4	.090
				29	A3	1570	6.2	100	99	178	51	0.32	.325
				25	DRw13	1375	5.0	21	24	159	47		.183
701	US2	BAC	MIN 14173	57	DQw1	3681	6.9	1736	432	110	81	3.2	.716
				*57	DRw14	3681	7.1	791	79	1055	91	5.8	.454
				*57	DR2	3681	7.1	649	158	1197	81	3.4	.321
				*57	DR1	3681	6.7	307	145	1539	68	2.1	.133
				*57	DRw13	3681	6.6	305	185	1541	63	1.3	.095
				*57	DRw10	3681	6.6	47	16	1799	75	2.7	.065
				22	DRw8	1513	5.9	39	113	71	26	0.70	.237
				19	Bw54	1357	5.2	12	62	59	17	0.054	.118
				20	DRw13	1277	5.0	8	44	50	16		.107

9wNo.:	REG	LAB.	SERUM-ID	STR	ANTIGEN	No.REAC.	AVE	+/+	MISS. +/-	EXTRA -/+	%INCL	Q-SCORE	R-VALUE
702	US8	LEE	GOLD	54	DQw1	3908	6.8	1649	662	55	72	2.9	.673
				*54	DRw14	3908	7.0	852	76	852	92	6.9	.542
				*54	DR2	3908	6.9	575	282	1129	68	2.9	.251
				*54	DRw13	3908	6.6	307	211	1397	60	1.9	.123
				*54	DR1	3908	6.6	253	236	1451	52	1.4	.062
				*54	DRw10	3908	6.4	44	26	1660	63	1.6	.052
				27	DRw13	1597	5.6	10	50	45	17		.143
				31	DRw8	1537	5.5	12	147	33	8	0.27	.093
				31	DR3	1376	6.2	17	295	15	6	0.27	.112
703	US6	BRN	CCB 1044	64	DQw1	3855	7.2	2037	254	109	89	4.2	.810
				*64	DRw14	3855	7.5	896	28	1250	97	6.8	.467
				*64	DR2	3855	7.2	713	134	1433	85	3.5	.305
				*64	DRw13	3855	6.8	421	95	1725	82	2.7	.205
				*64	DR1	3855	7.0	386	95	1760	81	2.6	.187
				*64	DRw10	3855	6.9	62	8	2084	89	2.6	.090
				21	DRw13	1563	5.7	22	37	86	38		.237
				20	B51	1500	5.9	42	156	44	22		.260
704	US5	CMC	1683 KZ	56	DRw52	3723	6.9	1598	1163	90	58	1.2	.427
				*56	DRw14	3723	7.2	628	262	1060	71	2.4	.284
				*56	DRw13	3723	7.0	374	115	1314	77	2.4	.243
				*56	DRw11	3723	6.6	614	398	1074	61	1.8	.188
				30	DRw8	962	6.1	17	24	73	42	1.8	.233
705	US6	BRN	CCB 976	40	DQw1	3878	6.3	1224	1080	56	54	1.9	.518
				*40	DRw14	3878	6.4	670	254	610	73	3.7	.470
				*40	DR2	3878	6.4	477	372	803	57	1.5	.261
				*40	DRw13	3878	6.2	250	271	1030	48	0.59	.125
				28	DRw13	1574	5.6	9	52	47	15		.121
706	US5	SWE	PARISIEN	52	DQw1	3851	6.7	1594	695	82	70	2.8	.638
				*52	DR2	3851	7.1	724	119	952	86	3.2	.452
				*52	DRw14	3851	6.6	721	208	955	78	2.8	.388
				*52	DRw13	3851	6.6	288	226	1388	57	0.50	.099
707	LAT	PRI	PR 100 D6	27	DR3	3725	6.0	204	305	428	41	0.90	.245
				26	DRw14	3216	5.9	225	551	203	29	0.71	.260
				22	DRw52	2440	5.6	174	1320	29	12	0.48	.151
708	LAT	GOR	BMB 0070	41	DRw52	3882	6.4	1328	1546	146	47	0.56	.287
				*41	DRw11	3882	6.5	616	422	858	60	1.1	.266
				*41	TA10	3881	6.5	922	916	551	51	0.36	.239
				*41	DRw8	3882	7.0	244	79	1230	76	2.3	.233
				*41	DRw12	3882	6.4	227	189	1247	55	0.60	.118
				26	DRw8	1008	6.4	20	22	126	48		.196

9wNo.:	REG	LAB.	SERUM-ID	STR	ANTIGEN	No.REAC.	AVE	+/+	MISS. +/-	EXTRA -/+	%INCL	Q-SCORE	R-VALUE
709	BEN	ROO	vR 133224	51	DRw52	3824	6.7	1837	1002	96	65	1.7	.481
				*51	DRw11	3824	6.8	795	244	1138	77	2.3	.317
				*51	DRw14	3824	7.2	681	221	1252	76	2.3	.277
				*51	DRw13	3824	6.7	416	102	1517	81	1.9	.236
				16	Cw5	985	5.6	29	86	67	26	0.076	.190
710	JAP	NAI	FD 1366	46	DR4	2985	6.7	506	302	382	63	1.2	.438
				39	DRw53	2177	6.3	179	435	203	30	0.77	.191
				36	DRw14	1545	6.2	79	379	119	18	0.045	.086
711	IT2	FER	FE-65	36	DR2	3840	6.4	421	413	209	51	1.3	.485
				24	DRw14	3006	5.8	99	765	110	12	0.068	.113
712	ANZ	CSH	AH 2996	43	TA10	3546	6.5	867	818	252	52	0.81	.407
				*43	DRw11	3548	6.6	581	398	538	60	2.4	.369
				*43	DRw12	3548	6.5	263	100	856	73	3.8	.297
				35	DR3	1863	6.3	152	156	100	50	2.4	.466
				28	DRw52	1555	5.8	91	827	9	10	1.7	.170
713	FRA	MAY	FST-16	59	DRw52	3829	6.9	1818	1020	40	65	2.9	.526
				*59	DR3	3829	7.8	511	12	1347	98	5.9	.391
				*59	DRw14	3829	7.0	706	200	1152	78	2.6	.328
				*59	DRw12	3829	6.9	325	82	1533	80	2.4	.216
				*59	DRw13	3829	6.4	347	166	1511	68	1.2	.150
				27	DRw13	991	5.6	5	5	35	50		.236
714	US8	NSF	SCF 1884	43	DRw52	3805	6.5	1419	1407	20	51	2.3	.434
				*43	DRw14	3805	6.5	590	315	849	66	2.1	.315
				*43	DR3	3805	6.8	395	135	1044	75	2.5	.305
				*43	DRw11	3805	6.6	510	532	929	49	0.80	.141
715	US7	DUP	NJ 3873-515	44	DRw14	3887	6.7	661	265	789	72	2.1	.394
				37	DR3	2961	6.7	334	93	455	79	2.9	.479
				29	DRw52	2534	5.9	366	1184	89	24	1.2	.185
				28	B44	984	5.4	33	169	56	17	0.0052	.129
716	US5	ALA	WH-6-ALA	MULTISPECIFIC									
717	FRA	GRA	FGR 126	69	DQw2	3685	7.5	898	62	1606	94	2.4	.325
				*69	DR7	3685	7.7	558	16	1946	98	1.7	.269
				*69	DR3	3685	7.2	393	106	2111	79	0.40	.092
				63	DRw12	2725	7.2	248	85	1358	75	0.42	.118
				62	DQw1	2354	7.1	984	624	346	62	0.27	.139
				53	DRw9	746	7.0	80	43	266	66	0.24	.166
				51	DQw3	623	6.8	223	250	43	48	0.38	.160

Table 1 (continued)

9wNo.:	REG	LAB.	SERUM-ID	STR	ANTIGEN	No.REAC.	AVE	+/+	MISS. +/-	EXTRA -/+	%INCL	Q-SCORE	R-VALUE
719	GER	BRA	BRA-950	59	DQw2	3707	7.2	776	163	367	83	2.8	.653
				*59	DR7	3707	7.5	541	26	602	96	4.6	.594
				*59	DR3	3707	6.6	270	230	873	54	0.74	.198
				34	A2	2765	5.9	243	1202	123	17	0.0072	.111
				43	A28	1301	5.7	28	132	95	18	0.039	.103
				46	Bw62	1142	6.9	25	112	70	19	0.027	.133
720	UKI	DIC	HUTTON	59	DQw2	3845	7.3	938	46	415	96	4.7	.739
				*59	DR7	3843	7.5	580	10	773	99	6.7	.563
				*59	DR3	3843	6.8	396	123	957	77	2.8	.340
				33	DRw12	2861	6.5	144	196	271	43	0.92	.290
				26	DRw9	2521	5.9	83	122	188	41	1.4	.286
				25	DR3	2316	5.2	60	95	128	39		.300
				32	Bw55	2157	5.5	22	55	106	29	0.27	.184
721	FRA	FAU	FRE 565	68	DQw2	3902	7.4	880	116	481	89	2.9	.657
				*68	DR7	3902	7.8	582	5	779	100	7.1	.567
				*68	DRw9	2906	7.6	261	25	1100	92	4.5	.333
				*68	DR3	3902	6.5	315	220	1046	59	1.2	.201
				53	DRw9	2609	7.5	211	21	270	91		.590
				33	DRw12	2674	6.4	126	205	144	39		.349
				29	DR3	2343	5.6	34	124	110	22		.172
				31	Bw53	2185	7.0	10	39	100	21	0.037	.106
722	FRA	MAY	FST-18	59	DQw2	3780	7.5	923	44	635	96	4.0	.646
				*59	DR7	3780	7.6	568	11	990	99	5.5	.491
				*59	DR3	3780	7.0	408	101	1150	81	2.0	.312
				32	Cw7	2809	6.2	399	494	234	45	0.28	.362
				21	DRw9	1920	5.9	55	127	181	31	0.31	.177
				20	DRw11	1728	5.6	87	417	88	18	0.10	.152
				15	DR3	1224	5.5	11	35	77	24		.128
723	NCY	CAR	BOS/HER	69	DQw2	3855	7.5	931	51	234	95	6.1	.822
				*69	DR7	3855	7.9	579	5	586	100	7.5	.634
				*69	DR3	3855	7.0	376	155	789	71	2.6	.353
				23	DRw53	2856	5.8	132	945	98	13	0.58	.120
				18	DR3	1779	5.1	27	106	71	21		.184
724	IT2	FER	FE-210	62	DQw2	3874	7.4	920	85	597	92	3.2	.635
				*62	DR7	3874	7.7	567	23	950	97	6.0	.494
				*62	DR3	3874	6.7	365	175	1152	68	2.2	.234
				40	DRw9	2869	7.3	183	39	414	83	4.1	.440
				27	DRw53	2647	6.0	271	583	143	32	1.2	.306
				20	DR3	1793	5.1	34	107	109	25		.174
726	BEN	ENG	EB-26	51	DQw2	3935	6.9	704	308	182	70	2.8	.663
				*51	DR3	3935	6.9	415	128	471	77	4.0	.516
				*51	DR7	3935	6.8	363	232	523	62	2.6	.389
				16	DR3	2923	5.7	64	100	118	40		.331
				16	DRw11	2759	5.4	62	712	56	9	0.11	.115
727	FRA	FAU	FRE 566	61	DQw2	3927	7.6	955	58	634	95	5.1	.646
				*61	DR7	3927	7.8	574	23	1015	97	5.8	.480
				*61	DR3	3927	7.1	439	105	1150	81	3.0	.329
				30	DRw53	2914	6.3	373	736	261	34	0.61	.226
				22	DRw12	1641	5.8	67	148	121	32	0.43	.240
729	ANZ	DAW	ARCHER M 25319	66	DRw53	3894	7.4	1468	379	357	80	2.2	.621
				*66	DR4	3894	7.7	1041	35	784	97	4.6	.618
				*66	DRw9	3894	7.3	257	24	1568	92	3.0	.249
				*66	DR7	3894	6.8	305	286	1520	52	0.29	.040
				33	DR4	2047	7.2	48	9	309	85		.298
				28	A2	1989	5.9	231	729	78	25	0.14	.227
				28	Bw54	1029	7.4	7	10	71	42	0.62	.165
				23	A11	1012	6.0	23	135	48	15	0.047	.127
730	FRA	FAU	FRE 527	69	DRw53	3899	7.6	1767	89	1045	96	2.1	.491
				*69	DR4	3899	7.7	1047	35	1765	97	3.6	.341
				*69	DRw9	3899	7.8	281	7	2531	98	3.8	.160
				*69	DR7	3899	7.3	525	66	2287	89	1.7	.158
				45	DQw3	2043	6.8	612	173	433	78	1.2	.424
				*45	TA10	2042	6.7	658	278	387	71	0.20	.352
				36	DR4	1258	7.3	17	0	416	100		.162
				35	Cw4	1241	6.5	97	118	319	46	0.017	.112
540	US5	MIT	C5313.1	56	DR2	3769	7.3	679	155	427	82	3.2	.610
				30	DRw53	2935	5.9	311	1274	116	20	0.048	.156
				*30	DR4	2935	6.0	157	734	270	18	0.028	.058
				*30	DR7	2935	5.7	104	436	323	20		.063
				*30	DRw9	2935	5.9	48	196	379	20	0.15	.044
				28	DR1	1299	6.0	47	239	62	17	0.25	.154
				27	Cw5	1012	5.8	18	110	44	15	0.023	.126
731	FRA	FAU	FRE 510	68	DQw3	3903	7.5	2082	114	731	95	2.0	.575
				*68	DR4	3903	7.7	1061	18	1752	99	4.3	.362
				*68	DR7	3903	7.0	496	97	2317	84	0.97	.109
				*68	DRw9	3903	7.6	271	15	2542	95	3.1	.142
				*68	DRw11	3903	7.1	893	150	1920	86	1.6	.182
				*68	DRw12	3903	7.4	375	37	2438	92	2.1	.145
				43	DRw53	1707	6.9	373	70	358	85	1.8	.495
				*43	DR4	1707	7.3	36	0	695	100		.170
				*43	DR7	1707	6.6	265	90	466	75		.330
				*43	DRw9	1707	7.3	88	12	643	88		.228
				29	DRw10	1246	6.2	26	13	314	67	1.1	.159
733	US8	FOT	FOT-STRA	52	DQw2	3903	7.2	840	163	534	84	4.1	.598
				*52	DR7	3903	7.5	575	15	799	98	6.3	.550
				*52	DR3	3903	6.5	263	273	1111	50	0.82	.116
				27	DRw53	2900	6.0	453	648	81	42	1.6	.459
				*27	DR4	2900	6.0	333	566	201	38	0.90	.322
				*27	DRw9	2900	6.1	119	110	415	52	2.5	.253

9wNo.:	REG	LAB.	SERUM-ID	STR	ANTIGEN	No.REAC.	AVE	+/+	MISS. +/-	EXTRA -/+	%INCL	Q-SCORE	R-VALUE
734	FRA	DAU	FPA-BOUZ	66	DRw53	3911	7.3	1674	177	322	91	3.7	.747
				*66	DR4	3911	7.1	946	131	1050	88	3.1	.454
				*66	DR7	3911	7.7	582	8	1414	99	5.5	.401
				*66	DRw9	3911	7.6	274	14	1722	96	4.5	.249
				27	DR7	2060	7.0	41	4	281	92		.311
				23	DRw10	2015	6.0	17	36	264	33	0.12	.086
735	FRA	DAU	FPA-2879	72	DRw53	3919	7.6	1755	105	479	95	3.3	.717
				*72	DR4	3919	7.4	997	83	1237	93	4.4	.440
				*72	DR7	3919	7.7	580	8	1654	99	6.2	.353
				*72	DRw9	3919	7.8	275	13	1959	96	5.6	.219
				35	DQw2	2059	7.0	225	29	254	89	1.9	.580
				*35	DR3	2059	6.7	226	122	253	65	2.0	.445
				*35	DR7	2059	6.4	39	3	440	93		.238
				14	DRw12	1805	5.6	72	152	182	33	0.43	.196
				14	DR4	1581	5.5	25	31	157	45		.199
				14	DR3	1525	5.2	37	99	120	28		.174
736	ANZ	FON	HUNT 19592	52	DRw53	3757	6.8	1261	496	158	72	2.7	.657
				*52	DR4	3757	7.1	837	177	582	83	3.5	.562
				*52	DR7	3757	6.6	321	245	1098	57	1.1	.165
				*52	DRw9	3757	6.8	163	101	1256	62	1.5	.136
				14	DRw14	2000	5.4	64	526	94	11	0.036	.071
737	UKI	BAT	PUGH	56	DRw53	3525	6.9	932	668	61	59	2.4	.610
				*56	DR4	3525	7.0	605	321	388	66	2.4	.493
				*56	DR7	3525	6.5	195	300	798	40	0.76	.101
				*56	DRw9	3525	7.5	206	50	787	81	4.3	.325
739	JAP	SEK	KS-53	47	DRw53	3842	6.7	885	926	354	49	0.59	.336
				*47	DRw9	3842	7.0	229	46	1010	84	2.3	.303
				*47	DR4	3842	6.6	504	549	735	48	0.42	.205
				*47	DR7	3842	6.6	186	391	1053	33	0.055	.080
				36	B7	2031	6.3	196	189	158	51	0.54	.427
				29	Bw60	1645	6.2	49	77	109	39	0.61	.286
740	US3	GRU	SPEERLING	55	DQw3	3835	6.9	1569	590	117	73	2.8	.656
				*55	DR4	3835	7.2	901	152	785	86	3.7	.516
				*55	DRw11	3835	6.7	588	443	1098	58	1.3	.160
				*55	DRw12	3835	6.8	281	124	1405	70	1.7	.176
741	FRA	ARN	FAR-8	56	DR7	3735	7.7	549	18	1331	97	3.3	.393
				44	DRw53	3168	6.6	734	499	597	56	0.87	.283
				37	B51	1935	6.5	104	107	493	50	0.17	.140
				36	Bw52	1724	6.9	50	48	443	52	0.19	.122

9wNo.:	REG	LAB.	SERUM-ID	STR	ANTIGEN	No.REAC.	AVE	+/+	MISS. +/-	EXTRA -/+	%INCL	Q-SCORE	R-VALUE
743	US8	NSF	NSF-1001	64	DRw53	3852	7.1	1423	388	131	79	3.1	.734
				*64	DR7	3852	7.7	570	18	984	97	6.0	.490
				*64	DR4	3852	6.7	739	308	815	71	2.1	.377
				*64	DRw9	3852	7.5	261	14	1293	95	5.2	.308
				43	DQw2	2041	6.4	79	175	52	32	1.2	.380
744	US1	DUQ	RINNELS	46	DQw2	3852	6.6	1599	554	171	75	0.0085	.640
				*46	DR4	3852	6.6	723	329	1047	69	1.7	.280
				*46	DRw11	3852	6.6	721	317	1049	70	2.0	.287
				*46	DRw12	3852	6.8	332	69	1438	83	3.1	.252
				21	DRw9	1699	5.4	32	66	139	33	1.2	.186
745	US1	DUQ	PETFALSKY	54	DQw3	3894	6.9	1804	384	239	83	2.8	.680
				*54	DR4	3894	7.3	959	111	1084	90	4.3	.458
				*54	DRw11	3894	6.7	737	309	1306	71	1.9	.218
				*54	DRw12	3894	6.8	329	81	1714	81	2.3	.191
				22	DRw53	1706	5.7	121	324	118	28	0.95	.226
				*22	DRw9	1706	5.7	34	67	205	34	0.98	.142
				*22	DR4	1706	5.5	16	20	223	45		.129
				*22	DR7	1706	5.7	66	288	173	19	0.091	.068
				*22	Bw60	1247	5.9	21	81	93	21	0.043	.119
				20	DR4	1145	6.3	6	6	87	50		.158
746	ANZ	DAW	M 33028	68	DQw3	3847	7.3	1888	275	218	88	3.2	.741
				*68	DRw11	3847	7.2	877	162	1229	85	3.7	.363
				*68	DR4	3847	7.3	819	230	1287	79	2.6	.287
				*68	DRw12	3847	7.5	389	19	1717	96	5.5	.281
				32	DRw9	1684	6.2	49	49	169	50	2.6	.274
				31	DRw12	1586	6.1	19	5	150	80		.275
				32	Bw57	1559	6.7	32	46	118	42	0.22	.244
				27	DRw11	1484	5.6	42	101	76	30		.259
				36	TA10	1341	6.6	13	52	63	20	1.6	.140
				*36	DR7	1341	6.5	29	245	47	11	0.21	.108
747	BEN	BRX	CINIGLIO-2	60	DQw3	3616	7.1	1753	279	329	87	2.8	.658
				*60	DR4	3616	7.2	836	159	1246	85	2.7	.330
				*60	DRw11	3616	7.1	784	193	1298	81	2.2	.279
				*60	DRw12	3616	7.2	339	41	1743	90	2.7	.219
				32	Cw8	1581	6.5	97	96	230	51	0.18	.272
				25	DRw9	1391	5.5	32	58	200	36	1.0	.133
				26	DRW12	1301	4.9	11	8	189	58	2.7	.144
				26	DRw14	1282	6.1	94	378	95	20	0.068	.111
				16	DRw11	810	5.7	27	88	68	24		.149
				*16	TA10	810	5.6	32	122	63	21	1.0	.136

Table 1 (continued)

9wNo.:	REG	LAB.	SERUM-ID	STR	ANTIGEN	No.REAC.	AVE	+/+	MISS. +/-	EXTRA -/+	%INCL	Q-SCORE	R-VALUE
748	ANZ	DAW	SMITH R 8323	63	DQw3	3850	7.3	1871	304	250	87	3.1	.709
				*63	DRw11	2850	7.3	901	136	1220	87	3.7	.388
				*63	DRw12	2850	7.5	397	13	1724	97	6.1	.290
				*63	DR4	2850	7.1	798	263	1323	76	1.8	.250
				20	TA10	1675	5.7	95	135	155	42	2.1	.295
				18	DR3	1445	5.6	69	212	86	25	0.57	.220
				19	DRw12	1164	6.8	5	1	81	84		.209
				18	DRw53	1158	5.3	44	299	37	13	0.33	.148
750	US3	PER	1135 B	64	DQw3	3908	7.3	1835	366	337	84	2.6	.635
				*64	DR4	3908	7.7	1057	22	1115	98	5.3	.527
				*64	DRw11	3908	6.9	868	181	1304	83	2.2	.331
				29	DRw11	1707	5.9	75	71	262	52		.243
				30	DR4	1561	7.7	29	6	233	83		.268
752	JAP	KAS	K-2417	72	DRw53	3793	7.5	1547	242	679	87	1.5	.533
				*72	DR4	3793	7.5	959	77	1270	93	3.0	.421
				*72	DRw9	3793	7.8	262	10	1964	97	3.8	.212
				*72	DR7	3793	7.1	451	129	1775	78	1.1	.165
				58	DR1	2004	6.8	233	108	446	69	1.2	.330
				61	DRw10	1663	7.7	46	2	400	96	3.1	.296
				58	DR4	1615	6.6	30	22	370	58		.139
				60	DR7	1563	6.6	19	22	351	40		.088
				63	DRw8	1446	7.1	58	118	275	33	0.058	.088
753	UKI	MOR	BRADSHAW	74	DRw53	3805	7.7	1734	70	773	97	2.9	.605
				*74	DR4	3805	7.8	1033	22	1474	98	5.5	.418
				*74	DR7	3805	7.4	508	62	1999	90	2.8	.161
				*74	DRw9	3805	7.8	274	7	2233	98	4.4	.135
				46	DQw3	2001	6.6	560	206	213	74	1.6	.558
				*46	DRw11	2001	6.5	396	232	377	64	1.5	.339
				*46	DRw12	2001	6.7	170	67	603	72	1.8	.249
				*46	DR4	2001	7.6	54	3	719	95		.197
				36	DR1	1218	6.1	79	175	117	32	0.79	.210
				35	DRw9	964	5.7	6	0	111	100		.213
				36	DRw11	958	5.5	22	80	89	22		.108
754	NCY	GOE	GRINNER	70	TA10	3699	7.6	1699	82	511	96	3.4	.700
				36	DQw3	1918	6.4	294	224	217	57	2.2	.414
				*36	DR4	1918	6.4	249	222	262	53	1.4	.338
				*36	DRw12	1918	6.8	15	2	496	89	4.6	.132
				*36	DRw11	1918	7.0	6	4	505	60	4.4	.055
				28	DRw8	1400	6.0	42	83	175	34	0.58	.157
				27	DRw12	1249	6.5	4	0	165	100		.143

9wNo.:	REG	LAB.	SERUM-ID	STR	ANTIGEN	No.REAC.	AVE	+/+	MISS. +/-	EXTRA -/+	%INCL	Q-SCORE	R-VALUE
755	US5	CMC	4016 KZ	84	DRw52	3737	7.8	2706	80	424	98	2.6	.620
				*84	DRw11	3737	7.8	978	24	2152	98	3.6	.227
				*84	DRw14	3737	7.8	884	17	2246	99	3.7	.219
				*84	DR3	3737	7.6	515	13	2615	98	2.8	.152
				*84	DRw12	3737	7.9	390	5	2740	99	3.9	.140
				*84	DRw8	3737	7.7	303	5	2827	99	3.4	.119
				*84	DRw13	3737	7.7	464	33	2666	94	2.2	.102
				50	B44	951	6.8	150	48	274	76	0.14	.322
				48	DRw8	753	7.2	36	1	238	98		.288
				46	DR2	716	6.2	117	141	121	46	0.60	.193
				49	DRw13	458	7.3	9	1	112	90		.215
				48	TA10	448	6.9	43	56	69	44	0.58	.227
756	US5	SIN	15886.1	79	DRw52	3802	7.6	2710	106	174	97	4.6	.805
				*79	DRw11	3802	7.7	978	39	1906	97	2.6	.287
				*79	DRw14	3802	7.8	869	30	2015	97	2.8	.271
				*79	DR3	3802	7.7	513	16	2371	97		.198
				*79	DRw13	3802	7.4	478	28	2406	95	2.0	.170
				*79	DRw12	3802	7.6	384	16	2500	96	2.3	.161
				*79	DRw8	3802	7.4	302	21	2582	94	1.8	.126
				36	DRw8	986	5.9	34	10	140	78		.338
				38	DRw11	934	6.2	10	7	126	59		.171
				38	DRw14	917	7.5	8	4	118	67		.177
				36	DRw13	905	6.0	5	4	113	56		.127
757	US2	BAC	MN 3534	69	DRw52	3782	7.3	2394	421	155	86	2.7	.642
				*69	DRw11	3782	7.7	1004	25	1545	98	6.1	.394
				*69	DRw14	3782	7.1	786	124	1763	87	3.5	.228
				*69	DRw12	3782	7.5	379	21	2170	95	5.0	.201
				*69	DRw8	3782	7.6	298	15	2251	96	5.4	.178
				*69	DR3	3782	7.2	433	91	2116	83	2.1	.130
				40	DRw8	967	7.2	37	4	118	91		.426
				33	DRw11	926	6.4	17	1	101	95		.345
				31	DRw12	875	6.0	5	1	89	84		.195
				32	DRw13	869	6.5	4	4	85	50	1.2	.126
758	US5	ALA	WH-8-ALA	87	DRw52	3755	7.8	2705	77	703	98	1.1	.378
				*87	DRw14	3755	7.9	867	21	2541	98	1.8	.132
				*87	DRw11	3755	7.8	989	31	2419	97	1.5	.131
				*87	DR3	3755	7.8	499	5	2909	100	2.0	.112
				*87	DRw12	3755	7.9	394	7	3014	99	1.9	.089
				*87	DRw13	3755	7.7	474	22	2934	96	1.0	.065
				*87	DRw8	3755	7.7	304	12	3104	97	0.93	.057
				69	DQw3	973	7.4	460	83	243	85	0.15	.313
				*69	DR4	973	7.3	406	97	297	81	0.23	.196
				60	DRw8	430	6.9	25	4	218	87		.161

9wNo.:	REG	LAB.	SERUM-ID	STR	ANTIGEN	No.REAC.	AVE	+/+	MISS. +/-	EXTRA -/+	%INCL	Q-SCORE	R-VALUE
759	US6	BRN	CCB-1035	48	DQw2	3872	6.8	660	332	251	67	2.4	.595
				*48	DR3	3872	6.8	389	141	522	74	3.1	.468
				*48	DR7	3872	6.7	336	246	575	58	2.0	.339
				32	DR3	2880	6.0	63	98	188	40		.262
				32	DRw11	2719	6.1	118	647	70	16	0.29	.210
				32	DQw3	1954	5.9	54	969	16	6	0.037	.096
761	NCY	CAR	BOS-ING	51	DQw3	3844	6.8	1631	515	89	77	3.4	.707
				*51	DR4	3844	7.0	851	190	869	82	3.7	.454
				*51	DRw11	3844	6.6	695	346	1025	67	2.4	.270
				*51	DRw12	3844	6.7	315	86	1405	79	3.1	.232
				25	TA10	1698	5.8	32	200	57	14	1.0	.153
				24	DRw11	1466	6.0	2	3	55	40		.109
763	US7	HAN	SEA 1114	34	DRw8	3884	6.4	172	153	164	53	1.9	.476
				27	DRw53	3559	5.7	105	1638	59	7	0.0025	.066
764	ANZ	CSH	AH 3516	28	B8	3863	6.0	148	280	205	35	0.60	.312
				*28	DR3	3863	5.9	116	418	237	22		.175
				24	DRw14	3435	5.7	76	741	129	10	0.036	.079
765	ANZ	BSH	LANCASHIRE B223	46	DRw14	3175	6.7	298	438	775	41	0.027	.078
				*46	DQw2	3171	6.6	330	499	741	40	0.81	.076
				44	DQw3	2435	6.4	509	961	264	35	0.42	.076
				45	DQw1	599	6.5	118	286	16	30	0.67	.236
766	ANZ	TAI	SOONG	35	TA10	3510	6.1	305	1335	57	19	0.33	.255
767	ANZ	CSH	AH 3549	44	DRW14	3639	6.6	441	425	1059	51	0.070	.110
				42	TA10	2751	6.4	645	853	406	44	0.017	.109
				41	DQw1	1253	6.3	280	477	126	37	0.082	.121
				43	DQw2	1130	6.7	131	182	239	42	0.12	.120
768	ANZ	CSH	AH 3556	34	DR2	3824	6.4	428	409	299	52	1.0	.433
				26	DRw14	2987	5.7	113	743	186	14	0.017	.067
769	ANZ	CSH	AH 3736	42	DRw14	3748	6.6	516	380	1285	58	0.13	.107
				40	DQw2	2852	6.5	413	348	872	55	1.2	.112
				*40	DR7	2852	6.6	247	214	1038	54	0.067	.075
				38	DQw1	2091	6.4	551	608	321	48	0.88	.132
				*38	DR2	2091	6.4	343	359	529	49	0.016	.103
				36	DQw3	932	6.3	301	461	20	40	0.55	.225
770	ANZ	CSH	AH 3727	47	DRw14	3713	6.7	557	329	1434	63	0.090	.104
				46	DQw3	2827	6.6	985	762	449	57	0.91	.144
				42	DQw1	1080	6.4	352	395	97	48	0.67	.169
				45	DQw2	333	6.6	64	90	33	42	0.51	.254

9wNo.:	REG	LAB.	SERUM-ID	STR	ANTIGEN	No.REAC.	AVE	+/+	MISS. +/-	EXTRA -/+	%INCL	Q-SCORE	R-VALUE
771	ANZ	CSH	AH 3657	50	DRw14	3795	6.8	587	314	1454	66	0.16	.127
				48	DQw3	2894	6.7	876	676	578	57	1.1	.133
				45	DQw1	1109	6.5	357	406	82	47	0.87	.219
				*45	DR2	1109	6.6	198	235	241	46	0.0043	.101
				46	DQw2	346	6.8	57	104	25	36	0.55	.257
				*46	DR3	346	6.4	39	70	43	36	0.025	.193
772	ANZ	CSH	AH 3624	20	Bw4	3788	5.7	259	1963	76	12	0.066	.118
773	US5	TER	NO-11801	32	TA10	3784	6.2	556	1244	97	31	0.67	.344
				23	DR3	1984	5.8	28	287	69	9	0.049	.081
774	US5	TER	JO-33401	57	DQw2	3772	7.4	897	73	726	93	4.3	.588
				*57	DR7	3772	7.5	537	39	1086	94	3.4	.430
				*57	DR3	3772	7.1	401	109	1222	79	1.6	.284
				34	DRw53	2802	6.3	512	547	214	49	0.90	.399
				24	DQw3	1609	5.7	109	577	50	16	1.9	.174
775	US5	TER	L-73541 Z	54	DQw2	3842	7.4	815	176	769	83	3.5	.491
				*54	DR3	3842	7.3	431	96	1153	82	3.0	.328
				*54	DR7	3842	7.3	446	138	1138	77	3.0	.302
				33	DQw3	2851	6.2	683	1045	86	40	0.61	.351
776	US5	TER	NO 2861 Z	50	DQw1	3807	6.7	1486	776	108	66	2.1	.584
				*50	DRw14	3807	6.9	710	194	884	79	2.8	.415
				*50	DR2	3807	6.8	572	267	1022	69	1.7	.284
				*50	DRw13	3807	6.5	272	237	1322	54	0.64	.092
				*50	DRw10	3807	6.5	44	26	1550	63	0.50	.058
				27	DRw8	1545	6.1	28	127	80	19	0.49	.145
777	US5	TER	461.1 Z	50	DQw3	3820	6.8	1471	662	153	69	2.0	.602
				*50	DRw11	3820	6.9	716	321	908	70	2.0	.328
				*50	DRw12	3820	6.9	333	71	1291	83	2.9	.278
				*50	DR4	3820	6.6	604	427	1020	59	0.81	.198
				15	TA10	1687	5.3	46	183	107	21	1.7	.152
778	US5	TER	L-68521 Z	59	DQw1	3739	7.0	1662	563	885	75	1.5	.171
				*59	DR2	3739	7.2	684	151	1863	82	0.50	.159
				*59	DRw11	3739	7.0	763	254	1784	76	0.29	.091
				*59	DRw12	3739	7.0	300	95	2247	76	0.22	.058
				52	DQw3	1514	6.8	777	385	108	67	1.0	.310
				33	B7	352	6.3	15	8	93	66	0.30	.198
779	US5	TER	N 1945	52	DQw3	3794	6.9	1453	671	191	69	1.7	.571
				*52	DRw11	3794	7.0	720	312	924	70	2.1	.326
				*52	DRw12	3794	7.1	345	57	1299	86	3.2	.295
				*52	DR4	3794	6.7	563	460	1081	56	0.67	.143
				21	TA10	1670	5.8	47	177	144	21	1.5	.118
				21	DR7	1425	6.0	56	264	85	18	0.068	.137

Table 1 (continued)

9wNo.:	REG	LAB.	SERUM-ID	STR	ANTIGEN	No.REAC.	AVE	+/+	MISS. +/-	EXTRA -/+	%INCL	Q-SCORE	R-VALUE
780	FRA	ARN	FAR-9	67	DQw2	3662	7.4	814	135	2024	86	1.3	.117
				*67	DR7	3662	7.4	478	80	2360	86	0.21	.083
				64	DQw3	2713	7.2	332	717	357	80	0.85	.146
				60	DQw1	1074	7.0	649	239	68	74	0.50	.293
781	FRA	BET	FLY-901	51	DRw14	3865	6.9	429	486	412	47	0.97	.339
				43	DRw11	2950	6.4	225	667	187	26	0.53	.214
				36	DRw12	2058	6.4	64	235	123	22	0.31	.177
				34	TA10	1759	6.0	44	369	79	11	0.10	.080
				34	DR7	1346	6.6	28	227	51	11	0.026	.105
785	IT2	FER	FELD2	30	DRw12	3731	5.9	91	295	320	24	0.18	.136
786	JAP	JUJ	T-383	65	DQw3	3814	7.3	1838	307	463	86	2.6	.588
				*65	DRw11	3814	7.3	828	191	1473	82	1.7	.258
				*65	DRw12	3814	7.5	375	26	1926	94	3.2	.233
				*65	DR4	3814	7.2	824	226	1477	79	1.1	.229
				36	DQw2	1669	6.3	238	307	225	44	0.32	.248
				34	DRw9	1124	6.1	44	30	181	60	1.5	.262
				34	TA10	1050	6.1	71	98	110	43	1.1	.287
				36	DRw8	881	6.6	28	93	82	24	0.12	.129
787	JAP	OKO	KYC 1031	48	DRw14	3785	6.8	351	528	321	40	0.70	.319
				41	DRw12	2906	6.3	58	295	263	17	0.11	.064
788	JAP	OKO	KYC 947	60	DRw52	3768	7.0	1695	1090	73	61	2.1	.470
				*60	DR3	3768	7.1	440	84	1328	84	3.4	.298
				*60	DRw14	3768	7.3	643	245	1125	73	2.4	.284
				*60	DRw13	3768	7.0	396	109	1372	79	2.4	.248
				*60	DRw12	3768	7.0	236	162	1532	60	1.5	.085
				*60	DRw11	3768	6.8	506	493	1262	51	1.1	.045
789	JAP	OKO	KYC 110	65	TA10	3850	7.4	1649	178	671	91	2.1	.583
				42	DR3	2023	6.8	206	118	465	64	1.4	.282
				35	DRw14	1699	6.3	221	320	244	41	0.43	.207
				31	DQw3	1158	6.1	133	269	111	34	0.94	.215
				27	DRw52	756	6.0	84	272	27	24	0.83	.238
790	JAP	MAE	A10/83	70	TA10	3793	7.4	1487	314	251	83	2.7	.701
				33	DQw3	1992	6.4	115	443	136	21	1.4	.151
791	US2	BAC	MN 14455	67	DQw3	3712	7.3	1822	248	240	89	3.4	.734
				*67	DR4	3712	7.3	898	134	1164	88	3.2	.393
				*67	DRw11	3712	7.5	841	135	1221	87	3.2	.368
				*67	DRw12	3712	7.2	321	63	1741	84	2.4	.192
				30	TA10	1642	6.4	104	114	136	48	1.4	.366
				23	DRw53	1424	5.7	61	324	75	16	0.57	.130
792	NCY	FUL	MC-3	56	DQw2	3837	7.3	693	289	455	71	1.7	.521
				*56	DR3	3837	7.2	399	130	749	76	3.2	.397
				*56	DR7	3837	7.1	354	222	794	62	1.7	.289
				34	TA10	2855	6.2	368	1027	87	27	0.097	.279
				24	DR3	1460	5.7	35	66	52	35	3.2	.330
793	US1	AMO	JA 715	56	DQw1	3762	6.9	1509	723	113	68	2.4	.597
				*56	DRw14	3762	7.0	696	200	926	78	3.3	.390
				*56	DR1	3762	7.1	360	107	1262	78	3.4	.258
				*56	DR2	3762	6.8	510	308	1112	63	2.0	.205
				*56	DRw10	3762	7.3	59	11	1563	85	3.5	.114
				*56	DRw13	3762	6.6	266	241	1356	53	0.95	.075
794	US1	JOH	CMAY/1	67	DQw1	3804	7.3	1934	329	133	86	3.5	.757
				*67	DRw14	3804	7.5	846	71	1221	93	4.6	.429
				*67	DR2	3804	7.2	688	142	1379	83	3.0	.303
				*67	DR1	3804	7.1	369	102	1698	79	2.6	.181
				*67	DRw13	3804	7.0	386	121	1681	77	2.5	.172
				*67	DRw10	3804	7.2	64	6	2003	92	2.8	.102
795	US1	DUQ	PEER	37	DQw1	3798	6.3	1101	1143	51	50	1.5	.490
				*37	DRw14	3798	6.4	548	360	604	61	2.5	.366
				*37	DR2	3798	6.4	394	434	758	48	1.3	.198
				*37	DRw10	3798	6.2	47	23	1105	68	2.0	.110
				*37	DR1	3798	6.2	201	271	951	43	0.92	.100
				*37	DRw13	3798	6.2	193	304	959	39	0.72	.072
796	US7	HAN	SEA 1121	39	DQw1	3813	6.4	1426	836	248	64	2.4	.466
				*39	DRw14	3813	6.6	697	209	977	77	2.4	.372
				*39	DR2	3813	6.5	522	317	1152	63	1.1	.196
				*39	DRw10	3813	6.2	51	19	1623	73	0.37	.080
				*39	DR1	3813	6.2	242	230	1432	52	0.49	.056
				*39	DRw13	3813	6.3	264	251	1410	52	0.57	.059
				23	TA10	1550	5.6	213	785	34	22	0.0068	.199
797	GER	MUE	MUE 37133	42	DRw10	3867	7.3	64	6	379	92	5.3	.341
				38	TA10	3797	6.3	292	1521	87	17	0.12	.195
803	EAE	MYR	Control	58	DR1	3832	7.1	381	98	193	80	4.2	.684
				39	DRw10	3353	7.1	49	11	144	82	4.4	.440
				30	DRw11	3293	5.8	71	853	73	8	0.053	.101
804	US2	BAC	CHARTIER	70	B44	3747	7.8	782	28	1172	97	2.6	.467
				54	DRw53	2937	6.9	877	474	295	65	0.70	.471
				*54	DR7	2937	7.5	346	29	826	93	2.2	.409
				*54	DR4	2937	6.5	418	363	754	54	0.33	.167
				*54	DRw9	2937	7.0	166	83	1006	67	0.48	.166
				36	DQw2	1586	6.0	92	113	203	45	0.73	.260

9wNO.	REG	LAB	ANTIBODY-ID	STR	ANTIGEN	NO.REAC	AVE	+/+	MISS +/-	EXTRA -/+	%INCL	Q-SCORE	R-VALUE
901	JAP	TSU	SHI	64	DQw1	3396	7.2	1597	423	359	80		.526
				*64	DRw14	3396	7.3	673	121	1283	85		.304
				*64	DR2	3396	7.2	589	164	1367	79		.223
				*64	DR1	3396	7.1	304	117	1652	73		.111
				*64	DRw13	3396	7.0	312	141	1644	69		.089
				*64	DRw10	3396	7.4	54	13	1902	81		.066
				54	DRw8	1376	7.2	73	60	286	55		.215
				53	Bw54	1230	6.7	47	41	233	54		.203
902	JAP	TSU	FU-3	52	DQw1	3330	6.8	669	1307	224	34		.192
				*52	DRw14	3330	6.9	282	501	611	37		.115
				*52	DR2	3330	6.8	252	480	641	35		.091
				*52	DRw10	3330	6.4	27	36	866	43		.050
				*52	DR1	3330	6.6	129	290	764	31		.034
				*52	DRw13	3330	6.4	142	303	751	32		.045
903	JAP	TSU	FU-4	52	DQw1	3224	6.9	1236	665	401	66		.342
				*52	DRw14	3224	7.1	553	194	1084	75		.255
				*52	DR2	3224	7.0	478	224	1159	69		.183
				*52	DRw13	3224	6.8	279	153	1358	65		.109
				*52	DRw10	3224	6.8	32	26	1605	56		.012
				39	DR4	1323	6.4	233	312	168	43		.227
904	JAP	AIZ	HU-26	88	DRw52	3378	7.8	2383	103	802	96		.113
				86	DQw1	893	7.7	445	17	358	97		.220
				84	DR4	431	7.7	270	16	88	95		.425
905	JAP	AIZ	HU-29	72	TA10	3428	7.4	1443	149	1502	91		.127
				68	DQw1	1836	7.2	1136	193	366	86		.154
				64	DRw53	506	7.3	269	76	97	78		.185
906	JAP	AIZ	HU-25	70	DR2	3401	7.7	730	34	1289	96		.397
				61	DR7	2637	7.1	344	145	945	71		.205
				59	DRw9	2149	7.2	154	72	792	69		.167
				58	DR1	1923	7.1	207	126	585	63		.195
907	JAP	AIZ	HU-28	63	DR2	3408	7.5	654	99	1886	87		.151
				57	TA10	2625	7.0	987	305	871	77		.121
				54	DQw2	1332	6.9	339	121	531	74		.128
908	JAP	TSU	FU-2	61	DQw3	3147	7.1	1371	368	482	79		.451
				*61	DRw11	3147	7.2	671	189	1182	79		.239
				*61	DRw12	3147	7.3	276	39	1577	88		.195
				*61	DR4	3147	7.0	589	230	1264	72		.157
				51	DR2	1408	6.9	199	233	283	47		.166
				46	TA10	976	6.7	59	67	224	47		.151

9wNO.	REG	LAB	ANTIBODY-ID	STR	ANTIGEN	NO.REAC	AVE	+/+	MISS +/-	EXTRA -/+	%INCL	Q-SCORE	R-VALUE
909	JAP	AIZ	HU-23	69	TA10	3424	7.4	1331	260	519	84		.554
				54	DQw3	1833	6.7	178	340	341	35		.084
				55	DQw1	1281	6.8	292	747	37	29		.115
910	JAP	TSU	FU-9	56	TA10	3356	6.9	617	927	449	40		.163
				49	DQw1	1812	6.6	360	949	89	28		.102
911	JAP	TSU	FU-6	46	B7	3071	6.5	157	316	549	34		.103
				45	DQw1	2563	6.5	332	1082	201	24		.073
912	JAP	TSU	FU-8	70	DRw52	2900	7.3	1386	751	412	65		.099
				*70	DRw11	2901	7.3	539	247	1259	69		.083
				64	Cw8	746	7.3	67	29	332	70		.126
913	JAP	AIZ	HU-11	60	DQw1	3330	7.1	1611	369	545	82		.421
				*60	DRw14	3329	7.3	690	86	1466	89		.279
				*60	DR2	3329	7.0	593	160	1563	79		.158
				*60	DRw13	3329	7.0	345	100	1811	78		.105
				*60	DR1	3330	6.8	296	116	1860	72		.056
				*60	DRw10	3229	7.4	56	11	2100	84		.056
				51	DR4	1350	6.9	323	231	222	59		.305
				44	DRw8	796	6.7	54	42	168	57		.234
914	JAP	TSU	FU-1	62	DQw1	3380	7.1	1530	486	679	76		.269
				*62	DRw14	3379	7.2	656	140	1552	83		.199
				*62	DR2	3379	7.1	567	186	1641	76		.112
				*62	DRw13	3379	7.1	330	122	1878	74		.063
				54	DR4	1364	6.9	361	200	318	65		.244
				50	DRw8	803	6.9	62	34	256	65		.188
				49	A24	705	6.6	86	85	169	51		.166
915	JAP	AIZ	HU-18	65	DQw3	3400	7.3	1617	474	1029	86		.548
				*65	DRw11	3400	7.3	746	161	1345	83		.257
				*65	DRw12	3400	7.5	349	19	1742	95		.239
				*65	DR4	3400	7.3	698	205	1393	78		.195
				44	Bw57	1502	7.0	46	27	427	64		.153
916	JAP	AIZ	HU-36						MULTISPECIFIC				
917	JAP	AIZ	HU-42	81	B7	3352	8.0	460	11	1587	98		.303
				76	Bw54	2878	8.0	162	4	1423	98		.211
				73	Bw58	2712	7.9	147	4	1276	98		.218
				71	Bw57	2561	8.0	124	1	1152	100		.224
				68	B27	2436	7.9	142	11	1010	93		.236
				64	Bw55	2283	8.0	99	2	911	99		.233
				*64	Bw56	2283	7.9	70	1	940	99		.196
				*64	Bw42	2283	8.0	32	0	978	100		.134

Table 1 (continued)

9WNO.	REG	LAB	ANTIBODY-ID	STR	ANTIGEN	NO.REAC	AVE	+/+	MISS +/-	EXTRA -/+	%INCL	Q-SCORE	R-VALUE
918	JAP	AIZ	HU-43	78	DR4	3344	7.8	857	37	1509	96		.333
				72	DR1	2450	7.8	348	25	1161	94		.276
				67	DRw9	2077	7.8	185	2	976	99		.273
				62	DQw1	1890	7.0	679	546	297	56		.103
				62	Cw1	663	7.1	41	15	255	74		.175
919	JAP	AIZ	HU-44	58	Cw1	3385	7.1	264	224	950	55		.156
				56	DRw9	2866	7.1	91	82	837	53		.110
				55	DR4	2693	6.9	262	378	575	41		.119
				52	B7	2053	7.1	142	197	433	42		.137
920	JAP	AIZ	HU-45	59	B7	3352	7.2	245	242	817	51		.165
				56	Bw54	2862	7.5	92	69	725	58		.155
				52	Bw56	2701	7.3	51	27	674	66		.150
				51	Bw42	2623	7.3	30	6	644	84		.156
				50	Bw57	2587	6.6	57	74	587	44		.099
921	JAP	AIZ	HU-46	55	DRw8	3361	7.1	163	114	1021	59		.148
				54	DQw3	3034	6.8	668	1052	330	39		.147
				*54	DR4	3034	6.9	365	473	633	44		.141
				54	Bw42	1322	7.1	13	3	317	82		.144
922	JAP	AIZ	HU-47	82	A24	3340	8.0	839	25	1348	98		.393
				73	A3	2476	7.8	446	21	902	96		.398
				63	A11	2009	7.8	285	15	617	95		.422
				51	A1	1709	6.7	200	196	417	51		.165
923	JAP	AIZ	HU-48	67	DQw3	3385	7.2	1461	438	642	77		.345
				*67	DR4	3385	7.4	805	108	1298	89		.326
				*67	DRw11	3385	7.1	649	246	1454	73		.128
				60	A24	1485	7.4	207	111	434	66		.231
				54	B7	1168	6.9	100	94	335	52		.132
924	JAP	AIZ	HU-2801	63	DQw1	3375	7.1	1277	735	627	64		.173
				*63	DR1	3375	7.1	311	108	1593	75		.135
				*63	DRw14	3375	7.2	530	268	1373	67		.112
				61	A24	1361	7.0	230	135	396	64		.207
				60	A32	996	7.4	53	13	343	81		.221
				58	B27	930	7.6	45	19	298	71		.188
				54	DR4	868	6.8	157	189	142	46		.187
925	JAP	AIZ	HU-2901	64	DRw8	3389	7.2	234	46	1142	84		.263
				63	DRw12	3109	7.6	243	114	899	69		.234
				57	A24	2749	7.0	287	371	611	44		.131
926	JAP	AIZ	HU-49	79	A24	3242	7.9	806	24	741	98		.580
				61	A23	2412	7.9	111	1	630	100		.327
927	JAP	SH	SH-2	72	DQw1	3403	7.4	1748	275	680	87		.403
				*72	DRw14	3403	7.5	713	85	1714	90		.220
				*72	DR2	3403	7.4	659	100	1768	87		.184
				*72	DR1	3403	7.4	341	79	2087	82		.082
				67	A24	1378	7.4	287	80	392	79		.349
				58	DRw8	1013	7.4	62	32	331	64		.178
928	JAP	?	Y 62-C-10	76	DQw3	3408	7.6	1705	205	1120	90		.191
				*76	DR4	3408	7.7	865	52	1960	95		.184
				*76	TA10	3408	7.5	1375	207	1450	87		.099
				68	DR1	1498	7.4	250	22	870	92		.186
				66	DRw9	1226	7.6	92	2	778	98		.171
				64	DQw1	1132	7.2	634	245	144	73		.137
929	GER	JOS	16-23	58	DR3	3300	6.8	275	165	1173	63		.147
				59	Cw1	2859	7.0	242	218	931	53		.103
930	BEN	ROO	vR 7.3.19.1	75	DRw52	3258	7.5	2081	309	343	88		.482
				*75	DRw11	3258	7.5	766	95	1659	89		.200
				*75	DRw14	3258	7.7	675	78	1749	90		.191
				*75	DR3	3258	7.7	424	23	2000	95		.187
				*75	DRw13	3258	7.3	390	48	2034	90		.132
				*75	DRw12	3258	7.6	316	41	2109	89		.113
931	SCA	SVE	B8-12.2*	MULTISPECIFIC									
932	SCA	SVE	H-39-49.5*	MULTISPECIFIC									
933	SCA	SVE	H-40-394.2*	MULTISPECIFIC									
934	SCA	SVE	H-81-218.11*	MULTISPECIFIC									
935	SCA	SVE	H-81-208.22*	MULTISPECIFIC									
936	SCA	SVE	H-74-202.2*	MULTISPECIFIC									
937	SCA	SVE	H-82-246.3*	MULTISPECIFIC									
938	SCA	SVE	H-82-246.3 1:500*	MULTISPECIFIC									
939	IT1	MTT	C-5.17	MULTISPECIFIC									
940	IT1	GAN	XI-21.4	71	DRw53	3387	7.4	1373	222	1137	87		.258
				*71	DR4	3388	7.5	827	84	1684	91		.231
				*71	DRw9	3388	7.5	248	15	2263	95		.134
				71	DR1	1793	7.3	244	61	894	80		.155
				71	DRw10	1487	7.7	44	2	849	96		.130
				71	DR3	1441	7.1	195	74	654	73		.132
				71	DRw14	1172	7.2	243	127	411	64		.135

* produced by Dr. M. Pierres, Marseille

9wNO.	REG	LAB	ANTIBODY-ID	STR	ANTIGEN	NO.REAC	AVE	+/+	MISS +/-	EXTRA -/+	%INCL	Q-SCORE	R-VALUE
941	IT1	GAN	X-2.7	67	DRw53	3394	7.4	1362	241	1052	85		.289
				*67	DR4	3395	7.4	793	121	1622	87		.209
				*67	DRw9	3395	7.5	234	29	2181	89		.114
				*67	DR7	3394	7.2	404	115	2010	78		.063
942	IT1	GAN	X-44.8	64	DRw53	3179	7.1	792	718	687	53		.113
				*64	DR4	3179	7.1	458	415	1021	53		.073
				*64	DRw9	3179	7.3	142	111	1337	57		.057
943	NCY	BOS	JAF-77-34-10	53	DQw1	3112	6.8	1242	606	402	68		.348
				*53	DRw14	3112	7.0	659	161	1074	78		.279
				*53	DR2	3112	6.8	424	257	1219	63		.100
				*53	DRw13	3112	6.8	272	150	1371	65		.092
				*53	DR1	3112	6.9	248	146	1396	63		.077
				*53	DRw10	3112	6.9	48	15	1595	77		.067
				46	DQw3	1263	6.5	343	631	59	36		.134
				47	Bw57	1250	6.3	39	28	354	59		.137
944	NCY	BOS	J-2	MULTISPECIFIC									
945	UKI	BOD	JMS-DR4.1 1	59	DQw1	3314	7.0	1611	370	501	82		.446
				*59	DRw14	3313	7.2	654	122	1457	85		.236
				*59	DR2	3313	6.9	588	151	1523	80		.177
				*59	DR1	3314	7.3	344	71	1768	83		.151
				*59	DRw13	3313	6.9	350	98	1761	79		.118
				*59	DRw10	3313	7.3	56	11	2055	84		.059
946	UKI	BOD	8F-10	78	DRw52	3246	7.6	2114	269	337	89		.510
				*78	DRw11	3247	7.7	811	45	1641	95		.268
				*78	DRw14	3246	7.6	702	56	1749	93		.220
				*78	DR3	3246	7.6	413	27	2038	94		.169
				*78	DRw13	3246	7.6	404	37	2047	92		.148
947	UKI	BOD	JMS-DR8.1.1	80	DRw52	3360	7.6	2173	302	314	88		.525
				*80	DRw11	3361	7.8	680	39	1628	96		.298
				*80	DRw14	3360	7.7	721	68	1766	92		.219
				*80	DR3	3360	7.7	433	17	2054	97		.199
				*80	DRw13	3360	7.6	421	32	2066	93		.170
948	UKI	BOD	C-504	80	DRw52	3321	7.6	2141	307	331	88		.500
				*80	DRw11	3322	7.8	834	52	1639	95		.272
				*80	DRw14	3321	7.6	701	81	1771	90		.193
				*80	DR3	3321	7.6	436	21	2036	96		.192
				*80	DRw13	3321	7.6	419	35	2053	93		.163
949	UKI	BOD	17.3.3	65	DQw2	3389	7.5	752	119	1570	87		.226
				*65	DR7	3389	7.6	481	37	1841	93		.223
				*65	DR3	3389	7.2	339	119	1983	75		.047
				60	DRw52	2518	7.0	1293	551	277	71		.265
				*60	DRw11	2519	7.1	536	153	1035	78		.195
				*60	DRw14	2518	7.1	438	173	1132	72		.109
				*60	DRw12	2519	7.2	237	81	1334	75		.095
				*60	DRw13	2518	6.8	277	124	1293	70		.060
				53	DR4	675	7.0	180	190	98	49		.167
950	FRA	FAU	XX 13.6.2	61	DRw52	3353	7.0	1094	1379	274	45		.117
				*61	DRw11	3354	7.0	446	449	923	50		.111
				*61	DR3	3353	6.9	225	231	1143	50		.069
				58	DR7	880	7.1	89	105	185	46		.196
951	FRA	BET	FLY-BL-12	64	DRw9	3178	7.6	232	30	1365	89		.230
				61	DR4	2882	7.0	470	315	870	60		.164
				61	DRw10	2097	7.8	53	7	817	89		.163
				60	DRw14	2037	7.0	305	295	512	51		.141
				58	DR1	1437	6.9	146	128	366	54		.179
952	FRA	BET	FLY-BL-12 1:1000	47	DRw10	3297	7.0	51	14	900	79		.155
				46	DRw52	3232	6.5	730	1672	170	31		.097
				*46	DRw14	3232	6.5	253	512	647	34		.065
953	FRA	DAU	CHEV.-64.2	65	DRw52	3276	7.2	1857	561	342	77		.346
				*65	DRw11	3277	7.3	726	152	1473	83		.201
				*65	DRw14	3276	7.3	617	149	1582	81		.158
				*65	DR3	3276	7.4	363	88	1836	81		.114
				*65	DRw8	3277	7.2	220	48	1979	83		.095
				49	DR2	858	6.8	142	149	200	49		.131
954	FRA	DAU	CHEV - 249.3	MULTISPECIFIC									
955	FRA	DAU	MAJA-51.2	54	DQw1	3054	6.9	1120	697	419	62		.273
				*54	DR2	3053	6.8	487	206	1051	71		.216
				*54	DRw14	3053	7.1	468	237	1070	67		.175
				*54	DRw13	3053	6.7	276	124	1262	69		.145
				47	DRw52	1236	6.5	322	524	96	39		.132
				*47	DRw11	1237	6.6	186	277	233	41		.103
956	FRA	DAU	FPA-BM50	MULTISPECIFIC									
957	FRA	DAU	FPA-141	MULTISPECIFIC									
958	FRA	DAU	FPA-53	MULTISPECIFIC									
959	FRA	DAU	FPA-M18	MULTISPECIFIC									

Table 1 (continued)

9wNO.	REG	LAB	ANTIBODY-ID	STR	ANTIGEN	NO.REAC	AVE	+/+	MISS +/-	EXTRA -/+	%INCL	Q-SCORE	R-VALUE
960	US1	AMO	SFR-3	69	DRw11	3207	7.2	330	523	696	39		.086
962	US1	AMO	GAP-D-1	64	DR2	3209	7.5	650	62	1344	92		.321
				56	DRw14	2497	7.1	490	195	854	72		.218
				52	DR7	1812	6.8	241	135	613	65		.174
				51	DRw12	1437	7.2	149	72	464	68		.213
				45	DRw13	1215	6.4	113	84	351	58		.174
963	US1	ZMI	HPA-39-11-10	51	DQw1	3369	6.8	957	1047	313	48		.251
				*51	DR1	3369	6.8	273	142	997	66		.217
				*51	DRw14	3369	7.0	402	382	868	52		.154
				*51	DRw10	3369	6.3	45	19	1225	71		.094
				*51	DR2	3369	6.7	326	429	944	44		.061
				44	Bw48	1363	7.1	16	9	297	64		.133
964	US1	AMO	NFB-14.12	48	DQw1	3110	6.6	830	1030	279	45		.228
				*48	DRw14	3109	6.8	399	323	710	56		.225
				*48	DR2	3109	6.5	316	389	793	45		.103
				*48	DRw13	3109	6.4	176	241	933	43		.054
				48	DR4	1250	6.6	169	363	110	32		.195
965	IT2	TAN	MCS-7	71	DRw52	3193	7.4	2040	311	544	87		.252
				*71	DRw14	3197	7.5	686	84	1898	90		.118
				*71	DRw12	3198	7.5	317	33	2267	91		.087
				*71	DRw8	3198	7.5	239	32	2345	89		.057
				*71	DRw11	3198	7.4	716	133	1868	85		.054
				58	DR4	847	6.9	331	92	213	79		.292
				58	DR2	424	7.1	130	50	83	73		.378
				48	DRw8	244	7.1	13	3	70	82		.264
967	US1	THP	E5A7.3A	45	DRw52	3372	6.4	488	1994	126	20		.063
968	US5	TER	TER M	51	TA10	2709	6.9	855	411	325	68		.453
				36	DRw52	1442	6.3	232	689	93	26		.084
969	US7	HAN	17.15	70	DQw3	2702	7.4	1153	392	371	75		.425
				*70	DRw11	2702	7.3	517	183	1007	74		.208
				*70	DRw12	2702	7.5	254	59	1270	82		.181
				*70	DR4	2702	7.4	507	226	1017	70		.157
				53	DRw9	1157	6.4	41	32	330	57		.134
970	GER	WER	TUE-22	MULTISPECIFIC									
972	ANZ	TAI	RM-2.82	56	DRW52	3360	6.9	1116	1363	320	46		.077
973	ANZ	TAI	RM2-102	57	DRw52	3337	6.8	1162	1302	329	48		.084
974	ANZ	TAI	RM-3.29	MULTISPECIFIC									
975	ANZ	TAI	RM-3.170	67	A2	3226	7.3	1154	451	402	72		.471
976	ANZ	TAI	RM-5.79	87	Bw4	3236	7.8	1746	124	740	94		.460
				73	A24	1370	7.7	364	33	377	92		.482
977	ANZ	TAI	RM-7.25	52	DQw3	3384	6.8	1312	582	926			.075
				51	DQw1	1490	6.7	783	392	143			.179
978	ANZ	TAI	RM-7.89	54	DRw52	3374	6.8	1086	1392	302			.091
979	ANZ	MCK	19-26.1 1:500	68	DRw53	3317	7.2	1219	349	829	78		.312
				*68	DRw9	3318	7.8	239	10	1810	96		.201
				*68	DR4	3318	7.0	651	240	1398	74		.141
				*68	DR7	3317	7.2	388	121	1660	77		.127
				63	DR3	1749	7.3	228	61	601	79		.281
				61	DRw10	1460	7.8	39	7	562	85		.160
				59	DRw14	1414	7.3	207	205	355	51		.138
980	ANZ	MCK	203-F5 1:500	78	DQw1	3171	7.6	1735	146	955	93		.249
				*78	DRw14	3170	7.7	697	46	1992	94		.139
				*78	DR2	3170	7.5	640	63	2049	92		.092
				*78	DRw13	3170	7.5	392	35	2297	92		.077
				*78	DR1	3171	7.5	364	36	2326	91		.065
				*78	DRw10	3170	7.8	53	7	2636	89		.014
				72	DRw53	1289	7.4	701	175	253	81		.200
				*72	DR4	1290	7.4	443	99	512	82		.150
				*72	DRw9	1290	7.6	143	25	812	86		.098
				68	DRw8	414	7.5	59	7	195	90		.251
981	ANZ	MCK	203-F5 1:1000	79	DQw1	3021	7.6	1645	161	818	92		.300
				*79	DRw14	3020	7.7	657	50	1806	93		.162
				*79	DR2	3020	7.5	598	70	1865	90		.109
				*79	DRw13	3020	7.5	360	45	2103	89		.074
				*79	DR1	3021	7.5	339	50	2124	88		.056
				73	DRw53	1214	7.4	604	212	214	75		.203
				*73	DR4	1215	7.4	396	119	422	77		.175
				*73	DRw9	1215	7.4	119	27	699	82		.112
982	ANZ	MCK	326-2-D 2.4 1:2	46	DQw1	3183	6.6	1226	309	977	36		.121
983	ANZ	MCK	326-2-D 2.4 1:5		NEGATIVE								
984	ANZ	MCK	HO-19-1-D-12.2 1:2	53	DRw52	3305	6.7	983	1449	254	41		.103
985	ANZ	MCK	HO-19-1-D-12.2 1:10	54	DRw52	3270	6.7	933	1483	246	39		.090
986	ANZ	MCK	HO-19-3D-11-G8 1:2	57	DRw52	2749	6.8	877	1140	262	44		.069

9wNO.	REG	LAB	ANTIBODY-ID	STR	ANTIGEN	NO.REAC	AVE	+/+	MISS +/-	EXTRA -/+	%INCL	Q-SCORE	R-VALUE
987	ANZ	MCK	HO-13-4-D-7.1 1:2	54	B7	3040	7.0	321	121	1227	73		.179
				53	Cw8	2572	6.9	182	60	1025	76		.183
				52	B8	2332	7.2	163	73	863	70		.169
				49	Bw62	2094	6.6	177	131	685	58		.138
988	ANZ	MCK	19-26.1 1:1000	65	DRw53	3214	7.2	1156	364	876	77		.252
				*65	DRw9	3215	7.8	240	14	1793	95		.190
				*65	DR4	3215	7.0	612	249	1421	72		.098
				*65	DR7	3214	7.1	352	135	1680	73		.079
				60	DR3	1694	6.9	213	70	663	76		.211
				61	DRw10	1411	7.9	40	4	623	91		.158
				59	DRw143	1367	7.4	235	171	388	58		.161
782	IT1	CAR	D4.90/5.56	MULTISPECIFIC									
783	IT1	CAR	D 7.69/9	62	DRw52	3262	7.1	1872	524	551	79		.147
				*62	DRw14	3262	7.3	645	120	1778	85		.127
				*62	DRw11	3263	7.3	684	177	1739	80		.071
				*62	DR3	3262	7.2	364	80	2059	82		.070
				54	DQw3	867	6.9	345	130	206	73		.208
784	IT1	CAR	AB 8.25/5	57	DR2	3341	7.1	587	154	1558	80		.167
				54	DQw3	2601	6.9	1065	508	494	68		.196
				*54	DRw11	2601	7.3	551	196	1008	74		.179
				*54	DRw14	2600	7.0	486	243	1072	67		.086
				49	DRw14	1028	6.8	261	164	233	62		.224
992	SAF	HAM	I-B-6	MULTISPECIFIC									
993	GER	WER	TUE-34	MULTISPECIFIC									
994	GER	WER	TUE-35	MULTISPECIFIC									
995	GER	WER	TUE-37	MULTISPECIFIC									
996	GER	WER	TUE-39	MULTISPECIFIC									
660	UKI	BOD	DR4.1.10	70	DQw1	3231	7.3	1600	337	568	83		.404
				*70	DRw14	3230	7.3	671	94	1497	88		.244
				*70	DR2	3230	7.3	577	156	1591	79		.134
				*70	DR1	3231	7.4	331	64	1837	84		.133
				65	DRw8	1294	6.8	77	51	491	61		.109
1102	US7	DUP	C-11	92	A2	3696	7.8	1771	106	259	95		.805
				89	A28	1818	7.8	218	22	40	91		.857
1103	US7	DUP	FH B-3	98	A2	3758	8.0	1860	42	287	98		.832
				90	A28	1855	8.0	234	8	52	97		.872
				50	DRw13	1613	7.1	17	219	36	8		.091

9wNO.	REG	LAB	ANTIBODY-ID	STR	ANTIGEN	NO.REAC	AVE	+/+	MISS +/-	EXTRA -/+	%INCL	Q-SCORE	R-VALUE
1104	US7	HAN	P-5-1	91	A2	3733	7.8	1789	106	176	95		.849
				76	A28	1837	7.7	104	130	71	45		.454
1105	US7	HAN	P-5.3	87	B7	3766	8.0	550	17	1777	98		.305
				84	Cw1	3199	7.8	399	89	1378	86		.224
				81	Bw58	2711	8.0	154	4	1224	98		.232
				79	Bw57	2553	8.0	140	1	1084	100		.249
				76	B27	2412	8.0	110	4	974	97		.231
				74	Bw65	2298	7.5	154	38	820	81		.231
				*74	Bw55	2298	7.9	62	2	912	97		.187
1106	US7	HAN	P-5.4	95	A2	3769	8.0	1870	37	1371	99		.352
				92	A3	1862	7.9	417	13	954	97		.290
				90	A28	1431	8.0	212	4	741	99		.282
				87	Aw33	1215	8.0	178	6	563	97		.310
				83	A31	1032	7.9	107	3	457	98		.296
				80	A30	917	7.9	102	3	349	98		.345
1107	US7	HAN	P-4.2.2	79	B27	3681	7.9	192	10	1701	96		.210
				77	A24	3479	7.2	608	312	1093	67		.206
				79	A32	2559	7.8	124	22	969	85		.210
				78	B13	2413	7.5	88	24	881	79		.173
				78	B37	2301	7.8	53	11	828	83		.155
				77	A23	2237	7.5	76	30	752	72		.160
1108	JAP	TSU	FU-10	90	A2	3731	7.9	1773	112	440	95		.715
				71	A28	1845	7.8	231	11	208	96		.654
1109	JAP	SH	SH-3	79	A1	3741	7.8	630	31	1387	96		.385
				72	A26	3080	7.7	303	28	1084	92		.324
				68	A11	2749	7.6	337	74	747	82		.364
				62	A24	2338	6.8	344	364	403	49		.235
				66	A25	1630	7.4	56	9	347	87		.290
				64	A23	1565	7.1	62	36	285	64		.256
1110	JAP	FU	FU-11	50	B8	3738	6.8	253	156	649	62		.309
				47	Aw33	3328	6.6	129	154	519	46		.201
1111	SCA	SVE	H-97-76.7*	69	B7	3714	7.6	497	59	425	90		.627
				52	B27	3158	7.2	107	79	318	58		.323
1112	SCA	SVE	H-97-102.11*	87	B7	3700	7.9	528	35	1001	94		.451
				82	Bw61	3137	7.6	303	61	698	84		.399
				81	Bw60	2773	7.8	214	41	484	84		.431
				77	B27	2518	7.8	151	18	333	90		.477
				69	B13	2349	7.4	60	56	273	52		.245
				67	Bw48	2233	7.4	29	13	244	70		.240

* produced by Dr. M. Pierres, Marseille

Table 1 (continued)

9WNO.	REG	LAB	ANTIBODY-ID	STR	ANTIGEN	NO.REAC	AVE	+/+	MISS +/-	EXTRA -/+	%INCL	Q-SCORE	R-VALUE
1113	SCA	SVE	H-81-257.11.3*	79	B7	3766	7.9	544	19	709	97		.564
				66	B27	3203	7.8	170	19	539	90		.409
				58	Bw60	3014	6.9	185	88	354	68		.411
				56	Bw61	2741	6.8	172	168	182	51		.423
1116	FRA	FAU	XIX-20.1	76	A3	3769	7.5	505	139	331	79		.614
				69	B7	3125	7.5	148	212	183	42		.358
1117	FRA	FAU	XXIII-23.1	75	B8	3732	7.7	384	28	1722	94		.261
				72	Cw8	3320	7.7	283	14	1439	96		.272
				*72	Bw65	3320	7.7	217	9	1589	97		.239
				*72	Bw64	3320	7.8	79	6	1643	93		.133
				69	B51	3023	7.6	345	55	1094	87		.302
				65	B18	2623	7.7	186	12	908	94		.303
				61	A28	2424	7.3	180	50	728	79		.273
				57	Aw33	2194	7.1	131	62	597	68		.229
1118	FRA	FAU	XXII-34.5	62	Bw54	3686	7.5	143	16	1214	90		.234
				60	B51	3527	7.1	271	143	943	66		.238
				58	Cw8	3113	7.3	210	111	733	66		.259
				*58	Bw64	3113	7.5	82	17	861	83		.207
				*58	Bw65	3113	7.3	136	98	807	59		.173
				53	Bw52	2792	7.2	93	36	640	73		.229
1119	FRA	DAU	OCH-126.7	58	A29	3709	7.5	154	33	216	87		.557
1120	FRA	DAU	OCH-71.1	57	A29	3582	6.9	105	67	231	62		.398
1121	FRA	DAU	OCH-184.1	48	A29	3618	6.9	100	79	72	56		.548
1122	FRA	DAU	FPA-GH-3-1	37	A11	3739	5.7	75	395	147	16		.161
				40	A3	3269	6.2	60	535	87	11		.127
1124	FRA	DAU	FPA-ber-3.74 1:10	68	Bw60	3120	7.7	212	33	883	87		.315
				63	Bw61	2875	6.9	208	114	675	65		.261
				64	Aw32	2553	7.4	100	27	575	79		.271
				62	A31	2426	7.3	96	44	479	69		.261
				59	A30	2285	7.0	115	83	364	59		.281
				58	A29	2088	7.1	81	50	283	62		.303
1127	FRA	DAU	FPA GH3		NEGATIVE								
1128	US3	GRU	B27-M1	52	B27	3746	6.7	101	106	275	49		.312
				50	B7	3539	6.1	111	431	164	21		.202
1129	US3	GRU	B27-M2	55	B27	3763	6.7	86	119	328	42		.237
				55	Bw47	3558	6.9	18	21	310	47		.134
1130	US3	GRU	A28,2-M1	48	A2	3768	6.6	834	1075	143	44		.411
				45	A28	1858	6.6	92	152	51	38		.438
				*45	Aw68	1858	6.6	88	138	55	39		.436
1131	IT1	GAN	GAN-X-15.4	76	A3	3759	7.5	560	78	77	88		.854
1132	IT1	CAR	AB-10.58/4	73	A2	3688	7.4	1403	475	358	75		.551
				55	B39	1810	7.0	65	23	291	74		.308
				53	Bw54	1722	6.8	58	36	233	62		.287
				54	B38	1628	7.2	57	35	176	62		.333
1134	NCY	BOS	SY-1	73	B13	3713	7.9	137	7	89	96		.748
1135	NCY	BOS	P-4-C-2	74	B7	3730	7.5	460	93	1224	84		.319
				71	B60	3177	7.4	244	43	980	86		.301
				70	B27	2890	7.7	164	13	816	93		.317
				65	B61	2713	7.3	244	94	572	73		.346
				63	A32	2375	7.4	97	7	475	94		.346
				60	B13	2271	7.5	83	33	392	72		.289
				*60	B38	2271	7.1	66	71	409	49		.170
				*60	B42	2271	7.4	26	9	449	75		.164
1136	NCY	BOS	4-D-12	70	Bw62	3655	7.6	350	84	1174	81		.290
				66	B51	3221	7.3	276	121	898	70		.258
				64	Bw52	2824	7.3	108	26	790	81		.234
				62	Bw72	2690	7.7	88	12	702	88		.253
				59	B35	2590	6.9	271	255	431	52		.277
				58	B49	2064	7.1	46	18	385	72		.224
1137	NCY	BOS	3C-6.1	48	Bw62	3625	6.7	117	314	297	28		.182
1138	NCY	BOS	4-F-12.3	59	A29	3746	7.4	157	30	198	84		.583
1139	UKI	BOD	BB 7.2	86	A2	3630	7.7	1623	208	107	89		.828
1140	UKI	BOD	LC-385	77	B8	3728	7.8	369	28	304	93		.672
1141	UKI	LAW	M-3.63-14	81	A2	3655	7.6	1670	177	246	91		.769
				75	A28	1807	7.5	209	27	36	89		.849
1142	UKI	LAW	CBRI-M1-20/86	95	A2	3740	7.9	1866	31	298	99		.832
				86	A28	1842	7.9	234	4	63	99		.861
1143	US1	AMO	SFR8.B6	90	Bw6	3548	7.8	2653	267	229	91		.532
				86	A2	628	7.6	166	179	63	49		.267

* produced by Dr. M. Pierres, Marseille

9wNO.	REG	LAB	ANTIBODY-ID	STR	ANTIGEN	NO.REAC	AVE	+/+	MISS +/-	EXTRA -/+	%INCL	Q-SCORE	R-VALUE
1146	US1	AMO	GAP-A3	86	A3	3573	7.9	583	25	563	96		.619
1147	US1	ZMI	PhR 9-17.7.1	78	B39	3731	7.8	180	14	1275	93		.258
				*78	B38	3731	7.7	158	13	1297	93		.240
				76	Cw8	3537	7.6	250	79	1025	76		.266
				*76	Bw64	3537	7.7	86	16	1189	85		.173
				*76	Bw65	3537	7.6	174	66	1101	73		.205
				72	A2	3057	7.3	606	978	280	39		.212
				*72	B18	3057	6.9	120	103	766	54		.154
				65	Bw42	1473	7.4	21	4	259	84		.218
1148	US1	ZMI	K 2.7.2	51	A2	3675	6.7	422	1428	207	23		.152
1150	ANZ	MCK	ABC-M3	59	B27	3333	7.7	143	19	378	89		.452
				48	B7	3171	6.5	165	321	213	34		.289
				50	Bw42	2685	6.9	19	17	194	53		.193
1151	FRA	FAU	ACMo XI 1413	90	A2	3765	7.8	1787	124	249	94		.803
				77	A28	1853	7.6	189	52	59	79		.739
1152	FRA	FAU	ACMO XI 231	85	A3	3749	7.9	617	22	289	97		.767
				61	A2	3110	6.9	233	1451	56	14		.170
1153	US5	TER	TER-M-B13	72	B13	3640	7.8	134	7	442	96		.436
				65	A3	3499	7.5	194	403	248	33		.271
1154	US5	TER	TER-M-B8	72	B8	3681	7.8	387	19	465	96		.603
				55	Bw59	3275	6.7	14	21	451	40		.077
1155	GER	WER	TÜ 48	92	Bw4	3629	7.9	2019	116	603	95		.596
				85	A24	1495	7.7	398	48	206	90		.649
				79	A32	1049	7.9	55	3	151	95		.458
				74	A23	991	7.9	35	3	116	93		.427
				67	B13	953	7.3	9	1	107	90		.427
				66	B27	943	8.0	8	2	99	80		.224
1156	GER	WER	TÜ 101	93	A2	3607	7.9	1755	70	427	97		.738
				80	A28	1781	7.9	219	14	207	94		.637
1157	GER	WER	TÜ 109	78	Bw4	3500	7.5	1417	629	482	70		.357
				74	A2	1454	7.3	369	343	117	52		.389
				68	A28	741	7.3	49	41	64	62		.445
1158	GER	WER	TÜ 110	71	B13	3624	7.8	125	19	470	87		.387
1159	GER	WES	MOAB Bw6	64	Bw6	3636	7.1	1440	1538	74	49		.290
1160	US7	HAN	8.1	80	B8	3671	8.0	386	13	231	97		.746

9wNO.	REG	LAB	ANTIBODY-ID	STR	ANTIGEN	NO.REAC	AVE	+/+	MISS +/-	EXTRA -/+	%INCL	Q-SCORE	R-VALUE
1125	FRA	VIV	F-BACATA-1	71	A32	3709	7.8	177	10	678	95		.392
				65	A25	3522	7.7	86	9	592	91		.301
1126	FRA	DAU	FPA-AUF 5.13 1:10	63	A11	3609	7.2	322	135	695	71		.358
				60	A3	3152	6.8	249	313	446	45		.250
1133	IT1	CAR	FIO.13/13	76	B7	3693	7.7	497	53	1707	91		.262
				73	B8	3143	7.6	318	44	1389	88		.243
				70	Bw61	2781	7.5	278	76	1111	79		.218
				68	Bw60	2427	7.5	180	57	931	76		.199
				66	Aw33	2170	7.6	154	62	762	72		.196
				*65	A31	2170	7.1	109	41	808	73		.168
				*65	A30	2170	7.3	101	41	816	72		.155
				*65	A32	2170	7.4	71	21	846	78		.149
				*65	A29	2170	7.3	84	40	833	68		.127
				*65	Bw48	2170	7.4	36	4	881	90		.132
1144	US1	MET	RM-2-B2,D2	87	A2	3503	7.7	1572	201	347	89		.689
				77	Bw58	1730	7.8	91	6	256	94		.449
				72	Bw57	1633	7.8	78	3	178	97		.507

Table 2. Pattern analysis program showing heterogeneity of DR5 in Caucasians

HLA-DR5 positive Number of positive cells: 242

Absolute no.	Percent	9w0598 DR5	9w0601 DR5	9w0597 DR5	9w0599 DR5	9w0611 DR5 sh.	9w0612 DR5 sh.	9w0613 DR5 sh.	9w0610 DR5 sh.	9w0609 DR5 sh.	
42	17.4	+	+	+	+	+	+	+	+	+	
11	4.5	+	+	+	+	+	+	+	+	+	
10	4.1	+	+	+	+	+	+	+	+	−	
10	4.1	+	+	+	+	−	−	−	+	−	Patterns suggesting a "short" DR5
9	3.7	+	+	+	+	−	+	+	+	+	
8	3.3	−	−	−	−	−	−	−	−	−	← Miscoded cells
7	2.9	+	+	+	+	−	+	+	+	+	
7	2.9	+	+	+	+	+	+	−	+	+	
7	2.9	+	+	+	+	+	+	−	+	+	
6	2.5	+	+	+	+	+	−	−	+	−	
5	2.1	+	+	+	+	−	−	−	−	−	Patterns suggesting a "short" DR5
5	2.1	+	+	+	+	+	+	+	+	−	
5	2.1	+	+	+	+	+	+	−	+	−	
4	1.7	+	+	−	+	−	−	−	−	−	Patterns suggesting a "short" DR5
4	1.7	+	+	+	+	−	+	−	+	−	
4	1.7	+	+	+	+	+	−	−	+	−	
4	1.7	+	+	+	+	+	−	+	+	−	
4	1.7	+	+	+	+	+	+	−	+	−	
4	1.7	+	+	+	+	−	+	−	+	+	
4	1.7	+	+	+	+	+	−	+	+	+	
3	1.2	+	+	+	+	−	−	+	+	+	
3	1.2	+	+	+	+	−	+	−	+	−	

Cells that do *not* match the condition: HLA-DR5 positive Number of cells: 758

Absolute no.	Percent	9w0598 DR5	9w0601 DR5	9w0597 DR5	9w0599 DR5	9w0611 DR5 sh.	9w0612 DR5 sh.	9w0613 DR5 sh.	9w0610 DR5 sh.	9w0609 DR5 sh.
461	60.8	−	−	−	−	−	−	−	−	−
41	5.4	−	−	−	+	−	−	−	−	−
37	4.9	−	−	+	−	−	−	−	−	−
21	2.8	−	+	−	−	−	−	−	−	−
16	2.1	−	+	−	+	−	−	−	−	−
13	1.7	−	+	−	−	−	−	−	−	−
12	1.6	−	−	+	+	−	−	−	−	−
11	1.5	−	−	−	−	−	+	−	−	−
11	1.5	+	−	−	−	−	−	−	−	−
9	1.2	+	−	−	+	−	−	−	−	−
7	0.9	−	−	−	−	−	−	−	+	−
5	0.7	−	−	−	−	−	−	+	−	−
5	0.7	+	−	+	−	−	−	−	−	−
5	0.7	+	+	−	−	−	−	−	−	−

sh. = short

Table 3. Family pattern program showing the segregation of a short DR5 (=DRw12)

HLA antigens coded on cards 02 – 05

Typing	Fa	Mo	C1	C2	C3
A11	8	8	8	1	8
B39	8	1	8	1	8
DRw6	8	1	8	1	8
Aw33	8	1	1	8	1
Cw3	8	1	1	8	1
Bw58	8	1	1	8	1
DR5	8	1	1	8	1
A11	8	8	8	1	8
Cw1	1	8	8	1	1
Bw54	1	8	8	1	1
DR4	1	8	8	1	1
A24	1	8	1	8	8
Bw52	1	8	1	8	8
DR2	1	8	1	8	8

Reaction patterns of long and short anti-DR5 sera

Serum no.	Specificity	Fa	Mo	C1	C2	C3
9w0598	DR5	8	1	1	8	1
9w0601	DR5	8	1	1	8	1
9w0597	DR5	8	1	1	6	1
9w0599	DR5	8	1	1	8	1
9w0611	DR5 short	1	1	1	1	1
9w0612	DR5 short	1	1	1	1	1
9w0613	DR5 short	1	1	1	1	1
9w0610	DR5 short	0	1	1	1	1
9w0609	DR5 short	1	1	1	1	1

Fa = father; Mo = mother; C = child

Analysis of HLA-DR Typing Sera Used in the Workshop Transplant Study

A. Amoroso[1], E. S. Curtoni[1], G. Opelz[2], A. Piazza[1], and S. Rendine[1]

1 Istituto di Genetica Medica, Università di Torino, Via Santena 19, 10126 Torino and Centro C.N.R. Immunogenetica ed Istocompatibilita, Torino, Italy
2 Institute of Immunology, University of Heidelberg, Im Neuenheimer Feld 305, 6900 Heidelberg, Federal Republic of Germany

Specificity of the Sera. Only cells with satisfactory positive and negative controls were evaluated (positive controls scores 6 or 8, negative control scores 1 or 2). These criteria were met by 85% of the recipient typings and 87% of the donor typings. A 2×2 table analysis was made taking into consideration the antigen assignment made by each submitting laboratory (Table 1). It shows that most DR antigens were defined by strong and monospecific sera, except for the following antigens, for which monospecific sera were not present in the set: DRw6, DRw8, DRw9, and DRw10.

As far as the DRw52, DRw53 and DQw1, DQw2, DQw3 specificities were concerned, a 2×2 comparison with antigens assigned by the submitting laboratories was not possible because DRw52, 53 and DQ phenotype assignments had not been requested. However, it appears from our preliminary analysis that the transplant serum set allows the assignment of these antigens based on their subtypic DR associations (Table 2). A more complete analysis will be carried out in the future and a possible relationship with graft survival will be investigated. The most recently recognized specificities, e.g., TA10, splits of DR2, DR4, DR5, and DRw6, can be identified with the genetic set of Workshop sera. Parallel tests were carried out in the laboratories of Drs. Albert (Munich), Mayr (Vienna), and Van Rood (Leiden) to establish the correspondence of transplant set sera with new splits as identified by the genetic set. This appears particularly interesting with respect to DRw6, which seems to identify a special responder status. We are planning to carry out a detailed analysis as soon as the cross-reference data can be made available to us by the three reference laboratories.

```
                                                                      FREQ.   CUM.   PERCENT    CUM.
                                                                              FREQ.             PERCENT
          I
     0.6  I                                                              0       0     0.00      0.00
          I
     1.2  I000000000000000000000000000000000000000000000000000        2538    2538    55.79     55.79
          I
     1.8  I00000000000                                                 561    3099    12.33     68.12
          I
     2.4  I000000                                                      346    3445     7.61     75.73
          I
     3.0  I00                                                          106    3551     2.33     78.06
          I
     3.6  I001                                                         119    3670     2.62     80.68
          I
     4.2  I01                                                          115    3785     2.53     83.21
M         I
E    4.8  I1                                                            73    3858     1.60     84.81
A         I
N    5.4  I011                                                         135    3993     2.97     87.78
          I
S    6.0  I1                                                            83    4076     1.82     89.60
T         I
R    6.6  I11                                                          115    4191     2.53     92.13
E         I
N    7.2  I11                                                          117    4308     2.57     94.70
G         I
T    7.8  I11111                                                       241    4549     5.30    100.00
H         I
          -------+-------+-------+-------+-------+-------+---
                400     800    1200    1600    2000    2400

                              FREQUENCY
```

Fig. 1. Distribution of mean reaction strengths for HLA-DR1 sera. The mean strength was calculated as the mean of single sera reactions against each cell sample. *1* indicates positive reactions with cells that had the DR1 antigen; *0* indicates reactions against cells without DR1

Histocompatibility Testing 1984
Edited by E. D. Albert et al.

Table 1. Specificity of HLA-DR typing sera

Serum	Antigen	+ +		+ −		− +	− −	Tot.	*r*	Strongest correlations of the extra reactions
		ST	WK	ST	WK					(no. of positive cells)
501	DR1	497	160	120	79	193	3458	4512	0.72	DRw10 (19), DRw8 (23)
503	DR1	692	79	250	181	82	3236	4520	0.70	DRw10 (24)
506	DR1	590	107	39	58	145	3534	4473	0.82	DRw10 (10)
513	DR1	544	138	133	115	172	3417	4520	0.71	DRw10 (21), DRw6 (85), DR2 (78)
517	DR1	701	64	226	142	67	3165	4365	0.73	
	DRw10	57	11	169	131	19	3213	3600	0.35	DR2 (141)
519	DR1	682	86	367	192	86	3120	4533	0.64	
	DRw10	50	18	317	174	19	3187	3765	0.27	DR2 (171), DRw6 (98)
520	DR1	604	113	137	109	133	3427	4523	0.74	
	DRw10	48	13	89	95	27	3533	3806	0.39	DR4 (89)
526	DRw10	62	17	196	215	16	4027	4533	0.34	DR1 (153)
528	DRw10	71	7	166	138	19	4127	4528	0.33	DR1 (143)
532	DR2	1048	114	71	79	91	3017	4420	0.87	DRw10 (9)
536	DR2	1125	92	67	53	51	3127	4515	0.91	DRw10 (10)
539	DR2	1112	91	299	227	46	2705	4480	0.74	DRw6 (170), DR5 (136), DR7 (89)
544	DR2	954	146	99	85	120	2963	4367	0.83	DRw6 (91)
556	DR3	996	60	213	233	71	2965	4538	0.74	DRw6 (147), DR5 (121)
558	DR3	799	140	61	92	168	3206	4466	0.81	
560	DR3	926	74	63	76	73	3163	4375	0.87	
562	DR3	856	138	93	90	121	3197	4495	0.82	
566	DR3	917	107	205	165	98	3030	4522	0.75	DRw6 (113), DR1 (83)
577	DR4	866	219	134	133	282	2825	4459	0.71	DRw9 (24), DR7 (76)
579	DR4	1228	91	105	127	78	2903	4532	0.85	DR5 (95)
583	DR4	1212	108	139	119	65	2850	4493	0.84	DRw9 (35), DR7 (75)
586	DR4	1114	153	153	143	110	2800	4473	0.80	DRw10 (15)
588	DR4	1101	126	48	60	139	2949	4423	0.87	
600	DR5	810	111	176	174	124	3079	4474	0.73	DR4 (169), DRw10 (10)
602	DR5	900	82	423	313	70	2706	4494	0.63	DRw8 (142), DRw6 (201), DR3 (189)
604	DR5	647	181	261	222	225	2957	4493	0.60	DRw6 (214), DRw8 (53), DR2 (125)
606	DR5	572	189	65	107	288	3273	4494	0.70	
615	DR5	900	66	393	169	82	2880	4490	0.68	
	DRw8	201	18	192	151	41	2921	3524	0.53	DR4 (183), DRw10 (11)
617	DR5	722	102	290	105	184	2951	4354	0.66	
	DRw8	186	25	104	80	41	3094	3530	0.64	DRw10 (10)
622	DRw8	162	67	95	114	64	4022	4524	0.61	DR5 (106)
625	DRw8	241	31	1063	381	17	2777	4510	0.30	DRw6 (328), DR4 (430), DR5 (243), DR7 (169)
628	DRw8	180	54	225	172	53	3774	4458	0.51	DR5 (148)
631	DR7	721	88	307	174	87	2927	4304	0.67	DR4 (204), DRw6 (85)
632	DR7	557	148	106	108	230	3367	4516	0.70	
635	DR7	820	55	39	48	46	3472	4480	0.91	
641	DR7	865	33	66	52	33	3425	4475	0.90	
648	DRw9	105	16	325	201	23	3794	4464	0.36	DR1 (128), DR7 (105), DR4 (128)
649	DRw9	112	18	520	257	12	3474	4893	0.32	DR4 (466), DR7 (166)

Cell phenotypes were defined by the participating laboratories
Strong reactions (ST): score 8 or 6; weak reactions (WK): score 4
Extra reactions were investigated by tail analysis [1]
Significant extra reactions were indicated only when the serum reacted against at least 10% of the cells carrying the antigen

Table 2. Assignment of MT and MB specificities

Sera related with DRw52

Serum	Positive reactions (%) Strong	Weak	Proportion (%) of samples positive with the serum on all samples possessing the antigens DR3	DR5	DRw6	DRw8	Number of extra reactions	Strongest association(s) of extra reactions
675	28	9	79	13	74		107	
676	25	10	60	39	74	12	127	DRw9 (13)
686	43	9	88	72	86	15	188	DR4 (94)
690	46	7	94	76	84	25	157	DRw9 (17)
695	55	6	90	90	89	82	218	DRw9 (24)
760	49	8	90	83	85	65	205	DRw9 (28)
725	28	10	79	33	44	45	230	DR7 (156), DRw9 (14)

Sera related with DRw53

Serum	Positive reactions (%) Strong	Weak	Proportion (%) of samples positive with the serum on all samples possessing the antigens DR4	DR7	DRw9	Number of extra reactions	Strongest association(s) of extra reactions
728	26	6	83	9	63	129	
738	39	6	90	77	75	141	DR1 (58)
742	39	6	79	93	75	139	

Sera related with DQw1

Serum	Positive reactions (%) Strong	Weak	Proportion (%) of samples positive with the serum on all samples possessing the antigens DR1	DR2	DRw6	DRw10	DRw8	Number of extra reactions	Strongest association(s) of extra reactions
651	32	10	54	75	76	53	9	89	
658	38	9	58	83	83	60	13	183	DR5 (78)
659	35	10	50	85	79	48	12	110	
665	46	10	78	88	90	73	23	231	DR3 (105), DR7 (57)
666	50	11	84	88	92	67	9	388	DR4 (230), DR5 (86), DRw9 (17)
673	44	9	79	83	88	75	18	171	DR5 (92)

Sera related with DQw2

Serum	Positive reactions (%) Strong	Weak	Proportion (%) of samples positive with the serum on all samples possessing the antigens DR3	DR7	Number of extra reactions	Strongest association(s) of extra reactions
718	27	8	50	85	333	DR5 (130), DRw8 (28)
732	32	7	53	93	444	DRw9 (89), DR4 (162)

Sera related with DQw3

Serum	Positive reactions (%) Strong	Weak	Proportion (%) of samples positive with the serum on all samples possessing the antigens DR4	DR5	DRw9	Number of extra reactions	Strongest association(s) of extra reactions
749	29	11	64	75	24	233	DR7 (95), DRw8 (27)
751	33	11	69	70	47	380	DR7 (156), DRw8 (38)

Quality of Tissue Typing. The "average strength of reaction" against each cell sample was calculated for each group of sera determining the same main specificity. The average strength was calculated as the mean of the reaction scores of all sera used for the definition of an antigen.

The distribution of the mean reaction strengths for each group of sera was compared with the antigen assignment. An example is given in Fig. 1. Further investigations are planned to check the antigen assignments in the presence of a low mean reaction strength. This should

(a) provide a criterion for evaluating technical problems in certain laboratories;
(b) allow to discriminate between high and low-quality antisera;
(c) help to recognize the presence of heterogenous antigen phenotypes; and
(d) make it possible to reassign, if necessary, a different phenotype to some individuals.

Because data collection for the transplant study was continued to the latest possible moment prior to the Workshop conference, the raw data on HLA typings could not be analyzed extensively for this report. Additional analyses are planned to test whether further improvements in HLA matching correlations can be achieved with in-depth consideration of HLA serology.

Acknowledgment. Computer time was donated by CSI-Piemonte

Reference

1. Piazza A, Sgarmella-Zonta L, Gluckmann P, Cavalli-Sforza LL (1975) The Fifth Histocompatibility Workshop gene frequency data: a phylogenetic analysis. Tissue Antigens 5:445

Antigen Report: HLA-A1

H. Festenstein[1], C.B. Carpenter[2], A. Alonso[1], and E. Williams[1]

1 Department of Immunology, The London Hospital Medical College. London E1, U.K.
2 Immunogenetics Laboratory, Brigham and Women's Hospital, Boston, MA 02115, USA

HLA-A1 was originally defined by Payne et al. [2] as LA-1 and by Dausset et al. [1] as Da-11 and was given its present designation at the Sixth International Histocompatibility Workshop.

Table 1. Anti-HLA-A1 sera

9W serum no.	Average score[a]	% Reactions missed	% Extra reactions	Serum strength[b]	Quality score
001	7.0	17	2	63	7.0
002	7.4	7	3	76	9.5
003	7.8	1	3	87	11.0
006	7.9	0	4	94	11.0
007	7.9	0	6	90	11.0
009	7.7	2	6	83	10.0

[a] For antigen-positive cells
[b] Percentage of score "8" reactions among the positive reactions

HLA-A1 is common in Caucasoids, less frequent in Negroids and rare in Mongoloids.

Six anti-A1 sera were submitted to the 9th Workshop. Sera 003, 006, 007, and 009 showed strong anti-A1 activity, whereas 001 and 002 were weak (Table 1). Sera 006, 007, and 009 also had anti-Aw36 activity.

The most significant two-locus haplotypes in Caucasoids carrying this antigen were: A1-B8, A1-Bw57, A1-Cw6, A1-Cw7, and A1-C4AQ0.

HLA-A1 remains a clearly defined antigen and there is no evidence of heterogeneity in the Ninth Workshop results.

References

1. Dausset J, Ivanyi P, Colombani P, Feingold N, Legrand L (1967) The Hu-1 system. Histocompatibility testing 1967. Munksgaard, Copenhagen, p 189
2. Payne R, Tripp M, Bodmer W, Bodmer J (1964) A new leucocyte isoantigen system in man. Cold Spring Harbor Symp Quant Biol 29:285–295

Histocompatibility Testing 1984
Edited by E. D. Albert et al.

Antigen Report: HLA-A2

E. S. Curtoni [1], S. D. Lawler [2], L. J. Kennedy [3], W. H. Marshall [4], and W. Wakeling [2]

1 Istituto Genetica Medica, Università di Torino, Via Santena 19, 10126 Torino, Italy
2 Dept of Cytogenetics and Immunology, Royal Marsden Hospital, London SW3, U.K.
3 Tissue Antigen Laboratory, Imperial Cancer Research Fund, P.O. Box 123, Lincolns Inn Fields, London WC2A 3PX, U.K.
4 Immunology Laboratories, Faculty of Medicine, M.U.N., St Johns, Newfoundland, Canada A1B 3V6

A2, one of the first HLA antigens to be recognized, was split early on into A2 and A28. Although at the time of the 1980 workshop it seemed to be a well-characterised entity, even then nonserological techniques (cytotoxic T cells) were beginning to show that there are variants of A2. At the present workshop A2, as studied with classic antisera, remains clearly defined. Among seven antisera, which primarily reacted with A2 positive cells, there were five with Q-scores of over 9. These gave results which were about as good as one could hope for. They detected some 99% of cells designated A2 by the submitting laboratories and gave 0–3% of extra reactions, a proportion of which may have been due to carry- over as judged by collateral evidence (for example, the first A2 antiserum after the A1 sera had a tail of A1 reactions). The assignment of A2 to specific cells by the submitting laboratories was in almost perfect agreement with the subsequent computer assignment; it was the antigen with the highest level of concordance in this regard ($r = 0.99$).

For further serological information on the definition of a new epitope on A2 cells, named A2/ 28 which is also found on Aw69 (28)-positive cells, the reader is referred to sections on A28 and on ABC monoclonal antibodies in this volume.

Monoclonal antibodies have also been shown in the data discussed at this workshop to react differentially with A2 cells in rare cases, and so far they define two rare variants of A2. These are found in the Japanese and Chinese populations and were first noted by Japanese workers [1]. These variants have been found to segregate in families; the full data will be published elsewhere.

Although not part of the serum analysis of this workshop, it is worth noting that A2 has now been shown to be heterogeneous in studies involving cytotoxic T cells and a corresponding monoclonal antibody [2] and by isoelectric focussing and aminoacid sequencing. Recent data on the three-dimensional structure of a class I antigen have also involved A2 [3].

With further polymorphism now being found in such a previously well-defined antigen as A2, we can look forward to a very considerable increase in the complexity of the HLA system.

References

1. Kusama M, Sato K, Yamashita Y, Nose Y, Sukegawa T, Tsuji K (1984) Further observation of monoclonal antibody 1139 [in Japanese]. Workshop Newsletter 6.
2. Russo C, Ah-Kaung, Pellegrino M, Ferrone S (1983) The monoclonal antibody CR11-351 discriminates the HLA-A2 variants identified by T-cells. Immunogenetics 18:23–35.
3. Vega AM, Bragado R, Ezquerra A, Lopez de Castro JA (1984) Variability and conformation of HLA class 1 antigens. Biochemistry 23:823.

Antigen Report: HLA-A3

F. Kissmeyer-Nielsen [1] and R. L. Walford [2]

1 Department of Clinical Immunology, Tissue Typing Laboratory, University Hospital of Århus, Denmark
2 Department of Pathology, UCLA School of Medicine, Los Angeles, CA 90024, USA

Workshop analysis of the HLA-A3 antigen has not yet revealed new information. There were no completely monospecific antisera included in the workshop, and Table 1 lists only the three best antisera as judged from the 1000 Caucasian cells included in the workshop analysis.

Pattern analysis has not given any further information. The results of analysis of other ethnic groups are essentially in accordance with those obtained in Caucasians.

Table 1. Best antisera according to workshop analysis

WS-serum No.	Average score	% Missed Reactions	% Extra Reactions	"Tail"
9w060	8.0	0	5	A11
9w057	7.9	0	5	A24
9w059	7.6	2	16	A11

Antigen Report: HLA-A11

F. Kissmeyer-Nielsen[1] and R. L. Walford[2]

1 Department of Clinical Immunology, Tissue Typing Laboratory, University Hospital of Århus, Denmark
2 Department of Pathology, UCLA School of Medicine, Los Angeles, CA 90024, USA

Pattern analysis has not given further information, but generally speaking the quality of the anti-HLA-A11 sera included in the workshop has been rather poor (Table 1), and they show marked cross-reactivity (although rather weak reactions with HLA-A3 and HLA-A1).
The results of analysis of other ethnic groups are essentially in accordance with those obtained in Caucasians.

Table 1. Quality of anti-HLA-A11 sera and cross-reactivity

WS serum	Average serum score	% Missed Reactions	% Extra Reactions	"Tail"
9w067	7.9	1	42	A1 A3
9w065	7.7	3	29	A3 A1
9w063	7.6	8	38	A3 A1

Antigen Report: HLA-A23

D. P. Singal[1], H. Bétuel[2], M. D'Souza[1], and L. Gebuhrer[2]

1 Department of Pathology, McMaster University, 1200 Main St. W., Hamilton, Ontario, Canada L8N 3Z5
2 Blood Transfusion Center, 69007 Lyon, France

History

Dausset [4] reported the existence of two subtypes of HLA-A9. Data analyzed at the Fifth International Histocompatibility Workshop held in Evian in 1972 confirmed these two subtypes, and these were designated Aw23 and Aw24 [2]. At subsequent workshops, A23 has been easy to define with sera giving high correlation coefficients [1, 3, 5]. A23 has the highest frequency in Negroids and is virtually absent in Mongoloids and Amerindians. A23 showed positive linkage disequilibrium with B44 and DR7 in Caucasians, and low positive linkage disequilibrium with B7-DR1 in Negroes [1].

Serology

In Caucasians, A23 is defined by positive reactions with A9 (036, 038, 039) and A23 (041, 042, 044, 043) sera and negative reactions with A24 sera. Serum 043 was weak and missed 13% reactions. Serum 041 missed 4% reactions, but gave 73% extra reactions. Sera 042 and 044 were good, giving 8% and 5% false-negative reactions and 25% and 32% false-positive reactions, respectively. Extra reactions with all A23 sera were predominantly with A24 cells.
Pattern analysis for sera defining A23 is given in Table 1.

Table 1. Pattern analysis for A23 sera

9w041	9w042	9w044	9w043	Antigen-positive cells (%)	
				Caucasians	Negroes
+	+	+	+	73	71
+	+	+	–	12	4
+	–	+	+	6	0
+	+	–	+	3	0
+	+	–	–	3	0

Conclusion

As in the previous workshops, A23 was well defined with the submitted sera.

Histocompatibility Testing 1984
Edited by E. D. Albert et al.

References

1. Arnaiz-Villena A (1980) Aw23. In: Terasaki PI (ed) Histocompatibility testing 1980. Tissue Typing Lab, Los Angeles, p 302
2. Bodmer JG (1972) HL-A9. In: Dausset J, Colombani J (eds) Histocompatibility testing 1972. Munksgaard, Copenhagen, p 637
3. Bodmer JG (1975) The ABC of HLA. In: Kissmeyer-Nielsen F (ed) Histocompatibility testing 1975. Munksgaard, Copenhagen, p 21
4. Dausset J (1971) The genetics of transplantation antigens. Transplant Proc 3:8–14
5. Dick HM (1977) HLA-A, B and C serology and antigen reports. In: Bodmer WF, et al (eds) Histocompatibility testing 1977. Munksgaard, Copenhagen, p 157

Antigen Report: HLA-A24

D. P. Singal [1], M. D'Souza [1], H. Bétuel [2], and L. Gebuhrer [2]

1 Department of Pathology, McMaster University, 1200 Main St. W., Hamilton, Ontario, Canada L8N 3Z5
2 Blood Transfusion Center, 69007 Lyon, France

History

HLA-A24 was first identified as a split of A9 by Dausset in 1970 [4]. It was confirmed by the data analyzed at the 1972 Histocompatibility Workshop held in Evian [2]. At the last three workshops, A24 has been well defined with sera giving high correlation coefficients [3, 5, 6]. In addition, there was a good agreement between laboratories on the definition of this antigen in cell exchange [1]. A24 has the highest frequency in Orientals and the lowest in Negroids. In Caucasians, A24-Bw61-DR2 showed significant positive linkage disequilibrium, and in Orientals, A24-B7-DR2 showed strong negative linkage disequilibrium [6].

Serology

In Caucasians, A24 is defined by positive reactions with A9 (036, 038, 039) and A24 (047, 050, 048, 051) sera and negative reactions with A23 (042, 044) sera. Of the A24 sera, serum 047 gave the least number of false-positive reactions. The majority of extra reactions with these sera were with A23-positive cells.

Pattern analysis for sera defining A24 is given in Table 1.

Table 1. Pattern analysis for A24 sera

9w047	9w050	9w048	9w051	Antigen-positive cells (%)	
				Caucasians	Negroes
+	+	+	+	74	89
+	+	+	–	10	4
+	+	–	+	1	7
–	+	+	+	1	0

Conclusion

As in the previous workshops, A24 was well defined using submitted sera.

References

1. Bernoco D, Terasaki PI, Perdue S, et al (1980) International cell exchange report. In: Terasaki PI (ed) Histocompatibility testing 1980. UCLA Tissue Typing Laboratory, Los Angeles, p 215.
2. Bodmer JG (1972) HL-A9. In: Dausset J, Colombani J (eds) Histocompatibility testing 1972. Munksgaard, Copenhagen, p 637
3. Bodmer JG (1975) The ABC of HLA. In: Kissmeyer-Nielsen F (ed) Histocompatibility testing 1975. Munksgaard, Copenhagen, p 21
4. Dausset J (1971) The genetics of transplantation antigens. Transplant Proc 3:8–14
5. Dick HM (1977) HLA-A, B and C serology and antigen reports. In: Bodmer WF, et al (eds) Histocompatibility testing 1977. Munksgaard, Copenhagen, p 157
6. Tait DB (1980) Aw24. In: Terasaki PI (ed) Histocompatibility testing 1980. UCLA Tissue Typing Laboratory, Los Angeles, p 305

Histocompatibility Testing 1984
Edited by E. D. Albert et al.

Antigen Report: A9.3

D. P. Singal [1], M. D'Souza [1], H. Bétuel [2], and L. Gebuhrer [2]

1 Department of Pathology, McMaster University, 1200 Main St. W., Hamilton, Ontario, Canada L8N 3Z5
2 Blood Transfusion Center, 69007 Lyon, France

During the Sixth International Histocompatibility Workshop, a third subset of A9 (A9.3) was described in Caucasians and African Blacks [2]. However, A9.3 was no longer considered valid at the last two workshops [1, 3]. Gebuhrer et al. [4] recently described a variant of A9 that is distinct from A23 and A24 in an Arab family. This subtype is defined by positive reactions with two A9 (038, 039) and two A24 (047, 048) sera and negative reactions with all anti-A23, two anti-A24 (050, 051), and two A9 (036, 037) sera. They named this variant A9.3, although it is not certain that it corresponds to the subset defined in 1975 [2].

References

1. Arnaiz-Villena A (1980) Aw23. In: Terasaki PI (ed) Histocompatibility testing 1980. UCLA Tissue Typing Laboratory, Los Angeles, p 302
2. Bodmer JG (1975) The ABC of HLA. In: Kissmeyer-Nielsen F (ed) Histocompatibility testing 1975. Munksgaard, Copenhagen, p 21
3. Dick HM (1977) HLA-A, B and C serology and antigen reports. In: Bodmer WF, et al (eds) Histocompatibility testing 1977. Munksgaard, Copenhagen, p 157
4. Gebuhrer L, Betuel H, Labonne MP, et al (1983) A third subset of HLA-A9. Ninth International Histocompatibility Workshop Newsletter 3:9–13

Antigen Report: HLA-A25

L.P. de Waal [1], G.G. de Lange [1], V. Joysey [2], C.P. Engelfriet [1], and A. Amoroso [3]

1 Central Laboratory of the Netherlands Red Cross, Blood Transfusion Service, P.O. Box 9190, Amsterdam, The Netherlands
2 Tissue Typing Laboratory, Addenbrooke's Hospital, Cambridge, U.K.
3 Istituto di Genetica Medica, Università di Torino, Via Santena 19, 10126 Torino, Italy

History

During the Fifth International Histocompatibility Workshop [1] the subdivision of HLA-A10 into A25 and A26 was established.
In the Sixth Workshop [2] A10 and its splits were clearly defined in Caucasians, whereas A25 was not found in Japanese. Aw34, a newly defined antigen belonging to the A10 cross-reacting group, was defined and shown to have a high frequency in Malays. During the Seventh and Eighth Workshops [3, 4] the definition of A25 and the distinction from A26 became firmly established. A25 is common in the Caucasian population (gene frequency 3.8%) but is essentially absent in Orientals and Negroes.
A25 was found to be in linkage disequilibrium with B18 and DR2 in Caucasians.

Serology

The population sample used for serum analysis consisted of approximately 5300 individuals from different races. In this population, A25 was defined by 13 sera (072, 075, 076, 077, 078, 079, 081, 085, 087, 090, 091, 114, 147) (Table 1). In a group of 570 Negroes the frequency of A25 was too low to allow any conclusions. Analysis of the total population revealed three relatively good A25 sera (085, $r = 0.882$; 087, $r = 0.638$; 090, $r = 0.817$).
The best A25 and A26 sera were 072 and 075 (containing in addition anti-Aw43), 078 (+Aw34), 077, 079 and 081 (+Aw34+Aw43). It is important to distinguish A25 from A26, Aw34, and Aw43 (Table 2). Seven sera distinguished A25 from A26, viz. 085, 087, 090 and 114 (positive with A25, negative

Histocompatibility Testing 1984
Edited by E. D. Albert et al.

Table 1. Selection of best Ninth Workshop sera with reactivity for A25

9w no.	Specificity	Q score	% 8 score	% Misses
072	A25	9.2	83	5
	A26	8.8	90	5
	Aw43	6.4	67	6
075	A25	10.0	87	5
	A26	13.0	97	3
	Aw43	8.6	100	6
	Tail: A3[a]			
076	A25	7.7	77	13
	A26	7.6	81	10
	Aw34	7.8	79	12
077	A25	9.6	87	3
	A26	11.0	90	3
	Aw43	5.3	86	12
	Aw34	4.6	73	37
078	A25	7.6	78	8
	A26	9.2	89	4
	Aw34	9.0	90	7
079	A25	8.5	77	6
	A26	11.0	88	2
	Aw34	7.5	92	18
	Aw43	7.6	100	7
081	A25	10.0	91	6
	A26	12.0	98	2
	Aw34	10.0	87	11
	Aw43	8.3	100	7
085	A25	9.1	93	6
	Tail: A26[a]			
087	A25	7.5	89	7
	Tail: A26 + A1[a]			
090	A25	7.0	62	20
	Tail: A26[a]			
091	A25	9.5	94	7
	A26	4.0	17	50
114	A25	8.7	71	19
	A32	11.0	84	8
	Tail: A26[a]			
147	A25	9.8	98	6
	A26	11.0	97	3
	A28	2.8	41	45
	A32	1.2		
	Aw33	1.8	43	70
	Aw34	7.8	97	9
	Aw43	1.5	50	83

[a] Tail: Q score < 1
The table is based on data from approximately 5300 individuals of different races

Table 2. Selection of Ninth Workshop sera defining A25, A26 and Aw34

Antigen	Ninth Workshop sera																	
	072	075	077	078	079	081	085	087	090	094	095	114	147	148	149	101	103	104
A25	+	+	+	+	+	+	+	+	+	–	–	+	+	–	+/–	–	–	–
A26	+	+	+	+	+	+	–	–	–	+	+	–	+	+	+/–	–	–	–
Aw34	–	–	+/–	+	+/–	+	–	–	–	–	+/–	–	+	+	+	–	+/–	–
Aw43	+	+	+	–	+	+	–	–	–	–	+/–	–	+/–	+	+/–	+	+	+

+/–, inconsistent reaction

with most A26) and 094, 095, and 148 (negative with A25, positive with A26). Seven sera distinguish between A25 and Aw34: 072, 075, 085, 087, 090, and 114 (positive with A25, negative with Aw34) and 148 (negative with A25, positive with Aw34). Finally the distinction from Aw43 can be made by means of 078, 085, 087, 090, and 114 (positive with A25, negative with Aw43) and 101, 103, 104, and 148 (negative with A25, positive with Aw43). For the definition of LN (= Aw66) the reader is referred to the Aw66 antigen report.

Conclusion

A25 is a clearly defined antigen, which can be clearly distinguished from A26, Aw34 and Aw43 in Caucasians. A25 was essentially absent in the Negroes studied in this Workshop.

References

1. Joint Report (1972) In: Dausset J, Colombani J (eds) Histocompatibility testing 1972. Munksgaard, Copenhagen
2. Joint Report (1975) In: Kissmeyer-Nielsen F (ed) Histocompatibility testing 1975. Munksgaard, Copenhagen
3. Joint Report (1978) In: Bodmer W, et al (eds) Histocompatibility testing 1977. Munksgaard, Copenhagen
4. Joint Report (1980) In: Terasaki PI (ed) Histocompatibility testing 1980. UCLA Tissue Typing Laboratory, Los Angeles

Antigen Report: HLA-A26

L. P. de Waal[1], G.G. de Lange[1], V. Joysey[2], C.P. Engelfriet[1], and A. Amoroso[3]

1 Central Laboratory of the Netherlands Red Cross Blood Transfusion Service, P.O. Box 9190, Amsterdam, The Netherlands
2 Tissue Typing Laboratory, Addenbrooke's Hospital, Cambridge, U.K.
3 Istituto di Genetica Medica, Università di Torino, Via Santena 19, 10126 Torino, Italy

History

The Fifth International Histocompatibility Workshop resulted in the designation of HLA-A25 and HLA-A26 as two subtypes of HLA-A10 [1]. Aw34, which belongs to the A10 cross-reacting group, was defined during the Sixth Workshop [2]. The existence of A26 was confirmed in various races, such as Caucasians, Orientals, and Negroes, at the Sixth (1975) and Seventh (1977) Workshops [2, 3]. During the Eighth Workshop (1980) [4] A26 was well defined. The gene frequency observed in Caucasians was 3.2%; in Israeli Jews, 10.5% (1980); in Orientals, 7.2%; and in Negroes, 4.5%. In the last population the suggestion of a short variant was put forward. A26 was found to be in linkage disequilibrium with B38 in several races.

Serology

During the Ninth Workshop 13 A26-reactive sera of high quality (072, 074, 075, 076, 077, 078, 079, 081, 082, 094, 095, 147, 148) were found (Table 1). An excellent almost A26-specific serum is 095 ($r = 0.915$; only a few extra reactions with Aw34 and Aw43). In addition, serum 148 recognizes A26, Aw34, and Aw43 (with residual activity against Aw33).

The other sera can be grouped as follows: A25 + A26 + Aw43 specificity (072, 074, 075); A25 + A26 + Aw34 specificity (076, 078); A10 + Aw34 + Aw43 specificity (077, 079, 081, 082). Serum 147 is complex and reacts with A25 + A26 + Aw34, with residual reactivity against A28, Aw33, Aw43, and Aw32.

Table 1. Selection of best Ninth Workshop sera with reactivity for A26

9w no.	Specificity	Q square	% 8 score	% Misses
072	A26	8.8	90	5
	A25	9.2	83	5
	Aw43	6.4	67	6
074	A26	8.1	82	12
	A25	4.0	57	42
	Aw43	7.5	87	6
	Tail: Aw34[a]			
075	A26	13.0	87	5
	A25	10.0	97	3
	Aw43	8.6	100	6
	Tail: A3[a]			
076	A26	7.6	81	10
	A25	7.7	77	13
	Aw34	7.8	79	12
077	A26	11.0	90	3
	A25	9.6	87	3
	Aw43	5.3	86	12
	Aw34	4.6	73	12
078	A26	9.2	89	4
	A25	7.6	78	8
	Aw34	9.0	90	7
079	A26	11.0	88	2
	A25	8.5	77	6
	Aw34	7.5	92	18
	Aw43	7.6	100	7
081	A26	12.0	98	2
	A25	10.0	91	6
	Aw34	10.0	87	11
	Aw43	8.3	100	7
082	A26	5.7	90	7
	A25	4.3	71	23
	Aw43	5.1	100	7
	Aw34	4.7	91	21
094	A26	7.9	65	17
	Tail: A25 A1 A29[a]			
095	A26	12.0	90	4
	Aw34	2.8	39	58
	Aw43	3.6	0	71
	Tail: A25[a]			
147	A26	11.0	97	3
	A25	9.8	98	6
	Aw34	7.8	97	9
	A28	2.8	41	45
	A32	1.2		
	Aw33	1.8	43	70
	Aw43	1.5	50	83
148	A26	8.5	98	2
	Aw34	5.1	92	12
	Aw43	5.7	100	7
	Aw33	3.8	17	28

[a] Tail: Q score < 1. The table is based on the data from approximately 5300 individuals of different races

Histocompatibility Testing 1984
Edited by E. D. Albert et al.

Analysis of the patterns obtained in 570 Negroes revealed that serum 072 did not react with 7.2% of A10-positive and Aw34, Aw32, Aw43, and Aw66-negative cells ($n = 42$). Since none of the A25-specific sera reacted, whereas sera 079 and 095 did react with these cells, the reaction pattern of serum 072 might suggest a "short" A26 variant in Negroes. A26 can be discriminated from A25 by sera 094, 095, and 148 (positive with A26, usually negative with A25) and by sera 085, 087, 090, and 114 (negative with A26, positive with A25) (see Table 2 in presentation on A25). Distinction between A26 and Aw34 can be made by sera 072 and 075 (positive with A26, negative with Aw34). Distinction from Aw43 is possible by serum 078 (positive with A26, negative with Aw43) and sera 101, 103, and 104 (negative with A26, positive with Aw43). The definition of Aw66 is given in the Aw66 antigen report.

Conclusion

A26 could be clearly defined and distinguished from A25, Aw34, and Aw43 in Caucasians and Negroes.

References

1. Joint Report (1972) In: Dausset J, Colombani J (eds) Histocompatibility testing 1972. Munksgaard, Copenhagen
2. Joint Report (1975) In: Kissmeyer-Nielsen F (ed) Histocompatibility testing 1975. Munksgaard, Copenhagen
3. Joint Report (1978) In: Bodmer W, et al (eds) Histocompatibility testing 1977. Munksgaard, Copenhagen
4. Joint Report (1980) In: Terasaki PI (ed) Histocompatibility testing 1980. UCLA Tissue Typing Laboratory, Los Angeles

Antigen Report: HLA-A28

E.S. Curtoni[1], S.D. Lawler[2], L.J. Kennedy[3], W.H. Marshall[4], and W. Wakeling[2]

1 Istituto Genetica Medica, Università di Torino, Via Santena 19, 10126 Torino, Italy
2 Dept. of Cytogenetics and Immunology, Royal Marsden Hospital, London SW3, U.K.
3 Tissue Antigen Laboratory, Imperial Cancer Research Fund, P.O. Box 123, Lincolns Inn Fields, London WC2A 3PX, U.K.
4 Immunology Laboratories, Faculty of Medicine, M.U.N., St Johns, Newfoundland, Canada A1B 3V6

A28, which is related serologically to A2, was accorded full antigen status after the Sixth Workshop. It has remained well defined, although data from Italy have repeatedly suggested that A28 could be split (see below).

At the Ninth Workshop the serological definition of A28 was satisfactory, but, provided carry-over has not been a problem (see A2 report), the sera that can be used to define A28 all contain significant amounts (by the chi-square test on 2 × 2 table data) of A2 reactivity and none is particularly strong (percentage of scores of 8 in the positive reactions with A28 cells). The strongest antiserum (str 70%) was 9w024, which reacted with 92% of cells designated A28 by submitting laboratories; however, some 15% of its positive reactions were with cells that were A28 negative and A2 positive. With other sera there were either more misses or more reactions with A2, or both. Because of these A2-tails the definition of A28 in the presence of A2 is still a problem.

A recent advance with A28 is the definition of a new antigenic determinant. The key to understanding this is that two monoclonal antibodies directed against A2 actually also react with a small subset of A28 cells, now called Aw69 (28). Thus, on rare A28 cells there is an antigen which is normally found on A2 cells but which is not detected by the best A2 sera. This has been named A2/28 [= A2 + Aw69 (28)].

This finding led to the realization that some A2 sera with A28 tails also recognized A2/28. The serologic reactions given in Table 1 suggest that A2/28 is the same antigen that has apparently defined a split in A28 in the Italian population. The essential data are given in Table 1.

It will be interesting to see whether this new epitope A2/28 is formed by a structure based on amino acid and DNA sequence homology between these alleles. In unpublished data from Parham's laboratory it is suggested that A2/28 resulted from an intragenic recombination, with about half the new gene deriving from each of A2 and A28.

Histocompatibility Testing 1984
Edited by E. D. Albert et al.

Table 1. Split of A28 into two subtypic specificities (Aw68 and Aw69) with Ninth Workshop reagents

Cells	9WS Sera [a]			9WS Moabs [a]		
	A2	A2+ Aw69	A28	A2 and A28	A2	A2+ Aw69
	0 0 0	0 0 0 0	0 0 0 0 0 0 0	1 1 1 1 1 1 1 1	1 1	1 1
	0 0 0	0 0 0 0	0 0 0 0 0 0 0	1 1 1 1 1 1 1 1	1 1	1 1
	1 1 1	1 1 1 2	2 2 2 2 2 3 3	0 0 0 3 4 4 5 5	3 4	0 3
Bodmer lab data	1 3 4	7 8 9 1	3 4 5 7 9 1 2	2 3 8 0 1 2 1 6	2 4	4 9
A2 Homozygotes	+ + +	+ + + +	? – – ? – – –	+ + + + + + + +	+ +	+ +
A2 Heter (most)	+ + +	+ + + +	– – – – – – –	+ + + + + + + +	+ +	+ +
Aw68 (28) (Regular)	– – –	– – – –	+ + + + + + +	+ + + + + + + +	– –	– –
Aw69 (28) (Rare)	– ? –	+ + + +	+ + + + + + –[b]	+ + + + + + + +	– –	+ +
Italy 1 reg. data (refers to families)						
Aw69 (28) (Less common)	– – –	0 + + +	+ + + + ? + ?	+ + + + + + + +	– –	+ +
Aw68 (28) (Common type)	– – –	0 – – –	+ + + + ? + ?	+ + + + + + + +	– –	– –

[a] Details of other reactivities not given
[b] Serum 32 appears to lack Aw69 reactivity

References

1. Kennedy LJ, Bodmer JG (1983) A2 variants. Ninth International Histocompatibility Workshop Newsletter 5
2. Richiardi P, Amoroso A, Conighi C, Menicucci A, Savi M, Marsico D, Fina C, Curtoni ES (1984) Further splits of A28. Ninth International Histocompatibility Workshop Newsletter 6

Antigen Report: HLA-A29

M.G. Hammond[1], H. Bétuel[2], and L. Gebuhrer[2]

1 Natal Institute of Immunology, Durban 4000, South Africa
2 Blood Transfusion Center, 69007 Lyon, France

The A29 antigen has been well defined since 1975 [1], and the five sera submitted as monospecific A29 sera for this workshop gave a clear definition in all races.

All five sera have high Q scores (Table 1), and the average strength scores show that nearly all positive reactions with A29 were very strong. Sera 9w104 and 9w108 had some extra reactions with A11 and A1 cells, respectively.

Table 1. A29 serum analysis

Serum	Q score	Ave strength with A29	Extras
9w102	9.9	7.6	
9w103	10.0	7.6	Aw43, Th, (A11)[a]
9w104	9.7	7.9	Aw43
9w106	12.0	7.7	Aw43
9w108	11.0	7.4	(Aw43), (A1)

[a] Antigens in parentheses show that only some cells were positive

The other extra reactions were only seen in the Negroid populations. Three sera, 9w103, 9w104, and 9w106, reacted with Aw43 cells, and serum 9w104 also reacted with cells carrying Th. Several broad Aw19 sera also recognized A29: 9w149, 9w150, 9w062, and 9w301. There were no discrepancies in the segregation patterns of 45 families.

A29 was not found in Chinese or Japanese cells but was present at low frequency in some southeast Asian populations.

As at previous workshops, A29 and B44 showed a positive linkage disequilibrium in Caucasoid and Negroid populations.

Reference

1. Bodmer T, Curtoni ES, van Leeuwen A, et al (1975) The ABC of HLA. A serological report of the Sixth Histocompatibility Testing Workshop. In: Kissmeyer-Nielsen F (ed) Histocompatibility testing 1975. Munksgaard, Copenhagen, p 21

Histocompatibility Testing 1984
Edited by E. D. Albert et al.

Antigen Report: HLA-A30/HLA-A31

C. Raffoux[1] and M. Savi[2]

1 INSERM U 93, Hôpital Saint Louis, 10 Place Docteur Fournier, 75010 Paris, France
2 Clinica Medica e Nephrologia, Cattedra di Genetica Medica, Parma, Italy

These two components of the Aw19 complex were first described at the Fourth International Workshop. During the Fifth Workshop Aw19 was subdivided into the following components: A29 (19.1), A30 (19.3), A31 (19.4), A32 (19.5), and residual reactions (19.6). A30 and A31 were considered to be the most difficult to define, because for a long time no monospecific sera were available. During the Eighth Workshop, distinction between these two specificities was possible only by pattern analysis and family segregation studies. A30 was mainly found in Negroes and was virtually absent in Orientals. A31 was mainly present in Orientals and rare in Negroes. In Caucasians both specificities were found. The most important linkage disequilibria were between A30 and B13 in Caucasians and between A30 and Bw42 in Negroes. No significant linkage disequilibrium was found with A31 in any population.

Serology

In the present Workshop there were 20 sera selected by computer as capable of identifying A30 and/or A31 antigens. Four out of 11 of these sera (9w126, 123, 122, and 119) recognized both specificities, clearly defining A30/A31 with $r = 0.95 - 0.79$. Five sera defined exclusively A30, and three of these (9w128, 129, and 138) showed good correlation ($r = 0.76 - 0.65$). Four sera recognized A31 and not A30, and two of these (9w140 and 135) were quite good sera for A31, with $r = 0.51$ and $r = 0.43$, respectively. The following sera recognized, in addition, other specificities: 9w138 (B13), 135 (Aw33) and 140 (Aw33 + Aw34). A30 was defined by two monospecific sera. There were no A31-monospecific sera, but A31 can be easily defined when sera A30/31 and A31 are positive in the absence of reactivity of the A30- and Aw33-specific sera (Table 1). The reactions of 9w133 (A30 + Cw5) suggest that there may be heterogeneity of A30, as emerged from studying segregation within 34 A30-positive families that are negative for A31 and Cw5. This serum segregates (strength 7.5) within 13 families (6 Negroid and 7 Caucasoid), being negative in 21 families (5 Negroid and 16 Caucasoid). Within the 9w133-positive Negroid families, A30 is associated three times out of five with the Bw58 antigen. In Caucasoid families that are 9w133 negative, A30 is associated with B13 twelve times out of sixteen.

Conclusion

There is no evidence that A31 can be subdivided. One serum (9w133) indicates that A30 might be split.

Table 1. Pattern distinguishing A30 from A31

	A30+A31	A30	A31	Aw33
	9 9 9 9 w w w w 1 1 1 1 2 2 2 1 6 3 2 9	9 9 9 w w w 1 1 1 2 2 3 8 9 8	9 9 w w 1 1 4 3 0 5	9 9 w w 1 1 4 4 3 6
A30	+ + + +	+ + +	– –	– –
A31	+ + + +	– – –	+ +	– –
Aw33	– – – –	– – –	+ +	+ +

References

1. Hawkins BR, Falk J (1980) Aw30. In: Terasaki PI (ed) Histocompatibility testing 1980. Munksgaard, Copenhagen, p 325
2. Rodey G (1980) Aw31. In: Terasaki PI (ed) Histocompatibility testing 1980. Munksgaard, Copenhagen, p 328

Histocompatibility Testing 1984
Edited by E. D. Albert et al.

Antigen Report: HLA-A32

J. Vives [1], H. Neumeyer [2], and J. Martorell [1]

1 Servicio de Inmunologia, Hospital Clinico y Provincial, c/Villarroel 170, 08006 Barcelona, Spain
2 Dept. of Immunology, University of Göttingen, Tissue Typing Laboratory, 3400 Göttingen, Federal Republic of Germany

History

The antigen A32 has been described as part of the Aw19 complex. In the Fifth [1], Sixth [2], and Seventh [3] Workshops, most sera recognizing A32 antigen reacted with A25 (A10). Some other sera did not present any cross-reactivity, but in general were too short and weak, as was the case with serum 419, which was presented at the Eighth Workshop [4].
These facts, together with the recent production of a monoclonal antibody reacting with A32 + A25 antigens (CATA1), led some authors to suggest as a possibility that A32 has no specific epitopes [5]. This hypothesis has not been confirmed at the present workshop, for a serum has been presented (9w130) which reacts specifically with A32.

Serology

During the Ninth Workshop, four sera (9w111, 9w112, 9w113, and 9w130) have been proposed as specific for A32. Only serum 9w130 gives clear-cut reactions specific for this antigen. This serum does not react with A25-positive cells. The other three sera give some extra reactions or are weak. Serum 9w111 is almost specific, but has extra reactions, especially with 20% of the A25-positive cells. 9w112 presents many extra reactions, especially with A25 and A24 cells. Serum 9w113 is short and weak but does not present extra reactions. Serum 9w118 is short and weak and gives some extra reactions. Since the short sera are generally weak there is no basis for postulating a subdivision of this antigen. Although sera 9w114 and 9w117 react with A25, they are very useful to define A32 in absence of A25 antigen.

Linkage Disequilibrium

A32 was in positive linkage disequilibrium with Cw2, Bw51, Bw61 and DR5 in European Caucasians; with Cw5 and Bw62-DR7 in North American Caucasians, and with Aw32-Cw1 in Negroes [4].

Conclusions

The data obtained at the present Workshop allow us to conclude that A32 is a well-defined antigen with at least one specific antigenic determinant defined by serum 9w130, which could be considered as a reference serum. In A25-positive cells, serum 9w130, and sometimes also 9w113, permit the assignment of A32. In A25-negative cells, sera 9w111, 9w114, 9w117, and 9w130 detect the presence of A32.

References

1. Bodmer JG (1972) w19 (w29, w30, w31, w32). In: Dausset J, Colombani J (eds) Histocompatibility testing 1972. Munksgaard, Copenhagen, p 641
2. Bodmer JG (1975) The ABC of HLA. In: Kissmeyer-Nielsen F (ed) Histocompatibility testing 1975. Munksgaard, Copenhagen, p 40
3. Dick M (1977) HLA-A, B and C serology and antigen reports. In: Bodmer WF et al (eds) Histocompatibility testing 1977. Munksgaard, Copenhagen, p 157
4. Pollock C, Rittner C (1980) Aw32 (joint report). In: Terasaki PI (ed) Histocompatibility testing 1980. UCLA Tissue Typing Laboratories, Los Angeles, p 331
5. Vilella R, Yague J, Vives J (1983) Monoclonal antibody against HLA-Aw32 + A25. Hum Immunol 6:53–62.

Histocompatibility Testing 1984
Edited by E. D. Albert et al.

Antigen Report: HLA-Aw33

M. C. Mazzilli [1], T.M. Neri [2], D. Adorno [3], A. Amoroso [4], S. Barocci [5], J. Martorell [6], G. B. Ferrara [7,8], E. Gandini [1], M. Savi [9], J. Vives [6], and A. Longo [7]

1 Cattedra di Genetica Medica, Università "La Sapienza", Via Portuense 292, 00149 Roma, Italy
2 Istituto di Clinica Medica e Nefrologia, Parma, Italy
3 Istituto C.N.R. di Tipizzazione Tissutale e Dialisi, L'Aquila, Italy
4 Istituto di Genetica Medica, Università di Torino, Via Santena 19, 10126 Torino, Italy
5 Servizio di Immunologia, XIII U.S.L., Genova, Italy
6 Servicio de Inmunologia, Hospital Clinico y Provincial, c/Villarroel 170, 08006 Barcelona, Spain
7 Istituto Nazionale per la Ricerca sul Cancro, Genova, Italy
8 Centro Ricerche Immunologiche, Avis, Bergamo, Italy
9 Cattedra di Genetica Medica, Università di Parma, Parma, Italy

History

At the 6th Workshop Aw33 was recognized as a single antigen in spite of some evidence for the existence of two specificities: the first Fe55 is present in Caucasian populations in linkage disequilibrium with B14; the second is present in the Malay population, showing no linkage disequilibrium with B14 [3, 6]. At the Seventh Workshop a split of Aw33 was suggested: Aw33.1 (in linkage disequilibrium with B14.2 antigen) and Aw33.2 (in linkage disequilibrium with B44 and cross-reacting with A28 [2, 4]). At the Eight Workshop Aw33 was well defined and the pattern of reaction of sera did not show any splitting of the antigen.

Serology

The antigen Aw33 is well defined by the Ninth Workshop antisera 9w141, 9w143, 9w062, 9w149, and 9w150, of which 9w141 and 9w143 seem to be the best; they have only occasional extra reactions. Sera 9w149 and 9w150 recognize almost all Aw33 cells but are also positive with A10 and Aw19 cells. Note, however, that 9w149 does not react with A30. Serum 9w062 is very strongly positive with some Aw19-positive cells (Table 1).

Split

Indications for an Aw33 split were shown in the Ninth Histocompatibility Workshop Newsletters [1, 5, 7]. From the general pattern analysis of the segregating families, two sera, 9w142 and 9w147, identify a part of Aw33 that corresponds to the old split designated Aw33.1. The cells that are negative with these sera but positive for antigen Aw33 are designated Aw33.2. Of fourteen informative families, Aw33.1 segregates with Bw65 (14.2) in three and with Bw52 in one family; Aw33.2 segregates with Bw58 in five families and with B44 in five.

Table 1. Properties of 9w141, 9w143, 9w150, 9w062, and 9w149

9w no.	Serum strength (% scores 8)	Q score	% Pos. Aw33	Tail	Other specificities
141	47	7.2	89	39	
143	34	5.4	77	39	
150	84	5.3	97	85	A10, Aw19
062	85	4.6	93	92	A3, A11, (Aw19)
149	84	4.7	92	86	A10, Aw 19, (A30 neg.)

Table 2. Properties of 9w142 and 9w147

9w no.	Serum strength (% scores 8)	Q score	% Pos. Aw33	Tail	Other specificities
142	49	1.5	29	42	
147	37	1.8	31	92	A10

Histocompatibility Testing 1984
Edited by E. D. Albert et al.

The properties of the two sera, 9w142 and 9w147, as judged by Q scores are summarized in Table 2.

Conclusions

Aw33 antigen was well defined by the Ninth Workshop antisera. Two antisera, 9w142 and 9w147, give evidence for a split that corresponds to the old Aw33.1.

References

1. Chandanayingyong D (1984) Further split of antigen Malay. Ninth Histocompatibility Workshop Newsletter 3, p 18
2. Dick HM (1977) HLA-A, B and C serology and antigen reports. In: Bodmer WF, et al (eds) Histocompatibility testing 1977. Munksgaard, Copenhagen, p 163
3. Ferrara GB, Tosi RM, Azzolina G, Carminati C (1973) A new antigen at the LA locus positively associated with the W14 (Maki) specificity of the four locus. Tissue Antigens 3:130
4. France OT (1977) Regional reports I and II. In: Bodmer WF, et al (eds) Histocompatibility testing 1977. Munksgaard, Copenhagen, p 441
5. Hammond MG (1984) The HLA-A10 and Aw19 complex in South African Indians and Negroes. Ninth Histocompatibility Workshop Newsletter 7, p 6
6. Joysey VC, Roger JH, Abbas A, Bland C, et al (1972) Study of Malay population. In: Dausset J, Colombani J (eds) Histocompatibility testing 1972. Munksgaard, Copenhagen, p 251
7. Mesman B, de Lange GG, Engelfriet CP, de Waal LP (1984) HLA-Aw33 subtypes. Ninth Histocompatibility Workshop Newsletter 7
8. Vives J (1980) Aw33 (joint report). In: Terasaki PI (ed) Histocompatibility testing 1980. UCLA Tissue Typing Laboratories, Los Angeles, p 334

Antigen Report: HLA-Aw34

A. Amoroso[1], C.P. Engelfriet[2], V. Joysey[3], G.G. de Lange[2], and L.P. de Waal[2]

1 Istituto di Genetica Medica, Università di Torino, Via Santena 19, I-10126 Torino, Italy
2 Central Laboratory of the Netherlands Red Cross Blood Transfusion Service, P.O. Box 9190, Amsterdam, The Netherlands
3 Tissue Typing Laboratory, Addenbrooke's Hospital, Cambridge, U.K.

History

During the Sixth International Histocompatibility Workshop the formerly determined "long Malay," HLA-A10.3, and F26 antigens were designated Aw34 [1]. At the Eighth Workshop Aw34 could only be defined by complex "A10-cross-reactive" sera containing Aw34 reactivity. Moreover, it appeared difficult to define Aw34 in the presence of A25 or A26 [2]. The frequency was 1.0% in Caucasoids, 12.5% in Negroes, and 1.9% in Orientals in the Eighth Workshop material.

Serology

At this Workshop Aw34 was defined by ten sera (029, 076, 078, 079, 081, 082, 147, 148, 149, and 151) reacting with Aw34-positive cells. Unfortunately, no Aw34-specific sera were available.
The sera can be grouped as follows: A25 + A26 + Aw34 sera (076, 078, 151); A25 + A26 + Aw34 + Aw43 sera (079, 081, 082); (A25) + A26 + Aw34 (+ Aw43) + Aw19 sera (147, 148, 149); A28 + Aw33 + Aw34 serum (029).

Sera 076, 077, 078, 079, 081, 082, 147, and 148 are described in the A25 and A26 antigen reports. For the remaining sera see Table 1. To establish the definition of Aw34 with Ninth Workshop sera and to distinguish Aw34 from other A10-cross-reacting

Table 1. Remaining Aw34-reactive Ninth Workshop sera

9w no.	Specificity	Q score	% 8 scores	% Misses
029	A28	6.0	86	17
	Aw33	3.0	51	41
	Aw34	6.0	73	19
149	A26	6.0	91	4
	A25	6.4	99	6
	A32	6.1	92	5
	A29	5.7	91	6
	Aw34	6.0	92	2
	Th	4.5	88	7
	A31	4.7	94	14
	Aw33	4.7	81	8
151	A26	2.4	50	49
	A25	2.9	58	33
	Aw33	1.1		
	Aw34	6.6	85	13
	Tail: A31[a]			

[a] Tail: Q score < 1

Histocompatibility Testing 1984
Edited by E. D. Albert et al.

antigens, we have investigated the reaction pattern of relevant sera with all Aw34-positive families in which the observed pattern segregated.

Twenty-four families of different races were analyzed (Table 2). One consistent reaction pattern was observed with most of the sera (Table 3). Reactions due to the presence of a second cross reacting antigen (especially Aw33 is troublesome in individual analyses) could be identified in the families. Distinction between Aw34 and A25 is possible for sera 029, 148 (positive with Aw34, negative with A25) and sera 072, 075, 085, 087 (negative with Aw34, positive with A25). Distinction from A26 and Aw66 is possible for sera 029 (positive with Aw34, negative with A26) and sera 072, 074, 075, 093, 094, 098, 099 (negative with Aw34, positive with A26).

Table 2. Ninth Workshop Aw34 and Aw66 families

	Aw34	Aw66
Caucasian	5	24
Mongoloid	7	22
Negro	9	1
Not known	3	–
Total	24	47

Finally, distinction from Aw43 is indicated by sera 029, 078, 147 (positive with Aw34, negative with Aw43), and sera 072, 074, 075, 101, 103, 104 (negative with Aw34, positive with Aw43). Thus, in the presence of A25, A26, or Aw66, Aw34 can still be distinguished by sera 029 and 148.

Comparison of the distribution of Aw34 and Aw66 suggests a remarkable difference in the races: only 1 of the 47 Aw66-positive families belonged to the Negro population, while 9 of the 24 Aw34-positive families were of Negroid origin.

Conclusion

Despite the fact that no Aw34-specific sera were available, Aw34 is rather well defined in all races studied and can be distinguished in most cases from the A10-cross-reacting antigens.

References

1. Bodmer J (1975) The ABC of HLA. In: Kissmeyer-Nielsen F (ed) Histocompatibility testing 1975. Munksgaard, Copenhagen, p 38
2. Joint report (1980) In: Terasaki PI (ed) Histocompatibility testing 1980. UCLA Tissue Typing Laboratory, Los Angeles

Table 3. Selection of Ninth Workshop sera defining Aw34, A25, A26, Aw66, and Aw43

Antigen	Ninth Workshop sera															
	029	072	074	075	076	078	081	085	087	093	094	098	099	147	148	149
Aw34	w/+	–	–	–	+	+	+	–	–	–	–	–	–	+	+	+
A25	–	+	+/–	+	+	+	+	+	+	–	–	–	+/–	+	–	+
A26	–	+	+	+	+	+	+	–	–	+/–	+	+	+	+	+	+
Aw66	–	+	+	+	+	+	+	–	–	○	○	○	○	+	+	+
Aw43	–	+	+	+	–	–	+	–	–	–	–	–	–	–	+	+
Aw33	+/–	–	–	–	–	–	–	–	–	–	–	–	–	+/–	+/–	+

○, different patterns observed (see Aw66 antigen report)
+/–, inconsistent results

Antigen Report: HLA-Aw36

H. Festenstein[1], C.B. Carpenter[2], A. Alonso[1], and E. Williams[1]

1 Department of Immunology, The London Hospital Medical College, London E1, U.K.
2 Immunogenetics Laboratory, Brigham and Women's Hospital, Boston, MA 02115, USA

HLA-Aw36 was originally defined during the Fifth International Histocompatibility Workshop and was called Mo* [1] and LT [2].

After the Sixth Workshop the WHO-IUIS Terminology Committee of HLA nomenclature officially designated this specificity Aw36.

This antigen is mainly found in Negroids. Aw36 is closely related to A1 and it is normally defined by a subset of A1 sera. At the Sixth Workshop, the A locus assignment of this antigen was confirmed by segregation patterns in a large Zambian family [4]. Although Aw36 is observed mainly in Negroids, sera with anti-Aw36 activity commonly originate from Caucasoids with no apparent Negroid ancestry. Anti-Aw36 activity is only found in anti-A1 sera and not in combination with any other single A locus specificity.

Three anti-Aw36 plus anti-A1 sera were submitted to the Ninth Workshop: 006, 007 and 009 (Table 1), with which Aw36 can be easily assigned in cells which are negative for A1.

Table 1. Anti-HLA-Aw36 sera

9W serum no.	Average score	% Reactions missed	% Extra reactions	Serum strength	Quality score
006	7.1	11	83	88	7.7
007	6.5	38	89	83	3.1
009	6.4	11	84	80	7.3

Although the majority of cells typed in this workshop as Aw36 reacted with all three anti-Aw36 sera, five cells were positive with 006 and 009 and negative with 007. However, the patterns of reactions were variable and probably do not signify a split of this specificity.

In a recent study of Nigerian cells, Aw36 was found in linkage disequilibrium with Bw53 and Cw4 [3].

References

1. Festenstein H, Adams E, Brown J, Burke J, Lincoln P, Oliver RTD, Rondiak G, Sachs JA, Welch SG, Wolf E (1973) The distribution of HL-A antigens and other polymorphisms in Bantu-speaking Negroids living in Zambia. In: Dausset J, Colombani J (eds) Histocompatibility testing 1972. Munksgaard, Copenhagen, p 359
2. Lawler SD, Klouda PT (1973) West Indian Negroes immigrant in the United Kingdom. In: Dausset J, Colombani J (eds) Histocompatibility testing 1972. Munksgaard, Copenhagen, p 415
3. Okoye R et al (1984) HLA polymorphism in the Nigerian population (submitted)
4. Wolf E, Festenstein H, Pritchard J, Watson B, Sachs J, Traub N (1975) Further HLA heterogeneity in Zambian and Caucasoids populations. In: Kissmeyer-Nielsen F (ed) Histocompatibility testing 1975. Munksgaard, Copenhagen, p 179

Antigen Report: HLA-Aw43

E.M. Campbell [1], E.D. du Toit [1], M.G. Hammond [2], and M. Oudshoorn [1]

1 Provincial Laboratory for Tissue Immunology, Private Bag 4, Observatory 7935, South Africa
2 Natal Institute of Immunology, P.O. Box 2356, Durban 4000, South Africa

History

In 1972, the occurrence of apparent triplets associated with HLA-A10 and A29 in the Khoisan populations of Namibia was reported [1]. In 1975 [6], an HLA-A10/A29 allele was defined in terms of the Fifth International Histocompatibility Workshop antisera and designated BK. The Sixth and Seventh Workshops [2, 3] provided further opportunities for studying BK. At both these workshops BK was serologically well defined with reactions involving HLA-A10, A26, and A29 antisera and was shown to segregate clearly within families. During the Eighth Workshop a monospecific HLA-Aw43 antibody was used for the first time, simplifying the assignment of this antigen [4]. Although at the time of the Eighth Workshop, HLA-Aw43 had only been found in Khoisan, Cape Colored, Xhosa, and South African Caucasoid individuals in Cape Town [4], we felt that HLA-Aw43 would eventually be detected in other Southern African groups. The assumption that Aw43 could be present in Southern African Negroes other than the Xhosa was based on the finding of Jenkins et al. [5] that there was a considerable San admixture in most Southern African Negroes.

Serology

The Ninth International Histocompatibility Workshop antisera allow good definition of the allele HLA-Aw43. No splits are apparent, and problems of identification should not arise. In our hands

Histocompatibility Testing 1984
Edited by E. D. Albert et al.

Table 1. Serum analysis in South African Negroes

9W Serum	Antigens	r	χ^2	% Missed	% Extras
072	Aw43	0.67	54	0	44
	A26	0.91	86	7	0
074	Aw43	0.65	52	0	46
	A26	0.95	96	0	0
075	Aw43	0.65	51	0	46
	A26	0.95	95	0	0
079	Aw43	0.62	47	0	50
	A26	0.87	82	0	13
081	Aw43	0.62	47	0	50
	A26	0.87	82	0	13
082	Aw43	0.61	44	0	51
	A26	0.79	66	7	20
100	Aw43	0.68	55	6	39
	A26	0.65	45	38	11
101	Aw43	0.92	102	6	0
103	A29	0.70	59	0	37
	Aw43	0.91	81	0	7
106	A29	0.69	57	0	39
	Aw43	0.87	74	0	13

9w101 is an excellent anti-Aw43 serum, with an r value of 0.92, as shown in Table 1. Four families, with 15 individuals positive for HLA-Aw43, were submitted from South Africa. The serum analysis of the ten best antisera for identifying HLA-Aw43 is shown in Table 1.

Gene Frequencies and Linkage Disequilibrium. The gene frequencies of HLA-Aw43 in various Southern African Negroid population groups ranges between 0.02 (Zulu) and 0.10 (Central!Kung) Aw43 is in linkage disequilibrium with B7, Bw70, and Cw4.

Conclusion

The antigen HLA-Aw43 was seen in South Africa during the Ninth Workshop. It was again well defined, particularly with antiserum 9w101.

References

1. Botha MC, du Toit ED, Jenkins T, van Leeuwen A, D'Amaro J, Meera Khan P, van der Steen G, van Rood JJ, van der Does J (1972) The HL-A system in Bushmen (San) and Hottentot (Khoikhoi) populations of South West Africa. In: Dausset J, Colombani J (eds) Histocompatibility testing 1972. Munksgaard, Copenhagen, p 421
2. Botha MC, Campbell E, Briggs BR, du Toit ED (1975) Further observations on BK, an African SD-1 antigen. In: Kissmeyer-Nielsen F (ed) Histocompatibility testing 1975. Munksgaard, Copenhagen, p 261
3. Dick H (1977) Joint Report. HLA-A, B and C serology and antigen reports. In: Bodmer WF, Batchelor JR, Bodmer JG, Festenstein H, Morris PJ (eds) Histocompatibility testing 1977. Munksgaard, Copenhagen, p 164
4. Du Toit ED, Briggs BR, Botha MC, Campbell EM (1980) Joint Report. HLA-Aw43. In: Terasaki P (ed) Histocompatibility testing 1980. UCLA Tissue Typing Laboratory, Los Angeles, p 344
5. Jenkins T, Zoutendyk A, Steinberg AC (1970) Gammaglobulin Groups (Gm and Inv) of various Southern African Populations. Am J Phys Anthropol 32:197–218
6. Nurse GT, Bodmer JG, Bodmer WF, van Leeuwen A, van Rood JJ, du Toit ED, Botha MC (1975) A reassessment of HL-A system in Khoisan populations in South West Africa. Tissue Antigens 5:402

Antigen Report: HLA-Aw66

L.P. de Waal [1], G.G. de Lange [1], V. Joysey [2], C.P. Engelfriet [1], and A. Amoroso [3]

1 Central Laboratory of the Netherlands Red Cross Blood Transfusion Service, P.O. Box 9190, Amsterdam, The Netherlands
2 Tissue Typing Laboratory, Addenbrooke's Hospital, Cambridge, U.K.
3 Istituto di Genetica Medica, Università di Torino, Via Santena 19, 10126 Italy

History

During the Eighth International Histocompatibility Workshop [3] it was agreed that HLA-A25, A26, and Aw34 were well defined, without evidence for further splits.

Recently, however, a new HLA-A antigen, called LN (= Aw66), was described, which is closely related to A25, A26, and Aw34 [4]. The definition of Aw66 was based on the reaction pattern of "monospecific" A25 and A26 sera and more complex "A10 cross-reacting" sera containing Aw66 reactivity and on segregation in families. Especially important for defining Aw66 were sera reacting with both A11 and Aw66. Linkage disequilibrium of Aw66 with Bw41 was observed [4].

Histocompatibility Testing 1984
Edited by E. D. Albert et al.

Table 1. Selection of Ninth Workshop sera defining A25, A26, Aw34, and Aw66 accommodated from Ninth Workshop newsletters

Antigen	Ninth Workshop sera																
	072	075	077	078	079	081	085	087	095	147	148	149	093	094	098	099	
A25	+	+	+	+	+	+	+	+	–	+	–	+/–	+/–	+/–	+/–	+/–	
A26	+	+	+	+	+	+	–	–	+	+	+	+/–	+	+	+	+	
Aw34	–	–	+/–	+	+/–	+	–	–	+/–	+	+	+	–	–	–	–	
Aw66	+	+	+	+	+	+	–	–	+	+	+	+	–	–	+	w	[5]
	+	+	+	+	+	+	–	–	+	+	+	+	+	w	–	–	[2]
	+	+	+	+	+	+	–	–	+	+	+	+	–	–	–	–	[1, 6]

+/–, inconsistent reaction; w, weak reaction

Table 2. Selection of four Ninth Workshop sera used to define Aw66

9w	Specificity	Q score	% 8 scores	% Misses
093	A26	2.9	47	50
	Tail: A28, A29			
094	A26	7.9	65	17
	Tail: A25, A1, A29			
098	A26	5.5	54	35
	Aw43	3.7	0	62
099	A26	6.9	56	31
	A25	1.6	35	78
	Aw43	3.1	0	56

Tail: Q score < 1

Table 3. Reaction pattern of selected Ninth Workshop sera tested against "A26/Aw66"-positive Workshop families

Pattern	Ninth Workshop sera					Family number ($n=47$)[a]		
	093	094	095	098	099	C	M	N
1	–/+	–/+	+	–	–	13	16	0
2	–	–/+	+	+/w	+/w	5	3	1
3	–	–/w	+	+/w	–	3	1	0
4	+	+/w	+	–	–	2	0	0
5	–	+	+	+/w	–	0	2	0
6	–	w	+	–	w	1	0	0

[a] C, Caucasian families; M, Mongoloid families; N, Negro families; w, weak reaction

Serology

Table 1 lists a summary of the reaction patterns of Ninth Workshop sera with Aw66-positive cells, as described in the Workshop Newsletters [1, 2, 5, 6]. All sera except the last four (093, 094, 098, 099) are described in the A25, A26, or Aw34 antigen reports (Table 2). On the basis of these selected sera, Aw66 can be distinguished from A25 by sera 095 and 148 (positive with Aw66, negative with A25) and sera 085 and 087 (negative with Aw66, positive with A25). Aw66 can also be distinguished from Aw34 by sera 072 and 075 (positive with Aw66, negative with Aw34). However, it is very difficult to distinguish Aw66 from A26. Nevertheless, sera 093, 094, 098, and 099 seem to distinguish between these two antigens.

Table 1 shows that on the basis of Ninth Workshop Newsletter data three distinct Aw66 patterns were observed.

Therefore we selected the Aw66 families on the basis of nonreactivity with two or more of the following sera: 093, 094, 098, 099. Forty-seven families in which the observed patterns segregated were investigated. The results in Table 3 suggest two major patterns. The more frequent pattern was characterized by negative reactions of sera 098 and 099. This pattern was found in 13 Caucasian families and 16 Mongoloid (mostly Japanese) families.

Table 4. Q scores of sera involved in the definition of antigens of the A10-cross-reactive group

9w	A25	A26	Aw34	Aw66	Other specificities
029			6.0		A28
071	4.9	5.1		0.9	A3, A29
072	9.2	8.8		4.5	Aw43
074	4.0	8.1	< 1	3.4	Aw43
075	10.0	13.0		6.4	Aw43, A3
076	7.7	7.6	7.8	4.6	
077	9.6	11.0	4.6	4.6	Aw34, Aw43

Table 4 (continued)

9w	A25	A26	Aw34	Aw66	Other specificities
078	7.6	9.2	9.0	4.3	
079	8.5	11.0	7.5	5.9	Aw43
081	10.0	12.0	10.0	7.8	Aw43
082	4.3	5.7	4.7	3.7	Aw43
083		< 1	3.3		
084	< 1	< 1	3.6	1.2	
085	9.1	< 1			
086	7.3			< 1	
087	7.5	< 1		1.3	A1
090	7.0	< 1		1.2	
091	9.5	4.0		1.8	
093		2.9			A28, A29
094	< 1	7.9			A1, A29
095	< 1	12.0	2.8	3.3	Aw43
098		5.5			Aw43
099	1.6	6.9			Aw43
112	6.4			< 1	A32, A24
114	8.7			1.3	A32
117	5.5				A32
141	< 1		1.7		A29, A31, A32, Aw33
143	< 1	< 1	3.6	1.5	A29, Aw33
144		1.4	3.6		Aw33
146			2.2		Aw33
147	9.8	11.0	7.8	5.6	A28, A32, Aw33, Aw43
148	< 1	8.5	5.1	3.9	A29, Aw33, Aw43
149	6.4	6.0	6.0	4.1	A29, A31, A32, Aw33, Th
150	5.6	5.1	5.1	2.5	A29, A30, A31, A32, Aw33, Aw43, Th
151	2.9	2.4	6.6	1.1	A31, Aw33, Th

Table 5. Q scores of sera involved in the discrimination of antigens Aw33 and Aw34

9w	Aw33	Aw34	Serum defined specificities
029	3.0		A28, Aw33, Aw34
032	2.1		A2, A28, Aw33
062	4.6		A3, A11, A29, A30, A31, Aw33, Aw34
063	< 1		A1, A3, A11, A31, Aw33
076		7.8	A25, A26, Aw34, Bw70
077		4.6	A25, A26, Aw34, Aw43, Bw70
078		9.0	A25, A26, Aw34, Bw70
079		7.5	A25, A26, Aw34, Aw43, Bw70
081		10.0	A25, A26, Aw34, Aw43, Bw70
082		4.7	A25, A26, Aw34, Aw43, Bw70
083		3.3	A26, Aw34
084		3.6	A25, A26, Aw34, Bw70
095		2.8	A25, A26, Aw34, Aw43, Bw70
135	< 1		A31, Aw33
140	5.5		A30, A31, Aw33
141	7.2	1.7	A25, A29, A31, A32, Aw33, Aw34
142	1.5		A3, A28, Aw33
143	5.4	3.6	A25, A26, A29, Aw33, Aw34, Bw70
144	2.7	3.6	A26, Aw33, Aw34
146	4.2	2.2	Aw33, Aw34
147	1.8	7.8	A25, A26, A28, A32, Aw33, Aw34, Aw43, Bw70
148	3.8	5.1	A25, A26, A29, Aw33, Aw34, Aw43, Bw70
149	4.7	6.0	A25, A26, A29, A31, A32, Aw33, Aw34, Bw70, Bw71
150	5.3	5.1	A25, A26, A29, A30, A31, Aw33, Aw34, Aw43, Bw70, Bw71
151	1.1	6.6	A25, A26, A31, Aw33, Aw34, Bw70, Bw71

The second pattern was characterized by positive reactions of sera 098 and 099 and negative reactions with 093 and 094. This pattern was found in 5 Caucasian and 3 Japanese families and 1 Negro family. Cells originally described [4] as Aw66 positive followed this second pattern. The other patterns in Table 3 were less frequent.

Thus, the possibility arises that besides Aw66 another subtype of the A10 cross-reacting group exists. However, for the definition of Aw66 and the distinction from A26 other sera are required. Unfortunately, no such sera (analogous to the anti-A11 and -Aw66 sera, as originally described [4]) were submitted to the Workshop.

Conclusion

Aw66 cannot be clearly defined by the Workshop sera (Tables 4, 5). It is especially difficult to distinguish it from A26. Family analysis suggests further heterogeneity of A26.

References

1. Gebuhrer L, Primard Y, Lalouse MP, Bétuel H (to be published) Recognition of antigen LN (locus A) in an informative family. Ninth International Histocompatibility Workshop Newsletter no. 3
2. Hammond MG (to be published) The HLA-A10 and Aw19 complex in South African Indians and Negroes. Ninth International Histocompatibility Workshop Newsletter no. 7
3. Joint report (1980) In: Terasaki PI (ed) Histocompatibility testing 1980. UCLA Tissue Typing Laboratory, Los Angeles
4. Mesman B, Lange GG, de Engelfriet CP (1983) A new HLA antigen, called LN, closely related to A25, A26 and Aw34. Tissue Antigens 21:192
5. Mesman B, Lange GG, de Engelfriet CP, Waal LP de (to be published) Definition of LN with 9th Workshop antisera. Ninth International Histocompatibility Workshop Newsletter no. 7
6. Moreno ME, Kreisler JM (to be published) Definition of antigen LN with Ninth Workshop sera in two informative families. Ninth International Histocompatibility Workshop Newsletter no. 5

Antigen Report: Th

T. Barbalho[1] and C. Raffoux[2]

1 HEMOPE (Centro de Hematologia e Hemoterapia de Pernambuco), Rua Joaquin Nabuco 171, 50 000 Recife, Brazil
2 INSERM U 93, Paris, France

The antigen Th is a specificity that was proposed by Wolf et al. [5] at the Eighth International Workshop as a Negro variant of A32. Since 1975, in Zambian Negroes, she had found concordant reactions with serum Li (5w69): A10 + A29 + A30 + A31 + A32 + Aw33 + Aw34 + Aw43 and serum Thompson (5w70): A31 + weak A32; and negative reactions with all Seventh Workshop Aw19 sera. Testing 6 Th-positive negroid cells against the Eighth Workshop sera, she found strong reactions only with serum 8w526 (A30, A31, Aw33; weak A29 and Aw34), which did not contain A32 antibodies. None of the other Aw19 and A10 sera gave any reaction with these cells. During the present Workshop, C. Dehay et al. [3] have described a Th-like antigen with the sera 9w148, 149, and 150 plus local sera against cells carrying Th-like or A32 specificities.

Serology

Five sera, 9w062, 104, 148, 149, and 150, defined the Th specificity, but only the last two gave strong reactions. Th has been found at this Workshop only in Negroid populations. There were 27 Negroid cells, which reacted strongly with sera 9w149 and 9w150.

Discussion

Th is different from the antigen Aw66 described by Mesman et al. [4] (Table 1), as Th cells do not react with A10 and A10 + 34 sera. Th is perhaps identical with the 19 BAC reported by Campbell et al. [1], since Th cells gave weakly positive reactions with serum 9W104. Th is probably different from the "Aw19 short" described by Chiewslip [2] because Th gave negative reactions with sera 9W029, 9W032, and 9W141.

Conclusions

Th has so far been defined only in Negroid populations. At this Workshop it has been identified by sera which also contain other specificities of the

Histocompatibility Testing 1984
Edited by E. D. Albert et al.

Table 1. Pattern of Th, A10, and Aw19 complex in Negroids

	A10	A10 + Aw34	Aw34	Aw19 + Aw66	A32	Aw19
	9 9 9 9	9 9 9 9 9 9	9 9	9 9 9 9 9	9 9 9 9	9 9 9 9 9
	w w w w	w w w w w w	w w	w w w w w	w w w w	w w w w w
	0 0 0 0	0 0 0 0 0 0	0 0	1 1 1 1 1	1 1 1 1	1 0 0 0 1
	7 7 7 7	7 7 7 7 8 8	8 8	4 4 4 5 5	1 1 1 3	0 6 2 3 4
	1 2 4 5	6 7 8 9 1 2	3 4	7 8 9 0 1	1 2 3 0	4 2 9 2 1
A10	+ + + +	+ + + + + +	– –	+ + + + +	– – – –	– – – – –
A32	– – – –	– – – – – –	– –	w w + + –	+ + + +	– – – – –
Aw66	+ + + +	+ + + + + +	– –	– – + + –	– – – –	– – – – –
Th	– – – –	– – – – – –	– –	– w + + –	– – – –	w w – – –

Aw19 complex. Although all the Th antisera also contained A32, we cannot conclude that Th is a variant or is included in A32.

References

1. Campbell EM, Taljaard DG, du Toit ED (to be published) 19 BAC; A possible new negroid HLA-A locus specificity. Ninth International Histocompatibility Workshop Newsletter no. 5:8
2. Chiewsilp P, Sujirachato K (1983) New Short Aw19. Ninth Workshop Newsletter 2:5–6
3. Dehay C, Raffoux C et al (1984) Th-like, a variant of Aw32 in Negroid populations. Ninth International Histocompatibility Workshop Newsletter no. 8:1–3
4. Mesman B, de Lange GG, Engelfriet CP (1983) A new HLA-antigen called L.N., closely related to A25, A26 and Aw34. Tissue Antigens 21:192–197
5. Wolf E, Prichard J, Watson B, Festenstein H (1980) Characterization of a new negroid A locus specificity Th. In: Terasaki PI (ed) Histocompatibility testing 1980. Munksgaard, Copenhagen, p 744

Antigen Report: HLA-B7

M. Kreisler and M.E. Moreno

Servicio de Inmunologia, Clinica Puerta de Hierro, Madrid, Spain

Since HLA-B7 can be considered as a "classical" specificity, we shall omit any introduction or general data [for review see 1].

At the Ninth Workshop, B7 has been well defined by several sera. Serological patterns did not show any possible splits. Of the 41 sera reacting with B7-positive cells, only 7 sera had a quality score > 5; 79% of 137 positive cells reacted with six of these. Sera 9w207, 9w203 and 9w205 were "monospecific," whereas sera 9w246, 9w245, 9w247, and 9w239 were highly efficient in defining B7 only in certain phenotypes since they had positive reactions with other B7 cross-reactive antigens (B7 CREG) [2].

The most frequent serological patterns of reaction for B7 cells are shown in Table 1. Caucasians had a

Table 1. Serological patterns

Type of cells	%	w207	w205	w203	w246	w247	w245	w239
In 172 Caucasian	63.4	+	+	+	+	+	+	+
B7 + 27 – w22-cells	5.8	+	+	–	+	+	+	+
	5.2	+	+	+	+	+	+	–
	4.7	+	–	+	+	+	+	+
	3.5	+	–	–	+	+	+	+
In 102 Negro	86.9	+	+	+	+	+	+	+
B7 + 27 – w22-cells								

Table 2. Serological features of seven sera defining B7

Serum	Origin	Q Score	Extra reactions	% Strength	Observations
w207	Richter	8.9	Bw73, 27	82	3% Extra reactions
w246	Richter	8.8	B27, w22, w73, w60, w42	92	41% Extra reactions
w205	Ferrara	8.4	Bw60, w73	60	6% Extra reactions 10% B7 Misses
w203	Paris	7.8	–	67	11% B7 Misses
w247	Richter	8.0	B27, w22, w73	92	47% Extra reactions
w245	Mayr	7.9	B27, w22, w48, w60	87	48% Extra reactions
w239	Amsterdam	6.2	Bw55, w42	78	13% Extra reactions

more heterogeneous pattern than Negroes. The most characteristic features for each individual serum are given in Table 2. In conclusion, B7 has been confirmed as a well-defined specificity during the Ninth International Workshop.

References

1. Nyulassy S, Hirschova V, Buc M, Kreisler M (1980) HLA-B7. In: Terasaki PI (ed) Histocompatibility testing. UCLA Tissue Typing Laboratory, Los Angeles, pp 353–355
2. Darke C (1983) A reanalysis of the HLA-B7 cross-reactive group. Tissue Antigens 22:326–334

Antigen Report: HLA-B8

M.M. Tongio, Y. Mitsuishi, G. Hauptmann, and S. Mayer

Institut d'Hématologie, Centre de Transfusion Sanguine, 10, rue Spielmann, 67085 Strasbourg Cedex, France

History

The HLA-B8 antigen has been known since 1965 and its characteristics were summarized in 1980 [4]. Of all the class I antigens studied by Vasilov et al. [8] it has the most acidic isoelectric point. Healthy individuals carrying HLA-B8 (but not all of them) have particular features not found in non-B8 individuals. These concern the decrease of some peripheral blood cell subsets (lymphocytes or monocytes [3, 5]); their IgG secretion when stimulated with PWM [9]; and their response in vitro when cultured with PHA, or Con A [5], with allogeneic or autologous cells [7] or with wheat antigen [2]. However, these features are probably not due to the presence of HLA-B8 itself, but rather to a gene or a set of genes in linkage disequilibrium with HLA-B8 [3, 5].

Serology

The Workshop antisera made it possible to define HLA-B8 very clearly.
Of the three sera described as "monospecific" anti-B8 (9w248, 9w249, 9w250), the best were 9w248 (average grade 7.9; quality score 11.0) and 9w250 (average grade 7.6; quality score 9.6). Serum 9w249 was weak and showed false-negative reactions. None of these sera contained extra antibodies except for 9w248, which reacted with a few B7 cells.
Of the three sera described as anti-B8 + Bw59 (9w253, 9w255, 9w259) 9w255 was the best, despite some extra reactions attributed to Aw32 in the Workshop analysis and to B14 in the French analysis. Serum 9w259 had many extra reactions (mostly HLA-A1), and 9w253 did not contain B8 antibodies.
Finally, the serum 9w240 described as anti-Bw46 + B8 defined the B8 specificity very well and the Bw46 specificity less well.
Other sera not indicated as such were found to contain anti-HLA-B8 antibodies; (a) Anti-DR sera 9w529, 9w574, and 9w694, which proved once more that platelet absorption cannot easily remove HLA-B8 antibodies; (b) a few other sera, which showed some anti-B8 extra reactions in addition to their given specificities (anti-B18, B14, Bw59, Cw7).

Linkage Disequilibrium

HLA-B8 is in very strong linkage disequilibrium with the following antigens in class I, A1, Cw7; in

Histocompatibility Testing 1984
Edited by E. D. Albert et al.

class II, DR3, and DPw1 [6]; in class III, complotype SCO1 [1]; and probably with GLO2 and the t allele of the T/t-like complex [1], as well as the gene or genes mentioned in the history section.

References

1. Awdeh ZL, et al (1983) Extended HLA/complement allele haplotypes: Evidence for T/t-like complex in man. Proc Natl Acad Sci USA 80:259–263
2. Cunningham-Rundles S, et al (1978) Response to wheat antigen in in vitro lymphocyte transformation among HLA-B8-positive normal donors. Transplant Proc 10:977–979
3. Lawley TJ, et al (1981) Defective Fc-receptor functions associated with the HLA-B8/DRw3 haplotype. Studies in patients with dermatitis herpetiformis and normal subjects. N Engl J Med 304:185–192
4. Mayer S, Tongio MM (1980) B8 report. In: Terasaki PI (ed) Histocompatibility testing 1980. Munksgaard, Copenhagen, pp 358–360
5. McCombs CC, Michalski JP (1982) Lymphocyte abnormality associated with HLA-B8 in healthy young adults. J Exp Med 156:936–941
6. Shaw S, et al (1981) Population studies of the HLA-linked SB antigens. Immunogenetics 14:153–162
7. Singal DP, Fagnilli L (1982) Proliferation of alloantigen sensitized human peripheral blood lymphocytes by autologous cells associated with the HLA-B8/DR3. Clin Exp Immunol 49:652–656
8. Vasilov RG, et al (1983) Analysis of human class I antigens by two-dimensional gel electrophoresis. Immunogenetics 17:333–356
9. Vuento R, et al (1983) Increased immunoglobulin production in vitro in healthy HLA-B8 positive persons. Scand J Immunol 18:551–555

Antigen Report: HLA-B13

W.B. Bias [1], C. Rohowsky-Kochan [2], E. Reed [2], and N. Suciu-Foca [2]

1 Dept. of Medicine, Johns Hopkins University School of Medicine, 720 Rutland Avenue, Baltimore, MD 21205, USA
2 Dept. of Pathology, Columbia College of Physicians and Surgeons, New York, NY, USA

HLA-B13 is unambiguously defined by sera submitted to the Ninth International Histocompatibility Workshop.

Table 1 shows (a) the internal correlation between sera that had no antibodies to B locus antigens other than B13; (b) the correlation between sera with antibodies against B13, Bw60 and Bw61; and (c) the correlation between three murine monoclonal antibodies detecting this specificity. This analysis was performed on a restricted panel of Caucasian cells.

Table 2 summarizes the data derived by tail analysis of these sera for the complete Workshop material. Reactions that were scored 1 or 2 were considered negative, while scores of 4, 6, and 8 were considered positive.

The average serum score and strength, as estimated from the Workshop analysis of the results obtained on the Caucasian panel, is shown in Table 3.

In conclusion, HLA-B13 is a well-defined specificity on the international panel of cells.

Table 1. Internal correlations

B13 Antisera					
138	99				
346	58	99			
348	69	86	99		
352	69	86	99	99	
350	69	86	99	99	99
	138	346	348	352	350
B13 + Bw60 + Bw61 Antisera					
356	99				
372	93	99			
373	93	99	99		
374	93	99	99	99	
376	82	88	88	88	99
	356	372	373	374	376
B13 Monoclonal					
1134	99				
1153	86	99			
1158	81	70	99		
	1134	1153	1158		

Table 2. Analysis of the correlation between serum reactivity and antigenic specificity of the sera

Ninth Workshop no.	HLA Specificity	+ +	+ −	− +	− −	*r* value
346	B13	305	36	6	5207	0.9326
348	B13	303	25	7	5237	0.9472
352	B13	296	29	25	5261	0.9113
350	B13	299	44	12	5233	0.9102
138	A30	347	165	15	4567	0.7893
	B13	281	291	30	4999	0.6417
	A31	50	165	308	4567	0.1332
356	Bw60	473	101	17	3632	0.8768
	Bw61	674	101	96	3632	0.8460
	B13	163	101	115	3632	0.8728
	Bw47	12	101	16	3632	0.2021
357	Bw60	439	75	64	3925	0.8459
	Bw61	327	75	46	3925	0.8294
	B13	97	75	182	3925	0.4134
	Bw47	7	75	21	3925	0.1360
372	B13	311	138	2	3853	0.8147
	Bw60	445	138	32	3853	0.8235
	Bw61	340	138	26	3853	0.8563
	Bw47	23	138	5	3853	0.3337
373	Bw60	473	96	21	3715	0.8773
	Bw61	371	96	5	3715	0.8732
	B13	267	96	9	3715	0.8311
	Bw47	26	96	2	3715	0.4382
	Bw48	17	96	18	3715	0.2589
374	Bw60	438	62	35	3850	0.8883
	Bw61	350	62	7	3850	0.9042
	B13	258	62	3	3850	0.8851
	Bw47	26	62	1	3850	0.5287
376	Bw60	465	146	38	3759	0.8162
	Bw61	369	146	5	3759	0.8239
	B13	273	146	8	3759	0.7788
	Bw47	27	146	1	3759	0.3800
	Bw41	37	146	62	3759	0.2500

Table 3. Analysis of Ninth Workshop anti-B13 sera in the Caucasian population

Serum serial no.	Ninth Workshop no.	Specificity from 2×2	Average serum score	% Misses	% Extra	Serum strength	Absolute no. of extras
254	346	B13	7.7	2	8	81	15
255	348	B13	7.9	3	9	88	18
256	352	B13	7.5	9	12	70	21
381	350	B13	7.9	3	10	87	20
94	138	A30	7.7	4	38	79	111
		B13	7.5	14	36	65	143
		A31	6.6	82	90	90	263
259	356	Bw60	7.9	2	43	73	177
		Bw61	6.4	25	83	73	331
		B40	7.6	8	28	74	135
		B13	6.5	49	40	47	55
260	357	B40	7.5	8	18	72	80
		B13	6.2	74	49	49	40
270	372	B13	8.0	0	73	84	471
		Bw60	7.8	2	58	85	333
		Bw61	7.6	10	85	85	475
		Bw47	7.9	12	95	84	572
271	373	B40	7.9	2	37	88	219
		B13	7.6	4	30	76	68
		B47	7.7	6	94	88	507
272	374	B40	7.9	2	36	93	205
		B13	7.7	1	24	85	50
		Bw47	7.9	3	94	93	495
273	376	B40	7.9	2	45	84	303
		B13	7.9	1	47	70	143
		Bw47	7.9	3	95	84	593

Antigen Report: HLA-B14: Definite Splitting into Bw64 (14.1) and Bw65 (14.2)

G. Mueller-Eckhardt[1], C. Darke[2], R. Fauchet[3], and P. J. Dewar[4]

1 Institute of Clinical Immunology and Blood Transfusion, Justus Liebig University, Langhansstr. 7, 6300 Giessen, Federal Republic of Germany
2 Tissue Typing Laboratory, Welsh Regional Blood Transfusion Centre, Cardiff, Wales, U.K.
3 Tissue Typing Laboratory, Regional Blood Bank, Rennes, France
4 Tissue Typing Laboratory, National Blood Transfusion Service, Newcastle upon Tyne, U.K.

History

The earliest report concerning the partition of the previously well defined HLA-B14 antigen came from Dewar et al. [4], who also introduced the first 14.1 antiserum, 7w392 (= 9w261), to the Seventh International Workshop. A few sera defining the 14.2 subtype only were included in the Eighth Workshop, but their serological analysis yielded inconclusive results [5, 7]. However, considerable support for the splitting of B14 has come from absorption/elution studies [1, 8] and, in particular, from linkage disequilibrium analyses with alleles of the HLA-A and DR loci [1–4, 10], with Bf [2] and, more recently, with C4 allotypes [11].

Serology

A pattern analysis of 108 unrelated B14 individuals (77 Caucasian, 31 Negro) is shown in Table 1. It appears that the split designation is based mainly on the positive (= Bw64) or negative (= Bw65) reactions of sera 9w260 and/or 9w261, while the sera defining Bw65 all show some false-positive and/or -negative reactions. However, the subtype of the majority of B14 cells can be clearly defined by the sera of the Ninth Workshop. Only a few B14-positive cells typed as Bw64 and Bw65 negative. Whether this pattern accounts for a weak Bw64 or Bw65, respectively, or another subtype of B14, remains unclear.

Table 2 shows the segregation of serum reactions in 14 families.

Linkage Disequilibrium

Since 1977, several investigators have reported strong linkage disequilibrium between Bw64, A32, and DR7 on the one hand, and Bw65, Aw33, and DR1 on the other [1–4, 10]. A significant association of Bw65 with HLA-A3, A28, A30, and BfF was observed in a large population in Wales [1, 2], but not among German and Austrian individuals [10, 11]. In a recent report C4 allotyping revealed the strongest associations with B14 subtypes observed so far, i.e., C4A3 with Bw64 and C4A2,B2 with Bw65 [11]. Distinct complotypes were also shown to be characteristic for Bw64 (BfS, C2C, C4A3B1) and Bw65 (BfS, C2C, C4A2B2 or BfF, C2C, C4A3B1). This observation was clearly confirmed in Ninth Workshop families. In 10 of 13 families Bw64 segregated with the S31 complotype, whereas among 22 families of the Bw65 subgroup S22 was found in 9 and F31 in 8 cases. Both B14

Table 1. Pattern analysis in 108 B14-positive Ninth Workshop cells

Absolute no.	%	9w Serum no. and specificity							Definition of subtype
		B14		Bw64		Bw65			
		270	272	261	260	262	263	264	
6	5.6	+	+	+	+	–	–	–	
6	5.6	+	+	+	–	–	–	–	
5	4.6	+	+	+	+	–	–	+	
3	2.8	+	+	+	+	–	+	–	Bw64
3	2.8	+	+	+	+	–	+	+	
1	0.9	+	+	–	+	–	–	–	
7	6.5	+	+	–	–	–	–	–	?
42	38.9	+	+	–	–	+	+	+	
7	6.5	+	+	–	–	+	–	–	Bw65
4	3.7	+	+	–	–	+	–	+	
2	1.9	+	+	–	–	–	+	+	
5	4.6	+	+	+	+	+	+	+	Bw64 + Bw65

Histocompatibility Testing 1984
Edited by E. D. Albert et al.
Springer-Verlag Berlin Heidelberg 1984

Table 2. Segregration pattern in B14-positive family members

9WS Family no.	family member	9w Serum 260	261	262	263	264	267	270	272	275	Assigned specificity
GER MUE 03	M	6	8	1	1	6	4	8	8	8	Bw64
	C3	6	8	1	4	1	1	6	8	8	(14.1)
GER MUE 02	M	1	8	1	1	1	6	6	8	8	
	C1	6	8	1	4	1	8	8	8	4	
	C2	1	6	1	1	1	0	8	8	1	
UK I DRK 14	M	6	8	1	2	2	8	8	8	8	
	C1	6	8	2	2	1	8	8	8	8	
ANZ DAW 11	M	6	8	1	1	1	8	8	8	8	
	C1	8	8	2	2	4	8	8	8	8	
	C2	1	8	1	1	1	8	8	8	8	
ANZ ROB 02	F	6	6	1	2	0	8	8	8	8	
	C1	8	1	1	1	0	8	8	8	8	
	C3	6	4	1	1	0	8	8	8	8	
	C4	6	6	1	1	0	8	8	8	8	
UK I AMO 05	M	2	8	4	1	1	8	8	8	8	
	C2	8	8	8	1	4	8	8	8	8	
FRA FAU 16	F	6	8	1	1	1	8	8	8	8	
	C1	6	8	1	1	1	8	8	8	8	
BEN ENG 01	F	1	1	8	8	8	8	8	8	8	Bw65
	C2	1	1	8	8	8	8	8	8	8	(14.2)
	C3	1	1	8	8	8	8	8	8	8	
US8 RUB 06	F	1	1	8	8	8	8	8	8	8	
	M	1	1	8	8	8	8	8	8	8	
	05	1	1	8	8	8	8	8	8	8	
	06	2	2	8	8	8	8	8	8	8	
IT2 GAN 03	F	1	1	8	8	8	8	8	8	8	
	C1	1	1	8	8	8	8	8	8	8	
	C4	1	2	8	8	8	8	8	8	8	
IT2 GAN 05	F	1	1	8	8	8	8	8	8	8	
	C1	1	1	8	8	8	8	8	8	8	
	C2	1	1	8	8	8	8	8	8	8	
	C6	1	1	8	8	8	8	8	8	8	
IT2 GAN 13	F	1	2	8	8	8	8	8	8	8	
	C1	1	1	8	8	8	8	8	8	8	
	C2	1	1	8	8	8	8	8	8	8	
	C3	1	1	8	8	8	8	8	8	8	
ANZ SER 04	F	1	1	8	8	8	8	8	8	8	
	M	1	1	8	8	8	8	8	8	8	
	C2	1	1	8	8	8	8	8	8	8	
FRA DAU 27	M	1	1	6	8	8	8	8	8	8	
	C1	1	1	4	8	8	8	8	8	8	
	C2	1	1	8	8	8	8	8	8	8	
	C3	1	1	8	8	8	8	8	8	8	

subspecificities are Bw6 positive. Cw8 appears to be equally associated with the Bw64 and the Bw65 subtype [10].

Special B14 Study

A special study was undertaken by three laboratories (MUE, DRK, DEW) to broaden the overall experience with B14 splits during the Ninth Workshop. With the generous support of many other laboratories (ALB, BAC, BAS, BRA, DAU, FER, FOT, GRU, JER, MIT, MYR, SUD, SUF, TER, YUN), a special B14 tray (card 18) was created which included (a) all the B14 sera selected for the Workshop; (b) sera showing a split tendency from the prescreening results; and (c) local specific absorbates (DRK). In all, 140 unrelated B14 individuals and 20 families were investigated. The quality of Ninth Workshop B14-splitting sera and the reaction pattern of B14 cells were clearly confirmed. Two specific absorbates (9w1928, 9w1836) proved to be particularly valuable as typing reagents for Bw64 and Bw65, respectively. A total of 33 B14 cells were exchanged among the three laboratories, with excellent agreement of split designation [9].

Conclusions

The Ninth Workshop is the first to provide a selection of antisera allowing a convincing serological definition of both B14 splits, Bw64 and Bw65. Only a few B14 cells remain serologically unclassified, yielding negative reactions with split sera of both subtypes. Linkage disequilibrium with determinants of the HLA-A and DR loci as well as Bf, C4A, and C4B provide strong additional evidence for the existence of at least two B14 subdivisions, Bw64 (14.1) and Bw65 (14.2).

References

1. Darke C (1980) Further evidence for the partition of B14. Tissue Antigens 15:25–30
2. Darke C (1984) Linkage disequilibrium between HLA-B14 subdivisions and HLA-A, DR and properdin factor B alleles. Tissue Antigens 23:68–71
3. Dewar PJ (1983) HLA-B14.1 in linkage disequilibrium with HLA-DR7. Tissue Antigens 22:310–311
4. Dewar PJ, Coates E, Murray S (1977) Subdivision of the antigen HLA-B14. Tissue Antigens 10:345–347
5. Fauchet R (1980) B14 Joint Report. In: Terasaki PI (ed) Histocompatibility testing 1980. UCLA Tissue Typing Laboratory, Los Angeles, pp 366–367
6. Fauchet R, Dejour C, Jalais E, Bouhallier O (1983) Defining B14 subtypes. Ninth International Histocompatibility Workshop Newsletter 1
7. Mueller-Eckhardt C, Mueller-Eckhardt G (1980) 8w63 Joint Report. In: Terasaki PI (ed) Histocompatibility testing 1980. UCLA Tissue Typing Laboratory, Los Angeles, pp 368–369
8. Mueller-Eckhardt G, Kunert B, Mueller-Eckhardt C (1980) Further studies on HLA B14 splits. In: Terasaki PI (ed) Histocompatibility testing 1980. UCLA Tissue Typing Laboratory, Los Angeles, pp 765–766
9. Mueller-Eckhardt G, Darke C, Dewar PJ (1983a) HLA B14 cell exchange. Ninth International Histocompatibility Workshop Newsletter 5:9–11
10. Mueller-Eckhardt G, Mayr WR, Prel L, Mueller-Eckhardt C (1983b) New evidence for the existence of HLA B14 subtypes. Tissue Antigens 21:58–61
11. O'Neill GJ, Mueller-Eckhardt G, Prel L, Schendel DJ (1984) C4 allotyping distinguishes HLA-B14.1 and B14.2 subgroups. Immunogenetics 19:335–341

Antigen Report: HLA-B18

W. Braun[1], E. Gandini[2], A. Zachary[1], N. Murphy[1], S. Cappellacci[2], G. Carminati[3], and G.B. Ferrara[4]

1 Cleveland Clinic Foundation, 9500 Euclid Ave., Cleveland, Ohio 44106, USA
2 Catedra di Genetica Medica, Università La Sapienza, Roma, Italy
3 Centro Ricerche Immunoematologiche Avis, Bergamo, Italy
4 Instituto Nazionale Per La Ricerca Sul Cancro, Genova, Italy

The seven sera used to define B18 were 9w189, 190, 193, 194, 196, 197, and 198 (Table 1). Serum 9w177 was also included in the central analysis, though it was primarily reactive with B35 and B51. On the basis of the 2 x 2 analyses, the most specific sera were 196 and 198, the other five sera having extra reactions with B35, B51, B14, and Cw8, and various parts of the haplotypes A1, B8, DR3, and Cw7. DR3 reactivity was noted in sera 189 and 197.

No distinctive patterns suggestive of a split were detected in the 93 positive Caucasian or 39 positive Negroid cells (Table 2). The three most common Caucasian patterns were: (a) all eight sera positive (77%); (b) all positive except 190 (9%) and (c) all positive except 189 (4%) (Table 2). With Negroid cells also three patterns were apparent: (a) all eight sera positive (92%); (b) all positive except 177 (5%); and (c) all positive except 198 (3%). Single antiserum differences were insufficient to warrant consideration of any split, especially without any supporting family data.

Linkage disequilibrium with A25 was noted. Deficiency of C2 has been reported with the A25-B18 haplotype. A decrease in B18 frequency was found with the DRw6 split DRw13.

Table 1. Ninth Workshop sera used for the identification of B18

	Average serum score	Percent missed reactions	Percent extra reactions	Serum strength	Other specificities
9w189	7.7	4	32	69	A1, B8, DR3
190	7.4	6	11	68	B51, B35
193	7.7	4	10	80	B51
194	7.9	3	39	71	B14, Cw8
196	7.6	2	7	80	
197	7.8	2	12	83	B8, DR3, Cw7
198	7.4	7	7	75	

Table 2. Pattern analysis in 93 B18-positive Caucasians

n	Percent	9w: 177	189	190	193	194	196	197	198
72	77.4	+	+	+	+	+	+	+	+
8	8.6	+	+	–	+	+	+	+	+
4	4.3	+	–	+	+	+	+	+	+
3	3.2	+	+	+	+	+	+	–	–
2	2.2	–	+	+	+	+	+	+	+
2	2.2	+	+	–	+	+	+	+	–
2	2.2	+	+	+	–	+	+	+	+

Conclusion

The B18 specificity may be viewed either as ideal, because it has not succumbed to splitting, or as dreary, because it is too simple. At present B18 is still best described, as in previous Workshops, as a single specificity with no reliable evidence for a split.

Histocompatibility Testing 1984
Edited by E. D. Albert et al.

Antigen Report: HLA-B27

B.S. Breur and P. Ivanyi

Division of Hematology, Central Laboratory of the Netherlands Red Cross Blood Transfusion Service,
P.O. Box 9190, Amsterdam, The Netherlands

As in the previous Workshops, HLA-B27 appears to be one of the best defined antigens. Four sera are very good or excellent (Table 1) as, indicated by their quality scores based on the formula of Mickey and Terasaki. The few extra reactions of the above-mentioned sera are cross-reactions, mostly with B7. Other sera with broader reactivity confirm the existence of the B7-related CREG: B7, B27, Bw22, B40 and Bw47. However, it should be noted that the existence of excellent anti-B27 sera and the absence of data for a B27 split are in sharp contrast with other published data about subtypes of B27. Subtypes of B27 were detected by MoAb B27M2 [1] and by CTLs [2]. Further analysis of the Ninth Workshop MoAbs may possibly help to solve this problem. Indications of the possibility of identifying subtypes of B27 with conventional sera were also found (see De Waal et al., this volume).

References

1. Grumet FC, et al (1982) Subtypes of HLA-B27 defined by monoclonal antibody. Hum Immunol 5:61–72
2. Breuning MH, et al (1982) Subtypes of HLA-B27 detected by cytotoxic T lymphocytes and their role in self recognition. Hum Immunol 5:259–268

Table 1. Qualities of four anti-B27 monospecific typing sera (conventional)

Serum no.	9w210				9w215				9w211				9w209			
Population	C	N	J	CH	C	N	J	CH	C	N	J	CH	C	N	J	CH
% Misses	1	0	0	0	0	0	0	0	0	1	0	0	4	0	0	0
% Extra reaction	6	1	9	0	5	1	9	2	12	4	9	0	26	8	13	3
QS	11.0				13.0				11.0				8.7			

C, Caucasian; N, Negro; J, Japanese; CH, Chinese

Antigen Report: HLA-B35

P. Rubinstein and M. Walker

Laboratory of Immunogenetics, Lindsley F. Kimball Research Institute of the New York Blood Center,
310 East 67th Street, New York, NY, 10021, USA

B35 is part of the antigenic cluster designated "4c" by Bodmer and Payne [1]. 4c displayed a significant but not absolute positive relationship to Bw4, then called 4a. The 4c cluster has been split successively: B5 was identified as a distinct entity in the 1967 Workshop; B18, B35, and Bw53 were well recognized in 1972 [2, 3]; and even splits of B5 were suggested by the data presented at the 1972 Workshop. Further definition of B35 took place at the 1975 Workshop, especially in the report of Payne et al. [4].

Serological identification of B35 is complicated by extensive cross-reactivity with other members of the 4c group, particularly Bw53. B35 is associated with Bw6: data presented at the 1980 Workshop failed to provide any convincing examples of Bw4-associated B35 haplotypes in Caucasoids, Negroes, or Japanese. Significant linkage disequilibrium exists between B35 and Cw4, B35 and DR1, and B35 and DR5, and probably with BfF, which may be secondary to the much stronger delta associating BfF and Cw4 [5].

Histocompatibility Testing 1984
Edited by E. D. Albert et al.

Table 1. Most specific B35 sera

No. 9w	Q score Strength	% Positive with cells positive for:				
		B35	Bw53	B51	Bw62	Bw70
181	8.6/76	96	90	16	–	–
180	8.5/81	96	–	–	29	42
172	8.0/92	95	96	95	–	–
182	6.9/56	86	77	4	–	–
171	7.9/87	96	96	95	–	–
177	7.7/91	95	100	96	–	–
179	6.1/66	89	35	–	28	51
199	5.2/85	89	98	90	–	–
184	2.5/41	51	–	–	–	–

The most specific of the Ninth Workshop B35 sera, according to the central analysis, are shown in Table 1. The only serum that appears to be "monospecific" is 9w184 (the weakest of the set), which showed 16% extra reactions but missed almost half the Bw35-positive cells. Two distinct patterns of cross-reactions are apparent in these sera; (a) Bw53 and B51, and (b) Bw62 and Bw70, w71, w72 (formerly 8w59) CREG. This difference facilitates the assignment of B35.

From population frequency data, the disequilibrium of B35 in the different ethnic groups appears to be the same as that reported at the Eighth Workshop. This is particularly interesting for the inclusion of this antigen in the Bw6 group. At this Workshop, there might be four exceptions: one in family FRABET 20, where two HLA-identical sibs who typed Bw4+, Bw6– were assigned both Bw35 and Bw53 (this family belongs to the "Other Caucasoid" group); the others were an Italian family with two HLA-identical Bw6-negative sibs typing for B38, a Swiss Bw6– individual also typing for B51, and a Japanese individual with a possible but not completely clear-cut B35, who also typed for Bw61. Since these were all the possible exceptions to the inclusion of B35 in the Bw6 group of specificities in a total of over 5000 parents (sorted as "NPR with serological data"), the nature of these apparent exceptions still needs clarification.

There was one monoclonal antibody with specificity for B35: 9w1136. It reacted with cells expressing Bw62, B51, Bw52, Cw3, and A26 with relatively low χ^2. After exclusion of Bw62, B51, and Bw52, the correlation coefficient (r) for B35 was only 0.234.

References

1. Bodmer WF, Payne R (1965) Theoretical consideration of leukocyte grouping using multispecific antisera. In: Balner H, Cleton FJ, Ermisse JG (eds) Histocompatibility testing 1966. Munksgaard, Copenhagen, p 1941
2. Albert ED, Mickey MR, Terasaki P (1972) Serology and genetics of Te58 (w18) and other specificities included in the 4c complex. Tissue Antigens 1:47
3. Engelfriet CP, Veenhoven von Riesz E, Kort-Bakker M, van den Berg-Loonen PM (1972) Some studies with anti-4c, anti-R, anti-HL-A5, anti-w5, w18 and description of a new antigen of the FOUR segregant series, called H.R. In: Dausset J, Colombani J (eds) Histocompatibility testing 1973. Munksgaard, Copenhagen, p 475
4. Payne R, Amos DB, Kostyu D, et al (1978) Subdivisions of the HLA-B5 and Bw35 complex. Tissue Antigens 11:302
5. Baur MP, Danilovs JA (1980) Joint Report: Frequency reference tables. In: Terasaki PI (ed) Histocompatibility testing 1980. UCLA Tissue Typing Laboratory, Los Angeles, p 955

Antigen Report: HLA-B37

K. Gelsthorpe[1], D. Smillie[1], and P.T. Klouda[2]

1 Regional Blood Transfusion Centre, Longley Lane, Sheffield S5 7JN, U.K.
2 UK Transplant Service, Southmead, Bristol BS10 4ND, U.K.

History

The HLA antigen B37 was first described as 'TY' by Gelsthorpe and Doughty [1]. The original serum defining B37 (TY) has now been included in four Workshops as: 6w111; 7w380; 8w450 and 9w329. B37 has an antigen frequency in Caucasians of approximately 3%.

Serology

In this Workshop four sera were included in the definition of B37: 324, 325, 327 and 329. The majority of B37-positive cells reacted clearly with all four antisera (Table 1). Sera 327 and 329 were the strongest but had longer "tails" (Table 2). Extra specificities in sera 324 and 327 are possibly direct-

Histocompatibility Testing 1984
Edited by E. D. Albert et al.

Table 1. Pattern analysis in HLA-B37-positive individuals (35/1000 Caucasian)

											Q Score
9w0324	B37	+	–	+	+	–	+	+	–	+	9.1
0325	B37	+	+	+	+	–	–	–	–	–	9.6
0327	B37	+	+	+	–	+	+	+	+	+	9.1
0329	B37	+	+	+	+	+	+	–	+	+	9.1
0447	TCN-1	+	+	–	+	+	–	–	–	+	4.8
Absolute no.		19	4	3	2	2	2	1	1	1	
%		54.3	11.4	8.6	5.7	5.7	5.7	2.9	2.9	2.9	

Table 2. Ninth Workshop data on HLA-B37-positive individuals (Caucasian)

	Serum strength %	A ++	B +–	C –+	D ––	% Extra reactions	% Misses
9w0324	59	93	36	19	3352	28	17
0325	59	98	16	11	3375	14	10
0327	60	105	101	3	3291	49	3
0329	67	108	58	2	3232	35	2
0447	58	92	391	16	3001	81	15

ed against B18 and B27, respectively. Serum 447 (submitted specificity TCN-1) also reacted with the majority of B37-positive cells, the apparent specificity of this serum now being B38 + B37 + other extras. If the pattern of reactivity of sera 425–428 is accepted as a good definition of Bw4, then B37 is included in Bw4 with the possible exception of two cells from a total of 116 B37-positive individuals.

Linkage Disequilibrium

HLA-B37 is in linkage disequilibrium with A1, Cw6 and DRw10 [2–4].

Conclusion

HLA-B37 is a well-defined Bw4-type antigen in linkage disequilibrium with A1, Cw6 and, possibly, DRw10. It has an antigen frequency of 3.1% in Caucasians and is rare in Oriental and Negro populations.

References

1. Gelsthorpe K, Doughty RW (1973) A new HL-A antigen: TY. Tissue Antigens 3:316
2. Colombe B, Payne R, Cann H (1980) Reactivity to a new DR specificity ST1 in selected 8th International Workshop antisera. In: Terasaki PI (ed) Histocompatibility testing 1980. UCLA Tissue Typing Laboratory, Los Angeles, p 841
3. Jacobsen BK, Svejgaard A (1979) A 'private' DR antigen associated with HLA B37. Tissue Antigens 14:361
4. Klouda PT (1980) B37. In: Terasaki PI (ed) Histocompatibility testing 1980. UCLA Tissue Typing Laboratory, Los Angeles, p 318

Antigen Report: HLA-B38

A. Alonso[1], R. Altshuler[2], S. Batat[3], C. Brautbar[3], H. Festenstein[1], E. Gazit[2], M.J. Latimer[4], D. McCloskey[1], P. Stastny[4], and E. Williams[1]

1 Department of Immunology, The London Hospital Medical College, London E1 2AD, U.K.
2 Chaim Sheba Medical Center, Tel-Hashomer, Israel
3 Hadassa Hebrew University Medical Center, Jerusalem, Israel
4 Department of Internal Medicine, Health Science Center, South Western Medical School, Dallas, TX 72235, USA

HLA-B16 was first defined at the Fifth International Histocompatibility Workshop. At the Sixth Workshop B16 was split into B38 (B16 long) and B39 (B16 short) [1]. In addition, B38 was found to be associated with Bw4 and B39 with Bw6 [2]. These Bw4 and Bw6 associations were confirmed at the Seventh Workshop.

At the Ninth Workshop B38 was identified by the following sera: 332, 333, 335, 340, 337, 339, and 447 (Tables 1 and 2).

Histocompatibility Testing 1984
Edited by E. D. Albert et al.

Table 1. Most specific Ninth Workshop sera defining B38

Serum serial no.	Ninth WS serum no.	Sub-lab	Ave. serum score[a]	Quality score[b]	Other specificities
244	332	JER	7.7		JAP Bw67; A3; B39
245	333	BAR	7.9		JAP Bw67; B8; Bw55; B39
246	335	BRU	7.6		JAP Bw67; B39
249	340	KOE	7.9	10.0	JAP Bw67; B49
247	337	DEW	7.3	7.4	B39 wk
248	339	BRA	7.3	5.5	JAP Bw67
322	447	CAC	7.7	6.5	B44; B37

[a] Average serum score is the average score for all the positive reactions for cells of the stated specificity
[b] Quality score as defined by Mickey and Terasaki [4]

Table 2. Pattern analysis for B38 (Caucasoid; $n = 1000$)

Absolute no.	Percent	9w0332 B38+39	9w0333 B38+39	9w0335 B38+39	9w0340 B38	9w0337 B38	9w0339 B38	9w0342 B39	9w0343 B39	9w0344 B39	9w0341 B39
29	54.7	+	+	+	+	+	+	−	−	−	−
6	11.3	+	+	+	+	−	+	−	−	−	−
2	3.8	−	+	+	+	+	+	−	−	−	−
2	3.8	+	+	−	+	+	+	−	−	−	−
2	3.8	+	+	+	+	−	−	−	−	−	−
2	3.8	+	+	+	+	+	+	−	−	+	−

The pattern of reactivity with 1000 randomly chosen Caucasoids clearly demonstrated that B38 can be dissociated from B39. As seen in Table 2, 55% (29) of B38 cells reacted positively with all sera defining B16 and B38 and did not react with the sera identifying B39.
The remaining 14 cells reacted in different combinations with the anti-B16 and anti-B38 sera, but were uniformly negative with the anti-B39 sera (excluding two cases that reacted positively with serum 344).

Linkage Disequilibrium

The most significant two-locus haplotypes in Caucasoids carrying this antigen were: B38-A26, B38-Cw7 and B38-C4A2.

Conclusion

B38 remains a clearly defined antigen. There is, however, an indication of an unusual B16 antigen [3] segregating in a Thai family (ANZ DCHO3), which has been submitted to this Workshop. This specificity, which is Bw4 associated, was defined by positive reactions with only the broad Bw16 sera (332, 333, and 335).

References

1. Histocompatibility Testing 1972, 1975, 1977. Munksgaard, Copenhagen
2. Schreuder I, D'Amaro J, Sandberg L, van Rood JJ (1975) Partition of the antigen w16 into subtypic determinants. Tissue Antigens 5:142
3. Chandanayingyong D (1983) Further splits of HLA-Bw16. Workshop Newsletter 2:15
4. Mickey MR, Terasaki PI (1980) The serological data of the 8th Workshop and summary analyses. In: Terasaki PI (ed) Histocompatibility testing 1980. UCLA Tissue Typing Laboratory. Los Angeles, p 25

Antigen Report: HLA-B39

A. Alonso[1], R. Altshuler[2], S. Batat[3], C. Brautbar[3], H. Festenstein[1], E. Gazit[2], M.J. Latimer[4], P. Stastny[4], and E. Williams[1]

1 Department of Immunology, The London Hospital Medical College, London E1 2AD, U.K.
2 Chaim Sheba Medical Center, Tel-Hashomer, Israel
3 Hadassa Hebrew University Medical Center, Jerusalem, Israel
4 Department of Internal Medicine, Health Science Center, South Western Medical School, Dallas, TX 72235, USA

At the Fifth International Histocompatibility Workshop, HLA-B16 was defined on the basis of several local designations, including U18, Te64, Ao81, and Da31. Two splits of B16 were reported during the Sixth International Histocompatibility Workshop [1]. These splits, B38 and B39, were later reported to be strongly associated with Bw4 and Bw6, respectively [2].

At the present Workshop, sera 9w332, 333, 335, 341, 342, 343, 344 and 446 were found to be reliable for the definition of B39 (Table 1). However, the distinction between B38 and B39 can only be made with sera 341, 342, 343, 344 and 446 (Table 2). It should be noted that these sera also contain activity against other specificities, in particular Bw67.

Data from this Workshop suggest that B39 may be heterogeneous. A new Bw6-associated subtype, ST-16 [3], was demonstrated in four Mexican-American families (US4 STA01, US4 STA03, US3 GRU09 and US3 GRU13) and two Chinese families (US8 SLE03 and US8 SLE14) with Ninth Workshop sera. ST-16 gives a shorter reaction pattern when compared with Bw39, being consistently negative with serum 344 (Table 2).

Another subtype of B39, designated B39B, has been encountered in Negroids (Nigerian and West Indian) and Saudi Arabian Caucasoids [4]. The B39B specificity reacts with B16 and B39 sera but is negative with MoAb 9w1132 (Table 2). A group of sera with activity for the B7 CREG antigens are also positive with B39B (data not shown).

Table 1. Most specific Ninth Workshop sera defining B39

Serum serial no.	9th WS serum no.	Sub lab	Ave. serum score[a]	Quality score[b]	Other specificities
244	332	JER	7.7		Bw67; A3; B38
245	333	BAR	7.9		Bw67; B38; B8; Bw55
246	335	BRU	7.6		Bw67; B38
250	341	TOK	7.3	5.7	Bw67
251	342	OSA	7.4	9.6	Bw67
252	343	NAI	7.5	7.7	Bw67
253	344	DUP	7.3	7.3	Bw67; B38 wk
321	446	HAN	7.7	6.5	Bw67; B38 wk

[a] Average serum score is the average score for all the positive reactions for cells of the stated specificity
[b] Quality score as defined by Mickey and Terasaki [5]

Table 2. Pattern analysis for B39 and new variants

9th WS serum no.	B39	B38	ST-16	B39B
332	+	+	+	+
333	+	+	+	+
335	+	+	+	+
341	+	–	±	+
342	+	–	+	+
343	+	–	+	+
344	+	–	–	+
446	+	–	+	+
1132[a]	+	+	NR	–

NR; not reported; ± variable reactivity
[a] Not based on Workshop analysis

Conclusion

HLA-B39 can be clearly distinguished from HLA-B38 by means of the Ninth Workshop sera. It is nonetheless difficult to define B39 in the presence of Bw67 on the basis of the reactivity of these sera. However, strong evidence has been presented for the heterogeneity of B39, especially when several ethnic populations were studied.

Histocompatibility Testing 1984
Edited by E. D. Albert et al.

References

1. Bodmer J (1975) The ABC of HLA, HLA-Bw16. In: Kissmeyer-Nielsen F (ed) Histocompatibility testing 1975. Munksgaard, Copenhagen, p 53
2. Schreuder I, D'Amaro J, Sandberg L, van Rood J (1975) Partition of the antigen w16 into two subtypic determinants. Tissue Antigens 5:142
3. Ness DB, Watson AK, Grumet FC (1982) ST-16: A new Bw16 subtype present in Mexican Americans. Hum Immunol 4:55
4. Williams E, Alonso A, Doyle P, Okoye R, Ollier W, Festenstein H (to be published) A new HLA-Bw16 subtype defined in both Negroids and Saudi Arab Caucasoids. Hum Immunol
5. Mickey MR, Terasaki PI (1980) In: Terasaki PI (ed) Histocompatibility testing 1980. UCLA Tissue Typing Laboratory, Los Angeles, p 27

Antigen Report: HLA-Bw41

H. Mervart[1], C. Taylor[2], and A. Ting[2]

1 National Reference Laboratory, Canadian Red Cross Society, Toronto, Canada
2 Nuffield Department of Surgery, Oxford, U.K.

Four sera (nos. 380, 381, 384, and 386) were submitted as monospecific anti-Bw41. Serum 378 defined Bw41, B40 and B12. Serum 241 defined Bw41 and Bw42.

For each serum the Q-score, percent of "correct" positive reactions, and "tail" antigens are shown in Table 1. Sera 380 and 381 proved to be monospecific, although the reactions were often weak. The other sera reacted with the majority of Bw41 positive cells, but all sera had extra reactivity, as shown in Table 1. Overall, Bw41 could be well defined with the Ninth Workshop sera and could be distinguished from Bw60 and Bw61.

Table 1. Q score, percent correct reactions with the listed antigen, and additional specificities in each serum. The sera are listed in order of quality

9WS no.	Antigen	Q score	% Correct	% 8's	Other specificities
384	Bw41	6.9	86	42	(B40)
360	Bw41	5.1	89	40	Bw60, (B7)
380	Bw41	5.9	82	53	
386	Bw41	5.3	84	45	(B13)
381	Bw41	4.3	76	34	
359	Bw41	2.3	51	82	Bw60, w61, w48, (B7, w42)
241	Bw41	1.4	44	25	Bw42

Table 2. A possible split of Bw41 as defined by serum 241

		359	360	380	381	384	386	241
Family W	Father	1	8	6	6	6	8	6
	C3	4	8	8	8	8	8	8
	C4	2	8	8	8	8	8	8
	C5	1	8	4	6	6	8	8
Family R	Father	8	8	8	8	8	8	8
	C1	6	8	8	8	8	8	8
	C2	8	8	8	4	8	8	8
	C3	8	8	8	8	8	8	8
	C4	4	8	4	6	8	8	8
Family D	Mother	2	8	6	4	8	8	8
	C1	6	8	8	8	8	8	8
	C2	8	8	8	2	8	8	6
Family M	Father	8	8	6	8	8	4	1
	C1	6	8	8	8	8	8	1
	C2	2	8	4	8	8	6	1
	C3	2	8	4	8	8	2	1

Serum 241 reacted strongly with all Bw42-positive cells and also with some, but not all, Bw41-positive cells. In Newsletters 3 and 8 of this Workshop a possible variant of Bw41 based on the reactivity of this serum 241 was reported from two laboratories (Mervart, Hammond). The reactions of this serum compared with the other Bw41 sera in four families from Mervart are shown in Table 2. Serum 241 was reactive in three families but nonreactive in the fourth family. The same pattern of reactivity was seen in the family reported by Hammond. An analysis of 13 Workshop families showed that serum 241 reacted in 3 families and negative in 6 families, and gave equivocal reactions in the other families. Therefore, there is some evidence that Bw41 may be split although the evidence is based on only one serum and obviously must be confirmed by more studies before it can be accepted as a split.

Histocompatibility Testing 1984
Edited by E. D. Albert et al.

Antigen Report: HLA-Bw42

J.R. Moraes [1], M.E. Moraes [1], H. Festenstein [2], A. Alonso [2], and E. Williams [2]

1 Hospital dos Servidores do Estado, Clinica Medica-Imunologia, Rua Sacadura Cabral 178, 20.226 Rio de Janeiro, Brazil
2 The London Hospital Medical College, London E1, U.K.

HLA-Bw42, previously called MWA, was defined during the Fifth International Workshop [1]. It is an antigen primarily found in Negroes, but it can be defined with some Caucasian sera whose main activity is usually with some other B7 CREG antigen [2, 3]. Definition of Bw42 was poor at the Sixth Workshop. A good agreement was established at the Seventh Workshop, when African Negroes were tested. During the Eighth Workshop definition of Bw42 was considered good although all sera contained additional reactivities with cells having B7 CREG antigens. Very similar results were found with sera submitted to the Ninth Workshop. As shown in Table 1, when sera with anti-Bw42 activity were analysed only with the Negroid populations it was possible to show that six reacted with more than 75% of the cells having the antigen; three, 9w237, 9w238, and 9w241, were particularly useful as they did not react frequently with other cells. Extra reactions were mainly observed in these sera when they were tested against cells positive for B7 and/or Bw55. The sole exception was serum 9w241, which did not react with any B7 CREG antigen, although probably defines a Bw41 split in Negroids and Caucasoids (Bw41 Report, p. 149 this volume) [4–6].

Table 1. Pattern of reactions of Bw42 in Negroes

Sera	Bw42	B7	Bw55	Bw41
9w236	####	oooo	####	
9w239	####	####		
9w237	####	oooo		
9w238	####	oooo		
9w230	####		####	
9w241	####			oooo
9w231	////		####	
9w240	////	oooo	////	
9w216	////	oooo		
9w229	////		####	
9w232	oooo		####	
9w218	oooo		####	
9w219	oooo		####	
9w217	oooo		####	
9w227	oooo		####	

\# Reactions with more than 75% of cells having the antigen
/ Reactions with 40% – 75% of cells having the antigen
o Reactions with less than 40% of cells having the antigen

Conclusions

Bw42 antigen was relatively well defined by Ninth Workshop sera. Again, no serum was found to be monospecific. Definition of the antigen was possible when account was taken of a special pattern of reactions with a cluster of six sera.

References

1. Festenstein H, Adams E, Brown J, et al (1973) In: Dausset J, Colombani J (eds) Histocompatibility testing 1972. Munksgaard, Copenhagen, p 397
2. Bodmer J, Curtoni ES, van Leeuwen A, Mickey MR, Kjerbye L, Degos L, Botha MC, Wolf E, Mayr WR, Staub-Nielsen L, Piazza A (1975) In: Kissmeyer-Nielsen F (ed) Histocompatibility testing 1975. Munksgaard, Copenhagen, p 21
3. Johnson A (1980) In: Terasaki PI (ed) Histocompatibility testing 1980. UCLA Tissue Typing Laboratory, Los Angeles, p 395
4. Tibensky D, Morochove L, Mervart H (1984) Ninth International Histocompatibility Workshop Newsletter 3:26
5. Hammond MG (1984) Short Bw41. Ninth International Histocompatibility Workshop Newsletter 8:9
6. Moraes ME, Salatiel I, Faria L, Zamolyi M, Zamolyi G, Moraes E, Moraes JR (1984) Ninth International Histocompatibility Workshop Newsletter 8:10–11

Histocompatibility Testing 1984
Edited by E. D. Albert et al.

Antigen Report: HLA-B44

K.K. Mittal

Transplantation Biology Branch, Office of Biologics Research and Review, Food and Drug Administration, 8000 Rockville Pike, Bldg. 29, Rm 232, Bethesda, MD 20205, USA

History

Antigen HLA-B12 was recognized by the WHO Nomenclature Committee in 1971 [1], and its subdivision B44 in 1975 [2]. B44 occurs with a phenotype frequency of 13%–22% among Orientals, Negroes, and Caucasoids; and its association with Bw4 and allelic segregation as a B locus allele have been shown by family studies [3, 4].

Serology

At this Workshop, antigen B44 was defined by sera 9w398, 9w394, 9w396, and 9w399 (Table 1). It was best defined by serum 9w398. While sera 9w394 and 9w396 were somewhat "shorter", sera 9w398, 9w396 and 9w399 produced extra reactions. The tail analysis of extra reactions revealed no consistent pattern. The phenotype frequency of B44 among Caucasians was 22.2% (as in 1980), and in Negroes 15.6% (13.7% in 1980).

Table 1. Reaction patterns of B44 sera

Pattern[a]	B44 sera				Number of persons	
	9w398	9w394	9w396	9w399	Caucasian	Negro
B12-positive	+	+	+	+	151	65
	+	+	–	+	37	3
	+	–	+	+	3	3
B12-negative	+	–	+	+	4	8
	+	–	–	+	7	6
	+	–	+	–	4	3
	+	–	–	–	0	5
	–	–	+	–	8	3
	–	–	–	+	13	8
Average serum score	7.9	7.5	7.6	7.9		

[a] Pattern as defined by B12 sera 9w388, 9w387 and 9w393

Summary

In families, B44 segregated as an allele of the B locus, and was associated with Bw4. It was clearly defined by the Ninth Workshop sera. A possible correlation of any of the shorter B44 patterns with subdivisions of B44 as suggested by cell-mediated lympholysis [5] needs further study.

References

1. Svejgaard A, Kissmeyer-Nielsen F, Thorsby E (1970) HLA typing of platelets. In: Terasaki PI (ed) Histocompatibility testing 1980. Munksgaard, Copenhagen, p 153
2. Bodmer J (1975) The ABC of HLA. In: Kissmeyer-Nielsen F (ed) Histocompatibility Testing 1975. Munksgaard, Copenhagen, p 48
3. Mittal K (1980) Joint Report – Bw44. In: Terasaki PI (ed) Histocompatibility testing 1980. UCLA Tissue Typing Laboratory, Los Angeles, p 398
4. Mittal K (1980) Allelic sub-divisions of the HLA-B12-Bw21 complex: Association with Bw4 and Bw6. Vox Sang 38:241
5. Tekolf W, Biddison W, Aster R, Shaw S (1982) Two subgroups of HLA-Bw44 defined by cell-mediated lympholysis that differ in Bw44 expression on platelets and in patterns of genetic linkage disequilibrium. J Immunol 129:1474

Histocompatibility Testing 1984
Edited by E. D. Albert et al.

Antigen Report: HLA-B45

E. Möller

Dept. of Clinical Immunology, Karolinska Institute, Huddinge Hospital, 14186 Huddinge, Sweden

History

As long ago as 1970 [1] it was recognized that HLA-B12 consisted of at least two distinct subgroups, defined by serum TT from Aarhus. They were referred to then as B12-non-TT and B12-TT*, and are now designated B44 and B45. During the Eighth International Histocompatibility Workshop in 1980, B45 was well defined by sera 192 and 397 (original TT).

Serology

Several sera used at the Ninth Workshop contained B45 reactivity, but most reagents also contained B44 (Table 1). However, there were three B45-specific sera, these being sera 400 (original TT*) from Aarhus, 401 from US1 (New Orleans), and 402 from US1 (Duquesnoy). Of these three sera, no. 401 showed *extensive* reactivity with B44 also, reacting with approximately 50% of all B44-assigned cells (Table 1).

In Caucasians there were three distinct reactivity patterns, which correlated well with local B45 assignment. The frequency of B45 in this population group is 1.3% (2.0% in 1980).

In the Caucasian pattern analysis, serum 402 did not react with any B44-positive cells, whereas serum 400 gave positive reactions with 13/238 B44 cells.

B45 is more frequent in the Negro population, with a frequency of 6.0% (7.7% in 1980).

As in Caucasians, most Negro cells react with all the B45 reagents and fail to react with the B44-specific sera. Serum 401 reacted with about 50% of B44-positive cells, but serum 402 did not react with any Negro B44 cells and serum 400 only with 2/83 B44 cells.

Conclusion

B45 is well defined by six sera in the present Workshop material, two of which are B45 monospecific. The serological definition of B45 is similar in the two populations studied, Caucasians and Negro. There is no indication of further splits of B45.

References

1. Svejgaard A, Kissmeyer-Nielsen F, Thorsby E (1970) HLA typing of platelets. In: Terasaki PI (ed) Histocompatibility testing 1970. Munksgaard, Copenhagen
2. Goldman SF, Kissmeyer-Nielsen F (1977) Definition of an antigen (TT*) closely related to HLA-B12 with monospecific antisera. Tissue Antigens 9:177
3. Pazderka F, Dossetor JB (1980) Bw45. In: Terasaki PI (ed) Histocompatibility testing 1980. UCLA Tissue Typing Laboratory, Los Angeles

Table 1. B45

Serum no.	Region	Laboratory	Frequency (%)		Q score	Extras
			Cauc.	Negro		
9w387	NCY	Yunis	20	21	6.0	B44
388	EAE	Zaretskaya	20	17	5.7	B44
393	US6	Braun	15	16	5.9	B44
400	SCA	Aarhus	2	4.9	11.0	
401	US1	New Orleans	12	15	7.3	B44
402	US1	Duquesnoy	1.5	5.6	7.1	

Histocompatibility Testing 1984
Edited by E. D. Albert et al.

Antigen Report: **HLA-Bw46**

S. H. Chan[1] and S. Naito[2]

1 WHO Immunology Centre, Faculty of Medicine, National University of Singapore, Sepoy Lines, Singapore 03.16
2 2nd Department of Medicine, Fukuoka University, Fukuoka, Japan

History

Bw46 is an oriental antigen first reported in 1975 as Singapore 2 (Sin 2) [1] and independently as HSIEH (Hs) [2]. It is in linkage disequilibrium with A2; with a Cw1/Cw3 complex [3–5] designated as Cw Bangkok (CwBk) at the Second Asia and Oceania Histocompatibility Workshop Conference (2 AOHWS), with DRw9 among the Chinese, and DRw8 among the Japanese (2 AOHWS). During the Sixth International Workshop several ANZ regional Caucasian anti-B15 sera reacted with Bw46 cells, suggesting that Bw46 may be related to B15 [6].

Evidence of Split

During the Second AOHWS serum 2AOHWS 506 (Singaporean Southern Chinese in origin) reacted "short" with Thai and Northern Chinese cells [7], suggesting that Bw46 may be split into a long Bw46 in Thai and Northern Chinese, and a short Bw46 occurring mainly among Southern Chinese.

Ninth International Workshop

Bw46 was detected in three ethnic groups, Chinese, Japanese and Thais, at this Workshop. There were three operationally monospecific antisera, 9w420, 421, and 422. Serum 420 had B8 activity but since B8 is absent or present only in very low frequency in these three ethnic groups, it could be considered operationally monospecific. Among the three monospecific sera there were some differences in reaction in different ethnic groups (Table 1). 9w421 was the best serum for definition of Bw46 among the Japanese, Northern Chinese, and Thais, but reacted poorly among Southern Chinese. There is a suggestion of heterogeneity in Bw46, based on the reaction of 9w422 and to a lesser extent of 9w421 among Chinese and Thai cells. 9w422 reacted well in some Bw46 cells, mainly from Northern Chinese and Thais. In contrast, 9w422 was nonreactive among Southern Chinese (Singapore and Hong Kong) Bw46 cells. Since Bw46 is associated with Bw6 it is interesting to note that two Bw6 sera, 9w436 and 9w431, reacted with 9w422 positive Bw46 cells (Thai, Northern Chinese) and did not react with 9w422-negative Bw46 cells (Southern Chinese). The 9w422-negative Bw46 cells were more likely to be associated with A2 than 9w422-positive Bw46 cells ($P = 0.025$). However, we must be cautious in the interpretation of a split in Bw46 because, while 9w422 segregated in Chinese families, its reaction pattern was inconsistent and lacked clear segregation patterns among the Japanese.

Conclusion

Bw46 was defined by 9w420, 421, and 422; and by 308, 310, 307, and 309 in the absence of B15 and B17. There was a suggestion of heterogeneity in Bw46 based on the restricted reactivity of serum 9w422, but this will have to be confirmed.

Table 1. BW46 and related serum reaction patterns in different ethnic groups

	Bw46	Bw6	Cw1	Cw3 (Bk)
	4 4 4 2 2 2 0 1 2	4 4 4 4 4 3 3 3 3 3 3 4 9 6 1	4 4 4 4 4 4 4 4 5 5 5 5 8 9 1 2 3 4	4 4 4 6 6 6 1 3 5
Thai, Shanghai Chinese	+ + +	+ + + + +	± ± ± ± ± ±	+ + +
Southern Chinese; Singapore/Hong Kong	+ ± –	+ + + – –	+ + + + + +	+ + +
Japanese	+ + ±	+ + + – ±	+ + + + + +	± ± +

Histocompatibility Testing 1984
Edited by E. D. Albert et al.

References

1. Simons MJ, Wee GB, Chan SH, Shanmugaratnam K, Day NE, de The, GB (1975) Probable identification of an HL-A second-locus antigen associated with a high risk of nasopharyngeal carcinoma. Lancet I:142
2. Payne R, Radvany R, Grumet C (1975a) A new second-locus HL-A antigen in linkage disequilibrium with HL-A2 in Cantonese Chinese. Tissue Antigens 5:69
3. Payne R, Radvany R, Grumet FC, Fieldman M, Cann H (1975b). Two third series antigens transmitted together. A possible fourth SD locus? In: Kissmeyer-Nielsen F (ed) Histocompatibility testing 1975. Munksgaard, Copenhagen, p 345
4. Chan SH, Wee GB (1979) Association of Bw46 and Cw1/Cw3 in Chinese. Tissue Antigens 14:179
5. Aizawa M, Yakura H, Wakisaka A, Maruyama N, Kimura S, Moriuchi J, Kuroda M, Hamatake K, Itakura K (1975) Analysis of the Workshop sera against Japanese permanent panel. In: Kissmeyer-Nielsen F (ed) Histocompatibility testing 1975. Munksgaard, Copenhagen, p 136
6. Bashir H, Bradley J, Chan SH, Cross R, D'Apice A, Dawkins R, Douglas R, Fong R, Hay J, Honeyman M, Innis M, Simons M, Tait B (1977) Australian-Singapore Regional Report. In: Bodmer WF, Batchelor JR, Bodmer JG, Festenstein H, Morris JT (eds) Histocompatibility testing 1977. Munksgaard Copenhagen, p 380
7. Chandanayingyong D (1983) Bw46. In: Simons MJ, Tait BD (eds) Proceedings of the Second Asia and Oceania Histocompatibility Workshop Conference, p 127

Antigen Report: HLA-Bw47

P. Reekers[1], L.J. Kennedy[2], and G.M.T. Schreuder[3]

1 Laboratory of Transplantation Serology, Blood Transfusion Service, Radboud Hospital, University of Nijmegen, Geert Grooteplein Zuid 12, Nijmegen, The Netherlands
2 Imperial Cancer Research Fund Laboratories, London, U.K.
3 Dept of Immunohematology, Blood Bank, University Hospital, Rijnsburgerweg 10, 2333 AA Leiden, The Netherlands

Serology

Bw47 was identified with the following 9WS sera: 243, 242, 377, 244, 1129 (monoclonal), 376, 374, 373, 372 and 356 (Table 1). None of these sera was specific for Bw47. The antigen Bw47 could be clearly distinguished from B27, Bw60, Bw61, Bw41, Bw48, B13, B7, Bw42, and Bw73 by comparison of the reaction patterns with the more or less specific reagents for these antigens (Table 2).

Table 1. 9WS sera with anti-Bw47 specificity

Serum no.	Submitting laboratory	Q score[a]	% 8's	Other specificities
9w243	Braun	3.4	84	B27
9w242	Arizona	4.3	54	B27, B12
9w377	Nijmegen	2.6	49	B27, A32 (B12)
9w244	Mervart	2.9	27	B27
9w376	Osaka	6.8	96	B40, B13
9w374	Paris	8.4	80	B40, B13
9w373	Rennes	6.4	80	B40, B13 (Bw48)
9w372	Bremen	5.7	76	B40, B13
9w356	Lyon	3.9	34	Bw60, Bw48 (Bw61)
9w1129	Grumet (monoclonal)		34	B27

[a] Q score assignment according to Mickey et al. [1] and Deppe et al., Cell Typing by Computer (this volume)

All local assignments were checked for the reaction patterns given in Table 2. A total of 74 Bw47-positive cells were identified, 12 from random individuals (all Caucasians) and 62 cells in 20 families (17 Caucasoid, 1 Mexican, 1 Asian Indian and 1 Cape Colored; no disease code). The gene frequency of this antigen is low in all populations: 0.2% in Caucasians; 0.0% in Negroes; 0.4% in Orientals. Bw47 was completely included in Bw4.

Linkage Disequilibrium

Bw47 has been reported to be in linkage disequilibrium with A3, Cw6, and DRw6. Table 3 indicates that A3-Cw6-Bw47 is a haplotype associated with either DRw6 or DR7. Two-locus haplotype frequencies have been calculated for A3-Bw47 (Δ rel. 0.59; $\chi^2 = 26.5$) and Bw47-Cw6 (Δ rel. 0.73; $\chi^2 = 52.5$; see also Baur et al., Population Analysis, this volume).

Conclusion

Bw47 has a serologic pattern distinct from that for antigens of B40-CREG, is included in Bw4, and

Histocompatibility Testing 1984
Edited by E. D. Albert et al.

Table 2. Distinctive patterns for Bw4 and B40-CREG

	1							
	2 2 3 2 1	3 3 3 3 3	2 2	3 3 3	3 3	2 2	3 3	3 3
	4 4 7 4 2	7 7 7 7 5	1 1	6 6 6	5 5	4 4	8 8	4 4
	3 2 7 4 9	6 4 3 2 6	0 5	1 3 5	3 5	5 6	4 0	6 8
Bw47	+ + + ± ±	+ + + + ±	– –	– – –	– –	– –	– –	– –
B7	– – ± –	– – – – –	– –	– – –	± ±	+ +	– –	– –
B13	– – – –	+ + + + –	– –	– – –	± –	– –	– –	+ +
Bw22	– – – –	– – – – –	– –	– – –	– –	+ +	– –	– –
B27	+ + + + +	– – – – –	+ +	– – –	– –	+ +	– –	– –
Bw41	– – – –	– – – – –	– –	– – –	– –	– –	+ +	– –
Bw48	– – – –	– – – – +	– –	– – +	+ +	+ +	– –	– –
Bw60	– – – –	+ + + + +	– –	+ + +	+ +	+ +	– –	– –
Bw61	– – – –	+ + + + ±	– –	– – –	+ +	– –	– –	– –
Bw73	– – – –	– – – – –	– –	– – –	– –	+ +	– –	– –
	Bw47 + B27	Bw47 + B13 + B40	B27	Bw60	B40 + Bw48	Bw73	Bw41	B13

Table 3. Linkage disequilibrium of Bw47 with Cw6, A3, and DR locus antigen

	A3	Cw6	DRw6	DR7
Familial haplotypes ($n = 20$)	10 (50%)	18 (90%)	9 (45%)	7 (35%)
Random population ($n = 12$)	9 (75%)	11 (90%)	3 (25%)	5 (40%)

shows linkage disequilibrium with A3, Cw6 and either DRw6 or DR7.

Reference

1. Mickey MR, Terasaki PI (1980) The serological data of the 8th Workshop and summary analyses. In: Terasaki PI (ed) Histocompatibility testing 1980. UCLA Tissue Typing Laboratory, Los Angeles, p 25

Antigen Report: HLA-Bw48

F. Kissmeyer-Nielsen [1], B. Graugaard [1], L.U. Lamm [1], H. Festenstein [2], A. Alonso [2], and E. Williams [2]

1 Department of Clinical Immunology, Tissue Typing Laboratory. University Hospital of Arhus C, Denmark
2 Department of Immunology, The London Hospital Medical College, London E1, U.K.

This specificity was originally described by our group [1, 2] with an antiserum, JA, which also contained Bw40. The specificity is found in 12% of Eskimos, but is very rare in Caucasians. Several sera in this workshop show reactivity with Bw48, but they all have many extra reactions. Based on

Table 1. Reaction pattern of anti-Bw48 sera

9w number	347	349	351	204	206	208	212	213	214	224	247	245	246	371*	362	365	369	370*
Bw48	–	–	–	–	–	–	–	–	–	–	–	+	+	+	+	+	+	+
Bw61	–	–	–	–	–	–	–	–	–	–	–	–	–	–	–	–	–	–
Bw60	–	–	–	–	–	–	–	–	–	–	–	–	+	+	+	+	+	+
Bw47	–	–	–	–	–	–	–	–	–	–	–	–	–	–	–	–	–	–
B27	–	–	–	–	–	–	+	+	+	+	+	w	+	–	–	–	–	–
B13	+	+	+	–	–	–	–	–	–	–	–	–	–	–	–	–	–	w
B7	–	–	–	+	+	+	–	–	–	–	+	+	+	–	–	–	–	–

9w number	367	359	368	353	355	360	373	356	372	374	376	357	366	377	354	358	364	363
Bw48	+	+	+	+	+	+	+	w	–	–	–	–	–	–	–	–	–	–
Bw61	w	+	+	+	+	+	+	+	+	+	+	+	+	–	+	w	–	–
Bw60	w	+	+	+	+	+	+	+	+	+	+	+	+	+	+	+	w	+
Bw47	–	–	–	–	–	w	+	+	+	+	+	+	+	+	–	–	–	–
B27	–	–	–	–	–	–	–	–	–	–	–	–	–	+	–	–	–	–
B13	–	–	–	+	+	w	+	+	+	+	+	w	w	w	+	–	–	–
B7	–	+	+	w	w	+	–	–	–	–	–	–	–	+	–	–	–	–

*, Sera in the transplant serum set; w, weak reaction

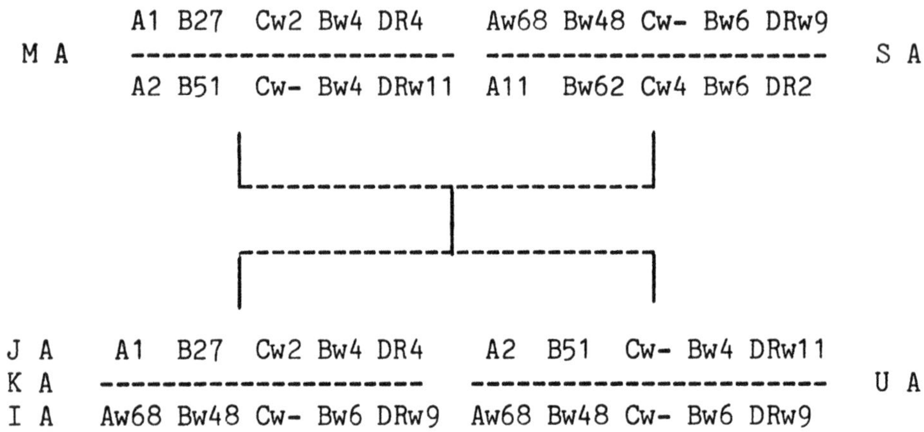

Fig. 1. Pedigree of a Kashmir family

Table 2. Reactivity of selected Bw48 sera in Japanese panel

Serum reactions 9w369	9w368	9w359	n	%	Cell selection criteria
+	+	+	15	93.7	Bw48-positive Bw60-negative and Bw61-negative cells
+	+	–	1	6.3	
other			0		Conclusion: all sera react against Bw48
+	+	+	106	92.2	Bw60-positive cells
+	+	–	2	1.9	Conclusion: all sera cross-react with Bw60
–	–	–	3	2.6	
other			3	2.6	
–	–	–	468	86.8	Bw48-negative; B40-negative cells
–	+	–	71	13.2	Conclusion: only 9W368 has activity in addition to B40
–	+	+	113	91.9	B40-positive, Bw48-negative and Bw60-negative cells
+	+	+	10	8.1	
					Conclusion: 9W369 reacts with some B40-positive and Bw60-negative cells

Japanese data, the serum 9w369, with a Q score of 9.6, can best be used to define Bw48, but also contains anti-Bw60 activity. Thus, Bw48 can only be assigned in the absence of Bw60. Two more sera, 9w368 and 369, may be helpful; both react strongly with nearly all Bw48-positive cells, but include reactions with some B7-positive and B40-positive cells.

In conclusion, Bw48 can be assigned with reasonable certainty in Bw60-negative cells and only with absolute certainty in cells negative for both B7 and B40 (Tables 1, 2).

A family from Kashmir positive for Bw48 was tested at the London Hospital with Ninth Workshop sera (Fig. 1).

References

1. Kissmeyer-Nielsen F, Andersen H, Hauge M, Kjerby KE, Mogensen B, Svejgaard A (1971) HL-A types in Danish Eskimos from Greenland. Tissue Antigens 1:74–80
2. Kissmeyer-Nielsen F, Kjerbye KE, Lamm LU, Jørgensen J, Petersen GB, Gürtler H (1972) Study of the HL-A system in Eskimos. In: Dausset J, Colombani J (eds) Histocompatibility testing 1972. Munksgaard, Copenhagen, pp 317–324

Antigen Report: HLA-B49

D. Ness[1], F. C. Grumet[1], B. Graugaard[2], and F. Kissmeyer-Nielsen[2]

1 Department of Pathology, Stanford University School of Medicine, Stanford, CA 94304, USA
2 Tissue Typing Laboratory, University Hospital of Århus, 8000 Århus, Denmark

History

B21 has been known since 1971 to be composed of at least two subtypes. The more common subtype, designated Bw49 at the Seventh Workshop [1], was originally described by Thorsby and co-workers as SL-ET and later given the name Bw21.1 at the First HLA Workshop of the Americas. This antigen is uniformly Bw4 associated; it has been reported to be in linkage disequilibrium with A26 and DRw8 [2] and to date has been found in all ethnic groups except Chinese [3]. Historically, the sera recognizing B49 are rarely monospecific, cross-reacting with Bw50, B44, or Bw52.

Serology

The reactivities of the anti-B49 sera relative to the approximately 175 B49+ cells tested are given in Table 1. The most specific sera were 410 and 413. The former was strong but reacted with Bw52+ cells, while the latter was more specific but rather weak. Serum 414 had the fewest misses but the longest tail. All other sera cross-reacted with either B44 or the B5 group.

Conclusions

B49 could be clearly distinguished from Bw50 in this Workshop. Significant linkage disequilibrium exists with A23 and Cw7 in the Caucasian population.

References

1. Bodmer FW, Batchelor JR, Bodmer JG, Festenstein H, Morris P (eds) (1977) Nomenclature for factors of the HLA-system. In: Histocompatibility testing 1977. Munksgaard, Copenhagen, p 14
2. Kastelan A, Kerhin-Brkljacic V, Brkljacic L, Zmijewski CM, Liberi H (1980) Joint report: Bw49. In: Terasaki PI (ed) Histocompatibility testing 1980. UCLA Tissue Typing Laboratory, Los Angeles, p 416
3. Baur MP, Danilovs JA (1980) Population analysis of HLA-A, B, C, DR, and other genetic markers. In: Terasaki PI (ed) Histocompatibility testing 1980. UCLA Tissue Typing Laboratory, Los Angeles, p 959

Table 1. Correlation (*r*) of anti-B49 sera with B49 cells

Serum	*r*	Missed reactions	Extra reactions	Other antibodies in the serum	Extras not accounted for by other antibodies
410	0.73	16	102	Bw52	41
413	0.70	50	51	–	51
409	0.64	15	181	Bw50, B44	60
405	0.63	34	131	Bw50, B44	42
407	0.53	14	323	Bw50, B44	109
404	0.49	56	193	Bw50, B44	88
416	0.48	17	405	B44	94
414	0.46	9	489	B51, Bw52	74
411	0.44	15	494	B44, B13	175
176	0.26	14	981	B51, w52, w53, w63, w15.3	35
175	0.25	17	976	B51, w52, w53, w15.3	50
174	0.24	31	1070	B51, w52, w53	150
173	0.12	64	1008	B51, w52, w15.3	102

Histocompatibility Testing 1984
Edited by E. D. Albert et al.

Antigen Report: HLA-Bw50

D. Ness[1], F.C. Grumet[1], B. Graugaard[2], and F. Kissmeyer-Nielsen[2]

1 Department of Pathology, Stanford University School of Medicine, Stanford, CA 94304, USA
2 Tissue Typing Laboratory, University Hospital of Åarhus, 8000 Århus C, Denmark

History

B21 has been known since 1971 to be composed of at least two subtypes. The less frequent subtype, designated Bw50 at the Seventh Workshop [1], was originally described by Thorsby and co-workers as ET* and later given the name Bw21.2 at the First HLA Workshop of the Americas. Bw50 is consistently associated with Bw6 [2] and has been found in all ethnic groups except Japanese, Chinese, and American and Asian Indians to date. Monospecific antisera to Bw50 are rare, and the antigen is thus often defined by subtraction, i.e., Bw6 cells reactive with broad anti-B21 sera and unreactive with anti-B49 sera are designated as Bw50 positive. This may be erroneous, however, since possibly a third subtype of B21 exists, which is Bw6 associated and characterized by reactivity with broad anti-B21 sera but not with specific anti-B49 or anti-Bw50 sera. This subtype has been found in American Indians [3; Kostyu D, personal communication] and in our own Mexican American population (unpublished observations). Bw50 has previously been shown in Caucasians to be in linkage disequilibrium with HLA-A2 and Cw6, with BfS1, and with DR7 and DQw2 [4, 5].

Serology

Because the broad anti-B21 sera are important in defining Bw50 and the possible third subtype, the reactivities of these sera relative to the combined approximately 249 B49- or Bw50-positive cells are given in Table 1. No data are available as to the number of B21-positive B49-negative Bw50-negative cells tested at the Ninth Workshop. Reactivities for the anti-Bw50 sera (including the broad B21 sera) relative to the approximately 74 Bw50-positive cells are given in Table 2. As observed at earlier Workshops, the correlation coefficients (r) are low for the anti-Bw50 sera, primar-

Table 1. Correlation (r) of anti-B21 sera with B21 (B49 or Bw50) cells

Serum	r	Missed reactions	Extra reactions	Q scores for Bw50	Other antibodies in the serum	Extras not accounted for by other antibodies
409	0.78	16	110	9.0	B44	60
405	0.77	43	70	7.3	B44	42
407	0.65	16	253	7.8	B44	109
404	0.58	79	146	4.0	B44	88

Table 2. Corrrelation (r) of anti-Bw50 sera with Bw50 cells

Serum	r	Missed reactions	Extra reactions	Q scores for Bw50	Other antibodies in the serum	Extras not accounted for by other antibodies
418	0.64	10	65	5.0	–	65
409	0.44	1	272	9.0	B49, B44	60
405	0.43	9	210	7.3	B49, B44	42
417	0.41	36	66	2.4	Bw52	42
419	0.37	10	294	5.7	Bw62	174
407	0.36	2	414	7.8	B49, B44	109
404	0.30	23	266	4.0	B49, B44	88

Histocompatibility Testing 1984
Edited by E. D. Albert et al.

ily due to the extra antibodies in each serum. Serum 418 was the most specific anti-Bw50 serum; in Caucasians it was also unreactive with 28/31 B49-positive cells tested. Sera 407 and 409 had the fewest "misses" but could not distinguish Bw50 from B49.

Conclusions

Bw50 could be distinguished from B49 with the sera used in this workshop. In the absence of specific anti-Bw50 sera, caution should be used in assigning Bw50, by subtraction, to cells which are Bw6-positive, because a third subtype of B21, which would also react in the same fashion may exist in some ethnic groups.

References

1. Bodmer WF (rapporteur) (1977) Nomenclature for factors of the HLA-system. In: Bodmer WF, Batchelor JR, Bodmer JG, Festenstein H, Morris P (eds) Histocompatibility testing 1977. Munksgaard, Copenhagen, p 14
2. Baur MP, Danilovs JA (1980) Population analysis of HLA-A, B, C, DR, and other genetic markers. In: Terasaki PI (ed) Histocompatibility testing 1980. UCLA Tissue Typing Laboratory, Los Angeles, p 959
3. Enseroth AF, Mann DL, Johnson AH, Knowler WC, Pettitt DJ, Bennett PH (1983) HLA and B lymphocyte alloantigens in Gila River Indians. Tissue Antigens 21:198
4. Ness DB, Cann HM, Grumet FC (1981) Strong linkage disequilibrium among HLA-Bw50, BfS1, and HLA-DR3/DR7, and mapping of the Bf locus. Hum Immunol 2:225
5. Wernet P, Mueller C, Mueller G, Schunter F (1980) Bw50 Joint Report. In: Terasaki PI (ed) Histocompatibility testing 1980. UCLA Tissue Typing Laboratory, Los Angeles, p 420

Antigen Report: HLA-B51 and HLA-Bw52

N. Kashiwagi[1], C. Taylor[2], and A. Ting[2]

1 Dept. of Transplantation, Kitasato University, Kanagawa, Japan
2 Nuffield Dept of Surgery, John Radcliffe Hospital, Oxford U.K.

Some sera were submitted to the Workshop as monospecific for B51 or Bw52, but the majority submitted contained other specificities in addition to B51 and/or Bw52. For each of the submitted sera the Q score, percent "correct" positive reactions based on laboratory-assigned antigens, and "tail" antigens derived from 2 x 2 comparisons are shown in Table 1.

The correlations among the nine sera submitted as monospecific for B51 in the Caucasian, Japanese, and Negro populations are shown in Table 2. Six sera (Workshop nos. 153, 152, 157, 156, 159, and 158) had r values of greater than 0.75 with each other and with B51 as assigned by the laboratory submitting the cell. Table 3 shows the analogous analysis for the ten Bw52 sera submitted to the Workshop. Four sera (164, 166, 167, 253) had high correlations among each other but the values were relatively low with Bw52-assigned cells. Thus, it appears that there are no monospecific sera for Bw52. These four sera had a "common" extra specificity, which, as can be seen in Table 1, was B51 in all cases.

Table 1. Q score, percentage of "correct" reactions with the listed antigen (% Correct), and additional specificities in each serum

9W no.	Antigen	Q score	% Correct	% 8's	Other specificities
175	B51	9.4	98	80	B49
	Bw52	8.3	98	80	
164	B51	8.9	92	84	(B18)
	Bw52	7.2	97	83	
169	B51	8.4	98	87	
	Bw52	7.9	93	87	
170	B51	9.6	96	81	
	Bw52	5.5	84	81	
173	B51	8.3	98	72	(B49, 8w66)
	Bw52	6.3	95	72	
176	B51	8.5	97	88	B49, w53, w63, 8w66
	Bw52	7.2	93	88	

Histocompatibility Testing 1984
Edited by E. D. Albert et al.

Table 1 (continued)

9W no.	Antigen	Q score	% Correct	% 8's	Other specificities
174	B51	8.2	97	80	B49, w53
	Bw52	6.6	94	79	
166	B51	6.9	95	67	
	Bw52	5.0	84	67	
167	B51	7.8	94	76	
	Bw52	2.9	59	75	
177	B51	8.2	97	91	B35, w53, 18
	Bw52	7.8	96	92	
253	B51	7.7	95	78	(Bw59)
	Bw52	6.8	94	78	
201	B51	7.8	95	76	B13
	Bw52	7.8	98	76	
172	B51	8.6	95	92	B35, w53
156	B51	6.2	82	56	
153	B51	6.6	87	69	
171	B51	7.9	95	87	B35, Bw53
157	B51	6.0	86	57	
152	B51	6.1	82	61	
160	B51	6.3	80	72	
158	B51	4.0	77	57	
159	B51	4.7	70	41	
414	Bw52	6.1	84	66	B49, (B51)
162	Bw52	4.7	75	46	(B51, B49)

Table 2. r values (×100) among sera submitted for B51

	Workshop no.	r (×100)								
Caucasian	153[a]									97[b]
	152[a]	95								92
	157[a]	93	91							93
	156[a]	93	88	89						94
	159[a]	90	88	86	84					88
	158[a]	85	84	85	82	83				86
	170	82	81	83	79	74	73			84
	169	82	81	83	78	74	72	91		82
	160	78	71	77	76	66	65	67	67	79
Japanese	156[a]									91
	158[a]	92								91
	157[a]	89	89							89
	153[a]	89	83	83						87
	159[a]	86	83	80	80					82
	152[a]	84	80	81	93	77				85
	160	80	78	71	80	83	76			75
	170	58	58	65	55	52	54	48		61
	169	52	54	60	50	47	49	42	83	57
Negro	157[a]									97
	153[a]	97								100
	152[a]	97	94							94
	156[a]	94	97	91						97
	159[a]	90	88	87	85					88
	158[a]	84	81	81	84	95				81
	160	78	81	81	78	70	64			81
	170	65	67	63	65	58	54	54		67
	169	51	53	52	51	45	39	48	58	53

[a] Most specific sera for the definition of B51
[b] r value (×100) with B51 as assigned by the local laboratory

Table 3. r value (×100) among sera submitted for Bw52

	Workshop no.	r (×100)									
Caucasian	170										39
	169	96									37
	253[a]	92	88								37
	167[a]	92	87	85							27
	164[a]	90	86	82	82						30
	166[a]	89	85	81	84	81					31
	201	86	82	80	78	76	75				35
	162	48	48	46	37	41	42	43			51
	414	31	31	31	25	26	26	27	34		38
	161	28	28	27	27	30	24	24	41	16	18
Japanese	164[a]										64
	253[a]	99									64
	166[a]	98	97								61
	170	97	96	95							58
	201	93	93	92	90						64
	169	91	91	89	87	87					56
	167[a]	86	85	87	89	80	77				40
	414	70	70	68	67	69	62	52			79
	162	61	60	59	58	59	51	46	75		77
	161	39	39	38	40	37	29	34	54	5	49
Negro	253[a]										72
	166[a]	99									72
	164[a]	91	91								65
	167[a]	85	85	77							41
	162	72	72	65	58						69
	170	69	69	62	81	47					33
	169	68	68	61	66	30	53				46
	201	67	67	61	58	49	56	45			49
	161	42	42	37	44	53	35	24	26		39
	414	33	33	29	25	36	28	16	32	2	36

In conclusion, there were a number of monospecific B51 sera, the most specific being nos. 152, 153, 156, 157, 158, 159. Other useful B51 sera without Bw52 (but with B35 and Bw53) were 171 and 172. There were no monospecific Bw52 sera, the best being nos. 162 and 414. No. 162 was a weak Bw52 serum containing weak B51 and B49 activity. Serum 414 did not react with B51-positive cells but had an anti-B49 reactivity. Despite the lack of monospecific sera, Bw52 could be easily defined with a combination of the B5 and B51 sera (see Table 1 in the Bw53 report, Taylor et al., this volume). There was no evidence of splits or variants of B51 or Bw52 at this Workshop.

Antigen Report: HLA-Bw53

C. Taylor[1], A. Ting[1], M.G. Hammond[2], L.P. de Waal[3], G.G. de Lange[3], and P. Engelfriet[3]

1 Nuffield Dept. of Surgery, John Radcliffe Hospital, Oxford, U.K.
2 Natal Institute of Immunology, P.O. Box 2356, Durban 4000, South Africa
3 Central Laboratory, Netherlands Red Cross Blood Transfusion Service, Amsterdam, The Netherlands

Only one serum (Workshop no. 163) was submitted as a monospecific anti-Bw53 serum. Other sera submitted as having anti-Bw53 as well as other antigens were: 170 (B5); 171, 172 (B5, B35); and 177 (B5, B35, B18).

For each serum the Q score, number of "correct" positive reactions, and "tail" antigens derived from 2 x 2 comparisons are shown in Table 1.

Serum no. 163 was submitted as a monospecific anti-Bw53 serum but the Workshop data did not confirm this. Bw53 could be differentiated from B51, Bw52, B35, and Bw70 with the Workshop sera, but there was no monospecific serum for Bw53. However, there are still some problems when the above-mentioned antigens are present. The definition of Bw53 is shown in Table 2: sera 174 and 176 reacted with B51, Bw52, and Bw53; sera 312, 181, and 182 with B35, and Bw53; sera 171 and 172 with B51, B35, and Bw53; and sera 199, 315, and 317 with B51, Bw52, B35, Bw70, and Bw53.

Table 1. Q score, percentage of "correct" to reactions with the listed antigen (% Correct), and additional specificities in each serum. The sera are listed in order of quality

9WS no.	Antigen	Q score	% Correct	% 8's	Other specificities
177	Bw53	8.3	100	89	B35, 51, w52, 18
172	Bw53	7.9	98	92	B35, 51
199	Bw53	4.8	98	84	B35, 51, (w52)
171	Bw53	6.7	96	89	B35, 51
176	Bw53	5.5	91	86	B51, w52, 49, (w63), 8w66
181	Bw53	7.0	90	79	B35, (51)
182	Bw53	6.5	91	84	B35 (51, w52)
174	Bw53	5.1	89	78	B51, w52, 49
317	Bw53	4.6	96	73	B35, 51, w52, 18, w62, +
312	Bw53	4.4	92	76	B35, w62, 50, w70 (w57)
315	Bw53	5.8	92	84	B35, 51, w52, w62, w70
316	Bw53	2.6	78	56	Bw62, 35, (w63, 51, w57, w46)

Table 2. Definition of B51, Bw52, Bw53, B35, and Bw70 with the Ninth Workshop sera

	153	156	157	160	202	180	179	316	311	318	199	315	317	312	181	182	171	172	177	174	176	201	164	169	173	175	253	170	167	162	414
B51	+	+	+	+	−	−	−	?	−	−	+	+	+	−	−	−	+	+	+	+	+	+	+	+	+	+	+	+	+	−	−
Bw52	−	−	−	−	−	−	−	−	−	−	+	+	+	−	−	−	−	−	+	+	+	+	+	+	+	+	+	?	?	?	+
Bw53	−	−	−	−	−	−	−	−	−	−	+	+	+	+	+	+	+	+	+	+	+	−	−	−	−	−	−	−	−	−	−
B35	−	−	−	−	+	+	+	+	+	?	+	+	+	+	+	+	+	+	+	−	−	−	−	−	−	−	−	−	−	−	−
Bw70	−	−	−	−	+	+	+	+	+	+	?	+	+	+	?	?	−	−	−	−	−	−	−	−	−	−	−	−	−	−	−

?: weak reaction

Histocompatibility Testing 1984
Edited by E. D. Albert et al.

Antigen Report: HLA-Bw54, HLA-Bw55, and HLA-Bw56

Y. Konoeda[1], M.S. Park[1], A. Barbetti[1], A. Wakisaka[1], P.I. Terasaki[1], S. Sekiguchi[2], and T.C. Fuller[3]

1 UCLA Tissue Typing Laboratory, University of California, Los Angeles, CA 90024, USA
2 National Defense Medical College, Tokorozawa, Saitama, Japan
3 Massachusetts General Hospital, Boston, MA, USA

History

Heterogeneity of the antigen Bw22 has been reported at the previous Workshops and was confirmed in different populations by many investigators.

Bw54 was initially discovered by several Japanese centers independently, and designated as J1, SAP1, and SN1 [1–3]. Splits of Bw22 in Caucasians were suggested mainly by the associations with different C locus antigens (Cw1 and Cw3). The specificity designated Bw55 (originally BT22 and Te22) was reported to be associated with Cw3 and Bw56 (originally DA30) with Cw1.

At the Sixth Workshop, two new B locus specificities were designated SN-2 and IM-2. At the Seventh Workshop, Bernoco and Wolf reported two new B locus specificities, designated Te90 and BF, both showing a similar reaction pattern. At the Eighth Workshop, SN-2 (= IM-2, = Te90, = BF) was designated 8w57 and at the Ninth Workshop this antigen was named Bw67.

Serology

Many of the antisera submitted and selected for the Ninth Workshop recognized specificity of the Bw22-complex antigens. The following sera formed clusters identifying Bw54 (222, 224, 225, and 223), Bw55 (232, 227, 236, 226, and 231) and Bw56 (233, 234, and 235). Serum 236 which, in the analysis of Caucasians, seemed to recognize Bw22, also recognized Bw42 and Bw67 in Negroes and Orientals. It must be stated that antisera for Bw55 and Bw56 often contain Bw42 specificity.

At the Ninth Workshop, Bw67 (8w57, SN-2, BF, IM-2 and Te90) proved to be well defined by the Workshop sera. Bw67 was defined by ten sera, one Bw55-Bw42 serum (236), seven broad Bw22 sera (217, 218, 230, 1105, 247, 245, and 246), and two B16 sera (332 and 333). Other Bw22 and B16 sera did not react positively. In addition, two sera (445 and 443) gave strong reactions with Bw67 and did not react with Bw42.

Conclusions

Distinct patterns of the Bw22-complex antigens are shown in Table 1. The data analysis from this workshop provides evidence for the existence of the new B-locus specifity, Bw67, that will be described elsewhere in this volume.

References

1. Juji T, Hagino Y, Tamura M, et al (1973) A possibly new Japanese specific HLA antigen (J-1). Jpn Exp Med 43:447
2. Nakayama E, Itakura K, Yakura H, et al (1974) Sa-1, a possible new HLA specificity found in the Japanese population. Vox Sang 27:134–140
3. Saito S, Naito S, Toyoda K, et al (1975) A study on HLA system in Japanese. Tissue Antigens 5:217
4. Bodmer J (ed) (1975) Joint Report: ABC of HLA. In: Kissmeyer-Nielsen F (ed) Histocompatibility testing 1975. Munksgaard, Copenhagen, p 48
5. Laundy GJ, Entwistle CC (1975) The HLA antigen: W22. In: Kissmeyer-Nielsen F (ed) Histocompatibility testing 1975. Munksgaard, Copenhagen, p 278
6. Danilovs J, Terasaki PI, Gjertson D, Bernoco D (1978) Five subtypic specificities of the Bw22 complex in four racial groups. Transplant Proc 10:725
7. Naito S, Saito S, Toyoda K, et al (1975) A study of anti-W22 complex sera in the Japanese population and the characterization of a possible new antigen of second segregant series, called SN-2. In: Kissmeyer-Nielsen F (ed) Histocompatibility testing 1975. Munksgaard, Copenhagen, p 289
8. Bodmer W, et al (eds) (1978) Histocompatibility testing 1977. Munksgaard, Copenhagen, p 175
9. Terasaki PI (ed) (1980) Histocompatibility testing 1980. UCLA Tissue Typing Laboratory, Los Angeles, p 433

Table 1. Reaction pattern of Bw22 complex antigens

9W / Antigen	222 225 224 223	227 232 236 231 226	233 234 235	445 443	216 229 219 217 218 230	1105 247 245 246	332 333	Key sera
Bw54	+ + + ±	– – – – –	– – –	– –	± + + + + ±	± – – –	– –	222, 225, 224, 223
Bw55	– – – –	± + + ± ±	– – –	– –	+ + + + + +	+ + + +	– –	227, 232, 231, 226
Bw56	– – – –	– – – – –	+ + +	– –	+ + ± + + +	+ + ± –	– –	233, 234, 235
Bw67	– – – –	– – + – –	– – –	+ +	– – – ± ± ±	+ + + +	+ +	445, 443, 236
Other		+				+ + + +	+ +	B7, Bw42, B16

 Histocompatibility Testing 1984
Edited by E. D. Albert et al.

Antigen Report: HLA-Bw57

A. Cambon-Thomsen [1], H. Festenstein [2], A. Alonso [2], M. Thomsen [1], and E. Williams [2]

1 INSERM U. 100, CHU Purpan, 31052 Toulouse Cedex, France
2 Dept. of Immunology, The London Hospital, London E1 2AD, U.K.

History

Data from the Seventh International Histocompatibility Workshop suggested the existence of two alleles subtypic to HLA-B17 [3, 8], and this was confirmed during the Eighth Workshop [4, 5]. These alleles are designated HLA-Bw57 and Bw58 and are included in Bw4. During the 72nd International Cell Exchange of Terasaki, another split of B17 was suggested on a cell from a Negro donor (cell 288).

Serology

In this workshop, 26 sera with strong reactivity to Bw57 were submitted: one was monospecific: 9w303; eight reacted with Bw57 and Bw58 only: 9w293, 296, 298, 290, 291, 306, 292, 304, with Q scores from 12.0 to 7.2; two reacted with Bw57, Bw58 and Bw63: 9w305, which had a Q score for Bw57 of 11.0, and 9w299 (Q score 8.4); five were positive with Bw57, Bw62, Bw63, and sometimes Bw46, and negative with Bw58: 9w302, 309, 307, 308, 310 with Q scores from 9.6 to 7.4; one reacted with the same antigens plus B35, Bw53, Bw50, and Bw71, Bw72: 9w312; nine sera recognizing interlocus specificities reacted mainly with Bw57 and various HLA-A antigens: 9w318 with A1, 9w323 with A9, 9w033, 034, 319, 320, 321, and 322, with A2, and 9w301 with A29. This frequent involvement of Bw57 in interlocus specificities must be emphasized. The antigen Bw57 could easily be defined with these sera, and assignment of Bw57 was possible in the presence of Bw58, Bw62 or Bw63 in the same individual, based on the reactions with 9w305, which never reacted with Bw62, and with 9w303, reacting only with Bw57. In addition, 15 antisera showed some anti-Bw57 and, to a lower extent, anti-Bw58 activity in the tail analysis: 9w017, 041, 217, 218, 219, 277, 278, 316, 378, 396, 398, 399, 451, 465, and 469. Segregation was clear in informative families [1], and at least in one Caucasoid family the independent segregation of Bw57 and Bw58 from one Bw57/w58 heterozygous parent could be observed. There was no evidence of further splits of B17 in any racial group, and Bw57 was always associated with Bw4.

Linkage Disequilibrium

The gene frequency of Bw57 was 0.026 in Caucasoids and 0.012 in Mongoloids; this gene was more frequently found in Negroids, but the number of individuals tested was too small to allow calculations. The alleles most frequently found on the same haplotype as Bw57 were A1, Cw6, DR7, Bf*S, C4*A6, B1, with strong linkage disequilibrium in Caucasoids; A2, A1, Cw6, Cw3, DR7, Bf*S, C4*A6, B1 in Mongoloids; and A29, Cw7, DRw9, DRw6 in Negroids. The alleles associated with Bw58 were different. The nonhemolytic rare C4 variant A6 has previously been found to be associated with Bw57 but not with Bw58 in various populations [2, 6, 7], and the workshop data confirmed this association, although Bw57 was also often found together with C4A3.

Conclusion

Bw57 was well defined with the 9W sera, even in the presence of cross-reacting antigens, and it was clearly different from Bw58. These two antigens differ in their association with products from other loci, in particular C4 allotypes. Of special interest is the frequent involvement of Bw57 in interlocus specificities.

References

1. Cambon A, Thomsen M, Sommer E, Abbal M, Calot M, Ohayon E (1983) Definition of Bw57 and Bw58 with 9W sera and their association with C4 allotypes. Ninth Workshop Newsletter 5:20–23
2. Cambon-de Mouzon A, Ohayon E, Hauptmann G, Sevin A, Abbal M, Sommer E, Vergnes H, Ducos J (1982) HLA-A, B, C, DR antigens, Bf, C4 and glyoxalase I (GLO) polymorphisms in French Basques with insulin-dependent diabetes mellitus (IDDM). Tissue Antigens 19:366–379
3. Dick HM (1978) Joint report. HLA-A, B, and C serology and antigen reports. In: Bodmer WF, Batchelor JR, et al (eds) Histocompatibility testing 1977. Munksgaard, Copenhagen, pp 157–204
4. Goldmann SF, Bittighofer PM (1980) Joint report. Bw57. In: Terasaki PI (ed) Histocompatibility testing 1980. UCLA Tissue Typing Laboratory, Los Angeles, pp 444–446

5. Gyodi E, Petranyi GG (1980) Joint report. Bw58: In: Terasaki PI (ed) Histocompatibility testing 1980. UCLA Tissue Typing Laboratory, Los Angeles, pp 447–449
6. O'Neill GH, Miniter P, Pollack MS, Dupont B (1980) Different HLA antigen associations for the functionally active and inactive products of the complement C4F1 allele. Hum Immunol 1:23–30
7. O'Neill GH, Nerl C, Pollack MS (1983) Analysis of active and inactive complement C4 complotypes associated with subtypes of HLA-B17 in different racial groups. Am J Hum Genet 35:309–317
8. Westphal E, Mueller-Eckhardt G, Goldmann SF (1977) HLA-Bw15 and Bw17 in the German populations. Tissue Antigens 10:173

Antigen Report: HLA-Bw58

A. Cambon-Thomsen[1], A. Alonso[2], H. Festenstein[2], M. Thomsen[1], and E. Williams[2]

1 INSERM U. 100, CHU Purpan, 31052 Toulouse Cedex, France
2 Dept. of Immunology, The London Hospital, London E1 2AD, England

History

Data from previous workshops allowed definition of two splits of the B17 antigen: Bw57 and Bw58, both Bw4 associated. No monospecific serum to Bw58 was available.

Serology

Among the 26 sera submitted to this workshop that allowed a clear definition of B17 (see Bw57 report), none was monospecific for Bw58. This antigen could, however, be clearly defined by positive reactions with (a) the sera reacting with both Bw57 and Bw58: 9w293, 296, 291, 292, 306, 290, 298, and 299, with Q scores from 12 to 5.9; (b) the sera reacting with Bw57, w58, and w63: 9w305 and 299, with Q scores of 9.2 and 5.9, respectively; and (c) by negative reactions with the sera reacting either with Bw57 only: 9w303, or with Bw57, w62, w63 and w46: 9w302, 309, 307, 308, and 310 (Table 1). The nine antisera that recognized interlocus specificities involving B17: 9w301, 318, 323, 319, 322, 320, 321, 033, and 034, were generally more closely correlated to Bw57 than to Bw58. Finally, among the sera exhibiting some anti-B17 activity in the tail analysis, those reacting with Bw58 were 9w017, 217, 218, 219, 304, 451, and 469. The antigen Bw58 so defined segregated clearly in families; at least in one family the specificities Bw57 and Bw58 segregated independently from a heterozygous parent. It could be defined in the presence of Bw62 or Bw63 in the same individual. The key sera in such cases were 9w305, reacting with Bw57, w58, w63 and never with Bw62; 9w303, which was monospecific for Bw57; and the anti-Bw62 sera 9w285, 282, and 284, which did not react with Bw63, Bw57, and Bw58.

Linkage Disequilibrium

The gene frequency of Bw58 is 0.017 in Caucasoids and 0.020 in Mongoloids. It is higher in Negroids, but the number of individuals tested was too small to allow precise calculations. The most frequent

Table 1. Pattern of reactions of 9W sera with Bw57, w58, w62, and w63 cells[a]

	303	293	296	298	290	291	306	292	304	295	305	302	309	307	308	310	312	301	318	319	322	033	034	323	320	321	378	316	218
	↓									↓	↓							*i*	*i*	*i*	*i*	*i*	*i*	*i*	*i*	*i*			
w57	+	+	+	+	+	+	+	+	+	+	+	+	+	+	+	+	+	+	+	+	+	+	+	±	±	±	+	±	−
w58	−	+	+	+	+	+	+	+	+	+	+	−	−	−	−	−	−	+	±	±	±	±	±	±	±	±	−	−	±
w62	−	−	−	−	−	−	−	−	−	−	−	+	+	+	+	+	+	−	−	−	−	−	−	−	−	−	+	−	−
w63	−	−	−	−	−	−	−	−	−	+	+	+	+	+	+	+	+	−	−	−	−	−	−	−	−	−	+	−	−

[a] See also table in the Bw62 report by Chandanayingyong et al., this volume
↓, key sera for definition of Bw57, w58 in the presence of Bw62 in the same individual; *i*, sera recognizing interlocus specificities

Histocompatibility Testing 1984
Edited by E. D. Albert et al.

haplotypes involving Bw58 also carried the alleles A2, Aw33, Cw6, Cw blank, Cw3, DR2, Bf*F, C4*A3,B1 in Caucasoids; Aw33, Cw3, DR5, DR3, DRw6, Bf*S, C4*A3,4,12 or Q0 and C4*B1 in Mongoloids; A30, A28, Cw6, Cw3, DR5, or DRw6 in Negroids. It must be stressed that A29 was never found together with Bw58 in the Negroids, and C4*A6 was never associated with Bw58 in Mongoloids, while these alleles were frequently on the same haplotype as Bw57 in the same populations. The alleles showing the most significant linkage disequilibrium with Bw58 were Aw33 in Caucasoids and Aw33, Cw3, DR3, and DRw6 in Mongoloids. At this workshop Cw3 was subdivided into Cw3.1 (9w467 positive) and Cw3.2 (9w467 negative): it is only the Cw3.2 variant that is associated with Bw58.
In conclusion, Bw58 was clearly defined by Ninth Workshop sera although no monospecific serum was available. It segregated independently of Bw57 in families. Linkage disequilibria for Bw57 were different from those observed for Bw57.

Antigen Report: HLA-Bw59

H. Kunikane, T. Okuyama, M. Kasahara, and M. Aizawa

Department of Pathology, Hokkaido University School of Medicine, Sapporo 060, Japan

History

HLA-Bw59 was first reported by Nakai et al. [1] as a new HLA-B locus antigen (HOK-1) found in the Japanese on the basis of extra reactions of some HLA-B8 typing antisera. During the Eighth International Histocompatibility Workshop, this antigen was proposed as 8w69 and given an official designation Bw59 [2]. However, Bw59 was strongly cross-reactive with B8, and no monospecific sera defining Bw59 were available at that time. Two years later, two antisera monospecific for Bw59 were found at the Eighth Japan HLA Workshop (Tokyo, 1982), confirming the existence of this antigen [3].
At this Workshop, four monospecific antisera defining Bw59 were found.

Serology

Of the eight antisera with anti-Bw59 activity, four (9w254, 256, 257, and 258) were specific for Bw59 (Table 1). In general, the serum-to-serum and serum-to-antigen correlations of these sera were relatively low (Table 1 and Fig. 1). However, this

	9W254	9W256	9W257	9W258	9W253	9W255	9W259
9W256	0.56						
9W257	0.42	0.66					
9W258	0.45	0.62	0.65				
9W253	0.35	0.13	0.06	0.03			
9W255	0.54	0.68	0.58	0.55	0.08		
9W259	0.50	0.59	0.47	0.52	0.10	0.65	
9W447	0.19	0.48	0.35	0.39	0.03	0.45	0.48

(Boxed: Bw59-monospecific sera — 9W256, 9W257, 9W258 × 9W254, 9W256, 9W257)

Fig. 1. Serum-to-serum correlation coefficient in the Japanese

Table 1. List of antisera with HLA-Bw59 activity

Serum no.	Region	Laboratory	Original name	Specificities	Correlation coefficient (*r*)		
					Cauc. + Jap.	Jap.	S.I.[a]
9W253	US3	Grumet	AQ-9540	Bw59 + B51 + Bw52	–	0.94	0.88
9W254	JAP	Tokunaga	50-92	Bw59	0.47	0.52	0.48
9W255	JAP	Sakura	20616	Bw59 + B8	0.88	0.71	0.94
9W256	JAP	Juji	1-519	Bw59	0.67	0.71	0.68
9W257	JAP	Shirai	A2420	Bw59	0.48	0.56	0.50
9W258	JAP	Kyoto	35PK-18	Bw59	0.61	0.63	0.49
9W259	US4	Stastny	JUNGMANN	Bw59 + B8	0.84	0.75	0.96
9W447	US5	CMC	11008-K	Bw59 + B37 + B38	–	0.49	0.82

[a] S.I., Strength Index

Histocompatibility Testing 1984
Edited by E. D. Albert et al.

Table 2. Reaction patterns of seven antisera in a panel of 25 Bw59-positive but B5-negative Japanese individuals[a]

Absolute no.	Percent	9w253	9w254	9w255	9w256	9w257	9w258	9w259
10	40.0	–	+	+	+	+	+	+
7	28.0	+	+	+	+	+	+	+
1	4.0	+	+	+	+	–	–	+
1	4.0	–	+	+	+	+	+	–
1	4.0	–	+	–	+	+	+	+
1	4.0	–	–	+	+	+	+	+
1	4.0	–	+	+	+	–	–	+
1	4.0	–	–	+	+	+	–	+
1	4.0	–	–	+	+	–	+	+
1	4.0	–	–	+	+	+	–	–

[a] Of a total of 1000 Japanese individuals, 25 were Bw59 positive but B5 negative

Table 3. HLA haplotypes with significant linkage disequilibria

Haplotype	H.F.[a]	Delta value	t
Bw59, Cw1	1.7%±0.4%	1.3%±0.3%	4.10
Bw59, DR4	1.3%±0.5%	0.8%±0.3%	2.62

[a] H.F., Haplotype frequency

was not due to the splitting of Bw59, but to the relatively weak cytotoxic activity of these antisera (Table 1). All individuals thought to be positive for Bw59 were positive for at least two of these four sera (Table 2).

Bw59 is cross-reactive with B8, B5, B16, and the Bw22 complex. The four antisera 9w253, 255, 259, and 447 were multispecific for Bw59 and these antigens.

The reactivity with Bw4 and Bw6 sera is helpful in distinguishing Bw59 from B8, because Bw59 is Bw4 positive whereas B8 is Bw6 positive.

No split of Bw59 was identified at this Workshop.

Family Segregation

Proper segregations of Bw59 were confirmed in all families in which this antigen was assigned.

Antigen Frequency

The antigen frequency of Bw59 in the Japanese population was 3.96%. This figure is quite similar to that (4.2% in the Oriental) reported at the last Workshop [2]. This antigen was not found in Caucasoids and is very rare in Negroes.

Linkage Disequilibria

Statistically significant linkage disequilibria between Bw59 and Cw1 and between Bw59 and DR4 [2] were confirmed in the Japanese population (Table 3).

Conclusions

(a) Four antisera specific for Bw59 were found at the present Workshop. Thus, the identification of this antigen was much easier than at the Eighth International Histocompatibility Workshop.

(b) The distribution of Bw59 is virtually restricted to Orientals. Bw59 is in linkage disequilibrium with Cw1 and DR4.

References

1. Nakai Y, Kano T, Asanuma T, Moriuchi J, Wakisaka A, Itakura K, Aizawa M (1979) A new HLA-B antigen (HOK-1) found in the Japanese. Tissue Antigens 14:47–51
2. Aizawa M, Itakura K (1980) Joint Report: Bw59 (8w69). In: Terasaki PI (ed) Histocompatibility testing 1980. UCLA Tissue Typing Laboratory, Los Angeles, p 450
3. Saji H, Maruya E (1982) Bw59. Ishoku: 495–496 (in Japanese)

Antigen Report: HLA-Bw60

S.F. Goldmann[1], D. Middleton[2] and L.J. Kennedy[3]

1 Dept. of Transplantation Immunology, Red Cross Blood Bank, Oberer Eselsberg 10, 7900 Ulm, Federal Republic of Germany
2 Belfast City Hospital, Belfast, Northern Ireland
3 Tissue Antigen Laboratory, Imperial Cancer Research Fund, P.O. Box 123, Lincolns Inn Fields, London WC2A 3PX, U.K.

History

Bw60 was serologically defined as a split of Bw40 at the Eighth International Histocompatibility Workshop 1980 [1]. It could be clearly recognized with monospecific sera, and separated from Bw61, the other Bw40 split, and from the cross-reacting antigen Bw48.

Serology

Of the sera included in the Ninth Workshop, 17 reacted strongly with Bw60 cells. Three of them (9w363, 9w365 and 9w361) were Bw60 specific; one serum (9w362) also reacted with Bw60 cells but with less strong reactions; one serum (9w360) demonstrated a high score with Bw60 and Bw41 cells; and sera 9w369 and 9w370 reacted strongly with Bw60 and Bw48 cells (Table 1). Two sera (9w356, 9w357) clearly lysed Bw60 and Bw61 cells, and sera 9w355, 9w368 and 9w353 lysed Bw60, Bw61 and Bw48 cells. Sera 9w372, 9w373, 9w374 and 9w376 showed a high score of reactivity with Bw60, Bw61, B13, and Bw47 cells. Serum 9w359 reacted strongly with Bw60, Bw61 and Bw48 and weakly with Bw41.

Linkage Disequilibrium

The known linkage disequilibrium between Bw60, Cw3, and DR4 could be confirmed [1]. There were, however, some differences in the different ethnic groups.

Conclusions

Bw60 can be clearly defined with the 9ws specific sera 9w363, 9w365, 9w361, and 9w362. The antigen is well distinguished from the other Bw40 split Bw61 and also from the crossreacting antigen Bw48 and the antigens B13, Bw41, and Bw47 in the workshop sera.

Reference

1. Dawkins RL, Houliston JB (1980) Joint Report: Bw60. In: Terasaki PI (ed) Histocompatibility testing 1980. UCLA Tissue Typing Laboratory, Los Angeles, pp 453–457

Table 1. Reactivity[a] of Ninth Workshop sera defining Bw60

9w sera	Bw60	Bw61	Bw48	Bw47	Bw41	B13	B7
365	++++	–	–	–	–	–	–
370	++++	–	++++	–	–	+	–
369	++++	–	++++	–	–	–	–
363	++++	–	–	–	–	–	–
360	++++	–	–	–	++++	–	–
362	+++	–	+	–	–	–	–
361	+++	–	–	–	–	–	–
356	++++	+++	+	–	–	+	–
355	++++	+++	++++	–	–	–	–
368	++++	++++	++++	–	–	–	+
357	+++	+++	–	–	–	–	–
353	++++	++++	++++	–	–	–	–
359	++++	++++	++++	–	++	–	–
372	++++	++++	–	+++	–	++++	–
373	++++	++++	–	+++	–	++++	–
374	++++	++++	–	++++	–	++++	–
376	++++	++++	–	++++	+	++++	–

[a] Q scores: >6: ++++, 4–5.9: +++, 3–3.9: ++, 1–2.9: +, <1: –

Histocompatibility Testing 1984
Edited by E. D. Albert et al.

Antigen Report: HLA-Bw61

S.F. Goldmann[1], D. Middleton[2], and L.J. Kennedy[3]

1 Dept. of Transplantation Immunology, Red Cross Blood Bank, Oberer Eselsberg 10, 7900 Ulm, Federal Republic of Germany
2 Belfast City Hospital, Belfast, Northern Ireland
3 Tissue Antigen Laboratory, Imperical Cancer, Research Fund, P.O. Box 123, Lincolns Inn Fields, London WC2A 3PX, U.K.

History

The subdivision of Bw40 in two subtypic antigens Bw60 and Bw61 was first described in an African Indian population by Hammond et al [1]. The two Bw40 splits were later also found in Caucasians and Japanese [2, 3]. However, monospecific Bw40 subtype sera were found only for the definition of Bw60 and not for Bw61 [3]. Therefore Bw61 could only be recognized by subtraction.

Serology

Of the sera included in the Ninth Workshop, 16 showed a high score for reactivity with Bw61 cells. However, only serum 9w366 reacted mainly with Bw61; the other 10 sera defined the two Bw40 subtypes Bw60 and Bw61. Two sera, 9w356 and 9w357, were duospecific for Bw61 and Bw60; sera 9w353, 9w355, 9w359, and 9w368 reacted with Bw61 and Bw60, and also with Bw48; and sera 9w372, 9w373, 9w374, and 9w376 reacted equally strong with Bw61, Bw60, B13 and Bw47 cells (Table 1). Though no specific reagents were found, definition of Bw61 was possible by subtraction when the four Bw60-specific sera (9w361, 9w362, 9w363, and 9w365), three duospecific sera (9w369, 9w370 and 9w360) were negative, and the sera containing Bw60 and Bw61 were positive.

Linkage Disequilibrium

Linkage disequilibrium with Cw2 was again found in Caucasians, and with Cw3 in Orientals.

Conclusions

Only one serum (9w366) was found to react mainly with Bw61 cells. Although there were no specific sera detecting Bw61 at this Workshop, Bw61 was rather well defined when the operational specific Bw60 sera or duospecific Bw60 sera not containing Bw61 antibodies were negative and the other sera reacting with Bw60 and Bw61 cells were positive. Definition was, therefore, impossible when both Bw60 and Bw61 were present on the same cell. Bw61 is associated with Cw2 in Caucasians and with Cw3 in Orientals.

Table 1. Reactivity[a] of Ninth Workshop sera defining Bw61

9w sera	Bw61	Bw60	Bw48	B13	Bw47	Bw41	B7
366	+++	+	–	–	–	–	–
356	+++	++++	+	–	–	+	–
357	+++	+++	–	–	–	–	–
353	++++	++++	++++	–	–	–	–
355	+++	++++	++++	–	–	–	–
368	++++	++++	++++	–	–	–	+
359	++++	++++	++++	–	–	–	–
372	++++	++++	–	++++	+++	–	–
373	++++	++++	–	++++	+++	–	–
374	++++	++++	–	++++	++++	–	–
376	++++	++++	–	++++	++++	+	–
365	–	++++	–	–	–	–	–
363	–	++++	–	–	–	–	–
362	–	+++	–	–	–	–	–
361	–	+++	+	–	–	–	–
369	–	++++	++++	–	–	–	–
370	–	++++	++++	–	–	–	–
360	–	++++	–	–	–	++++	–

[a] Q scores: >6: ++++, 4–5.9: +++, 3–3.9: ++, 1–2.9: +, <1: –

Histocompatibility Testing 1984
Edited by E. D. Albert et al.

References

1. Hammond MG, Appado B, Brain P (1972) HLA antigens and antibodies in South African Indians. Tissue Antigens 2:389
2. Dick HE, Bodmer WF (1977) Joint report 4: HLA-A, -B and -C serology. In: Bodmer WF, Batchelor JR, Bodmer JG, Festenstein H, Morris PJ (eds) Histocompatibility testing 1977. Munksgaard, Copenhagen, pp 178–180
3. Thompson JP (1980) Joint report: Bw60. In: Terasaki PI (ed) Histocompatibility testing 1980. UCLA Tissue Typing Laboratory, Los Angeles, pp 458–461

Antigen Report: HLA-Bw62 and Other Bw6-Associated Variants of B15

D. Chandanayingyong [1], A. Cambon-Thomsen [2], and M.G. Hammond [3]

1 Blood Bank, Siriraj Hospital, Bangkok 10700, Thailand
2 INSERM U. 100, Unité de Recherches d'Immunologie et de Cytogénétique, 31052 Toulouse Cedex, France
3 P.O. Box 2356 Natal Institute of Immunology, Durban, South Africa

History

Subdivisions of B15 were suggested at the Fourth International Workshop [18] and were reported at the Sixth Workshop to be found often in Malay and Chinese populations [11]. Sera against these variants were described as early as 1974 [14]. During the Seventh Workshop, one component appeared to be associated with Bw4 and another with Bw6 [9]. At the Eighth Workshop, two splits were defined: Bw62, which is Bw6 associated [17], with one exception recently published [1], and Bw63, which is Bw4 associated [19]; a third split was proposed in Negroids: 8w66, which is Bw4 associated [7]. During the Seventy-second International Cell Exchange, further splits of B15 were suggested: B15.3 in Chinese [12] and a new B15 variant in Vietnamese [13], both of which are Bw6 associated. At the Second Asia-Oceania Histocompatibility Workshop, an antigen report on B15 described a short pattern of reaction within Bw62, called Bw62.1 [15].

Serology

During this Workshop, the complexity of B15 has been described in nine newsletters [2–6, 8, 10, 16, 20], and the different patterns of reactions are shown in Table 1. Bw62 was clearly defined by positive reaction with four monospecific sera: 9w285, 9w286, 9w284, and 9w289, with Q scores of 8.9, 8.5, 7.4, and 5.3 respectively. Bw62.1 or sh (short) was defined by negative reaction with these four key sera for Bw62. Twenty-five families in this Workshop, six from Japan, four from Thailand and China, 11 from South Africa and four from the USA, with 28 informative sibs, showed clear segregation of this split. B15.3 and B15 SL were negative with the above-mentioned sera and also with a number of other sera (see Table 1). B15 G and B15 Sau seem to be rather similar, and further data are needed in order to support a clear difference between the two. B15 S (Siamese), in contrast, seems to have a pattern different from that of other splits mentioned and to react with some Bw45 sera. Separate segregation of B15 S (Siamese) and B15 T (Thai; see report on Bw63) was also seen in one family (FAM ANZ DCH 06; Fig. 1).

Linkage Disequilibrium

The gene frequencies of Bw62 as calculated in the Workshop Central Analysis were 0.06 for Caucasoids and 0.08 for Mongoloids. A strong linkage disequilibrium was noted with Cw3.1 and with Cw3.2, and an association with DR4 in Caucasoids and DRw9 in Mongoloids.

Conclusion

Bw62 was well defined in this Workshop and a number of other Bw6-associated B15 components were defined. Bw62.1 or sh (short) seems to be well defined, but the other splits need further studies.

Histocompatibility Testing 1984
Edited by E. D. Albert et al.

Table 1. Reaction pattern of B15 on Ninth Workshop sera

	173	174	175	179	180	276	277	278	281	282	284	285	286	289	299	305	307	308	309	310	311	312	313	401	402
Bw62				–	–	+	+	+	+	+	+	+	+	+	–	–	+	+	+	+	+	+	+		
Bw62.1 (sh):																									
Ts-1 [16]				+	+	+	+	+	+	+	–	–	–	–	0	–	+	+	+	+	+	+	+		
B15 Short Thai [5]				+	+	+	+	+	+	+	–	–	–	–	–	–	+	+	+	+	+	+	+		
B15 KEMP [3]				+	0	+	+	+	+	w	–	–	–	–	0	–	+	+	+	+	+	+	+		
SH 7 [20]				+	+	+	+	+	+	+	–	–	–	–	0	0	+	+	+	+	+	+	+		
Bw62 S [10]				0	0	+	+	+	+	+	–	–	–	–	0	0	+	+	+	+	+	+	+		
B15.3				0	0	–	–	–	w	–	–	–	–	–	–	–	+	+	+	+	w	+	+		
B15 SL1 [2]				–	–	–	w	–	w	–	–	–	–	0	0	–	+	+	+	+	+	+	+		
B15 S (Siamese) [4]				–	–	–	–	+	+	+	0	–	–	+	–	–	+	+	+	–	–	–	–	+	+
B15 Sau [2]				–	+	–	–	–	–	+	–	–	–	–	0	–	–	+	+	+	+	+	+		
B15 G [2]				+	+	–	–	–	+	+	w	–	–	–	0	w	+	+	+	+	+	+	+		
Bw63	+	+	±	–	–	+	+	+	+	–	–	–	–	w	+	+	+	+	+	+	–	w	w		
8w66	+	+	+	–	–	±	±	±	±	–	–	–	–	–	–	+	+	+	+	+	–	+	+		
B15 T (Thai) [4]	–	–	–	–	–	+	+	+	–	–	0	–	–	–	–	–	+	+	+	–	+	+	+		

(0: not tested; w: weak reaction)

FAM ANZ, DCH 06

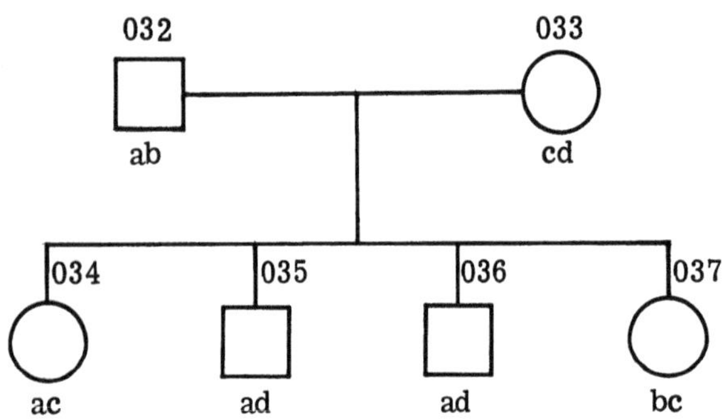

a = A2, B15S, Cw3 BW6 b = A2, B15T, Cw-, BW4

c = A11, B51, Cw -, BW4 d = Aw19, Bw44, Cw7, BW4

References

1. Alonso A, Ollier W, Doyle P, Williams E, Festenstein H (1983) Family investigation demonstrating the association of HLA-Bw62 with HLA-Bw4. Tissue Antigens 22:32–36
2. Alonso A, Doyle P, Williams E, Festenstein H (1984) Further splits of HLA-B15. Ninth Workshop Newsletter V
3. Campbell EM, Taljaard DG, Du Toit ED (1984) B15 Kemp/B15 short Thai. Ninth Workshop Newsletter V
4. Chandanayingyong D (1983) A possible new Thai variant of B15. Ninth Workshop Newsletter II
5. Chiewsilp P, Chandanayingyong D, Sujirachato K (1983) B15 short Thai. Ninth Workshop Newsletter II
6. Coates E, Stratton A, Dewar PJ (1983) Definition of Bw62, Bw63 and B15.3. Ninth Workshop Newsletter IV
7. Danilovs J, Pollock C (1980) 8w66. In: Terasaki PI (ed) Histocompatibility testing 1980. UCLA Tissue Typing Laboratory, Los Angeles, pp 477–479
8. Dejour G, Fauchet R, Jalais E, Bouhallier O, Genetet B (1983) B15.3 (Chinese) specificity. Ninth Workshop Newsletter III
9. Dick HB (1978) HLA-A, B and C serology and antigen reports. In: Bodmer W et al (eds) Histocompatibility testing 1977. Munksgaard, Copenhagen, p 157
10. Hammond MG (1984) HLA-B15 complex in South African Indians. Ninth Workshop Newsletter VIII
11. Joysey VC, Roger JH, Bland C, et al (1975) Further studies on a Malay population. In: Kissmeyer-Nielsen F

(ed) Histocompatibility testing 1975. Munksgaard, Copenhagen, p 251
12. Loon J, Bernoco D, Terasaki P, Takemura S (1981) Report of the 72nd International Cell Exchange. UCLA Tissue Typing Laboratory, Los Angeles
13. Loon J, Terasaki PI, Takemura S (1981) Report of the 73rd Cell and 1st Serum Exchange. UCLA Tissue Typing Laboratory, Los Angeles
14. Richiardi P, Castagneto M, D'Amarro J, et al (1974) Four new HLA allelic factors subtypic to HLA-12 and W15. Their correlation with W4 and W6. J Immunogenet 1:323
15. Saueracker G, Christiansen FT, Dawkin RL (1981) Antigen Report ABC B15. In: Simmons MJ, Tait BD (eds) Proceedings of the Second Asia and Oceania Histocompatibility Workshop Conference 1981. Immunopublishing, Victoria, Australia, p 80
16. Shiraki T, Akasa T, Asami M, Ueda Y, Morishima Y, Hasegawa I, Yoshida TO (1983) A study of a new HLA-B locus antigen TS-1 with 9th workshop sera. Ninth Workshop Newsletter III
17. Singal DP, Lung P (1980) Bw62. In: Terasaki PI (ed) Histocompatibility testing 1980. UCLA Tissue Typing Laboratory, Los Angeles, pp 462–464
18. Thorsby E, Kissmeyer-Nielsen F, Svejgaard A (1970) New alleles of the HLA system: serological and genetic studies. In: Terasaki PI (ed) Histocompatibility testing 1970. Munksgaard, Copenhagen, p 137
19. Troup GM (1980) Bw63. In: Terasaki PI (ed) Histocompatibility testing 1980. UCLA Tissue Typing Laboratory, Los Angeles, pp 465–468
20. Zhao TM, Lee TD, Bu KJ, Zhang GL, Rubinstein P (1984) Definition of the HLA-B antigen SH 7, identical to TS-1 in the Chinese population. Ninth Workshop Newsletter VII

Antigen Report: HLA-Bw63 and Other Bw4-Associated Variants of B15

A. Cambon-Thomsen [1], D. Chandanayingyong [2], M. Thomsen [1], and M.G. Hammond [3]

1 INSERM U. 100, Hôpital Purpan, 31052 Toulouse Cedex, France
2 Blood Bank, Faculty of Medicine and Siriraj Hospital, Mahidol University, Bangkok 10700, Thailand
3 Natal Institute of Immunology, P.O. Box 2356, Durban 4000, South Africa

History

Bw63 was clearly defined at the Eighth International Histocompatibility Workshop as a Bw4-associated subdivision of B15, as had been suggested at previous workshops [3]. At the same workshop another component of B15, also included in Bw4, and found preferentially in Negroids, was also described: 8w66, which had been first suggested in the 31st International Cell Exchange of Terasaki [2].

Serology

At the Ninth Workshop, among the 25 sera reacting strongly with at least one component of B15, none was monospecific for Bw63. This antigen was defined by positive reaction with sera directed against B15 + B17: 9w310, 307, 309, 308, 305, 278, and 299, with Q scores from 9.6 to 5.0, or against B15 alone: 9w276, 281, and 277, with Q scores of 6.3, 4.8, and 4.8, respectively. Among these sera, 9w305 and 299 did not react with Bw62-positive cells. Serum 9w278 was negative on Negroid Bw63-positive cells and positive on Caucasoid Bw63-positive cells. Some sera reacted only with cells from Bw63-homozygous individuals: 9w289, 290, 314. Bw63 was also defined by negative reactions with the Bw62-specific sera (9w282, 284, 285, 286, and 289). The following sera also had some Bw63 activity in the tail analysis: 9w176, 316, 323, 306, 234, 286, 163, and 302. Antigen 8w66 was assigned only to seven cells in the Negroid population. The pattern of reactivity was shorter than that of Bw63: negative reaction with 9w299 and variable pattern with 9w276, 277, 278, and 281. In addition, three sera directed against B5 and B49 reacted with 8w66-positive cells: 9w173, 174, and 175; 9w173 and 174 also contained some anti-Bw63 activity. Another pattern of B15: B15T was described in a Thai family: ANZ DCH 06 [1]: this variant had the same pattern as 8w66, but sera 9w173, 174, and 175 were negative. All the reaction patterns are tabulated in the report on Bw62 in this volume.

Linkage Disequilibrium

The gene frequency of Bw63 is 0.006 in Caucasoid and Mongoloid populations. The most frequent associations were with A24, A32, Cw7, Cw-, DRw6, and BfF in Caucasoids, while Bw63 was associated with A26, Cw3, and DR5 in Mongoloids.

Histocompatibility Testing 1984
Edited by E. D. Albert et al.

Conclusion

Bw63 was clearly defined at the Ninth Workshop although no monospecific serum was available. The other variants of B15 associated with Bw4 need further confirmation.

References

1. Chandanayingyong D (1983) A possible new Thai variant of B15. Workshop Newsletter no. 2
2. Danilovs J, Pollock C (1980) Joint report: 8w66. In: Terasaki PI (ed) Histocompatibility testing 1980. UCLA Tissue Typing Laboratory, Los Angeles, pp 477–479
3. Troup GM (1980) Joint report: Bw63. In: Terasaki PI (ed) Histocompatibility testing 1980. UCLA Tissue Typing Laboratory, Los Angeles, pp 465–468

Antigen Report: HLA-Bw67

P.L. Mattiuz[1], T.O. Yoshida[2], E.D. du Toit[3], C. Conighi[1], E.M. Campbell[3], and T. Akaza[4]

1 Institute of Medical Genetics, Via L. Borsari 46, 44100 Ferrara, Italy
2 Hamamatsu University School of Medicine, 3600 Harida-Cho, Hamamatsu City 431-31, Japan
3 Provincial Laboratory for Tissue Immunology, Private Bag 4, 7935 Observatory, Cape Town, South Africa
4 Nagoya Daini Red Cross Hospital, 2–9 Myokencho, Shoowaku, Nagoya 466, Japan

History

During the Sixth and Seventh Workshop, new HLA-B specificities (SN-2, BF, Te90) intermediate between B16 and Bw22 were described [1, 2]. During the Eighth Workshop, these specificities were coded as 8w57: the antigen could be defined by sera belonging to the B16 or Bw22 cross-reacting groups [3]. At the Ninth Workshop, 8w57 received the official designation of Bw67.

Serology

During the Ninth Workshop, some sera recognizing specificities belonging to B16 (sera 9w333, 332, 443, and 444) and/or to Bw22 (sera 9w445, 236, and 444) cross-reacting groups also recognized the specificity Bw67 in the Japanese population. The presence of this antigenic specificity can be easily detected by means of sera 9w333 (Q score [4] 6.7), 332 (Q score 5.1), 445 (Q score 5.8), and 443 (Q score 5.9); serum 445 seems to be monospecific (although the reaction is not very strong) and it is of Japanese origin. The patterns of reaction of these sera with B38, B39, B7, Bw42, Bw54, Bw55, Bw56, and Bw67 are shown in Table 1. The reaction pattern indicating the presence of Bw67 segregates together with a B locus "blank" allele in ten families of Japanese origin (Table 2). It is noteworthy that four of the ten Bw67 haplotypes carry A11 and six carry DR2, whereas the frequencies of these alleles, estimated from population data [5], are respectively 0.09 and 0.20; an increased frequency of A11 in individuals carrying Bw67 (then called SN-2 or 8w57) was observed by Naito et al. [1] and by Wolf [3]. All the haplotypes with Bw67 carry the supertypic antigen Bw6.

Table 1. Serum reaction patterns

Specificity	9w serum no.			
	332	333	443	445
B38	+	+	–	–
B39	+	+	±	–
B7	–	–	±	–
Bw42	–	±	±	–
Bw54	–	–	–	–
Bw55	–	±	±	–
Bw56	–	–	–	–
Bw67	+	+	+	+

Table 2. HLA alleles segregating with Bw67

Family no.	HLA alleles at locus			
	A	C	B	DR
JAP MIY 01	2	–	– w6	2
JAP MIY 82	–	–	– w6	–
JAP SEK 54	–	–	– w6	2
JAP SEK 84	w33	–	– w6	2
JAP TOK 09	11	–	– w6	–
JAP TOK 10	24	–	– w6	4
JAP TSU 44	11	–	– w6	2
JAP TSU 55	11	–	– w6	2
JAP YOS 07	2	w7	– w6	–
UK5 PAK 18	11	–	– w6	2

Histocompatibility Testing 1984
Edited by E. D. Albert et al.

Conclusions

Some of the sera submitted to the Ninth Workshop clearly identify the specificity Bw67 (formerly SN-2, BF, Te90, 8w57), which is subtypic to Bw6. This antigen, observed only in families of Japanese origin, is probably in positive linkage disequilibrium with A11, and perhaps with DR2.

References

1. Naito S, Saito S, Toyoda K, Konomi K, Yamamoto H, Okochi K (1975) A study of anti-w22 complex sera in the Japanese population and the characterization of a possible new antigen of the second segregant series, called SN-2. In: Kissmeyer-Nielsen F (ed) Histocompatibility testing 1975. Munksgaard, Copenhagen, pp 289–298
2. Ivaskova E, Mackintosh P, Radvany R (1977) Bw16 (Bw38, Bw39). In: Bodmer WF, Batchelor JR, Bodmer JG, Festenstein H, Morris PJ (eds) Histocompatibility testing 1977. Munksgaard, Copenhagen, p 175
3. Wolf E (1980) 8w57. In: Terasaki PI (ed) Histocompatibility testing 1980. UCLA Tissue Typing Laboratory, Los Angeles, pp 469–472
4. Mickey MR, Terasaki PI (1980) The serological data of the 8th Workshop and summary analyses. In: Terasaki PI (ed) Histocompatibility testing 1980. UCLA Tissue Typing Laboratory, Los Angeles, pp 21–25
5. Baur MP, Danilovs JA (1980) Population analysis of HLA-A, B, C, DR and other genetic markers. In: Terasaki PI (ed) Histocompatibility testing 1980. UCLA Tissue Typing Laboratory, Los Angeles, pp 955–993

Antigen Report: HLA-Bw70, HLA-Bw71, and HLA-Bw72

G.J. Laundy[1], C. Raffoux[2], G.M.T. Schreuder[3], and P.T. Klouda[1]

1 U.K. Transplant Service, S.W. Regional Transfusion Centre, Southmead, Bristol BS10 4ND, U.K.
2 INSERM U. 93, Hôpital St. Louis, 2, place du Dr. Fourniers, 75010 Paris, France
3 Dept. of Immunohematology, Blood Bank, University Hospital, Rijnsburgerweg 10, 2333 AA Leiden, The Netherlands

The antigens Bu (= Bw71) and SV (= Bw72) were originally identified in 1977 in English and Dutch populations [1, 2]. Both were recognised as low-frequency Bw6-associated antigens included in the tail of some multispecific sera defining the B5, 35, 18, 15, 21 (7b) cross-reactive group. A two-centre collaborative study established that Bu and SV were two independent, though closely related and cross-reactive, specificities [3].

At the Eighth Histocompatibility Workshop, Bw71 and Bw72 were included in the 8w59 specificity [4], which probably corresponds to the Da(6) residue of Da6 originally defined by platelet complement fixation [5, 6]. Data from the Eighth Workshop confirmed the existence of these two discrete, independently segregating specificities [4]. Bw71 was shown to be associated with A28 and, particularly in Negroes, with Cw3. Bw72 was shown to be in moderate association with A1 in Caucasians and in strong association with A23 and Cw2 in Negroes. These associations were confirmed in a study of an East African Black population [7].

Reported antigen frequencies vary from 0.9% Bw70 (Bu + SV) in 2800 Dutch and English Caucasoids [3], with a ratio of 2 : 1 for Bw72 : Bw71, to a combined frequency of over 30% in East African Black subjects, with Bw72 again representing the majority [7]. This corresponds to Da(6), which was found to by very common in Negroes but which occurred in less than 1% of Caucasians [8].

Reappraisal of laboratory antigen assignments in the workshop raw data file identified 99 examples of Bw70 in 93 families (out of a total of 2102 families) and a further 29 examples amongst 1208 unrelated donors used in the workshop cellular studies. In the absence of informative family, studies Bw71 and Bw72 could not be reliably assigned in the presence of B35 or B15. Six cells were excluded from the final pattern analysis because of incomplete data.

Eleven sera identified all or part of Bw70; six of these were submitted as recognizing this antigen. The distinction between Bw71 (Bu) and Bw72 (SV) is based primarily on the reaction patterns of four sera (9w180, 179, 186, 317). Five others proved useful in defining the Bw70 antigen (9w313, 312, 311, 315, 202).

Several reaction patterns were evident (Table 1). These could be divided into two groups. The first is characterized by strong positive reactions with serum 9w180 and mostly positive reactions with serum 9w179 (30/44 cells). Of the 44 cells in this group, 12 do not react with either 9w179 or 9w186; 8 of these are Caucasoid. The first group includes five previously reported Bw71-positive families.

Table 1. Serological definition Bw71 and Bw72

		Ninth Workshop sera 180	179	186	317	313	312	311	315	202	338	1136	No.	Race C	N	M	O
Bu (Bw71)	1	+	+	+	+	+	+	+	+	+	+	+	14	4	7	1	2
	2	+	+	–	+	+	+	+	+	+	+	+	10	2	4	2	2
	3	+	–	–	+	+	+	+	±	+	±	+	10	7	2	1	
	4	+	–	+	+	+	+	+	+	+	+	+	2		1		1
	5	+	+	+	±	+	+	±	+	+	+	+	2		1	1	
	6	+	–	–	–	+	+	+	+	±	–	+	2	1		1	
	7	+	+	–	–	+	+	–	–	+	–	+	4			4	
SV (Bw72)	1	–	–	–	+	+	+	+	+	+	+	+/0	34	5	23	1	5
	2	–	–	–	+	+	+	+	+	+	–	+	20	11	5	1	3
	3	–	–	–	+	+	+	±	+	±	±	±	14	9	2	2	1
	4	–	–	–	–	+	+	+	+	±	–	+	6	4			2
	5	–	+	–	±	+	+	+	±	+	+	+	4	1	2		1
B5					+	+			+			+					
Bw53			±		+	+	+		+			+					
B35		+	+	±	+	+	+	+	+	+	±	+	Cross-				
B18					+	+							reactive				
B15		±	±	±	+	+	+	+	+	+	±	±	antigens				
B17							±										
B49					+		+		±			+					
Bw50				±		+	+	+	+	+							
Bw22						±	+			+	+	±					

C, Caucasoid; N, Negroid; M, Mongoloid; O, other; ±, positive or negative reaction; +/0, positive or not tested

The second group of 78 cells is characterized by negative reactions with sera 9w180, 179, and 186. This group includes four previously reported Bw72-positive families. The majority of Negroid Bw72 cells react with all the remaining sera (Bw72 pattern 1). Caucasoid cells tend to have more variable reactivity and are generally negative with serum 9w338 (Bw72 patterns 2, 3, and 4). A monoclonal antibody, 9w1136, reacts with all Bw71 cells but was negative with 10 of 70 cells classified as Bw72-positive (8 cells were not tested).

Bw71 shows a moderate association with A28 and Cw3, whereas Bw72 strongly associated with A9 and Cw2, particularly in Negroes. Both Bw71 and Bw72 are included in Bw6.

Three Negroid families had either Bw71 or Bw72 in each parent and showed good serological segregation of the two specificities. In one other family, Bw71 and Bw72 were identified in one parent. Due to the presence of B35 in the other parent, this family was not informative. The proportions of Bw72 and Bw71 found in Caucasians (30 and 14) and Negroes (32 and 15) agrees with that previously observed [3, 7]. Of 14 Bw70-positive Mongoloid families, 10 were Bw71 positive. Of these, 4 showed an unusual reaction pattern in which they were negative with sera 9w317, 311, 315, and 338 (Bw71, pattern 7). All four families were from the ANZ region; one was Maori and the others unclassified Mongoloid.

The combined frequency of Bw71 and Bw72 in random families varied from 29% in black Africans and 11% in black Americans to 2% in Japanese and 0.9% in West European Caucasoids.

Bw71 and Bw72 are well recognised antigens, which show good serological segregation. In the absence of B35 and, in most cases, B15, Bw71 and Bw72 can be readily assigned with the aid of the 9W serum set even though it does not include a monospecific reagent. The Bu-SV antigen was given workshop recognition (see: Nomenclature for factors of the HLA system 1984, this volume) as Bw70 with the splits Bw71 (w70) = Bu and Bw72 (w70) = SV.

References

1. Laundy GJ, Entwistle CC (1977) Bu – A new antigen at the HLA-B locus. Tissue Antigens 10:180
2. Schreuder I, Bos A, van de Berg-Loonen E (1977) SV = PR. A new B-locus antigen discovered. In: Bodmer WF, et al (ed) Histocompatibility testing 1977. Munksgaard, Copenhagen, p 408

3. Schreuder I, Nieman HG, Laundy GJ, Entwistle CC (1980) Bu and SV: Two closely related B-locus specificities. Tissue Antigens 16:169–175
4. Entwistle CC, Laundy GJ (1980) 8w59: Joint Report. In: Terasaki PI (ed) Histocompatibility testing 1980. UCLA Tissue Typing Laboratory, Los Angeles, p 475
5. Colombani J, Colombani M, Dausset J (1970) Cross reactions in the HL-A system with special reference to the Da6 cross-reacting group. In: Terasaki PI (ed) Histocompatibility testing 1970. Munksgaard, Copenhagen, p 79
6. Degos L, Colombani J, Kissmeyer-Nielsen F, Svejgaard A, Mueller-Eckhardt C, van Rood JJ, Oliver RTD (1975) Joint report on platelet complement fixation workshop. In: Kissmeyer-Nielsen F (ed) Histocompatibility testing 1975. Munksgaard, Copenhagen, p 348
7. Hall PJ, Levin AG, Entwistle CC, Knight SC, Wasunna A, Kung'n A, Brubaker G (1982) HLA antigens in African black patients with Burkitt's lymphoma or nasopharyngeal carcinoma and in controls: A pilot study. Hum Immunol 5:91–105
8. Oliver RTD, Festenstein H (1975) Platelet complement fixation and HL-A typing of Zambian negroids. In: Kissmeyer-Nielsen F (ed) Histocompatibility testing 1975. Munksgaard, Copenhagen, p 354

Antigen Report: HLA-Bw73

F. Kissmeyer-Nielsen[1], B. Graugaard[1], P. Kühnl[2], and W.R. Mayr[3]

1 Department of Clinical Immunology, Tissue Typing Laboratory, University Hospital of Århus, 8000 Århus C, Denmark
2 Institute of Immunohematology, University of Frankfurt, 6000 Frankfurt, Federal Republic of Germany
3 Institute of Blood Group Serology, University of Vienna, 1090 Vienna, Austria

This antigen, originally described by Mayr and Kirnbauer [1], has been assigned in 17–21 cells of the 5000 cell panel. Three sera, 9w245, 9w246 and 9w247, have Q scores between 7.5 and 6.0. They all miss approximately 20% of Bw73-positive cells, but at least two of these three sera react with all the cells. The three sera all contain anti-B7, anti-B27, and anti-Bw22 components. Thus, Bw73 can only be properly assigned on cells negative for these antigens. Serum 9w479 may be helpful, since in addition to Bw73 it contains anti-Cw4 and anti-Cw6 components, but not B7, B27 and Bw22 components. Furthermore, in some laboratories serum 9w440 behaved as an operationally specific anti-Bw73. Similar patterns were found in Caucasians and Negroes.

In the Second Workshop Newsletter we showed in family studies that the Bw73 antigen segregated as an HLA-B antigen. We also reported on a local antiserum (9963/81), which contained anti-Bw73 + anti-Cw4. During and after the Ninth Workshop, we have found four additional antisera reacting with the Bw73 antigen – all originating from multiparous women. Most often the Bw73 antigen is found on Cw7-positive cells. This antigen can also be identified on thrombocytes.

We will report later on details of about these antisera, but can state briefly that we could not demonstrate the Bw73 antigen on cells from any of the husbands. Lymphocytes from three husbands were tested in absorption experiments and were all able to remove the Bw73 activity in the serum, as could all leucocytes of different HLA phenotypes tested so far, but not leucocytes from the serum donors.

We can conclude that anti-Bw73 is very peculiar, and we cannot give any accurate explanation except to postulate:

1. It is not an auto-antibody
2. It may be a very special cross-reactive antibody

Table 1. Serum reaction patterns for assignment of Bw73

Selected antisera	Selected cells: B7–; B27–; ($n = 724$)						
9w245	+	+	+	+	–	–	–
9w246	+	+	–	–	+	–	–
9w247	+	–	+	–	–	+	–
n	26	35	21	12	10	19	601
Bw73 assigned	+	+	+	–	–	–	–
Percent	3.6	4.8	2.9	1.7	1.4	2.6	83.0

Histocompatibility Testing 1984
Edited by E. D. Albert et al.

3. Anti-Bw73 antibodies have so far been found only in pregnancy antisera

We attempted to establish patterns of serum reactions for the assignment of Bw73 = 9w81 = 8w40 = KA = IEH. There is no isolated pattern output for Bw73-positive cells, but they are included in the pattern shown in Table 1 and can thus be assigned when two or three sera react.

Cells selected were B7-negative and B27-negative cells ($n = 724$).

Reference

1. Mayr WR, Kirnbauer M (1981) Rare HLA-A, B, C antigens in Caucasoids. In: Steinberg C, Lefkovits L (eds) The immune system, vol 2. Karger, Basel, pp 217–223

Antigen Report: HLA-Bw4 and HLA-Bw6

J. D'Amaro[1], R. Fauchet[2], and E. Westphal[3]

1 Dept. of Immunohematology, University Hospital, Rijnsburgerweg 10, 2333 AA Leiden, The Netherlands
2 Laboratoire d'Histocompatibilité, Centre Regional de Transfusion Sanguine, Rennes, France
3 Tissue Typing Laboratory, Institute of Hygiene, Kiel, Federal Republic of Germany

Five Bw4 and five Bw6 sera were provided in the serum set. Their reaction patterns were highly concordant with at least four positive sera in 72% of the Bw4 cells and 76% of the Bw6 cells. Extra reactions ranged from 3% to 6% for the Bw4 sera and from 1% to 5% for the Bw6 sera. As observed in previous workshops, A9 was the most common extra specificity for the Bw4 sera, although A2, A28, and A32 were also observed. An overview of the performance of the Bw4 and Bw6 sera is shown in Table 1.

Four monoclonal antibodies demonstrated Bw4 and Bw6 specificities: 9w1155 and 9w1157 for Bw4, and 9w1143 and 9w1159 for Bw6. 9w1155

Table 1. Summary of the performance of the Ninth Workshop Bw4 and Bw6 sera

Specificity	Serum	% STR[a]	% Extra reactions	% Misses
Bw4	9w423	82	8	6
Bw4	9w425	92	3	3
Bw4	9w427	77	14	4
Bw4	9w428	90	2	7
Bw4	9w430	79	22	4
Bw6	9w431	88	7	2
Bw6	9w433	86	3	2
Bw6	9w434	85	6	5
Bw6	9w436	74	18	1
Bw6	9w439	94	1	2

[a] Percentage scores of 8 of the positive reactions

Table 2. HLA-B antigen inclusions

Bw4		*Bw6*
B5 : B51, Bw52		
Bw53		B35
		B18
		Bw70: Bw71, Bw72
Bw63 ←	B15	→ Bw62
8w66		
B17 : Bw57		Bw46
: Bw58		
B49 ←	B21	→ Bw50
B44 ←	B12	→ B45
B13		Bw73
Bw47		B40 : Bw60, Bw61
		Bw48
		Bw41
B27		B7
		Bw42
		Bw22 : Bw54, Bw55, Bw56
		Bw67
		B14 : Bw64, Bw65
Bw59		B8
B38 ←	B16	→ B39
B37		

Horizontal lines separate cross-reactive clusters

Histocompatibility Testing 1984
Edited by E. D. Albert et al.

Table 3. Segregation of a B35 (Bw4) variant in two families

Family 10, submitted by IT1CON

	Phenotype						Genotype							Code
Mother	23	30	35	41	4	6	30	35	4	/	23	41	6	CD
Father	24	11	35	38	4	6	24	38	4	/	11	35	6	AB
Child	11	30	35		4	6	11	35	6	/	30	35	4	BC
Child	11	30	35		4	6	11	35	6	/	30	35	4	BC
Child	24	30	35	38	4	–	24	38	4	/	30	35	4	AC
Child	23	11	35	41	–	6	11	35	6	/	23	41	6	BD
Child	24	30	35	36	4	–	24	38	4	/	30	35	4	AC
Child	11	30	35		4	6	11	35	6	/	30	35	4	BC
Child	23	24	38	41	4	6	24	38	4	/	23	41	6	AD

Familiy 20, submitted by FRABET

	Phenotype						Genotype							Code
Mother	32	34	8	35	4	6	32	35	4	/	34	8	6	CD
Father	11	28	53	39	4	6	11	39	6	/	28	53	4	AB
Child	28	34	8	53	4	6	28	53	4	/	34	8	6	BD
Child	11	32	53	35	4	–	11	53	4	/	32	35	4	A/B C
Child	11	34	8	39	–	6	11	39	6	/	34	8	6	AD
Child	28	32	53	35	4	–	28	53	4	/	32	35	4	BC
Child	11	34	35	39	4	6	11	39	6	/	34	35	4	AC/D

was a good Bw4 reagent but, just as in the Bw4 sera, it had extra reactions with A2, A9, and A32. 9w1157 missed many Bw4 cells and had many extra reactions. 9w1143 reacted well with Bw6 and gave extra reactions with A2 and A28 in most Caucasoids and African Negros, with A2 and A11 in Asian Indians, and with A2, A9, and Aw33 in Mongoloids, A9 being clearly the most common extra specificity. 9w1159 appears to have Bw6 reactivity but it is frequently negative or weakly positive with cells which are Bw4 and Bw6 positive.
An inclusion analysis revealed no significant deviations with previous reports. An updated report is set out in Table 2 and it includes the provisional Ninth Workshop specificities. Finally, two families with a B35 (Bw4) variant are presented in Table 3.

Antigen Report: HLA-Cw1

L.P. de Waal[1], G.G. de Lange[1], T. Sasazuki[2], and C.P. Engelfriet[1]

1 Central Laboratory, Netherlands Red Cross Blood Transfusion Service, P.O. Box 9190, Amsterdam, The Netherlands
2 Dept. of Human Genetics and Medical Research, Tokyo Medical and Dental University, Tokyo 113, Japan

History

The HLA-Cw1 antigen was well defined in 1970 at the Fourth International Histocompatibility Workshop [1].
At the Eighth Workshop [2] the gene frequency of Cw1 was determined for Caucasians to be 3.92%; for Orientals, 15.74%; and for Negroes, 0.99%. Linkage disequilibrium was observed in Caucasians with B27, B51, and Bw56 and in Orientals with the Bw22 antigens.
Especially in Orientals, Cw1 and Cw3 can be coded for by one haplotype in strong linkage disequilibrium with Bw46 [3].

Serology

Seven excellent Cw1-reactive sera (448, 449, 450, 451, 452, 453, 454) were submitted (Table 1). Two sera only reacted with Cw1-positive cells (448, 452). Serum 452, however, which was not a very strongly reactive serum, gave negative reactions

Histocompatibility Testing 1984
Edited by E. D. Albert et al.

Table 1. Selection of most specific Ninth Workshop sera with reactivity for Cw1

9W no.	Specificity	*r*	Q score	% 8 score	% Misses
448	Cw1	0.889	9.7	94	8
449	Cw1 Tail[a]: B51	0.872	10.0	93	5
450	Cw1 Tail: Cw3	0.814	8.0	94	11
451	Cw1 Tail: B51, Bw57, Bw58 Cw6	0.885	9.3	92	5
452	Cw1	0.849	6.8	69	15
453	Cw1 B27 Cw2	0.833	9.8 2.2	96	4
454	Cw1 Tail: B51, A2	0.776	8.0	94	3

[a] Tail, Q score < 1

with 15% of the Cw1-positive cells. The remaining sera had residual activity against other antigens (a Q score of < 1 was called residual activity). Pattern analysis among 1000 Japanese and 295 Chinese individuals confirmed the above data.

Conclusion

Cw1 is well defined by Ninth Workshop sera in Caucasians, Japanese, and Chinese populations.

References

1. Sandberg L, Thorsby E, Kissmeyer-Nielsen F, Lindsholm A (1970) Evidence of a third sublocus within the HLA-chromosomal region. In: Terasaki PI (ed) Histocompatibility testing 1970. Munksgaard, Copenhagen, p 165
2. Gelsthorpe K (1980) Cw1 Joint Report. In: Terasaki PI (ed) Histocompatibility testing 1980. UCLA Tissue Typing Laboratory, Los Angeles, p 482
3. Goodfellow PN, Payne R (1977) Serological studies on Cw1 and Cw3. A possible gene duplication in Oriental populations. Tissue Antigens 10:181

Antigen Report: HLA-Cw2

B.K. Jakobsen[1], C.P. Engelfriet[2], and A. Svejgaard[1]

1 Tissue Typing Laboratory, State University Hospital (Rigshospitalet), Tagensvej 20, 2200 Copenhagen Ø, Denmark
2 Central Laboratory, Netherlands Red Cross Blood Transfusion Service, P.O. Box 9190, Amsterdam, The Netherlands

Six alloantisera contained anti-Cw2: 9w455 –9w460. In the combined analysis, serum 9w458 had the lowest number of extra reactions and the fewest false negatives, whereas the other sera tended to give some extra reactions, usually associated with Cw7, B27, and/or B7. In our experience, sera 9w457, 9w458, and 9w460 behaved perfectly well as anti-Cw2 reagents, while 9w455, 9w456, and 9w459 were difficult to read because of turbidity. There was no evidence that Cw2 may be split.

The Cw2 antigen showed the same linkage disequilibria as described in previous workshops.

Histocompatibility Testing 1984
Edited by E. D. Albert et al.

Antigen Report: HLA-Cw3

E.M. Campbell[1], E.D. du Toit[1], M.M. Tongio[2], A. Urlacher[2], S. Mayer[2], and W.R. Mayr[3]

1 Provincial Laboratory for Tissue Immunology, Falmouth Rd., Observatory 7925, Cape Town, South Africa.
2 Centre de Transfusion Sanguine, 10, rue Spielmann, 67095 Strasbourg, Cedex, France
3 Institute for Blood Group Serology, University of Vienna, Spitalgasse 4, 1090 Vienna, Austria

History

Cw3 was first described by means of two sera, UPS from Copenhagen and Sa-50 from Gothenburg [9]. This antigen was confirmed as belonging to the third HLA series at the 1975 Workshop [8], where it was called Cw3. As early as 1974, Mayr [5] suggested that this antigen could be split into two parts, T3.1 and T3.2. This was confirmed at the Second Asia and Oceania Histocompatibility Workshop [2], where serum 537 from Dr. Aizawa showed that Cw3 could be split into Cw3.1 and Cw3.2.

In 1975, Payne et al. [7] noted that in some Oriental families Cw3 could occur concurrently with Cw1 on the same haplotype. Additional information at the Second Asia and Oceania Workshop showed that it was the Cw3.2 split that occurred with Cw1 on the same haplotype in strong linkage disequilibrium with Bw46. The question was thus raised as to whether this Cw1-Cw3 co-segregating phenotype was the consequence of a gene duplication in Orientals, as suggested by Goodfellow and Payne [4], or whether it was in fact a new C locus antigen (CWB) that could be recognized by most anti-Cw1 and Cw3 sera.

Serology

Sera 9w461, 9w462, 9w463, 9w464, 9w465, 9w466, and 9w467 were distributed as anti-Cw3 sera. They all had a high average reaction score (> 7).

The classic Cw3 specificity was best defined by sera 9w465 and 9w466 (quality score = 11.0 and 8.9), despite a few extra reactions. Sera 9w463 and 9w461 produced almost as good a definition despite a few false-negative reactions (quality score = 8.6 and 7.7). When serum 9w462 was tested, 19% of Cw3-positive cells reacted negatively, and, although serum 9w464 was a good anti-Cw3 serum, it gave additional B35 reactions. The pattern analysis of the sera defining Cw3 showed that in 80% of Cw3-positive Caucasoids and Mongoloids there was a positive reaction with at least five of the six sera.

Serum 9w467 allowed a split to be defined in Cw3. Individuals found positive with this serum were called Cw3.1, and those found negative, Cw3.2 (Table 1) [1]. Taking into account the results obtained in 5500 individuals of different racial backgrounds; Cw3.1 and Cw3.2 had almost the same frequency. The fact that Cw3 and Cw3.1 were co-capping [6] demonstrated that Cw3.1 was a true subtypic factor of Cw3. It would be very interesting to compare the splits of Cw3 as described by Mayr [5] and Chandangayingyong et al. [2] and the present Workshop split Cw3.1 as defined by serum 9w467.

Very few of the Oriental Bw46, Cw1-Cw3 cells reacted with serum 9w467, showing that these cells are usually not Cw3.1. Their reactivity to the six other anti-Cw3 sera depended on the Bw46 families tested. The cells of some families reacted positively to all six sera, others to only some of them. In this case, sera 9w461 and 9w465 were the best as both their strength and their segregation in families were

Table 1. Reaction patterns of the splits of Cw3

	461	462	463	464	465	466	467
Cw3.1	+	+	+	+	+	+	+
Cw3.2	+	+	+	+	+	+	–
Cw3.3	+	(+)	(+)	–	+	–	–

Table 2. Absorption of serum 9w467 with platelets of Cw3.1, Cw3.2, and Cw1/3.2, Cw6-positive individuals

Sera / Cells	Cw3.1	Cw3.2	Cw1/3.2, Cw6
Unabsorbed serum titer	8	Neg	Neg
Serum absorbed with Cw3.1-positive platelets (2 cases)	Neg	Neg	Neg
Serum absorbed with Cw3.2-positive platelets (2 cases)	Neg	Neg	Neg
Serum absorbed with Cw1/3.2, Cw6 platelets (1 case)	4	Neg	Neg

Histocompatibility Testing 1984
Edited by E. D. Albert et al.

very good. Thus, the possibility of a *third split of Cw3*, Cw3.3 (see Table 1), defined by sera 9w461 and 9w465 exists, which would be most frequently found on Bw46 Cw1-Cw3 cells. Absorptions of serum 9w467 with Cw3.1, Cw3.2, and Bw46 Cw1-Cw3 platelets showed that the anti-Cw3.1 reactivity could be clearly absorbed with Cw3.1 or Cw3.2 platelets but only partially with Bw46 Cw1-Cw3 platelets (Table 2). This suggests that, at least in some cases, the Cw3 part of Cw1-Cw3 could behave differently from Cw3.1 and Cw3.2.

Linkage Disequilibrium

When first described in 1972, Cw3 specificity was found to show a linkage disequilibrium with HLA-B40, HLA-B15 and HLA-Bw22 in Caucasoids [9] and later with the A2, Cw1-Cw3, Bw46 haplotype in Mongoloids [3]. At the present Workshop (Grangé et al., this volume), the following linkage disequilibria were found: A2, Cw3, Bw60, DRw6; A24, Cw3, Bw62, BfF; A2, Cw3, Bw62; Cw3, Bw55 in Caucasoids and Aw33 or A–, Cw3, Bw58; Cw3 Bw60, DRw9; Cw3, B35 in Mongoloid populations. There were too few Negroid haplotypes for investigation. The final Workshop data necessary for the study of linkage disequilibrium with the splits of Cw3 were not available, but some were obtained from laboratories in France, Spain, South Africa, Austria, and Japan (Dr. Makoto Kuroda). These data suggested that Cw3.1 is in linkage disequilibrium with Bw55 and Bw62, and Cw3.2 with Bw60, Bw58, and Bw62 in Caucasoids; and that Cw3.1 is in linkage disequilibrium with Bw62 and B35, and Cw3.2 with Bw60 and Bw61 in Mongoloids.

References

1. Campbell EM, du Toit E (1983) Possible splits of Cw3. Ninth Workshop Newsletter I:10–13
2. Chandanayingyong D, Tait B, d'Apice A (1981) Serum 537: Does it recognize a subtype of Cw3? In: Simons MJ, Tait BD (eds) Proceedings of the Second Asia and Oceania Histocompatibility Workshop Conference, Melbourne, pp 424–427
3. Chandanayingyong D: Bw46 report. In: Simons MJ, Tait BD (eds) Proceedings of the Second Asia and Oceania Histocompatibility Workshop Conference, Melbourne, pp 127–129
4. Goodfellow PN, Payne R (1978) Serological studies of Cw1 and Cw3 expressed on the same haplotype. Tissue Antigens 11:350–356
5. Mayr W (1974) Neue Untersuchungen im Bereich des HLA Systems: ein dritter Locus mit serologisch nachweisbaren Merkmalen. Fol Haematol 101:401–411
6. Mayr WR, Kirnbauer M (1984) Cw3.1, a split of Cw3. Ninth Workshop Newsletter VI:13–14
7. Payne R, Radvany R, Grumet FC, Feldmann M, Cann H (1975) Two third series antigens transmitted together. A possible fourth SD locus? In: Kissmeyer-Nielsen F (ed) Histocompatibility testing 1975. Munksgaard, Copenhagen, pp 343–347
8. Staub-Nielsen L, Ryder LP, Svejgaard A (1975). The third (AJ) segregant series. In: Kissmeyer-Nielsen F (ed) Histocompatibility testing 1975. Munksgaard Copenhagen, pp 324–329
9. Svejgaard A, Staub-Nielsen L, Ryder LP, Kissmeyer-Nielsen F, Sandberg L, Lindholm A and Thorsby E (1972) Subdivisions of HLA-A antigens. Evidence of a "new" segregant series. In: Dausset J, Colmbani J (eds) Histocompatibility testing 1972. Munksgaard, Copenhagen, pp 465–473

Antigen Report: HLA-Cw4*

S. Scholz[1] and A. Wakisaka[2]

1 Laboratory for Immunogenetics, University Children's Polyclinic, Pettenkoferstraße 8a, 8000 Munich 2 Federal Republic of Germany

2 Tissue Typing Laboratory, University of California at Los Angeles, Los Angeles, CA, USA

As in the earlier workshops, Cw4 is very well defined at in the Ninth Workshop by six monospecific antisera (9w472, 9w470, 9w469, 9w471, 9w473, and 9w468) which are all positive in 77.4% of the Cw4-positive cells. Four additional Cw4 antisera with a tail of Cw6 react in 64.6% simultaneously with the monospecific Cw4 antisera (9w479, 9w480, 9w482, and 9w481). The quality scores for the sera are 10.0 for serum 9w470, 10.0 for serum 9w472, 9.2 for serum 9w471 and 11.0 for serum 9w482. The lowest quality score of 4.6 among these ten sera was found for serum 9w481.

There are no splits and so far no variation in the ethnic groups tested for antigen Cw4.

* Supported by DFG grants AI 92/13-1, 13-2

Antigen-Report: HLA-Cw5

J. Hay and W.R. Mayr

1 Red Cross Blood Centre, 301 Pirie Street, Adelaide 5000, South Australia
2 Institute for Blood Group Serology, University of Vienna, Spitalgasse 4, 1090 Vienna, Austria

The excitement surrounding this antigen at the Eighth Workshop was dashed at the Ninth, basically because of the frequency with which the one allele in a family sometimes gave a long reaction pattern and sometimes a short one. Coupled with this was the fact that the short pattern was as variable in these families as in those in which the pattern was always short: in the ANZ regional analysis the numbers of these two groups of families were equal.

Ten sera reacted with Cw5, three of which were anti-Cw5 + 8 (Table 1).

There was very clear distinction between positive and negative patterns, all Cw5 cells reacting with at least four, and 28% with all eight of the primary anti-Cw5 sera, 9w483–490, while 86% of Cw5-negative cells were completely unreactive to all Cw5 antisera. The quality of the sera was high, with Q scores of around 6.0 for six (sera 483–488).

Table 1. Reaction patterns in Caucasians

9ws Serum	*r*	% False positives	% False negatives	Other possible specificities
483	0.83	13	16	Cw4, B44
484	0.81	20	6	B44
485	0.77	10	26	
486	0.85	8	16	
487	0.85	8	18	
488	0.80	10	23	Cw4
489	0.61	42	22	Cw8, B14
490	0.36	22	52	B14
133	0.59	31	36	A30
274	0.45[a]	42	14	B14, Cw8

[a] *r*Cw(5 + 8) for 9w274 is 0.80

There was no strong indication of the existence of a split of Cw5, since the various short patterns varied within one family. The linkage disequilibrium between Cw5 and B44 and B18 was confirmed.

Antigen-Report: HLA-Cw6

S. Scholz[1] and A. Wakisaka[2]

1 Laboratory for Immunogenetics, University Children's Polyclinic, Pettenkoferstraße 8a, 8000 Munich Federal Republic of Germany
2 Tissue Typing Laboratory, University of California at Los Angeles, Los Angeles, CA, USA

The situation regarding definition of the Cw6 antigen with the Ninth Workshop serum set has improved but is still not completely satisfactory. There is now a better change of identifying Cw6 even if Cw4 is also present, although the reaction patterns of the sera for Cw6 are as heterogeneous as before and the quality score is greater than 1 in only 9 of 17 sera. Only four Cw6 antisera show a homogeneous reaction pattern with about 50% of the Cw6 positive cells. These sera are 9w474, 9w475, 9w476, and 9w479. The last, serum 9w479, is a Cw4 + Cw6 antiserum. The highest quality scores are: 7.3 for 9w474; 6.4 for 9w479; 6.4 for 9w475; 5.6 for 9w476; and 5.9 for 9w477. The extra reactivity against Cw4 in the four best Cw6 antisera is weak but still present. The strength of the reaction in all of these sera is over 50%. In the population pattern analysis and family segregation analysis we found no sign of any splits.

* Supported by DFG grants AI 92/13-1, 13-2

Antigen Report: HLA-Cw7

V. Lepage[1], W.R. Mayr[2], M. Busson[1], and L. Degos[1]

1 Hôpital Saint Louis, Centre Hayem, Place du Dr. A. Fournier, 75010 Paris, France
2 Institut für Blutgruppenserologie der Universität Wien, Spitalgasse 4, 1090 Wien, Austria

History

The antigen Cw7 was first defined by Dehay et al. [1] as CVE. They reported (a) that it was an allele of the HLA-C series; (b) that it was independent of HLA-A and B antigens in capping experiments; (c) that gene frequency was 0.163 in Caucasoids; and (d) that the linkage disequilibrium was found with B7 and B8. During the Eighth Workshop, Cw7 was defined by two sera with good segregation in the families, and a split into two parts was suggested [2].

Serology

Six sera were submitted to the Ninth Workshop as defining Cw7: 9w494, 495, 496, 497, 498, and 499. Two other sera are in association with Cw7: 9w314 and 9w442, submitted as defining a new ABC specificity.

The percentage of scores of 6 and 8 in the positive reactions and the specificity of the sera are shown in Table 1.

In the Caucasoid population the first six sera reacted concordantly. At least five of the six Cw7 sera were positive in 69.9% of the Cw7-positive cells. A further 10.5% of these cells react with four of the six sera.

All sera have nearly the same number of "extra" reactions, except for 9w499, 314, and 442.

In the Japanese, the six Cw7 sera were reactive concordantly in only 22% of the Cw7-positive cells; in 39% five of six sera were positive.

The segregation of Cw7 in families was good.

Table 1. Analysis of sera defining Cw7

Serum identity	Percentage of scores of 6 and 8	Percentage of missed reactions	Percentage of extra reaction
9w494	87.2	7	11
9w499	78.2	13	17
9w497	77.6	17	10
9w498	75.3	19	10
9w496	73.6	25	9
9w495	76.6	21	14
9w314	77.0	30	17
9w442	67.4	54	25

Split of Cw7

Two sera react with a part of Cw7: 9w314 and 9w442. In the French region, serum 9w442 submitted as "new ABC" gave the following results:

	+/+	+/−	−/+	−/−	Total
9w442 × Cw7	45	76	16	260	397

Among the 16 extra reactions, 12 are Cw blank (confirmed by family data). A satisfactory segregation of Cw7-9w442 positive or negative specificities is found.

Serum 9w314 includes all the Cw7 cells positive with the 9w442 serum plus some other Cw7 cells (Fig. 1). The segregation of this specificity is fairly good.

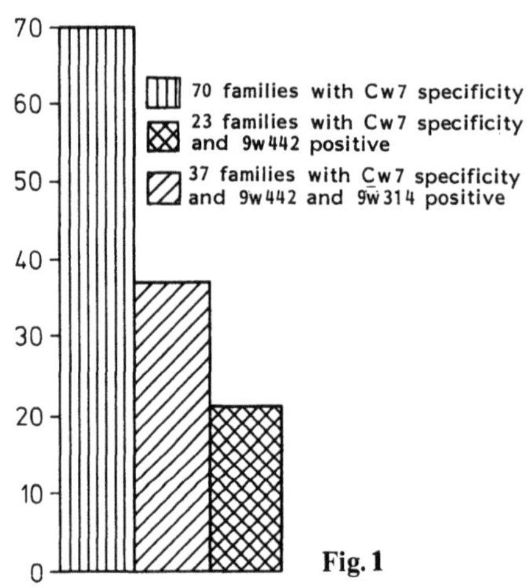

Fig. 1

Linkage Disequilibrium

The known linkage disequilibrium of Cw7 with B7 and B8 is confirmed.

Conclusion

Cw7 is well defined in Caucasoid and Japanese populations. A split is suspected (by serum 9w442 and perhaps 314).

References

1. Dehay C, Schmid M, Benajam A, Legrand L, Dausset J (1979) Seventh allele of the HLA-C series (Cve). Transplant Proc 11:613
2. Sasazuki T, Dausset J, Tokunaga K, Sato H, Okochi K, Naito S (1980) Cw7 Joint report. In: Terasaki PI (ed) Histocompatibility testing 1980. UCLA Tissue Typing Laboratory, Los Angeles, p 501

Histocompatibility Testing 1984
Edited by E. D. Albert et al.

Antigen Report: HLA-Cw8

J. Hay [1] and W.R. Mayr [2]

1 Red Cross Blood Centre, 301 Pirie Street, Adelaide 5000, South Australia
2 Institut für Blutgruppenserologie der Universität Wien, Spitalgasse 4, 1090 Wien, Austria

The definition of Cw8 was difficult, because of the cross-reactivity between Cw5 and Cw8 and the strong linkage disequilibrium with B14.
Five sera were submitted as anti-Cw8: three containing no anti-Cw5 (9w491 – 493) and two with anti-Cw5 (489, 490) (Table 1). Furthermore, serum 274 reacted as anti-Cw5 + w8. It was not clear whether these sera also reacted with B14: the analysis of a restricted material, however, indicated that sera 490 and 274 did contain anti-B14, while 493 seemed to react with B14 but not with Cw8.

Table 1. Reaction patterns in Caucasians

9WS Serum	*r*	% False positive	% False negative	Other possible specificities
489	0.60	10	0.8	Cw5
490	0.69	8	0.1	Cw5
491	0.65	0.8	4	
492	0.65	6	2	B14, Cw3, B40Ch., B15Ch.
274	0.49 [a]	11	0.4	B14

[a] r Cw(8 + 5) for 9w274 is 0.80

Fifty-four cells in the ANZ region, designated neither B14 nor Cw8, reacted with serum 492; of these cells 94% were Mongoloid, and 86% of them were designated B15/Cw blank: 25 of 25 Thai and 12 of 14 Chinese cells. These extra reactions of 492 with cells showing at most one known HLA-C antigen were confirmed in other regions. This reaction pattern segregated with haplotypes carrying C blank and therefore suggested that serum 492 recognizes a new allele at the C locus besides Cw8.
In summary, it can be concluded that Cw8 is still not very well defined, essentially because of cross-reactivity with Cw5 and strong gametic association with B14.

Antigen Report: New HLA-C

L. Degos [1] and G. Mueller-Eckhardt [2]

1 Hôpital Saint Louis, 2, Place du Dr. Fournier, 75010, Paris, France
2 Institute of Clinical Immunology and Blood Transfusion, 6300 Giessen, Federal Republic of Germany

History

Among the new C antigens proposed during the Eighth International Histocompatibility Workshop [1 – 5] one, previously called T8 or T9, was newly designated Cw8, in linkage disequilibrium with B14 in the Caucasian population. T10 and T11 (in linkage disequilibrium with B16) were not well defined.
From the new set of Cw sera studied for prescreening at the Ninth International Histocompatibility Workshop, serum N858 (Hammond) could be a candidate for a new C specificity in linkage disequilibrium with the B5 antigen [6]. This serum was not included in those submitted to the Ninth International Histocompatibility Workshop. A combined antigen, Cw1-Cw3, with both specificities transmitted together, has also been described in previous papers [7, 8].

Serological Splits of Cw3

Several reports in the Newsletters [9 – 15] described a split of Cw3, observed with serum 9w467, into *Cw3.1* (positive with serum 467); and *Cw3.2* (negative with serum 467).
An equal proportion of each subgroup exists in Caucasians (Cw3.1 = 46%) while Cw3.2 is more common in Negroes and Mongoloids.

Histocompatibility Testing 1984
Edited by E. D. Albert et al.

Familial segregation confirms the existence of these two alleles in the three populations [15]. Lysostrip experiments confirmed that Cw3.1 is carried by the Cw3 gene product [12].
Linkage disequilibria are different for the two splits in Caucasians (Cw3.1/Bw55 and Bw62; Cw3.2/Bw60, Bw58, and Bw62).

Cwl.Cw3 or Cw3 SHI: A positive reaction with three Cw3 sera (9w461, 463, 465) and negative reactivity with the other Cw3 (9w462, 464, 466, 467) is often associated with a positive reactivity with six Cwl sera (9w448, 441, 451, 452, 453, 454). This Cwl-Cw3 specificity is found mainly in Chinese and Thai cells. A strong positive linkage disequilibrium is found with Bw46. This Cwl-Cw3 specificity is transmitted as a unique specificity in family data.

Cw7 Splits

Two sera (9w314 and 9w442) subdivided the Cw7 specificity (see V. Lepage et al., Cw7 report, this volume).

Serum 447

In the French region, this serum reacted with 34 of 330 cells from unrelated individuals. No defined Cw specificity was found in 9 cases, and only one Cw specificity in 19 cases. Thus, in 28 cases it corresponds to a Cw blank. The 6 other cells which possess two Cw specificities were typed as Cw4 (4/6) and Cw6 (3/6).
Thirty-nine families were studied for the Workshop in various laboratories. In 25 families serum 9w447 segregated as a Cw blank. It was associated 15 times with Bw38. In 6 families it reacted with Cw6 sera, and in 4 families with Cw7. In 4 families the segregation did not follow HLA haplotypes.

References

1. Trabace S, Belvedere M, Richiardi P, Olivetti E (1980) Possible new HLA-C antigens. In: Terasaki PI (ed) Histocompatibility testing 1980. UCLA Tissue Typing Laboratory, Los Angeles, p 787
2. Zachary A, Murphy N, Braun E (1980) New C locus in linkage disequilibrium with B14. In: Terasaki PI (ed) Histocompatibility testing 1980. UCLA Tissue Typing Laboratory, Los Angeles, p 788
3. Julin M, Kokimies S, Lokki M (1980) Possible New HLA-C locus antigens. In: Terasaki PI (ed) Histocompatibility testing 1980. UCLA Tissue Typing Laboratory, Los Angeles, p 789
4. Mayr WK, Kirnbauer M, Mayr D (1980) New HLA-C antigens defined by 8w antisera. In: Terasaki PI (ed) Histocompatibility testing 1980. UCLA Tissue Typing Laboratory, Los Angeles, p 798
5. Mervart H, Tibensky D (1980) Possible new C locus antigen TII. In: Terasaki PI (ed) Histocompatibility testing 1980. UCLA Tissue Typing Laboratory, Los Angeles, p 791
6. Raffoux C, Lepage V, Dehay C, Degos L, Busson M, Dausset J (1983) Cw new. Ninth Workshop Newsletter I:14–15
7. Payne R, Radvany R, Grumet F, Feldman M, Cann H (1975) Two third series antigens transmitted together. A possibility for the SD locus? In: Kissmeyer-Nielsen F (ed) Histocompatibility testing 1975, Munksgaard, Copenhagen, pp 343–347
8. Chan SH and Wee GB (1979) Association of Bw46 and Cwl/Cw3 in Chinese. Tissue Antigens 14:179–180
9. Campbell EM, Du Toit ED (1983) Possible splits of Cw3. Ninth Workshop Newsletter I:10–13
10. Fauchet R, Dejour G, Jalais E, Bouhallier O, Genetet B (1983) Linkage disequilibrium with splits of Cw3. Ninth Workshop Newsletter IV:13–14
11. Tongio MM, Mayer S (1983) Further information on the Cw3 split. Ninth Workshop Newsletter II:22
12. Mayr WR, Kirnbauer M (1984) Cw3.1, a split of Cw3. Ninth Workshop Newsletter VI:13–14
13. Chiewsilp P, Sujirachato K (1983) Cw3.1 and Cw3.2. Ninth Workshop Newsletter II:23
14. Rani R, Mittal K (1984) Segregation of Cw3.1 and Cw3.2 in an intercross family. Ninth Workshop Newsletter VII:20–21
15. Tait BD, Boyle A (1983) Possible subtypes of Cw3. Ninth Workshop Newsletter III:27–28

Antigen Report: HLA-DR1

R. Fauchet[1], A. van Leeuwen[2], E.J. Yunis[3], and G.M.T. Schreuder[2]

1 Histocompatibility Laboratory, Blood Bank 35000 Rennes, France
2 Dept. of Immunohematology, University Medical Center, 2333 AA Leiden, The Netherlands
3 Sidney Farber Cancer Institute, Harvard Medical School, Boston, Mass, USA

DR1 was defined at the Seventh Histocompatibility Workshop by five sera [1], and at the Eighth Workshop it was clearly identified by 10 sera. There was no evidence for a split of DR1 [2]. At the Ninth Workshop, the frequency of DR1 was 14.7% in Caucasians and 9.45% in Negroes.

Histocompatibility Testing 1984
Edited by E. D. Albert et al.

Table 1. Anti-DR1 sera

Serum no.	Caucasian: 14.7% $n = 1000$				Negro: 9.45% $n = 571$			Other specificities
	% Frequency		Correlation coefficient		% False		Percentage of strong reactions	
	C	N	C	N	+	–		
9w502	14.3	10.15	0.98	0.96	13	12	81	
9w504	17.8	14.88	0.89	0.77	32	3	91	DRw6 + DRw10
9w505	14.3	10.15	0.98	0.96	16	8	85	
9w507	16.8	12.95	0.92	0.83	26	8	85	DR3
9w508	15.1	11.38	0.91	0.84	26	13	73	
9w510	16.1	9.45	0.94	1	17	8	82	DRw10
9w511	14.3	10.68	0.94	0.89	14	10	81	
9w512	13.7	9.10	0.96	0.98	11	17	67	
9w515	16.7	11.20	0.85	0.91	23	10	81	DRw10
9w521	14.3	12.25	0.93	0.86	21	14	71	DRw10

C, Caucasoid; N, Negroid

Table 2. DR1 pattern analysis

9w sera	502	505	512	508	511	510	515	507	504	Populations
Pattern 1	+	+	+	+	+	+	+	+	+	50% Caucasian 65% Negro
2	+	+	+	⊟	+	+	+	+	+	4.8% Caucasian 5.6% Negro
3	+	+	+	+	⊟	+	+	+	+	3.4% Caucasian 3.7% Negro

Serology

Caucasian data (147 DR1 cells) and Negro data (54 DR1 cells) showed that DR1 was clearly defined by ten sera (Table 1). Five of them appeared to be anti-DR1 exclusively: 502, 505, 512, 508, 511, with a high correlation coefficient of ≥ 0.85. The others contained additional antibodies: anti-DRw10 in sera 510, 515, and 521; anti-DRw6, DRw10 in serum 504; and anti-DR3 in serum 507. Three frequent patterns of reactions were observed (Table 2). The first is defined by the positive reactions of all the above sera. The second and third patterns depend on negative reactions of sera 508 or 511: serum 508 failed to react with 4.8% of the Caucasian and 5.6% of the Negro DR1-positive cells. Serum 511 missed 3.4% of Caucasian and 3.7% of Negro DR1-positive cells.

Conclusions

DR1 is well defined. There is no clear evidence for DR1 splits, although negative reactions of serum 508 or 511 have been noted in Caucasian and Negro DR1-positive cells.

References

1. Bodmer JG, Pickbourne P, Richards S (1978) In: Bodmer WF, et al (eds) Histocompatibility testing 1977. Munksgaard, Copenhagen, pp 35–84
2. Batchelor JR (1980) DR1 joint report. In: Terasaki PI (ed) Histocompatibility testing 1980. UCLA Tissue Typing Laboratory, Los Angeles, p 508

Antigen Report: HLA-DR2

J.R. Batchelor[1], J. Hors[2], I.A. Dodi[1], H. Bétuel[3], and I. Borelli[4]

1 Department of Immunology, Royal Postgraduate Medical School, Hammersmith Hospital, Ducane Road, London W12 OHS, U.K.
2 INSERM U.93, Hôpital St Louis, 2 Place du Dr. Fournier, 75010 Paris, France
3 Centre de Transfusion Sanguine, Lyon, France
4 Istituto de Genetica Medica Università di Torino, via Santena 19, 10126 Torino, Italy

History

At the Eighth International Histocompatibility Workshop, Lawler and Dewar [7] concluded that DR2 was a well-defined antigen, and claims of splits awaited further confirmation. Since then, heterogeneity of DR2 has been further documented [8]. Gebuhrer et al. [4] divided DR2 into a long DR2 identified by positive reactions with all the Ninth Workshop DR2 sera including 9w555, and a short variant, DR2S, defined by positive reactions with all the DR2 antisera except 9w555. These findings have been confirmed in other laboratories [5, 9]. Two other variants have been claimed. DR2 Lum [9] was identified in South African Negroes by positive reactions with all the Ninth Workshop DR2 sera except 9w542 and 543. The other split, FT31 [5], has been observed in Chinese and was identified by positive reactions with all the Ninth Workshop DR2 sera except 9w546–550.

Heterogeneity of DR2 is also indicated by the number of HTC-defined specificities associated with it. These include Dw2 and Dw12 [2, 11], FJO and DB9 [3, 4], and MN2 [10]. These HTC specificities appear to be distinct from each other, although their interrelationships have not been fully explored.

The relationships of the serologically defined splits of DR2 to the HTC-defined associated specificities also remains to be examined. Freidel et al. [3] concluded that FJO corresponds to DR2S.

Preliminary work on restriction DNA fragment length polymorphisms of DR2-positive cells derived from normal individuals and from patients with insulin-dependent diabetes mellitus or multiple sclerosis has further shown heterogeneity of DR2 [1].

The heterogeneity of DR2 has been further underlined by the results of studies with monoclonal antibodies [6].

Serology

DR2 was readily identified. The five most specific sera, judged by consistency, Q scores, and strength of reactions, are listed in Table 1. These five sera behaved equally well in Caucasoid, Japanese, and Negroid populations.

The variant DR2S was also confirmed by the Ninth Workshop data. A subset of 48 Caucasoid, 40 Japanese, and 29 Negroid families in which DR2 segregated was analyzed for the presence of the putative DR2S variant. Table 2 shows that it was found in 22 of these families; only 1 anomalous result was observed in the segregation pattern of DR2S amongst the 58 children of these families. It is, therefore, concluded that DR2S is a genuine variant of DR2, and that the negative reactions of 9w555 are not merely attributable to technical factors.

Four other sera, 9w552 and 9w548–550, also showed patterns of reactivity on cell panels from unrelated subjects which indicated the possibility of further variants of DR2. However, inspection of the subset of 48 Caucasoid families did not provide any strong evidence in support of further variants. Several examples were found of positive reactions on the children's cells with negative reactions on the parents. It was concluded from this first analysis that these antisera did not permit definitive identification of further variants of DR2.

Table 1. Ninth Workshop antisera for HLA-DR2

Serum no.	Q score	% Misses	% Extra reactions	*r*	% Score 8
534	9.8	4	10	0.91	66
541	9.2	4	4	0.92	67
535	9.3	3	8	0.92	72
542	8.5	8	8	0.87	57
530	7.1	7	9	0.85	60

Table 2. Families analyzed for inheritance of DR2S

Race	Caucasoids	Japanese	Negroids
No. of families informative for segregation of DR2S	5	9	8
No. of children	10	25	23

Histocompatibility Testing 1984
Edited by E. D. Albert et al.

Conclusion

DR2 is clearly defined serologically. Although heterogeneous by HTC analysis, only one variant form (DR2S) has been definitively identified by serological methods.

References

1. Cohen D, Cohen O, Marcadet A, Massart C, Lathrop M, Deschamp I, Hors J, Schuller E, Dausset J (1984) HLA Class II B DC DNA restriction fragments differentiate among HLA-DR2 individuals in insulin-dependent diabetes and multiple sclerosis. Proc Natl Acad Sci USA (in press)
2. Dupont B, Braun DW, Yunis EJ, Carpenter CB (1980) HLA-D by cellular typing. In: Terasaki PI (ed) Histocompatibility testing 1980. UCLA Tissue Typing Laboratory, Los Angeles, p 229
3. Freidel AC, Betuel H, Gebuhrer L, Fabre A, Lambert J (1984) Distinct subtypes of HLA-D associated with DR2. Ninth Histocompatibility Newsletter no. 7, p 24
4. Gebuhrer L, Bétuel H, Lambert J, Friedel AC, Favre M (1983) Division of HLA DR2 in two splits. Ninth Histocompatibility Newsletter no. 2
5. Honeyman M, Hakos G, Doran T, Bashir HV (1984) Splits of DR2 and associated HLA-D in various ethnic groups. Ninth Histocompatibility Newsletter no. 8, p 14
6. Kasahara M, Takenouchi T, Ikeda H, Ogasawara K, Okuyama T, Ishikawa N, Wakisaka A, Kikuchi Y, Aizawa M (1983) Serologic dissection of HLA-D specificities by the use of monoclonal antibodies. Immunogenetics 18:525
7. Lawler SD, Dewar PJ (1980) DR2 (joint report). In: Terasaki PI (ed) Histocompatibility testing 1980. UCLA Tissue Typing Laboratory, Los Angeles, p 511
8. Mervart H, Kalovsky E, Moore PBL (1983) Splits of the HLA DR2 antigen. Tissue Antigens 22:29
9. Oudshoorn M, Campbell EM, Du Toit ED (1983) Splits of HLA-DR2. Ninth Histocompatibility Newsletter no. 5, p 29
10. Reinsmoen NL, Bach FH, Layrisse Z (1983) HLA-DW/LD subtypes of HLA-DR2. Hum Immunol 81:302
11. Sasazuki T, Kaneoka H, Tsuji K, Nose Y, Kashiwagi N, Kaneko T (1980) HLA-D in Japan. In: Terasaki PI (ed) Histocompatibility testing 1980. UCLA Tissue Typing Laboratory, Los Angeles, p 274

Antigen Report: HLA-DR3

T.C. Fuller[1], M.S. Park[2], and E. Thorsby[3]

1 Massachusetts General Hospital, Boston, MA 02114, USA
2 UCLA School of Medicine, Los Angeles, CA 90024, USA
3 Rikshospitalet Oslo, Norway

History

HLA-DR3, as originally described by the Leiden group in 1973, was clearly defined by high-quality sera at both the Seventh and Eighth International Workshops (WS).

Serology

At the present Workshop, 46 sera were associated with DR3 in that the serum quality scores were greater than 1. The 11 most specific sera defining this specificity are listed in Table 1, The most

Table 1. Best-quality sera defining HLA-DR3

9WS ID#	Serum name	Laboratory	Quality score	r^a	% Extras	% Scores of 6+8 s
564	WILLIAMS	LAW	8.5	0.96	13	94.4
570	STILLWELL	DUP	5.7	0.83	12	89.6
565	NYBC 002	RUB	7.2	0.82	5	84.4
567	BOS/BUR	CAR	5.7	0.73	8	78.4
569	N-310	HAM	5.4	0.69	11	83.9
557	IA-35	AMO	4.0	0.67	24	85.6
561	WATSON	WOO	4.3	0.66	13	73.5
559	CCB 1045.1	BRN	4.1	0.62	8	72.2
568	10895	MRV	3.4	0.53	12	71.1
573	EVINK	THP	2.9	0.47	10	65.0
571	HAYWARD	DUQ	3.4	0.45	15	64.2

[a] Derived from random population; 6 and 8 scores only were considered positive

Histocompatibility Testing 1984
Edited by E. D. Albert et al.

reliable sera (strong reactivity, highest correlation and quality scores) are 9w564, 570, and 565. In comparison with the sera at the Eighth Workshop, only one of which was accepted in the present study (9w557 = 8w565), there is no overall improvement in the quality of the reagents.

The pattern analyses provided yielded no evidence for ethnic variation in this antigen. However, there is a suggestion of a split ("short") in DR3 in that three sera (9w571 and 573, and possibly 568) had a high percentage of DR3 misses (54%, 52%, and 32%, respectively). Several families were found in which this "short" DR3 segregated. Since all three sera involved (9w568, 571, 573) are quite weak, it is still possible that this "short" DR3 is due to a serological artifact.

As expected, strong linkage disequilibrium of DR3 with HLA-B8, Dw3, DRw52, and DQw2 was found.

Conclusion

HLA-DR3 was well defined at this Workshop.

Antigen Report: HLA-DR4

J. Williamson[1], B. Tait[2], P. Richiardi[2], J. Awad[3], R. Fauchet[4], E.S. Curtoni[5], H. Festenstein[3], R.L. Dawkins[1]

1 Dept. of Clinical Immunology, Royal Perth Hospital, Perth, Australia
2 Tissue Typing Laboratory, Royal Melbourne Hospital, Melbourne, Australia
3 Dept. of Immunology, The London Hospital, London E1 2AD, U.K.
4 Laboratoire d'Histocompatibilité, Centre Regional de Transfusion Sanguine, 35000 Rennes, France
5 Instituto de Genetica Medica, Università di Torino, via Santena 19, 10126 Torino, Italy

History

DR4 (WIA4) was first described at the Seventh International Workshop with two sets of sera (anti-WIA4 and -WIA4x7). The correlations for the sera were not high. Although the antigen was better defined at the Eighth Workshop there were several reports of DR4 subtypes.

Further evidence of heterogeneity was shown at the Second Asia and Oceania Histocompatibility Workshop, with at least one family clearly demonstrating the segregation of two subtypes. Several Ninth Workshop Newsletters have provided still further examples.

The analysis of DR4 is complicated by the difficulty in distinguishing between DR4, DQw3, and DRw53. It is likely that the final resolution of this problem will have to await the further elucidation of the contribution of the various class II antigens by biochemical and DNA techniques.

Serology

The Ninth Workshop data reveal at least 12 different serum patterns of DR4 after assigning DR5, DQw3, and DRw53, and after excluding some sera which reacted principally with these specificities. It is noteworthy that some of these patterns are only found within individual laboratories, but all segregated in at least one family. Undoubtedly some of the complexity is related to technical problems which are reproducible within families. Some illustrative patterns are shown in Table 1.

It appeared possible to identify three major groups of patterns, including two short inclusions, and to make tentative assignments to the sera (Table 2). Some of the monoclonal antibodies were especially valuable, as illustrated by 9w940, which allowed recognition of 4.3 in *some* laboratories (Table 3).

Relationship Between DR4 Subtypes and Other HLA Loci

Several Workshop reports suggested that there might be serological differences between DR4-Dw4, DR4-Dw15, DR4-Dw14, DR4-Dw13 and DR4-Dw10. It was only possible to examine this issue using pre-Workshop HLA-D assignments on very limited material, but a tentative summary is given in Table 4.

In conclusion, DR4 has been reasonably well defined at this workshop. There is evidence for three different splits, which are largely based on negative reactions of a number of weak sera.

Histocompatibility Testing 1984
Edited by E. D. Albert et al.

Table 1. Patterns of DR4 with alloantisera

Pattern no.	9w sera														
	589	576	575	580	585	595	581	590	587	592	594	582	591	593	578
1	+	+	+	+	+	+	+	+	+	+	+	+	+	+	+
2	+	+	+	+	+	+	+	+	+	+	W	W	W	W	+
3	+	+	+	+	+	+	+	+	+	+	–	–	+	–	+
4	+	+	+	+	+	+	+	+	–	–	–	–	–	–	+
5	+	+	+	+	+	+	+	+	+	–	–	–	–	+	–
6	+	+	+	+	+	+	+	+	+	–	–	–	–	–	–
7	+	+	+	+	+	+	+	+	–	–	–	–	–	–	–
8	+	+	+	+	+	+	+	–	+	–	–	–	–	–	–
9	+	+	+	+	+	+	W	–	W	W	–	–	–	W	W
10	–	+	+	+	+	W	–	–	–	–	–	–	–	W	W
11	–	+	+	+	–	–	W	–	–	–	–	–	–	W	W
12	–	+	+	+	–	–	–	–	–	–	–	–	–	–	–

W, weaker reactions, which did not necessarily segregate well with families

Table 2. Characteristics of alloantisera

Pattern no.	9w sera														
	589	576	575	580	585	595	581	590	587	592	594	582	591	593	578
Reactivity 4.1	+	+	+	+	+	+	+	+	+	+	+	+	+	+	+
4.2	+	+	+	+	+	+	+	+	+	+	–	–	–	+	+
4.3	W	+	+	+	W	W	W	–	W	W	–	–	W	W	W
Indices															
% Misses	14	13	14	5	9	23	13	19	18	31	48	35	44	36	25
% Extra-reactions	9	22	14	32	22	13	29	11	9	11	12	22	35	28	14
Q score	6.8	5.6	6.1	5.2	5.3	3.7	4.6	5.5	5.6	4.5	3.1	2.9	1.7	2.4	4.1
Other	–	–	–	–	DR5	–	DR5	–	–	–	–	–	DR5	–	–
Strength	51	43	54	58	50	43	46	49	46	38	28	31	34	35	37

W, weak or variable reactivity in some laboratories

Table 3. Segregation of 4.1/4.3 and potential value of 9w940 in Family CRB12

Haplotype	589	576	575	580	585	595	581	590	587	592	594	582	591	593	578	940	
ab	1	8	8	8	6	4	1	1	1	1	1	1	6	1	6	1	4.3
cd	6	8	8	8	8	4	6	8	4	8	4	6	6	8	6	8	4.1
ac	6	4	8	8	8	6	6	6	6	8	4	6	6	4	6	8	4.1+4.3
bc	6	4	8	6	6	6	6	8	6	6	6	6	6	6	6	8	4.1
ad	1	6	6	8	6	6	1	1	1	1	1	1	8	1	4	1	4.3
bd	1	1	1	1	1	1	1	1	1	1	1	1	1	1	1	1	

Table 4. Tentative summary of relationships between DR4 splits and alleles at other loci

Subtype	9w serum patterns				
	576, 575, 580, 585, 595	589, 581, 590, 587	592, 594, 582	DQw3	Associations
4.1	+	+	+	+	Dw14
	+	+	±	+	?Dw4
	+	+	+	–	Dw15
4.2	+	+	–	+	Dw13 B51
4.3	+	–	–	+	?Dw10 B35, 38

Antigen Report: HLA-DR5 and Its Subtypes HLA-DRw11 and HLA-DRw12

H. Bétuel[1], L. Gebuhrer[1], G.M.T. Schreuder[2], S.F. Goldmann[3], A. Arnaiz Villena[4], and Z. Layrisse[5]

1 Histocompatibility Laboratory, Blood Transfusion Center, 1 – 3 Rue du Vercors, 69007 Lyon, France
2 Dept. of Immunohematology, Blood Bank, University Hospital, Rijnsburgerweg 10, 2333 AA Leiden, The Netherlands
3 Dept. of Transplantation Immunology, Red Cross Blood Bank, Oberer Eselsberg 10, 7900 Ulm, Federal Republic of Germany
4 Sce. Imuno. Cent. Especial Ramon y Cajal, Madrid, Spain
5 Instituto Venezolano de Investigaciones Cientificas, Caracas, Venezuela

The existence of splits of HLA-DR5 were not accepted during the Eighth Histocompatibility Workshop, although some laboratories had claimed the existence of subsets [1]. At the present Workshop, difficulties in the distinction of DR5 from DRw6 and DRw8-related specificities led us to analyze several groups of sera differentiating these specificities. The segregation pattern of the sera mentioned in Table 1 were studied in informative families. Further details are given in the Joint Report on DRw6 (Schreuder et al., this volume). In brief, families were selected in which serum reactions appeared sufficiently strong and clearly segregated from parents to offspring. Such segregation patterns were termed haplotypes. Examples of such haplotypes are shown in Table 2. Several DR5-related patterns were observed in which all DRw52, DR5+w13 (6.6) and DR5+w8+w13 sera were positive. DR5 sera were invariably found positive in all haplotypes of patterns a, b, and c in Table 2.

Pattern a represents the DQw3-associated DRw11 (DR5), which is the most frequently encountered combination [3]. The Dw5 HTCs type with this serological pattern corresponding to DRw11 in the new nomenclature. (See also Report on HTC serology.)

Pattern b shows the DQw1-associated DRw11, which is rare in Caucasoids but has been found in other populations, e.g., Cape Coloreds and South American Negroes. In such families, DR3 + w6 sera were occasionally found to be positive.

Pattern c was observed in two Italian families, where DRw11 segregated with DQ blanks (DQw1-, DQw3-negative as well as DQw2; data not shown). Such a DRw11-DQ blank association is probably very rare.

Patterns d and e (DRw12 or DR5 sh, LB 5x8) are characterized by negativity of DR5 sera, but the DR5 + w13 + (w8) sera were positive in both patterns. In addition, in pattern d, TA 10 + DR5 sera are consistently positive.

Pattern d represents the DQw3-associated DRw12 (DR5 sh). It is observed in HTC Herluf (9w1503) and in several other families.

Pattern e was observed in only one Italian family, where DQ blank segregated with the DRw12 pattern. DRw12 is easily confused with the DRw13 (6.6), DQw3-associated specificity. Further details are given in the Joint Report on DRw6 (Schreuder et al., this volume). The serological pattern of this DRw13 is shown for HTC 1802 in Table 2 (f). The only way to separate them is by considering the reactivity of the DR3 + w6 sera which are usually negative with DRw12. Due to the inconsistent reactions of these "3 + w6" sera, many haplotypes could not be assigned as DRw12 or DRw13, DQw3. In Table 2, reactions of DQw3 and TA 10 sera are grouped together. TA 10 as described by Maeda [2] is probably included in DQw3, and is said to reside on DQ molecules. Two sera recognize this specificity clearly: 9w790 (a monoclonal antibody) and 9w607. Sera that were originally thought to detect long DR5 now appear as mixtures of TA 10 and DR5. The different patterns just described are summarized in Table 3. It must be added that DQw3 and TA 10 can sometimes be found in combination with other DR specificities, e.g., DR2, DR3, and DR4. However, DR4 can also be associated with DQw3-positive, TA 10-negative and DQ blank (Table 3).

Table 1. Ninth Workshop sera used for the analysis of DR5 related specificities

DRw52	699, 756, 697,
DR5 + DRw13 (6.6)	681, 709,
DR5 + DRw13 + DRw8	616, 682, 618,
DRw14 (6.9)	787, 781,
DR3 + DRw6	678, 679, 680, 713, 714,
DRw8	619, 763 (weak), 621,
DRw11 (DR5 – LB5)	611, 612, 613, 609, 596, [610]
TA10 + DR5	599, 598, 601, 603, 597,
TA10	790, 607, 789 (+ DR3)
DQw3	761, 745, 746, 744, 748,
DQw1	654, 655, 661,

[ ] Other specific sera whose reactions do not appear in Table 2

Conclusion

Two main subgroups of DR5 can be defined, DRw11 and DRw12, which are clearly distinct and

Histocompatibility Testing 1984
Edited by E. D. Albert et al.

Table 2. Serum reaction patterns of DR5, (DRw11 and DRw12) haplotypes (and DRw13 for comparison)

	HLA-DR							HLA-DQ				
	w52	5+ w13	5+w8 +w13	w14	3+w6	w8	DRw11	TA10 +DR5	TA10	DQw3	DQw1	
9w Family codes	676 959 967	67 80 19	666 181 628	77 88 71	66677 77811 89034	676 162 931	66665 11109 12396	55665 99009 98137	767 908 079	77777 64444 15648	666 656 451	Local assignment
	a. DRw11, DQw3 haplotypes											
IT2GAN 05	888	88	881	14	11816	111	88888	88888	888	88888	111	5
FRABET 09(5)	686	86	684	11	11122	114	66448	86888	468	86666	111	5/Dw5
GERGOL 17	888	81	888	14	11446	114	88888	88888	868	44446	111	5
ANZFON 02	888	81	888	11	11116	111	88888	88888	868	81888	111	5
ANZROB 01, 02	888	86	881	11	11111	111	88888	88888	888	86888	111	5
LATJRM 05	668	86	886	11	14166	111	88888	88888	888	66668	111	5
GERALB 01, 02	688	84	882	11	11144	111	48868	88868	666	46848	111	5
JAPTOK 06	888	61	886	11	11161	211	88888	88888	888	88888	111	5
ANZBSH 06	888	68	861	11	11111	112	68066	88888	866	66848	111	5/Dw5
ANZSER 03, 05	888	88	888	81	11111	111	88888	88888	888	88888	111	5
GERGSW 02	888	61	884	11	11111	111	88888	88888	166	66818	111	5/Dw5
	b. DRw11, DQw1 haplotypes											
US4RAD 14	888	88	888	12	14888	011	08888	88888	118	11141	888	5
LATJRM 01, 03	888	88	888	11	88888	111	88888	88888	111	11112	888	5
SAFDUT 01, 03	688	86	882	11	11821	111	88888	88888	111	11114	668	5/Dw5 negative
UK1FES 06	688	68	881	11	11411	111	88818	88888	111	11111	666	5
	c. DRw11, DQ blank haplotype											
IT2FER 04, 08	888	84	886	18	11011	111	66168	88888	118	11112	111	5
	d. DRw12, DQw3 haplotypes											
BENROO 1503 HTC	686	84	884	11	11111	116	41111	84616	486	48868	111	LB5x8/DHerl
BENROO 01	888	48	888	14	11111	118	11111	88882	888	88888	111	LB5x8/DHerl
FRABET 15	464	44	666	12	11222	116	11111	86626	426	64424	111	5sh/DHerl
ITAMTT 15	888	86	888	11	11111	111	11168	88868	188	11818	111	5
UK1FES 09	466	66	661	11	11111	112	41111	44646	626	46646	111	–
GERGSW 02	666	81	868	11	11111	111	81114	88868	888	88888	111	5/Dw5 negative
UK1MOR 04	886	41	886	11	11141	112	11111	82886	888	66808	111	5
US7HAN 01	648	81	881	11	11111	118	11122	88888	888	88888	000	5
	e. DRw12, DQ blank haplotype											
IT1MTT 06	888	88	888	11	11111	111	11111	11111	111	11111	111	–
	f. DRw13, DQw3 haplotypes											
BENROO 1802HTC	888	88	888	18	88881	111	11118	88818	888	88888	111	w6.2, LB 5x8
FRABET 09(2)	686	88	884	11	66668	112	21142	24662	146	41412	111	w6.2/D1802

Table 3. Summary of reaction patterns of DRw6, DR5, DRw8 and DQ antisera

DR, DQ haplotypes	Ninth Workshop antisera										
	HLA-DR							HLA-DQ			
	w52	5+w6	5+w6+w8	w14	3+w6	w8	w11	DR5+ TA10	TA10	DQw3	DQw1
DRw13, DQw1	+	+	+	–	+/–	–	–	–	–	–	+
DRw13, DQw3	+	+	+	–	+/–	–	–	+	+	+	–
DRw13, DQ –	+	+	+	–	+/–	–	–	–	–	–	–
DRw14, DQw1	+	–	–	+	+/–	–	–	–	–	–	+
DRw14, DQw3	+	–	–	+	+/–	–	–	+	+	+	–
DRw11, DQw3	+	+	+	–	–	–	+	+	+	+	–
DRw11, DQw1	+	+	+	–	+/–	–	+	+	–	–	+
DRw11, DQ –	+	+	+	–	–	–	+	+	–	–	–
DRw12, DQw3	+	+	+	–	–	–	–	+	+	+	–
DRw8, DQ –	+	–	+	–	–	+	–	–	–	–	–
DRw8, DQw3	+	–	+	–	–	+	–	+	+	+	–
DRw8, DQw1	+	–	+	–	–	+	–	–	–	–	+
DR4, DQw3, TA10	–	–	–	–	–	–	–	+	+	+	–
DR4, DQw3	–	–	–	–	–	–	–	–	–	+	–
DR4, DQ –	–	–	–	–	–	–	–	–	–	–	–
DR2, DQw3, TA10	–	–	–	–	–	–	–	+	+	+	–
DR3, DQw3, TA10	+	–	–	–	+	–	–	+	+	+	–

segregate in families. The majority of these DR5 specificities are in linkage disequilibrium with DQw3 and TA 10.

References

1. Engelfriet E, De Lange G, Hilterman T, Van den Berg-Lonen E (1980) DR5: Joint Report: In: Terasaki PI (ed) Histocompatibility testing 1980. UCLA Tissue Typing Laboratory, Los Angeles, pp 518–521
2. Maeda H (1984) Mouse monoclonal antibody detects a new polymorphic Ia determinant other than HLA-DR antigen: a possible allele of DC1. Tissue Antigens 23:163–170
3. Schreuder GMT, Van Leeuwen A, Termijtelen A, Parlevliet J, D'Amaro J, Van Rood JJ (1982) Cell-membrane polymorphisms coded for in the HLA D/DR region. I. Relation between D and DR. Hum Immunol 4:301–310

Antigen Report: HLA-DRw6 and Its Subgroups HLA-DRw13 and HLA-DRw14

G.M.T. Schreuder [1], L.J. Kennedy [2], L. Gebuhrer [3], J. Awad [4], H. Bétuel [3], L. Degos [5], and M. Jeannet [6]

1 Department of Immunohematology and Blood Bank, University Medical Center, 2333 AA Leiden, The Netherlands
2 Imperial Cancer Research Fund, London, U.K.
3 Centre de Transfusion Sanguine, Lyon, France
4 Department of Immunology, The London Hospital Medical College, London E1 2AD, U.K.
5 INSERM, Hôpital St. Louis, 2 Place du Dr. Fournier, 75010 Paris, France
6 Unité d'Immunologie de Transplantation, Hôpital Cantonal, Geneva, Switzerland

History

The specificity DRw6 was first described in 1977 during the Seventh Histocompatibility Workshop [1]. Since monospecific sera were not available, the DRw6 antigen was defined by two groups of sera, DR2 + w6 and DR3 + w6. The Eighth Histocompatibility Workshop did not clarify the definition of DRw6. During that Workshop, again, no monospecific sera could be identified. The definition of DRw6 was then predominantly based on positive reactions with DR3 + w6 sera. Due to this

Histocompatibility Testing 1984
Edited by E. D. Albert et al.

Table 1. Possible equivalents of locally assigned DRw6 subtypes

WHO nomenclature 1984	Ninth Workshop	Leiden	Bodmer	Other
DRw13, DQw1	DRw6.6-MB1	LB6.6	6Z	6.1, 6.6, 8w6Y
DRw13, DQw3	DRw6.6-MB3	LB6.2	6Y	6.2
DRw14, DQw1	DRw6.9-MB1	LB6.9	6X	6.3, 6.9, IaLad9, FT19, KD5, 901
DRw14, DQw3	DRw6.9-MB3	LB6.2	6A	6.2

restriction many individuals were reported as Dw6 positive, DRw6 negative. However, it was clear that DRw6 was always associated with DRw52 (MT2) and very often, but not always, with DQw1 (MB1 or DC1). Four different reports were devoted to DRw6 and several subgroups of this specificity were described [2–5]. In several papers published during the last 2 years the existence of three main subgroups of DRw6 has been discussed [6]:

1. DRw6.6, 6.1, 8wDRw6Y: DQw1 positive, associated with Dw6.
2. DRw6.9, 6.3: DQw1 positive, associated with Dw9. The serological definition of this Dw9-related DR specificity was first clearly described by Awad [7]. Later, a serum was described which almost monospecifically recognized this specificity, then called 901 (serum 9w781) [8].
3. DRw6.2: DQw1 negative, HLA-D unknown. This specificity has been confused with the DR5-related specificity LB5x8 (DRw12) [6]. A number of the previously used designations for DRw6-related specificities are indicated in Table 1.

Ninth Workshop DRw6 Analysis

The aim of our study was to provide a reliable definition of DRw6-related specificities.

It was necessary to include the DR5- and DRw8-related serum reactions in addition to DRw6, because of previous confusion of DRw6, DQw1-negative specificities and DRw12 (LB5x8) (H. Bétuel et al., joint reports on DR5 and DRw8, this volume).

Selection of the Ninth Workshop sera for this analysis was based on performance of the sera when tested with Ninth Workshop HTCs (G. Schreuder et al., "HLA-DR, DQ, LB, and TA10 Specificities of Ninth Workshop HTCs", this volume), some DRw6-positive families in Leiden, and on proven usefulness as reported in Ninth Workshop Newsletters.

The sera, which are listed in Table 2, represented the following (groups of cross-reacting) specificities: DRw52 (MT2), 5 + w6, 5 + w6 + w8, w14 (6.9), 3 + w6, w8, w11 (DR5), TA10 + DR5, TA10, DQw3 (MB3), DQw1 (MB1). Reactions of these sera were listed for all individuals for whom data was present on the workshop computer tape (provided by M. Baur), together with the locally assigned DR, MB, MT, and Dw specificities. Laboratories were selected where serum reactions appeared sufficiently strong and clearly segregated from parents to offspring. It was thus possible to study serum segregation patterns for DR5, w6, and w8 related specificities in informative families.

All DRw6 specificities are DRw52 positive.

Table 2. Ninth Workshop sera used for the analysis of DRw6-, DR5- and DRw8-related specificities

Specificity	9W Sera
DRw52 (MT2)	694, 697, 699, 756
DR5 + DRw13 (w6.6)	681, 709
DR5 + DRw13 + DRw8	616, 618, 682
DRw14 (w6.9)	781, 787
DR3 + DRw6	678, 679, 680, 713, 714
DRw8	619, 621, 763 (weak)
DRw11 (DR5-LB5)	596, 609, 611, 612, 613
TA10 + DR5	597, 598, 599, 601, 603
TA10	790, 607, 789 (+DR3)
DQw3 (MB3, MT4, DC4)	744, 745, 746, 748, 761 (LB-E13)
DQw1 (MB1, MT1, DC1)	652, 654, 655, 661

DRw13

DRw13 (see Table 3) is characterized by positive reactions with DRw52, 5 + w6, and 5 + w6 + w8 sera. DRw14 sera were negative with a few exceptions. The 3 + w6 sera showed variable reactivity and were not helpful for the definition of the DRw13 specificity. This type of DRw6 can be associated with different DQ types.

Table 3a deals with the DQw1-associated DRw13, which is the most frequently encountered combination. The Dw18 (Dw6A) and Dw19 (Dw6B) HTCs type with this serological pattern (Schreuder et al., this volume). Table 3b deals with the DQw3, TA10-associated DRw13. This combination is probably rare in Caucasoids. This serological pattern was also found with HTC 9w1802 (Schreuder et al., this volume). The DQw3-asso-

Table 3. Serum reaction patterns of DRw13 haplotypes (and DRw12 for comparison)

	HLA-DR							HLA-DQ				
	w52	5+ w13	5+w8 +w13	w14	3+w6	w8	DRw11	TA10 +DR5	TA10	DQw3	DQw1	
9w	6676	67	666	77	66677	676	66665	55665	767	77777	6666	Local
W	9959	80	181	88	77811	162	11109	99009	908	64444	5556	assignment
Family codes S	4967	19	628	71	89034	931	12396	98137	079	15648	2451	
	a. DRw13, DQw1 haplotypes											
FRABET 25	8888	88	888	11	48888	111	41111	11118	112	00000	6268	w6
SAFDUT 01	8888	88	888	11	48844	111	11111	11116	111	11111	8428	w6/Dw6
LATJRM 02	8888	88	888	11	88888	111	11111	11118	114	11111	1888	w6.1
US7HAN 01	8888	88	888	11	48888	118	11111	88118	816	16111	8888	w6
BENROO 03	8888	88	888	11	18821	111	11111	61211	418	11111	8888	w6.6/Dw6
EAEBRT 03	8888	88	888	11	88888	111	11111	11111	111	11111	8888	w6
UKIDRK 07	8888	88	886	11	61088	111	11111	11116	111	11111	6166	w6
UKIWOR 17	8888	88	881	14	88884	211	11111	44114	111	11111	8888	w6.1
JAPJUJ 03, 04	8888	88	801	14	88888	111	11111	11112	111	11111	8888	–
NCYYAG 05	8888	88	661	11	48484	111	11111	11114	111	11111	8888	w6
US5MIT 07	8884	88	681	16	62221	111	11111	11111	111	11111	6646	w6.2
US4STA 16	8888	88	884	11	48461	111	11111	11111	111	11111	8888	w6
IT2GAN 13, 16	8888	88	881	11	88048	111	11116	11116	111	11111	8888	w6
US8RUB 02, 03, 08	8888	88	882	11	84881	111	11111	11111	111	11111	1888	w6.1
US2BAC 12	6886	88	884	41	68461	111	11111	11111	111	11111	8888	w6.1
GERGSW 03	8828	88	881	11	88488	111	11111	11111	111	11111	8888	w6/Dw6
NCYMRV 03, 04, 06	8888	88	881	11	88168	111	11111	11112	111	11111	8888	w6.1
US5FTW 10, 11	8888	88	881	61	18888	111	11011	11111	111	11111	8888	w6.1
ANZBSH 11	8888	68	682	41	18861	111	01111	11111	111	11111	8888	w6.1
JAPYOS 01, 02	6888	88	881	11	18188	011	00100	11112	111	11111	8888	–
US1AMO 05	8884	88	881	11	48141	111	11111	11111	111	11111	8888	w6
GERALB 09	6888	88	881	21	18122	111	12222	11111	111	11211	8888	w6
UKIFES 09	6666	66	661	11	16421	111	11111	11112	111	11111	6646	w6Y
US2BAC 05, 09	6886	66	661	41	26641	111	11111	11116	112	11111	8666	w6.1/Dw6
JAPSEK 71	8888	88	888	11	16161	111	11111	11112	114	11111	8888	–
JAPJUJ 10	8888	86	881	11	14110	111	11111	11118	111	11111	1880	w6Y
IT1MCC 02	8888	66	664	11	16611	111	11111	11114	111	11111	8846	w6Y
	b. DRw13, DQw3 haplotypes											
BENROO 1802HTC	8888	88	888	18	88881	111	11118	88818	888	88888	1111	w6.2, LB5x8
ANZCHI 04	8868	46	684	41	14686	116	11112	84811	828	88868	1111	DR5
ANZTAI 06	8888	84	884	11	44881	116	11111	88814	888	88888	1111	DR5
LATJRM 02	8888	88	888	11	88818	118	81142	88888	888	88888	1111	DR5
UKIDRK 11	6886	86	888	11	66086	111	01144	66666	146	16626	1111	DR5
FRABET 09	6686	88	884	11	66668	112	21142	24662	146	41412	1111	w6.2
ANZBSH 02	8888	46	814	11	12681	116	11111	88820	848	68848	1111	–
SAFDUT 28	8888	41	886	11	14688	116	11114	88828	848	88888	1111	LB5x8
US3GRU 08	8886	88	881	11	18816	111	11118	88888	888	88888	1111	DR5
US4STA 01, 16	8888	88	888	18	88881	111	11011	88888	888	88888	1111	DR5
US5FTW 09	8888	84	888	11	88881	111	11014	88888	888	88888	0000	DR5
US1HEJ 09	8888	88	848	11	86181	111	11111	48822	888	66868	0000	DRw6
	c. DRw13, DQ blank haplotypes											
FRADAU 02	8888	88	401	11	16661	111	11111	11111	111	11111	1111	DRw6.2
IT1MCC 01	8888	41	861	11	18811	111	11111	11111	111	11111	1111	–
	d. DRw12, DQw3 haplotypes											
BENROO 1503HTC	4686	84	884	11	11111	116	41111	84616	486	48868	1111	LB5x8/DHerl
BENROO 01	6888	48	888	14	11111	118	11111	88882	888	88888	1111	LB5x8/DHerl

Table 4. Serum reaction patterns of DRw14 haplotypes

	HLA-DR							HLA-DQ				
	w52	5+ w13	5+w8 +w13	14	3+w6	w8	DRw11	TA10 +DR5	TA10	DQw3	DQw1	
9w	6676	67	666	77	66677	676	66665	55665	767	77777	6666	Local
W	9959	80	181	88	77811	162	11109	99009	908	64444	5556	assignment
Family codes S	4967	19	628	71	89034	931	12396	98137	079	15648	2451	
a. DRw14, DQw1 haplotypes												
US7HAN 07	8888	14	112	68	88888	111	11111	11111	111	11111	8888	w6Y
ANZCHI 03	8888	11	881	88	16888	111	11111	11111	114	11111	8888	w6
US4STA 13	8888	14	481	88	44848	111	11111	11111	111	11111	8888	w6
FRABET 22	8888	11	481	88	46866	111	11112	44211	116	11111	8888	901
JAPTOK 03	8888	10	101	88	88688	111	11111	24211	216	11111	8888	–
US3GRU 08	8886	16	111	68	16846	111	11111	11111	111	11111	8888	w6.1
US1WAR 01	8888	12	111	88	16884	111	11111	11110	118	11111	8888	w6
SAFDUT 20	8888	12	611	88	16888	111	11111	11116	118	11111	8888	w6Y/Dw9
US4RAD 10	8888	16	411	88	16868	111	11111	11111	111	11111	8888	w6.1
NCYMRV 20	8888	12	111	88	12888	111	11111	11116	114	11111	8888	w6.1
IT1MTT 02	8881	11	111	68	81111	111	11111	11111	111	11111	8888	w6.1
IT1CRB 06	6888	11	111	88	16166	211	11111	11111	111	11111	6468	w6.1
JAPYOS 01	8888	11	111	88	16168	011	11011	11111	111	11111	4448	–
LATJRM 05	8888	11	241	88	16128	111	11111	11111	111	11111	1888	w6.1
NCYMAR 02	4884	11	161	88	14011	111	11111	11111	111	11111	8888	w6
NCYMRV 04	8888	11	181	88	14088	111	11111	11112	111	11111	8888	w6.1
FRABET 02	8888	12	221	68	11442	111	11111	11111	214	11111	6686	901/Dw9
SCAKIS 03	8888	11	121	66	12644	111	11111	11111	111	11111	8118	w6
US5FTW 04	8888	11	111	88	11661	111	11011	11111	116	11111	8888	w6.1
US2BAC 05, 09	8888	11	141	88	11841	111	11111	11111	111	11111	8888	w6.1
BENROO 16	8888	11	411	88	11811	111	11111	11111	111	11111	8888	w6.9
IT2GAN 04	8888	11	111	88	11811	111	11111	11111	111	11111	8888	w6
ANZBSH 01	6686	11	161	66	12211	111	11111	11111	111	11111	8888	–/Dw9
JAPSEK 30	8888	11	111	88	11088	118	11111	10111	111	11111	8888	w6
ANZSER 04	8888	11	141	88	12110	111	11111	11111	111	11111	8888	w6.1
US8NSF 01	6888	11	141	66	11804	111	11111	11111	111	11111	8888	w6
UKIDRK 03	6886	42	111	46	11648	111	11111	11111	111	11111	6228	w6
JAPJUJ 02	8888	11	111	88	11860	111	11111	11111	111	00101	8888	–
JAPYOS 13	8888	11	111	88	11411	011	11011	11111	111	11111	8818	–
IT1MTT 07	8884	11	111	68	14111	111	11111	11114	111	11111	8888	w6Y
UKIFES 10	6828	11	111	16	12121	111	11111	12111	111	11111	0666	w6
JAPAIZ 06, 09	8888	11	210	08	11011	116	11111	11111	110	11111	8888	–
US3GRU 13	8888	11	141	88	11611	111	11111	11111	111	11111	8888	w6
b. DRw14, DQw3 haplotypes												
LATLAY 1701HTC	8188	41	641	68	88688	111	11111	88861	888	88888	1111	w6.2
BENROO 1702HTC	8886	16	411	28	88884	111	11111	68816	646	88688	1111	w6.2
US5ABS 01, 05	8888	11	111	88	88888	111	11111	88888	888	88888	1111	w6.2
US5ABS 11, 12	8888	11	111	88	88888	111	11111	88881	888	88888	1111	w6.2
IT2GAN 11	8888	11	881	88	11828	112	11111	88881	888	88888	1111	DR5
US3GRU 13	8881	11	111	18	18881	111	11111	18811	888	86868	1111	DR5
JAPTOK 04	6666	11	111	14	66666	111	11111	16611	616	11826	1111	–
LATLAY 06	6888	11	111	28	46886	111	11111	48861	888	88888	1111	DR5

Table 5. Summary of reaction patterns of DRw6, DR5, and DRw8 with HLA-DR and DQ antisera

	HLA-DR							HLA-DQ			
	DRw52	5+w6	5+w6 +w8	w14	3+w6	w8	w11	TA10 +DR5	TA10	DQw3	DQw1
DRw13(w6), DQw1	+	+	+	–	+/–	–	–	–	–	–	+
DRw13(w6), DQw3	+	+	+	–	+/–	–	–	+	+	+	–
DRw13(w6), DQ blank	+	+	+	–	+/–	–	–	–	–	–	–
DRw14(w6), DQw1	+	–	–	+	+/–	–	–	–	–	–	+
DRw14(w6), DQw3	+	–	–	+	+/–	–	–	+	+	+	–
DRw11(5), DQw1	+	+	+	–	–	–	+	+	–	–	+
DRw11(5), DQw3	+	+	+	–	+/–	–	+	+	+	+	–
DRw11(5), DQ blank	+	+	+	–	–	–	+	+	–	–	–
DRw12(5), DQw3	+	+	+	–	–	–	–	+	+	+	–
DRw8, DQw1	+	–	+	–	–	+	–	–	–	–	+
DRw8, DQw3	+	–	+	–	–	+	–	+	+	+	–
DRw8, DQ blank	+	–	+	–	–	+	–	–	–	–	–

Table 6. Reaction patterns of Ninth Workshop monoclonal antibodies with DRw6-, DR5-, and DRw8-related specificities

	HLA-DR						HLA-DQ			
	'3+5+w6'				DR3 +w6		DQw1		DQw3 +w7	
9w	946	947	948	930	925	929	945	960	915	969
DRw13, DQw1 a. (Dw18?)	+	+	+	+	–	+	+	+	–	–
b. (Dw19?)	+	+	+	+	–	–	+	+	–	–
DRw13, DQw3	+	+	+	+	(–)	–	–	–	+	+
DRw14, DQw1	+	+	+	+	–	–	+	+	–	–
DRw14, DQw3	+	+	+	+	(–)	–	–	–	+	+
DRw11, DQw3	+	+	+	+	–	–	–	–	+	+
DRw11, DQw1	+	+	+	+	–	–	+	+	–	–
DRw12, DQw3 (Herluf)	–	–	–	+	+	–	–	–	+	+
DRw8, DQ blank	–	–	–	–	+	–	–	–	–	–
DRw8, DQw3	–	–	–	–	+	–	–	–	+	+
DRw8, DQw1	–	–	–	–	+	–	+	+	–	–

Table 7. Associations of DRw13 and DRw14 and B locus specificities

	DRw13, DQw1			DRw14, DQw1	
	Caucasoid 196/1232[a]	Mongoloid 58/255	Negroid 35/143	Caucasoid 56/1232	Mongoloid 21/255
B12	–[b]	+++	–	–	–
B17	–	++	–	–	–
B35	–	–	–	+	–
B39	–	++	–	–	–
Bw55	–	–	–	++++	–
Bw56	–	–	–	–	+++
Bw60	++	–	–	–	++
Bw61	–	–	–	–	++

[a] Number of positive/total number of unrelated individuals

[b] –: no increase in frequency against controls; +: about 50% increase in frequency against controls; ++: two-fold increase in frequency against controls; +++: three fold increase in frequency against controls; ++++: four-fold increase in frequency against controls

ciated DRw13 is easily confused with the serological pattern for DRw12, based on HTC 9w1503 Herluf (Bétuel et al., Joint Report on DR5, this volume) and is shown in Table 3d. The only way to separate them, using alloantisera is by considering the reactivity of the 3 + w6 sera, which are usually negative with DRw12. Due to the inconsistency of the reactions of this group of sera (see Table 3a) many haplotypes could not be assigned either DRw12 or DRw13 when associated with DQw3. However, DRw12 and DRw13 can be distinguished using monoclonal antibodies (see below).
Table 3c deals with the same DRw13 specificity in association with DQ blank (DQw2 negative, data not shown). No HTC has been found with this serological pattern. It appears to be extremely rare, as it was only observed in two families.

DRw14

The second type of DRw6 (DRw14) is shown in Table 4. It is characterized by positivity of DRw52 and DRw14 sera and negativity to 5 + w6 and 5 + w6 + w8 sera. The 3 + w6 sera again showed variable reactivity.
DRw14 can also be found in association with different DQ types. Table 4a deals with the DQw1-associated DRw14, which is fairly frequent. Dw9 HTCs type with this serological pattern (Schreuder et al., this volume). Table 4b deals with the DQw3-, TA10-associated DRw14. It is less frequently encountered than the DQw1-associated DRw14. The Dw16 (DB8) HTCs 9W1701 and 1702 showed this type of reactions (Schreuder et al., this volume). As yet no other DQ associations with DRw14 have been found.

Summary

We have summarized the patterns of the DRw6 haplotypes of Tables 3 and 4 in Table 5, together with a simplified overview of the reaction patterns of DR5 and DRw8 haplotypes (Bétuel et al., this volume). The putative DR reagents can be used to define two types of DRw6, i.e., DRw13 and DRw14. These are clearly different from DR5 (DRw11 and DRw12) and DRw8. Each of these specificities can be found in association with different DQ types. When DRw6 is associated with DQw3, the TA10 specificity is always present. [For further discussion of TA10 see Joint Report on DR5 (Bétuel et al., this volume).]

Use of Monoclonal Antibodies (MCAs) in the Definition of DRw6

The MCAs shown in Table 6 can be used to distinguish some of the specificities discussed above. For example, DRw13, DQw3, and DRw12 can be distinguished using the MCAs 9w946, 947, 948, and 9w925. 9w946, 947, and 948 are positive with DRw13 but negative with DRw12, while 9w925 is negative with DRw13 but positive with DRw12 and with DRw8 (J. Bodmer et al., joint report on DR MCAs, this volume). These particular patterns have not been seen with alloantisera. The MCA 9w929, which reacts with DR3 and part of the DRw13, DQw1 cells, did not correlate with 3 + w6 alloantisera. However, it may correlate with the two types of Dw6, Dw18 being positive with 9w929 and Dw19 negative.

HLA-B Locus Associations with DRw6-Related Specificities

To estimate the degree of association between HLA-B and DRw6-related specificities, a computer assignment was made for DRw13, DQw1 and for DRw14, DQw1. The DQw3-associated DRw6 subgroups were too rare to be considered.
The analysis was performed in unrelated individuals from three ethnic groups. Only four DRw14, DQw1 Negroid individuals were found, so that this group had to be excluded. Control frequencies were obtained from the same populations. Table 7 indicates some notable associations between DRw6 and B locus specificities.

References

1. Bodmer JG, Pickbourne P, Richards S (1978) Joint report: Ia serology. In: Bodmer WF, et al (eds) Histocompatibility testing 1977. Munksgaard, Copenhagen, pp 35–84
2. Jeannet M (1980) DRw6. In: Terasaki PI (ed) Histocompatibility testing 1980. UCLA Tissue Typing Laboratory, Los Angeles, pp 524–525
3. Sekiguchi S, Kreisler M, Omori K, Nakata S, Park MS, Jeannet M (1980) 8wDRw6Y. In: Terasaki PI (ed) Histocompatibility testing 1980. UCLA Tissue Typing Laboratory, Los Angeles, pp 530–531
4. Kreisler M, Nakata S, Omori K, Park MS (1980) DRw6 (6.1 and 6.2) vs MT1. In: Terasaki PI (ed) Histocompatibility testing 1980. UCLA Tissue Typing Laboratory, Los Angeles, pp 526–528
5. Bodmer J, Park MS, Omori K (1980) 8wDRw6Y (5/6). In: Terasaki PI (ed) Histocompatibility testing 1980. UCLA Tissue Typing Laboratory, Los Angeles, pp 532–534
6. Schreuder GMT, Parlevliet J, Termijtelen A, Rood JJ van (1983) Reanalysis of the HLA-DRw6 complex. Tissue Antigens 21:62–74
7. Awad J, Jaraquemada D, Festenstein H (1982) Serological analogue of HLA-Dw9. Tissue Antigens 19:233–237
8. Bétuel H, Gebuhrer L, Lambert J, Freidel AC, Farre A (1983) A possible new HLA-DR allele. Hum Immunol 8:227–237

Antigen Report: HLA-DR7

B.K. Jakobsen[1], P.I. Terasaki[2], and A. Svejgaard[1]

1 Tissue Typing Laboratory, Division 7631, State University Hospital, Tagensvej 20, 2200 Copenhagen Ø, Denmark
2 UCLA Tissue Typing Laboratory, University of California, Los Angeles, CA, USA

The following sera (listed in order of quality) behaved as very good anti-DR7 typing reagents: 9w638, 640, 629, 630, 642, and 633. Each of these had very few extra reactions and few false negatives. In particular, there was no reactivity against DR4- or DRw9-positive cells. Sera 9w637 and 9w634 contained mainly anti-DR7 but gave some extra reactions with no obvious specificity. Serum 9w639 was a weak anti-DR7. Serum 9w636 contained anti-DR3 + 7. The same was true for 9w717, 719–724, and 727, which reacted with almost all DR7 cells. Other broad sera containing strong anti-DR7 activity were 9w731, 733–735, 741, and 743. In addition, 9w774 (submitted as new) contained anti-DR7. There was no evidence that DR7 may be split.

The DR7 antigen showed the same linkage disequilibria as described at previous workshops.

Antigen Report: HLA-DRw8

H. Bétuel[1], L. Gebuhrer[1], G.M.T. Schreuder[2], Z. Layrisse[3], A. Arnaiz Villena[4], and S.F. Goldmann[5]

1 Histocompatibility Laboratory, Blood Transfusion Center, 1–3 Rue du Vercors, 69007 Lyon, France
2 Dept. of Immunohematology, Blood Bank, University Hospital, Rijnsburgerweg 10, 2333 AA Leiden, The Netherlands
3 Instituto Venezolano de Investigaciones Cientificas, Caracas, Venezuela
4 Sce. Imuno. Cent. Especial Ràmon y Cajal, Madrid, Spain
5 Dept. of Transplantation Immunology, Red Cross Blood Bank, Oberer Eselsberg 10, 7900 Ulm, Federal Republic of Germany

The definition of DRw8 at the last Histocompatibility Workshop was based on the reactions of five sera with *r* values between 0.40 and 0.58 [1]. For this Workshop, analysis of DRw8 was studied in relation to DR5 and DRw6. More extensive serum reaction patterns are presented in all three reports to permit a better comparison of these cross-reacting specificities (Table 1). The segregation pattern of the sera shown in Table 1 were studied in informative Workshop families. The mode of selection is given in details in the Joint Reports on DR5 (Bétuel et al., this volume) and on DRw6 (Schreuder et al., this volume). Examples of such haplotypes are presented in Table 2. Several DRw8-related patterns were observed in which all DRw52 (MT2), DR5 + w8 + w13 (6.6) and DRw8 sera were positive.

Pattern a represents DRw8 associated with DQ (MB) blank, which is the most frequently encountered combination. It is mostly recognized by Dw8-HTCs. Since the set of reactions is almost the same in all populations, only a few examples are given.

Pattern b shows DRw8 in association with DQw1. HTC 9w806 of Japanese origin is given as an example, together with some informative haplotypes. This pattern is frequent in Orientals and can also be observed in other populations, as already described in Australian Aborigines [3].

Table 1. Ninth Workshop sera[a] used for the analysis of DRw8-related specificities

DRw52	699, 756, 697
DR5+DRw13 (6.6)	681, 709
DR5+DRw13+DRw8	616, 682, 618
DRw14 (6.9)	787, 781
DR3+DRw6	678, 679, 680, 713, 714
DRw8	619, 763 (weak), [624, 627]
DRw8+weak DR5	621, [620, 623, 626]
DRw11 (DR5-LB5)	611, 612, 613, 609, 596
TA10+DR5	599, 598, 601, 603, 597
TA10	790, 607, 789 (+DR3)
DQw3	761, 745, 746, 744, 748
DQw1	654, 655, 661

[a] The sera in brackets are specific sera; their patterns of reaction are not shown for the families in Table 2

Histocompatibility Testing 1984
Edited by E. D. Albert et al.

Table 2. Serum reaction patterns of DRw8 haplotypes

	HLA-DR							HLA-DQ				
	w52	5+ w13	5+w8 +w13	w14	3+w6	w8	DRw11	TA10 +DR5	TA10	DQw3	DQw1	
Family codes \ 9W	676 959 967	67 80 19	666 181 628	77 88 71	66677 77811 89034	676 162 931	66665 11109 12396	55665 99009 98137	767 908 079	77777 64444 15648	666 556 451	Local assignment
	a. DRw8, DQ blank haplotypes											
GERGSW 11	688	11	888	11	11111	868	11111	11111	246	11111	111	8/Dw8
ANZSER 04, 05	488	18	888	11	11111	818	11118	11118	111	11111	111	8
FRABET 16	868	14	666	11	11111	668	11112	21114	114	12112	111	8/Dw8
JAPSEK 81, 82	888	11	818	11	11111	848	11118	11118	111	11111	111	8
	b. DRw8, DQw1 haplotypes											
US7HAN 806 HTC	888	48	888	18	11118	888	11114	11118	181	11111	888	8/Dw8
JAPYOS 06	888	11	818	11	11111	068	11111	11111	111	11111	888	8
JAPJUJ 15	688	41	888	11	11112	828	14411	10114	114	11111	646	w6
ANZWOO 01, 02	888	14	646	16	11411	228	11114	11112	111	11111	888	8
JAPMIY 08, 09	488	11	888	11	11111	048	11111	11111	111	11111	888	8
GERMUE 27	888	11	888	11	11111	688	11116	11118	111	11111	888	8
JAPAIZ 06	488	11	888	01	11011	168	11111	11111	110	11111	888	–
	c. DRw8, DQw3 haplotypes											
BENROO 805 HTC	888	11	888	16	11111	868	11111	88811	888	86888	111	8/Dw8
GERGOL 13	888	82	888	16	11146	688	11111	88888	888	88848	111	5
JAPJUJ 20	888	11	888	11	44441	818	11011	66642	666	24848	000	8
JAPYOS 13	888	11	848	11	11111	018	01111	14811	828	11818	111	8
	d. DRw8 variant? DQw3 haplotypes (Japanese)											
JAPSEK 64	888	11	888	11	88184	114	11111	88881	888	88888	111	5
JAPAIZ 12, 13	848	11	680	01	11481	018	11011	18811	888	86888	111	5
JAPYOS 07	888	11	881	11	88181	016	11011	88888	818	88888	111	–
JAPOKO 02	888	11	888	11	86186	618	11111	88888	888	88888	111	8w17
JAPOKO 07	888	61	888	01	88182	018	11011	88888	888	88888	111	6.2
JAPSEK 50	848	11	888	11	66181	116	41116	88888	888	88888	111	8

Table 3. Schematic reaction patterns of DRw6, DR5, DRw8 and DQ antisera

DR, DQ haplotypes	Ninth Workshop antisera										
	HLA-DR							HLA-DQ			
	w52	5+w6	5+w6+w8	w14	3+w6	w8	5	DR5+ TA10	TA10	DQw3	DQw1
DRw13, DQw1	+	+	+	–	+/–	–	–	–	–	–	+
DRw13, DQw3	+	+	+	–	+/–	–	–	+	+	+	–
DRw13, DQ –	+	+	+	–	+/–	–	–	–	–	–	–
DRw14, DQw1	+	–	–	+	+/–	–	–	–	–	–	+
DRw14, DQw3	+	–	–	+	+/–	–	–	+	+	+	–
DRw11, DQw3	+	+	+	–	–	–	+	+	+	+	–
DRw11, DQw1	+	+	+	–	+/–	–	+	+	–	–	+
DRw11, DQ –	+	+	+	–	–	–	+	+	–	–	–
DRw12, DQw3	+	+	+	–	–	–	–	+	+	+	–
DRw8, DQ –	+	–	+	–	–	+	–	–	–	–	–
DRw8, DQw3	+	–	+	–	–	+	–	+	+	+	–
DRw8, DQw1	+	–	+	–	–	+	–	–	–	–	+
DR4, DQw3, TA10	–	–	–	–	–	–	–	+	+	+	–
DR4, DQw3	–	–	–	–	–	–	–	–	–	+	–
DR4, DQ –	–	–	–	–	–	–	–	–	–	–	–
DR2, DQw3, TA10	–	–	–	–	–	–	–	+	+	+	–
DR3, DQw3, TA10	+	–	–	–	+	–	–	+	+	+	–

Pattern c represents DRw8 in association with DQw3 and TA10. This pattern was defined by HTC 9w805 and found in one Caucasian family and in some Oriental families.

Some examples of haplotypes with a possible DRw8 variant associated with DQw3, TA10 are shown in Table 2d. This association is characterized by positivity of DR5 + w8 + w13 and DR3 + w6 sera, and weak or negative reactions of DRw8 sera. Since DR5 + w13 and DR5-sera were regularly negative, it excludes the possibility that this pattern belongs to DR5 or to DRw13 (w 6.6). This may correspond to the previously described specificity 8wDRw17 [2]. A schematic representation (Table 3) of these different patterns of DQw3-associated DR5, DRw13 (6.6), and DRw14 (6.9) is also given. The relationship between DQw3 and TA10 has been discussed in the joint report on DR5 (H. Bétuel et al., this volume).

Conclusion

DRw8 is mainly found in linkage disequilibrium with DQ blank. In the Workshop data, depending on the population studied, DRw8 was also found on haplotypes together with DQw1 or with DQw3.

References

1. Dausset J (1980) Drw8. Joint report. In: Terasaki PI (ed) Histocompatibility testing 1980. UCLA Tissue Typing Laboratory, Los Angeles, pp 538–540
2. Nakata S, Park MS, Terasaki PI, Omori K (1980) 8wDRw17. Joint report. In: Terasaki PI (ed) Histocompatibility testing 1980. UCLA Tissue Typing Laboratory, Los Angeles, pp 548–550
3. Termijtelen A, Boettcher B, Bradley BA, D'Amaro J, Van Leeuwen A, Van Rood JJ (1980) DR typing in Australian aborigines: an indication for a second locus in the HLA-D region defined by serology. Tissue Antigens 16:140

Antigen Report: HLA-DRw9

J. Williamson [1] and A. McNicholas [2]

1 Royal Perth Hospital, Perth, Western Australia
2 Immunogenetics Laboratory, University of Munich, Pettenkoferstr. 8a, 8000 Munich 2, Federal Republic of Germany

DRw9 was recognized as WIA4x7 at the Seventh Workshop, but was still not well defined at the Eighth Workshop.

In this Workshop, sera 9w644, 645, 646, 647, and 650 provided a clear definition, although there were extra reactions in some laboratories. Serum 647 was essentially monospecific in most laboratories, but was short in several Japanese families.

Pattern analysis in Caucasians, Negroes, and Japanese show that 100% of the DRw9-positive cells react with at least three of the five sera given above. None of the DRw9-negative cells is positive with more than two of the five sera. There is no convincing evidence for a split of DRw9. A listing of the most specific DRw9 sera is given in Table 1.

In general, DRw9 was associated with DQw3. In some cases, however, DRw9 was found on the same haplotype with DQw2.

Table 1. The most specific Ninth Workshop sera defining DRw9

9W sera	Average strength	Percent false negatives	Percent false positives	Percent strong reactions	Q score	Tail specificities
644	7.8	3	40	63	7.2	DQw2, DRw10
645	7.8	2	49	62	7.6	DRw10, DRw53
646	7.6	2	49	55	6.6	DR7, DRw53
647	7.4	7	20	64	6.4	–
650	7.7	1	53	55	7.4	DRw53

Histocompatibility Testing 1984
Edited by E. D. Albert et al.

Antigen Report: HLA-DRw10

R. Fauchet[1], A. van Leeuwen[2], E.J. Yunis[3], and G.M.T. Schreuder[2]

1 Histocompatibility Laboratory, Blood Bank, 35000 Rennes, France
2 Dept. of Immunohematology, University Medical Center, 2333 AA Leiden, The Netherlands
3 Sidney Farber Cancer Institute, Harvard Medical School, Boston, Mass, USA

At the Eighth Histocompatibility Workshop, DRw10 was defined by a single monospecific serum 8w1097 [1], which showed a reactivity identical to the previously described ST1 specificity [2]. The other six anti-DRw10 sera in the Eighth Workshop set contained additional antibodies against DRw9, DR1, and DR4. The Ninth Workshop prescreening showed good monospecific anti-DRw10 sera [3, 4].
At the present Workshop, the frequency is 2.1% in Caucasians and 3.5% in Negroes.

Serology

The serological analysis is based on 21 Caucasian and 20 Negro DRw10-positive cells. DRw10 was clearly defined by three monospecific sera: 524, 527, and 525, giving a correlation coefficient of over 0.85 and over 78% 8 and 6 reactions. All other good sera contained anti-DR1: 515, 516, 518, 521, 522, 523. Weak anti-DRw10 activity was found in 504, 510, and the anti-DQw1 sera 652, 653, 654, 655, 668, 669, 670, 700, 701, and 703. Three sera reacted with DRw9 and DRw10: 518 (DR1, w10, w9); 644, 645 (good anti-DRw9) (Table 1).

Table 1. Anti-DRw10 sera

Serum no.	DRw10							
	Caucasian: 2.1% $n=1000$				Negro: 3.50% $n=571$			
	% Frequency		Correlation r		% False		Percent strong reactions	Other specificities
	C	N	C	N	+	–		
9w523	2.7	12.76	0.71	0.41	78	1	96	DR1
9w525	2.6	3.50	0.89	1	62	3	87	
9w524	1.9	3.50	0.95	1	60	13	81	
9w527	1.6	3.50	0.87	1	57	21	78	
9w516	9.5	10.68	0.43	0.55	47	40	82	DR1
9w518	14.6	14.88	0.27	0.45	35	6	82	DR1+DR2 +DRw9+
9w521	4.8	10.85	0.49	0.51	21	14	71	DR1
9w515	12.5	9.63	0.28	0.58	23	10	76	DR1
9w522	11.9	8.93	0.27	0.47	18	19	60	DR1
9w529	14.4	5.77	0.32	0.77	89	8	90	B8

Table 2. Pattern analysis

9 w-sera / Pattern	DRw10			DR1+DRw10					DR1,2,w9,?		Population (%)	
	524	527	525	523	516	515	521	522	518	529	C	N
1	+	+	+	+	+	+	+	+	+	+	38.1	70
2	+	+	+	–	+	+	+	+	+	+	9.5	10
3	+	+	+	+	+	+	–	+	+	+	4.8	
	+	+	+	+	+	+	–	–	+	+		5.0

Histocompatibility Testing 1984
Edited by E. D. Albert et al.

Serological Pattern

The most frequent pattern is characterized by positive reactions of sera 524, 527, 525, 523, 516, 515, 521, 522, 518, and 529 (38.1% in Caucasian cells; 70% in Negro cells). A second pattern was defined by the negative reaction of serum 523, which failed to react in 9.5% of Caucasian and 10% of Negro DRw10-positive cells (Table 2).

Linkage Disequilibrium

The most frequent associations were with Bw62 in Negro families and with B37 in Caucasians.

Conclusion

Several good monospecific sera clearly defined DRw10. There is no evidence for a split of this specificity.

References

1. Grumet FC, Ness DB (1980) In: Terasaki PI (ed) Histocompatibility testing 1980. UCLA Tissue Typing Laboratory, Los Angeles, p 542
2. Colombe B, Payne R (1980) In: Terasaki PI (ed) Histocompatibility testing 1980. UCLA Tissue Typing Laboratory, Los Angeles, pp 543–545
3. Fauchet R, Bouhallier O, Jalais E, Genetet B (1983) Serological definition of DRw10 and DRw9 specificities. Ninth Workshop Newsletter 1
4. Gebuhrer G, Betuel H (1984) Definition of HLA-DRw10. Ninth Workshop Newsletter 7, p 41

Antigen Report: HLA-DRw52

C. Conighi [1], P.L. Mattiuz [1], and G.M.T. Schreuder [2]

1 Institute of Medical Genetics, University of Ferrara, Ferrara, Italy
2 Dept. of Immunohematology, Blood Bank, University Hospital, Rijnsburgerweg 10, 2333 AA Leiden, The Netherlands

History

During the Eighth International Workshop, Park et al. [1] described the specificity MT2 (= DRw52). According to their data, DRw52 includes DR3, 5, w6, and w8. These findings were confirmed by Juji et al. [2] in the Joint report on MT2 (= DRw52).

Serology

Many sera tested during the Ninth International Workshop are associated with DRw52: the majority of them have a quality score (Q score) [3] lower than 1, indicating that these reagents are of doubtful value as typing reagents. Among the remaining sera, 9W688, 692, 693, 694, 696, 697, 698, 699, and 756 showed a Q score higher than 2.5 and coefficients of correlation (r) with the antigen DRw52 (local assignment) ranging from 0.65 to 0.78. The r values between these sera ranged from 0.78 to 0.97 in Caucasians and from 0.66 to 0.98 in Negroes, indicating the consistency of the cluster. Considering the patterns of the reactions with the selected antisera, clear assignment of the antigen DRw52 is possible. Cells carrying the antigen reacted with all or all but one of the antisera in 98% of Caucasians and in 100% of Negroes. In the absence of the antigen, the cells showed negative reactions with all or all but one of the sera in 98% of both Caucasian and Negro cells.

DRw52 includes DR3, w6, w8, w11, and w12 almost perfectly. In Caucasians, the pattern analysis showed that 4% of the cells carrying one of these specificities (local assignment) gave negative reactions with the DRw52 sera; these "exceptions" may be due to miscoding. The pattern analysis also showed that in the absence of the above-mentioned DR specificities, 4% of the cells reacted with all the selected anti-DRw52 antisera. This could be due to miscoding or to the presence of a specificity recognized by the anti-DRw52 antisera in molecules not carrying DR specificities [4].

Conclusions

DRw52 can be defined clearly with a set of antisera tested during the Ninth International Workshop.

Histocompatibility Testing 1984
Edited by E. D. Albert et al.

References

1. Park MS, Terasaki PI, Nakata S, Aoki D (1980) Supertypic DR group: MT1, MT2 and MT3. In: Terasaki PI (ed) Histocompatibility testing 1980. UCLA Tissue Typing Laboratory, Los Angeles, pp 854–857
2. Juji T, Maeda H, Omori K (1980) MT2. In: Terasaki PI (ed) Histocompatibility testing 1980. UCLA Tissue Typing Laboratory, Los Angeles, pp 565–566
3. Mickey MR, Terasaki PI (1980) The serological data of the 8th Workshop and summary analyses. In: Terasaki PI (ed) Histocompatibility testing 1980. UCLA Tissue Typing Laboratory, Los Angeles, pp 21–25
4. Tanigaki N, Tosi R, Sagawa K, Minowada J, Ferrara GB (1983) The distribution of DR5, MT2 and MB3 specificities on human IA subsets. Immunogenetics 17:371

Antigen Report: **HLA-DRw53**

V. Lepage[1], F.C. Grumet[2], M. Busson[1], J. Colombani[1], D. Ness[2], and L. Degos[1]

1 Hôpital Saint Louis, Centre Hayem, 2 Place du Dr. Fournier, 75010 Paris, France
2 Stanford University, Stanford, CA 94304, USA

History

During the Seventh Workshop, WIA4x7 was described with a set of sera containing activity for both DR4 and DR7. During the Eighth Workshop, new facts were observed:

1. The specificity IA4x7 was defined by duo- or trispecific antisera [1]
2. The Japanese specificity 7J was considered to be equivalent to IA4x7 [2–4]
3. Whether IA4x7 belonged to the DR locus [5, 6] or not [7, 8] was controversial.
4. The WHO Nomenclature Committee designated a part of IA4x7 as DRw9 [9]
5. The determinant MT3 (DRw53) includes DR4, DR7, DRw9 and DRw10 [10]
6. Finally, the binding data show that "the DR4x7 determinant, previously described as being associated with all DR4-positive and most DR7-positive individuals tested so far is represented on a molecular subset differing from both the DR4 and DR7 molecular subset, and it is probably equivalent to the DRw53 specificity detected by cytotoxicity assay." [11].

Serology

During the Ninth Workshop two 2 subsets of sera were used to define the DRw53 specificity in Caucasians. The first group of antisera (9W734, 735, 736, 743) is positive with DR4 and/or DR7 and/or DRw9. Other sera were related to DR4, DRw9 and less to DR7 (9W729, 737, 739) or to DR7, DRw9 and less to DR4 (9W733). The second group (9W730, 731, 753) included the same specificities (DR4,7, w9) plus the DR5 specificity.
Table 1 shows the quality of the sera, i.e., their strength and specificity.
DRw53 is defined by seven sera reacting together (9W734, 735, 736, 743, 730, 731, 753) in 37% of DR4-, 7- or w9-positive cells.
It is important to note that all anti-DRw53 sera (no data for 9W733) were negative in 2.6% of DR4-positive DR7-positive, or DRw9-positive cells.
Conversely, DR4, 7 and DRw9-negative cells were never DRw53 positive. The segregation of DRw53 antisera in families was good, except for sera 9W733, 737, and 739.

Table 1. Qualtiy of the various sera

Serum identity / Specificity[a]	DRw53			DR4		DR7		DRw9	
	1	2	3	1	2	1	2	1	2
9w734	86	13	20	77	20	92	5	87	16
9w743	83	24	17	70	41	94	6	87	16
9w735	91	10	29	85	16	95	4	91	13
9w736	74	34	19	76	23	47	46	64	44
9w737	79	56	17	75	51	61	68	86	37
9w739	69	66	26	65	56	ND	ND	ND	27
9w729	ND	33	25	91	11	57	54	81	31
9w733	ND	ND	ND	53	60	89	7	64	48
9w730	ND	12	37	92	8	78	20	91	9
9w731	88	14	38	91	5	66	26	91	15
9w753	94	12	31	95	5	82	20	95	11

[a] 1, Percentage of scores of 6 and 8 reactions; 2, percentage missed reactions; 3, percentage extra reactions; ND, no data

Histocompatibility Testing 1984
Edited by E. D. Albert et al.

Conclusion

The DRw53 specificity is well defined with the Ninth Workshop sera. Some difficulties in the analysis are due to the presence of anti-DR antibodies in the anti-DRw53 sera. Two main points are noted:

1. Cells were detected that were positive for DR4, 7 or w9, but negative for MT3; the reverse was not observed.
2. Two groups of DRw53 antibodies were noted: one with and one without anti-DR5 activity.

Biochemical studies (of the genes and gene products) raise the question of whether the DRw53 specificity may be carried by a molecule similar to but different from the DR molecule (Tosi et al., this volume; Goyert et al., this volume; Cohen et al. this volume).

References

1. Colombe B, Payne R (1980) Evidence from family data for two specificities in 8W12. In: Terasaki PI (ed) Histocompatibility testing 1980. UCLA Tissue Typing Laboratory, Los Angeles, p 831
2. Maeda H, Juji T (1980) A new DR antigen crossreactive with DRw4 and DRw7. In: Terasaki PI (ed) Histocompatibility testing 1980. UCLA Tissue Typing Laboratory, Los Angeles, p 837
3. Sekiguchi S, Kobayashi K, Konoeda Y, Takata H (1980) Two components of the Ia4x7B lymphocyte antigen found in Japanese. In: Terasaki PI (ed) Histocompatibility testing 1980. UCLA Tissue Typing Laboratory, Los Angeles, p 836
4. Aizawa M, Wakisaka A, Morinchi J, Nakai Y, Kano T, Itakura K (1980) A new B cell allo-antigen characteristic for Orientals? In: Terasaki PI (ed) Histocompatibility testing 1980. UCLA Tissue Typing Laboratory, Los Angeles, p 826
5. Lung P, Hidalggo R, Giugal DP (1980) Ia4x7 B lymphocyte antigen in Caucasians. In: Terasaki PI (ed) Histocompatibility testing 1980. UCLA Tissue Typing Laboratory, Los Angeles, p 834
6. Kato M, Matsui C, Taniai S, Watanabe K, Kashiwagi N (1980) 7J specificity in HLA-DR antigens. In: Terasaki PI (ed) Histocompatibility testing 1980. UCLA Tissue Typing Laboratory, Los Angeles, p 839
7. Payne R, Colombe B (1980) On the trail of the 4x7 B lymphocyte antigen. In: Terasaki PI (ed) Histocompatibility testing 1980. UCLA Tissue Typing Laboratory, Los Angeles, p 829
8. Dewar PJ, Lawler SD (1980) Still on the trail of the Ia4x7 antigens. In: Terasaki PI (ed) Histocompatibility testing 1980. UCLA Tissue Typing Laboratory, Los Angeles, p 838
9. Colombe B, Payne R (1980) 8W12 (DRw9 + 10). In: Terasaki PI (ed) Histocompatibility testing 1980. UCLA Tissue Typing Laboratory, Los Angeles, 543
10. Nakata S, Park MS, Omori K (1980) MT3. Joint Report. In: Terasaki PI (ed) Histocompatibility testing 1980. UCLA Tissue Typing Laboratory, Los Angeles, p 569
11. Tosi R (1980) MT3. Joint Report. In: Terasaki PI (ed) Histocompatibility testing 1980. UCLA Tissue Typing Laboratory, Los Angeles, p 568

Antigen Report: New HLA-DR

T. Juji[1], L. Degos[2], and H. Bashir[3]

1 Blood Transfusion Service, Tokyo Women's Medical College, Tokyo, Japan
2 INSERM, Hôpital St. Louis, 2 Place du Dr. Fournier, 75010 Paris, France
3 Red Cross Blood Transfusion Service, Sydney, Australia

A new specificity, DRw14, defined by two sera (9w781 and 9w787), corresponds to the one previously termed DRw6.3 (at the Eighth Workshop) DRw6.9, 901, FT19, Bod X, or KD5. Detailed serological definition is described in the DRw6 antigen report (Schreuder et al., this volume).

Some DR specificities are in linkage disequilibrium with several DQ specificities. These various combinations do not represent DR subdivisions. For instance, DR4 is in linkage disequilibrium with DQw3 or with DQ blank (equivalent to Dw15 (DYT-HTC)), and DR7 is sometimes associated with DQw2 (corresponding to Dw7) or DQw3 (corresponding to Dw11).

A new DR antigen is suspected in cells positive for DQw1, but negative for the known DR antigens DR1-w14. This suspected specificity is sometimes called DR6.4, DR"BR", FT22, or BON. Family studies have confirmed the segregation of this DR blank DQw1-positive haplotype, which was also found in homozygous form in family BON from Toulouse.

The key sera for the definition of TA10 are 9w790, 9w599, and 9w601. TA10 was suggested to be a gene product of the DQ locus, possibly included in DQw3. It was confirmed to segregate on haplotypes with various DR antigens (DRw11, DRw12, DR4, DRw8, DRw9 and DR2). Serum 9w790 pre-

Histocompatibility Testing 1984
Edited by E. D. Albert et al.

Table 1. Splits of DR (see individual antigen reports) are shown in Table 1

Specificity	Serological definition	DW equivalent	DQ linkage disequilibrium
DR2 short	9w555 neg	FJO	DQw1
DR4.1	9w594 pos 582 pos 591 pos	Dw14 (LD40) Dw4	DQw3 neg TA10 neg
DR4.2	9w594 neg 582 neg 591 neg	Dw13 (DB3)	DQw3 pos TA10 pos
DRw11 DR5 long	9w609 to 9w613 pos	Dw5	DQw3 pos TA10 pos
DRw12 DR5 short	9w609 to 9w613 neg	DB6	DQw3 pos TA10 pos

cipitates class II antigen molecules in different positions from those of DR antigens in 2-D gel electrophoresis. TA10 was shown to be clearly defined at this Workshop. Significant linkage disequilibria were found between TA10 and DR5 [DRw11 and DRw12 (= NJ2)]. NJ2 is a DR antigen that has been well defined at Japanese workshops, and it is DQw3 positive and DQw1 negative. However, it was not defined at this workshop. TA10 may be identical with 8wDRw13 and Te22.

At this workshop, TB21, a short component of DQw3, was defined by a set of sera, i.e., 9w786, 9w744, 9w746, and 9w748. Some of the DR4-positive cells in Caucasians and Negroes and about 50% of Japanese DR4-positive cells are negative for TB21.

References

1. Maeda H (1984) Mouse monoclonal antibody detects a new polymorphic Ia determinant other than HLA-DR antigen; possible allele of DC-1. Tissue Antigens 23:167–170
2. Maeda H, Juji T (1981) New DR subtypes included in MT2. Transplant Proc 13:1985–1988
3. Maeda H, Juji T (1982) A new B-cell alloantigen, TB21, coded for in the HLA-D/DR region. Tissue Antigens 20:327–334

Antigen Report: HLA-DQw1

G.B. Ferrara[1,2], M.S. Park[4], N. Tanigaki[3], and P.I. Terasaki[4]

1 Istituto Nazionale per la Ricerca sul Cancro, Genova, Italy
2 Centro Ricerche Immunoematologiche A.V.I.S., Bergamo, Italy
3 Roswell Park Memorial Institute, Buffalo, NY, USA
4 UCLA Tissue Typing Laboratory, Los Angeles, CA, USA

History

The supertypic specificity DR1 + 2 + w6 (later called DQw1 = DC1 = MB1 = MT1 = LB12), was discovered at the Seventh Workshop [1]. This specificity was shown to reside on a subset of class II molecules called the DC subset [2], differing from the DR subset for both the alpha and the beta subunits [3, 4]. DQw1 has been shown more recently to be associated also with DRw10.

Serology

Best Sera for Definition

Table 1 summarizes the properties of the 11 most specific DQw1 antisera as judged by Q scores.

Presence of Antibodies Against Subtypic Specificities

Supertypic antisera often contain antibodies against subtypic components. These may account for some of the variation in the strength of antisera

Histocompatibility Testing 1984
Edited by E. D. Albert et al.

Table 1. DQw1 antisera

Antiserum	Q scores for DQw1	%+ DR1	%+ DR2	%+ DRw6	%+ DRw10	Percent extra-reactions	Serum strength (% scores 8)
9w662	6.2	90	97	81	68	7	64
9w661	6.6	86	97	88	71	9	63
9w664	6.8	86	92	87	70	10	59
9w669	7.0	84	94	87	78	10	57
9w674	6.3	83	92	86	75	10	57
9w663	5.7	85	87	84	70	9	57
9w668	6.6	81	82	81	66	8	50
9w654	5.7	62	93	76	59	8	54
9w657	5.5	75	96	84	67	12	62
9w667	5.6	72	93	73	62	8	54
9w672	5.1	85	87	87	74	11	53

against different cell classes. It is important to recognize the existence of subtypic components because they may hinder the recognition of "dissociated phenotypes." For instance, a DR1-positive + DQw1-negative phenotype will not be recognized if the DQw1 antiserum used contains anti-DR1 antibodies. Subtypic components can be detected either by cross-absorption tests or by the ability of the antiserum to bind the isolated molecules bearing the determinant to be tested, in this case DR1, DR2, or DRw6.
Table 2 shows the data obtained by a molecular binding test similar to that used for Eighth Workshop antisera [5]. Only binding above 5% is shown.

Table 2. Results of molecular binding test

Serum	DQw1	DR1	DR2	DRw6
9w662	32.6	10.3	8.0	
9w661	31.1	5.3	10.4	
9w664	10.2			
9w669	37.2		13.0	5.8
9w674	30.3	5.8		
9w663	39.2	13.6		
9w668	30.3			
9w654	31.5	9.2	7.2	
9w657	18.9		13.4	
9w667	21.3		13.6	
9w672	32.1			8.4

Possible DQw1 Splits

At the Eighth Workshop the specificity Te21 was described, which includes only part of DR1 and DR2 [6]. Possible candidates for this DQw1-included specificity are the antisera 9w518, 514, and 531. However, it is rather difficult to rule out the possibility that they are weak DQw1 antisera.
The DR1 + 10 pattern seems to emerge from several antisera: 504, 509, 510, 511, 515, 516, 518, 521, 522.
Another possible DQw1-included specificity which should be considered is the DR2 + w6 reactivity group. This is represented by four antisera, as shown in Table 3.
However, in this case too, the possibility of weak DQw1 reactivity is difficult to rule out. These four antisera are in fact rather weak (strength varying from 27 to 44). DQw1 in association with DR1 may be more difficult to detect judging by the generally lower strength (percent of scores of 8) of DQw1 antisera with DR1-positive individuals (see 2 × 2 analysis of this Workshop).

Conclusions

In general, DQw1 seems to be a very well-defined specificity according to a group of highly correlat-

Table 3. Antisera representing the DR2 + w6 group

Antisera	Q scores	%+ DR1	%+ DR2	%+ DRw6	%+ DRw10	Percent extra-reactions	Serum strength (% scores 8)
9w706	2.8	0	73	56	0	9	35
9w776	2.1	0	43	48	0	14	34
9w705	1.9	0	42	51	0	11	27
9w778	1.5	0	70	64	0	0	44

ed antisera. Specificities included in DQw1 and yet supertypic cannot be defined with confidence. Since structural differences have been demonstrated between DQ molecules associated with DR1, and DRw6 [4] it is possible that serological determinants corresponding to these differences will be found in the future.

References

1. Bodmer JG (1977) Ia Serology. In: Bodmer WF, et al (eds) Histocompatibility testing 1977. Munksgaard, Copenhagen, pp 351 – 357
2. Tosi R, Tanigaki N, Centis D, Ferrara GB, Pressman D (1978) Immunological dissection of human Ia molecules. J Exp Med 148:1592
3. Corte G, Calabi F, Damiani G, Bargellesi A, Tosi R, Sorrentino R (1981) Human Ia molecules carrying DC1 determinants differ both in alpha and beta subunits from Ia molecules carrying DR determinants. Nature 292:357
4. Shackelford DA, Mann DL, Van Rood JJ, Ferrara GB, Strominger JL (1981) Demonstration of structural polymorphism among HLA-DR light chains by two-dimensional gel electrophoresis. Proc Natl Acad Sci USA 78:4566
5. Tosi R, Tanigaki N (1980) Joint Report. In: Terasaki PI (ed) Histocompatibility testing 1980. UCLA Tissue Typing Laboratory, Los Angeles, pp 558 – 563
6. Park MS, Terasaki PI (1980) Second DR locus. In: Terasaki PI (ed) Histocompatibility testing 1980. UCLA Tissue Typing Laboratory, Los Angeles, pp 578 – 582

Antigen Report: HLA-DQw2

M. Marrari[1] and R.J. Duquesnoy[2]*

1 Section Head, HLA-D Serology, Central Blood Bank of Pittsburgh, 812 Fifth Avenue Pittsburgh, PA 15219, USA
2 University of Pittsburgh School of Medicine, Scaife Hall, Room 406, Pittsburgh, PA 15261, USA

DQw2 (MB2) was originally defined in 1979 by a cluster of five Seventh Workshop B-cell antisera as a new HLA-D region antigen associated with DR3 and DR7 [1]. This determinant is similar to Te24 [2] and DC3 [3]. During the Eighth Workshop, DQw2 could be defined by a serum cluster with high correlation values [4]. However, most sera in this cluster also contained DR7 antibodies, making DQw2 assignment on DR7 cells more difficult. Although DQw2 has been suggested to present a cross-reacting group of DR3 + DR7 antigens, recent biochemical data from different laboratories have demonstrated that DQw2 resides on class II molecules different from DR molecules and perhaps equivalent to the murine I-A molecules [5, 6]. This would suggest that DQw2 may be controlled by a distinct HLA-D gene. Disease association studies have shown strong associations of DQw2 with celiac disease and dermatitis herpetiformis.

A preliminary analysis of selected DQw2 antisera with data obtained from Region 17 (Amos) laboratories, including our own, showed significant correlations in the reactivity patterns of sera 719, 720, 721, 722, 723, 724, 726, 727, 759, 774, 775, and 792, with r values between 0.60 and 0.90 in North American Caucasoids and black panels.

* Work supported by AI-21410

The reaction patterns of DQw2 antisera were studied by family segregation analysis using the best data set selected by Albert and co-workers (Munich) for final analysis. Twelve DQw2 antisera were studied in three groups of 50 DQw2+ families with either DR3+ cells (as determined by positive reactions with the DR3 cluster 557, 561, 564, 565, 567, and 570), DR7+ cells (reacting with the DR7 cluster 629, 630, 633, 638, 640, and 642), or DR3–, DR7– cells. In the latter group, particular attention was given to DRw9+ cells reacting with DRw9 sera 644, 645, 647 and 650. We also studied two groups of families with a DR3+ or DR7+ parent who was DQw2– as indicated by computer antigen assignment. Only those reaction patterns which showed good family segregation with one haplotype were considered for analysis. In certain instances, we also included DQw2 antiserum reaction patterns for which no informative segregation was available in a given family, but nevertheless complemented patterns already defined by segregation in other families.

The most frequently observed reaction patterns for DQw2 antisera are shown in Table 1. The DR7 cells generally gave one of two patterns: the first reacting with all 12 sera, the second showing positive reactions with nine sera and negative reactions with sera 726, 792, and 759. The latter pattern was pre-

Histocompatibility Testing 1984
Edited by E. D. Albert et al.

Table 1. DQw2 antiserum reaction patterns

DR, DQ type of cells	726	792	759	775	727	719	723	721	724	720	774	722
DR7 + DQw2 +	+ +	+ +	+	+ +	+ +	+ +	+ +	+ +	+ +	+ +	+ +	+ +
DR7 + DQw2 – (B17 assoc. DQw3 +)	–	–	–	±	+	+	+	+	+	+	+	+
DR3 + DQw2 +	+ +	+ +	+ +	+ +	+ +	+	+ +	+ +	+ +	+ +	+ +	+ +
DR3 + DQw2 –	–	–	–	±	+	–	–	–	–	–	–	–
DRw9 + DQw2 – (DQw3 + , Japanese)	–	–	–	–	+ +	±	–	+ +	+ +	+	+ +	+

+ +, Almost always positive; +, frequently positive; ±, occasionally positive; –, generally negative

ferentially found with DR7 cells which also typed as B17. Previous cellular HLA-D data have shown that B17, DR7 cells are generally positive for Dw11 rather than Dw7 and that these cells are DQw2– [8]. The reactivity of the nine DQw2 antisera in the second pattern with DR7 cells could be due to the presence of extra DR7 antibodies in these sera. This explanation is compatible with the findings in several laboratories that most DQw2 antisera contain extra DR7 antibody activity.

Table 1 also shows two reactivity patterns of DQw2 antisera with DR3 cells. The first pattern consists of positive reactions with all 12 DQw2 antisera and suggest the presence of DQw2 on these DR3 cells. A second pattern with DR3 cells was recognized whereby most DQw2 antisera failed to react with these cells. The exception was serum 727 (and to some extent also 775), and the positive reactions of these DR3+, DQw2– cells might be due to the presence of extra DR3 specific antibody activity. On the other hand, serum 775 has been proposed by Tongio and Mayer [7] to recognize a DR3 and DR7 (or DQw2)-associated antigen, perhaps encoded by a gene located near DP.

The DR3+, DQw2– and DR7+, DQw2– cells were also analyzed for their reactivity with DQw1 and DQw3 specific antisera. The majority of DR7+, DQw2– cells gave generally positive reactions with DQw3 antisera (see Workshop report on DQw3 by R. J. Duquesnoy and M. Marrari, this volume). It is possible that this B17, DR7, DQw3 haplotype is associated with the cellularly defined Dw11 specificity [8]. On the other hand, most DR3+, DQw2– cells failed to give significant reactions with DQw1 or DQw3 specific sera segregation in informative families. M. Oudshoorn et al. (Segregation of DQ and DR: "Exceptions to the Rule," this volume) have demonstrated DR3, DQw1 haplotypes segregating in at least two black families. In this data set, we did not have access to these families. Nevertheless, it seems that many DR3+, DQw2– haplotypes type as DR3, DQ "blank". The DQ blank could mean the presence of an undefined DQ antigen associated with DR3 or that the DQw2 was missed because of possible weak expression leading to false-negative reactions with DQw2 antisera. For the latter, it should be noted that a considerable number of families showed one or more members exhibiting weak reactions with DQw2 antisera, while others carrying the same haplotype reacted strongly with these sera (this is also true for DQw1 and especially DQw3). In other words, a negative assignment for DQ may be related to a technical problem. Relevant to this might be the observations in several laboratories that monocytes have weak DQ antigen expression.

No DR3–, DR7– cells were identified in these groups of families that were DQw2+. One group of DRw9 cells of primarily Japanese origin reacted with several DQw2 antisera. The reaction pattern, shown in Table 1, showed some similarity with the pattern observed with the B17 associated DR7+, DQw2– cells. Since the key DQw2 antisera 726 and 792 were negative with DRw9 cells, it seems that these cells were DQw2–. The positive reactions with certain DQw2 antisera might be due to the presence of extra DR7 antibodies which cross-reacted with DRw9. As shown in the workshop report on DQw3, DRw9 associates with a short DQw3. Other investigators, including Nunez and Stastny [9] have demonstrated the DRw9+, DQw2+, DQw3– haplotype segregating in families.

In summary, this workshop serum set contained several DQw2 specific antisera, most of which appeared to contain extra DR7 antibody activity. The best DQw2 sera were 726, 792 and perhaps also 759. The strong DQw2 association of DR3 and DR7 was confirmed.

References

1. Duquesnoy RJ, Marrari M, Annen K (1979) Identification of an HLA-DR associated system of B cell alloantigens. Transplant Proc 11:1757

2. Park MS, Terasaki PI (1980) Second DR locus. In: Terasaki PI (ed) Histocompatibility testing 1980. UCLA Tissue Typing Laboratory, Los Angeles, pp 578–582
3. Tanigaki N, Tosi R (1982) The genetic control of human Ia alloantigens: a three-loci model derived from the immunochemical analysis of "supertypic" specificities. Immunol Rev 66:5
4. Duquesnoy RJ, Marrari M (1980) MB system joint report. In: Terasaki PI (ed) Histocompatibility testing 1980. UCLA Tissue Typing Laboratory, Los Angeles, pp 552–555
5. Tanigaki N, Tosi R, Duquesnoy RJ, Ferrara GB (1983) Three IA species with different structures and alloantigenic determinants in an HLA-homozygous cell line. J Exp Med 157:23
6. Shackelford A, Strominger JL (1984) Identification of three class II antigens, DR7, MB2, and MT3, from a homozygous human cell line. Hum Immunol 9:159
7. Tongio M, Mayer S (1983) Which is the antigen recognized by serum 9W775? Ninth Workshop Newsletter 2
8. Dupont B, Braun DW, Yunis EJ, Carpenter CB (1980) HLA-D by cellular typing: joint report. In: Terasaki PI (ed) Histocompatibility testing 1980. UCLA Tissue Typing Laboratory, Los Angeles, pp 229–267
9. Nunez G, Stastny P (1983) Different MB specificities are associated with DRw9. Ninth Workshop Newsletter 5

Antigen Report: HLA-DQw3

R.J. Duquesnoy [1] and M. Marrari [2] *

1 University of Pittsburgh School of Medicine, Scaife Hall, Room 406, Pittsburgh, PA 15261, USA
2 Section Head, HLA-D Serology, Central Blood Bank of Pittsburgh, 812 Fifth Avenue, Pittsburgh, PA 15219, USA

DQw3 (MB3) was originally defined in 1979 by clusters of Seventh International and Third American Workshop alloantisera as a new HLA-D region antigen associated with DR4 and DR5 [1]. This specificity is also similar to Te22 [2], TB21 [3], LB-E13 [4], DC4 [5], and MT4 [6]. During the Eighth Workshop, five sera were used to define DQw3 (MB3) [7]. However, many DQw3 antisera also contained DR4-specific antibodies. Several laboratories have recently generated monoclonal antibodies specific for DQw3, including IVD12 (Capra), 17.15 (Hansen), TA10, PLM2 and PLM12 (Maeda), Hu18 (Aizawa), and 2HB6 (Bodmer). Biochemical studies have indicated the existence of DQw3-carrying molecules distinct from DR4 and DR5 [8, 9]. The data suggest that DQw3 is encoded by a distinct HLA-D gene different from HLA-DR. Cellular studies with alloreactive T cell clones have demonstrated that T cells recognize DQw3-associated PLT and CML determinants [10].

A preliminary analysis of selected DQw3 antisera with data obtained from Region 17 (Amos) laboratories, including our own, showed significant correlations in the reaction patterns of sera 744, 745, 746, 747, 748, 750, and 791, with *r* values between 0.66 and 0.90 in North American Caucasoids and blacks. Additional DQw3 antisera included for this analysis were 584, 740, 745, 754, 761, and 777 as well as monoclonal antibodies 908, 915, and 969.

The reaction patterns of DQw3 antisera were studied by family segregation analysis using the best data set selected by Albert and co-workers (Munich) for the final analysis. The DQw3 antisera were studied in three groups of 50 DQw3+ families (primarily Japanese and South African blacks, some European and American) with either DR4+ cells (as determined by positive reactions with the DR4 antisera 575, 576, 580, 581, 585, 589, and 595), DR5+ cells (reacting with 597, 598, 599, 601, and 603), or DR4–, DR5– cells. In the latter group, particular attention was given to DRw6 and DRw8 cells as well as DR7 and DRw9 cells that were DQw2–. We also studied two groups of families with a DR4+ or DR5+ parent who was DQw3– as indicated by computer antigen assignment. The DQw3 antiserum reaction patterns were compared with those of DRw53 antisera (734, 735, 736, and 743) and with a serum cluster (730, 731, and 753) that reacted with DR4, DR5, and DR7 cells. Only those reaction patterns were considered for analysis which showed good family segregation with one haplotype. In certain instances, we also included reaction patterns for which no informative segregation was available in a given family, but nevertheless complemented patterns already defined by segregation in other families.

For this series of families, the most frequently observed reaction patterns for DQw3 antisera are shown in Table 1. Three patterns were observed with DR4 cells. The first pattern showed positive reactions with all DQw3 antisera including the monoclonals. These DR4 cells were considered DQw3+. The second pattern, primarily observed with Japanese DR4 cells, showed positive reactions

* Work supported by AI-21410

Table 1. DQw3 antiserum reaction patterns

	DQw3 antisera													DQw3 MoAb			DRw53 antisera				DR4, 5, 7 antisera		
	791	750	745	584	747	740	761	754	777	746	748	786	744	969	908	915	734	743	735	736	730	731	753
DR4+, DQw3+	+	+	+	++	+	±	+	+	±	++	+	+	++	++	+	+	++	++	++	++	++	++	++
DR4+, DQw3+ (Japanese)	++	++	++	++	±	++	±	±	–	–	–	–	–	±	±	±	+	+	+	+	++	++	++
DR4+, DQw3–	±	+	±	++	±	+	–	–	–	–	–	–	–	–	–	–	±	±	±	±	++	++	++
DR5+, DQw3+	++	++	++	++	++	+	+	+	+	++	++	++	+	++	++	++	–	–	–	–	++	++	++
DR5+, DQw3+ (Japanese)	++	++	++	++	+	++	+	++	–	–	–	–	–	±	±	±	+	+	+	+	++	++	++
DR5+, DQw3–	+	+	–	–	±	–	–	±	–	–	–	–	–	±	±	–	–	–	–	–	–	±	–
DR7+, DQw3+ (B17 Assoc. DQw2–)	++	±	±	++	+	±	–	±	+	++	±	++	+	++	++	++	++	++	++	–	++	++	++
DRw9+, DQw3+ (Japanese)	±	–	+	++	+	–	–	–	–	++	+	+	++	+	+	+	++	++	++	+	++	++	++
DR5&DRw6 Related, DQw3+	++	±	–	±	±	–	–	++	±	+	+	+	±	++	+	++	–	–	±	–	±	±	±

++, Almost always positive; +, frequently positive; ±, occasionally positive; –, generally negative

with about two-thirds of the DQw3 antisera, but only occasionally positive reactions with the DQw3 monoclonals. These DR4 cells were positive for DRw53 and reacted with the DR4 + 5 + 7 antisera. The third pattern showed positive reactions with less than half of the DQw3 antisera and with none of the monoclonals. Although each of these cells reacted strongly with the DR4 + 5 + 7 antisera, only half were positive for DRw53. This reaction pattern with DQw3 antisera was interpreted to mean negative assignment of DQw3 on these DR4 cells. The few positive reactions could be due to the presence of DR4 antibodies in these antisera.

Three major DQw3 antiserum reaction patterns were observed with DR5 cells. The first pattern showed positive reactions with all DQw3 antisera, including the monoclonals, suggesting that these DR5 cells were DQw3+. The second pattern was observed with Japanese DR5 cells and was practically identical to the short DQw3 pattern with Japanese DR4 cells. This suggests that the reactivity of these DQw3 antisera with DR4 or DR5 cells was not due to extra DR antibodies, but rather indicated the detection of a DQw3-related variant. This short DQw3 is similar to the DQw3 subtype reported by Maeda and Hirata [11].

The third pattern with DR5 cells showed generally positive reactions with only three DQw3 antisera. These DR5 cells were considered to be DQw3–, and it is possible that the DQw3 antisera contained extra DR5 antibodies. The DR5–, DQw3– cells also failed to react with the DQw3 monoclonals and the DR4, 5, 7 antisera. Many DR5+ DQw3– cells (especially of Negro origin) were positive for DQw1.

The workshop report on DQw2 (M. Marrari and R. J. Duquesnoy, this volume) describes DR7+, DQw2– and Japanese DRw9+, DQw2– cells which reacted with several DQw2 antisera presumably containing extra DR7 (and DRw9) antibody activity. These cells were generally DQw3+ as shown by positive reactions with DQw3 antisera (Table 1). The reaction pattern with DRw9 cells was shorter than that with DR7 cells. Several families showed segregation of DRw5 and DRw6-related specificities with DQw3. These specificities included LB5 (DRw11), DR5×8 (DRw12), and DRw6.9 (DRw14), and were always MT2+ (DRw52+). The serological definition of these specificities and their DQ associations have been studied by Schreuder et al. [12] (report on DRw6, this volume).

In summary, although several DQw3 antisera appeared to have extra DR4 antibody activity, DQw3 could be readily defined in this workshop. Several reaction patterns were observed, suggesting possible subtypes of DQw3. HLA-DR associations of DQw3 included DR4, DR5 (both DRw11 and

DRw12), DRw6 (DRw14 and possibly DRw13), DR7, and DRw9. This workshop analysis on DQw3 was done with a limited number of families of few racial origins. A more comprehensive study is necessary to fully analyze the complexity of DQw3.

References

1. Duquesnoy RJ, Marrari M, Annen K (1979) Identification of an HLA-DR associated system of B cell alloantigens. Transplant Proc 11:1757
2. Park MS, Terasaki PI, Nakata S, Aoki D (1980) Supertypic DR groups: MT1, MT2 and MT3. In: Terasaki PI (ed) Histocompatibility testing 1980. UCLA Tissue Typing Laboratory, Los Angeles, pp 854–857
3. Maeda H, Juji T (1982) A new B-cell alloantigen, TB21, coded for in the HLA-D/DR region. Tissue Antigens 20:327–334
4. Termijtelen A, Boettcher B, Bradley BA, D'Amaro J, van Leeuwen A, van Rood JJ (1980) DR typing in Australian aborigines. An indication for a second locus in the HLA-D region defined by serology. Tissue Antigens 16:140–146
5. Tanigaki N, Tosi R (1982) The genetic control of human Ia alloantigens: a three-loci model derived from the immunochemical analysis of "supertypic" specificities. Immunol Rev 66:5
6. Park MS, Terasaki PI, Bernoco D (1980) Relationship between MT and DR antigens. In: Terasaki PI (ed) Histocompatibility testing 1980. UCLA Tissue Typing Laboratory, Los Angeles, pp 572–573
7. Duquesnoy RJ Marrari M (1980) MB System. In: Terasaki PI (ed) Histocompatibility testing 1980. UCLA Tissue Typing Laboratory, Los Angeles, pp 552–555
8. Karr RW, Kannapell CC, Stein JA, Gebel HM, Mann DL, Duquesnoy RJ, Fuller TC, Rodey GE, Schwartz BD (1982) Molecular relationships of the human B cell alloantigens MT2, MB3, MT4 and DR5. J Immunol 128:1809
9. Hurley CK, Giles RC, Capra JD (1983) The human MHC: evidence for multiple HLA-D-region genes. Immunol Today 4:219
10. Zeevi A, Scheffel C, Annen K, Bass G, Marrari M, Duquesnoy RJ (1982) Association of PLT specificity of alloreactive lymphocyte clones with HLA-DR, MB and MT determinants. Immunogenetics 16:209
11. Maeda H, Hirata R (1984) MB3 and its related specificities: serological detection of its subtype and allelic antigen. Ninth Workshop Newsletter 7:49–52
12. Schreuder I, Parlevliet J (1983) HLA-DR, LB, MB, MT and "8w13" with 9W HTCs. Ninth Workshop Newsletter 5:41–45

Reports on Monoclonal Antibodies

HLA-A, B, C Monoclonal Antibodies

R. Fauchet[1], J.G. Bodmer[2], L.J. Kennedy[2], M.C. Mazzilli[3], C. Müller[4], C. Raffoux[5], and P. Richiardi[6]

1 Laboratoire d'Histocompatibilité, Centre Regional de Transfusion Sanguine, Rue Pierre Jean Gineste, 35000 Rennes, France
2 Imperial Cancer Research Fund, P.O. Box 123, Lincoln's Inn Fields, London WC2A 3PX, U.K.
3 Cathedra di Genetica Medica, Università la Spezia, Via Portuense 19, 00149 Rome, Italy
4 Immunologisches Labor, HLA-Serologie Abt. II, 7400 Tübingen, Federal Republic of Germany
5 Hôpital St. Louis, 2 Place du Dr. Fournier, 75010 Paris, France
6 Istituto di Genetica Medica, Università di Torino, Via Santena 19, 10126 Torino, Italy

Since Köhler and Milstein (1975) perfected the hybridroma technique, it has been possible to produce monoclonal antibodies (Mo Abs) which react against antigens of the human MHC. This technology allowed the production of some polymorphic reagents, of which 54 HLA-A and B Mo Abs were selected for the Ninth Workshop; 49 of these had clear HLA-A or B specificity assigned by the submitting laboratory. Two analyses were carried out. The first used 5000 unrelated individuals including 3000 Caucasoids, 1500 Japanese, and 500 Negroes. The second was performed on data from all British laboratories, selected European laboratories (ARN, BAR, FAU, FER, GAN, JEA, VIV, IT 1, CRB, CON, MTT, MEN, SAV), South African laboratories (DUT, HAM), and Japanese laboratories (TOK, KSH, OKO, SAS).

It is striking that in all the ethnic groups studied (Caucasoids, Negroes, and Japanese) a high number of reagents had additional specificities compared with the submitted specificity(ies) (28/49). There are two possible ways of explaining these results: the first, and most important, possibility is carry-over, which is responsible for these additional specificities at least 12 times out of 28, as shown in Table 1. This table (by Dr. M. Barthalo)

Table 1. Carry-over diagram

1103 A2, A28	1104 A2 ►A28	1113 B7, 27, 40, w47, 13	1116 A3 ►B7, B27
1121 A29 B7	1122 A3, A11 ►A29	1130 A2, A28 B39	1131 A3 ►A2, A28
1134 B13	1135 A32, B27 ►B7, 40, w41, w47	1142 A2, A28	1143 Bw6
1146 A3 A2, A28◄	1151 A2, A28	1152 A3 ►A2	1153 B13, B40 ►A3
1154 B8 B13, A2◄	1156 A2, A28	1157 Bw4, A23 ►A2, A28	1158 B13 ►A2
1160 B8	1125 A25, 32 ►A2, B8		

Top specificities as given by submitting laboratory, lower specificities additional (arrows = the additional carry over specificities)

indicates where carry-over has occurred, assuming serpentine distribution of reagents. The carry-over was observed with eight HLA-A Mo Abs (six A2, A28 reagents, one A3, and one A29) and four HLA-B Mo Abs (two B7, B27, one B13, B40, and one B8). These were probably the most concentrated Mo Abs used in this study. For example, the problem of carry-over is clearly demonstrated for the three HLA Mo Abs 9w1131, 9w1146, and 9w1152, which were all contaminated by anti-HLA-A2 activity from previous Mo Abs on the typing tray. These particular Mo Abs have been used extensively and exchanged several times and have never previously shown any activity other than HLA-A3 [1, 2, 3].

A second possibility is that, because a larger range of ethnic groups were studied in the Workshop than in the submitting laboratories, the extra activity might be due to ethnic differences not previously detected. Apart from 1137, which was weak, all the Mo Abs showed identifiable specificity and could be divided into three groups: group I, with 24 HLA-A Mo Abs; group II, with 22 HLA-B Mo Abs; and group III, with seven possible HLA-A + B Mo Abs.

Group I. The 24 anti-HLA-A Mo Abs could be subdivided into six subgroups, as shown in Table 2. In subgroups 1 to 5 the HLA-A specificities were well defined; subgroups 1 and 2 are the only HLA-A-monospecific Mo Abs, A3 and A29 respectively. Subgroups 3, 4, and 5 include well-known cross-reacting specificities: A3-A11, A32-A25, and A2-A28 respectively. The last subgroup contained broad polymorphic specificities.

Group II. The 22 anti-HLA-B Mo Abs can also be subdivided into six subgroups (Table 3). Subgroups 1 and 2 are the only HLA-B-monospecific Mo Abs, B8 and B13 respectively. Subgroup 3 includes the B7-B27-related Mo Abs with some discrepancies in different populations. Subgroup 4 contains the B14 CREG and B5 CREG. Subgroup 5 contains one broad polymorphic reagent, and subgroup 6 contains Bw6-Bw4 Mo Abs.

Group III. This includes seven Mo Abs reacting against HLA-A and B antigens, the so-called interlocus Mo Abs: 1107 (B7 + A32), 1124 (A23 + B40), 1132 (A2 + B16), 1133 (B7 + Aw19), 1135 (B7 + A32), 1144 (A2 + B17), and 1155 (Bw4 + A32).
The reaction frequencies of antibodies and a series of pattern analyses were carried out on selected sets of data. The comparison between the reaction frequencies of the antibodies showed no difference

Table 2. Anti-HLA-A Mo Abs

Group	Antigens	9W no.	
1	A3	1131, 1146, 1152	All populations
2	A29	1119, 1138, 1120, 1121	Caucasoid and Negro Not significant in Japanese
3	A3 – A11	1126, 1122	Caucasoid and Negro
4	A32 – A25	1125	Caucasoid and Negro
5	A2 – A28	1139, 1141, 1142, 1151	All populations
		1108, 1156	Only A2 in Japanese
		1102, 1103, 1104	A2 – A24 in Japanese
		1130	B39 in Japanese
6	A2, A3, 28, 30, A31, 32	1106	
	A1, 11, 23, 24 A25, 26	1109	

Table 3. Anti-HLA-B Mo Abs

Group	Antigens	9W no.	
1	B8	1140, 1154, 1160	
2	B13	1134, 1153, 1158	
3	B7 – B27	1128, 1129, 1150	Bw42 in Negro
	B7	1111	B40, B27 in Caucasoid
		1112	B40 in all populations B27, w47 in Caucasoid Bw48 in Japanese
		1113	B40 in all populations B27, w47 Caucasoid
4	CREG B14 B8, 14, 18, 51, 38, 39	1117, 1118, 1147	All populations
	CREG B5 B5, 15, 21	1136	
5	B27, B7 Bw22, 17, 15	1105	
6	Bw6	1159, 1143	Caucasoid
	Bw4	1157	

for the Mo Abs 1102, 1104, 1108, 1156 (A2, A28), 1116 (A3), 1134 (B13), and 1154 (B8), and very small differences for 1147 (CREG B14), 1151 (A2, A28), and 1126 (A3, A11); significant discrepancies were observed for 1107, 1112 (B7 related), 1109 and 1110 (broad antibodies), 1130 (A2, A28), and 1159 (Bw6), as well as for some polymorphic well-defined Mo Abs, 1160 (B8), 1119 (A29), 1131 and 1152 (A3). For other Mo Abs, there are great differences in reaction frequencies between laboratories. Either the sensitivity of the techniques used in the different laboratories or the choice of the selected complement could explain the different results.

Pattern Analyses

A2, A28. The A2, A28 Mo Abs (1102, 1103, 1104, 1108, 1130, 1132, 1139, 1141, 1142, 1144, 1151 and 1156) gave clear patterns defining A2, A28 and the new antigen Aw69 (previously A2/28), as shown in Table 4. Several A2 variants could also be defined occurring in reasonable numbers in more than one ethnic group. Pattern 1 in Table 4 is the normal A2, with all the Mo Abs positive. Pattern 2 is defined by the negative reaction of 1132. Two rare patterns, 3 and 4, were also identified. The former corresponded to the negative reactions of 1144, the latter to those of 1151 and 1156. The last pattern, 5, might be a Chinese variant of A2, as suggested by L. J. Kennedy. All of these variants have been shown to be inherited in more than one family. The new antigen Aw69, previously 2/28, was defined by the positive reactions of 1104 and 1139 plus the negative reactions of 1132 and 1144. This antigen was found in several laboratories [4, 5, 6], although it appears to be restricted to certain ethnic groups, namely Italians, Armenians, and Arabs. Table 4 also shows two clear patterns of Aw68 (28.1 and 28.2): the first one (probably 28.1) is negative with 1132, 1144, 1104 and 1139, while the second one (probably 28.2) is also negative with 1151 and 1156.

It is interesting to note that the only Mo Abs which are pure A2 with no A28 are, in fact, "interlocus" Mo Abs and contain B locus reactivity: 1132 is A2 plus B8, and 1144 is A2 plus B17.

A3, A11. There were four HLA-A3 antibodies, 1131, 1146, 1152, and 1116, and two A3 + A11 antibodies, 1122 and 1126, as shown in Table 5. There seemed to be several patterns for A3 but no clear pattern for A11. Antibodies 1146 and 1152 appeared to be the best A3 Mo Abs, as well as the most reproducible ones.

A25, A32. The antibodies 1127 and 1125 are related to A25 and A32, but only 1125 is a good reagent.

A29. Antibodies 1119, 1120, 1121, and 1138 gave a good definition of A29, with 1119 and 1138 giving the highest r values. It is interesting to note that 1119, 1120, and 1121 were produced from the same fusion but are three different hybridomas. 1138, a rat monoclonal antibody which has a specificity for Class I $RT1^{u}$ private antigen of the Lewis rat, did not react with Japanese A29 cells.

B7-Related Mo Abs. Seven Mo Abs, 1105, 1111, 1112, 1113, 1128, 1129, and 1150, defined B7 and the B7-related antigens B27 and B40. B7 appeared to be the main specificity in 1105, 1111, 1112, and 1113, with good average scores of 8 and few misses.

Table 4. Patterns of A2, A28 Mo Abs

														ALL U.K. LABS		ARN BAR FAU FER GAN JEA VIV		DUT HAM		TOK KSH OKO SAS	
	9W no. Local names	1102 CII	1103 FHB 3	1108 FU 10	1130 A28 2MI	1141 3.63 14	1142 MI 20	1151 XII 413	1156 TU 101	1132 AB 1058	1144 RM2	1104 P5.1	1139 BB 7.2	UK		Europe		Black		Japan	
														n	Spec.	*n*	Spec.	*n*	Spec.	*n*	Spec.
A2	pattern 1	+	+	+	+	+	+	+	+	+	+	+	+	123	A2	55	A2	16	A2	47	44/47 A2
A2	pattern 2	+	+	+	+	+	+	+	+	–	+	+	+			99	A2	12	A2	8	A2
A2	pattern 3	+	+	+	+	+	+	+	+	+	–	+	+	15	A2						
A2	pattern 4	+	+	+	+	+	+	–	–	+	+	+	+	2	A2 Chinese ?			8	A2	24	A2
A2	pattern 5	+	+	+	+	+	+	+	+	+	+	+	–	1	Chinese					20	A2
A28	Aw69 (2/28)	+	+	+	+	+	+	+	+	–	–	+	+	3	w69	5	w69	3		2	A2 (?)
A28	Aw68 A28.1	+	+	+	+	+	+	+	+	–	–	–	–	22	A28	4	A28	6	A28		
A28	Aw68 A28.2	+	+	+	+	+	+	–	–	–	–	–	–			3	A28				
	specificity	A2, 28, w69						A2, 28 w69 not A2 Chinese		A2 B8	A2 B17	A2, w69 not A28									

Table 5. Patterns of A3, A11 Mo Abs

	9W no. Local name	A3 1131 X-15.4	1146 GAP. A3	1152 XI-23.1	1116 XX20.1	A3, A11 1122 FPA GH3	1126 FPA-ARIF	No. of cells
A3		+	+	+	+	+	+	38
		+	+	+	+	–	+	76
		+	+	+	+	–	–	48
		+	+	+	–	–	–	71

Table 6. Patterns of B7- related Mo Abs

	9w no. Local name	B7 1105	1111 11-97	1112 11-97	1113 11-81	B27 1128 M1	1150 ABC M3	1129 M2	Cells U.K. *n.*	Spec.	Europe *n.*	Spec.	Black *n.*	Spec.	Japan *n.*	Spec.
B7	1	+	+	+	+	–	–	–	49	B7	27	B7	6	B7	20	16/20
	2	+	+	+	+	+	–	–	6	B7	6	B7				
	3	+	+	+	+	+	+	–	5	B7	6	B7	5	B7	2	B7
	4	+	+	+	+	–	+	–	10	[6 B7 3 B27	4	B7			7	5/7
B40	5	–	–	+	+	–	–	–	9	Bw60					10	B40
B27	6	+	–	+	+	+	+	±	10	B27						
	7	–	–	–	+	+	+	–	5	B27						
		B7 B27	B7	B7 B27	B7 B27 B40	B27 B7	B27 B7	B27								

In 1128, 1129, and 1150 the main specificity was B27, with a good average score and a few misses for 1150. As shown in Table 6, the patterns were complex, with four patterns clearly defining B7 and two defining B27. Antibody 1129 was weakly positive, but could subdivide B27. Splits of B27 have been shown previously by Grumet [7]. B40 could be characterized by the negative reaction of 1128, 1129, 1150, 1105, and 1111 and the positive reaction of 1112 and 1113.

B8-B14-Related Mo Abs. There were three monospecific B8 Mo Abs, 1140, 1154 and 1160 with good average scores and few misses. Table 7 shows these plus other reagents which could define B8 but also contained activity against the following: B37 (1110); B18 + B14, B51, B38 + B39 (1117); and B14 + B38 + B39 (1147). The Mo Ab 1118 reacted with most of these specificities except B8. Several patterns for B8 were observed, and one (the fifth in the table) only seemed to occur in the black population. There were possibly two patterns for B14 based on 1117, 1118 and 1147.

B13. Antibodies 1134, 1153, and 1158 seemed to identify B13 very clearly. Patterns with 1134 negative and 1153 negative were found in all populations (Table 8).

B5 CREG. Antibody 1136 appeared to be broad polymorphic, containing B5, B15 (w62), B35, Bw70, B17 and B21.

Bw4, Bw6. Two Mo Abs, 1155 and 1157, defined Bw4. Antibody 1155 seemed complex, as it reacted with A9 and A32 cells. Antibody 1157 was different in that it showed no correlation with HLA-A locus specificities. Antibody 1155 also reacted with some Bw6 cells which were A9 negative and A32 negative. Antibodies 1143 and 1159 defined Bw6 in most ethnic groups, although negative reactions were observed with Bw4-Bw6 heterozygous cells, perhaps linked with the low titer of Mo Abs and the loss of activity with storage. (See DR monoclonal antibody joint report, this volume.)

Ethnic Variations. Two Mo Abs, 1106 and 1109, had previously been considered as broad HLA-A

Table 7. Patterns of B8, B14 Mo Abs

	B8			B8 + B14					Cells			
9W no.	1140	1154	1160	1110	1117	1118	1147	1148	U.K.	Europe	Black	Japan
Local name	LBC 3B5	TERM B8	8.1	FU III	XXIII 23.1	XX.II 34.5	PHR 917.71	K27 2				
B8	+	+	+	+	+	+	+	+	10	2	1	3
	+	+	+	+	+	+	+	−	14	2	4	
	+	+	+	+	+	−	+	−	27	3		
	+	+	+	−	+	−	−	−	4	16		
	+	+	+	+	+	−	−	−			9	
	+	+	−	+	+	+	+	−	3			
	+	+	−	+	+	−	+	−	5			
B14	−	−	−	−	+	+	+	−	28	2	10	
	−	−	−	+	+	+	+	−	2			
					B8 B14	B8 B14	B8 B14					

Table 8. Patterns of B13 Mo Abs

9W no.	1134	1153	1158	No. of cells			
Local name	SY-1	TER MB13	TVE 110	U.K.	Europe	Black	Japan
				23	22	3	7
	+	+	+	19/23 B13	18/22 B13	2/3 B13	4/7 B13
	−	+	+	7	15	5	7
	+	−	+	3	1		2

antibodies. In the Japanese population, 1106 reacted with A2, Aw33, A31, and some A3 cells, whereas 1109 reacted mainly with A26, A11, some A1, and some A3 cells. Family studies confirmed the segregation patterns [8]. In the Caucasoid population, reactivity to these Mo Abs segregates with particular haplotypes, but also with a broader range of specificities.

Conclusion

The Ninth Workshop class I Mo Abs proved very interesting, and included several reagents for some HLA-A and B specificities: A3, A29, A25, B7, B27, B8, B13, Bw4, and Bw6. There were no HLA-C antibodies. For the first time, a new specificity, Aw69, has been defined with Mo Abs, and confirmation of a possible split of A28 has been indicated. B27 and B40 cannot be clearly identified, although B7 was well characterized. A B14 serological pattern was identified.

However, the discrepancies observed between the different laboratories still remain to be resolved. One explanation could be the variability caused by carry-over. Some ways of avoiding this are discussed in the HLA-D Region Monoclonal Antibodies joint report in this volume. A second explanation would be the titer of the Mo Abs and their storage conditions. Finally, the sensitivity of the technique used in each laboratory and the choice of the complement used could be responsible.

It is important to be aware of these risks and to take them into account when assessing the results of Mo Ab testing.

References

1. Berger AE, Davis JE, Cresswell P (1982) Monoclonal antibody to HLA-A3. Hybridoma 1:87–90
2. Bourel D, Fauchet R, Genetet B, Merdrignac G, Hurez D (1982) A monoclonal antibody to HLA-A3 allo-antigen. Immunol Letters 5:233–237
3. Trabace S, Mazzilli MC, Cascino I, Lulli SP, Costanzi S, Costanzi PS, Gandini E (1984) A mouse monoclonal antibody detecting the allospecificity HLA-A3. Tissue Antigens 23:12–16
4. Belvedere M, Richiardi P, Luciani G, Curtoni ES (1980) Crossreactions among HLA-A antigens particularly focused on HLA-A28. In: Terasaki PI (ed) Histocompatibility testing 1980. UCLA, Los Angeles, p 751

5. Kennedy LJ, Bodmer JG (1983) A2 variants including A2/A28 (a new A-locus antigen) defined by monoclonal antibodies (MCA). Ninth Workshop Newsletter V:1 – 3
6. Müller C, Liangru S, Schneider M, Ziegler A, Wernet P (1983) A cytotoxic monoclonal IgM antibody (Tü 101) directed against an antigenic determinant shared between the HLA-A allospecificities A2 and A28. Hum Immunol 6:189 – 197
7. Grumet FC, Fendly VM, Fish L, Foung S, Engleman EG (1982) A monoclonal antibody (B27M2) subdividing HLA-B27. Hum Immunol 5:61 – 72
8. Sato K, Kusama M, Yamashita Y, Nose Y, Sukegawa T, Tsuji K (1984) Possible supertypic HLA-A antigen detected by monoclonal antibodies in Japanese. Ninth Workshop Newsletter 6:26

HLA-D Region Monoclonal Antibodies

J.G. Bodmer[1], L.J. Kennedy[1], M. Aizawa[2], R.L. Dawkins[3], V. Lepage[4], M.C. Mazzilli[5], and P. Richiardi[6]

1 Imperial Cancer Research Fund, P.O. Box 123, Lincoln's Inn Fields, London WC2A 3PX, U.K.
2 Department of Pathology, Hokkaido University, School of Medicine, Kata 14 jo, Nishi 5, Kata-Ku, Sapporo, Japan
3 Tissue Typing Laboratory, Department of Clinical Immunology, Royal Perth Hospital, Perth, Western Australia 6000
4 Institut de Recherches Sur les Maladies du Sang, Hospital St. Louis, 2 Place du Docteur Fournier, 75475 Paris Cedex 10, France
5 Cattedra di Genetica Medica, Via Portuense 292, 00149 Rome, Italy
6 Istituto di Genetica Medica, Via Santena 19, 10126 Torino, Italy

Introduction

This is the first Histocompatibility Testing Workshop in which monoclonal antibodies have been featured as reagents separated from conventional antisera. In view of the virtually unlimited supply of a monoclonal antibody, its usually very high titre and its exquisite specificity for a particular epitope it appears to be an ideal reagent for the accurate definition of HLA specificity. The questions that this study was planned to answer were:

1. Do monoclonal antibodies work as well or better than conventional antisera for the definition of known antigens?
2. Can they identify new specificities?
3. Can they contribute extra information not easily obtainable with conventional antisera?
4. Can monoclonal antibodies be used in serological tissue typing in the same way as conventional antisera or do they need special handling?

Selection of Antibodies

Groups who had produced or had access to monoclonal antibodies to D region products were asked to submit them for a pre-Workshop screening. Details of published references and evidence of specificity were also requested. Since previous exchanges had suggested that there might be technical problems involved in the handling of monoclonal antibodies it was suggested (a) that the antibodies should not be frozen, but should be shipped and stored at +4 °C with the addition of 0.1% sodium azide; and (b) that different concentrations of the antibodies should be submitted, to see which proved the most robust when submitted to the inevitably disturbing conditions of shipping, resorting, shipping again and testing in different laboratories.
The 110 D region antibodies submitted were then screened by five laboratories and the results centrally analysed. On the basis of this analysis 93 D region monoclonal antibodies were selected, 92 of which were on plates 31 and 32, the DR monoclonal plates, and one on the DR serum plates (nos. 975 and 976 were ABC antibodies). The antibodies selected for the Workshop study are listed in Table 1 with their submitted specificities.

Analysis of the Data

Because of the technical problems of handling monoclonal antibodies involving carry-over and lack of reactivity (discussed elsewhere in this report), an analysis based on pooled combined data from unselected laboratories failed to show specificity for most of the antibodies. As a result, it was decided to carry out two steps of selection to produce data relatively free from technical problems on which to carry out the analysis. As there were few controls in the data, the selection was not

Histocompatibility Testing 1984
Edited by E. D. Albert et al.

Table 1. D region monoclonal antibodies

9w no.	Local name	Submitted by	Submitted specificity
901	SH-1	TSU	DR1, 2, w8
902	FU3	TSU	DR2, 4, w8
903	FU4	TSU	DR2, 4, w8
904	HU26	AIZ	All except DR7, w9
905	HU29	AIZ	DR polymorphic
906	HU30	AIZ	DR2 + weak DR1, 7, w9
907	HU28	AIZ	DR polymorphic
908	FU2	TSU	TB21
909	HU23	AIZ	DR4, 5, w8 (TA10)
910	FU9	TSU	
911	FU6	TSU	
912	FU8	TSU	
913	HU11	AIZ	DQw1-like
914	FU1	TSU	
915	HU18	AIZ	DQw3-like (TB21)
916	HU36	AIZ	DR polymorphic
917	HU42	AIZ	DR polymorphic
918	HU43	AIZ	DR1, 4, w9
919	HU44	AIZ	DR polymorphic
920	HU45	AIZ	DR polymorphic
921	HU46	AIZ	DR2, 4, w9 (+Dw15 part of DR4)
922	HU47	AIZ	DR polymorphic
923	HU48	AIZ	DR4
924	HU33	AIZ	DR polymorphic
925	HU39	AIZ	DR polymorphic (? DRw6 · 2)
926	HU49	AIZ	DR polymorphic
927	SH2	SH	DR1, 2, 4, w8
928	Y62C10	?	All except DRw6
929	16-23	JOH	DR3 plus some DRw6
930	VR7319 · 1	ROO	DRw52
931	B8-12 · 2	SVE	Positive with most B cells
932	H39-49 · 5	SVE	Broad polymorphic
933	H40-394 · 2	SVE	B cell polymorphic
934	H81-218 · 11	SVE	B cell polymorphic
935	H81-208 · 22	SVE	B cell polymorphic
936	H74-202 · 2	SVE	B cell polymorphic
937	H82-246 · 3	SVE	B cell polymorphic + some T cells
938	H82-246 · 3 (1/500)	SVE	B cell polymorphic
939	C-5.17	MTT	Broad polymorphic
940	XI-21 · 4	GAN	DR4, 7, w9
941	X-2 · 7	GAN	DR4, 7 and some DR3
942	X-44 · 8	GAN	DR7?
943	JAF77 · 34-10	FAL	DQw1
944	I-2	YUN	All but DR7
945	JMSDR4 · 1 · 1 (10X)	BOD	DQw1
946	8F10 (JMSDR8 · 1 · 1 (2X))	BOD	DR3, 5, w6
947	JMSDR8 · 1 · 1 (4X)	BOD	DR3, 5, w6
948	C5D4 (JMSDR8 · 1 · 1 (1X))	BOD	DR3, 5, w6
949	17 · 3 · 3 (5X)	BOD	DR7
950	XXI-3 · 6 · 2	FAU	Broad polymorphic
951	FLY-BL-12	BET	DR4, w9, w10
952	FLY-BL-12 (1/100)	BET	DRw9, w10
953	CHEV 642	DAU	DR5 short
954	CHEV 249 · 3	DAU	DR polymorphic
955	MAJA 51 · 2	DAU	DR polymorphic
956	FPA-BM50	DAU	DR polymorphic, all but DR7?
957	FPA-141	DAU	DR polymorphic
958	FPA-53	DAU	DR polymorphic
959	FPA-M18	DAU	$\beta 2M$
960	SFR-3	AMO	DR5
962	GAP-D1	AMO	Unknown: misses DR1, 3 cells
963	HPA49 · 11 · 10	ZMI	DR1
964	NFB-14 · 12	AMO	Polymorphic
965	MCS7	TAN	DR3, 5, w6 + weak DR2 and DR4

Table 1 (continued)

9w no.	Local name	Submitted by	Submitted specificity
967	E5A7 · 3A	THO	DQw1, neg to DRw14
968	TER-M	TER	DR5
969	17 · 15	HAN	DR4, 5, some DR7
970	Tue 22	WER	DQ monomorphic
972	RM-2 · 82	TAI	DR monomorphic
973	RM-2 · 102	TAI	DR monomorphic
974	RM-3 · 29	TAI	All except DR7
975	RM-3 · 170	TAI	ABC A2, Bw57
976	RM-5 · 79	TAI	ABC Bw4 + A24
977	RM-7 · 25	TAI	Monomorphic
978	RM-7 · 89	TAI	Monomorphic
979	19 · 26 · 1 (1/500)	ANZ	
980	203-F5 (1/500)	ANZ	
981	203-F5 (1/1000)	ANZ	
982	326 · 2 · D2 · 4	ANZ	
983	326 · 2 · D2 · 4 (1/5)	ANZ	
984	HO-19 · 1 · D · 12 · 2	ANZ	
985	HO-19 · 1 · D · 12 · 2 (1/10)	ANZ	
986	HO-19 3D.H.G.8	ANZ	
987	HO-134D71	ANZ	
988	19 – 26 · 1	ANZ	DR2, w6
782	D4 90 55/6	CRB	All but DR7
783	D7 · 69/9	CRB	All but DR7
784	AB8 · 25/5	CRB	DR2, 5, some DR4 und DRw6
992	IJ-B-6	HAM	DRw52
993	Tue 34	WER	DR monomorphic
994	Tue 35	WER	DR monomorphic
995	Tue 37	WER	DR monomorphic
996	Tue 39	WER	DR monomorphic
660	JMSDR4.1.1 (10X)	BOD	DR1, 2, w6, w10
790	A-10-83	MAE	TA10

simple. The two strategies tried were:

1. Selection of data from some of the laboratories who produced monoclonal antibodies, on the assumption that they would be accustomed to handling monoclonal antibodies
2. A much more rigorous selection involving agreement of reaction on duplicate samples of the same antibody and positivity to known monomorphic antibodies.

First Stage

For the first selected analysis, data from some monoclonal antibody producing laboratories were arranged into six sets. Four of them were Caucasoid: from the UK (337 individuals), Australia (258 individuals), USA (157 individuals), and the mainland of Europe (653 individuals). One of the other two sets was from South Africa, with 153 selected black cells, and the other from Japan, with 238 Japanese cells.

A cluster analysis was then performed [as described in 1, p. 45] on each of the data sets separately. The clusters were then compared to see which antibodies showed similar patterns of clustering in more than one set of data and ethnic group. Table 2 shows the results of this analysis. With this very rough technique four clusters showed a high level of reproducibility, that of the DQw3 antibody cluster showing significance in all groups analysed and DQw1, DRw52, and "all except DR7 and DRw9" agreeing in five out of six of the groups.

The above analysis was deliberately carried out with a minimum selection of "good data", in order to identify the monoclonal antibodies which were really robust and specific and could be expected to give clear results in almost all circumstances. The monoclonal antibodies listed for DQw1, DQw3, DRw52, and "all except DR7 and DRw9" meet those criteria.

In addition, there were clear specificities defined in one or two sets of data shown in section B of the table. These will be discussed in more detail later.

Second Stage

The more rigorous selection of good data as a basis for analysis was carried out in a way similar to that used in the Seventh Workshop for the selection of

Table 2. Clusters of DR monoclonal antibodies based on comparison of six sets of data (see text)

Antigen	Antibodies clustered	Population group
A. Well-defined specificities in several groups		
DQw1	901, 927, 660, 945	UK, ANZ, US, EUR, SAF
DQw1	901	JAP
DQw3	909, 915, 969, (908)	All groups
DRw52	930, 946, 947, 948, (953)	UK, ANZ, US, EUR, SAF
All except DR7 + DRw9	904, 944, (974)	UK, ANZ, US, EUR, JAP
B. Specificities identified in one or two groups		
DR2	906	UK, US
DR1	924, 963	UK, US
DR3	929	UK
DRw12, DRw8	925	UK, JAP
DR7	949	UK

good B cell typing data for the newly defined DR antigens. Then, as in this study, analysis of the total pooled data failed to show specificity or coherent clustering of reactivity. Selection in that study was based on hidden positive and negative controls and exact serum duplicates. In the present study there were no exact duplicates, so *r* values between the following pairs of antibodies were examined: (a) 901 and 945; (b) 945 and 660; (c) 946 and 947; and (d) 947 and 948.

These pairs were chosen for the following reasons:

1. Antibodies 901 and 945 were two different DQw1 antibodies, which showed very similar reactivity in some laboratories.
2. Antibodies 945 and 660 were samples of the same antibody, 4.1 at the same dilution (x10 supernatant), but from different batches. In fact 660 was slightly weaker than 945, but, in cases where the *r* value between the two was low, 660 often showed a higher frequency of reactions, indicating probable carry-over from the monomorphic antibody 996 (TÜ39), which was next to it on the plate.
3. Antibodies 946 and 947 were the x 2 and x 4 supernatants of the same short DRw52 antibody 8.1. Here was the best chance of a good *r* value, since they were next to each other on the plate and carry-over would be a positive advantage. However, 23 laboratories (17%) had *r* values of 0.3 or less and 1 laboratory showed a negative value for the association.
4. Antibodies 947 and 948 were the x 4 and x 1 supernatants from the antibody 8.1. Here again, in laboratories where the *r* value was low, the x 1 supernatant often showed greater reactivity than the x 4 supernatant, possibly due to carry-over from its neighbour, 949 (17.3.3), the DR7 + Dw15 antibody.

The average value of these four pairs was calculated separately for each of the 138 laboratories in which the DR monoclonal antibodies had been tested, and the results are shown in Fig. 1, which shows that only 16 laboratories (12%) had *r* values of 0.65 or more between the selected pairs, and 48 laboratories (35%) had *r* values lower than 0.3. This is some indication of the extent of the technical problems that will be discussed later. However it seems clear that the good data are not randomly selected, because more detailed checks of the laboratories that had high *r* values showed that for other comparisons, e.g., the reactivity of the DQw3 antibodies 915 and 969, or the "all except DR7 and DRw9", 904 and 944, they also had high *r* values. It was therefore decided that the further analysis of the DR monoclonal antibodies should be carried out mainly with data from the best 16 laboratories.

For most of the analyses discussed, the data were organised into four sets, the first set supplied by the three laboratories with *r* values greater than 0.8 for the pairs compared, then the next four, the following three and the final six of the 16 laboratories. The results were compared for consistency between the groups.

The first analysis performed was a cluster analysis [1] to identify sets of antibodies with similar activity. These clusters are shown in Table 3. There are 20 clusters of antibodies shown here. The first six clusters all have three or more antibodies in them and the first five can be assigned to a previously described D region specificity. The next five clusters consist of one antibody which shows a high correlation with a defined antigen, and the final nine clusters have no clearly defined specificity, although there is sometimes an indication of relationship to a D region antigen. In the following discussion these clusters and the antibodies in them will be described with indications of variation in specificity where it is known.

Cluster 1 consists of four antibodies with DQw1 specificity. As is shown in Table 4, the *r* values be-

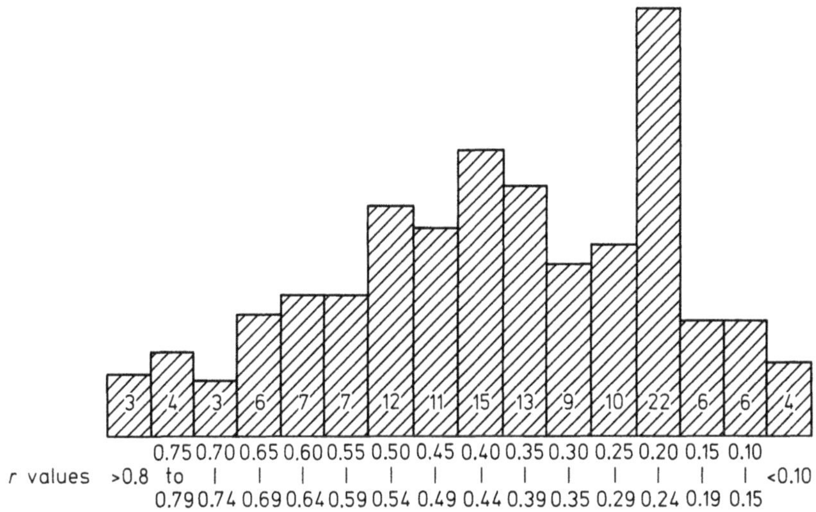

The *r* value is based on the average of the *r* values between:

901 and 945 both DQw1
945 and 660 same antibody
946 and 947 same antibody 4x & 2x
947 and 948 same antibody 2x & 1x

Fig. 1. Average *r* values between pairs of DR monoclonal antibodies used for the selection of "good" data in 138 laboratories

Table 3. Clusters of D region monoclonal antibodies based on selected data

Cluster	Antibodies	Specificity	Comments
1	901, 927, 945, 660	DQw1	
2	908, 915, 969	DQw3	
3	930, 946, 947, 948	DRw52	
4	904, 944, (935, 993, 994, 958, 957, 970)	All but DR7, DRw9	935 – 970 clustered with 904 and 944 but are weak mono. 904 and 944 are the best "all but DR7, DRw9"
5	909, 790, 968	TA10	Subset of DQw3
6	918, 940, 928	DR4, 1, w9	Allelic to DRw52?
7	906, DR2, DR2 short	> DR2	*r* with DR2 0.70
8	921, DRw8	DRw8 + YT (Dw15)	*r* with DRw8 0.50
9	923, DR4, DR4 short	DR4	*r* with DR4 0.60
10	941, DRw53	> DRw53	*r* with DRw53 0.50
11	949, DR7	DR7, YT (Dw15)	*r* with DR7 0.64
12	924, 963	?	963 related to DR1, *r* 0.54
13	936, 996	Mono	*r* 0.90 monomorphic
14	903, 943, 964, 914	~ DQw1	possibly kind of DQw1 associated with DR2
15	916, 931, 954, 980	Unknown	Frequency about 60%
16	919, 920	Unknown	*r* 0.75, frequency about 10%
17	932, 934, 992, 995, 937, 938	Unknown	Frequency 80%; some of these submitted as polymorphic and others monomorphic
18	984,978, 986	Unknown	Some relation with DR5 and DRw8
19	782, 974	Unknown	*r* 0.64. Negative *r* with DRw53
20	955, 962	Unknown	*r* 0.48. Related to DQw1

The lowest *r* value between any pair in the cluster is 0.39. Complete tables of *r* values for some of the clusters are given in subsequent tables

Table 4. Correlation between and patterns of reaction to DQw1 antibodies (928 individuals)

a) *r* values

660				
945	0.82			
927	0.78	0.81		
901	0.77	0.77	0.88	
	660	945	927	901

b) Reaction pattern

No. in pattern	901	927	945	660	
298	+	+	+	+	112 DRw6 (38%), 79 DR1 (27%), 54 DR2 (18%)
27	+	+	–	–	Only 6/27 DRw6 (22%)
8	–	–	+	+	2/8 DRw6 (37%)
222	–	–	–	–	

A further 70 individuals had other patterns of reactivity, but since many involved different reactivities to duplicates 945 and 660 they appear to give no significant information

Table 5. Correlation of DQw3 and TA10 antibodies (*r* values)

969						
915	0.83					
908	0.56	0.65				
909	0.57	0.57	0.35			
790	0.54	0.55	0.27	0.89		
968	0.39	0.32	0.32	0.54	0.45	
	969	915 DQw3	908	909	790 TA10	968

tween all pairs of these antibodies are very high (0.77 or greater), indicating great similarity of reaction. As mentioned above, two of the antibodies, 945 and 660, are duplicate samples of the same antibody. In addition to DQw1, antibody 901 also reacts to some DRw8 cells (both DQw3-positive cells and DQ blank cells) and to DR4 cells, which are Dw15 associated (see Table 7). The pattern analysis of these antibodies, shown in Table 4b, reveals a clear bimodal distribution indicating clear assignment of DQw1 antigen with these antibodies.

Cluster 2 shows the DQw3 antibodies, the best pair being 915 and 969. Table 5 gives the *r* values for the three DQw3 antibodies and also the three TA10 antibodies identified in cluster 5. The *r* values between the two sets of antibodies are shown in Table 5 as TA10 appears to be included in DQw3 as a DQ subregion subset. A pattern analysis shown in Table 6 shows that DR4, DQw3 cells do not appear to carry the TA10 specificity, whereas DR5, DQw3 cells usually do. This appears to be confirmed in a study of homozygous cell lines, as shown in Table 7. The DQw3, TA10 specificity is also seen on two DRw12, DQw3 cell lines including HERLUF.

Cluster 3 shows the DRw52 antibodies (Table 8). Three of them, 946, 947 and 948, are the same antibody at different dilutions and identify a "short DRw52" reacting only with DR3, 5 and w6 cells.

Table 6. Patterns of reaction in DR4- and DR5-positive cells

Total in pattern	DR4	DR5	DQw3		TA10		DQw1		
			915	969	909	790	901	945	
10	+	–	+	+	–	–	–	–	DR4, DQw3
15	–	+	+	+	+	+	–	–	DR5, DQw3, TA10 (4 of these are homozygous DR5 cell lines)
1	–	+	–	–	–	–	+	+	DR5, DQw1 (FPF, HTC 9w9901)
3	–	–	+	+	+	+	–	–	DQw3, TA10 with DRw6 e.g. AZL (DRw14, 9w1701) and DRw12, e.g., HERLUF (HTC 9w1503) and RPB (DR3, w12)

Table 7. Reactions of B cell lines on Ninth Workshop monoclonal antibodies

9W HTC no.	Cell name	DR	DQ	Dw[a]	9w sera: DRw52 (<w8)				5+w6		5+w6+w8			DRw8+DRw12	DR3+Dw18	DQw1			DQw3			TA10			DR7+Dw15	DRw8+Dw15	?DRw53	DR1+4		
					946	947	948	930	681	709	616	682	618	925	929	901	945	660	915	969	908	790	909	968	949	921	941	928	940	918
0605	WVB	w13	w1	18	8	8	8	8	8	8	4	8	1	1	8	0	8	8	0	1	0	1	0	1	1	1	1	8	8	1
	ARNT	w13	w1	18	8	8	8	0	8	8	8	8	1	0	8	0	8	8	0	1	0	1	0	0	1	0	0	0	0	0
0606	EMJH	w13	w1	19	8	8	8	8	8	8	8	8	1	1	1	8	8	8	1	1	1	1	1	1	1	1	4	6	1	8
0610	KT11	w13	w1	19	8	8	8	8	8	1	2	8	1	1	1	8	8	8	1	1	1	1	1	1	1	1	8	1	1	8
	WT46	w13	w1	19	8	8	8	8	8	8	8	8	1	1	1	8	8	8	1	1	1	6	1	1	1	1	1	1	1	1
	DAUDI	w13	w1	6	8	8	8	8	8	8	8	8	1	1	1	6	8	8	1	1	1	1	1	1	1	1	1	1	1	1
	WT52	w14	w1	9	8	8	8	8	1	1	4	1	1	1	1	8	8	8	1	1	1	1	1	1	1	1	1	8	8	8
	ABUC (WT9)	w14	w1	9	8	8	6	8	1	1	1	1	1	1	1	8	8	8	1	1	1	1	1	1	1	1	1	8	6	8
1701	AZL	w14	w3	16	8	8	8	8	1	4	1	1	1	1	1	1	1	1	8	8	1	8	1	1	1	1	1	8	8	8
1503	HERLUF	w12	w3	Herl	1	1	1	8	8	8	6	8	1	8	1	1	1	1	8	8	1	8	1	1	1	1	6	6	1	1
	RPB	3, w12	w2, w3		8	8	8	8	8	6	8	8	1	8	6	1	1	1	8	8	6	8	8	1	1	1	8	8	8	8
	WPB	1, w12	w1, w3		1	1	1	8	4	1	4	0	1	8	1	8	8	8	8	8	1	8	1	1	1	1	1	8	6	8
	MANN	7	w2	7	1	1	1	8	1	1	1	4	1	1	1	1	1	1	1	4	1	1	1	1	8	1	8	8	8	1
	IBW9	7	w2	7	1	1	1	1	1	1	1	8	1	1	1	1	1	1	1	1	1	1	1	1	8	1	8	8	8	1
	SC-CA	7	w3	11	1	1	1	8	1	1	1	1	1	1	1	1	1	1	8	8	1	1	1	1	8	1	8	1	1	8
	TF6	7, w12	w3		1	1	1	8	8	8	1	8	1	8	1	1	1	1	8	8	8	8	1	1	8	1	8	8	1	8
	KOZ	w9	w3		1	1	1	1	1	1	1	1	1	1	1	1	1	1	8	8	1	1	1	1	1	1	8	8	8	8
	KT14	w9	w3		1	1	1	1	1	1	1	1	1	1	1	1	1	1	8	8	8	1	1	1	1	1	8	8	8	8
	PRIESS	4	w3	4	1	1	1	1	1	1	1	1	1	1	1	1	1	1	8	8	1	8	1	1	1	1	8	8	8	8
	WT-51	4	w3	4	1	1	1	1	1	1	1	1	1	1	1	1	1	1	8	8	8	1	1	1	4	1	8	8	8	8
	LEIF-T	4	w3	4	1	1	1	1	1	1	1	1	1	1	1	1	1	1	8	8	8	1	1	1	1	1	8	8	8	8
	2046-SF	4	w3	10	1	1	1	1	8	1	1	8	1	1	1	1	1	1	8	8	6	1	1	1	1	1	8	4	1	1
	FSH4	4	w3	10	1	1	1	1	8	1	1	8	1	1	1	1	1	1	1	8	1	1	1	1	1	1	1	8	1	8
	SN-T	4	w3	?	1	1	1	1	1	1	1	1	1	1	1	1	1	1	8	1	8	6	1	1	1	1	8	8	8	8
	KT2	4	w3	KT2	1	1	1	1	1	1	1	1	1	1	1	1	1	1	8	6	1	4	1	1	1	1	8	8	8	8
	SJ-AH	4	–	15 (YT)	1	1	1	1	1	1	1	1	1	1	1	8	1	1	1	1	1	1	1	1	8	8	8	8	8	1
	KT9	4	–	15 (YT)	1	1	1	6	1	1	1	1	1	1	1	8	1	0	1	1	6	1	1	1	8	8	8	8	8	8
0808	MADURA-T	w8	–	8	1	1	1	1	4	8	8	8	4	8	1	8	1	1	8	1	1	1	1	1	1	8	1	8	8	8
	231	w8	–	8	1	1	1	1	1	1	8	8	1	8	1	8	1	0	1	1	1	1	1	1	1	8	1	8	6	8
	JOM-TC	w8, w12	w3		1	1	1	8	4	0	8	8	1	8	1	8	1	1	8	8	1	8	1	1	1	8	6	8	6	6
	SWEIG	5	w3	5	1	8	8	8	8	8	8	8	1	1	1	1	1	1	8	8	6	8	8	1	1	1	1	8	1	1
	WT48	5	w3	5	8	8	8	8	8	8	8	8	1	1	1	1	1	1	8	8	8	8	8	1	1	1	1	8	1	1
	WT50	5	w3	5	8	8	8	8	8	8	8	0	1	1	1	1	1	1	8	8	6	8	8	1	1	1	1	8	1	1
	IDF	5	w3	5	8	8	8	8	8	8	8	8	1	1	1	1	1	1	8	8	1	8	6	1	1	1	1	8	1	6
	DHF2	5	w3	5	8	8	8	8	8	8	8	8	1	1	1	1	1	1	8	1	1	8	8	1	1	1	1	8	1	8
	RAFF-T	5	?w1, w3		8	8	8	8	8	8	8	8	1	1	1	6	1	1	1	8	1	8	1	1	1	1	1	8	1	1
	SPO-H	5	w1		8	8	8	8	8	8	8	8	1	1	1	8	8	8	1	8	1	1	1	6	1	1	8	8	6	1
9901	FPF	5	w1		8	8	8	1	8	8	8	8	1	1	1	8	8	8	1	1	1	1	1	1	1	1	1	8	1	1
1803	RML	2	w3		1	1	1	1	6	1	2	8	1	1	1	0	1	1	0	8	0	8	0	0	1	1	0	8	0	0
	BR18	2, w14	w1		8	8	8	8	1	1	1	8	1	1	1	8	8	8	1	1	1	1	1	1	1	1	1	8	8	8

[a] A blank in this column indicates Dw typing has not been done

Table 8. Correlation between DRw52 antibodies (*r* values)

930				
946	0.75			
947	0.78	0.93		
948	0.81	0.93	0.95	
	930	946	947	948

Table 9. Correlation between "All except DR7 and DRw9" antibodies (*r* values)

970								
957	0.52							
958	0.64	0.73						
994	0.60	0.84	0.82					
993	0.60	0.84	0.82	0.96				
935	0.58	0.75	0.79	0.87	0.87			
944	0.52	0.64	0.52	0.62	0.62	0.55		
904	0.47	0.62	0.53	0.64	0.64	0.57	0.85	
	970	957	958	994	993	935	944	904
	Broad or monomorphic						All except DR7 and DRw9	

Table 10. Correlation (*r* values) between DR4 + DR1 + related antibodies: allelic to DRW52?

928			
940	0.50		
918	0.52	0.69	
	928	940	918

Antibody 930 has a slighter longer specificity, reacting also with DRw12 (e.g., HERLUF). Neither of these antibodies reacts with DRw8. These antibodies are extremely useful for identifying the difference between DRw12 on the one hand and DRw13 and w14 on the other as shown in Table 7.

Cluster 4 probably consists of two sets of antibodies, whose *r* values are shown in Table 9. Two of these antibodies, 904 and 944, have the specificity all but DR7 and DRw9, the other antibodies are a mixture of "broadly polymorphic" and monomorphic. It is interesting to speculate whether the lack of reactivity of these latter is associated with whatever the specificity of all but DR7 and DRw9 turns out to be.

Cluster 6 consists of an interesting group of three antibodies, which seem to identify a specificity previously seen in antisera with DR4 + DR1 specificity. In a study by Italian laboratories, informative families show 940 segregating with DR1 (7/7 haplotypes), DR4 (8/9 haplotypes), DRw10 (1/1 haplotypes), and DRw6 in 2/9 (haplotypes). Similar findings have been noted by V. Lepage et al. (HLA DR1 and DR4 Common Antigenic Epitope on the HLA-DR Molecule, this volume) and Gebuhrer et al. [2]. The *r* values in the Workshop study are shown in Table 10. Apart from the positive association noted with DR1, 4, and w9, an interesting indication was a negative association with the specificity DRw52.

This could indicate that the specificity identified by cluster 6 is allelic to DRw52, but in the data so far there is no clear evidence of this. It does not seem so far to be clearly related either to the presence or absence of DRw53 or DRw52 or the recognised DQ specificities DQw1 or DQw3.

The next five clusters each consist of a single antibody which shows an association with an assigned antigen:

Cluster 7 contains the association of the antibody 906 with DR2. The antibody also seems to react occasionally with DR1, DR7 and DRw9.

Cluster 8 contains the antibody 921 associating with DRw8 with an *r* value of 0.5. As is shown in the discussion on Japanese data later in this report, the antibody appears to react with a subset of DRw8 and Dw15 (DR4,YT).

Cluster 9 shows antibody 923 in association with DR4. In Caucasoids it also seems to react with some DR5 and DRw8 cells.

Cluster 10 shows the association of 941 with DRw53 with an *r* value of 0.5, although the antibody seems to be broader than the usual definition of DRw53 since it is also seen in the absence of either DR4 or DR7.

Cluster 11 shows the antibody 949 with an *r* value of 0.64 with DR7. This antibody is of great interest as it is a mouse anti-mouse antibody, made across an I-E difference in the mouse, and yet reacts clearly in humans with DR7 and, as is shown in Japanese cells, with Dw15 (DR4,YT). As shown in Table 11, 949 is seen segregating in the absence of DR7, with Dw15 (DR4,YT), in an Italian family with DR4 that is DQw1 and DQw3 negative and in a black family with DR3 and DQw2. Biochemical studies indicate that it is directed primarily against a DR product, but its precise specificity is not yet clear.

The remaining nine clusters are possibly not quite so clearly identified:

Cluster 12 contains two antibodies, one of which, 963, shows an *r* value of 0.54 with DR1, although the other does not.

Table 11. Patterns of reaction of 9w949 in the presence and absence of DR7 in families

	DR4	DQw3	DQw2	DQw1	↓		
9w Serum number	575 589 585 597 590	746 747 748 754 786 915 969	724 759 795 792 726 719	652 654 661 945 660	949	Antigens assigned to the cells:	
Serum Specificity (DR, DRw)	4 4 4 4 4	4+5 4+5 4+5 4+5+8 NEW – –	3+7 3+7 NEW NEW 3+7 3+7	2+6 2+6 1+2+6 – –		DR1 DR2 DR3 DR4 DR5 DRw6 DR7 DRw8 DRw9 DRw10	
Lab Cell Id.							
BOD 18 K R	8 8 8 8 8	1 1 1 1 1 1 1	1 1 1 1 6 1	8 8 8 1 8	1	1 8 1 8 1 1 1 1 1 1	DR4, DQw3
BOD 19 K V	1 8 8 8 0	6 0 6 0 0 0 0	1 0 8 0 4 0	0 0 1 0 0	0	1 1 1 8 1 1 8 1 1 1	Normal pattern
BOD 20 K I	8 8 8 8 8	8 8 8 8 1 8 1	6 1 1 1 4 1	8 8 8 8 8	1	1 8 1 8 1 1 1 1 1 1	Reaction to
BOD 21 K B	8 8 8 8 8	2 8 2 1 8 8 8	8 2 8 8 8 8	1 1 1 1 8	8	1 1 1 8 1 1 8 1 1 1	949 is due to
BOD 22 K L	0 6 8 6 0	6 0 8 0 0 1 2	0 0 1 0 8 0	0 0 1 1 1	2	1 1 1 8 1 1 8 1 1 1	presence of
BOD 23 K N	8 8 8 8 8	8 8 8 1 8 1 8	8 8 8 8 8 8	1 1 1 1 1	8	1 1 1 8 1 1 8 1 1 1	DR7.
BOD 24 K A	8 8 8 8 0	8 0 8 0 0 0 0	0 0 8 0 8 0	0 0 1 0 0	0	1 1 1 8 1 1 8 1 1 1	
CRB 70 D E	8 6 8 8 6	1 1 1 1 1 2 2	1 1 1 1 1 1	1 8 8 1 1	4	1 8 1 8 1 1 1 1 1 1	DR4,
CRB 71 D G	8 6 8 8 6	1 6 2 1 2 2 2	1 1 1 1 1 1	1 4 4 2 2	8	1 1 1 8 1 8 1 1 1 1	neg. to DQw3,
CRB 72 D R	8 6 6 6 6	1 1 1 1 1 1 2	1 1 1 1 1 1	1 1 6 2 1	6	1 1 1 8 1 8 1 1 1 1	pos. to 949
CRB 73 D S	8 8 8 6 8	1 6 1 1 1 2 2	1 1 1 1 1 1	1 1 1 1 1	8	1 1 1 8 1 1 1 1 1 1	(Dw15?)
CRB 74 D D	8 6 8 8 6	1 6 1 1 1 2 1	1 1 1 1 1 1	1 1 8 1 1	8	1 1 1 8 1 8 1 1 1 1	
CRB 75 D S	8 8 8 8 6	1 8 1 1 0 2 2	1 1 1 1 1 1	4 6 8 1 1	6	1 1 1 8 1 8 1 1 1 1	
DUT 18 W M	8 8 8 8 8	8 8 8 4 8 8 8	8 8 8 8 8 1	1 1 1 8 8	8	1 1 8 8 1 1 1 1 1 1	DR3, DQw2
DUT 19 W S	8 8 8 8 8	8 8 8 1 8 8 8	1 1 1 1 1 1	1 6 6 8 8	1	1 1 1 8 1 1 1 1 1 8	pos. to 949
DUT 33 W R	8 6 8 6 6	6 1 1 1 6 1 1	1 1 1 1 1 1	1 1 4 6 6	1	1 1 1 8 1 1 1 1 1 8	in absence of
DUT 118 W R	8 8 8 8 8	8 8 6 1 8 8 8	8 8 6 8 8 8	1 1 1 1 1	6	1 1 8 8 1 1 1 1 1 1	DR7.
DUT 307 W S	8 8 8 8 8	8 8 8 1 0 0 0	1 1 0 0 1 1	1 1 1 0 0	0	1 1 1 8 1 1 1 1 1 1	
RDS 335 S	6 8 8 2 8	1 1 1 1 1 1 1	1 1 1 1 1 1	1 1 1 1 1	8	1 1 1 8 1 1 1 1 1 1	Dw15 (DR4,YT)
RDS 336 K	8 8 8 8 8	1 4 1 1 1 0 0	6 1 1 1 1 1	1 1 8 0 0	8	1 1 1 8 1 1 1 1 1 1	

Cluster 13 contains possibly the two best monomorphic antibodies, with an *r* value between them of 0.9 and a frequency approaching 100%.

Cluster 14 contains four antibodies which have quite a high association with DQw1 but not a very high association with the antibodies in cluster 1, the main DQw1 cluster. Examination of the pattern of reaction indicates that a larger proportion of the cells are DR2 positive than for the cluster 1 antibodies. Possibly this cluster defines a type of DQw1 more associated with DR2 than DR1, DRw6 or DRw10.

Cluster 15 shows a group of four antibodies with *r* values, as shown in Table 12, of around 0.6. The frequency of the antibodies is around 60%, but examination of family and random data have not so far suggested a specificity for this cluster.

Table 12. Correlations between four antibodies with unidentified specificity (*r* values)

Unidentified				
980				
954	0.68			
931	0.65	0.66		
916	0.48	0.55	0.51	
	980	954	931	916

Cluster 16 has two antibodies with a high *r* value of 0.75, a low frequency, and no identified specificity.

Cluster 17 contains six antibodies of high frequency, some of them known to be monomorphic.

Cluster 18 contains three antibodies which have some specificity related to either DR5 or DRw8, as shown in Table 13.

Table 13. Correlations between antibodies related to DR5 or DRw8 (*r* values)

984			
978	0.49		
986	0.52	0.70	
	984	978	986

Cluster 19 contains two antibodies whose only identifiable association is a negative one with DRw53.

Cluster 20 contains two antibodies with an *r* value of 0.48, which have some relationship to DQw1.

In addition to the data obtained from the antibodies occurring in the above clusters, other antibodies in the Workshop had useful and clearly identified specificities, among these 925 and 929.

Antibodies 925 and 929

Antibody 925, which is also discussed in the section on Japanese results later in this report, reacts with most DRw8 and DRw12 cells. Antibody 929 is an antibody which was originally thought to react only with DR3 until it was noted that it also reacted with a subset of DRw13 cells corresponding to the Dw18 split of Dw6. These two antibodies, together with the DRw52, DQw1 and DQw3 MCAs discussed above, have been of great value in defining the splits of DRw6 and their relationship to the DQ subregion. This is discussed in the DRw6 antigen report in this volume. It is of interest, however, to look at the definition of DRw6 in the context of monoclonal antibodies, and Table 14 shows the pattern of reaction of monoclonal antibodies for the definition of DRw6. The points to note are:

1. The difference between DRw12 and the two other specificities, DRw13 and DRw14, is clearly shown by antibodies 946 and 930. While 930 reacts to all these specificities, 946 reacts only to DRw13 and DRw14 and not the DRw12, as discussed above in connection with DRw52.
2. Antibody 925 has a reciprocal pattern to 946 in that it reacts to DRw8 and DRw12, and not to DRw13 or DRw14. Since 925 was clearly negative in two of the families shown in the DRw6 report as carrying the DRw13, DQw3 specificity (GRU8 and STA1), it can be assumed that the specificity of 925 is related to the DR locus rather than the DQ locus. This is confirmed by the fact that the DRw8 cells which are 925 positive can be DQw3 or DQ blank.

Table 14. Definition of DRw6 and some related specificities using Ninth Workshop monoclonal antibodies

	Antigen designation			DR determinants				DQ determinants			
				DRw52 e.g.		"5 + w8 + w13" sera*	DRw8 + DRw12	DQw1 e.g.		DQw3 e.g.	DR3 + Dw18
	DR	DQ	Dw	946	930		925	945	901	969	929
DRw6	DRw13	DQw1	Dw18	+	+	+	–	+	+	–	+
DRw6	DRw13	DQw1	Dw19	+	+	+	–	+	+	–	–
DRw6	DRw13	DQw3	?	+	+	+	(–)	–	–	+	–
DRw6	DRw14	DQw1	Dw9	+	+	–	–	+	+	–	–
DRw6	DRw14	DQw3	Dw16	+	+	–	(–)	–	–	+	–
DR5	DRw11	DQw3	Dw5	+	+	+	–	–	–	+	–
DR5	DRw11	DQw1	?	+	+	+	–	+	+	–	–
DR5	DRw12	DQw3	D HerL	–	+	+	+	–	–	+	–
	DRw8	DQw3	Dw8	–	–	+	+	–	+	+	–
	DRw8	DQ blank	Dw8	–	–	+	+	–	+	–	–

( ) indicates result has not been confirmed
* Formerly designated "5 + w6 + w8" sera

3. To turn to the DQ-related determinants, we come to an immediate puzzle: Antibody 945, proved by biochemistry (see J. Bodmer et al., page 432, this volume) to identify a DQ specificity, reacts only with DQw1, while 901, also an anti-DQw1 antibody, has other reactions. In Table 14, 901 is shown to react with DRw8 as mentioned above, and Table 7 (above) shows that it also reacts with DRw15 (DR4, YT). As neither of these specificities is related to DQw1, it is interesting to speculate what the common epitope might be. Apart from this puzzle, the DQw1 and DQw3 antibodies react as expected in the definition of these specificities and help to resolve the difficulties in the definition of DRw6.
4. Antibody 9w929, the DR3 plus DRw6 subset antibody, adds a further degree of specificity, since as shown in Table 14, it reacts only with the Dw18 type of DRw13 and not with Dw19. These and other data are shown in more detail in Table 15 and Table 7, which show the different types of DRw6, DRw12, w13, w14 with DQw1 and DQw3 as well as the Dw18/Dw19 difference.

In this section we have described the results of analysis of some clusters of antibodies and some individual antibodies which have been identified as defining particular subsets of known specificities. Other antibodies have been mentioned whose specificity has not yet been clearly identified; further, more detailed study will be needed on these.

Subregion Specificity of the D Region Monoclonal Antibodies

It is clear, as is discussed in other reports in this volume (M. Crumpton et al., Biochemistry of Class II Antigens: Workshop Report; J. Dausset and D. Cohen, HLA at the Gene Level; E. D. Albert et al., The Serological Analysis of the Data of the Ninth Histocompatibility Workshop), that the HLA-D region is extremely complex. Three subregions have been identified, DR, DQ, and DP, with possibly three β-chains coding for polymorphism in the DR subregion, two β and at least one α polymorphic chains in the DQ subregion, and two polymorphic β and two α in the DP subregion. Speculations on the different functions of these subregions are supported by observations that in different stages of B cell development and T cell activation, and in leukaemia, melanoma and other malignant cells, products of the different subregions are differentially expressed. It is therefore of great interest to identify which subregion product a monoclonal antibody is directed against. This is studied in detail for a few antibodies using biochemical techniques as described in the Biochemistry Report in this volume. However, using a series of tumour cell lines which have been shown to lack the DQ product, and in some cases normal B lymphoblastoid cell lines from the same donor, it was possible to identify, for the majority of D region monoclonal antibodies, whether they were directed primarily against the DR or the DQ region. These results are shown in Table 16. As a complete set of cell lines for all specificities was not available, some antibodies, as shown in column 3 "DR or DQ", could not be characterised by this method. It was not possible to identify DP antibodies by this method since the presence or absence of DP has not yet been established on these cell lines. These studies were done primarily in BOD laboratory, and some confirmatory and complementary information was obtained from studies in NSF and DAW laboratories. As expected, DR antibodies and DRw52, 53 antibodies reacted in the absence of DQ. Of particular interest, and something that should be checked more carefully using biochemical techniques, is the suggestion that some of the "all but DR7 and DRw9" are directed against DR products (904, 944 and 958), whereas others are directed against the DQ products (974, 782 and 783). Table 17 shows, for the "all but DR7 and DRw9" and some of the monomorphic antibodies, the way in which assignment to a particular subregion, as listed in Table 16, was carried out. Some of the panel of cell lines used are shown, consisting of an HLA-D-negative T cell line, a series of normal B lymphoblastoid cell lines and a series of DQ-negative tumour cell lines. From the pattern of reaction of antibodies on cell lines lacking the DQ product it is possible to get some idea of whether an antibody is more probably directed to a DR or a DQ product. However, whereas positivity on a DQ-negative line almost certainly means that the antibody is not DQ, i.e., more likely to be DR, lack of reactivity does not necessarily mean that the antibody is directed to DQ. This is because the antibody may be weak and the tumour lines may have reduced amounts of some DR products as well as lacking DQ. Thus in Table 16 the assignment to subregion should be taken as indicative rather than definitive. Definitive assignments need biochemical studies, as discussed in the report of the biochemistry study elsewhere in this volume. It is important not to be too rigid in all cases in the assignment of the specificity of an antibody to a particular subregion as, for example, there is evidence from Hansen et al. [3] that an anti-DQw3 antibody, 969 (17.15), is directed primarily against the DQ product in DR5 cells and the DR product in DR4 cells.

Table 15. D region monoclonal antibodies in the definition of DRw6 in families and selected cell lines

	DRw52				DR 5,w6,w8 sera				DQ w1		DQ w3																	
9w Serum number:	946	947	948	930	616	709	681	682	945	660	915	969	929	925	Antigens assigned to the cells													
Serum specificity (DR, DRw):					5+6+8	6	5+6	5+6							DR1	DR2	DR3	DR4	DR5	DRw6	DR7	DRw8	DRw9	DRw10	DRw13	DRw14	DQw1	DQw3	
Lab Cell Id.																													
BOD 1 B W	8	8	8	8	1	1	8	6	4	2	1	1	1	1	1	1	1	1	1	8	8	1	1	1	8	1	1	1	DRw13, DQw1
BOD 2 B J	8	8	8	8	1	1	4	1	1	1	1	1	8	4	1	1	8	1	1	1	8	1	1	1	1	1	1	1	Normal pattern
BOD 3 B M	8	1	1	1	1	1	1	1	1	1	1	1	1	1	1	1	1	1	1	1	8	1	1	1	1	1	1	1	
BOD 4 B H	8	8	8	8	4	1	8	8	6	6	1	1	1	1	1	1	8	1	1	8	1	1	1	1	8	1	1	1	
DAU 112 G J	0	8	8	0	4	6	8	0	8	1	0	1	0	0	1	1	1	1	1	8	8	1	1	1	4	0	1	1	
DAU 113 G J	1	6	1	1	1	1	1	1	8	1	4	1	1	1	1	1	1	1	1	1	8	1	1	1	1	0	1	1	
DAU 114 G L	6	1	1	1	6	1	1	1	8	1	1	1	1	1	1	1	1	1	1	1	8	1	1	1	1	0	1	1	
DAU 115 G I	6	8	0	1	6	8	8	4	6	1	1	1	1	1	1	1	1	1	1	8	8	1	1	1	4	0	1	1	
DAU 116 G S	8	8	1	1	1	1	1	1	8	1	1	1	1	1	1	1	1	1	1	1	8	1	1	1	1	0	1	1	
DAU 117 G C	1	6	0	0	4	6	6	6	0	1	1	1	1	1	1	1	1	1	1	8	8	1	1	1	4	0	1	1	
DAU 118 G O	1	1	4	1	4	1	1	1	8	1	1	1	1	1	1	1	1	1	1	1	8	1	1	1	1	0	1	1	
AIZ 660 M Y	8	8	8	8	4	8	8	8	8	0	1	1	1	1	8	1	1	1	1	0	1	0	1	1	0	0	8	1	
AIZ 661 M K	6	1	1	1	1	1	1	1	8	0	1	1	1	1	8	1	1	8	1	0	1	0	1	1	0	0	8	8	
AIZ 662 M N	8	8	8	8	6	8	8	8	8	0	1	1	1	1	1	1	1	8	1	0	1	0	1	1	0	0	8	8	
AIZ 663 M Y	8	8	8	8	6	8	8	8	8	0	1	1	1	1	8	1	1	1	1	0	1	0	1	1	0	0	8	1	
AIZ 664 M S	8	8	8	8	4	8	8	0	8	0	1	1	1	1	8	1	1	1	1	0	1	0	1	1	0	0	8	1	
AIZ 665 M R	8	8	8	8	6	6	8	8	8	0	1	1	1	2	8	1	1	1	1	0	1	0	1	1	0	0	8	1	
RDS 342 WT46 Dw19	8	8	8	8	8	8	8	8	8	8	1	1	1	1	1	1	1	1	1	8	1	1	1	1	8	1	0	0	Dw19 cells
RDS 343 KT11 Dw19	8	8	8	8	2	1	6	8	8	8	1	1	1	1	1	1	1	1	1	8	1	1	1	1	8	1	0	0	negative to 929
RDS 344 ARNT Dw18	8	8	8	8	8	8	8	8	8	8	1	1	8	1	1	1	1	1	1	8	1	1	1	1	8	1	0	0	Dw18 cells
RDS 345 WVB Dw18	8	8	8	8	4	8	8	8	8	8	1	4	8	1	1	1	1	1	1	8	1	1	1	1	8	1	0	0	positive to 929
RDS 339 ABUC Dw9	8	8	6	8	1	1	1	1	8	8	1	1	1	1	1	1	1	1	1	8	1	1	1	1	1	8	0	0	DRw14, DQw1
RDS 340 WT52 Dw9	8	6	8	8	1	1	1	4	8	8	1	1	1	1	1	1	1	1	1	8	1	1	1	1	1	8	0	0	
BOD 25 P S	1	1	1	8	6	0	0	8	4	6	4	6	1	8	1	8	1	1	8	1	1	1	1	1	1	1	0	0	DRw12, DQw3
BOD 26 P V	8	8	8	8	1	0	0	1	4	6	1	1	1	1	8	1	8	1	1	1	1	1	1	1	1	1	0	0	Positive to 925
BOD 30 P W	2	2	8	8	4	0	0	8	8	4	6	8	1	8	8	1	1	1	8	1	1	1	1	1	1	1	0	0	Negative to
BOD 31 P S	8	8	8	8	4	0	0	8	1	1	8	8	4	8	1	1	8	1	8	1	1	1	1	1	1	1	0	0	946 - 948
BOD 32 P J	8	8	0	8	8	0	0	8	8	0	8	0	4	8	8	1	1	1	8	1	1	1	1	1	1	1	0	0	
AIZ 673 H S	1	1	1	8	4	1	4	8	1	0	8	8	1	8	1	1	1	8	8	0	1	0	1	1	0	0	1	8	DRw12
AIZ 674 H M	8	8	8	8	1	1	1	1	8	0	1	1	6	8	8	1	1	1	1	0	1	0	1	1	0	0	8	1	
RDS 346 Herluf	1	1	1	8	6	8	8	8	1	1	8	8	1	8	1	1	1	1	1	1	1	1	1	1	1	1	0	0	DRw12, DQw3 neg. to 946 - 948
RDS 347 AZL	8	6	8	8	1	4	1	1	1	1	8	8	1	1	1	1	1	1	1	4	1	1	1	1	0	0	0	0	DRw14, DQw3

For nomenclature see DRw6 antigen report in this volume.

Table 16. Subregion assignment based on reactivity with DQ-negative cell lines

DR	DQ	DR or DQ
906 DR1, 2, 7, w10	901 DQw1 + DRw8 + DR4 Dw15 assoc. 903	908 919 ? some T cell lines + ve
921 DR4-Dw15 assoc., w8	909 part of DQw3 (?TA10) 913 < DQw1	920 923 DR4, 5, w8 (not DRw12)
925 DRw8 + DRw12	914 < DQw1 915 DQw3	928 ? DR1 + 4 953 DR2, 3, 5, w6, w8
930 DR3, 5, w6, w12	927 DQw1 + DRw8 + DR4 – Dw15 assoc.	954 ? DR3 + 5 + w6
946 DR3, 5, w6	929 DR3 + some w6	962
947 DR3, 5, w6		972 DR7, 4+ +
948 DR3, 5, w6	940 DR1, 4, 7, w9	977
960 ? DR5	941 DR3, 4, 7±	978
968 DR5	943 weak DQw1 945 DQw1 949 DR7 + DR4 – Dw15 assoc. 951 ? DR1, 4, w10, 7 955 956 963 Wk DQw1 964 969 DQw3 + DR7 979 DR1, 3, 4, w6 988 DR1, 3, 4, w6, 7 660 DQw1 790 TA10 (< DQw3)	984 986 974 all but DR7 + DRw9 938 ? Mono
904 all but DR7, DRw9		
944 all but DR7, DRw9 ? w10	782 all but DR7 + DRw9	
958 ? all but DR7	783 weak, all but DR7	
992 ? Mono	905 ? Mono 907 ? Mono	
932 Mono	970 Mono	
934 Mono	784 Mono	
935 Mono		
957 Mono		
993 Mono		
994 Mono		
995 Mono		

Regional Reports

Apart from the data on the monoclonal antibodies derived from the general analysis as described above, there are three sets of data from individual regions which are relevant to this report. These reports are from Italy, France and Japan.

Italy. In the Italian study the D region monoclonal antibodies were examined to see how they segregated with HLA haplotypes in informative families. Table 18 shows how these data, dividing the antibodies into those segregating more than 75% with HLA, those segregating 50% – 75%, and those segregating less than 50%. Table 18 points out those antibodies which are most robust as typing reagents, either because of their inherent stability or possibly because of an advantageous position on the typing plate. It also highlights some of the technical problems, which will be discussed later, since antibody 660, in the less than 50% category, is the duplicate of 945, which is in the best category. Data from Italy also showed the activity of the DR4 + DR1 group (cluster 6) and their segregation as discussed above.

France. In study from France the antibodies were tested in the complement fixation assay. The results

Table 17. D subregion specificity of Ninth Workshop "All but DR7+DRw9" and monomorphic monoclonal antibodies

				All but DR7 +DRw9						Monomorphic									Cell type
				DR			DQ			DR							DQ		
		DR	DQ	904	944	958	974	782	783	932	934	935	957	993	994	995	970	784	
From same donor	HSB2	–	–	1	1	1	1	1	1	1	1	1	1	1	1	1	1	1	T cell line
	SB	2	w1	8	8	8	8	8	8	8	8	8	8	8	8	8	8	8	Normal B cell
	KOZ	w9	w3	1	1	8	4	8	4	8	8	8	0	8	8	6	8	0	
	MANN	7	w2	1	1	8	1	1	1	8	8	8	8	8	8	8	8	8	
From same donor	B85	3, 7	w2, w8	8	8	8	8	8	8	8	8	8	8	8	8	8	8	8	
	Nalm 6	3, 7	–	8	8	8	8	8	1	8	8	8	8	8	8	8	1	1	C-ALL lines
	Nalm 16	3, 7	–	8	8	8	6	1	1	8	8	8	8	8	8	8	1	1	
	Nalm 1w	13	–	8	8	8	8	4	1	8	8	8	8	8	8	8	1	1	
	Mapp	1	–	8	8	8	1	1	1	8	8	8	8	8	8	8	1	1	
	KM3	5	–	8	0	8	1	1	1	8	8	8	8	8	8	8	1	1	
	IGR3	1, 7	–	8	4	8	1	1	1	8	8	8	0	8	8	8	1	1	Melanoma cell line

[a] Reacts with DR7 homozygous cell lines but not with DR7 homozygous B cells

Table 18. Segregation HLA haplotypes in informative families in Italy

>75%		50% – 75%			<50%
901	928	902	948	974	911
906	930	903	949	975	914
907	940	905	950	976	925
909	942	908	951	978	952
912	943	910	953	980	958
915	944	913	954	981	964
917	945	916	955	982	967
918	946	919	956	985	977
921	957	920	960	987	983
922	962	923	963	782	988
926	965	924	968	783	660
927	969	929	970		
	979	939	972		
	784	947	973		
$n=26$		$n=39$			$n=11$

of this study are shown in Table 19. Other cytotoxic data from France agreed with the results discussed in the previous sections of this report.

Japan. A large number of the D region monoclonal antibodies used in this Workshop were submitted by Japanese groups who had conducted studies in a Japanese population. In studies performed with all the D region monoclonal antibodies the following observations were made. A list of D region polymorphic monoclonal antibodies whose reactivity correlates with known specificities [DR, DQ, or DR (MT)] in the Japanese population (AIZ, JUJ, MIY, OKO, SEK, and YOSI) is shown in Table 20. The r values for a new D region specificity (TB21; ≃DQw3) originally described by Maeda and Juji [6] are given in Table 21. Two monoclonal antibodies (9w908 and 915) and three TB21-specific alloantisera (9w744, 746, and 747) showed similar serologic reactivity.

Another new D region specificity (TA10) associated with DR5, DRw12, a part of DR4, and DR blank is defined by monoclonal antibody 9w909 and one monoclonal antibody (9w790) in the DR sera set ($r = 0.9$).

It should be noted that DRw9 is frequent in Japanese, but rare in Caucasoids. Thus, it would be interesting to compare the reactivity pattern of 9w904, 918, 928 and 951 in the two ethnic groups.

The reactivity of 9w915 and 9w909 on a panel of B cells from 105 Japanese individuals (AIZ, MIY, OKO, SEK and YOS) is shown in Fig. 2.

In a study using cells of Japanese origin, we found that the three DR4-associated D specificities – Dw15 (DYT), DKT2 and Dw4 – can be distinguished on the basis of serologic reactivity with 9w915 (HU-18) and 9w909 (HU-23) [5]. Briefly, cells homozygous for Dw15 are negative for both 9w915 and 9w909; those homozygous for DKT2, positive only for 9w915; and those homozygous for Dw4, positive for both. Thus, the pattern analysis of these two monoclonal antibodies in Caucasoids, Negroes, and other ethnic groups, where DR4-associated D specificities are expected to be present in different frequencies, will be of interest.

Reactivity of 9w925 in a panel of B cells from 105 Japanese individuals (JUJ and MIY) is shown in Fig. 3.

Table 19. Ninth Workshop monoclonal antibodies (MCAs) studied by complement fixation on PHA blasts (PHA-CF)[a]

MCAs with anti-MCA identity	Proposed	D Region specificity Found (*r*)
904	DR7, w9	Negative correlation with DR7 (−0.47)
908		DR5 (0.48)
909	DR4, 5, w8	DQw3 (0.68), DR5 (0.58)
917		DR2, w6 (0.58)
923	DR4	DR4, 5 (0.45)
929	DR3, w6	DR3 (0.66)
949	DR7	DR7 (0.66)
951	DR4, w9, w10	DR1 (0.61), DR1, 4 (0.58)
987		Negative correlation with DRw53 (−0.74)

[a] PHA-CF was performed by the CF fixation microtechnique using 20 000 cells obtained after 3 days culture with PHA. Ninety-four MCAs were studied

Monomorphic MCAs: 905, 919, 931, 934, 935, 936, 937, 939, 941, 954, 957, 958, 959, 969, 994, 996
Negative MCAs: 902, 903, 910, 911, 912, 913, 915, 918, 920, 921, 925, 944, 945, 946, 947, 948, 950, 964, 965, 967, 968, 974, 976, 978, 979, 980, 983, 984, 985, 988, 783, 993
MCAs with polymorphic pattern, but not correlated with HLA-D specificity: 901, 906, 907, 914, 916, 922, 924, 926, 927, 928, 930, 932, 933, 938, 940, 942, 943, 952, 953, 955, 956, 960, 962, 963, 970, 972, 973, 977, 981, 982, 986, 782, 784, 992, 995, 660
MCAs with ABC specificity: 975, A2 ($r = 1.00$)

Table 20. D region polymorphic monoclonal antibodies and their specificities in Japanese subjects [4, 5]

9w901	DQw1
9w904	All but DR7 + DRw9
9w906	DR2 (1)
9w908	TB21 (≃ DQw3)
9w909	TA10 (2)
9w915	TB21 (2)
9w918	DR1 + DR4 + DRw9
9w925	DRw52 short
9w928	DR1 + DR4 + DRw9
9w930	DRw52 short
9w940	DRw53
9w945	DQw1
9w946	DRw52 short
9w947	DRw52 short
9w948	DRw52 short
9w951	DRw9
9w962	DR1 + DR2
9w968	DR5
9w979	DRw53
9w660	DQw1

Table 21. Definition of TB21

9w908	0.85				
9w915	0.90	0.81			
9w744	0.80	0.66	0.75		
9w746	0.86	0.77	0.87	0.81	
9w747	0.68	0.62	0.71	0.75	0.70
	9w748	9w908	9w915	9w744	9w746

Table 22. Definition of short DRw52 by monoclonal antibodies

Group	9w925	9w930	9w946 9w947 9w948	no. of panel positive	DR
I	+	+	+	7	
II	+	+	−	17	DR5 (DRw12)
III	−	+	+	24	DR5 (DRw11)
IV	+	−	−	13	DRw8
V	−	+	−	8	
VI	−	−	−	4	

Most of the DRw8-positive and all of the DRw12-positive individuals are positive for 9w925 in our Japanese panels. This antibody is reported to detect a new DR specificity in Caucasoids [7]. (It is also discussed elsewhere in this report in relation to the definition of DRw6 and DRw12.)

Five monoclonal antibodies (9w925, 930, 946, 947, and 948) showed "DRw52 short" specificity. The pattern analyses of these five are shown in Table 22 (AIZ and JUJ).

DRw52-positive individuals were roughly divided into six groups (groups I–VI). Most individuals grouped as II or III were positive for DR5, whereas those grouped as IV were positive for DRw8. Three monoclonal antibodies (9w946, 947, and 948) had similar reactivity patterns. The reactivity of 9w921 is shown in Fig. 4.

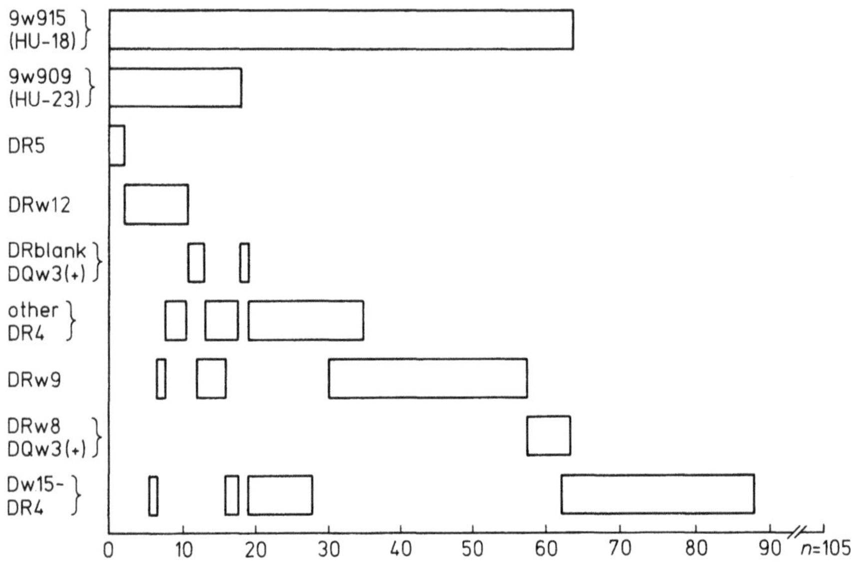

Fig. 2. Reactivity of 9w915 and 9w909 in Japanese subjects. *Bars,* individuals positive for corresponding reactivities shown on left. 9w915 is negative for Dw15 (DR4, DYT) except when DRw12, DR blank or DRw9 is present

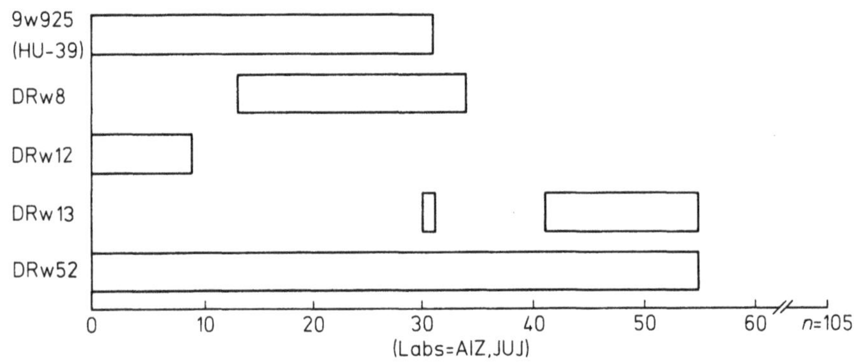

Fig. 3. Reactivity of 9w925 in Japanese. Reaction pattern is essentially the same in Caucasoids positive for DRw12 and negative for DRw13 or DRw14

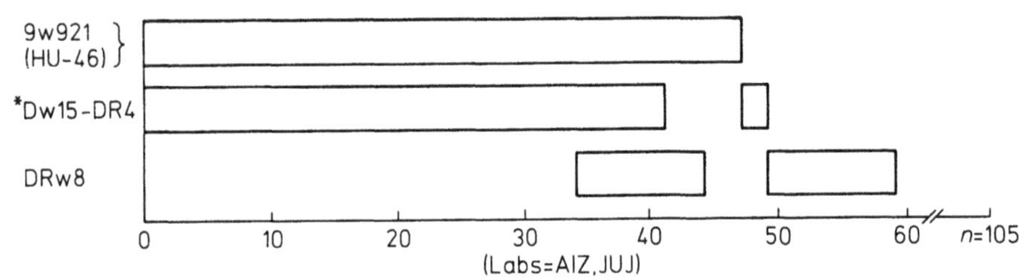

Fig. 4. Reactivity of 9w921 in Japanese. 9w921 reacts with most Dw15 (DR4, DYT)-positive cells and some of DRw8-positive cells in Japanese. In Caucasoids in which Dw15 (DR4, DYT) is absent, this MCA reacts mainly with DRw8-positive cells. Since amino acid sequences of 9w921-reactive molecules in Dw15 (Dr4, DYT) cells are homologous to DQ, this MCA may detect DQ allelic products associated with Dw15 (DR4, DYT) that are negative for DQw3. * Assigned by positive reactions to DR4, DR4.1 sera, DR4 short; 9w582, 587, 592, 594, and negative reactions to 9w915 = monoclonal antibody

Technical Problems of Handling Monoclonal Antibodies

It was clear, even at the pre-Workshop screening stage of the study, that technical considerations would play a large part in determining the quality of the data produced. Thus it may be helpful to discuss some of these problems and suggest some of the ways in which they may be handled in future.

The two major problems which confront a serologist planning to use monoclonal antibodies for cytotoxic tissue typing with the techniques developed for conventional antisera are (1) carry-over and (2) loss of reactivity.

Carry-over. This is a problem which has been seen with some high-titred conventional antisera. But, in general, with antisera whose titres rarely exceed 1 : 4 or 1 : 8, the carrying over of activity of one antibody from one well to the next has not caused major problems. However, many monoclonal antibodies, particularly the monomorphic antibodies, have titres reaching up to many thousands. It has been shown that with such an antibody, when the normal serological techniques are used, carry-over of antibody activity can extend over as many as five or six of the following wells.

There are some obvious solutions to this problem. One is to dilute the antibody with a suitable diluent so that it has a titre comparable with conventional antisera. A second would be to use a "no-touch" technique, not allowing the needle to touch the antibody and avoid carry-over in this way. A third is to put a large number of diluent spots between each of the antibody-containing wells, so that carry-over can be recognised and a clearly negative spot can be seen before the next antibody-containing well. It is clear that the last solution, that of additional diluent spots, is likely to be the most foolproof, but it is also the most expensive in terms of reagents and time needed to carry out the tests. The no-touch technique can be shown to be very risky, since aerosols can be produced which themselves may lead to more random carry-over. Therefore the first solution, that of sufficient dilution seems to be the best. This, however, leads on to the second major problem of the use of monoclonal antibodies, that of loss of reactivity.

Loss of Reactivity. It is possible to determine a working titre of monoclonal antibody, diluted in some form of diluent containing a suitable protein source. The antibody can then be diluted to this concentration for storage, shipping or putting on a typing plate. In many cases it will be noted that over a period of time, even if the antibodies are stored at +4 °C, but more quickly if they are frozen and thawed, the antibody activity will be reduced and eventually lost. Careful studies are needed to determine what happens to this activity. It seems probable, following preliminary studies with labelled antibodies, that if they are stored in plastic tubes or on plates the antibody sticks to the surface of the container. The way to combat this might be to coat the surface of the tubes and plates with a suitable protein source, such as BSA.

Experiments of adding different sources of protein to the diluted antibody have also been carried out. So far no clear recipe for success has been achieved, although two points have emerged:

1. Human serum inhibits the activity of the antibody and should be avoided.
2. Foetal calf serum is probably better in general than other protein sources in that it is neither toxic nor inhibitory, but at concentrations of 10% or 20% it does not seem to be sufficient to offset the problems of loss of activity.

More work will be needed in this area to identify a better carrier for the antibody.

Two other possible methods of handling the instability of cytotoxic antibodies can also be tried. One would be to add a sublytic amount of a monomorphic antibody, such as CA206, to give a synergistic effect. The other is a method used successfully to produce cytotoxic activity in IgG1 antibodies which are normally not cytotoxic. This is to add a rabbit anti-mouse (RAM) antibody to the test. RAM, freshly diluted, can be added to the antibody in the test well, either before or after the cells are added. With 1 μl of a dilution 1/5 of RAM three polymorphic IgG1 antibodies have been used successfully in a cytotoxic assay. This simple method, with or without a washing step before the addition of the second antibody, could well be applied to cytotoxic antibodies to see whether they can be stabilized at a workable concentration. This would help with the problems of both carry-over and loss of activity.

Two other possibly related problems are encountered in the use of monoclonal antibodies. One is that culture supernatant often works better and more reliably than purified immunoglobulin. The other is that some batches of complement work better than others with monoclonal antibodies. The question of complement was studied in detail in Dawkins' laboratory, where several batches of complement were tested. The answer to these two problems may be the same. If an antibody is of low affinity it may need another source of antibody to form the necessary complexes on the cell surface. This may be supplied by greater amounts of antibody in some batches of complement than in others. It may also be present in culture supernatant and absent in purified immunoglobulin preparations.

As shown in Table 23, complement batch 1693 gave excellent discrimination between strongly positive (9) and negative (1), with no evidence of carry-over even though adjacent typing wells were used. It was possible to assign many DR antigens without the need for allo-antisera.

With complement batch 3054, there was poor discrimination, with many false positives (e.g., 933) and the appearance of carry-over (e.g., 923 to 937).

Table 23. Effect of complement on reactivity of monoclonal antibodies

Complement	923	924	925	926	927	928	929	930	931	932	933	934	935	936	937	938	939	940	941	942	943
3054	9	8	7	3	3	9	4	6	9	9	9	9	9	9	9	9	2	9	9	7	1
1693	9	1	1	1	1	9	1	1	9	0	1	9	9	9	9	9	1	9	9	1	1

The cytotoxicity scores (1 = negative to 9 = positive) with two different batches of complement

At least some groups using 3054 found extreme hyperactivity with the monoclonal antibodies.

It may be relevant to the interpretation of these results that 3054 (unabsorbed) had substantial anti-human activity, whereas 1693 (buffy coat absorbed) was negative in this respect.

It is clear that the solution of these problems, either by the methods suggested above or by other methods, is a necessary next step in the development of monoclonal antibodies as typing reagents. It will of course, on a more direct level, be informative to look closely at the methods of those laboratories who produced good D region monoclonal data in this Workshop.

Conclusions

In the previous sections we have discussed selection of the data on which these analyses were based and the reasons why such selection was necessary. We have described the specificity of some of the antibodies, those for which clear patterns of reaction have so far emerged in these data. In Table 24 we attempt to give a summary of the activity of the antibodies based on the analyses discussed in the report. To answer the questions mentioned in the introduction as being the basis of this study, we can reach the following conclusions.

1. "Do monoclonal antibodies work as well or bet-

Table 24. Specificity of D region monoclonal antibodies based on selected "good" data

9W no.	Local name	1st spec.	*r*	2nd spec.	*r*	% Pos.	Comments
901	SH-1	DQw1	0.82			48	Also DRw8 + Dw15
902	FU 3	NS	–			1	
903	FU 4	DQw1	0.50			45	
904	HU 26	–	–			89	All except DR7 & DRw9
905	HU 29	NS				85	? Monomorphic
906	HU 30	DR2sh	0.81	DR2	0.74	41	+ Some DR1, 7, w10
907	HU 28	DQw1	0.54			66	
908	FU 2	DQw3	0.63	DR3	0.48	39	
909	HU 23	DQw3	0.61			26	? TA10
910	FU 9	NS				0	
911	FU 6	NS				0	
912	FU 8	NS				21	Some T cells positive
913	HU 11	DQw1	0.64	DRw8	0.39	64	
914	FU 1	DQw1	0.56			41	
915	HU 18	DQw3	0.97			48	Perfect fit
916	HU 36	NS				62	Some T cells positive
917	HU 42	DR2sh	0.36			40	Some T cells positive
918	HU 43	DR4	0.39	DR1	0.45	63	
919	HU 44	NS				10	Some T cells positive
920	HU 45	NS				8	Some T cells positive
921	HU 46	DRw8	0.50			5	Also Dw15
922	HU 47	NS				52	Some T cells positive
923	HU 48	DQw3	0.9			36	But DRw12 negative
924	HU 33	DR1	0.34			38	? Some T cells positive
925	HU 39	DRw8	0.39			14	+ DRw12
926	HU 49	NS				13	ABC-A9
927	SH 2	DQw1	0.80			48	+ DRw8 + Dw15
928	Y62C10	DR4sh	0.34			77	?DR1 + 4
929	16-23	DR3	0.30			21	+ Dw18
930	VR7319 · 1	DRw52	0.60			51	DR3, 5, w6 and w12 related
931	B8-12 · 2	NS				65	
932	H39-49 · 5	NS				89	? Monomorphic

Table 24. (continued)

9W no.	Local name	1st spec.	r	2nd spec.	r	% Pos.	Comments
933	H40-394 · 2	NS				79	? Monomorphic DR
934	H81-218 · 11	NS				90	Monomorphic DR
935	H81-208 · 22	NS				94	Monomorphic DR
936	H73-202 · 2	NS				72	
937	H82-246 · 3	NS				83	
938	H82-246 · 3 (1/500)	NS				72	Weak monomorphic
939	C-5.17	NS				47	
940	XI-21 · 4	DR4sh	0.46			59	DR4, 7, w9, 1
941	X-2 · 7	DRw53	0.50	DR5	0.31	60	? + DR7
942	X-44 · 8	NS				17	Some T cells positive
943	JAF77 · 34-10	DQw1	0.57			41	
944	I-2	NS				89	all except DR7 + DRw9
945	JMSDR4 · 1 · 1 (10X)	DQw1	0.78			48	
946	8F10 (JMSDR8 · 1 · 1 (2X))	DRw52	0.87			46	DR3, 5, w6 related DRw12 negative (946–948)
947	JMSDR8 · 1 · 1 (4X)	DRw52	0.87			46	
948	C5D4 (JMSDR8 · 1 · 1 (1X))	DRw52	0.87			47	
949	17 · 3 · 3 (5X)	DR7	0.64			35	+ Dw15
950	XXI-3 · 6 · 2	NS				5	
951	FLY-BL-12	DRw9	0.30	DR4sh	0.33	28	Also DR1, <7
952	FLY-BL-12 (1/100)	NS				1	
953	CHEV 642	DRw52	0.74			31	+ DR2
954	CHEV 249 · 3	NS				70	? DRw52
955	MAJA 51 · 2	DRw52	0.53			30	
956	FPA-BM50	DR4sh	0.51			76	Also DR1, 2, 5
957	FPA-141	NS				92	? Monomorphic
958	FPA-53	NS				93	? All but DR7
959	FPA-M18	NS				95	β2-microglobulin
960	SFR-3	NS				3	? Weak DR5
962	GAP-D1	DQw1	0.67			59	
963	HPA49 · 11 · 10	DR1	0.54	DQw1	0.34	21	
964	NFB-14 · 12	DQw1	0.51			32	
965	MCS7	DRw52	0.30			52	Also DR2, DR4
967	E5A7 · 3A	NS				1	
968	TER-M	DR5	0.44			14	
969	17 · 15	DQw3	0.97			47	
970	Tue 22	NS				88	Monomorphic (DQ)
972	RM-2 · 82	NS				8	
973	RM-2 · 102	NS				6	
974	RM-3 · 29	NS				83	All but DR7? + DRw8
975	RM-3 · 170	NS				20	ABC-A2 + Bw57
976	RM-5 · 79	NS				33	ABC-A24 + Bw4
977	RM-7 · 25	NS				52	
978	RM-7 · 89	NS				6	
979	19 · 26 · 1 (1/500)	DR3sh	0.46			56	+ Extras, DR1, 4, w6
980	203-F5 (1/500)	DQw1	0.45	DQw3	0.45	55	
981	203-F5 (1/1000)	DQw1	0.45	DQw3	0.45	80	
982	362 · 2 · D2 · 4	NS				11	
983	326 · 2 · D2 · 4 (1/5)	NS				6	
984	HO-19 · 1 · D · 12 · 2	NS				4	
985	HO-19 · 1 · D · 12 · 2 (1/10)	NS				1	
986	HO-19 3D.H.G.8	NS				5	
987	HO-134D71	DQw1	0.33			44	
988	19-26 · 1	DR3sh	0.4	DRw9	0.32	46	? + DR1, 4, 7, w6
782	D4 90 55/6	NS				78	All but DR7, w9
783	D7.69/9	NS				58	Weak, all but DR7
784	AB8.25/5	DR2sh	0.38			62	+ Weak DR5
992	I-B-6	NS				89	? Monomorphic DR
993	Tue 34	NS				95	Monomorphic DR
994	Tue 35	NS				95	Monomorphic DR
995	Tue 37	NS				92	Monomorphic DR
996	Tue 39	NS				93	Monomorphic
660	JMSDR4 · 1 · 1 (10X)	DQw1	0.97			53	Perfect fit
790	A-10-83	DQw3	0.61			30	? TA10

ter than conventional antisera for the definition of known antigens?"

The answer to this is certainly "yes" for some antigens. These antigens include DQw1, DQw3, DRw52, and DRw6. There are specific antibodies, or ones whose extra specificity is clearly identified, also for DR1, DR2, DR3, DR4, DR5, DR7 and DRw8, but as in most cases there is only one antibody for each of these specificities it would seem safer to wait for other antibodies of similar specificity before embarking on an "all monoclonal" tray.

2. "Can they identify new specificities?"

   Here again the answer is "yes". New specificities DRw11, w12, w13, w14 have all received official recognition after this Workshop mainly because the subtle and previously obscure differences between them have been clarified by the monoclonal antibodies in the Workshop. Other new specificities recognised include TA10, the split of DQw3 and the antigen identified by 925 described above.

3. "Can they contribute extra information not easily obtainable with conventional antisera?"

   The answer is "yes". An example of this demonstrated in this report is the clear definition of some specificities previously identified only by mixed lymphocyte culture or biochemical studies. These include the difference between Dw18 and Dw19 defined by 929 and Dw15 seen with antibodies 949, 901, and 921 as clearly different from Dw4. There is no doubt that closer examination of the data will reveal other instances of the discriminatory power of monoclonal antibodies as mentioned, for example, in the discussion of complement above.

4. "Can monoclonal antibodies be used in serological tissue typing in the same way as conventional antisera or do they require special handling?"

   The answer to this is that they cannot yet be used in the same way as conventional antisera and that up to now they do require special handling. These problems, relating to the high titres of the antibodies leading to carry-over and the instability of their activity on storing have been discussed in detail above. The answers to these problems lie either in stabilisation of the antibodies or possibly in the use of some other technique for assaying them. Such a method might be a micro-ELISA assay, which could have many advantages over cytotoxicity.

This Workshop has clearly demonstrated that monoclonal antibodies can play a valuable role in the definition of HLA specificity and can reveal new and exciting information about the region not previously available. It should be the challenge for the next Workshop to solve the technical problems so that all the data can reach the standard of the best data in this Workshop.

References

1. Bodmer JG, Pickbourne P, Richards S (1977) Ia serology. In: Bodmer WF, et al (eds) Histocompatibility testing 1977. Munksgaard, Copenhagen, pp 35–84
2. Gebuhrer L, Bétuel H, Lambert J, Freidel AC, Farre A (1983) Subtypes of HLA-DR4. Ninth Workshop Newsletter 3:41–48
3. Hansen JA, Martin PJ, Kamoun M, Nisperon B, Thomas ED (1981) A supertypic HLA-DR specificity (DR4 + 5) defined by murine monoclonal antibody. Hum Immunol 2:103–111
4. Kasahara M, Ogasawara K, Ikeda H, Okuyama T, Ishikawa N, Takenouchi T, Wakisaka A, Kikuchi Y, Aizawa M (1983) A monoclonal antibody that detects a polymorphic determinant common to HLA-DR1 and 2. Tissue Antigens 21:105–113
5. Kasahara M, Takenouchi T, Ogasawara K, Ikeda H, Okuyama T, Ishikawa N, Moriuchi J, Wakisaka A, Kikuchi Y, Aizawa M, Kaneka T, Kashiwagi N, Nishimura Y, Sasazuki T (1983) Serologic dissection of HLA-D specificities by the use of monoclonal antibodies. Immunogenetics 17:485–495
6. Maeda H, Juji T (1982) A new B-cell alloantigen, TB21, coded for in the HLA-D/DR region. Tissue Antigens 20:327–334
7. Park MS, Wakisaki A, Terasaki PI, Koneda Y, Barbetti A (1984) A new DR specificity (dn1) which is detected by a monoclonal antibody. Ninth Workshop Newsletter 6:17

HLA-A, B, Interlocus Specificities

P. Richiardi [1], A. Cambon-Thomsen [2], and A. Menicucci [3]

1 Istituto di Genetica Medica, Università di Torino e Centro CNR Immunogenetica e Istocompatibilità, via Santena 19, 10126 Torino, Italy
2 Unité de Recherches d'Immunologie et de Cytogénétique, INSERM U100, CHU Purpan, Toulouse Cédex, France
3 Centro Regionale Tipizzazione Tissutale, U.S.L. 10/D, Firenze, Italy

History

For a long time it was supposed that antigenic epitopes common to different HLA loci products did not exist. The first report of an A11 x Bw6 alloantibody was by Belvedere et al. [1], followed by two reports of cross-reacting A9-Bw4 by Legrand et al. [2] and Scalamogna et al. [3]. In 1980 Kostyu et al. [4] identified a public HLA antigen associated with A9, A32 and Bw4; finally in 1982 Claas et al. provided evidence of an antigenic determinant shared by A2 and B17. Thus, the existence of epitopes common to products of A and B loci can no longer be questioned. Monoclonal antibodies have quite definitely shown that interlocus epitopes are present on HLA-A, B molecules.

Serology

Analysis of Ninth Workshop alloantisera and MoAbs allows the identification of consistent groups of serologically associated HLA-A- and B antigens.

1. Alloantisera. Many sera reacting with products of A and B loci were submitted. Among the sera significantly correlated with A and B antigens, those reacting with antigens in positive linkage disequilibrium were discarded, as such antibodies are more likely to be a mixture. There is a remarkable involvement of B17 [5], which probably cross-reacts with A29 (9w301), A1 (9w318), A2 (9w33, 34, 319, 320, 321, 322), A23 (9w323, also correlated with Bw56 and Bw63). Correlation with Bw57 is generally higher than with Bw58. Among the B17-A2 sera, 34, 319, and 320 react with all A2-positive cells, while 33 and 321 miss. 20% of A2-positive cells and 322 is negative with 70% of the A2-positive cells. Families show that it reacts only with some A2 homozygotes. Absorptions of sera 033, 321, and 322 show that they contain a single interlocus antibody population. Moreover, Calot et al. [6] demonstrated that they react with a different epitope from those identified by other A2 and B17 subtypic and supertypic antibodies, as is recognized by the A2 x B17 MoAb MA2.1 [7]. Analogous results were obtained by Ahern et al. [8] for serum 033.
Further probable interlocus epitopes shown by tail analysis are: A32-Bw4 (423), A25-Bw4 (427), A1-A11-Bw6 (434), A23-B49 (411), A32-B27 (377, correlated also with B7 and B13).

2. Monoclonal Antibodies. Some consistent groups of interlocus specificities can be identified. Some of these are identical with those demonstrated with alloantisera.

Interlocus CREG	MoAb	Further correlated antigens
A32, B27	1107	A9, B37, Bw63
	1135	B7, B40, Bw41, Bw47
Aw19, B40, Bw41	1124	A23 (?)
	1133	B7, B8
Aw33, B8	1110	A31
	1117	A26, A28, B18, B14, B51, B16
A9, Bw4	1155	A32
	1157	
A2, B17	1144	
A2, B16	1132	
	1147	Note: A2 could be carry-over.

Conclusions

Preferential groups of cross-reacting interlocus specificities can be detected both with Ninth Workshop conventional alloantisera and with monoclonal xenoantibodies.

References

1. Legrand L, Dausset J (1975) The complexity of the HLA gene product. II. Possible evidence for a "public" determinant common to the first and second HLA series. Transplantation 19:177–180

Histocompatibility Testing 1984
Edited by E. D. Albert et al.

2. Belvedere M, Mattiuz PL, Curtoni ES (1975) An antibody cross-reacting with LA and FOUR antigens of the HLA system. Immunogenetics 1:538–548
3. Scalamogna M, Mercuriali F, Pizzi C, Sirchia G (1976) Cross-reactivity between the first and second segregant series of the HLA system. Tissue Antigens 7:125–127
4. Kostyu DD, Cresswell P, Amos DB (1980) A public HLA antigen associated with HLA-A9, Aw32 and Bw4. Immunogenetics 10:433–442
5. Claas F, Castelli-Visser R, Schreuder I, van Rood J (1982) Allo-antibodies to an antigenic determinant shared by HLA-A2 and B17. Tissue Antigens 19:388–391
6. Calot M, Cambon A, Herve G, Ohayon E (1983) Interlocus specificities to new allosera within an epitope shared by HLA-A2 and B17. Abstract, European Histocompatibility Training Conference, Strasbourg
7. McMichael AJ, Parham P, Rust N, Brodsky F (1980) A monoclonal antibody that recognizes an antigenic determinant shared by HLA-A2 and B17. Hum Immunol 1:121–129
8. Ahern AT, Phelan DL, Oldfather JW, Parham P, Fuller TC (1982) HLA-A2 and HLA-B17 antigens share an alloantigenic determinant. Hum Immunol 5:139

Specificity of the Ninth Workshop Anti Ia Alloantisera as Assessed by the Direct Binding Assay*

N. Tanigaki[1], P. Overturf[1], L. Rendina[1], J. Shaver[1], R. Tosi[2], and G. B. Ferrara[3]

1 Department of Molecular Immunology, Roswell Park Memorial Institute, 666 Elm Street, Buffalo, NY, 14263, USA
2 Laboratorio di Biologia Cellulare, CNR, 00196 Roma, Italy
3 Istituto per Studio et la Cura dei Tumori, 16132 Genova, and AVIS, Bergamo, Italy

Antibody specificity can be easily defined when the binding of antibody to antigen is measured directly. A sensitive determination of such direct binding is possible by the use of radiolabeled antigen. This is also the case for alloantigens [1, 2]. We have been using ^{125}I-labeled Ia antigens for specificity assay of the alloantisera and more recently of the monoconal antibodies. The assay method (we call it the direct binding assay) first allows reaction of a test alloantiserum or a monoclonal antibody with a radioiodinated Ia preparation, and then measures the extent of binding by the double-antibody technique [2]. When a panel of ^{125}I-labeled Ia preparations of different specificities is used, the major or putative antibody specificity can be deduced from the reaction pattern. This assay has been found particularly useful in the search for antibodies that can be used for Ia typing by the binding inhibition assay [2, 3] and also for immunospecific isolation of Ia molecules carrying different specificities [4].

We applied this assay method in analysing the Eighth Workshop anti-Ia alloantisera. As reported previously [5], the major specificity detected by the direct binding assay correlated, in most cases, with the specificity defined in population study by the cytotoxic test. Although the method was not suitable for the detection of antibodies with low binding affinity, it showed a clear advantage over the cytotoxic test in identifying "supertypic specificities".

The same assay has been applied to the Ninth Workshop anti-Ia alloantisera. All 236 antisera were tested against an improved antigen panel consisting of ^{125}I-labeled preparations of Ia antigens isolated from cells of the following cell lines; LG2 (DR1, 1), LG14 (DR3, 3), LG38 (DR5, 5), LG10 (DR7, 7), Daudi (DRw6, –), U698M (DR2, 4), BT1 (DR4, w9), and RPMI8392 (DRw6, w10). For assay of the supertypic alloantisera three DR-deleted Ia preparations (indicated as DR$^-$ in the Tables) derived from LG14, LG38, and Daudi were included in the antigen panel. The first two were prepared by absorption with MCS7, a monoclonal antibody possessing a high reactivity restricted to DR [6]. The DR-deleted Daudi-Ia was obtained by papain digestion and subsequent lentil-lectin chromatography and gel filtration [7]. An enhancement in the percent Ia binding (see Table 1) with these DR-deleted Ia preparations compared with the DR-undeleted original preparations indicates that the

* This work was supported in part by USPHS-grants AI20251 and CA17276, awarded by the National Institute of Allergy and Infectious Diseases and the National Cancer Institute, Department of Health and Human Services, and by a grant from Progetto Finalizzato CNR Ingegneria Genetica Sottoprogetto "Basi moleculari delle malattie ereditarie", CNR grants 820130504 and 820133696, and a grant awarded by the North Atlantic Treaty Organization

Table 1. Monospecific anti-DR antisera

9th Workshop serum no.	Percentage of Ia binding with								Deduced specificity
	LG2 (1, 1)	LG14 (3, 3)	LG38 (5, 5)	LG10 (7, 7)	U698M (2, 4)	BT1 (4, w9)	Daudi (w6, –)	8392 (w6, w10)	
504	38.7	−0.2	−1.1	−1.9	0.0	4.2	2.3	2.5	DR1
508	11.7	0.7	−0.1	−2.1	1.7	0.8	1.7	1.4	DR1
509	19.4	2.2	0.9	−1.2	−0.5	1.0	1.4	−0.8	DR1
510	11.8	0.3	−0.3	−2.3	0.0	−1.1	0.0	−2.1	DR1
512	42.0	1.3	−0.1	1.6	0.0	4.0	−0.4	0.0	DR1
514	51.3	0.2	0.9	−0.5	4.1	2.8	0.2	5.0	DR1
521	54.6	0.1	−0.4	−0.3	1.7	3.0	−2.5	1.5	DR1
522	49.3	1.9	1.1	−0.3	−0.4	0.4	−2.0	2.6	DR1
516	2.9	1.9	0.1	−1.7	−0.6	2.0	−1.3	22.0	DRw10
523	0.6	0.3	0.7	−1.9	−0.1	−0.7	0.3	18.1	DRw10
529	−1.0	−1.6	−0.6	−0.7	−1.6	1.6	1.3	19.0	DRw10
538	3.0	−0.3	3.2	2.9	20.0	4.4	−1.2	–	DR2
541	3.2	4.6	−0.2	−0.9	16.4	4.4	−2.1	–	DR2
552	1.7	0.0	3.9	−0.2	10.8	2.3	2.8	–	DR2
575	1.3	1.2	3.2	2.6	8.8	9.8	1.9	–	DR4
576	0.4	−1.8	2.1	1.1	9.8	8.1	0.4	–	DR4
578	−1.0	−0.4	1.4	4.1	10.8	14.1	1.0	–	DR4
587	0.7	0.5	2.2	1.4	10.6	7.8	3.9	–	DR4
589	0.4	1.1	3.4	4.2	14.7	11.9	0.4	–	DR4
592	1.4	1.5	−0.5	0.8	8.4	11.3	−1.7	–	DR4
629	0.8	1.2	−2.2	23.2	−0.6	4.3	1.0	–	DR7
634	4.8	0.8	3.9	14.1	1.1	3.0	−1.8	–	DR7
636	3.5	3.4	0.4	60.6	0.8	−0.2	2.1	–	DR7
638	1.4	0.5	−0.4	36.6	0.0	0.9	−2.1	–	DR7
630	1.1	0.4	−0.3	0.1	0.9	7.3	−1.8	–	DRw9
644	1.4	−1.2	0.8	1.2	1.7	10.3	0.2	–	DRw9
645	1.3	0.6	2.0	0.4	0.7	16.3	−3.2	–	DRw9
650	1.5	−0.8	1.7	0.9	2.2	6.6	−0.6	–	DRw9

antibody specificity is directed to DQ molecules or to DR-like molecules we call BR, rather than to DR molecules. Results, expressed as the percent Ia binding, i.e., the proportion of the maximum binding of each labeled Ia preparation obtained with an excess of rabbit anti-human Ia antiserum 7147 [2], are shown in Tables 1–7 for a limited number of antisera that gave the typical reaction patterns expected from the known Ia specificities.

Table 1 lists the antisera that showed a monoreactive pattern in the direct binding assay. They bound essentially to only one (two in the case of DR4) of the Ia preparations in the antigen panel. Their reactivities are probably directed to DR molecules. However, for the decisive specificity assignment, a structural analysis of the reacting molecules would be necessary, because our recent data indicate that there are DQ specificities that show single linkage disequilibrium with DR specificities [8].

Table 2 shows representative antisera possessing DRw52 specificity. Their reaction pattern corresponds to the known DR association of DRw52; they react with LG14, LG38, and Daudi, but not with others (the present antigen panel does not contain DRw8-positive and "8wDRw13"-positive Ia preparations). It is significant that these antisera can be classified into two groups, one reacting with the DR-deleted preparations (the last four) and another not binding to those Ia preparations (the first four). This "DRw52 splitting" supports our previous assumption that two different specificities underlie the DRw52 serological pattern, one carried by DR molecules and another located on BR molecules [4]. Most of the anti-DRw52 antisera so far analyzed belong to the second group, although they often have additional anti-DQ activity. The molecules isolated from the DR-deleted LG38-Ia preparation with one such anti-DRw52 antiserum K3010 lacking anti-DQ activity (Katagiri) has been shown to share a very similar α-chain with DR molecules, and the population distribution of the specificity has been found to conform to the DRw52 pattern [6]. The question as to whether the specificity detected by the first group of antisera also follows the DRw52 pattern remains to be investigated.

Table 2. Representative anti-DRw52 antisera

9th Workshop serum no.	Percentage of Ia binding with								
	LG2 (1, 1)	Daudi (w6, –)	LG14 (3, 3)	LG38 (5, 5)	LG14 (DR⁻)	LG38 (DR⁻)	LG10 (7, 7)	U698M (2, 4)	BT1 (4, w9)
681	−0.6	21.4	20.7	17.1	2.6	3.0	−1.2	−1.0	−1.2
684	−0.5	37.4	47.6	33.6	5.5	4.1	−0.4	−0.4	−2.0
694	0.1	16.1	32.5	33.3	6.3	6.3	−1.1	0.9	2.9
709	0.2	26.7	34.8	32.8	5.1	7.3	−0.9	2.2	0.8
687	0.7	41.3	60.0	53.7	25.4	35.7	1.6	1.0	1.9
689	0.4	31.5	72.7	51.7	34.6	30.6	0.7	1.9	2.5
697	1.0	45.1	51.1	48.8	22.8	21.6	0.9	3.2	0.6
758	−0.6	33.5	64.3	60.3	30.1	34.0	−1.1	−1.6	2.2

Table 3. Monospecific anti-DQw1 antisera

9th Workshop serum no.	Percentage of Ia binding with								
	LG2 (1, 1)	U698M (2, 4)	8392 (w6, w10)	Daudi (w6, –)	Daudi (DR⁻)	LG14 (3, 3)	LG38 (5, 5)	LG10 (7, 7)	BT1 (4, w9)
668	6.4	0.7	4.7	9.4	33.4	0.0	−0.6	0.8	5.0
670	5.4	2.2	6.1	10.9	35.9	1.1	−0.9	−0.9	3.2
671	5.6	2.4	8.6	10.2	38.1	3.2	−0.8	−0.3	5.9
672	9.8	1.1	4.6	8.7	31.1	1.9	1.9	−0.5	6.1
674	7.1	4.3	0.5	6.4	21.9	1.4	0.7	2.3	4.0

Table 4. Antisera containing anti-DQw2 activity

9th Workshop serum no.	Percentage of Ia binding with								
	LG2 (1, 1)	LG14 (3, 3)	LG14 DR⁻)	LG38 (5, 5)	LG38 (DR⁻)	LG10 (7, 7)	U698M (2, 4)	BT1 (4, w9)	Daudi (w6, –)
721	0.9	2.9	6.4	3.4	2.2	62.4	−0.3	4.3	0.9
722	0.6	3.7	7.6	0.7	0.3	69.5	0.8	9.2	1.4
723	1.5	6.2	12.4	0.4	0.0	67.9	−1.3	3.1	0.5
720	1.8	6.5	11.7	3.0	1.8	63.2	8.9	15.0	0.6
724	1.3	11.1	14.9	3.5	2.3	64.5	5.8	11.6	0.3
743	2.1	3.9	14.6	0.0	4.5	62.3	8.1	17.0	0.3

Table 5. Antisera which possibly have anti-DQw3 activity

9th Workshop serum no.	Percentage of Ia binding with								
	LG2 (1, 1)	LG14 (3, 3)	LG14 (DR⁻)	LG38 (5, 5)	LG38 (DR⁻)	LG10 (7, 7)	U698M (2, 4)	BT1 (4, w9)	Daudi (w6, –)
747	1.0	2.2	1.6	11.1	24.3	0.0	7.4	9.0	0.4
761	0.5	0.5	0.4	6.8	12.6	−0.1	16.8	12.3	0.2
731	1.3	1.9	1.3	12.2	19.9	3.7	21.4	24.5	−0.1
791	0.7	3.4	0.6	15.7	23.1	4.1	15.4	20.5	−1.6
730	1.6	2.0	2.3	14.8	23.5	8.7	38.8	33.8	−0.1
745	6.7	1.2	3.6	13.6	20.5	5.3	17.3	22.8	0.4
753	13.8	3.2	4.1	11.8	26.4	9.3	38.8	32.2	−0.2

Table 3 lists monospecific anti-DQw1 (DC1, MB1, MT1, LB12) antisera. The association of DQw1 with DR1, 2, w6, and w10 is well known. The reaction pattern leading to this specificity is low binding with LG2, U698M, Daudi and RPMI8392, coupled with no or only a negligible reaction with LG14 and LG38. The lack of reactivity with the last two Ia preparations eliminates anti-DRw52 activity. Since DQw1 reactivity varies from one Ia preparation to another, the most reliable criterion is a higher binding with DR-deleted Daudi-Ia preparation than with the non-DR-deleted original preparation. All antisera shown by the cytotoxic assay to have a 2 + w6 pattern or a 1 + 2 + w6 pattern indeed contained anti-DQw1 antibody. However, many of them also possessed antibody against DR1, 2, or w10, as assessed by the too high binding with Ia preparations carrying these DR specificities. Only those listed in Table 3 were regarded as monospecific by the present assay, although clarification is needed for the binding with BT1-Ia.

Table 4 gives antisera containing anti-DQw2 (DC3, MB2) antibody. This specificity is found in 63% of DR3-positive individuals and also in 63% of DR7-positive ones [9]. In addition, it is detected in DRw9-positive cells. The relatively loose association with DR3 and DR7 is thought to permit frequent occurrence of antisera having this specificity, and yet only a few were found in the Ninth Workshop antisera tested. LG14 and LG10 are DQw2 positive. Therefore, a positive binding with these two Ia preparations coupled with an enhanced binding with the DR-deleted LG14-Ia can be interpreted as indicative of DQw2 specificity. Those listed are not monospecific; their major reactivity is directed to DR7 and three antisera apparently contain anti-DRw53 (BR4, MT3) activity [10] as assessed by the binding with U698M and BT1. Anti-DR3 antisera possessing anti-DQw2 activity presumably exist. In fact, the Fe96/19 we used for isolation of the molecules carrying the DQw2 specificity from LG10-Ia preparation belonged to this category [9]. No such antisera were found in the present assay. DQw2 appears to be the primary HLA specificity associated with celiac disease [11].

Table 5 lists antisera that may have anti-DQw3 (DC4, MB3, MT4) activity. This specificity is detected in all DR4-positive and DR5-positive individuals and in a small fraction of DR7-positive cases [6]. DRw9 is also the associated DR specificity. The reaction pattern supporting this specificity is a positive binding with LG38 and with U698M and BT1. This must then be accompanied by enhanced binding with the DR-deleted LG38-Ia. This requirement is crucial for identification of anti-DQw3 antibody by the present antigen panel, because the positive reaction with U698M or BT1 may reflect merely their reactivity with DR4 or DRw9, and not with DQw3. The DR-linkage pattern suggests that three groups of anti-DQw3 antisera must exist, each group carrying anti-DR4 or -DR5 or -DRw9 activity. All the antisera shown in Table 5 are classified to the anti-DR4 group. In addition, five antisera appear to contain anti-DRw53 (MT3) antibody [10], as indicated by a low but significant reaction with LG10. A considerable number of antisera of nominal specificity DR5 or DRw52 have been found to contain anti-DQw3 antibody. Detection would be facilitated if a DR-deleted Ia preparation from DR4 (or DRw9)-homozygous cells were added to the present antigen panel.

Table 6 shows antisera that may contain anti-DC5 activity. This specificity was recently found [12]. It is present on DQ molecules and behaves like a split specificity of DQw3. The distribution in the population is restricted to DR5-positive and/or "8wDRw13"-positive individuals and to a small proportion of DR4-positive individuals. The reaction pattern suggesting this specificity is a clear positive binding with LG38-Ia preparation and with the DR-deleted preparation. Those showing a

Table 6. Antisera which possibly contain anti-DC5 activity

9th Workshop serum no.	Percentage of Ia binding with								
	LG2 (1, 1)	LG14 (3, 3)	LG14 (DR⁻)	LG38 (5, 5)	LG38 (DR⁻)	LG10 (7, 7)	U698M (2, 4)	BT1 (4, w9)	Daudi (w6, -)
607	4.4	3.1	3.9	10.7	22.5	−0.8	0.7	4.2	3.0
773	1.4	0.6	−0.9	5.5	9.2	0.6	2.3	4.9	−0.7
777	−0.7	−0.9	−1.2	5.2	10.7	−0.1	−0.1	0.4	0.0
786	−0.3	−0.7	3.0	6.7	13.0	−1.2	−2.8	2.4	−1.7
596	4.2	0.5	1.0	20.4	11.3	0.8	2.8	3.5	−4.9
599	5.1	2.0	2.7	37.9	21.5	1.0	6.0	3.6	9.4
601	2.6	1.0	3.8	32.2	28.1	1.7	2.8	1.5	1.8
603	−0.2	1.0	4.0	17.0	18.1	−0.1	1.6	−0.9	−0.1
608	0.2	2.2	−2.8	32.6	8.6	−2.5	0.0	5.9	−1.0

Table 7. Antisera which possibly possess anti-DCα3 activity

9th Workshop serum no.	Percentage of Ia binding								
	LG2 (1, 1)	LG14 (3, 3)	LG14 (DR^-)	LG38 (5, 5)	LG38 (DR^-)	LG10 (7, 7)	U698M (2, 4)	BT1 (4, w9)	Daudi (w6, –)
612	2.3	2.1	12.3	−0.2	6.9	−0.2	−0.4	1.0	−3.9
789	−0.1	3.0	12.2	14.3	23.1	−0.4	−3.1	1.4	3.2
775	3.4	5.0	13.2	8.6	16.7	9.2	−2.3	0.3	−3.6
792	0.9	6.5	19.3	12.1	22.9	10.8	3.1	1.9	0.8

reduced binding with the latter must contain anti-DR5 antibody, whereas those giving an enhanced binding could be "pure" anti-DC5 antisera. 8w670 (Curtoni) is the only such pure antiserum so far found. Since the antigen panel does not include Ia preparations from either "8wDRw13" positive cells or DR4-positive, DC5-positive cells, these antisera should be further evaluated for specificity by a population study. The fact that the DC5 specificity is carried by a fraction of DR4-positive individuals may have an implication for further characterization of the primary HLA-association of various DR4-associated diseases.

Table 7 lists antisera that may possess anti-DCα3 activity. This specificity is designated so because its Ia-α-chain localization has been demonstrated by the direct binding with isolated α-chains [13]. It is tightly associated with DR5 and "8wDRw13" and somewhat loosely with DR3. The characteristic reaction pattern is an enhanced binding with both DR-deleted LG14-Ia and LG38-Ia preparations. Here again, the lack of a DR-deleted "8wDRw13" positive Ia preparation makes it necessary to confirm the specificity by a population analysis.

In conclusion, the present study has found excellent antisera against "subtypic" DR specificities and also sorted out antisera containing antibodies directed to "supertypic" DR specificities. However, the specificities defined by the direct binding assay alone are only putative. The final specificity assignment has to be made on the basis of data obtained by the binding inhibition assay which reveals the population distribution of a specificity, and also by the sequential binding assay which decides the molecular localization of a specificity [2]. It should be supported by a structural analysis of the reacting molecules. The detection of antisera highly specific for DR1 and DRw10, along with the availability of antisera monospecific to DQw1, would facilitate the dissection of DR-like specificities tightly linked to these DR specificities. More important, the identification of antisera containing anti-DCα3 activity or anti-DC5 activity would contribute to a further study of the primary HLA association of various DR3 or DR4-associated diseases.

References

1. Tanigaki N, Miyakawa Y, Yagi Y, Kreiter VP, Pressman D (1973) Radioiodinated soluble HLA antigens: HLA alloantigenic characterization and use in radioimmunoassay. J Immunol Methods 3:109–126
2. Tanigaki N, Tosi R (1982) Assessment of the specificity of human Ia alloantisera and alloantigens by the use of radioiodinated human Ia antigens. Tissue Antigens 20:1–21
3. Tosi R, Tanigaki N, Centis D, Rossi PL, Alfano G, Ferrara GB, Pressman D (1980) HLA-DR typing by radioimmunoassay. Transplantation 29:302–305
4. Tanigaki N, Tosi R (1982) The genetic control of human Ia alloantigens: A three-loci model derived from the immunochemical analysis of 'supertypic' specificities. Immunol Rev 66:5–37
5. Tosi R, Tanigaki N, Centis D (1980) Analysis at molecular level of the specificity of 8th workshop antisera. In: Terasaki PI (ed) Histocomatibility testing 1980. UCLA Tissue Typing Laboratory, Los Angeles, pp 903–906
6. Tanigaki N, Tosi R, Sagawa K, Minowada J, Ferrara GB (1983) The distribution of DR5, MT2, and MB3 specificities on human Ia subsets. Immunogenetics 17:371–386
7. Tosi R, Tanigaki N, Centis D, Ferrara GB, Pressman D (1978) Immunological dissection of human Ia molecules. J Exp Med 148:1592–1611
8. Tanigaki N, Tosi R, Katagiri M, Ferrara GB (to be published) A DC specificity associated with DR4 in single linkage disequilibrium. Immunogenetics (submitted)
9. Tanigaki N, Tosi R, Duquesnoy RJ, Ferrara GB (1983) Three Ia species with different structures and alloantigenic determinants in an HLA-homozygous cell line. J Exp Med 157:231–247
10. Tanigaki N, Tosi R, Pressman D, Ferrara GB (1980) Molecular identification of human Ia antigens coded for by a gene locus closely linked to HLA-DR locus. Immunogenetics 10:151–167
11. Tosi R, Vismara D, Tanigaki N, Ferrara GB, Cicimarra F, Buffalano W, Follo D, Auricchi S (1983) Evidence that celiac disease is primarily associated with a DC locus allelic specificity. Clin Immunol Immunopathol 28:395–403
12. Tanigaki N, Tosi R, Centis D, Ferrara GB (to be published) DR5-associated DC molecules carry three different allospecificities. Hum Immunol (in press)
13. Tosi R, Tanigaki N, Sorrentino R, Centis D, Ferrara GB (1984) Serologically detectably polymorphism of the HLA-DC α-subunit. J Immunol 132:277–282

HLA-DR, DQ, and Dw Relationships

G.M.T. Schreuder [1] and L. Degos [2]

1 Department of Immunohematology and Blood Bank, University Hospital Leiden, Rijnsburgerweg 10, 2333 AA Leiden, The Netherlands
2 Hôpital Saint Louis, 2 Place du Dr. Fournier, 75010 Paris 10, France

It is well established that HLA-DR and DQ (MB, DC) series correspond to DR and DQ molecules, respectively. Their equivalents in mice are IE and IA, which are considered to have stimulatory capacity in mixed lymphocyte culture. Aside from the DR stimulatory molecules, the DQ molecules are also stimulatory. This is demonstrated by a recombinant DR/DQ, which shows positive MLR with the ABCDR-identical, DQ-different sib (Carlsson et al., this volume).

Thus, if it is not to be a stimulator in primary MLR, a cell most probably has to be identical with the responding cell for both HLA-DR and DQ. Thus, an HTC might only give a typing response (negative response) when DR and DQ are identical with the cell to be typed.

Certain HLA-DR and DQ combinations occur frequently due to linkage disequilibrium, which can be specific for the population under study.

For many HLA-DR and DQ combinations for which examples have been presented at this Workshop, HTC have been found. They are shown in Table 1, by their Dw specificity, their 9w number or their local name (if they were not included in the Workshop). For some serologically defined HLA-DR-DQ combinations, although they have been observed to segregate in families, HTC have not yet been reported. They are denoted marked ▲ in Table 1. It can be expected that all possible DR and DQ combinations will be observed in the future.

(For clarification of the DR, DQ and D nomenclature see the appropriate joint reports.)

Table 1. HLA-DR and DQ combinations

	DQw1	DQw2	DQw3		Blank
			TA10+	TA10−	
DR1	Dw1				
DR2	Dw2, w12				
DR2sh.	FJO		DB9		
DR3		Dw3	▲		▲
DR4			Dw4 Dw13	Dw10 Dw14	Dw15
DRw11	9901		Dw5		▲
DRw12			DB6		▲
DRw13	Dw6		1802		▲
DRw14	Dw9		Dw16		
DR7		Dw7		Dw11	
DRw8	Dw8.2		Dw8.2		Dw8
DRw9		▲		DB5	
DRw10	SHY				
Blank	BON				

HLA-DR, DQ, LB, and TA10 Specificities of Ninth Workshop Homozygous Typing Cells

G.M.T. Schreuder [1], I. Doxiadis [2], J. Parlevliet [1], and H. Grosse-Wilde [2]

1 Department of Immunohematology and Blood Bank, University Hospital Leiden, Rijnsburgerweg 10, 2333 AA Leiden, The Netherlands
2 Department of Immunogenetics, University Hospital of Essen, 4300 Essen, Federal Republic of Germany

Homozygous typing cells (HTC) are the reference reagents for the cellular definition of HLA-D [1] and originally formed the basis for the definition of HLA-DR [2]. The serological definition of HLA-DR is improving through the availability of better techniques and an increasing number of reagents. With the exception of DRw6, the specificities DR1-w10 are quite well defined [3]. In the meantime, several DR specificities have been reported as probably heterogeneous. Very little data is available as to whether such serologically defined new groups correlate with the established and new

Histocompatibility Testing 1984
Edited by E. D. Albert et al.

Table 1. HLA typing of Ninth Workshop HTC

9WS Nr.	HLA-	Local ID	From	HLA -A	-B	-C	-DR	-DQ	Other
0101	Dw1	AL	BSH	3	51, 35	4	1	1	
0102	Dw1	HEN	GSW	2, 29	44	5	1	1	
0103	Dw1	MAM	BET	31	44, 14		1	1	
0104	Dw1	MDE	STA	3, 31	27, 35	2, 4	1	1	
0105	Dw1	WOE	GSW	3, 25	18, 35	4	1	1	
0201	Dw2	CI	BUC	3, 25	7, 18	7	2	1	
0202	Dw2	HOF	GSW	3, 25	7, 18	7	2	1	
0203	Dw2	KER	MYR	2	7	7	2	1	
0204	Dw2	PIL	WAN	3	7	7	2	1	
0301	Dw3	AVL	ROO	1	8	7	3, 52	2	
0302	Dw3	CHR	GSW	1	8	7	3, 52	2	
0303	Dw3	COX	DTO	1	8	7	3, 52	2	
0304	Dw3	GSM	STA	1	8	7	3, 52	2	
0305	Dw3	LHM	HAN	1	8	7	3, 52	2	
0401	Dw4	HBH	BSH	2	44, 62	3, 5	4 (4.1), 53	3	LB-E13, TA10
0402	Dw4	HIM	MYR	2	62	3	4 (4.1), 53	3	LB-E13, TA10
0403	Dw4	JAH	HAN	2	62	3	4 (4.1), 53	3	LB-E13
0404	Dw4	SUD	GSW	2	44	5	4 (4.1), 53	3	LB-E13
0501	Dw5	BAU	MYR	2	18	7	11, 52	3	LB-E13, TA10
0502	Dw5	BRI	FER[a]	9	5		not tested		
0503	Dw5	DHI	FES		not tested				
0504	Dw5	HVB	BSH	1, 32	35, 41	4	11, 52	3	LB-E13, TA10
0505	Dw5	KRO	WER	2	44	7	11, 52	3	LB-E13, TA10
0506	?	SM	BUC	24	35	4	11, 52	1, 3	LB-E13, TA10
0601	Dw18	HBS	BET	2, 28	27, 39	2	13, 52	1	
0602	Dw18	HHK	ROO	3	7	7	13, 52	1	
0603	Dw18	JTED	STA	2, 29	35, 27	1, 4	13, 52	1	
0604	Dw18	SCL	GSW	2	44	5	13, 52	1	
0605	Dw18	WDV	ROO	2	38	–	13, 52	1	
0606	Dw19	EMJ	HAN	2, 3	60	3	13, 52	1	
0607	Dw19	KRA	GSW	2	60	3	13, 52	1	
0608	Dw19	SLE	HAN	2	60	3	13, 52	1	
0609	?	KSH	FES	3, 28	14, 27	2, 8	13, 52	1	
0610	Dw19	KT11	KSH	33	44	–	13, 52	1	
0611	Dw19	STEP	HSU	11	60	3	13, 52	1	
0701	Dw17	BOR	GSW	30	13	6	7, 53	2	
0702	Dw7	BUP	HSU[a]	2	14	–⊕	7, 53	2	
0703	?	MMF	YUN	2, 33	14	–⊕	7, 53	2	
0704	Dw17	PIT	DTO	29	44	4	7, 53	2	
0705	Dw17	WET	WER	28, 29	44	7	7, 53	2	
0801	Dw8	BTB	TSB	2	7, 27	1, 7	8, 52	–	
0802	Dw8	MMR	ROO	3, 24	7, 18	7	8, 52	–	
0803	?	OLG	LAY	31	62	1, 3	8, 52	–	
0804	Dw8	SEC	LAY[a]	31	62	1	not tested		
0805	Dw8.2	LUY	ROO	2	51	–	8, 52	3	LB-E13, TA10
0806	Dw8.2	TAB	HAN	2	46	1, 3	8, 52	1	
0807	Dw8	BAE	GSW	2	51	–	8, 52	–	
0808	Dw8	MAD	SVE	2	60	3	8, 52	–	
0901	Dw9	BRU	WAN[a]	2, 28	39, 60	3	14, 52	1	
0902	Dw9	CHN	BET	1, 3	8, 41	–	14, 52	1	
0903	Dw9	GECL	BET	28	44, 55	3, 7	14, 52	1	
0904	Dw9	GEV	FES	3, 26	55, 62	3	14, 52	1	
0905	Dw9	OH	TSB	2	44	5	14, 52	1	
1001	Dw10	AL10	BAC	26	38	–	4 (4.2), 53	3	LB-E13
1002	Dw10	LE10	BAC	26	38, 35	4	4 (4.3), 53	3	LB-E13
1003	Dw10	MAY	BRA	26	38	–	4 (4.2), 53	3	LB-E13
1004	?	RLO	STA[a]	3, 26	38, 41	–	4 (4.1), 53	3	LB-E13
1005	Dw10	TS10	BAC	26	38	–	4 (4.2), 53	3	LB-E13
1101	Dw11	BEI	HSU	2	57	6	7, 53	3	
1102	Dw11	GRO	GSW	2	57	6	7, 53	3	
1103	Dw11	KIA	HSU[a]	2	17		7, 53	3	
1104	Dw11	KIJ	HSU[a]	2	17		7, 53	3	
1105	Dw11	SM11	YUN	1, 25	44, 57	4	7, 53	2, 3	

Table 1. (continued)

9WS Nr.	HLA-	Local ID	From	HLA -A	-B	-C	-DR	-DQ	Other
1201	Dw12	BGE	BRA	1, 2	52	–	2	1	
1202	Dw12	TOK	SAS	24	52	–	2	1	
1301	?	JHA	FES	31	51	–	4 (4.2), 53	3	LB-E13, TA10
1302	Dw13	PEA	GSW	31	51	–	4 (4.2), 53	3	LB-E13, TA10
1303	Dw13	SSTO	HSU	32	44	5	4 (4.2), 53	3	LB-E13
1401	?	BIN4	BAC	2, 31	60, 14	3	4 (4.1), 53	3	LB-E13
1402	Dw14	KY	BSH	31	60	3	4 (4.1), 53	3	LB-E13
1403	Dw14	LS40	BAC	1, 26	27, 60	2, 3	4 (4.1), 53	3	LB-E13
1404	Dw14	MT	BSH[a]	31	60	3	not tested		
1405	?	PEM	BET	2	35, 60	3, 4	4 (4.1), 53	3	LB-E13
1406	Dw14	THO	HAN	2, 3	60	3	4 (4.1), 53	3	LB-E13
1501	DB6	BM16	FER	2	18	7	12, 52	3	LB-E13, TA10
1502	?	BM24	FER[a]	1	41		2, 11, 52	1, 3	LB-E13, TA10
1503	DB6	HERL	SVE	2	35, 44	4, 5	12, 52	3	LB-E13, TA10
1504	?	HRL	FAU	2, 3	52, 39	1,7	8, 11, 52	3	LB-E13, TA10
1601	Dw8.2	HI-2	FUK	not tested					
1602	Dw8.2	SHIM	SAS	2	46	1, 3	8, 52	1	
1701	Dw16	AMAL	LAY	2	62	3, 7	14, 52	3	LB-E13, TA10
1702	Dw16	CRIS	LAY	2, 31	51, 62	3	14, 52	3	LB-E13, TA10
1801	DB9	BASI	LAY[a]	2	51		2 short	3	LB-E13, TA10
1802	?	HAG	WER	2	41	7	13, 52	3	LB-E13, TA10
1803	DB9	REMI	LAY	2	51	–	2 short	3	LB-E13, TA10
1901	Dw17	BH13	YUN	2	13	6	7, 53	2	
1902	Dw9	DJ	ONO	1, 23	8, 50	6, 7	3, 14, 52	1, 2	
1903	?	LBU	FES	30	13	6	7, 53	2	
1904	Dw9	SI	ONO	1, 30	8, 13	6, 7	14, 52	1	
9901	Dw5	FPA	FES	1	35	4	11, 52	1	
9902	Dw15	HAS	BAC[a]	2	54, 62	1, 3	4 (4.1), 53	n.t.	LB-E13 ?
	DB5	DKB	local	24	60	3	9, 53	3	

[a] HLA-ABC typing not performed in Leiden, typing as given by laboratory of cell origin; ?, undefined HLA-D specificity; ⊕, not tested for Cw8

HLA-D specificities. Even less is known about the influence of the recently defined MB, DC, or LB-E (now DQ) locus products in cellular techniques.

The Ninth Workshop (9W) offered us the possibility of studying a large number of HTC provided by laboratories from all over the world with the extensive set of 9w DR typing sera.

All 9w HTC are listed in Table 1, together with their 9w and local identification, their origin, and HLA-D specificities as defined by the Workshop (H. Grosse-Wilde et al., Definition of HLA-D with HTC, this volume).

One ampoule of the majority of the 9w HTC was tested with our local set of 80 DR typing sera and with as many as possible of the 9W DR trays 10–13. Due to technical problems, the workshop set of monoclonal antibodies could not be tested. The two-color fluorescence test was used. When enough cells were available, HLA-ABC typings were performed with our local set of 120 typing sera in the standard NIH technique. The viability of the HTCs was generally good (70%–100% viable B cells). The number of cells per ampoule varied considerably: 12 HTCs could not be tested on all DR trays. The HLA-ABC, DR, and DQ typings of the HTC tested are given in Table 1. None of the HTC typed serologically as DRw9 or DRw10. Our local DB5/DRw9 HTC DKB was included in this study to give a more complete impression of DR specificities of the HTC.

From our local serum analysis, performed with the 9W sera on 170 cells tested for the Workshop, sera were selected that correlated well with each other and with the assigned DR, DQ, LB-E13, and TA10 specificities. Moreover, the reports in the 9W Newsletters enabled us to select sera that defined possible DR splits in more than one laboratory. The serum clusters which we obtained, with their *r* values, are given in Table 2.

When HTC were ordered according to their DR and DQ types, the serum patterns set out in Fig. 1 were observed. Due to lack of space, it is not possible to show the reactions of each serum towards each HTC. The 9w numbers of the HTC included in each pattern are listed in Table 3. Some cells, although serologically identical to a certain HTC

HTC[⊗]	DR1	DR2	DR2 s	DR3	3+6	DR4 1+2+3	DR4 1+2	DR4 1	w11	5+ w13	w14	DR7	DR8	DR9	w52	w53	DQ1	DQ2	DQ3	LB-E13	TA10	TYPING[⊕] DR	TYPING[⊕] DQ
Dw1	+++																+++					1	1
	+++																+++						
Dw2		++	+														+++					2	1
		++	+														+++						
Dw12		++	+														+++						
		++	+														+++						
DB9		++																	+++	+++	++++	2 sh	3
		++																	+++	+++	++++		
Dw3				+++	+++										+++			+++				3	2
				+++	+++										+++			+++					
Dw4 a						+++++	+++	++								+++			+++	+++	++++	4.1	3
Dw4 b						+++++	+++	++								+++			+++	+++			
1004						+++++	+++	++								+++			+++	+++			
Dw10 b						+++++										+++			+++	+++		4.3	3
Dw10 a						+++++	+++									+++			+++	+++		4.2	3
1301						+++++	+++									+++			+++	+++	++++		
Dw13 a						+++++	+++									+++			+++	+++	++++		
Dw13 b						+++++	+++									+++			+++	+++			
Dw14						+++++	+++	++								+++			+++	+++		4.1	3
						+++++	+++	++								+++			+++	+++			
1401,1405						+++++	+++	++								+++			+++	+++			
Dw15						+++++	+++	++								+++			NT	(+)		4.1	?
						+++++	+++	++								+++							
Dw5 a									+++	+++					+++				+++	+++	++++	11	3
									+++	+++					+++				+++	+++	++++		
Dw5 b									+++	+++					+++		+++					11	1
DB6										+++					+++				+++	+++	++++	12	3
										+++					+++				+++	+++	++++		
Dw6 Dw18					+/-					+++					+++		+++					13	1
Dw6 Dw19					+/-					+++					+++		+++						
609					+/-					+++					+++		+++						
1802					+++					+++					+++				+++	+++	++++	13	3
Dw9 a					-/+						+++				+++		+++					14	1
					-/+						+++				+++		+++						
Dw9 b				+++	+++						+++				+++		+++	+++				14,3	1,2
Dw16					+++						+++				+++				+++	+++	++++	14	3
					+++						+++				+++				+++	+++	++++		
Dw17												+++				+++		+++				7	2
												+++				+++		+++					
Dw7												+++				+++		+++					
703,1903												+++				+++		+++					
Dw11 b												+++				+++		+++	+++			7	2,3
Dw11 a												+++				+++			+++			7	3
												+++				+++			+++				
Dw8													+++		+++							8	-
													+++		+++								
803													+++		+++								
Dw8.2 a													+++		+++				+++	+++	++++	8	3
Dw8.2 b													+++		+++		+++					8	1
DB5														+++		+++			+++			9	3
														+++		+++			+++				
506									+++	+++					+++		+++		+++	+++	++++	11	1,3
1502		++	+						+++	+++					+++		+++		+++	+++	++++	11,2	1,3
1504									+++	+++			+++		+++				+++	+++	++++	11,8	3

Fig. 1. Ninth Workshop serum clusters with Ninth Workshop HTC. X, see Table 2 for serum clusters; ⊗, see Table 3 for HTC numbers; ⊕, see Table 1 for complete HLA typing; +, sera positive in cluster; +/–, sera mostly positive in cluster; –/+, sera sometimes positive in cluster; blank, sera negative in cluster; NT, sera of cluster not tested

cluster, did not type for that HLA-D specificity and were omitted from further analysis (H. Grosse-Wilde et al., Definition of HLA-D with HTC, this volume). Such cells are indicated with their respective 9w numbers in Fig. 1. Whenever serological heterogeneity was observed within the HLA-D HTC groups, this is indicated in Table 3 and Fig. 1.

HLA-DR Typing of HTC

Reaction patterns of the serum clusters with the HTC clusters are shown in Fig. 1.

The following DR specificities were only represented by one HLA-D specificity: DR1-Dw1, DR3-Dw3, DRw11-Dw5, DRw9-DB5. Both Dw2 and Dw12 typed as DR2, whereas DB9 cells typed as DR2 short.

DR4 appeared heterogenous and could be subdivided into DR4.1, 4.2, and 4.3. DR4.1 was found on HTC Dw4, Dw14, and Dw15. DR4.2 was observed on Dw10 and Dw13. Only one Dw10 HTC, 9w1009, typed as DR4.3.

The DRw13 subtype of DRw6 was observed on both Dw18 and Dw19 (Dw6) HTC as well as on HTC 9w1802, the only difference being that "3 + 6"

Table 2. Clusters of Ninth Workshop DR sera (and *r* values) used in Fig. 1

DR1 (*r*>.7)	: 502, 511, 512, 505, 507, 509, 510, 514
DR2 (*r*>.7)	: 541, 542, 535, 545, 533, 534, 543
DR2 short	: 555
DR3 (*r*>.8)	: 557, 561, 565, 567, 568, 569, 570
DR3+w6 (*r*>.6)	: 678, 679, 680, 713, 714
DR4.1+4.2+4.3 (*r*>.7)	: 589, 595, 576, 581
DR4.1+4.2 (*r*>.8)	: 590, 592, 578, 587
DR4.1 (*r*>.5)	: 591, 594, 582
DRw11(5) (*r*>.6)	: 613, 596, 609, 611, 612, 610
DR5+w13 (*r*=.8)	: 681, 709
DRw14 (*r*=.4)	: 787, 781 (+weak DRw13)
DR7 (*r*>.8)	: 638, 639, 629, 630, 633, 636, 640, 642
DRw8 (*r*>.5)	: 619, 763, 621 (+DRw12)
DRw9 (*r*>.7)	: 644, 647, 650
DRw52 (*r*>.7)	: 683, 689, 692, 693, 694, 696, 697, 698, 699, 756, 757
DRw53 (*r*>.6)	: 734, 735, 743
DQw1 (*r*>.7)	: 652, 672; 670, 671 (+DR3, 4 and 7)
DQw1+DR2 (*r*>.8)	: 653, 654, 655, 661, 662, 664, 667, 668, 669, 674, 657, 701, 702, 703
DQw2 (*r*>.6)	: 726, 792, 775 (+DR5)
DQw3 (*r*>.7)	: 744, 746, 748, 745 (+DR4)
LB-E13	: 761 (+DR4)
TA10 (*r*>.5)	: 790, 607, 789 (+DR3)
TA10+DR5 (*r*>.6)	: 597, 598, 601, 603

Table 3. HLA-D clusters and the respective HTC numbers with which the serum patterns of Fig. 1 were obtained

HLA-D	HTC
Dw1	: 101, 102, 103, 104, 105.
Dw2	: 201, 202, 203, 204.
Dw3	: 301, 302, 303, 304, 305.
Dw4	: a-401, 402; b-403, 404.
Dw5	: a-501, 504, 505; b-9901
Dw6 – Dw18 (6A)	: 601, 602, 603, 604, 605
– Dw19 (6B)	: 606, 607, 608, 610, 611
Dw7 (7AB)	: 702
Dw8	: 801, 802, 807, 808
Dw8.2	: a-805; b-806, 1602
Dw9	: a-901, 902, 903, 904, 905, 1904; b-1902
Dw10	: a-1001, 1003, 1005; b-1002
Dw11 (Dw7B)	: a-1101, 1102, 1103, 1104; b-1105
Dw12	: 1201, 1202
Dw13 (DB3)	: a-1302; b-1303
Dw14 (LD40)	: 1402, 1403, 1406
Dw15 (DYT)	: 9902
Dw16 (DB8)	: 1701, 1702
Dw17 (Dw7A)	: 701, 704, 705, 1901
DB5	: DKB
DB6	: 1501, 1503
DB9	: 1801, 1803
D undefined	: 506; 609; 703; 803; 1004; 1301; 1401; 1405; 1502; 1504; 1802; 1903

sera reacted often weakly with Dw6 cells but very strongly with 9w1802.

DRw14, the other subtype of DRw6, was found on Dw9 and Dw16 HTC. One Dw9 HTC, 9w1902, typed as DR3, DRw14. Again, "3 + 6" sera showed different reactivity towards Dw9 and Dw16 HTC.

DR7 was present on all Dw7 cells, including Dw11 and Dw17 HTC. DRw8 was observed on Dw8 and Dw8.2 HTC.

The DRw12 (LB5 × 8) specificity, originally defined with HTC Herluf (9w1503), was also observed on 9w1501. Both cells were provisionally designated as DB6.

DRw52 (MT2) was present on all DR3-, w8-, w11-, w12-, w13-, and w14-positive HTC, whereas DRw53 (MT3) was found on all DR4-, 7-, and w9-positive HTC.

HLA-DQ (Previously MB, DC, LB-E) on HTC

DQw1 was present on DR1-Dw1, DR2-Dw2, DR2-Dw12, DRw13-Dw6 (Dw18, Dw19), and DRw14-Dw9 HTC. Within the DRw11-Dw5 cluster one HTC, 9w9901, was DQw1 positive. DQw1 was also present on two DRw8-Dw8.2 HTCs (9w806, 1602).

DQw2 was found on DR3-Dw3, DR7-Dw7 (Dw17), and one DR7-Dw11 HTC, 9w1105. Moreover, it was observed on the DR3, DRw14 heterozygous cell 9W1902.

DQw3 was present on DR2-DB9, all DR4-positive HTC (Dw15 not tested for DQw3), DRw11-Dw5 (except 9w9901), DRw12-DB6, DRw14-Dw16, all DR7-Dw11 HTC, and the DRw9-DB5 HTC. It was also observed on the DRw13 HTC 9w1802 and the DRw8-Dw8.2 HTC 9w805.

The specificity LB-E13 [4] is included in DQw3, but absent on DR7-Dw11 and DRw9-DB5 cells.

Another DQw3-related specificity is TA10 [5], which appears to be included in LB-E13. The distribution of TA10 seems heterogeneous in the DR4-positive HTC. Two DR4.1-Dw4 HTC (9w401, 402) and one DR4.2-Dw13 HTC (9w1302) were TA10 positive. All Dw10 and Dw14 HTC were TA10 negative.

Many DQ antisera appeared to contain anti-DR antibodies, which complicated the definition of DQ specificities.

As shown in Table 2, many DQw1 antisera probably also contained anti-DR2 antibodies, as they were reactive toward the DR2 short-DQw3-DB9 HTC.

Only three anti-DQw2 antisera did not react with the DR7-Dw11 and/or DRw9-DB5 HTC and thus did not contain additional DR7 and/or DRw9 activity. Neither did these sera contain extra DR3 activity (M. Oudshoorn et al., Segregation of DQ and DR: "Exceptions to the Rule," this volume).

The four DQw3 sera listed in Table 2 did not contain additional DR5 activity, since they did not react with the DRw11-DQw1 HTC 9w9901.

Both local and the 9w761 anti-LB-E13 sera probably contain extra DR4 activity, and are thus not informative for the typing of the Dw15 cell 9w9902. Many TA10 sera also contained additional DR5 antibodies which could be demonstrated by positive reactions with the 9w9901 HTC.

Summary

The relationship between D, DR and DQ is intriguing. The serological analysis of HTCs reveals the following:

1. All HTC express only one DR specificity, with the exception of the Dw9 cell 9w1902. Moreover, the majority of the HTC express only one DQ specificity, exceptions being cells 9w1902 and 9w1105 (Dw11). This suggests a strong association of HLA-D determinants with DR and probably DQ determinants.
2. Different HLA-D specificities can express the same HLA-DR and DQ determinants without further serological distinction as yet (for example Dw2 and Dw12).
3. Further serological subdivision of DR groups, in combination with different DQ (sub)groups, can be associated with different HLA-D specificities: this is demonstrated with DR4. Dw4, Dw14 and Dw15 are DR4.1, and Dw10 HTCs are DR4.3 (and 4.2), whereas Dw13 HTCs are DR4.2. Moreover, Dw4 and Dw13 can be associated with TA10, whereas Dw15 (DYT) cells are probably DQw3-TA10 negative [6].
4. HTC, identical for DR, but expressing different DQ specificities, appeared to cluster into the same HLA-D specificities.

In conclusion, expression of the same DR or DQ antigenic determinant does not result in a prediction of the HLA-D determinant in the HTC. The HLA-D determinants are more strongly associated with DR than with DQ antigenic determinants.

References

1. Thorsby E, Piazza A (1975) Joint report from the sixth International Histocompatibility Workshop Conference. II Typing for HLA-D (LD-1 or MLC) determinants. In: Kissmeyer-Nielsen F (ed) Histocompatibility testing 1975. Munksgaard, Copenhagen, pp 414–458
2. van Rood JJ, van Leeuwen A, Keuning JJ, Blussé van Oud Alblas A (1975) The serological recognition of the MLC determinants using a modified cytotoxicity technique. Tissue Antigens 5:73–79
3. Terasaki PI, Park MS, Bernoco D, Opelz G, Mickey MR (1980) Overview of the 1980 International Histocompatibility Workshop. In: Terasaki PI (ed) Histocompatibility testing 1980. UCLA, Los Angeles, pp 1–17
4. Schreuder GMT, van Leeuwen A, Termijtelen A, Parlevliet J, D'Amaro J, van Rood JJ (1983) Cell membrane polymorphisms in the HLA-D/DR region. Hum Immunol 4:301–312
5. Maeda H (1984) Mouse monoclonal antibody detects a new polymorphic Ia determinant other than HLA-DR antigen: a possible allele of DC-1. Tissue Antigens 23:163–170
6. Kasahara M, Takenouchi T, Ogasawara K, et al (1983) Serologic dissection of HLA-D specificities by the use of monoclonal antibodies. Immunogenetics 17:485–495

Definition of HLA-D with HTC*

H. Grosse-Wilde[1], I. Doxiadis[1], and H. Brandt[2]

1 Department of Immunogenetics, University Hospital of Essen, 4300 Essen, Federal Republic of Germany
2 Department of Medical Computer Science and Biomathematics, University Hospital of Essen, 4300 Essen, Federal Republic of Germany

Introduction

This report summarizes the fourth collaborative effort in conjunction with the International Histocompatibility Workshop to use a common scheme to type for HLA-D determinants with homozygous typing cells (HTC) in the mixed lymphocyte culture (MLC) test. This method, now more than ten years old, was originally proposed by us [1] and subsequently incorporated into the Sixth, Seventh, and Eighth International Histocompatibility Workshops [2, 3, 4]. The results of these three Workshops can be summarized as follows:

1. At least 12 distinct HLA-D determinants (Dw1 through w12) can be recognized in the population.
2. Some of these determinants are heterogeneous or cross-reactive.
3. There is an HLA-D "blank" gene frequency of approximately 30% as evidence for additional, still unrecognized determinants.
4. The HLA-D determinants are in linkage disequilibrium, especially with HLA-DR and HLA-B alleles.
5. As for the serologically defined HLA antigens, the gene frequencies of the individual HLA-D determinants vary between different ethnic groups.

In addition, the following problems, partly inherent to cellular typing, were encountered:

1. The assignment of an HLA-D specifity to a given responder is based on non-/low reactivity (positive typing response) towards a given set of HTC; such nonreactivity may result from technical difficulties arising from such problems as handling of frozen cells, which varies from laboratory to laboratory.
2. Although the MLC test used for HLA-D typing is miniaturized, the number of typing cells needed remains an obstacle to testing a sufficient number of individuals, for example when rare HLA-D specificities or splits have to be defined.
3. In contrast to serological HLA reagents, which are able to recognize single epitopes, the HTC stimulates as a complete cell expressing both (presumably identical) HLA-D haplotypes.
4. The individual HTC typing response results from all the (in)compatibilities recognized by the responding cell on the HTC in reference to its own HLA-D determinants.

In an attempt to clarify some of the above-mentioned points, the participating laboratories agreed upon a division of the cellular part (HTC) into two consecutive levels. The first level, performed by a selected number of laboratories, focused on a better definition of typing reagents for HLA-D determinants presumed to be heterogeneous (Dw1, Dw6, Dw7 + w11, Dw8) and on the definition of HTC clusters defining new determinants. The second level involved 30 participating laboratories performing family segregation studies with the final Workshop set of HTC. The selection of these HTC was based on the first-level results as well as on data from previous Workshops and published data [5].

First Level Studies

The call for HTC resulted in a total offer of 259 individual HTC, from which 175 were finally tested in the first level. The participating laboratories had to submit two identical sets of their offered HTC plus cells heterozygous for the respective specificity.

Figure 1 identifies the laboratories which performed the actual typing experiments and the HLA-D specificities studied. These reference typings comprised an HTC checkerboard and typing of a selected panel including the heterozygotes of the submitting laboratories. The inclusion of defined heterozygotes for a given HTC (e.g., family members of the reference donor) was done to facilitate the identification of HTC clusters defining possible splits, rare specificities, or new specificities among the group of HTC submitted as blank.

* This work was supported by the Deutsche Forschungsgemeinschaft (AL-92/13-1) and by SFB102 TPB4

Histocompatibility Testing 1984
Edited by E. D. Albert et al.

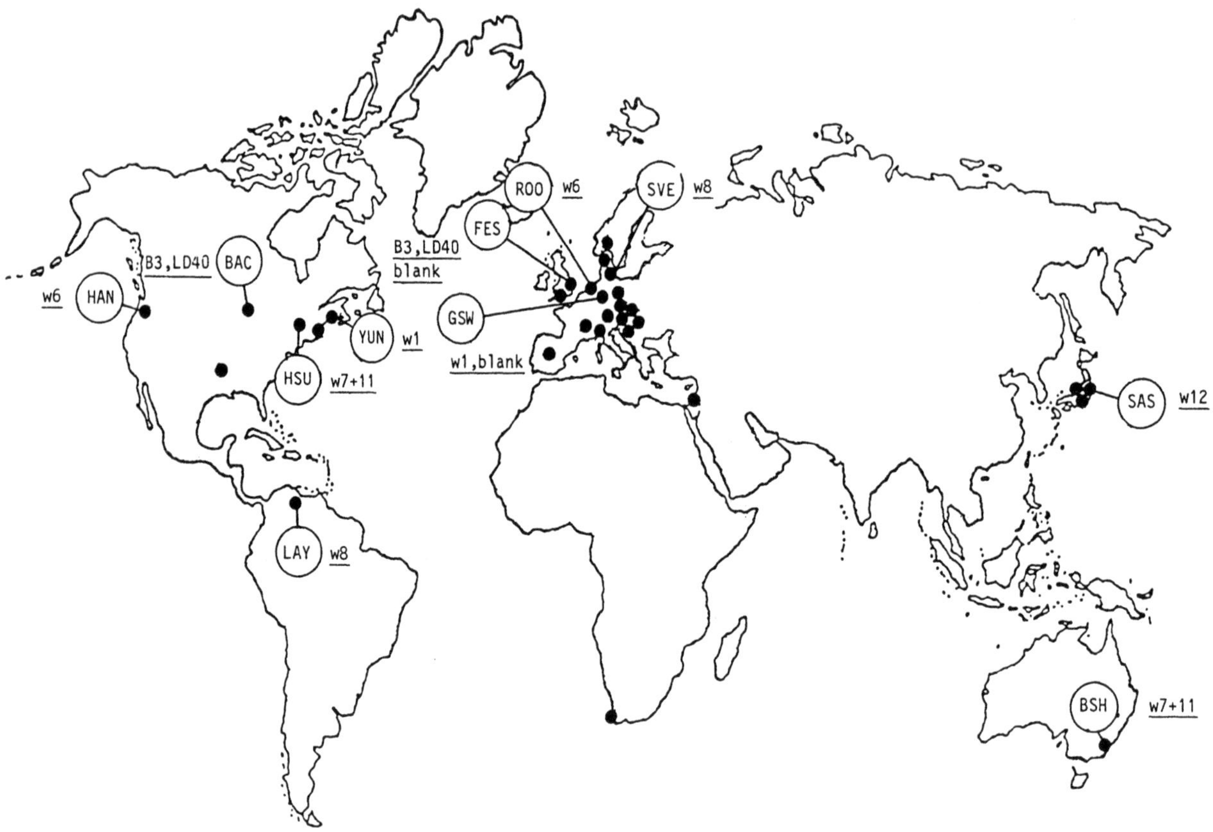

Fig. 1. Distribution of the participating laboratories in the first level

Table 1. Summary of final set of Workshop HTC

					0611														
					0610														
					0609														
					0608		0808												
					0607		0807												
				0506	0606		0806						1406						
0105		0305		0505	0605	0705	0805	0905	1005	1105			1405						
0104	0204	0304	0404	0504	0604	0704	0804	0904	1004	1104			1404	1504				1904	
0103	0203	0303	0403	0503	0603	0703	0803	0903	1003	1103		1303	1403	1503			1803	1903	
0102	0202	0302	0402	0502	0602	0702	0802	0902	1002	1102	1202	1302	1402	1502	1602	1702	1802	1902	9902
0101	0201	0301	0401	0501	0601	0701	0801	0901	1001	1101	1201	1301	1401	1501	1601	1701	1801	1901	9901
w1	w2	w3	w4	w5	w6	w7	w8	w9	w10	w11	w12	w13	w14	B6	B7	w16	B9	B10	blank
					6.1		8.1					(B3)	LD40			(B8)			
					6.2		8.2												
					6.3		8.3												

The data from this first level study were analyzed locally (see accompanying reports) and centrally. For the central analysis the median cpm values of each experiment were submitted to Essen together with the relevant information on the actual MLC matrix size, the individual responses, and HTC studied. The data were fed into a computer (IBM 4341) and calculated to stabilized relative responses (SRR; for details see data analysis section). An overall analysis was then performed by calculating the multiple correlation coefficients between the SRR values obtained and subsequently clustered according to a statistical analysis system (SAS) cluster analysis program. The unbiased clusters defined by this program are graphically depicted in Fig. 2 as a dendrogram where the allocation of the individual HTC either to established or tentatively labeled (DB3, LD40, DB6 through DB10) determinants is given. Based on this analysis, on previous Workshop data, including recently published

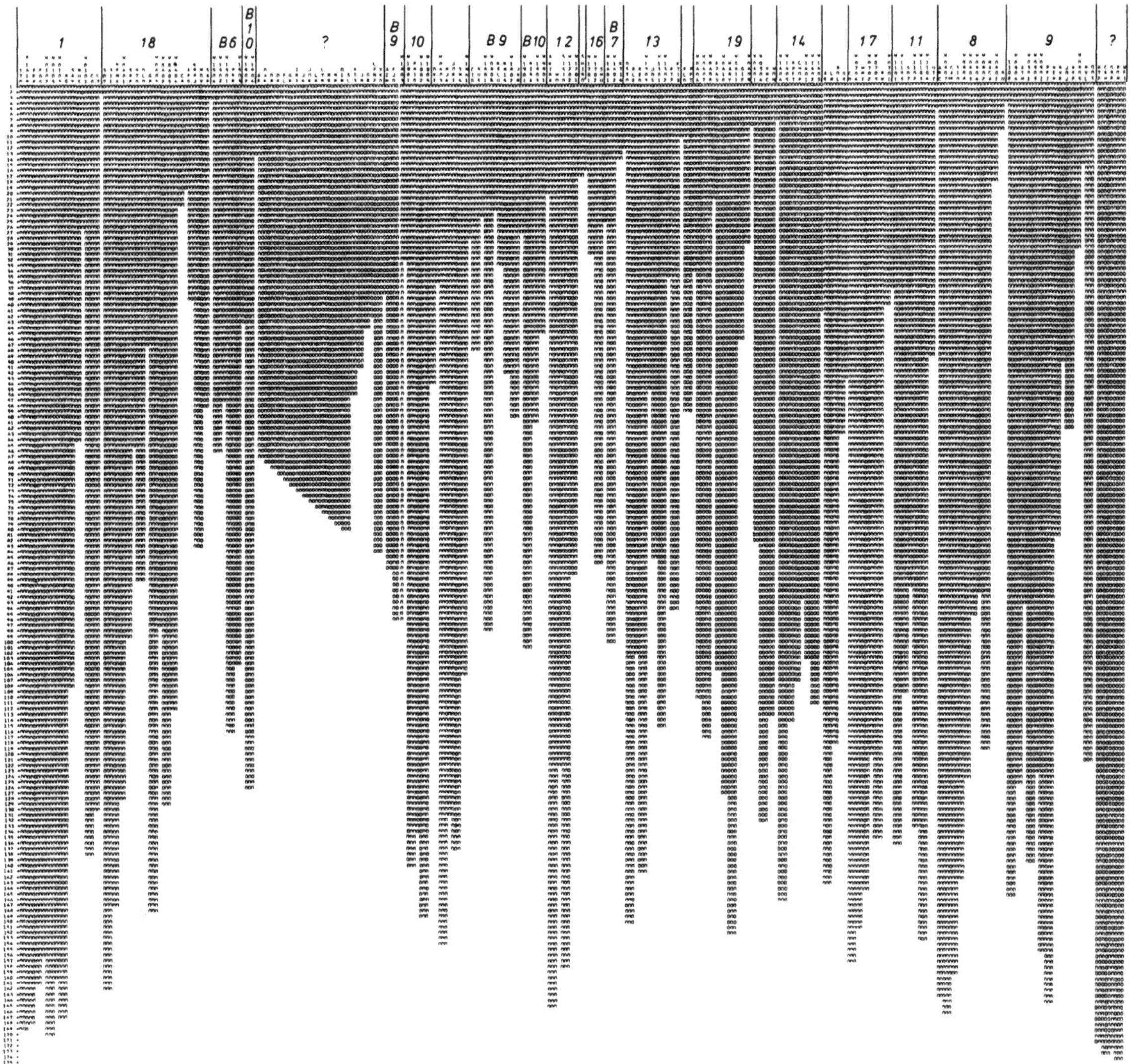

Fig. 2. Allocation of the individual HTC to established (*Dw*) or tentatively labeled (*B*) HLA-D specificities

data [5], and on the actual availability of a sufficient amount of cells (200 ampoules, 5×10^6 cells per ampoule), 91 HTC were selected as the final set for the second level (Table 1).

Second Level Studies

Experimental Design

With regard to the MLC technique to be used by the laboratories, the standards set by the organizers of the cellular part of the Eighth International Histocompatibility Workshop 1980 were followed [4]. A total number of 200 ampoules of each HTC had to be submitted centrally to Essen where the individual Workshop sets were compiled and then returned to the participating laboratories. It was decided not to divide the 30 participating laboratories into two hemispheres (Fig. 3), as was done in the previous Workshop, but to supply each participant with the same set of typing reagents. Only for those HTC where not enough ampoules were submitted did only some of the laboratories receive the reagents. Table 2 summarizes the origin of the Workshop HTC, the local identification, and the number of ampoules received per laboratory. The design of the studies to be performed by each laboratory was to type, using the Workshop HTC set and on two different occasions, at least four complete families (parents plus four or more offspring) as well as the own HTC submitted. For the splits of Dw6 and Dw7, as well as for the tentatively labeled new determinants, those labs who had submitted HTC for these determinants should include one family positive for the respective determinant. All individuals tested should be typed in addition with the complete Workshop sera set and, where possible, for other HLA-linked markers.

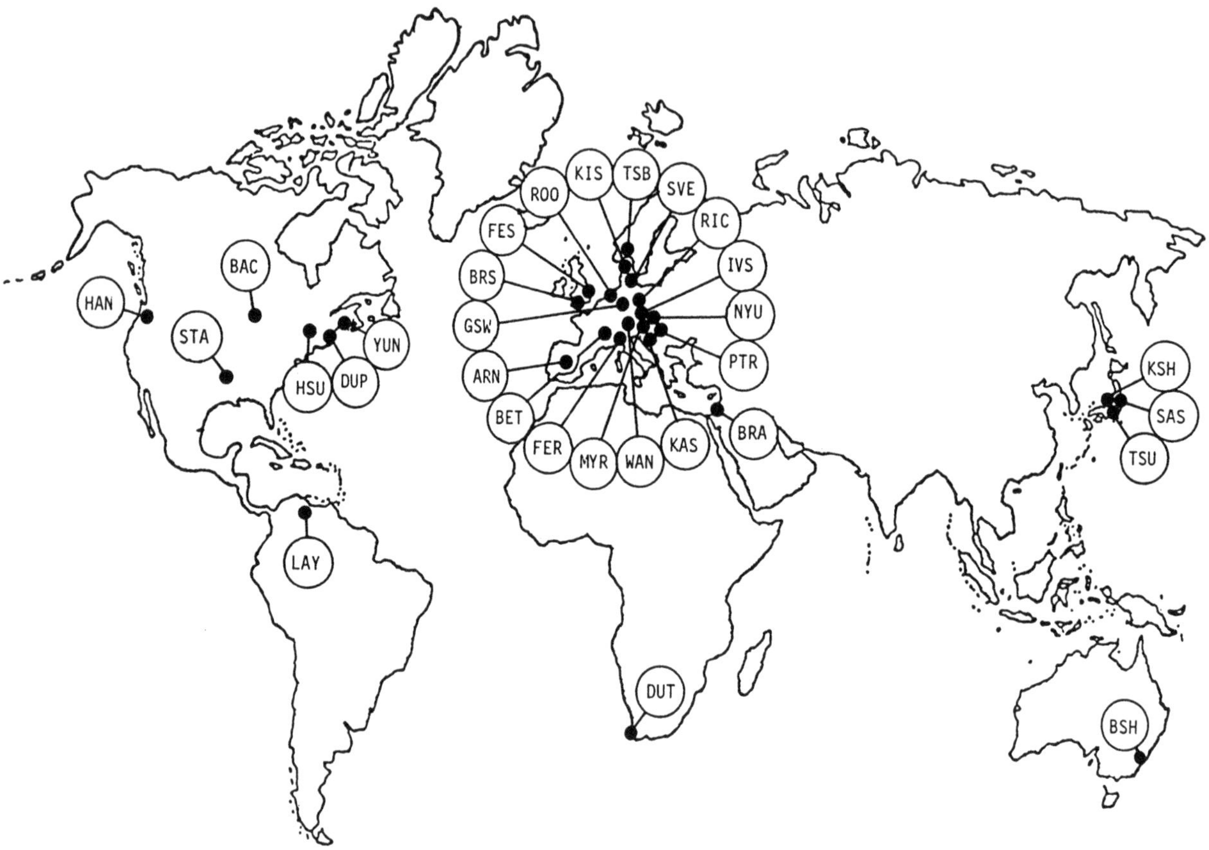

Fig. 3. Distribution of the 30 participating laboratories in the Cellular Part (HTC)

Central Data Analysis

The data submission format was identical to that used in the Eighth Workshop [4]. The experimental results (median cpm values) were submitted through the regional center to Düsseldorf and there checked for formal errors. The data were then transferred to Essen, where the final analysis of the cellular part (HTC) was performed. Printouts from each experiment were generated in Essen and returned to each participating laboratory for corrections (Fig. 4). It should be mentioned that no laboratory, including our own, had no corrections. The corrected data were computed and calculated to SRR values. The individual steps in this computation are depicted in Fig. 5. High values within each row (responder) or each column (stimulator) were distinguished from low values using the Wilcoxon ranking test as previously described [6]. The mean of the high value group was set to 100% reference for calculating the individual RR and SRR values. Where the Wilcoxon ranking test failed to identify the high value group, the mean of all values in each row or column was taken as 100% reference.
Prior to further data processing, the distribution of all SRR values in each experiment was compared to the summarized distribution derived from all experiments. Experiments showing obvious deviations in the two distributions were excluded from contributing to the generation of SRR histograms per each HTC (Fig. 6).
To optimize the HTC typing it was intended to assign individual cut-off points to each HTC. Two examples of successful assignments are shown in Fig. 7a, b. The identification of bimodality as the basis for assigning individual cut-off points was done by a nonlinear regression program (SAS). This program identifies and plots the distribution of the SRR values within each mode. A scoring system was applied based on the following cut-off points:

- The peak of the high value mode was taken as the cut-off between scores 1 and 2.
- The end point of the low value mode was taken as the cut-off between scores 2 and 4.
- The intersection of both modes was taken as the cut-off between scores 6 and 8.
- The midpoint between cut-off points 2/4 and 6/8 was taken as the cut-off point between positive and negative typing responses, i.e., between scores 4 and 6. In Fig. 7a this cut-off point is 49% SRR, in Fig. 7b 43% SRR.

Table 2. Workshop number, specificity, local identification, and number of ampoules sent by organizers

WSNO	SPEC	LOCID	LABID	ARN	BSH	BET	BRA	BUC	DUP	FER	FES	MYR	GSW	HAN	HSU	KIS	KSH	LAY	ONO	BAC	SAS	STA	SVE	ROO	TSB	DUT	TSU	WAN	YUN	BRS	WER	RIC	IVS	KAS
9W0101	DW1	AL	BSH	6	6	6	6	4	6	6	6	5	6	6	6	6	6	6	6	6	6	6	6	6	6	6	6	6	6	6	6	6	4	5
9W0102	DW1	HEN	GSW	6	6	6	6	4	6	6	6	5	6	6	6	6	6	6	6	6	6	6	6	6	6	6	6	6	6	6	6	6	4	5
9W0103	DW1	MAM	BET	6	6	6	6	4	6	6	6	5	6	6	6	6	6	6	6	6	6	6	6	6	6	6	6	6	6	6	6	6	4	5
9W0104	DW1	MDE	STA	6	6	6	6	4	6	6	6	5	6	6	6	6	6	6	6	6	6	6	6	6	6	6	6	6	6	6	6	6	4	5
9W0105	DW1	WOE	GSW	6	6	6	6	4	6	6	6	5	6	6	6	6	6	6	6	6	6	6	6	6	6	6	6	6	6	6	6	6	4	5
9W0201	DW2	CI	BUC	6	6	6	6	4	6	6	6	5	6	6	6	6	6	6	6	6	6	6	6	6	6	6	6	6	6	6	6	6	4	5
9W0202	DW2	HOF	GSW	6	6	6	6	4	6	6	6	5	6	6	6	6	6	6	6	6	6	6	6	6	6	6	6	6	6	6	6	6	4	5
9W0203	DW2	KER	MYR	6	6	6	6	4	6	6	6	5	6	6	6	6	6	6	6	6	6	6	6	6	6	6	6	6	6	6	6	6	4	5
9W0204	DW2	PIL	WAN	6	6	6	6	4	6	6	6	5	6	6	6	6	6	6	6	6	6	6	6	6	6	6	6	6	6	6	6	6	4	5
9W0301	DW3	AVL	ROO	6	6	6	6	4	6	6	6	5	6	6	6	6	6	6	6	6	6	6	6	6	6	6	6	6	6	6	6	6	4	5
9W0302	DW3	CHR	GSW	6	6	6	6	4	6	6	6	5	6	6	6	6	6	6	6	6	6	6	6	6	6	6	6	6	6	6	6	6	4	5
9W0303	DW3	COX	DUT	6	6	6	6	4	6	6	6	5	6	6	6	6	6	6	6	6	6	6	6	6	6	6	6	6	6	6	6	6	4	5
9W0304	DW3	GSM	STA	6	6	6	6	4	6	6	6	5	6	6	6	6	6	6	6	6	6	6	6	6	6	6	6	6	6	6	6	6	4	5
9W0305	DW3	LHM	HAN	6	6	6	6	4	6	6	6	5	6	6	6	6	6	6	6	6	6	6	6	6	6	6	6	6	6	6	6	6	4	5
9W0401	DW4	HBH	BSH	6	6	6	6	4	6	6	6	5	6	6	6	6	6	6	6	6	6	6	6	6	6	6	6	6	6	6	6	6	4	5
9W0402	DW4	HIM	MYR	6	6	6	6	4	6	6	6	5	6	6	6	6	6	6	6	6	6	6	6	6	6	6	6	6	6	6	6	6	4	5
9W0403	DW4	JAH	HAN	6	6	6	6	4	6	6	6	5	6	6	6	6	6	6	6	6	6	6	6	6	6	6	6	6	6	6	6	6	4	5
9W0404	DW4	SUD	GSW	6	6	6	6	4	6	6	6	5	6	6	6	6	6	6	6	6	6	6	6	6	6	6	6	6	6	6	6	6	4	5
9W0501	DW5	BAU	MYR	6	6	6	6	4	6	6	6	5	6	6	6	6	6	6	6	6	6	6	6	6	6	6	6	6	6	6	6	6	4	5
9W0502	DW5	BRI	FER	6	6	6	6	4	6	6	6	5	6	6	6	6	6	6	6	6	6	6	6	6	6	6	6	6	6	6	6	6	4	5
9W0503	DW5	DHI*	FES	3	3	3	3	2	3	3	3	3	3	3	3	3	3	3	3	3	3	3	3	3	3	3	3	3	3	3	.	.	2	2
9W0504	DW5	HVB	BSH	6	6	6	6	4	6	6	6	5	6	6	6	6	6	6	6	6	6	6	6	6	6	6	6	6	6	6	6	6	4	5
9W0505	DW5	KRO	WER	6	6	6	6	4	6	6	6	5	6	6	6	6	6	6	6	6	6	6	6	6	6	6	6	6	6	6	6	6	4	5
9W0506	DW5	SM	BUC	6	6	6	6	4	6	6	6	5	6	6	6	6	6	6	6	6	6	6	6	6	6	6	6	6	6	6	6	6	4	5
9W0601	DW6.1	HBS	BET	6	6	6	6	4	6	6	6	5	6	6	6	6	6	6	6	6	6	6	6	6	6	6	6	6	6	6	6	6	4	5
9W0602	DW6.1	HHK	ROO	6	6	6	6	4	6	6	6	5	6	6	6	6	6	6	6	6	6	6	6	6	6	6	6	6	6	6	6	6	4	5
9W0603	DW6.1	JTED	STA	6	6	6	6	4	6	6	6	5	6	6	6	6	6	6	6	6	6	6	6	6	6	6	6	6	6	6	6	6	4	5
9W0604	DW6.1	SCL	GSW	6	6	6	6	4	6	6	6	5	6	6	6	6	6	6	6	6	6	6	6	6	6	6	6	6	6	6	6	6	4	5
9W0605	DW6.1	WDV	ROO	6	6	6	6	4	6	6	6	5	6	6	6	6	6	6	6	6	6	6	6	6	6	6	6	6	6	6	6	6	4	5
9W0606	DW6.2	EMJ	HAN	6	6	6	6	4	6	6	6	5	6	6	6	6	6	6	6	6	6	6	6	6	6	6	6	6	6	6	6	6	4	5
9W0607	DW6.2	KRA	GSW	6	6	6	6	4	6	6	6	5	6	6	6	6	6	6	6	6	6	6	6	6	6	6	6	6	6	6	6	6	4	5
9W0608	DW6.2	SLE	HAN	6	6	6	6	4	6	6	6	5	6	6	6	6	6	6	6	6	6	6	6	6	6	6	6	6	6	6	6	6	4	5
9W0609	DW6.3	KSH*	FES	4	4	4	4	3	4	4	4	3	4	4	4	4	4	4	4	4	4	4	4	4	4	4	4	4	4	4	4	.	3	3
9W0610	DW6.3	KT11	KSH	5	5	5	5	3	5	5	5	5	5	5	5	5	5	5	5	5	5	5	5	5	5	5	5	5	5	5	5	5	3	4
9W0611	DW6.3	STEPH	HSU	5	5	5	5	3	5	5	5	5	5	5	5	5	5	5	5	5	5	5	5	5	5	5	5	5	5	5	5	5	3	5
9W0701	DW7	BOR	GSW	6	6	6	6	4	6	6	6	5	6	6	6	6	6	6	6	6	6	6	6	6	6	6	6	6	6	6	6	6	4	5
9W0702	DW7	BUP	HSU	6	6	6	6	4	6	6	6	5	6	6	6	6	6	6	6	6	6	6	6	6	6	6	6	6	6	6	6	6	4	5
9W0703	DW7	MMF	YUN	6	6	6	6	4	6	6	6	5	6	6	6	6	6	6	6	6	6	6	6	6	6	6	6	6	6	6	6	6	4	5
9W0704	DW7	PIT	DUT	6	6	6	6	4	6	6	6	5	6	6	6	6	6	6	6	6	6	6	6	6	6	6	6	6	6	6	6	6	4	5
9W0705	DW7	WET	WER	6	6	6	6	4	6	6	6	5	6	6	6	6	6	6	6	6	6	6	6	6	6	6	6	6	6	6	6	6	4	5
9W0801	DW8.1	BTB/MB	TSB	.	3	3	3	2	3	3	3	2	3	3	3	3	3	3	3	3	3	3	3	3	3	3	3	3	3	.	.	.	.	2
9W0802	DW8.1	MMR	ROO	5	5	5	5	3	5	5	5	5	5	5	5	5	5	5	5	5	5	5	5	5	5	5	5	5	5	5	5	5	3	4
9W0803	DW8.1	OLG	LAY	6	6	6	6	4	6	6	6	5	6	6	6	6	6	6	6	6	6	6	6	6	6	6	6	6	6	6	6	6	4	5
9W0804	DW8.1	SEC	LAY	6	6	6	6	4	6	6	6	5	6	6	6	6	6	6	6	6	6	6	6	6	6	6	6	6	6	6	6	6	4	5
9W0805	DW8.2	LUY	ROO	3	3	3	3	2	3	3	3	3	3	3	3	3	3	3	3	3	3	3	3	3	3	3	3	3	3	3	3	3	2	3
9W0806	DW8.2	TAB	HAN	4	4	4	4	3	4	4	4	3	4	4	4	4	4	4	4	4	4	4	4	4	4	4	4	4	4	4	4	4	3	3
9W0807	DW8.3	BAE	GSW	5	6	6	6	4	6	6	6	5	6	6	6	6	6	6	6	6	6	6	6	6	6	6	6	6	6	6	6	6	4	5
9W0808	DW8.3	MAD	SVE	.	.	.	.	.	.	.	3	3	3	3	3	3	3	3	3	3	3	3	3	3	3	.	.	3	.	.	.	.	.	.
9W0901	DW9	BRU	WAN	6	6	6	6	4	6	6	6	5	6	6	6	6	6	6	6	6	6	6	6	6	6	6	6	6	6	6	6	6	4	5
9W0902	DW9	CHN	BET	6	6	6	6	4	6	6	6	5	6	6	6	6	6	6	6	6	6	6	6	6	6	6	6	6	6	6	6	6	4	5
9W0903	DW9	GECL	BET	6	6	6	6	4	6	6	6	5	6	6	6	6	6	6	6	6	6	6	6	6	6	6	6	6	6	6	6	6	4	5
9W0904	DW9	GEV*	FES	3	3	3	3	2	3	3	3	3	3	3	3	3	3	3	3	3	3	3	3	3	3	3	3	3	3	3	3	3	2	3
9W0905	DW9	OH/EK	TSB	3	.	3	3	2	3	3	3	2	3	3	3	3	3	3	3	3	3	3	3	3	3	3	3	3	3	.	.	.	.	2
9W1001	DW10	AL10	BAC	6	6	6	6	4	6	6	6	5	6	6	6	6	6	6	6	6	6	6	6	6	6	6	6	6	6	6	6	6	4	5
9W1002	DW10	LED10	BAC	6	6	6	6	4	6	6	6	5	6	6	6	6	6	6	6	6	6	6	6	6	6	6	6	6	6	6	6	6	4	5
9W1003	DW10	MAY	BRA	6	6	6	6	4	6	6	6	5	6	6	6	6	6	6	6	6	6	6	6	6	6	6	6	6	6	6	6	6	4	5
9W1004	DW10	RLO	STA	6	6	6	6	4	6	6	6	5	6	6	6	6	6	6	6	6	6	6	6	6	6	6	6	6	6	6	6	6	4	5
9W1005	DW10	TS10	BAC	6	6	6	6	4	6	6	6	5	6	6	6	6	6	6	6	6	6	6	6	6	6	6	6	6	6	6	6	6	4	5
9W1101	DW11	BEI	HSU	6	6	6	6	4	6	6	6	5	6	6	6	6	6	6	6	6	6	6	6	6	6	6	6	6	6	6	6	6	4	5
9W1102	DW11	GRO	GSW	6	6	6	6	4	6	6	6	5	6	6	6	6	6	6	6	6	6	6	6	6	6	6	6	6	6	6	6	6	4	5
9W1103	DW11	KIA	HSU	6	6	6	6	4	6	6	6	5	6	6	6	6	6	6	6	6	6	6	6	6	6	6	6	6	6	6	6	6	4	5
9W1104	DW11	KIJ	HSU	6	6	6	6	4	6	6	6	5	6	6	6	6	6	6	6	6	6	6	6	6	6	6	6	6	6	6	6	6	4	5
9W1105	DW11	SM11	YUN	6	6	6	6	4	6	6	6	5	6	6	6	6	6	6	6	6	6	6	6	6	6	6	6	6	6	6	6	6	4	5
9W1201	DW12	BGE	BRA	6	6	6	6	4	6	6	6	5	6	6	6	6	6	6	6	6	6	6	6	6	6	6	6	6	6	6	6	6	4	5
9W1202	DW12	TOK	SAS	6	6	6	6	4	6	6	6	5	6	6	6	6	6	6	6	6	6	6	6	6	6	6	6	6	6	6	6	6	4	5
9W1301	DB3	JHA*	FES	3	3	3	3	2	3	3	3	2	3	3	3	3	3	3	3	3	3	3	3	3	3	3	.	3	3	.	.	.	.	2
9W1302	DB3	PEA	GSW	6	6	6	6	4	6	6	6	5	6	6	6	6	6	6	6	6	6	6	6	6	6	6	6	6	6	6	6	6	4	5
9W1303	DB3	SSTO	HSU	6	6	6	6	4	6	6	6	5	6	6	6	6	6	6	6	6	6	6	6	6	6	6	6	6	6	6	6	6	4	5
9W1401	LD40	BIN40	BAC	6	6	6	6	4	6	6	6	5	6	6	6	6	6	6	6	6	6	6	6	6	6	6	6	6	6	6	6	6	4	5
9W1402	LD40	KY	BSH	.	3	3	.	.	.	3	3	.	3	3	3	.	.	3	.	3	3	.	3	3	3	.	.	3	.	.	.	.	.	.
9W1403	LD40	LS40	BAC	6	6	6	6	4	6	6	6	5	6	6	6	6	6	6	6	6	6	6	6	6	6	6	6	6	6	6	6	6	4	5
9W1404	LD40	MT	BSH	3	3	3	3	2	3	3	3	3	3	3	3	3	3	3	3	3	3	3	3	3	3	3	3	3	3	3	3	3	2	3
9W1405	LD40	PEM	BET	6	6	6	6	4	6	6	6	5	6	6	6	6	6	6	6	6	6	6	6	6	6	6	6	6	6	6	6	6	4	5
9W1406	LD40	THO-070	HAN	6	6	6	6	4	6	6	6	5	6	6	6	6	6	6	6	6	6	6	6	6	6	6	6	6	6	6	6	6	4	5
9W1501	DB6	BM16	FER	6	6	6	6	4	6	6	6	5	6	6	6	6	6	6	6	6	6	6	6	6	6	6	6	6	6	6	6	6	4	5
9W1502	DB6	BM24	FER	6	6	6	6	4	6	6	6	5	6	6	6	6	6	6	6	6	6	6	6	6	6	6	6	6	6	6	6	6	4	5
9W1503	DB6	HERLUF	SVE	.	.	3	.	.	.	3	3	.	3	3	3	3	.	3	3	.	3	.	3	3	3	.	.	.	3	.	.	.	.	.
9W1504	DB6	HRL-2171	FAU	6	6	6	6	4	6	6	6	5	6	6	6	6	6	6	6	6	6	6	6	6	6	6	6	6	6	6	6	6	4	5
9W1601	DB7	HI-2	FUK	4	4	4	4	2	4	4	4	3	4	4	4	4	4	4	4	4	4	4	4	4	4	4	4	4	.	.	.	.	.	3
9W1602	DB7	SHI	SAS	6	6	6	6	4	6	6	6	5	6	6	6	6	6	6	6	6	6	6	6	6	6	6	6	6	6	6	6	6	4	5
9W1701	DB8	AMA	LAY	6	6	6	6	4	6	6	6	5	6	6	6	6	6	6	6	6	6	6	6	6	6	6	6	6	6	6	6	6	4	5
9W1702	DB8	CRI	LAY	6	6	6	6	4	6	6	6	5	6	6	6	6	6	6	6	6	6	6	6	6	6	6	6	6	6	6	6	6	4	5
9W1801	DB9	BAS	LAY	6	6	6	6	4	6	6	6	5	6	6	6	6	6	6	6	6	6	6	6	6	6	6	6	6	6	6	6	6	4	5
9W1802	DB9	HAG	WER	6	6	6	6	4	6	6	6	5	6	6	6	6	6	6	6	6	6	6	6	6	6	6	6	6	6	6	6	6	4	5
9W1803	DB9	REM	LAY	6	6	6	6	4	6	6	6	5	6	6	6	6	6	6	6	6	6	6	6	6	6	6	6	6	6	6	6	6	4	5
9W1901	DB10	BH-13	YUN	6	6	6	6	4	6	6	6	5	6	6	6	6	6	6	6	6	6	6	6	6	6	6	6	6	6	6	6	6	4	5
9W1902	DB10	DJ	ONO	5	5	5	5	4	5	5	5	4	5	5	5	5	5	5	5	5	5	5	5	5	5	5	5	5	5	5	5	5	3	4
9W1903	DB10	LBU*	FES	.	3	3	.	.	3	3	3	.	3	3	3	3	3	3	.	3	3	3	.	3	3	.	3	3	3	.	.	.	3	.
9W1904	DB10	SI	ONO	5	5	5	5	3	5	5	5	5	5	5	5	5	5	5	5	5	5	5	5	5	5	5	5	5	5	5	5	5	3	5
9W9901	DBL	FPA*	FES	3	3	3	3	2	3	3	3	3	3	3	3	3	3	3	3	3	3	3	3	3	3	3	3	3	3	3	3	3	2	3
9W9902	DBL	HAS-15	BAC	6	6	6	6	4	6	6	6	5	6	6	6	6	6	6	6	6	6	6	6	6	6	6	6	6	6	6	6	6	4	5

DB3 = Dw13, LD40 = Dw14

The data from only 30 HTC allowed an unambiguous assignment; that from the remaining HTC precluded such an assignment (example in 7c). In those cases an arbitrary assignment was made based on the mean of the SRR values estalished as cut-off points in the 30 HTC (Table 3).

The next step in the data analysis involved the assignment of both an HLA-D specificity to each HTC and an HLA-D determinant to each individual tested (Fig. 8). For the former, multiple correlation coefficients between the SRR values obtained from each HTC were calculated, clustered in an unbiased manner, and plotted in a dendrogram (Fig. 9) as described above for the first level. The order of HTC within each cluster reflects the degree of similarity in their typing patterns; likewise, the order of the clusters reflects the degree of similarity in relation to each other. For example, the Dw1 cluster to the left is most similar to its neighboring Dw3 cluster but least similar to the Dw7 cluster, which in turn is further divided into two subgroups (splits) Dw17 and Dw11. A further example of a subgroup is found in the neighbouring cluster for Dw6, which can be divided into Dw18 and Dw19.

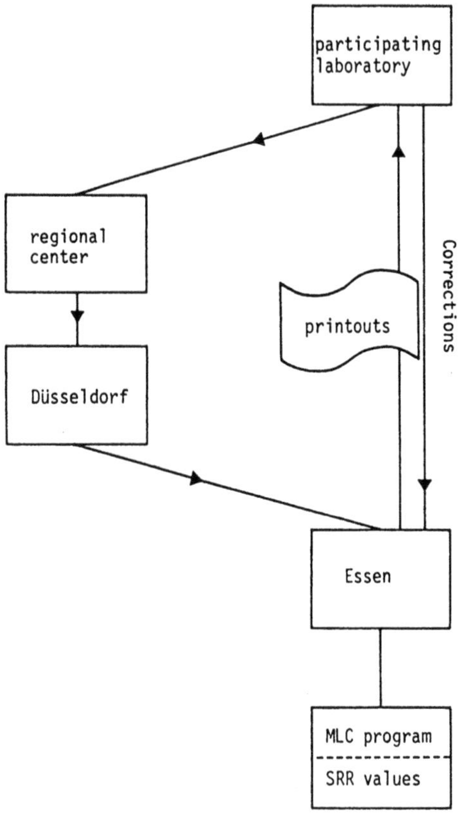

Fig. 4. Central data analysis: data flow

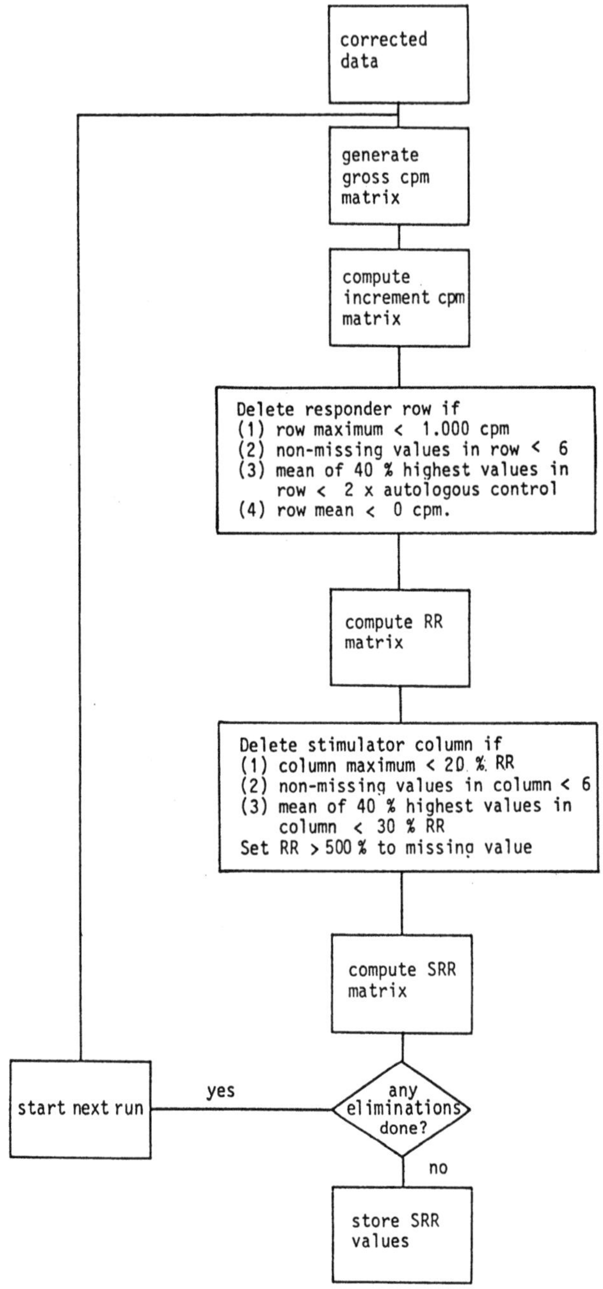

Fig. 5. Central data analysis: data processing I

Fig. 6. Example of an exclusion of an individual experiment. This experiment was excluded from further analysis because the experimental SRR distribution (---) did not match the reference SRR distribution (—)

▼

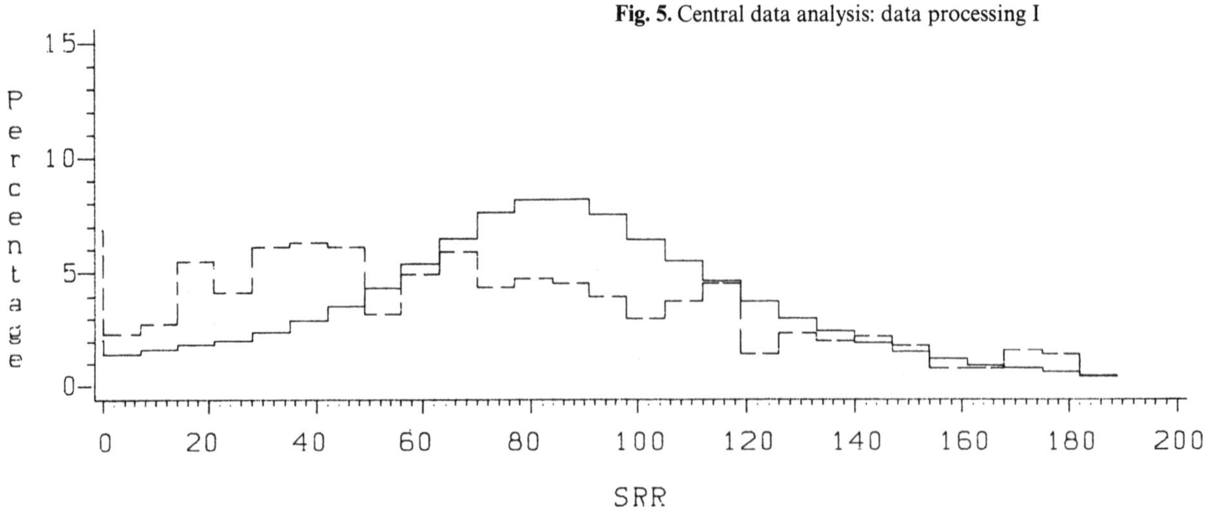

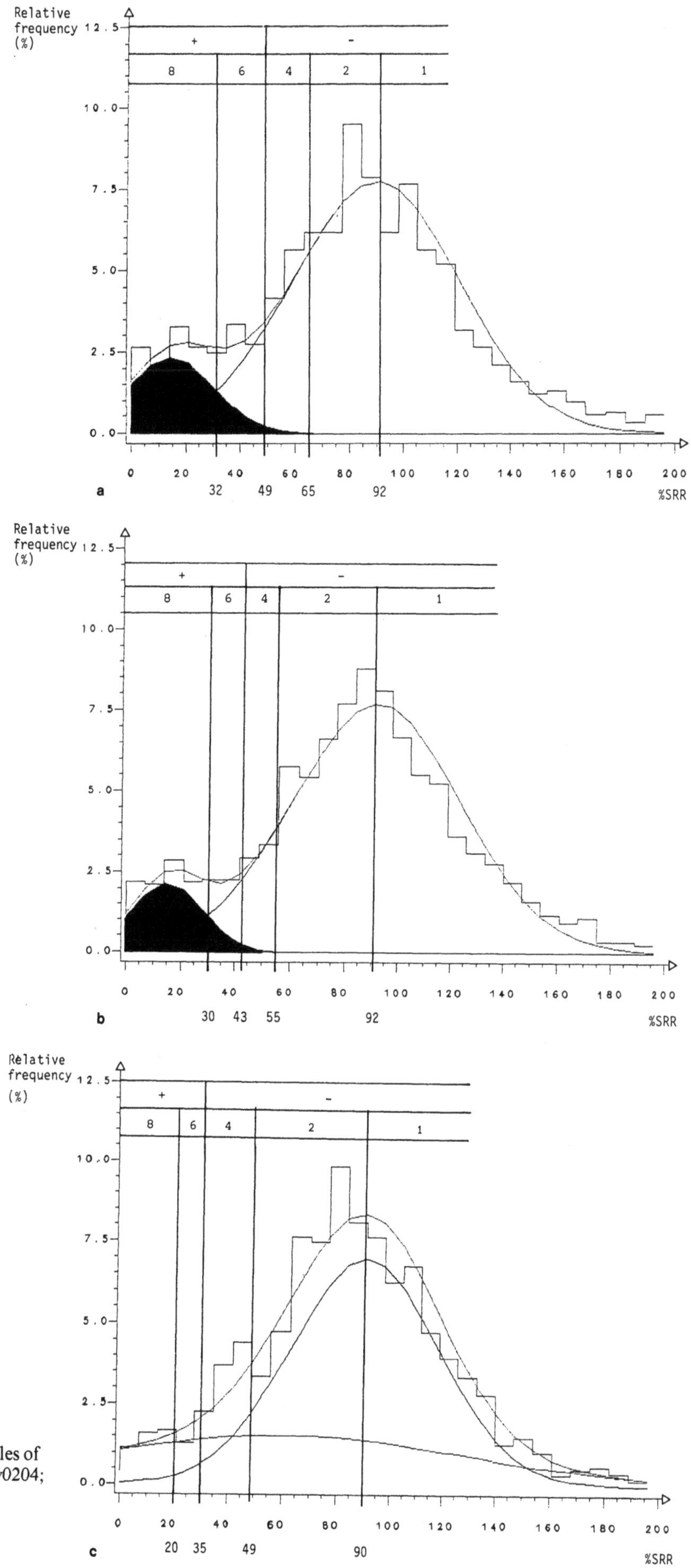

Fig. 7 a – c. Central data analysis: examples of cut-off point definitions. **a** 9w0101; **b** 9w0204; **c** 9w0404

Table 3. Summary of cut-off points for the 91 HTC

WS HTC no.	Score 8/6	6/4	4/2	2/1
9w0101	32	49	65	92
9w0102*	20	35	49	90
9w0103	25	42	59	95
9w0104*	20	35	49	90
9w0105	34	48	62	93
9w0201	15	27	38	90
9w0202	27	37	47	98
9w0203*	20	35	49	90
9w0204	30	43	55	92
9w0301	21	44	67	91
9w0302	17	49	80	92
9w0303*	20	35	49	90
9w0304	20	29	38	92
9w0305	19	30	40	90
9w0401*	20	35	49	90
9w0402	19	32	45	90
9w0403*	20	35	49	90
9w0404*	20	35	49	90
9w0501*	20	35	49	90
9w0502*	20	35	49	90
9w0503	21	37	53	90
9w0504	18	29	40	89
9w0505*	20	35	49	90
9w0506	12	22	31	91
9w0601*	20	35	49	90
9w0602*	20	35	49	90
9w0603*	20	35	49	90
9w0604	6	10	14	83
9w0605*	20	35	49	90
9w0606*	20	35	49	90
9w0607*	20	35	49	90
9w0608*	20	35	49	90
9w0609*	20	35	49	90
9w0610*	20	35	49	90
9w0611*	20	35	49	90
9w0701	12	33	53	90
9w0702	24	49	74	90
9w0703[a]				
9w0704*	20	35	49	90
9w0705*	20	35	49	90
9w0801*	20	35	49	90
9w0802	22	35	47	90
9w0803*	20	35	49	90
9w0804*	20	35	49	90
9w0805*	20	35	49	90
9w0806*	20	35	49	90
9w0807*	20	35	49	90
9w0808*	20	35	49	90
9w0901*	20	35	49	90
9w0902	10	24	38	87
9w0903	27	47	67	91
9w0904*	20	35	49	90
9w0905*	20	35	49	90
9w1001*	20	35	49	90
9w1002*	20	35	49	90
9w1003	23	42	59	90
9w1004*	20	35	49	90
9w1005*	20	35	49	90
9w1101*	20	35	49	90
9w1102*	20	35	49	90
9w1103	22	35	48	91
9w1104	18	32	45	90
9w1105*	20	35	49	90
9w1201*	20	35	49	90
9w1202*	20	35	49	90
9w1301	16	27	38	90
9w1302	8	20	31	90
9w1303*	20	35	49	90
9w1401*	20	35	49	90
9w1402*	20	35	49	90
9w1403*	20	35	49	90
9w1404*	20	35	49	90
9w1405	20	36	52	90
9w1406*	20	35	49	90
9w1501*	20	35	49	90
9w1502	15	27	39	87
9w1503*	20	35	49	90
9w1504*	20	35	49	90
9w1601*	20	35	49	90
9w1602*	20	35	49	90
9w1701	23	35	46	90
9w1702*	20	35	49	90
9w1801	14	30	46	90
9w1802*	20	35	49	90
9w1803*	20	35	49	90
9w1901*	20	35	49	90
9w1902*	20	35	49	90
9w1903*	20	35	49	90
9w1904*	20	35	49	90
9w9901	18	36	53	90
9w9902*	20	35	49	90

[a] Deleted due to low stimulatory ability

*, No individual cut-off points given; means ± SD of the cut-off points derived from the 30 HTC with good bimodal distribution were assigned. Cut-off point 6/8: 19.6 ± 6.7; cut-off point 4/6: 34.6 ± 9.7; cut-off point 2/4: 48.7 ± 14.4; cut-off point 1/2: 90.4 ± 2.5

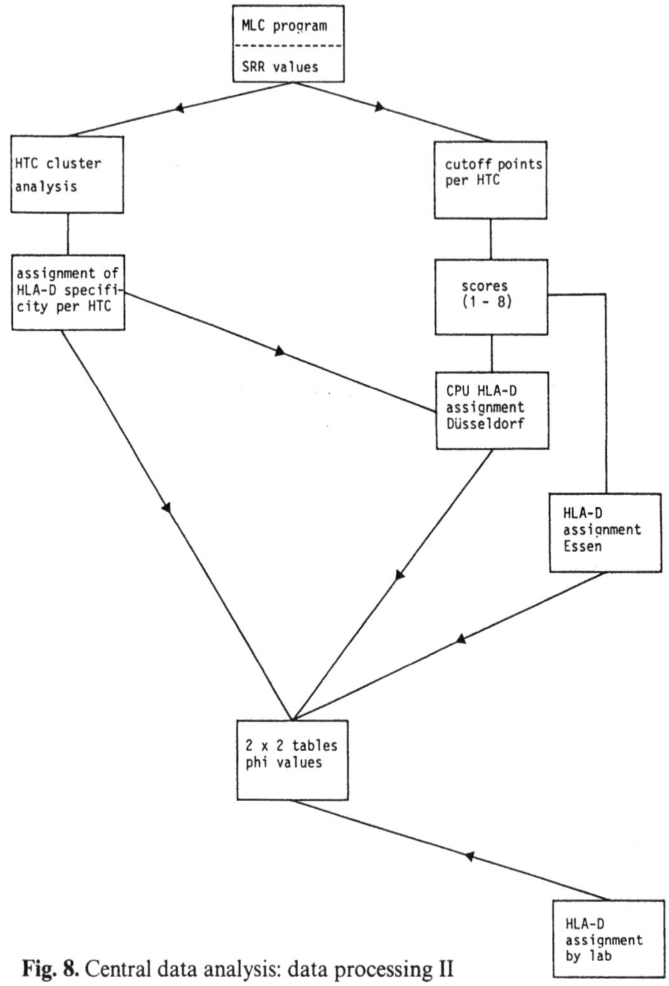

Fig. 8. Central data analysis: data processing II

Based on the order depicted by the cluster analysis (Fig. 9), the correlation coefficients of the SRR values for all the HTC are listed in Table 4.

For the assignment of HLA-D types to individuals, two approaches were used: (a) cell typing by computer (H. Deppe et al., Cell Typing by Computer, this volume), and (b) assignment by inspection. The program for cell typing by computer utilized the scores for each responder against each HTC as well as information on the HLA-D specificity assigned to each HTC as described above.

The HLA-D assignment by inspection was based on the majority of positive typing responses, i.e., scores 6 and 8, toward HTC of a given cluster. Assignments made to specificities defined by only two HTC (e.g. Dw12, Dw13, and Dw16) were confirmed by family segregation (see accompanying report on segregation analysis.)

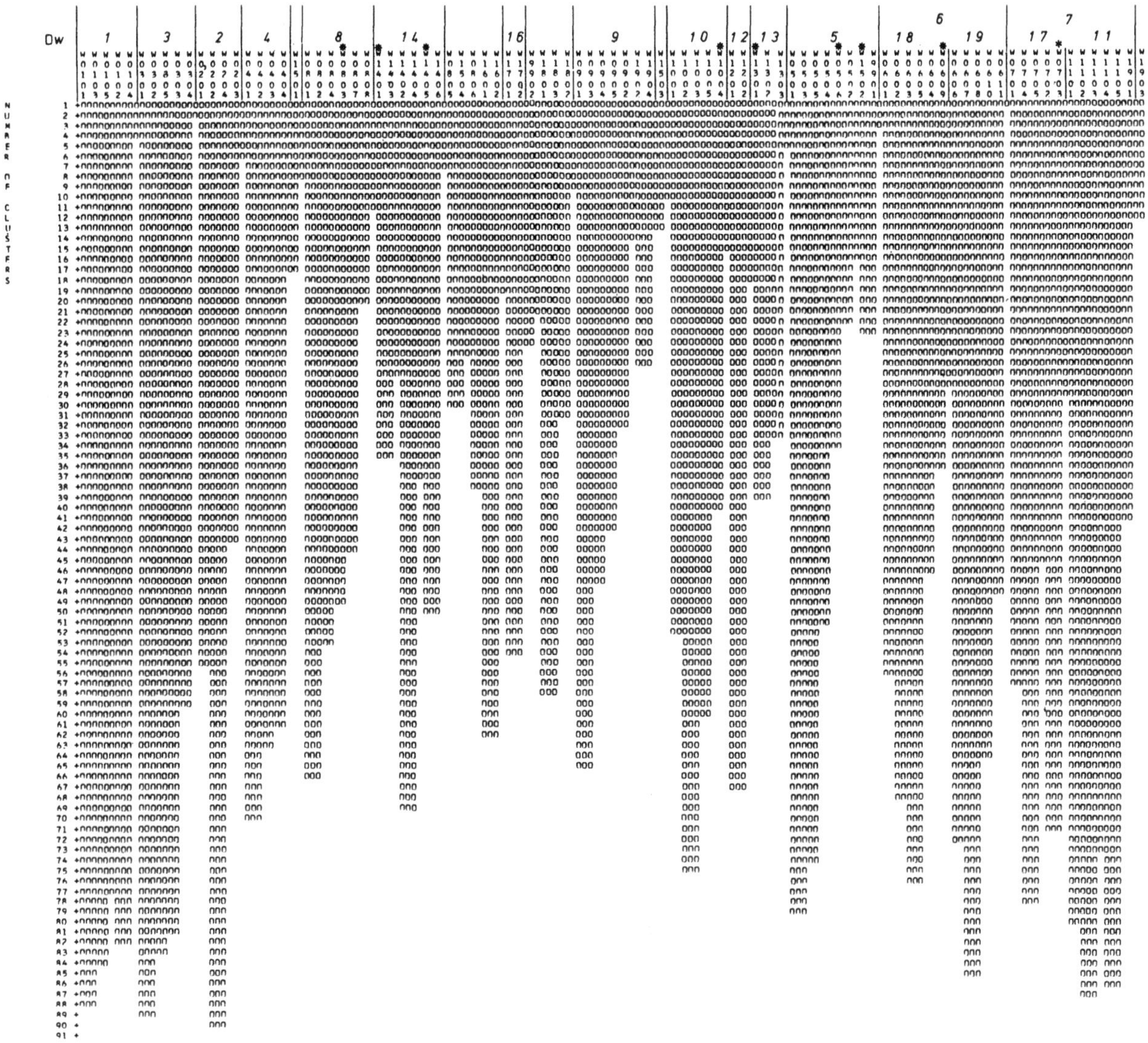

Fig. 9. Unbiased clustering of the Workshop HTC based on the multiple correlation coefficients of the SRR values. At head of figure, *stars* (*) identify HTC subsequently excluded from the cluster; the *cross* shows the HTC deleted due to low stimulatory ability

Table 5 summarizes the correlation between the HLA-D assignments by computer with the typing results obtained by HTC belonging to defined clusters (see above). Except for Dw5, the individual HTC typing results are in good agreement with the D locus assignment by computer. In addition, this table compares results obtained from repeat testings, in that the highest value was considered "maximum score" and the lowest value "minimum score." For the 17% tested only once, the same value had to be used as maximum and minimum score due to the dictates of the program. The comparison of the *r* values obtained for maximum and minimum score indicated an acceptable level of reproducibility.

Similarly, Table 6 summarizes the correlation between HLA-D assignments by inspection with the HTC typing results. In contrast to the computer assignment, all correlations, including that for Dw5, show good overall agreement. The level of reproducibility based on the comparison of maximum and minimum scores proved to be comparable to that obtained with the computer assignment data. On the basis of these comparisons it was decided to accept the inspection method for the final Workshop HLA-D assignments.

As already indicated in Fig. 9 and Table 4, HLA-Dw6 could be split into two distinct subgroups, Dw18 and Dw19 (Table 7). The subgroup Dw19 appeared to be more homogeneous than Dw18. Only 14 individuals could not be assigned to one of these groups and were therefore typed as Dw6. By segregation analysis, two individuals could be identified as heterozygous for Dw18 and Dw19, mimicking the typing pattern of the Dw6 positives. The previously recognized cross-reacting group

Table 4. Multiple correlation coefficients between Workshop HTCs (SRR)

• value 0.00 – 0.25;
– negative value;
* blank HTC

Table 5. Correlation between HLA-D determinants (computer method) and typing results (+ ≙ score 8, 6/– ≙ score 4, 2, 1) of HTC

		maximum Score						minimum Score					
D	WS HTC	++	+-	-+	--	X^2	r	++	+-	-+	--	X^2	r
w1	9W0101	137	10	79	691	471.5	.72	128	19	67	703	452.8	.70
	9W0102	86	21	24	638	442.6	.76	73	34	18	644	378.8	.70
	9W0103	104	35	49	754	411.3	.66	96	43	41	762	390.0	.64
	9W0104	95	24	35	700	447.2	.72	86	33	31	704	401.1	.68
	9W0105	115	20	26	772	604.1	.80	107	28	19	779	584.2	.79
w2	9W0201	66	62	31	751	261.7	.54	58	70	30	752	216.6	.49
	9W0202	104	27	31	790	530.7	.75	99	32	29	792	503.8	.73
	9W0203	44	18	25	340	160.8	.61	42	20	24	341	151.7	.60
	9W0204	113	13	42	786	575.3	.78	105	21	34	794	551.5	.76
w3	9W0301	115	13	79	724	428.4	.68	99	29	63	740	371.0	.63
	9W0302	117	8	85	656	403.4	.68	96	29	60	681	341.8	.63
	9W0303	72	50	34	752	306.3	.58	59	63	30	756	237.0	.51
	9W0304	44	46	22	487	154.9	.51	43	47	22	487	149.3	.50
	9W0305	83	51	10	800	477.1	.71	73	61	9	801	412.8	.66
w4	9W0401	51	44	20	851	332.2	.59	44	51	17	854	285.0	.54
	9W0402	58	47	24	796	315.3	.58	48	57	24	796	237.4	.51
	9W0403	39	55	19	778	211.3	.49	28	66	14	783	147.1	.41
	9W0404	64	33	45	767	300.0	.57	51	46	36	775	232.0	.50
w5	9W0501	35	19	95	627	96.1	.35	33	21	82	640	98.5	.36
	9W0502	21	23	84	389	22.3	.21	18	26	74	399	17.6	.18
	9W0503	28	23	69	599	80.6	.33	24	27	67	601	58.8	.27
	9W0504	15	57	72	779	11.9	.11	15	57	63	788	15.5	.13
	9W0505	30	31	75	761	88.9	.31	24	37	56	780	74.6	.29
	9W9901	6	49	62	646	0.3	.02	6	49	55	653	0.7	.03
w18	9w0601	33	68	30	787	118.3	.36	30	71	29	788	102.2	.33
	9W0602	59	47	68	747	176.6	.44	53	53	61	754	156.3	.41
	9W0603	45	58	33	762	179.7	.45	39	64	25	770	166.1	.43
	9W0604	25	78	24	744	76.5	.30	23	80	23	745	67.9	.28
	9W0505	49	61	59	789	137.5	.38	45	65	55	793	123.4	.36
w19	9W0606	47	55	19	857	279.9	.53	39	63	16	860	228.2	.48
	9W0607	57	42	29	766	294.5	.57	47	52	27	768	225.3	.50
	9W0608	40	53	25	818	207.8	.47	35	58	21	822	183.9	.44
	9W0610	61	35	45	771	281.6	.56	56	40	42	774	253.3	.53
	9W0611	49	46	63	724	145.2	.41	42	53	56	731	118.1	.37
w7	9W0702	141	46	70	639	352.9	.63	121	66	55	654	304.0	.58
w17	9W0701	48	110	24	699	126.5	.38	35	123	19	704	85.9	.31
	9W0704	84	68	40	659	245.8	.54	70	82	36	662	191.2	.47
	9W0705	77	85	30	735	249.0	.52	70	92	23	742	239.4	.51
	9W1901	40	128	50	670	42.5	.22	32	136	43	677	30.1	.18
w11	9W1101	36	14	59	850	227.9	.49	30	20	48	861	189.0	.45
	9W1102	36	17	48	800	228.7	.50	34	19	41	807	230.0	.50
	9W1103	41	10	71	828	243.9	.51	35	16	63	836	198.1	.46
	9W1104	36	17	56	809	209.1	.48	31	22	48	817	178.0	.44
	9W1105	25	23	68	809	98.9	.33	19	29	54	823	69.9	.27
w8	9W0801	32	16	18	668	289.8	.63	31	17	17	669	283.1	.62
	9W0802	42	17	47	802	268.9	.54	42	17	47	802	268.9	.54
	9W0804	30	18	51	713	156.7	.44	25	23	43	721	127.0	.40
	9W0807	35	22	26	845	297.3	.57	30	27	25	846	237.6	.51
	9W0808	28	15	59	427	80.7	.39	27	16	59	427	74.4	.37
w9	9W0901	24	19	42	701	133.0	.41	22	21	31	712	142.7	.43
	9W0202	26	29	21	899	228.9	.48	22	33	14	906	216.1	.47
	9W0903	58	2	79	807	349.4	.61	52	8	64	822	329.6	.59
	9W0904	27	11	42	683	186.9	.49	27	11	42	683	186.9	.49
	9W0905	38	7	66	608	190.0	.51	38	7	63	611	197.0	.52
	9W1902	21	27	98	638	32.4	.20	20	28	88	648	33.5	.21
	9W1904	28	25	50	800	139.3	.39	26	27	44	805	131.9	.38
w10	9W1001	24	6	72	712	139.3	.41	20	10	68	716	100.8	.35
	9W1002	25	4	41	843	278.6	.55	23	6	33	851	278.6	.55
	9W1003	28	10	74	815	159.0	.41	25	13	68	821	136.5	.38
	9W1005	30	7	66	755	190.1	.47	29	8	60	761	192.3	.47
w12	9W1201	18	5	48	888	187.3	.44	17	6	45	891	177.3	.43
	9W1202	18	5	56	814	152.1	.41	15	8	51	819	115.3	.36
w13	9W1302	8	5	24	846	126.7	.38	7	6	21	849	110.3	.39
	9W1303	13	0	56	845	161.5	.42	11	2	47	854	135.9	.39
w14	9W1402	21	6	22	448	172.6	.59	16	11	21	449	111.2	.47
	9W1403	28	8	54	842	165.6	.42	24	22	51	845	129.0	.37
	9W1404	25	16	24	885	263.5	.53	23	18	19	860	261.6	.53
	9W1406	19	21	32	843	139.7	.39	18	22	27	848	143.7	.40
w16	9W1701	11	6	28	886	158.0	.41	11	6	24	890	177.8	.44
	9W1702	15	3	48	835	164.6	.43	14	4	43	840	158.2	.42

Table 6. Correlation between HLA-D determinants (inspect. method) and typing results (+ ≙ score 8, 6/– ≙ score 4, 2, 1) of HTC

		maximum Score						minimum Score					
D	WS HTC	++	+-	-+	--	X^2	r	++	+-	-+	--	X^2	r
w1	9W0101	91	12	45	403	276.2	.71	88	15	37	411	284.4	.72
	9W0102	63	17	17	361	252.5	.74	54	26	10	368	231.0	.71
	9W0103	74	24	26	425	262.9	.69	67	31	21	430	242.8	.66
	9W0104	66	17	23	402	263.9	.72	59	24	20	405	232.8	.68
	9W0105	75	16	13	431	347.2	.81	67	24	11	433	306.9	.76
w2	9W0201	41	26	19	433	185.4	.60	33	34	28	434	135.0	.51
	9W0202	67	7	26	452	331.3	.77	64	10	25	453	312.8	.75
	9W0203	24	3	23	191	93.2	.62	23	4	22	192	88.6	.61
	9W0204	72	7	27	459	344.4	.78	69	10	21	465	349.7	.79
w3	9W0301	65	7	42	435	264.6	.69	57	15	27	450	260.8	.69
	9W0302	72	5	57	362	215.8	.66	60	17	35	384	203.3	.64
	9W0303	46	22	20	442	218.0	.64	37	31	17	445	166.7	.56
	9W0304	30	22	8	305	145.3	.63	29	23	8	305	138.6	.62
	9W0305	55	16	8	468	348.2	.80	48	23	7	469	298.8	.74
w4	9W0401	40	18	15	496	260.0	.67	33	25	15	469	196.4	.59
	9W0402	42	20	21	447	209.1	.63	33	29	21	447	142.1	.52
	9W0403	27	30	12	449	146.0	.53	18	39	11	450	81.8	.40
	9W0404	44	16	29	432	198.1	.62	34	26	25	436	138.8	.52
w5	9W0501	48	37	12	370	176.6	.61	41	19	36	371	134.4	.54
	9W0502	34	14	25	245	102.3	.57	28	20	21	249	79.9	.50
	9W0503	56	18	15	358	237.3	.73	52	22	14	359	217.1	.70
	9W0504	50	30	8	451	261.9	.70	44	36	7	452	227.4	.65
	9W0505	52	30	20	437	209.4	.62	38	44	15	442	145.2	.52
	9W9901	24	53	19	381	54.9	.34	23	54	19	381	50.7	.33
w18	9W0601	15	21	21	485	76.3	.37	15	21	19	487	82.1	.39
	9W0602	29	10	49	465	125.7	.48	25	14	45	469	100.4	.43
	9W0603	18	14	32	465	87.1	.41	14	18	25	472	66.0	.35
	9W0604	16	16	17	469	108.8	.46	16	16	15	471	117,4	.48
	9W0605	24	14	33	491	125.7	.47	24	14	26	498	148.0	.51
w19	9W0606	29	18	19	507	199.0	.60	24	23	12	512	173.7	.55
	9W0607	35	14	21	451	207.6	.63	27	22	19	453	143.9	.52
	9W0608	24	19	18	435	155.4	.53	20	23	15	498	127.8	.48
	9W0610	36	11	31	450	190.2	.69	32	15	29	452	161.4	.55
	9W0611	27	16	48	426	88.2	.41	22	21	43	431	63.5	.35
w7	9W0702	82	13	67	379	199.5	.61	75	20	57	392	192.7	.60
w17	9W0701	13	18	24	455	59.0	.34	8	23	17	462	31.9	.25
	9W0704	49	16	33	416	196.0	.62	40	20	29	420	148.2	.54
	9W0705	51	22	24	453	226.0	.64	44	29	18	459	202.1	.61
	9W1901	25	46	19	447	79.4	.38	19	52	15	451	57.6	.33
w11	9W1101	46	21	18	486	251.7	.66	39	28	12	492	226.6	.63
	9W1102	37	24	14	440	199.8	.62	31	30	12	442	163.1	.56
	9W1103	49	16	28	467	235.5	.63	44	21	24	471	212.7	.62
	9W1104	48	17	27	469	238.4	.65	46	17	25	469	223.5	.61
	9W1105	37	26	11	442	187.1	.59	33	27	10	444	176.9	.56
w8	9W0801	19	6	20	402	150.5	.60	18	7	19	403	141.6	.56
	9W0802	23	4	26	477	195.5	.61	22	5	24	479	190.2	.60
	9W0804	11	8	36	389	46.9	.32	7	12	28	397	22.9	.23
	9W0807	22	4	15	502	260.3	.69	18	8	15	502	190.8	.59
	9W0808	15	5	34	253	55.6	.43	15	5	34	253	55.6	.43
W9	9W0901	14	14	20	408	78.2	.41	11	17	16	412	59.6	.36
	9W0902	18	17	13	532	156.4	.52	14	21	10	535	120.8	.46
	9W0903	35	1	39	484	236.3	.65	35	1	29	494	279.2	.71
	9W0904	15	6	21	413	121.9	.52	15	6	21	413	121.9	.52
	9W0905	21	3	31	349	126.7	.56	20	4	31	349	115.7	.53
	9W1902	16	13	53	372	38.4	.29	15	14	5	380	40.0	.30
	9W1904	21	12	30	470	118.8	.47	20	13	27	473	117.3	.47
w10	9W1001	17	4	34	407	109.5	.49	17	4	30	411	120.6	.51
	9W1002	14	6	17	502	158.2	.54	13	7	12	507	171.1	.56
	9W1003	15	5	43	486	91.2	.41	15	5	37	492	103.9	.43
	9W1005	17	4	23	444	154.4	.56	17	4	20	447	168.6	.59
w12	9W1201	16	9	23	513	131.6	.48	15	10	21	515	125.1	.47
	9W1202	14	10	24	497	102.2	.43	11	13	22	499	69.8	.36
w13	9W1302	3	3	9	498	60.4	.34	3	3	8	499	66.3	.36
	9W1303	10	1	28	492	118.6	.47	8	3	24	496	88.2	.41
w14	9W1402	11	3	12	267	101.6	.59	8	6	10	269	66.3	.48
	9W1403	13	6	24	504	118.6	.47	11	8	20	508	100.4	.43
	9W1404	12	6	13	522	166.5	.55	12	6	8	527	212.2	.62
	9W1406	11	9	17	515	107.4	.44	10	10	15	517	99.2	.42
w16	9W1701	7	1	15	535	149.6	.52	7	1	15	535	149.5	.52
	9W1702	8	1	22	511	121.6	.47	8	1	19	514	136.1	.50

Table 7. Subdivision of Dw6 into Dw18 and Dw19, and of Dw7 into Dw11 and Dw17

REGLAB	CELLID	HLA-DW	9W0601 9W0602 9W0603 9W0604 9W0605	9W0611 9W0608 9W0610 9W0606 9W0607
GERGSW	03005	6	+++++	+++++
NCYYUN	09123	6	+++++	++++
FAFPTR	11006	6	++++	+++++
BENROO	02010	6	-+++-	+++++
GERGSW	01003	6	+-+++	+++++
FAFPTR	11005	6	++++	+-+++
GERGSW	03002	6	-++++	-++++
GERGSW	03004	6	-++++	-++-+
GERWAN	08071	6	+++--	+++-+
FAFPTR	11002	6	++-+	+--++
FAFRIC	13002	6	++-+-	-+++-
GERGSW	03006	6	-++-+	--+++
NCYBIA	05006	6	++ +	+-++
NCYYUN	09122	6	-++-+	+-+-
SCATSB	18117	18,19	++++-	+++++
SCATSB	18119	18,19	-+-++	+++++
GERGSW	01001	18	+++++	+-+--
SAFDUT	04022	18	+++++	-+--+
SCASVE	02109	18	+++-+	-----
SCATSB	25151	18	+++-+	-----
SCASVE	02113	18	+++-+	-----
US2BAC	17008	18	+++-+	-----
SCATSB	25153	18	++-++	-----
SCAKIS	01001	18	-++++	-- --
UKIBRS	03036	18	++-++	+----
FAFPTR	10002	18	+++--	-----
UKIFES	20111	18	+++--	-----
UKIFES	20112	18	++ -+	-----
FAFKAS	16164	18	++- +	----
UKIFES	05027	18	++-+-	-----
UKIBRS	03243	18	+++	-----
UKIBRS	06514	18	-+++-	-----
SCAKIS	01006	18	-++-+	-- --
US2BAC	09004	18	-++-+	-----
FAFKAS	16162	18	-++ +	----
FAFKAS	16165	18	-++ +	----
SAFDUT	04021	18	-+-++	-----
FAFKAS	16163	18	++- +	+---
SAFDUT	04029	18	-+-++	-+---
SCASVE	02110	18	-++-+	+----
SCAKIS	04027	18	-+ ++	+- --
UKIFES	05030	18	-+-++	----+
FAFPTR	10005	18	-+-++	--+--
UKIBRS	06533	18	++---	-----
SCASVE	02112	18	-++--	-----
US2BAC	09005	18	-++--	-----
FAFKAS	16166	18	--+ +	----
US7HAN	02017	19	-----	+++++
SAFDUT	01003	19	-----	+++++
FRABET	07007	19	-----	+++++
US7HAN	02008	19	-----	+++++
GERWAN	12096	19	-----	+++++
SAFDUT	01002	19	-----	+++++
US4STA	16003	19	-----	+++++
US7HAN	02012	19	-----	+++++
FAFPTR	09007	19	-+---	+++++
GERWAN	12093	19	-+---	+++++
US7HAN	07048	19	----+	+++++
BENROO	02013	19	--+--	+++++
US7HAN	02015	19	----+	+++++
GERWAN	12098	19	-----	+++++
US7HAN	07055	19	-+--+	+++++
FAFPTR	09002	19	--++-	+++++
FRABET	07002	19	-----	-++++
JAPKSH	05005	19	-----	+-+++
US4STA	16002	19	-----	+++-+
JAPTSU	93005	19	-----	++-++
JAPTSU	94003	19	----+	-++++
BENROO	02011	19	+----	++++-
GERWAN	08063	19	-+---	+++-+
US4STA	16007	19	---+-	-++++
US7HAN	07053	19	----+	+-+++
GERWAN	12095	19	--+-+	++-++
JAPTSU	94004	19	+---+	-++++
GERWAN	08072	19	-----	+-++-
JAPTSU	93004	19	-----	-++-+
UKIFES	00001	19	-- --	+-+-+
NCYBIA	05002	19	-- -	+++-
SCATSB	18118	19	---+-	+-+-+
JAPKSH	03001	19	----+	+-++-
JAPTSU	94001	19	----+	+-+-+
JAPKSH	05004	19	-----	+-+--
GERWAN	12094	19	-----	-+-+-
GERWAN	08073	19	-----	-+--+
FRABET	07006	19	-----	--+-+
JAPTSU	93003	19	-----	---++

REGLAB	CELLID	HLA-DW	9W0702	9W1105 9W1104 9W1103 9W1102 9W1101	9W0701 9W1901 9W0705 9W0704
FAFPTR	08001	7	+	+++++	++++
GERGSW	02005	7	+	+++++	++++
GERGSW	04001	7	+	+++++	++++
GERGSW	04002	7	+	+++++	++++
GERGSW	04003	7	+	+++++	++++
GERGSW	04004	7	+	+++++	++++
GERGSW	04005	7	+	+++++	++++
SCATSB	18118	7	+	+++++	+++-
GERGSW	02002	7	+	+++++	+-++
NCYYUN	07109	7	+	+++++	+-++
NCYYUN	07110	7	+	+++++	+-++
US7HAN	07056	7	+	+++++	+-++
FAFPTR	08005	7	+	+++++	-+++
FAFPTR	08006	7	+	+++++	-+++
GERGSW	01005	7	+	+++++	-+++
GERGSW	01002	7	+	+++++	--++
US7HAN	05033	7	+	+++++	--++
FRAARN	15002	7	+	+++-+	++++
NCYYUN	06103	7	+	-++++	+-++
FRAARN	15005	7	+	+-+++	+-++
SAFDUT	01006	7	-	+-+++	++-+
NCYYUN	06107	7	+	+-+++	+-++
BENROO	01001	7	+	+++--	++++
SAFDUT	10057	7	+	-++++	-+-+
FAFPTR	08007	7	+	++++-	-++
SAFDUT	10056	7	+	+-+++	-+-+
FAFPTR	09002	7	+	++++-	-+-+
BENROO	01006	7	+	++-+-	+-++
GERGSW	02006	7	+	+-+-+	+-++
US7HAN	05034	7	+	+-+-+	-+++
GERGSW	02008	7	+	-++-+	+-++
FRAARN	15003	7	+	-+-++	+-++
SAFDUT	01001	7	+	+-++-	++--
US7HAN	05036	7	+	+-+-+	--++
US7HAN	07049	7	+	+--++	+-+-
FAFPTR	08004	7	+	-+++-	--++
FRAARN	15004	7	+	-+-++	--++
UKIBRS	01502	7	+	---++	+-++
NCYYUN	07112	7	-	-++-+	---+
BENROO	01007	7	+	++---	++--
BENROO	01004	7	+	++---	-++-
BENROO	01008	7	+	++---	-+-+
BENROO	01005	7	+	++---	-+--
SCAKIS	02008	11	+	+++++	----
SCAKIS	02010	11	+	+++++	----
SCAKIS	02012	11	+	+++++	----
NCYYUN	04091	11		+++++	--
US7HAN	07050	11	+	+++++	-+--
AN7BSH	03016	11	+	+++++	--+-
US7HAN	07048	11	+	+++++	--+-
NCYYUN	04093	11		-++++	--+
NCYYUN	04094	11		-++++	--+
AN7BSH	03019	11	+	-++++	----
NCYYUN	04092	11		-+-++	+-
AN7BSH	03014	11	+	-++-+	----
UKIFES	04024	11	+	-++-+	----
UKIFES	04023	11	+	--+++	----
UKIFES	05031	11	-	-+-++	+---
UKIFES	00001	11	+	-+-+-	----
UKIFES	04025	11	-	-- ++-	----
FAFPTR	07012	17	+	----+	++++
SAFDUT	01003	17	+	+-+--	++++
UKIBRS	08218	17	+	--+ +	++++
UKIBRS	08080	17	+	-+---	++-+
SCAKIS	01002	17	+	-----	+++-
FAFMYR	16003	17	+	-----	-+++
FAFMYR	05004	17	+	-----	+-++
UKIFES	12069	17	+	-----	+-++
US2BAC	17001	17	+	--+--	-+++
SCAKIS	13077	17	+	--+-	+-++
UKIBRS	08217	17	+	--+-+	+-++
SCAKIS	01005	17	+	-----	+-+-
US2BAC	17004	17	+	-----	+--+
US7HAN	07055	17	+	+----	--++
FAFMYR	16001	17	+	+----	--++
UKIFES	12071	17	-	+----	+-+-
UKIFES	12070	17	-	-----	+-+-
FAFMYR	05006	17	-	-----	-+-+

Table 8. Final allocation of Workshop HTC to respective HLA-D specificities

w1	w2	w3	w4	w5	w7	w8	w9	w10	w11 (w7)	w12	w13	w14	w15	w16	w17 (w7)	w18 (w6)	w19 (w6)	blank
																		1802 'HAG'
																		1803 'B9'
																		1801 'B9'
																		1602 'B7'
																		1601 'B7'
																		0806 'B7'
																		0805 'B7'
																		1503 'B6'
																		1903
																		1504
																		1502
																		1501 'B6?'
							1904											1405
				9901			1902											1401
0104		0304		0502		0808	0902		1105							0604	0611	1301
0102	0203	0303	0404	0504		0807	0905	1005	1104			1406			1901	0605	0608	1004
0105	0204	0305	0403	0505		0804	0904	1003	1103			1404			0705	0603	0610	0803
0103	0202	0302	0402	0503		0802	0903	1002	1102	1201	1302	1403		1702	0704	0602	0607	0609
0101	0201	0301	0401	0501	0702	0801	0901	1001	1101	1202	1303	1402	9902	1701	0701	0601	0606	0506

Table 9. Antigen and gene frequencies of the Workshop-defined HLA-D specificities among the parents of the selected families ($n = 200$)

HLA-	*n*	af	gf
Dw1	38	19.0	10.0
Dw2	29	14.5	7.5
Dw3	29	14.5	7.5
Dw4	16	8.0	4.1
Dw5	34	17.0	8.9
Dw6	4	2.0	1.0
Dw7	21	10.5	5.4
Dw8	14	7.0	3.6
Dw9	13	6.5	3.3
Dw10	7	3.5	1.8
Dw11	7	3.5	1.8
Dw12	8	4.0	2.0
Dw13	5	2.5	1.3
Dw14	9	4.5	2.3
Dw16	4	2.0	1.0
Dw17	7	3.5	1.8
Dw18	17	8.5	4.3
Dw19	18	9.0	4.6
DB9	1	0.5	0.3
B7	1	0.5	0.3
B6	2	1.0	0.5
HAG	3	1.5	0.8
D-blank	111	55.5	33.3

HLA-Dw7 + w11 [4] could be further clarified to the extent that one set of HTC typed for Dw11 while a second set typed for Dw17 (Table 7). Interestingly, one HTC (9w0702) typed for both splits, possibly recognizing a cellular analogue to the serologically defined supertypic specificities (e.g., A9 for A23 and A24). The majority of the tested individuals, however, typed positive with both sets of HTC and were therefore assigned to the Dw7 specificity.

The assignment of each Workshop HTC to one of the 19 HLA-D specificities is shown in Table 8. The 19 HTC classified as HLA-D blank, because their typing pattern failed to correlate with the other specificities, include, in addition to two probable heterozygous cells, those cells most likely representing new, as yet undefined HLA-D types [B6 (Herluf), B7 (8.2), B9, and HAG]. Unfortunately, the Workshop set for the second level included only one HTC (9w9902) for the well-characterized, DR4-related specificity, DYT, known to be present in the Oriental population [7], which is now officially recognized as Dw15 (Nomenclature for Factors of the HLA System 1984, this volume).

In keeping with previous joint reports of HLA-D typing the antigen and gene frequencies of the HLA-D specificities defined in this Workshop were calculated (Table 9). However, these figures are not representative for a random population since the panels typed were not randomly selected.

As mutual MLC non-/low reactivity indicates HLA-D compatibility, the participating laboratories were requested to use their own submitted HTC as responder(s) against the Workshop HTC set. This HTC cross-check resulted in the checkerboard matrix given in Table 10. As expected, HTC belonging to the same cluster showed mutually low or negative reactions. The heterogeneity in Dw7 is also evident from this cross-check. Interestingly, the cross-check revealed an obvious coding error, in that 9w0303 and 9w0704 originating from the same lab were inadvertently mislabeled. In addition, 9w1004, submitted as a Dw10

Table 10. Checkerboard matrix of the HTC cross-check

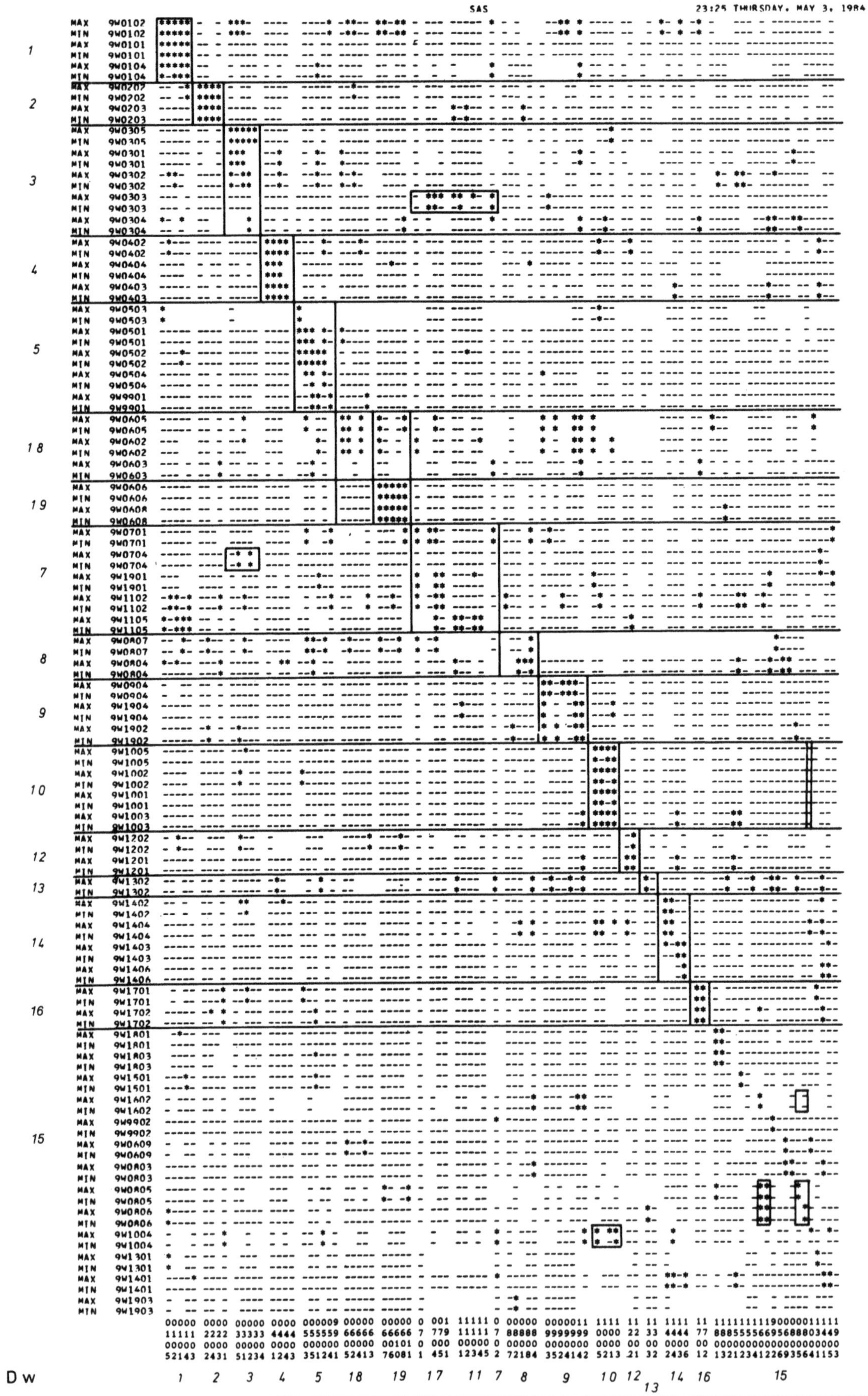

*, score 6 or 8; –, score 1 – 4; empty space, untested or deleted combination

HTC, proved to be heterozygous. The cross-check between 9w1601, 9w1602 and 9w0805, 9w0806 gave tentative evidence that 0805 and 0806 are heterozygous for a determinant defined by 1601 and 1602.

Summary

In contrast to the frequently expressed skepticism concerning the cellular typing of D-region-encoded antigens, these data demonstrate that D typing is feasible, allowing even a further delineation of established specificities (i.e., Dw6) as well as a definition of new specificities (i.e., Dw13, Dw14, Dw15, and Dw16). The decision to carry out these studies on two levels (first level: identification of discriminating typing reagents as well as new clusters on a highly selected panel; second level: confirmation of the data by family segregation on an extended Workshop basis) proved to be justified, although the workload for some of the participating laboratories bordered on the unreasonable. Here we would like to express our special thanks to those labs as well as to all other participants in this enterprise. There is still room for further cellular studies focusing on the specificities not officially designated, such as B6, B7, B9, and HAG. Furthermore, while the relationship between the Workshop-defined D specificities and the serologically defined class II (DR, DQ) antigens, as discussed in more detail by G. Schreuder et al. (HLA-DR, DQ, LB, and TA10 Specificities of the Ninth Workshop Homozygous Typing Cells, this volume), is not yet clarified, we feel justified in suggesting that D, DR, and DQ are distinct antigenic systems. Finally, these thoroughly studied Workshop HTC will serve as reference for further biochemical and molecular genetic analysis of the HLA-D region.

Acknowledgements. The authors are grateful to Ms. A. Czeczatka, Ms. B. Kostka, and Ms. M. Limper for excellent technical assistance and Ms. S. Richter for typing the manuscript.

References

1. Mempel W, Grosse-Wilde H, Albert E, Thierfelder S (1973) Atypical reactions in HL-A-typed related and unrelated pairs. Transplant Proc 5:401–408
2. Thorsby E, Piazza A (1975) Joint report from the Sixth International Histocompatibility Workshop Conference. II. Typing for HLA-D (LD-1 or MLC) determinants. In: Kissmeyer-Nielsen F (ed) Histocompatibility testing 1975. Munksgaard, Copenhagen, pp 414–458
3. Festenstein H, Oliver RTD, Sachs JA, McMichael AJ, Bodmer WF (1978) Overall analysis of the HTC data based on clusters, patterns and antigen reports. In: Bodmer WF, Batchelor JR, Bodmer JG, Festenstein H, Morris PJ (eds) Histocompatibility testing 1977. Munksgaard, Copenhagen, pp 115–141
4. Dupont B, Braun DW Jr, Yunis EJ, Carpenter CB (1980) Joint report: HLA-D by cellular typing. In: Terasaki PI (ed) Histocompatibility testing 1980. UCLA Tissue Typing Laboratory, Los Angeles, pp 229–267
5. Mickelson EM, Nisperos B, Layrisse Z, Se Jong Kim, Donnall Thomas E, Hansen JA (1983) Analysis of the HLA-DRw8 haplotype: recognition by HTC typing of three distinct antigen complexes in Caucausians, native Americans and Orientals. Immunogenetics 17:399–410
6. Ruppelt W, Grosse-Wilde H, Netzel B (1976) Computer program for the evaluation and interpretation of MLC data. Z Immun Forsch 152:293–297
7. Sasazuki T, Kaneoka H, Tsuji K, Nose Y, Kashiwagi N, Kaneko T (1980) Joint report: HLA-D in Japan. In: Terasaki PI (ed) Histocompatibility testing 1980. UCLA Tissue Typing Laboratory, Los Angeles, pp 274–276

Appendix A. List of participating HLA-D laboratories (data submission)

Lab	Code	Participants	Institutions
ANZ	BSH	Bashir, Honeyman	Red Cross Blood Transfusion Service, Sydney, New South Wales, Australia
BEN	ROO	van Rood, Termijtelen	Academisch Ziekenhuis Leiden, Leiden, The Netherlands
EAE	NYU	Nyulassy, Buc	Medical Faculty, Department of Medical Microbiology and Immunology, Bratislava, CSSR
EAE	IVS	Ivaskova, Rychlikova	Czechoslovak Academy of Sciences, Praha, CSSR
EAE	KAS	Kastelan, Gerenćer	Tissue Typing Center KBC REBRO, Zagreb, Yugoslavia
EAE	MYR	Mayr, Hajek	Institut für Blutgruppenserologie der Universität Wien, Austria
EAE	PTR	Petranyi, Onody	National Institute of Haematology and Blood Transfusion, Budapest, Hungary

Appendix A (continued)

Lab	Code	Participants	Institutions
EAE	RIC	Richter, Menzel	Bezirksinstitut für Blutspende- und Transfusionswesen, Berlin, DDR
FRA	ARN	Arnaiz-Villena, Requeiro	S. de Immunologia, Centro Ramon y Cajal, Madrid, Spain
FRA	BET	Betuel, Freidel	CTS de Lyon, Miribel, France
GER	BRA	Brautbar, Amar	Hadassah Medical Center, Lab. for Immunohematology, Jerusalem, Israel
GER	GSW	Grosse-Wilde, Doxiadis	Abteilung f. Immungenetik, Universitätsklinikum Essen, Germany
GER	WAN	Wank, Schendel	Immungenetisches Labor, Institut für Immunologie der Universität München, Germany
IT2	FER	Ferrara	Istituto Scientifico per lo Studio e la Cura dei Tumori, Genova, Italy
JAP	KSH	Kashiwagi	Kitasato University School of Medicine, Dept. of Transplantation, Kanagawa-Ken, Japan
JAP	SAS	Sasazuki	Tokyo Medical & Dental University, Medical Research Institute, Department of Human Genetics, Tokyo, Japan
JAP	TSU	Tsuji	Tokai University School of Medicine, Department of Transplantation, Kanagawa, Japan
LAT	LAY	Layrisse	Instituto Venezolano de Investigaciones Cientificas, Caracas, Venezuela
NCY	BIA	Bias, Hsu	The Johns Hopkins University Department of Medicine, Baltimore, U.S.A.
NCY	YUN	Yunis	Sidney Farber Cancer Institute, Division of Immunogenetics, Boston, U.S.A.
NCY	ZIE	Zier	Children's Hospital of Philadelphia, Philadelphia, Pennsylvania, U.S.A.
SAF	DUT	du Toit, Oudshoorn	Provincial Laboratory for Tissue Immunology, Observatory, Capetown, South Africa
SCA	KIS	Kissmeyer-Nielsen, Kristensen	Tissue Typing Laboratory, University Hospital, Aarhus, Denmark
SCA	SVE	Svejgaard, Platz, Ryder	Tissue Typing Laboratory, Righospitalet, København, Denmark
SCA	TSB	Thorsby	Tissue Typing Laboratory, Rikshospitalet, Oslo, Norway
UKI	BRS	Bradley, Stichcombe	U.K. Transplant Service, South Western Regional Transfusion Centre, Bristol, U.K.
UKI	FES	Festenstein, Jaraquemada, Ollier	The London Hospital Medical College, Department of Immunology, London, U.K.
US2	BAC	Bach, Reinsmoen	University of Minnesota, Histocompatibility Labs, Minneapolis, U.S.A.
US4	STA	Stastny	Southwestern Medical School, Dept. of Internal Medicine, Dallas, U.S.A.
US7	HAN	Hansen, Mickelson	Puget Sound Blood Center, Fred Hutchinson Cancer Research Center, Seattle, U.S.A.

Total no. families tested	145	
Total no. family members tested	906	
Total no. unrelated individuals tested (including 64 HTC as responders)	132	
	Family	Unrelated
Total no. HLA-D lab assignments	389	0
Total no. HLA-D computer assignments (max.)	819	126
(min)	809	119
Total no. HLA-D workshop assignments	635	0

Segregation Analysis (HTCs) *

I. Doxiadis[1], H. Grosse-Wilde[1], and E. Valentine-Thon[2]

1 Department of Immunogenetics, University Hospital of Essen, 4300 Essen, Federal Republic of Germany
2 Department of Human Genetics, University Hospital of Essen, 4300 Essen, Federal Republic of Germany

For the fourth time in conjunction with the International Histocompatibility Workshop the segregation of HLA-D determinants in families was investigated [1, 2, 3]. One hundred forty-five families were typed by the participating laboratories (see Appendix A) using the Workshop HTC set as described in the accompanying Cellular Part (HTC) and the data submitted to Essen. From these 145 families, 100 were selected for inclusion in the final Workshop set based on the following criteria:

1. The family was tested with most of the Workshop homozygous typing cells (HTC), and the data were not deleted by the computer analysis [see Data Analysis section in accompanying Cellular Part (HTC)].
2. No family member showed positive (score 6 – 8) typing responses to all the HTC.
3. No family member showed negative (score 1 – 2) typing responses to all the HTC, except in families where either one parent had two blank haplotypes or both parents shared a blank haplotype.

The scoring system (1 – 8) for response to each HTC described in the accompanying Cellular Part (HTC) was used. The following rules were applied for HLA-D assignment (inspection method) for each family member, where the entire pattern of reaction to all HTC was taken into consideration:

1. The majority of HTC defining an HLA-D determinant were positive (scores 6 – 8). When the cluster was defined with an even number of HTC (e.g., Dw2, Dw4, etc.), the decision whether to assign the determinant was made relative to the other reactions. For example, it was assigned when the scores with the other HTC were low (1 – 2), but not when the other scores were high (4 – 6).
2. In those few cases where an individual showed scores of less than 6, a score of 4 was accepted as a positive typing response when most other scores were 1 and 2.
3. When a family member failed to type for the expected determinant (scores 1 – 2 with the respective HTC), the assignment was considered as "missing."
4. Triplets were assigned when a family member showed high scores (6 – 8) with three independent HLA-D determinants. In those cases where in a family the assignment to either Dw17 or Dw11 failed, the family was typed as Dw7. The same holds for Dw18 and Dw19, where the assignment Dw6 was made.

Because of the quantity of data, only selected families can be shown. Table 1 lists the segregation of HLA-D determinants in 11 families selected to represent all specificities, as well as examples of triplets. Within each family the parents are presented first, followed by the children. Positive scores are underlined. The assignment of the respective HLA-D specificities is also given. The following comments can be made.

The Dw1 specificity clearly segregates in family FRABET 13. The same holds for Dw2 in this family and in SCAKIS 01 and SCATSB 12. Dw2 shows no cross-reactivity with Dw12. The latter specificity cross-reacts, however, in family SCAKIS 02, where a positive reaction segregates with the Dw2 haplotype (one HTC). The parent of this family carrying the Dw2 haplotype represents one of the three cases of triplets found in the Workshop set.

Dw3 segregates nicely in SCAKIS 01 and US7HAN 02.

The DR4-related D specificities, such as Dw4, Dw10, Dw13, and Dw14, are inherited in the same mendelian way as all specificities analyzed, without any cross-reactivity to each other. This is demonstrated for Dw4 in GERWAN 04, Dw10 in EAEKAS 18, Dw13 in SCATSB 12, and Dw14 in GERWAN 08.

None of those positive reactions cross-reacted with the Dw15 (9w9902) HTC which is also DR4-related.

Dw5 was assigned to members of EAEKAS 18, GERWAN 04, SCAKIS 02, and LATLAY 21, where the segregation is clearly shown.

Dw8 segregates in SCATSB 12, GERWAN 04, and US7HAN 04. Similar results can be demonstrated for Dw9 in US7HAN 02.

The oriental DR2-related Dw12 specificity is shown in GERWAN 08 and FRABET 13. In the former family it can clearly be assigned even in the presence of Dw2 (e.g., members 066, 067, 068, 070) as demonstrated by segregation; in the latter, it

* This work was supported by the Deutsche Forschungsgemeinschaft (AL-92/13-1) and by SFB102 TPB4

Table 1. Eleven families selected to represent all Workshop-defined HLA-D specificities

		HLA-Dw	1	2	3	4	5	7	8	9	10	11	12	13	14	15	16	17	18	19	87	B6	HAG	B9	
R	C	H	99999	9999	99999	9999	999999	9	99999	9999999	9999	99999	99	99	9999	9	99	9999	99999	99999	9999	9	9	99	99999999
E	E	L	WWWWW	WWWW	WWWWW	WWWW	WWWWWW	W	WWWWW	WWWWWWW	WWWW	WWWWW	WW	WW	WWWW	W	WW	WWWW	WWWWW	WWWWW	WWWW	W	W	WW	WWWWWWWW
G	L	A	00000	0000	00000	0000	000009	0	00000	0000011	1111	11111	11	11	1111	9	11	0100	00000	00000	0011	1	1	11	01111100
L	L	-	11111	2222	33333	4444	555559	7	88888	9999999	0000	11111	22	33	4444	9	77	7977	66666	66666	8866	5	8	88	59443086
A	I	D	00000	0000	00000	0000	000000	0	00000	0000000	0000	00000	00	00	0000	0	00	0000	00000	10100	0000	0	0	00	00000000
B	D	W	13542	1243	12534	1234	135421	2	48127	1425324	3125	54321	12	23	6342	2	12	1154	12345	18067	5612	3	2	13	63511439
SCAKIS	01001	2,18	22222	883-	12111	11-2	211224	4	21222	224-4-2	442-	12111	26	62	242-	2	26	2111	28686	42-22	1222	2	2	24	21222212
SCAKIS	01002	3,17	42124	212-	66618	21-1	111212	6	21222	222-2-2	222-	22222	22	22	222-	2	22	6882	12112	21-11	2122	2	1	22	16241222
SCAKIS	01003	2,3	42212	883-	88828	21-2	111112	1	12212	221-2-2	222-	11122	26	22	222-	2	22	1121	12221	41-21	1212	2	1	22	11221122
SCAKIS	01004	2,3	22412	888-	68828	11-2	111111	1	11112	222-1-1	212-	11111	24	12	222-	2	12	1111	24111	11-11	1221	2	1	22	11221211
SCAKIS	01005	17,18	12112	212-	41212	11-1	621212	6	22212	111-1-1	211-	21122	12	11	211-	2	11	6462	24624	42-12	2221	1	2	21	28112122
SCAKIS	01006	17,18	22114	221-	21111	21-1	211112	6	11122	112-1-2	422-	22121	22	12	212-	2	12	4342	46626	42-21	2222	2	1	22	28221124
SCATSB	12088	2,8	22222	8888	4222-	2222	622121	4	46888	111-642	2221	12111	22	22	2212	2	24	2122	12222	11111	2622	2	2	22	12112262
SCATSB	12089	2,13	42221	6888	1622-	2224	222121	6	24222	212-422	1222	22112	12	48	1122	1	22	4124	14422	12111	1421	1	2	24	12114121
SCATSB	12091	3,13	21122	1244	2422-	1112	112121	4	16236	111-621	1211	11111	11	44	1111	2	11	1121	12416	11111	2212	1	1	11	21112111
SCATSB	12093	2,8	64424	4888	2422-	2222	422221	6	88688	221-424	2222	12122	22	12	2622	2	42	2222	22424	12411	2622	2	2	22	22222261
SCATSB	12094	2,13	21222	4888	2421-	1222	811111	2	12121	211-622	2122	12212	12	48	1212	1	12	2122	11212	11111	1211	1	1	42	11112211
EAEKAS	18181	5,-	11-2-	222-	2-11-	2-2-	-64664	1	-----	-2222--	2622	622-2	11	-2	222-	2	12	-212	121-1	1221-	1211	-	2	44	--222111
EAEKAS	18182	5,10	11-1-	111-	1-11-	1-1-	-84482	1	-----	-1224--	8828	222-1	22	-1	112-	2	12	-211	111-2	1141-	4121	-	1	12	--111121
EAEKAS	18183	5,10	11-1-	111-	2-11-	1-1-	-84284	2	-----	-2221--	8348	412-1	12	-2	122-	2	14	-611	111-2	1111-	2111	-	1	26	--121422
EAEKAS	18184	5,10	11-1-	111-	1-21-	1-2-	-42284	1	-----	-1121--	8326	212-1	22	-1	211-	1	12	-211	111-1	1111-	1111	-	1	12	--212411
EAEKAS	18185	5,-	11-1-	111-	1-12-	2-1-	-88882	1	-----	-1112--	2611	111-1	11	-1	111-	2	12	-811	111-1	1121-	1161	-	2	26	--111211
EAEKAS	18186	10,-	11-1-	111-	1-12-	1-1-	-42111	1	-----	-1124--	8848	212-1	22	-2	112-	4	11	-411	111-2	2121-	2111	-	1	24	--112221
US7HAN	02008	9,19	11111	2212	21212	1122	4111-2	2	22121	3549623	2111	22211	22	12	2111	1	11	2121	21222	89888	1212	2	1	12	21122222
US7HAN	02009	3,-	21122	2121	88368	1222	2121-1	1	11121	1222111	2122	22221	12	22	2211	1	22	2221	12222	41221	1222	2	2	22	21221122
US7HAN	02011	9,-	21222	2211	22211	2122	2122-1	1	21121	6623645	4222	21212	21	22	2211	2	11	2121	22222	41221	2222	2	2	12	21221212
US7HAN	02012	19,-	21421	2222	12221	2242	4122-1	1	21122	1111121	2111	22222	11	22	2211	2	22	2122	22222	36888	1212	2	2	22	12211222
US7HAN	02013	3,9	22222	2221	88868	2222	2122-1	2	22122	6249688	2111	22242	22	22	4211	2	22	2222	22222	12222	1422	2	2	22	22211222
US7HAN	02015	19,-	22212	2222	26224	1126	2112-2	2	22122	1221121	2222	22222	24	11	2111	1	22	2121	24422	88839	1211	2	1	12	21111422
US7HAN	02017	3,19	22422	2224	69692	2242	4222-1	1	21222	2221221	2222	11222	21	22	2222	2	11	2221	42224	68835	2222	2	2	22	22212124
GERWAN	08063	12,19	21212	221-	11222	1121	421122	2	-6212	62226-1	2422	22222	68	22	2224	1	11	2122	12214	86866	2211	-	1	11	81222212
GERWAN	08064	2,14	21422	438-	12212	2222	121221	1	-1422	12111-1	6122	22212	22	11	8664	1	11	2122	22212	22222	2211	-	1	11	81441421
GERWAN	08065	14,19	11211	212-	12212	2122	121421	2	-2222	11112-1	4222	22222	12	11	6458	1	11	2221	12222	44842	2211	-	1	11	12241222
GERWAN	08066	2,12	22222	632-	22222	2111	121222	1	-2222	21222-2	1222	22222	86	24	2222	2	11	1121	22222	22222	1222	-	2	22	12222226
GERWAN	08067	2,12	24222	453-	21122	1111	121421	1	-4224	22244-1	2222	22221	84	22	2222	1	12	2121	22222	22222	2222	-	1	11	18222222
GERWAN	08068	2,12	22422	588-	24122	1111	411221	2	-2222	22224-1	2121	22221	86	22	4424	2	22	2221	22111	12222	2224	-	2	11	11222122
GERWAN	08069	12,14	22424	222-	22222	1221	121221	2	-2622	22222-1	4222	22221	88	22	8668	1	11	4224	21221	12222	2222	-	2	21	21641242
GERWAN	08070	2,12	11222	688-	42221	2212	111222	1	-2122	22222-2	2222	12122	96	22	2412	2	22	1211	11212	22422	2224	-	4	22	12122226
GERWAN	08071	2,19	12422	685-	41222	2221	122222	1	-2214	42222-1	4242	22121	24	22	4222	1	11	2122	22424	88646	2222	-	2	21	11222268
GERWAN	08072	14,19	21212	211-	21212	2211	121221	1	-1222	22211-1	2222	12221	11	22	6645	2	11	2212	22221	62382	1211	-	1	21	12221226
GERWAN	08073	14,19	22221	212-	11112	1221	121221	1	-2222	14222-1	2222	21121	22	22	6666	1	21	2221	12222	26426	2222	-	2	21	12461222
GERWAN	04020	4,8	22422	211-	21222	6668	122211	4	-8638	24222-1	4222	22222	22	22	2212	2	21	1221	22222	14122	6212	-	1	22	22122242
GERWAN	04021	5,-	22222	211-	21222	2221	688864	1	-2212	21221-2	2122	22212	22	21	2111	1	12	4222	22422	22122	4211	-	1	21	21112211
GERWAN	04022	4,-	42241	222-	11212	6866	222442	4	-2242	22122-4	4222	12222	41	22	1212	2	22	2222	22422	22222	4221	-	1	62	21112222
GERWAN	04023	4,-	12221	221-	42422	6888	622242	6	-2222	24122-1	6242	22842	22	11	2222	1	28	4224	11422	22222	2222	-	2	14	81112222
GERWAN	04024	4,-	21421	221-	21222	8368	222141	4	-2242	42142-8	2242	22222	21	22	2212	1	12	2122	22242	12222	2211	-	1	24	81121122
GERWAN	04026	4,-	21222	212-	24222	8826	224221	2	-2222	28221-1	2222	22212	22	22	2122	1	11	2122	22411	12222	2211	-	1	11	81221221
GERWAN	04027	5,8	21212	211-	21222	2121	654262	2	-6868	46242-1	2222	22221	22	22	2122	1	21	2121	12211	62424	2222	-	2	22	11222242
GERWAN	04028	5,8	11221	211-	11222	2112	442154	1	-8848	22222-1	1242	22221	42	42	1111	1	21	1121	21212	22121	2242	-	2	41	61112282
US7HAN	04026	8,16*	11124	1112	26112	2211	8222-2	4	36482	6222121	6625	22224	24	22	2611	2	88	2121	11122	11121	2212	1	1	22	21121282
US7HAN	04027	8,16	11124	1112	42212	2221	2222-1	1	68488	2111121	2121	22222	22	21	1111	1	88	1111	12212	21222	2212	1	2	11	21121242
US7HAN	04028	16,-	11122	1212	22211	1221	2222-4	2	22121	2221222	4122	12111	22	22	2211	1	88	2211	11112	21221	1222	2	2	22	21211222
US7HAN	04029	8,-	42222	1221	46222	2242	2222-2	2	68686	1221222	2221	22222	22	22	2222	2	24	2122	22222	12222	2422	2	2	22	22222262
US7HAN	04030	8,16	11211	1221	22222	2222	2221-1	2	86285	1121112	2221	22222	21	22	4211	2	88	2222	22222	22222	1422	1	2	22	22221222
US7HAN	04031	16,-	21126	2112	22211	1122	4112-4	1	14122	2124122	2244	12222	22	21	1211	2	88	2111	11222	11221	2222	4	2	24	21211222
SCAKIS	02007	2,5*	22162	188-	42121	22-2	888888	1	22222	241-1-2	222-	11121	68	82	212-	2	22	6211	28122	11-12	1112	2	2	12	82112128
SCAKIS	02008	5,11	22212	111-	14112	12-1	864861	6	22111	112-1-1	121-	68888	12	21	141-	1	12	4222	22121	21-11	2111	1	1	12	41111111
SCAKIS	02009	5,-	22111	212-	42212	12-1	638685	1	12112	222-2-2	222-	21112	22	21	242-	2	22	1111	21211	42-22	2224	4	2	22	21212212
SCAKIS	02010	5,11	22212	221-	11212	12-2	886621	6	12221	112-1-1	212-	86898	11	11	221-	1	11	1222	11111	22-11	2212	2	1	11	61111111
SCAKIS	02011	2,5	11112	668-	11111	12-1	858885	4	21122	122-1-1	212-	11111	16	21	212-	1	12	1211	12222	42-22	1122	2	1	22	61111111
SCAKIS	02012	2,11	22224	648-	14112	22-2	111112	6	21211	2-2-4-2	222-	68888	26	22	444-	2	22	1222	22222	21-11	2122	1	1	24	2242-212
SCAKIS	02013	2,11	11122	444-	42222	12-2	111111	4	22221	1-1-1-2	211-	22245	28	21	261-	2	12	4221	12222	12-22	1212	1	2	12	1-22-112
US7HAN	07048	7,19	12114	1226	42212	1221	2112-1	6	22122	2111211	2461	65898	42	21	1111	2	11	2264	22222	88888	1111	1	1	11	11211216
US7HAN	07049	7,-	24224	2222	24222	1121	1112-1	4	22121	2221421	2641	62466	22	22	2122	2	21	6464	11212	11222	1211	2	4	11	22222222
US7HAN	07050	7,-	12122	2222	21122	1111	4111-1	8	16121	2221422	2244	88868	22	22	2212	1	22	2244	11112	11221	2112	2	6	11	12221212
US7HAN	07053	19,-	22122	2226	24224	2222	4122-1	2	42122	2222221	2241	21122	22	22	2122	1	21	2211	42222	82866	2221	2	4	12	11222424
US7HAN	07055	7,19	12122	2228	22122	1112	4112-2	8	21121	2121211	2446	42224	22	22	2112	2	11	4266	24222	86886	2121	1	1	21	12221414
US7HAN	07056	7,-	24424	2221	22448	1222	2122-1	3	28124	2221211	4241	88888	22	11	1111	1	21	4266	24222	21222	1111	1	1	11	22121222
FRABET	13001	2,12	22212	688-	22222	2226	242221	4	1-211	4222221	2222	21122	88	12	2211	2	11	2211	22222	22222	2111	1	2	12	2-221212
FRABET	13002	1,-	88888	111-	12211	2122	112111	2	2-111	2222422	2222	22222	11	11	1211	2	11	2222	21121	11112	1211	1	1	22	1-221211
FRABET	13003	12,-	11211	222-	21111	2222	222222	1	1-112	2222422	2222	22222	84	22	1111	1	11	2212	22222	11111	1211	1	2	12	2-111221
FRABET	13004	1,2	85648	688-	21222	1124	221111	4	--111	2111122	2212	21211	22	12	2122	2	21	1221	12111	12111	1111	2	1	12	1-121211
FRABET	13005	1,2	88868	685-	24221	22-4	212121	2	--121	2122221	2222	21222	22	1-	22-1	1	21	1211	22111	11111	1122	1	1	11	2-221211
FRABET	13006	2,-	11111	588-	22221	2222	222211	1	--112	2222422	2212	22222	24	22	2212	2	21	2222	22122	11111	2112	2	2	22	2-222212
LATLAY	21025	5,16	21241	1241	21122	2221	886886	2	22442	221-122	8124	22144	22	21	2222	2	28	2111	2-422	21222	2222	4	2	42	24242122
LATLAY	21022	16,-	21121	1141	1-111	1111	1-11--	2	14-12	224-612	2-64	11222	11	11	181-	2	88	1112	-4626	42626	2121	1	2	21	2-14-21-
LATLAY	21016	16,-	24242	2242	6-222	2222	212122	4	22622	4221211	6222	22242	22	21	2422	2	88	2222	21422	21121	1221	4	2	22	16462221
LATLAY	21017	5,16	22412	4224	2-111	1212	884662	2	24421	2212411	2116	22222	21	21	1222	2	88	2422	21222	21222	2221	4	2	42	22262222
LATLAY	21023	16,-	66222	2241	6-242	2222	112122	6	21212	4221422	2212	22224	21	62	2212	2	84	2122	21224	22222	1211	2	2	21	12222112
LATLAY	21024	16,-	84224	4262	24242	2422	421121	1	21212	642-412	1121	12112	24	22	2222	2	88	2121	1-121	12212	6222	2	2	22	24122122

segregates independently from Dw2 which is present in the same individual (parent).

The Dw6 subgroups Dw18 and Dw19 are shown in SCAKIS 01 and US7HAN 07 respectively. Both subgroups are clearly defined, showing no cross-reactivity with each other and segregating independently in the respective families.

The new determinant Dw16 is demonstrated in two families US7HAN 04 and LATLAY 21. Although this specificity is defined by only two HTC, it clearly segregates in both cases.

The most difficult specificity in the present Workshop was Dw7 and its subgroups Dw17 and Dw11. In the families presented here, Dw17 segregates nicely in SCAKIS 01 and Dw11 in SCAKIS 02. On the other hand, Dw7 had to be assigned in family US7HAN 07 because of obvious cross-reactivity between the two subgroups. The latter case proved to be the most frequent when the analysis of the 100 families was performed.

Two cases of triplets are demonstrated here: SCAKIS 02007, with Dw2, Dw12, and Dw5, where the Dw12 determinant does not segregate according to the assignment rules mentioned above; and US7HAN 04026, reacting positively with Dw8, Dw16 and Dw10, where the latter determinant also does not segregate appropriately.

The 200 diplotypes of the 100 Workshop families are depicted in Fig. 1. Forty-four percent showed two HLA-D specificities, while 47% showed only

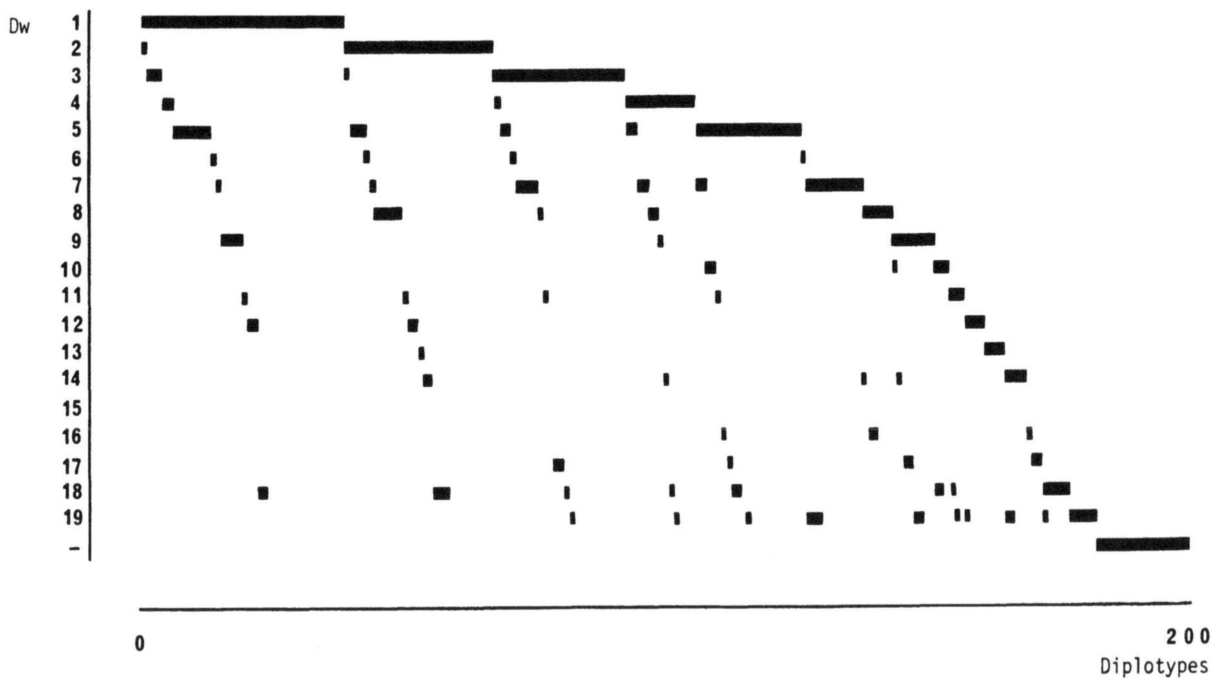

Fig. 1. HLA-D specificities in parents of 100 families included in the final analysis

Table 2. Segregation analysis in 100 (69%) of 145 families tested in the Workshop

HLA-D	w1	w2	w3	w4	w5	w6	w7	w8	w9	w10	w11	w12	w13	w14	w16	w17	w18	w19
Total no. parental haplotypes	38	29	29	16	34	4	21	14	13	7	7	8	5	9	4	7	17	18
Informative segregation	36	26	23	15	31	4	18	11	11	6	6	8	5	9	4	6	15	15

Total No. of family members typed: 635
Total No. of haplotypes: 1270
Total No. of "antigen(s) missing": 13 (≙ 2.05% of the individuals tested; 1.02% of the haplotypes defined)
Total No. of "triplets": 3

one and 8.5% none. The high number of blanks is due largely to deliberate selection of families with unknown specificities and to a lesser degree to experimental difficulties. The numbers, therefore, should not be compared with previous results [1, 2, 3].

Table 2 demonstrates the inheritance of the HLA-D specificities to the respective children in the Workshop families. Since most parental haplotypes could be indentified in the offspring, the respective HLA-D specificities represent well-defined entities. From a total of 635 individuals typed representing 1270 haplotypes, only 13 (≙ 1.02%) were set as "missing."

A comparison could be made between HLA-D and HLA-DR of the tested families. The HLA-DR data were based on the computer assignment of the Workshop (H. Deppe et al., Cell Typing by Computer, this volume). Only parental haplotypes were involved in this analysis. Haplotypes where no assignment could be made, either due to experimental problems for both HLA-D and/or HLA-DR or because of non-testing of the respective cells, were set as "blank.". As reported by G. Schreuder et al. (HLA-DR, DQ, LB, and TA10 Specificities of the Ninth Workshop Homozygous Typing Cells, this volume), it is at the moment still not possible to predict the HLA-D determinants based on HLA-DR and/or DQ typing of the tested cells. However, as shown in Table 3, HLA-D typing predicted without exception the HLA-DR type of the tested cells, when the haplotypes were informative for both HLA-D and DR (225 cases). These data, of course, require confirmation by more extensive family analyses.

In conclusion, in 69% of the submitted families and in 70% of the total family members, an HLA-D assignment could be made. 1.02% of HLA-D ha-

Table 3. Comparison between HLA-D and HLA-DR based on the Workshop data

HLA-D	HLA-DR 1	2	3	4	5	w6	7	8	w9	w10	blank[a]
w1	34	0	0	0	0	0	0	0	0	0	4
w2	0	27	0	0	0	0	0	0	0	0	1
w3	0	0	21	0	0	0	0	0	0	0	5
w4	0	0	0	16	0	0	0	0	0	0	0
w5	0	0	0	0	26	0	0	0	0	0	5
w6	0	0	0	0	0	3	0	0	0	0	1
w7	0	0	0	0	0	0	15	0	0	0	4
w8	0	0	0	0	0	0	0	12	0	0	2
w9	0	0	0	0	0	5	0	0	0	0	6
w10	0	0	0	7	0	0	0	0	0	0	0
w11	0	0	0	0	0	0	5	0	0	0	1
w12	0	5	0	0	0	0	0	0	0	0	2
w13	0	0	0	5	0	0	0	0	0	0	0
w14	0	0	0	7	0	0	0	0	0	0	2
w16	0	0	0	0	0	2	0	0	0	0	2
w17	0	0	0	0	0	0	6	0	0	0	1
w18	0	0	0	0	0	17	0	0	0	0	1
w19	0	0	0	0	0	12	0	0	0	0	5
blank[a]	3	14	4	19	19	7	6	4	9	7	29

[a] = not tested/not defined

plotypes could not be found in either parents or children. A total of three individuals showed "triplets".

Acknowledgements. The authors are grateful to Mr. H. Brandt for helpful discussions and advice on computer analysis and to Ms. S. Richter for typing the manuscript.

References

1. Thorsby E, Piazza A (1975) Joint report from the Sixth International Histocompatibility Workshop Conference. II. Typing for HLA-D (LD-1 or MLC) determinants. In: Kissmeyer-Nielsen F (ed) Histocompatibility testing 1975. Munksgaard, Copenhagen, pp 414–458
2. Lamm LU, Cullen P, Edwards JH, van Leeuwen A, Larsen B, Cann H, Thompson J, Albert E, Monk K, Richards S, Bodmer WF (1978) Family analysis. In: Bodmer WF, Batchelor JR, Bodmer JG, Festenstein H, Morris PJ (eds) Histocompatibility testing 1977. Munksgaard, Copenhagen, pp 279–293
3. Dupont B, Braun DW Jr, Yunis EJ, Carpenter CB (1980) Joint report: HLA-D by cellular typing. In: Terasaki PI (ed) Histocompatibility testing 1980. UCLA Tissue Typing Laboratory, Los Angeles, pp 229–267

Appendix A.

Lab.	Code	Participants	Institutions
ANZ	BSH	Bashir, Honeyman	Red Cross Blood Transfusion Service, Sydney, New South Wales, Australia
BEN	ROO	van Rood, Termijtelen	Academisch Ziekenhuis Leiden, Leiden, The Netherlands
EAE	NYU	Nyulassy, Buc	Medical Faculty, Department of Medical Microbiology and Immunology, Bratislava, CSSR
EAE	IVS	Ivaskova, Rychlikova	Czechoslovak Academy of Sciences, Praha, CSSR
EAE	KAS	Kastelan, Gerenčer	Tissue Typing Center KBC REBRO, Zagreb, Yugoslavia
EAE	MYR	Mayr, Hajek	Institut für Blutgruppenserologie der Universität Wien, Austria
EAE	PTR	Petranyi, Onodi	National Institute of Hematology and Blood Transfusion, Budapest, Hungaria
EAE	RIC	Richter, Menzel	Bezirksinstitut für Blutspende- und Transfusionswesen, Berlin, DDR
FRA	ARN	Arnaiz-Villena, Requeiro	S. de Immunologia, Centro Ramon y Cajal, Madrid, Spain
FRA	BET	Betuel, Freidel	CTS de Lyon, Miribel, France
GER	BRA	Brautbar	Hadassah Medical Center Lab. for Immunohematology, Jerusalem, Israel
GER	GSW	Grosse-Wilde, Doxiadis	Abteilung f. Immungenetik, Universitätsklinikum Essen, Germany
GER	WAN	Wank, Schendel	Immungenetisches Labor, Institut für Immunologie der Universität München, Germany
IT2	FER	Ferrara	Istituto scientifico per lo studio e la cura dei tumori, Genova, Italy
JAP	KSH	Kashiwagi	Kitasato University, School of Medicine, Dept. of Transplantation, Kanagawa-Ken, Japan

Appendix A (continued)

Lab	Code	Participants	Institutions
JAP	SAS	Sasazuki	Tokyo Medical & Dental University Medical Research Institute, Department of Human Genetics, Tokyo, Japan
JAP	TSU	Tsuji	Tokai University School of Medicine, Department of Transplantation, Kanagawa, Japan
LAT	LAY	Layrisse	Instituto Venezolano de Investigaciones Cientificas, Caracas, Venezuela
NCY	BIA	Bias, Hsu	The John Hopkins University Department of Medicine, Baltimore, U.S.A.
NCY	YUN	Yunis	Sidney Farber Cancer Institute, Division of Immunogenetics, Boston, U.S.A.
NCY	ZIE	Zier	Children Hospital of Philadelphia, Philadelphia, Pennsylvania, U.S.A.
SAF	DUT	du Toit, Oudshoorn	Provincial Laboratory for Tissue Immunology, Observatory, South Africa
SCA	KIS	Kissmeyer-Nielsen	Tissue Typing Laboratory, University Hospital, Aarhus, Denmark
SCA	SVE	Svejgaard, Platz, Ryder	Rigshospitalet, Tissue Typing Laboratory, København, Denmark
SCA	TSB	Thorsby	Rikshospitalet, Tissue Typing Laboratory, Oslo, Norway
UKI	BRS	Bradley, Stichcombe	U.K. Transplant Service, South Western Regional Transfusion Center, Bristol, U.K.
UKI	FES	Festenstein, Jaraquemada, Ollier	The London Hospital Medical College, Department of Immunology, London, U.K.
US2	BAC	Bach, Reinsmoen	University of Minnesota, Histocompatibility Labs., Minneapolis, U.S.A.
US4	STA	Stastny	Southwestern Medical School, Dept. of Internal Medicine, Dallas, U.S.A.
US7	HAN	Hansen, Mickelson	Puget Sound Blood Center, Fred Hutchinson Cancer Research Center, Seattle, U.S.A.

Total no. families tested	145	
Total no. family members tested	906	
Total no. unrelated individuals tested (including 64 HTCs as responders)	132	
	Family	Unrelated
Total no. HLA-D lab assignments	389	0
Total no. HLA-D computer assignments		
(max)	819	126
(min)	809	119
Total no. HLA-D workshop assignments	635	0

First Level Testing of HLA-DR4-Associated New HLA-D Specificities: Dw13 (DB3), Dw14 (LD40), Dw15 (DYT), and DKT2 *

D. Jaraquemada [1], N.L. Reinsmoen [2], W. Ollier [1], R. Okoye [1], F.H. Bach [2], and H. Festenstein [1]

1 Department of Immunology, London Hospital Medical College, Turner Street, London El 2AD, U.K.
2 Immunology Laboratory, Box 724, Mayo Memorial Building. University of Minnesota, Minneapolis, MN 55455, USA

HLA-DR4 is associated with several mixed lymphocyte culture (MLC)-defined HLA-D specificities. In addition to Dw4 and Dw10, four tentative Dw specificities were previously described: Dw13 [1, 2], Dw14 [3], Dw15 [4] and DKT2 [5]. Homozygous typing cells (HTC) defining these specificities were submitted to two reference laboratories (FES and BAC) for the first-level testing (Table 1). Checkerboard MLC experiments between all HTC were performed in both laboratories. A selected panel of previously HLA-D-typed heterozygous individuals were also tested with these HTC. The results in counts per minute (cpm) were sent to Essen where they were double-normalised to standardised relative responses (SRR). These were then pooled for each responder/stimulator combination and the mean SRR was calculated. In case of more than two testings, the median SRR was used. Scores were calculated from these mean/median SRR according to the criteria previously described [1]. Correlation coefficients were calculated from 2 × 2 contingency tables of the assigned scores.

* This work was generously supported by the Nuffield Foundation and the Arthritis and Rheumatism Council of Great Britain

Table 1. List of HTC

ID	Specificity [a]	Workshop no.	Lab. of origin	HLA type					
PEA	Dw13 (DB3)	9w1302	GSW	A31	B51	C –	DR4	DQw3	DPw4
FLE	Dw13 (DB3)	–	FES	A2	Bw63	Cw7	DR4	DQw3	DPw4
RED	Dw13 (DB3)	–	FES	A2	Bw63	Cw7	DR4	DQw3	DPw4
JHA	Dw13 (DB3)	9w1301	FES	A31	B51	C –	DR4	DQw3	DPw3
SSTO	Dw13 (DB3)	9w1303	HSU	A32	B44	Cw5	DR4	DQw3	
DSTO	Dw13 (DB3)	–	HSU	A32	B44	Cw5	DR4	DQw3	
JDS	Dw13 (DB3)	8w327	BET	A24	B51	Cw2	DR4	DQw3	
KT2	DKT2	–	KSH	A2	B51	C –	DR4		
KT13	DKT2	–	KSH	A24, 31	B7, 51	C –	DR4		
LS40	Dw14 (LD40)	9w1403	BAC	A1, 26	B27, w60		DR4	DQw3	
BIN40	Dw14 (LD40)	9w1401	BAC	A2, 31	B14, w60		DR4	DQw3	
MT	Dw14 (LD40)	9w1404	BSH	A31	Bw60	Cw3	DR4	DQw3	DPw2, 3
KY	Dw14 (LD40)	9w1402	BSH	A31	Bw60	Cw3	DR4	DQw3	
CHOP40	Dw14 (LD40)	–	BAC	A31, 32	Bw60		DR4	DQw3	
070A	Dw14 (LD40)	9w1406	HAN	A2, 3	Bw60	Cw3	DR4	DQw3	
PEM	Dw14 (LD40)	9w1405	BET	A2	B35, w60	Cw2, w4	DR4	DQw3	
BPET	Dw14 (LD40)	–	HSU				DR4	DQw3	
AL10	Dw10	9w1001	BAC	A26	B38		DR4	DQw3	
TS10	Dw10	9w1005	BAC	A26	B38		DR4	DQw3	DPw4
LEO10	Dw10	9w1002	BAC	A26	B35		DR4	DQw3	
EM10	Dw10	8w210	BAC	A26	B38		DR4	DQw3	
KT3	Dw15 (DYT)	–	KSH	A24	Bw54	Cw1	DR4		
HAS15	Dw15 (DYT)	9w9902	BAC	A2	Bw54, w62	Cw1, w3	DR4	DQw3	
JORI	Dw4	–	BAC				DR4	DQw3	
MJ4	Dw4	–	BAC	A2	B35, w62		DR4	DQw3	DPw4
SM4	Dw4	–	BAC	A2, 32	B44, 39		DR4	DQw3	DPw3, 4
NIN	Dw4	–	BAC	A24	Bw61		DR4	DQw3	
JAH	Dw4	9w0403	HAN	A2	Bw62	Cw3	DR4	DQw3	DPw3, 4

[a] Old nomenclature in parenthesis

Histocompatibility Testing 1984
Edited by E. D. Albert et al.

Table 2. Checkerboard MLC results between DR4-positive HTC

		Dw13 (DB3)	DKT2	Dw14 (LD40)	Dw10	Dw15 (DYT)	Dw4
Dw13 (DB3)	PEA[a]	3333333	33	12211111	311	12	21131
	FLE	133133.	33	3123....	...	1.	.....
	RED	3.333.3	..	12222113	322	13	23321
	JHA	3333323	11	12111111	211	11	11111
	SSTO	3332333	13	11111112	211	11	31111
	DSTO	233233.	33	11111...	...	1.	.....
	JDS	1.323.3	..	11111112	111	.2	11111
DKT2	KT2	121232.	33	23112...	...	1.	.....
	KT13	133333.	33	11111...	...	1.	.....
Dw14 (LD40)	LS40	1111111	31	33332321	111	11	11111
	BIN40	1112111	12	33333322	111	11	11111
	MT	1211111	11	33333332	212	11	11121
	KY	1111111	11	33332232	111	11	11111
	CHOP40	1.11..1	..	33113321	121	.1	11211
	070A	1.11..1	..	23233332	121	.1	11111
	PEM	1.11..1	..	33332333	111	.1	11111
	BPET	2.13..1	..	33333212	121	.1	21311
Dw10	AL10	2.33..1	..	11111111	333	.2	12121
	TS10	1.13..2	..	11111111	333	.1	11111
	LEO10	1.12..1	..	11111111	333	.1	11111
Dw15 (DYT)	KT3	111121.	11	21111...	...	3.	.....
	HAS15	1.111.1	..	11111111	111	.3	21111
Dw4	JORI	2.11..1	..	11111111	331	.1	33333
	MJ4	1.11..1	..	11111111	111	.1	33333
	SM4	1.11..1	..	11111111	111	.1	33333

[a] Scores: 1, SRR > 65; 2, SRR 45 – 64.9; 3, SRR < 45; ·, not tested

Checkerboard Analysis

Table 2 shows the results of checkerboard testing between all the HTC. Clear differences were seen between HTC defining the specificities Dw13, Dw14 and Dw15 when compared to each other as well as to Dw4 and Dw10. DKT2 HTC showed high cross-reactivity with the Dw13 HTC but not with any of the others.

Panel Studies

The results of typing a selected panel of heterozygous responder cells are given in Table 3. Some were tested in both reference laboratories. The definitions of the Dw13, Dw14 and Dw15 specificities were as clear as those of Dw10 and Dw4. The only DKT2 HTC tested showed no cross-reactions with Dw13 when typing heterozygous responders. No DKT2-positive heterozygous individuals were available.

Correlations

The significant ($p < 0.01$) correlation coefficients between the HTC are shown in Table 4. Most HTC showed clear clustering with those defining the same specificity and no association with the others: DSTO and JDS showed poor association with other Dw13 HTC, but were clearly associated with the definition of the specificity.

PEM and BPET also showed poor correlations with Dw14 HTC.

Dw15 HTC could not be correlated because no Dw15-positive heterozygous individuals were tested by both HTC. However, both clearly defined the specificity.

The DKT2 specificity could not be defined at the first level. Two cells tested, KT2 and KT13, showed clear cross-reactivity in checkerboard MLC but not in panel testings with Dw13. The relationship between these two specificities remains unclear. They have been described separately in different populations; however, previous reports have suggested that this cross-reactivity exists in Caucasoid and Mongoloid populations [6, 7, 8].

First-level data demonstrate the clear definition of three new HLA-DR4-related HLA-D specificities: Dw13, Dw14 and Dw15. All three have now been officially recognised by the Nomenclature Committee 1984. Four DR4-positive individuals (nos. 44–47, Table 3) were negative for all of them, indicating that more DR4-associated Dw specificities have yet to be defined.

Table 3. Heterozygous panel typing of DR4-positive HTC

	Dw13 (DB3)	DKT2[a]	Dw14 (LD40)	Dw10	Dw15 (DYT)	Dw4	Dw	DR
1	2333332	1	11111111	1111	11	11111	13 3	4 3
2	3133313	1	21111111	1111	12	21121	13 –	4 4
3	3233311	1	11111111	2333	11	11111	13 10	4 4
4	3313333	2	2123111.	1211	21	21111	13 5	4 5
5	3333312	1	12111111	1111	21	11111	13 7	4 7
6	3333211	1	1311111.	1111	11	11111	13 8	4 8
7	1.213.3	.	11111111	1111	.1	11111	13 8	4 8
8	2.233.3	.	11111111	1111	.1	11111	13 3	4 3
9	3.313.3	.	21111111	1221	.1	11121	13 1	4 1
10	1.323.3	.	11111111	1211	.1	11111	13 6	4 6
11	3.333.3	.	11111111	1111	.1	11121	13 3	4 3
12	2.313.3	.	11111111	1111	.1	11111	13 7	4 7
13	3.313.3	.	11311111	1111	.1	11111	13 –	. .
14	333313.	1	111.1...	...1	2.	.....	13 7	4 7
15	133133.	2	111.1...	...2	1.	.....	13 –	4 –
16	133233.	2	131.1...	...1	1.	.....	13 3	4 3
17	233133.	3	133.1...	...3	1.	.....	13 3	4 3
18	1.131.1	.	33331311	1111	.1	11111	14 3	4 3
19	1.111.1	.	32321311	1111	.1	11111	14 3	4 3
20	1.111.1	.	33311111	1111	.2	31111	14 –	4 –
21	1.111.1	.	23313323	1111	.1	11111	14 –	4 –
22	1.111.1	.	32321313	1111	.1	11111	14 8	4 8
23	1.111.1	.	33333313	1111	.1	11111	14 2	4 2
24	1.111.1	.	33333112	1111	.1	22111	14 3	4 3
25	1.111.1	.	33313321	1111	.1	33213	14 4	4 4
26	1111111	1	31331323	1111	21	11111	14 6	4 6
27	11.111.	1	333.3...	...3	2.	.....	14 2	4 2
28	11.131.	3	333.3...	...2	3.	.....	14 7	4 7
29	11.111.	1	333.2...	...1	2.	.....	14 1	4 1
30	11.11..	1	211.....	...3	2.	.....	10 5	4 5
31	1.111.1	.	11111211	3333	.1	11111	10 7	4 7
32	1.111.1	.	11111111	3333	.1	11111	10 2	4 2
33	2.131.1	.	11111111	3333	.1	11111	10 5	4 5
34	1.111.2	.	11111111	3333	.1	11111	10 5	4 5
35	1.111.1	.	11111111	3333	.1	11111	10 –	. .
36	1.111.3	.	11111111	3213	.3	11111	10 YT?	9 –
37	1.111.1	.	11111111	1111	.3	11111	15 5	4 5
38	1.111.1	.	11111111	1111	.3	11111	15 5	4 5
39	111111.	1	111.1...	...1	3.	.....	15 5	4 5
40	11.111.	1	111.1...	...2	3.	.....	15 B7	4 8
41	1.111.1	.	11111111	1111	.1	23133	4 7	4 7
42	1.111.1	.	11111111	1111	.1	33232	4 3	4 3
43	1.111.1	.	11111111	1111	.1	33133	4 5	4 5
44	1.111.1	.	11111111	1111	.1	11111	– 6	4 6
45	111111.	1	311.2...	...1	31	.....	– 3	4 3
46	3.131.1	.	11111111	1111	.1	11111	– 6	4 6
47	11.131.	2	131.1...	...1	1.	.....	– 1	4 1

Scores as in Table 2. Stimulators in the same order as in Table 1

[a] Only KT13 used

., not tested

Table 4. Significant correlation coefficients ($p < 0.01$) between DR4-positive HTC

Dw13 (DB3)	PEA	–																											
	FLE	.41	–																										
	RED	.55	.75	–																									
	JHA	.58	.48	.37	–																								
	SSTO	.40	.56	.78	.30	–																							
	DSTO	*	.81	.56	.51	.52	–																						
	JDS	.52	*	.59	*	.81	.52	–																					
DKT2	KT2	*	*	*	*	*		*	–																				
	KT13	*	*	*	*	.53	.48	*	.66	–																			
Dw14 (LD40)	LS40	*	*	*	*	*	*	*	*	*	–																		
	BIN40	*	*	*	*	*	*	*	*	*	.63	–																	
	MT	*	*	*	*	*	*	*	*	*	.79	.66	–																
	KY	*	*	*	*	*	*	*	*	*	.68	.59	.59	–															
	CHOP40	*	*	*	*	*	*	*	*	*	.53	.63	.51	.48	–														
	070A	*	*	*	*	*	*	*	*	*	.71	.62	.68	.53	.56	–													
	PEM	*	*	*	*	*	*	*	*	*	*	.45	*	.53	*	*	–												
	BPET	*	*	*	*	*	*	*	*	*	.37	*	.47	*	*	.42	*	–											
Dw10	AL10	*	*	*	*	*	*	*	*	*	*	*	*	*	*	*	*	*	–										
	TS10	*	*	*	*	*	*	*	*	*	*	*	*	*	*	*	*	*	.78	–									
	LEO10	*	*	*	*	*	*	*	*	*	*	*	*	*	*	*	*	*	.72	.92	–								
	EM10	*	*	*	*	*	*	*	*	*	*	*	*	*	*	*	*	*	.91	.91	.91	–							
Dw15 (DYT)	KT3	*	*	*	*	*	*	*	*	*	*	*	*	*	*	*	*	*	*	*	*	*	–						
	HAS15	*	*	*	*	*	*	*	*	*	*	*	*	*	*	*	*	*	*	*	*	*	NC	–					
Dw4	JORI	*	*	*	*	*	*	*	*	*	*	*	*	*	*	*	*	*	*	*	*	*	*	*	–				
	MJ4	*	*	*	*	*	*	*	*	*	*	*	*	*	*	*	*	*	*	*	*	*	*	*	.71	–			
	SM4	*	*	*	*	*	*	*	*	*	*	*	*	*	*	*	*	*	*	*	*	*	*	*	.48	.68	–		
	NIN	*	*	*	*	*	*	*	*	*	*	*	*	*	*	*	*	*	*	*	*	*	*	*	.62	.77	.52	–	
	JAH	*	*	*	*	*	*	*	*	*	*	*	*	*	*	*	*	*	*	*	*	*	*	*	.68	.84	.57	.74	–
Antigen definition	Dw13	.62	.80	.83	.37	.80	.62	.79	*	*	*	*	*	*	*	*	*	*	*	*	*	*	*	*	*	*	*	*	*
	DKT2	*	*	*	*	*	*	*	*	*	*	*	*	*	*	*	*	*	*	*	*	*	*	*	*	*	*	*	*
	Dw14	*	*	*	*	*	*	*	*	*	.86	.73	.86	.65	.68	.83	.42	.44	*	*	*	*	*	*	*	*	*	*	*
	Dw10	*	*	*	*	*	*	*	*	*	*	*	*	*	*	*	*	*	.77	.87	.94	.87							
	Dw15	*	*	*	*	*	*	*	*	*	*	*	*	*	*	*	*	*	*	*	*	*	.74	.78	*	*	*	*	*
	Dw4	*	*	*	*	*	*	*	*	*	*	*	*	*	*	*	*	*	*	*	*	*	*	*	.77	.95	.52	.83	.91

r values calculated from 2×2 contingency tables
*, Not significant; NC, not computable: no Dw15 positive responder tested with both HTC

Acknowledgment. We are grateful to Denny Williams for typing the manuscript.

References

1. Jaraquemada D, Ollier W, Okoye RC, Sachs JA, Festenstein H, Grosse-Wilde H (1983) Tissue Antigens 22:315
2. Dupont B, Braun DW Jr, Yunis EJ, Carpenter CB (1980) In: Terasaki PI (ed) Histocompatibility testing 1980. UCLA, Los Angeles, p 229
3. Reinsmoen NL, Bach FH (1982) Hum Immunol 4:249
4. Sasazuki T, McMichael A, Payne R, McDevitt HO, Yakura H, Wakisaki A, Aizawa M, Itakura K (1977) Tissue Antigens 9:62
5. Sasazuki T, Kaneora H, Tsuji K, Nose Y, Kashiwagi N Kaneko T (1980) In: Terasaki PI (ed) Histocompatibility testing 1980. UCLA, Los Angeles, pp 274–276
6. Jaraquemada D, Alonso A, Awad J, D'Amaro J, Ollier W, Doyle P, Okoye RC, Williams E, Festenstein H, Lian F, Gouangyan Z, Renbiao E, Jenchieh T (1984) Tissue Antigens 23:23
7. Nose Y, Sato K, Nakagawa M, Kondoh K, Inouye H, Tsuji K (1982) Hum Immunol 5:199
8. Nose Y, Inouye H, Tsuji K, Reinsmoen N, et al (1982) Jpn J Transplantation 17:3

First Level Testing of Dw6 HTC*

A. Termijtelen[1] and E.M. Mickelson[2]

1 Department of Immunohematology and Blood Bank, University Hospital, Rijnsburgerweg 10, 2333 AA Leiden, The Netherlands
2 Puget Sound Blood Center and Fred Hutchinson Cancer Research Center, Seattle, Washington, USA

The data obtained from the Seventh and Eighth Workshops indicated that Dw6 is a heterogeneous specificity, possibly consisting of three subtypes: Dw6.1, 6.2 and 6.3 [1, 2]. We prescreened all Dw6 homozygous typing cells (HTC) offered to the Ninth Workshop, thus allowing a selection of representative HTC for each provisionally defined Dw6 subgroup.

An MLC matrix was performed in Leiden between 25 Dw6 HTC, listed in Table 1, and 13 non-Dw6 HTC. Two clusters of typing reactions were observed (Fig. 1).

Results of a comparable experiment, performed in Seattle, showed the same two clusters (Fig. 2). Cluster 1 was provisionally referred to as Dw6A and Cluster 2 as Dw6B (later officially assigned as Dw18 and Dw19 respectively). The cells 97D and possibly DLO were heterozygous for Dw6A and Dw6B and thus no good as typing cells. The specificity of cell KSH (9w0609) was not clear from these experiments [3].

Typing a panel of Dw6/X heterozygous responder cells clearly showed, in both the Leiden and the Seattle experiments, the same division of typing cells into two clusters. The overall correlation coefficients for the Dw6 HTC are given in Table 2. Within the Dw6A subgroup, some HTC appeared to be "shorter" than the others, i.e., gave fewer typing reactions. Whether this is the result of differences in technique or implies further heterogeneity within Dw6 cannot be concluded from the present experiments. No serological distinction

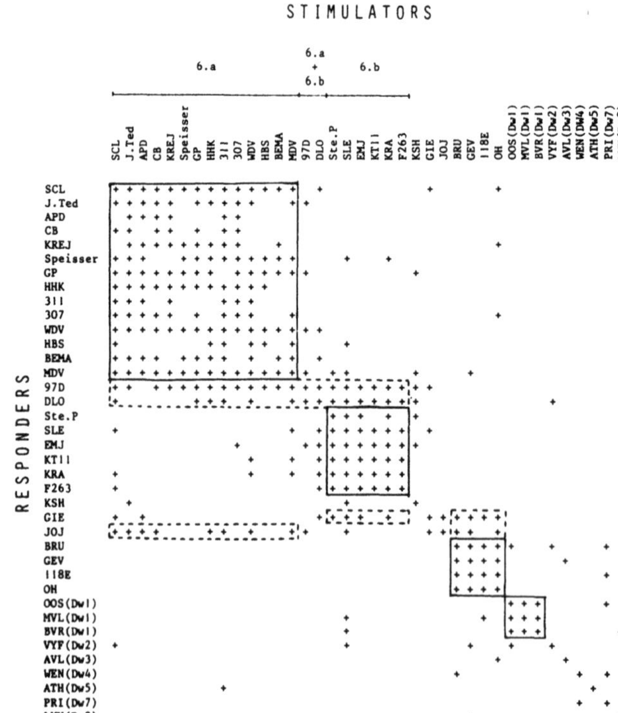

Fig. 1. Leiden MLC matrix of Dw6 HTC. +, typing reactions according to local analysis

* Supported in part by the Dutch Foundation for Medical Research (FUNGO), which is subsidized by the Dutch Organization for the Advancement of Pure Research (ZWO), and the J. A. Cohen Institute for Radiopathology and Radiation Protection (IRS)

Histocompatibility Testing 1984
Edited by E. D. Albert et al.

Table 1. Dw6 HTC submitted for first level testing

Label	Region	WS75	WS77	WS80	WS84	HLA-A, -B, -C[a]	-DP[a]	First-level assignment	New designation
HBS	BET				9w0601	A28, 2; B27, 39; Cw2	1	Dw6A	Dw18
HHK	ROO				9w0602	A3, B7, Cw7/A3, B7, Cw7	4	Dw6A	Dw18
J. Ted	STA			8w145	9w0603	A2, B27, Cw1/A29, B35, Cw4	n.t.	Dw6A	Dw18
SCL	GSW				9w0604	A2, B44, Cw5/A2, B44, Cw5	2, 4	Dw6A	Dw18
WDV	ROO	15006	7w512	8w149	9w0605	A2, B38/A2, B38	2, 4	Dw6A	Dw18
EMJ	HAN				9w0606	A2, Bw60, Cw3/A3, Bw60, Cw3	n.t.	Dw6B	Dw19
KRA	GSW				9w0607	A2, Bw60, Cw3/A2, Bw60, Cw3	n.t.	Dw6B	Dw19
SLE	HAN			8w146	9w0608	A2, Bw60, Cw3/A2, Bw60, Cw3	3	Dw6B	Dw19
KSH	FES				9w0609	A3, 28; B14, 27; Cw2, w8	n.t.	?	?
KT11	TSU			8w405	9w0610	Aw33, B44/Aw33, B44	2, 4	Dw6B	Dw19
Ste.P[b]	HSU				9w0611	A11, Bw60, Cw3/A11, Bw60, Cw3	n.t.	Dw6B	Dw19
311	KIS					A2; Bw60, w62; Cw3	4	Dw6A	Dw18
307	KIS					A2, 24; Bw62; Cw3	4	Dw6A	Dw18
Speiss	MYE					A2, B44, Cw5/A2, B44, Cw5	n.t.	Dw6A	Dw18
KREJ	IVS	8001	7w515	8w150		A2, Bw62, Cw3/A2, Bw62, Cw6	n.t.	Dw6A	Dw18
BEMA	BET					A3, 31; Bw47, w55; Cw3, w3	n.t.	Dw6A	Dw18
GP	SVE					A3, B38/A32, B38	n.t.	Dw6A	Dw18
CB	BSH					A1, Bw62, Cw3/A1, Bw62, Cw3	n.t.	Dw6A	Dw18
APD	ROO			8w148		A1, Bw60/A1, Bw60	4	Dw6A	Dw18
MDV	ROO					A2, B38/A2, B51	2, 4	Dw6A	Dw18
HRU	IVS	8008	7w514	8w151		A31, B8, Cw7/A31, B8, Cw7	n.t.	Dw6B	Dw19
F263	BET					A24, Bw55, Cw3/A31, B39	2, 4	Dw6B	Dw19
Mar.P[b]	HSU					A11, Bw60, Cw3/A11, Bw60, Cw3	n.t.	Dw6B	Dw19
97D	BET			8w326		A1, 3; B39, w64; Cw7, w8	n.t.	Dw6B	Dw19
DLO	HAN					A2, 30; B27, w60; Cw2, w3	2, 3	?	?

[a] HLA-A, -B, -C and -DP assignments are combined results of local assignments and typings performed in Leiden.
[b] HLA-identical siblings.

Table 2. Correlation coefficients for the Dw6 HTC

	SCL	WDV	MDV	HHK	APD	GP	BEMA	J.Ted	CB	Spei	HBS	311	307	KREJ	KSH	97D	Step	EMJ	KRA	Marp	KT11	F263	SLE	DLO
SCL	×	.5	.5	.5	.5	.5	.5	.4	.4	.4	.4	–	–	–	–	–	–	–	–	–	–	–	–	–
WDV		×	.7	.5	.5	.5	.5	.5	.4	–	.4	.6	.5	–	–	–	–	–	–	–	–	–	–	–
MDV			×	.5	.4	.6	.4	.4	.4	.4	.5	.4	–	–	–	–	–	–	–	–	–	–	–	–
HHK				×	.7	.6	.5	.6	.6	.4	.5	.6	.5	.5	–	–	–	–	–	–	–	–	–	–
APD					×	.6	.5	.8	.7	.5	–	.5	.5	.6	–	–	–	–	–	–	–	–	–	–
GP						×	.5	.6	.6	.6	.5	.5	.5	.5	–	–	–	–	–	–	–	–	–	–
BEMA							×	.4	.4	.4	.6	–	.4	–	.5	–	–	–	–	–	–	–	–	–
J.Ted								×	.7	.5	–	.6	.6	.6	–	–	–	–	–	–	–	–	–	–
CB									×	.4	.4	.6	.6	.6	–	–	–	–	–	–	–	–	–	–
Speis										×	.5	–	–	–	–	–	–	–	–	–	–	–	–	–
HBS											×	.4	–	–	–	–	–	–	–	–	–	–	–	–
311												×	.7	.5	–	–	–	–	–	–	–	–	–	–
307													×	.7	–	–	–	–	–	–	–	–	–	–
KREJ														×	–	–	–	–	–	–	–	–	–	–
KSH															×	–	–	–	–	.4	–	–	–	–
97D																×	–	–	–	–	–	–	–	–
Ste.P																	×	.8	.8	.7	.6	.6	.5	–
EMJ																		×	.8	.8	.8	.7	.5	–
KRA																			×	.8	.7	.7	.5	–
Mar.P																				×	.8	.6	.5	–
KT11																					×	.7	.5	–
F263																						×	.4	–
SLE																							×	–
DLO																								×

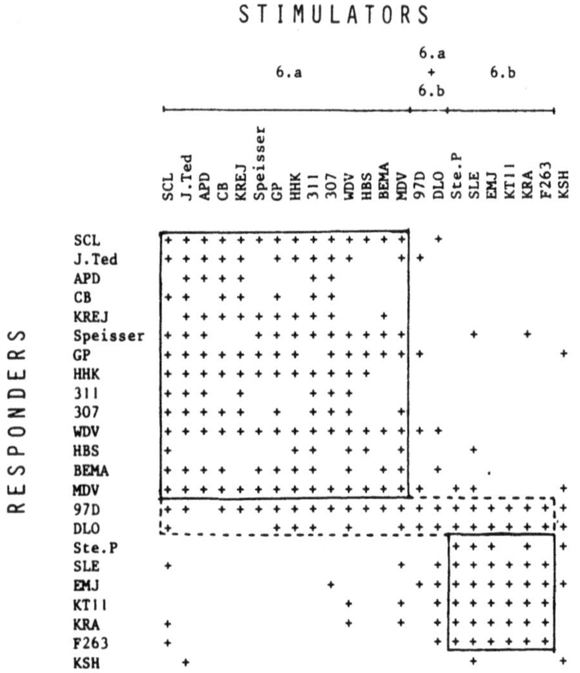

Fig. 2. Seattle MLC matrix of Dw6 HTCs. +, typing reactions according to local analysis

could so far be made between the two subgroups. All cells typed DRw13 (w6), DRw52, DQw1.

Comparing our data with the Eighth Workshop results we conclude that the subtype Dw18 may be identical to Dw6.3 and Dw19 to Dw6.1. The existence of Dw6.2 could in our experiments not be confirmed. This might be due to the fact that none of the Dw6.2 HTCs described in the previous workshop was included in the present experiments.

References

1. Festenstein H, Oliver RTD, et al (1978) Overall analysis of the HTC data based on clusters, patterns, and antigen reports. In: Bodmer WF, Batchelor JR, Bodmer JG, Festenstein H, Morris PG (eds) Histocompatibility testing 1977. Munksgaard, Copenhagen, p 115
2. Dupont B, Braun DW, Yunis EJ, Carpenter CB (1980) HLA-D by cellular typing. In: Terasaki PI (ed) Histocompatibility testing 1980. UCLA Tissue Typing Laboratory, Los Angeles, p 229
3. Termijtelen A, Schreuder GMT, Michelson EM, Van Rood JJ (1984) Ninth International Histocompatibility Preworkshop testing of Dw6 HTCs. Two subtypes of Dw6. Tissue Antigens 24:10

First Level Testing of Dw7 HTC

M. Honeyman[1], S.H. Hsu[2], G. Hakos[1], C. Rayment[1], M.M. Chan[2], and H. Bashir[1]

1 New South Wales Red Cross Blood Transfusion Service, 153 Clarence Street, Sydney, N.S.W. 2000, Australia
2 The John Hopkins University Department of Medicine Division of Medical Genetics, 807 Traylor, 720 Rutland Avenue, Baltimore, MD 21205, USA

First-level testing of the Dw7 homozygous typing cells (HTC) indicated in Table 1 was carried out in two laboratories, Sydney and Baltimore, in order to ensure a selection of HTC representative of any possible subgroups. The protocol for the Eighth International Histocompatibility Workshop [1] was followed for these tests.

Results of the checkerboard MLC tests between the HTC are indicated in Fig. 1 (Sydney) and Fig. 2 (Baltimore). Three major subgroups are apparent in Fig. 1, in close agreement with the results in Fig. 2. Several HTC tested were heterozygous for the Dw7 subgroups as follows: Sm11: 7.1, 7.2; AR: 7.2, 7.3; 2APO, 20657, WE5: 7.3, 7.4.

HTC of subgroups 7.2 and 7.3 typed on HTC of subgroup 7.1, but not vice versa. HTC of subgroup 7.2 were mutually stimulatory with those of subgroup 7.3.

The correlation matrix of r values ($x\ 10^{-2}$) derived from both checkerboard tests and typings of 40 heterozygous panel cells (Fig. 3) extends the observation of the three subgroups. Correlations were highest within subgroups 7.1, 7.2, and 7.3 (mean r 0.61, 0.55, and 0.47). Between subgroups 7.1 and 7.2 the mean r was 0.35 and between subgroups 7.1 and 7.3 it was 0.40, whereas between subgroups 7.2 and 7.3 it was only 0.12. Table 2 lists the salient features of each subgroup.

References

1. Dupont B, Braun DW, Yunis EJ, Carpenter CB: HLA-D by cellular typing. In: PI Terasaki, Ed., Histocompatibility testing 1980. Los Angeles, UCLA Tissue Typing Laboratory, 1980, p 229

Histocompatibility Testing 1984
Edited by E. D. Albert et al.

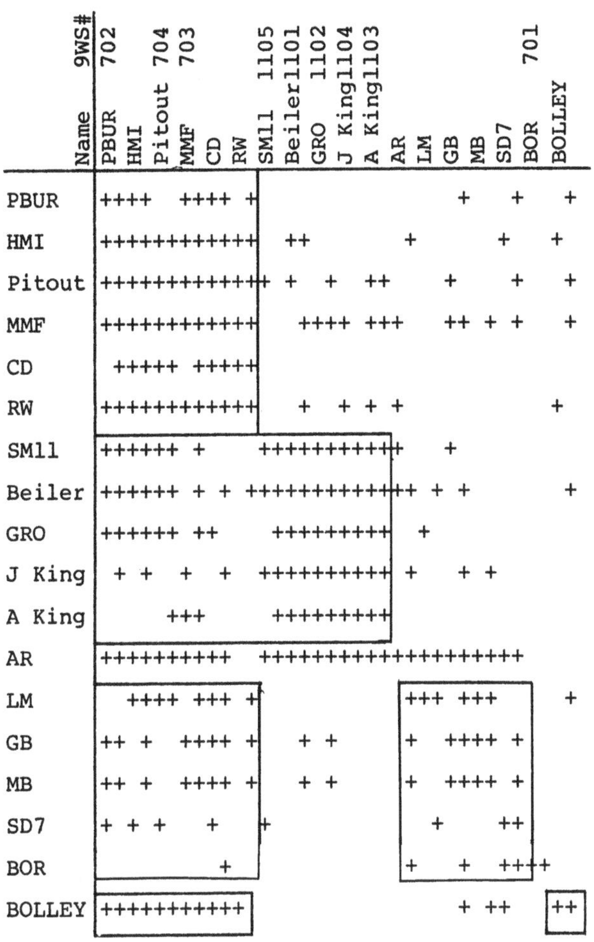

Fig. 1. MLC checkerboard of Dw7 HTC in Sydney

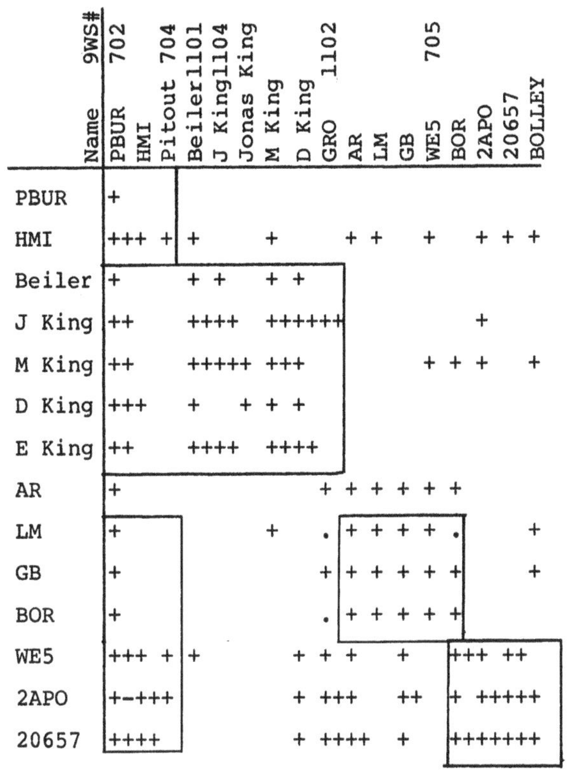

Fig. 2. MLC checkerboard of Dw7 HTC in Baltimore

Table 1. HTCs submitted to the Dw7 preworkshop

Label	Laboratory	Workshop no.	HLA		
			A	B	DR
Bolley	MYR		1, –	8, 12	7, –
BOR	GSW	9w701	30, –	13, –	7, –
Burkhardt	HSU	9w702, 8w156	1, 2	14, –	7, –
HMI	FES	8w157	23, –	44, –	7, –
MMF	YUN	9w703	2, –	14, –	7, –
Pitout	DTO	9w704, 7w557	29, –	44, –	7, –
SD7	YUN		2, 30	13, 44	7, –
SM11	YUN	9w1105	1, 25	44, w57	7, –
Beiler	HSU	9w1101, 8w164	2, –	w57, –	7, –
GRO	GSW	9w1102, 8w166	2, –	w57, –	7, –
John King	HSU	9w1104, 8w163	2, 24	w57, –	7, –
Aaron King	HSU	9w1103	24, –	w57, –	7, –
Jonas King	HSU		24, –	57, –	7, –
Moses King	HSU		24, –	57, –	7, –
20657	BET	8w159	23, 32	44, w63	7, –
2APO	BET		1, 29	12, 7	7, –
LAD	BRA		30, –	7, –	7, –
WE5(WET)	WER	8w158, 9w705	28, –	44, –	7, –
AR	BSH		1, 2	8, –	7, –
CD	BSH		28, 29	12, –	7, –
GB	BSH		2, 28	13, –	7, –
LM	BSH	8w303	2, 29	44. –	7, –
MB	BSH		2, 28	13, –	7, –
RW	BSH		2, 23	44, –	7, –

Table 2. Summary of subgroups of Dw7

Subgroup	8th WS name	Linkage disequilibrium		HTC
		HLA-B	DQ	
7.1	Dw7	B14, 44	w2	PBUR, HMI, Pitout, MMF, CD, RW
7.2	Dw11	Bw57	w3	Beiler, GRO, A King, J King
7.3	DB1	B13	w2	LM, GB, MB, BOR

r x 10^{-2}

	PBUR	HMI	Pitout	MMF	CD	RW	BOR	SM11	Beiler	GRO	J King	A King	AR	LM	GB	MB	Bolley	SD7
PBUR	*																	
HMI	64	*																
Pitout	59	65	*															
MMF	77	56	64	*														
CD	62	62	60	54	*													
RW	54	56	69	67	52	*												
BOR	60	64	60	59	58	54	*											
SM11	40	45	35	45	32	44	26	*										
Beiler	36	20	16	27	30	12	57	57	*									
GRO	48	57	52	50	44	42	45	45	49	*								
J King	52	34	24	30	22	21	39	39	56	59	*							
A King	32	23	29	22	18	34	34	34	47	56	63	*						
AR	55	48	37	40	33	26	34	34	20	30	31	14	*					
LM	50	26	26	38	28	24	15	15	17	23	23	14	47	*				
GB	44	50	46	47	49	50	28	28	01	26	07	05	52	56	*			
MB	44	43	54	51	48	38	14	14	08	35	14	13	29	39	36	*		
BOLLEY	41	46	55	31	49	34	51	01	-08	15	00	06	30	51	50	59	*	
SD7	23	21	15	19	18	26	02	51	34	14	50	20	11	17	14	-01	06	*

Dw7.1

7.1, 7.2

Dw7.2

7.2, 7.3

Dw7.3

Fig. 3. Correlation matrix of Dw7 HTCs

First Level Testing of Dw8 HTC

Z. Layrisse[1], B. Carreño[1], A. Svejgaard[2], P. Platz[2], L. P. Ryder[2], and T. Kristensen[2]

1 Laboratorio de Fisiopatología, Instituto Venezolano de Investigaciones Científicas, Caracas, Venezuela
2 Tissue Typing Laboratory, University Hospital, Copenhagen N., Denmark

At the invitation circulated by one of us (A.S.) from Copenhagen, nine laboratories (Table 1) submitted DRw8 homozygous typing cells (HTC) to the Ninth Workshop Dw8 First level testing phase which was to be carried out in Copenhagen and Caracas. Four of the laboratories included also several DRw8 heterozygous cells to be used as control responders in the mixed lymphocyte experiments

Histocompatibility Testing 1984
Edited by E. D. Albert et al.

(MLC). A total of 12 HTC and 19 DRw8+ controls were thus available. The HTC from Leiden and the heterozygous cells from Minneapolis, Oslo, and Lyon were not sent to Caracas.

With this material and several other local HTC and control panels, a total of seven large MLC experiments were carried out following the technique used during the Eighth Workshop [1]. The four experiments performed in Copenhagen used 26 or 31 cells as stimulators and 27 or 40 responders, while in Caracas 14–19 stimulators and 23–36 responders were used in three experiments. Details of the protocols and raw counts per minute (cpm) obtained in each experiment were submitted to the central laboratory in Essen where stabilized relative responses (SRR) were calculated. Data presented here are based on SRR values handed to participating laboratories during the pre-Workshop meetings in Munich.

Table 1. HTCs and heterozygous donors submitted for Ninth Workshop DW8 fist-level testing

Lab.	HTC Local Id.	9w	Heterozygous donors
BAC	ARC		SJ, MHB, KH
BET	SID		136E; F471
GSW	BAE	807	MB, FB, SB
HAN	TAB	806	GT
LAY	OLG	803	TR, LM
	SPA	804	
	CAB		
SUF	MACA		
ROO	MMR	802	
	LUY	805	
TSB	BTB	801	AB, AS, WQ, KH, TM
SVE	MAD		BAJ, PN, HS

Table 2 shows the condensed checkerboard results obtained from duplicate experiments performed in Copenhagen and Caracas. With the exception of combinations involving HTC MMR (9w802) and LUY (9w805), which were not tested in Caracas, and others indicated with an asterisk which could be tested only once for technical reasons, most values shown in the table represent results obtained from four experiments. Based on bidirectional typing responses (SRR between 0.and 38) three clusters as indicated by the boxes in the table could be identified; BAE (9w807), MAD (9w808), BTB (9w801), MACA, and ARC; SPA (9w804) and OLG (9w803); and TAB (9w806) and LUY (9w805). Bidirectional typing responses were also observed between other HTC pairs, such as SPA and MACA and SID and MACA. Several unidirectional typing responses were additionally evident.

A total of 25 DRw8+ and 27 DRw8– heterozygous panel cells were tested as responders in duplicate MLC experiments against the 12 Dw8 HTC either

Table 2. Ninth Workshop Dw8 first-level testing: MLC checkerboard with Dw8 HTC

	BAE 807	MAD 808	BTB 801	MACA	ARC	MMR 802	SID	CAB	OLG 803	SPA 804	LUY 805	TAB 806
BAE 807		+ + + +	+ + +[a]	+ + +	+ + +		–	+ + +	–	+ + +		–
MAD 808	+ + + +		+ +[a]	+ +	+ + + +		–	–	–	–	–	–
BTB 801	+ + +	+ + +		+ + + +	–[a]	+ + + +[a]	–	–	–	–	+ + + +[a]	–
MACA	+ + + +	+ + + +	+ + +[a]			+ + + +[a]	+ + +	+ +	–	+ +	–[a]	–
ARC	+ + + +	+ + + +	+ +[a]				+ + +	+ +	–	–	–	–
MMR 802				–[a]	–					+ + + +[a]		–
SID	+ + +	+ +	–[a]	+ +		+ + + +[a]		+ +	–	–	–[a]	–
CAB		–	–[a]	–	+ + +				+ + +	–		–
OLG 803	–	–	–[a]	–	–	–	–			+ + + +	–	–
SPA 804	–	+ +	–[a]	+ +	+ + + +				+ + + +			–
LUY 805	–	–[a]	–	–[a]	–	–[a]	–	–	–	+ +[a]		+ + +
TAB 806	–	–	–[a]	–	–	–	–	–	–	–	+ +	

Scores: + + + +, %SRR 0–20; + + +, %SRR 21–30; + +, %SRR 31–40; –, %SRR ≧ 41

[a] Tested in only one experiment

Table 3. Typing response patterns obtained with 18 of 20 DRw8-positive heterozygous cells tested with 12 Dw8 HTC submitted to Ninth Workshop first level testing

	DR	BAE 807	ARC	BTB 801	MACA	MAD 808	MMR 802	CAB	SID	SPA 804	OLG 803	TAB 806	LUY 805
HS[a]	3, 8	+	+	+	+	+		–	–	–	–	–	–
AB	3, 8	+	+	+	+	+		–	–		–	–	–
BAJ[a]	6, 8	+	+	–	+	+	–	–	–	–	–	–	–
MB[a]	5, 8	+	+	+	–	–	+		–			–	–
A5	1, 8	+	+	–		–	+	–	–			–	–
LM	2, 8	+	+	+	+	–						–	–
SB[a]	5, 8	+	–	+	–	–	–	–	–	–	–	–	–
FB[a]	7, 8	+	+	+	+	+	+	–		+		–	–
HK	4, 8			+	+	+			–	+	–	–	–
TM	3, 8	+		+		+	+	–	–	+		–	+
EQ	3, 8		+			+	+	+	+	+		+	
136E	4, 8	+	+	+	+	+	+	+		+	+	–	
TR[a]	2, 8	–	–	+	–		–		–	+	+	–	–
TA	2, 8	–			–		–	+	–	+	+	–	
CL	2, 8	–			–		–	–	–	+	+	–	
IZU	2, 8	–	–	–	–		–	–	–	–	–	+	
GT[a]	9, 8	–	–	–	–	–	–	–	–	–	–	+	+
D6512	2, 8	–		–	–	–	–	–	–	–	–	+	+

Scores: +, %SRR≦45; –, %SRR≧46
[a] Tested in Copenhagen and Caracas

in Copenhagen or Caracas. Twenty-one of the DRw8+ cells showed reproducible typing responses with at least two HTC, while none of the DRw8– cells did. If reproducible results obtained in at least two MLC experiments are compared, different patterns of typing responses (SRR < 45) are found. This is illustrated with 18 DRw8+ panel cells in Table 3. Note that each pattern was confirmed in Copenhagen and Caracas with seven of the responder cells which appear in the table.

Three patterns are clearly distinguished: cells which type only to HTC BAE (9w807), ARC, BTB (9w801), MACA, MAD (9w808), and MMR (9w802); those typing only to HTC TAB (9w806) and LUY (9w805); and those typing only to SPA (9w804) and OLG (9w803). A fourth group gives overlapping responses to at least one of the HTC forming each cluster. HTC CAB, originating from Caracas, has been confirmed to be DRw8 homozygous, but Dw8 heterozygous by family MLC and PLT typing performed recently in our laboratory.

The first-level HTC testing thus demonstrates the existence of at least two Dw8 subgroups, one defined by HTC 801, 802, 807, 808, ARC, and MACA, another defined by HTC 805 and 806. A third subgroup defined by HTC 9w803 and 9w804 is less clear due to cross-reactions of a subset of the DRw8+ panel cells with 9w804. Similar results have recently been reported by Mickelson et al. [2] based on data obtained with some of the HTCs submitted to this Workshop.

Although the existence of a third subgroup defined by HTCS SPA (9w804) and OLG (9w803) has been demonstrated using PLTs generated by sensitization of Caucasian Dw8 HTC with HTCs SPA and OLG [3] and family studies performed in Amerindians [4], further tests are necessary to find out its frequency among other Mongoloid groups.

The serological typing of HTCs with Ninth Workshop sera has shown that HTCs defining other D splits (L. Degos, HLA-DR Workshop Summary, this volume) may share the same DR specificity but differ in their DQ antigen, thus suggesting the involvement of a haplotypic combination (DR/DQ) in MLC responses. Regarding Dw8 HTC, it is of interest to point out that although HTC 9w805 and 806 (LUY and TAB) apparently define one Dw8 subgroup, the former is DRw8/DQ3 while the latter is DRw8/DQ1; on the other hand, HTC 801, 802, 803, 804, 807, and 808 share DRw8/DQ blank haplotypes [5]. Furthermore, while DRw8 is found in Caucasian cells associated either with DQ3 or DQ blank, in Amerindians it is almost exclusively found with DQ blank. It remains to be ascertained whether or not the so far unidentified DQ specificity of Caucasians and Amerindians is the same.

References

1. Dupont B, Braun DW, Yunis EJ, Carpenter CB (1980) HLA-D by cellular typing. Joint report. In: Terasaki PI (ed) Histocompatibility testing 1980. UCLA, Los Angeles, pp 229–267
2. Mickelson EM, Nisperos B, Layrisse Z, Kim SJ, Donnall Thomas E, Hansen JA (1983) Analysis of the HLA-DRw8 haplotype: recognition by HTC typing of three distinct antigen complexes in Caucasians, native Americans and Orientals. Immunogenetics 17:399–410
3. Herrera F, Layrisse Z, Carreño B, Quintero M, Honeyman M, Mickelson EM, Tsuji K (1984) Definition of HLA-Dw8.2 by primary and secondary mixed lymphocyte cultures. Hum Immun (submitted)
4. Layrisse Z, Heinen HD, Simoney N, Stoikow Z, Balbas O, Leets I, Garcia E (1982) HLA-D typing with homozygous cells identified in an American indigenous isolate. II. Family studies and D/DR relationship. Tissue Antigens 20:86–99
5. Schreuder I, Parlevliet J (1983) HLA-DR, LB, MB and 8w13 with 9w HTCs. Ninth International Workshop Newsletter 5, pp 41–51

First Level Testing of HLA-D "Blank" HTC*

W. Ollier[1], I. Doxiadis[2], D. Jaraquemada[1], R. Okoye[1], H. Grosse-Wilde[2], and H. Festenstein[1]

1 Department of Immunology, London Hospital Medical College, Turner Street, London E1 2AD, U.K.
2 Abteilung Immungenetik, Universitätsklinikum Essen, Virchowstraße 171, 4300 Essen 1, Federal Republic of Germany

A total of 28 HTC of undefined HLA-D specificities were sent to the two reference laboratories (FES and GSW), for first level testing (Table 1). Checkerboard MLCs and panel testings were performed in both laboratories. The panel consisted of 95 heterozygous individuals with one or two undefined HLA-D specificities. Some were submitted by the laboratories as positive for a given HTC. The results in counts per minute (cpm) were double-normalised to stabilized relative responses (SRR), and these were converted to scores as previously reported [1] (Table 2). Correlation coefficients were calculated from 2 × 2 contingency tables.

Checkerboard Analysis

Table 2 shows the results from the checkerboard testing of 24 of 28 HTC. The first two cells (DKB and KT14) define the DB5 specificity associated with DRw9, which has previously been described [2, 3]. The other HTC were tentatively clustered and given provisional names, i.e. DB6 to DB10. DB1, formed by the HTC BIBA, LBU and BH13, had been described in the Eighth Workshop as defining a subtype of Dw7 [4]. The last three HTC (FPA, JVM and BM15), were all DR5+/Dw−, but did not form a clear cluster. BJR and SHY could not be tested in checkerboard.

Panel Testing

A total of 96 heterozygous cells were typed with some or all of the HTC and the results are given in Table 3. Correlation coefficients between the HTC forming each cluster are also shown.

DB5: The DB5 cells stimulated each other in checkerboard MLC but seemed to clearly define a DRw9-related HLA-D specificity. Of eight DRw9 positive responders, seven typed DB5 and did not give extra typing responses with any of the other HTC clusters.

DB6: Only three HTC were tested against the panel, i.e. HERLUF, BM16 and 2171A. They typed a group of DRw12 positive responders. Except for one case (no. 13), they did not give extra typing responses with the DRw6-positive, Dw6 and DB8 (Dw16) HTC. However, correlation coefficients between all these cells were not always significant.

DB7: The DB7 cells are SAS-011, HI-2 and LUY. All are DRw8-positive and Dw8-negative, as are the group of responder cells that they type. These include four Japanese cells (nos. 16–19) and two European Caucasoid cells (20, 21). Cell 15 was sent as positive responder to LUY, but did not type with SAS and HI-2. Nevertheless, high correlation coef-

* This work was generously supported by the Nuffield Foundation and the Arthritis and Rheumatism Council of Great Britain

Table 1. List of HTC

ID	Specificity[a]	Workshop no.	Lab. of origin	HLA type						
DKB	DB5	8w324	ROO	A24	B40	Cw3	DRw9		DB5	
KT14	DB5	–	KSH	A24	B51	C –	DRw9		DB5	
PBR	DBL	–	FES	A1, 2	B35, w57	Cw4, 6	DRw12, w52	DQw3	DB6	DPw2, 4
HERLUF	DBL	9w1503	SVE	A2	B35, 44		DRw12		DB6	
BM16	DBL	9w1501	FER	A2	B18	C –	DRw12		DB6	
2171A	DBL	9w1504	FAU	A2	B5		DR –		DB6	
BM24	DBL	9w1502	FER	A1	Bw41	C –	DR –		DB6	
SAS-011	DShim	9w1602	SAS	A2	Bw46	Cw1, 3	DRw8	DQw1	DB7	
HI-2	DShim	9w1601	FUK	A2	Bw46	Cw4	DRw8	DQw1	DB7	
LUY	DBL	9w0805	ROO	A2	B51		DRw8		DB7?	
HAG	DBL	9w1802	WER	A2	Bw41	Cw7	DRw6, w52	DQw3	DBL	
BELU	DBL	–	IVS	Aw33	Bw57		DR –		Dw16?	
CRI	LD15	9w1702	LAY	A2, 31	Bw62	Cw3	DRw6, w52	DQw3	Dw16	
AMA	LD15	9w1701	LAY	A2	Bw62	Cw3	DRw6, w52	DQw3	Dw16	
BAS	DBL	9w1801	LAY	A2	B51	Cw8	DR2	DQw3	DB9	
REM	DBL	9w1803	LAY	A2	B51	C –	DR2	DQw3		
FJO	JOUV	–	BET	A2, 3	B7, 16		DR2			
AZH	DBL	–	BRA	A24	Bw22	Cw1	DR2		DBL	DPw3
BIBA	Ivad-3	–	PTR	A2	B13	C –	DR3, 7			
BH13	DB1	9w1901	YUN	A2	B13	Cw6	DR7	DQw2		
LBU	DB1	9w1903	FES	A30	B13	Cw6	DR7	DQw2		
SI	Ivad-1	9w1902	PTR	A1, 30	B8	Cw6, 7	DRw6, w52	DQw1		
DJ	Ivad-1	9w1904	PTR	A1, 23	B8, w50	Cw6, 7	DRw6, w52	DQw1		
FPA	'F5'	9w9901	FES	A1	B35	Cw4	DRw11	DQw1		
JVM	LDV11	–	ROO	A2	B18		DRw11	DQw3		
BM15	DBL	–	FER	A1	B49	C –	DRw11	DQw3		
KSH	6?	9w0609	FES	A3, 28	B14, 27	Cw2, 8	DRw6	DQw1	Dw6	
WDV	Dw18	9w0605	ROO	A2	B38	Cw6	DRw6	DQw1	Dw18	DPw1, 2
APD	Dw18	–	ROO	A1	Bw60	C –	DRw6	DQw1	Dw18	
SLE	Dw19	9w0608	HAN	A2	Bw60	C –	DRw6	DQw1	Dw19	
BJR	DBL	–	HAN	A2	B17		DR2			
SHY	DBL	–	BRA	A29	B7	C –	DRw10	DQw1	DBL	DPw4

[a] Locally assigned

ficients between these HTC indicate that they could be defining a new DRw8-related specificity.

Dw16: The Dw16 group is formed by AMA, CRI and BELU. The first two show a very high correlation coefficient. The positive responders show clear cross-reactions with Dw6 HTCs. However, the panel studied consisted mainly of Caucasoids, while these two HTC are from Amerindian donors.

DB9: The HTC included were BAS, REM and FJO, all DR2-positive. These HTC typed two of six DR2+/Dw2– responders. A fourth DR2-positive HTC, AZH, was excluded as it did not show the same pattern of reactions.

DB1: In the Eighth Workshop this specificity was found to be associated with DR7. In our data it defined a subtype within Dw7 (Dw17 and Dw11).

The DR5-positive HTC FPA, JVM and BM15 do not show any correlation. Although all are Dw5 negative, they do not seem to share the same HLA-D specificity. Cell FPA typed three DR5+/Dw5– individuals, but also some who were Dw5 positive.

HAG: This HTC clearly typed six of the 59 cells tested. All except one of them (no. 88) have at least one DR blank and one D blank. These results indicate that this HTC may be defining a new HLA-D specificity associated with an undefined HLA-DR antigen.

DB10: The two cells defining this cluster give a very high correlation coefficient ($r = 0.50$, $p < 0.001$), but did not seem to clearly type any group of responders tested. (They were later shown to be Dw9; see H. Grosse-Wilde et al., Definition of HLA-D with HTC, this volume.)

BL: The two cells (BJR and SHY) included in this group did not give any clear typing response patterns with the selected panel. The other HTC that could not be defined were AZH, FPA, JVM and BM15. On the other hand, several responders with blank DR and D specificities (nos. 89 – 96) did not type with any of these HTC.

Table 2. Checkerboard MLC results between HLA-D Blank HTC

		DKB	KT14	PBR	HERL	BM16	2171A	BM24	SAS	HI-2	LUY	HAG	BELU	CRI	AMA	BAS	REM	FJO	AZH	BIBA	BH13	SI	DJ	FPA	JVM	BM15
DB5	DKB	3	2	.	.	.	1	.	.	.	3	1	1	1	1	1	2	1	1	.	.	.	.	1	1	.
	KT14	1	3	.	3	.	1	.	.	.	1	1	1	1	1	2	1	2	1	1	3	1	1	1	2	.
DB6	PBR	.	.	3	3	3	1	1	1	1	2	1	1	1	2	1	1	1	1	1	1	1	3	1	1	2
	HERL	.	.	2	3	3	2	1	.	1	1	2	2	1	2	1	1	1	1	1	1	1	1	1	1	3
	BM16	.	.	3	3	3	3	2	.	1	1	2	1	2	1	2	1	1	1	1	2	3	3	1	3	2
	2171A	1	2	2	2	3	3	3	.	1	1	2	1	3	3	2	1	3	1	3	1	1	1	3	1	1
DB7	SAS	.	.	.	.	.	.	.	3	3	2	1	.	3	3	1	1	1	1	3	1	.	.	1	1	1
	HI-2	.	.	1	1	1	1	1	2	3	1	1	1	1	1	1	1	1	1	1	1	1	2	1	1	1
	LUY	1	1	1	1	1	1	1	2	3	3	1	2	2	1	1	1	2	1	1	1	2	1	1	1	1
Dw16 (DB8)	HAG	1	1	1	1	1	1	1	1	1	1	3	3	2	1	1	1	1	1	1	1	1	1	1	1	1
	BELU	1	1	1	1	1	1	2	.	1	1	1	3	2	1	1	2	1	1	1	1	1	1	1	1	3
	CRI	2	2	1	1	3	1	1	.	3	3	1	1	3	3	1	1	3	3	1	1	1	3	1	1	3
	AMA	1	3	1	3	1	1	1	.	1	1	1	1	3	3	3	3	1	1	1	1	1	1	1	2	1
DB9	BAS	1	1	1	1	1	1	1	1	1	1	1	1	1	1	3	3	3	1	1	1	1	1	1	1	1
	REM	1	3	1	1	1	2	2	1	1	1	1	1	1	1	3	3	3	2	1	1	1	1	1	1	1
	FJO	1	1	3	1	1	1	3	1	1	1	3	1	1	1	3	3	3	1	1	2	1	1	3	3	1
	AZH	1	1	1	1	1	1	1	1	1	1	1	1	1	1	1	3	2	3	1	1	1	1	1	1	1
DB1	BIBA	2	1	1	1	1	1	2	2	1	1	1	1	1	1	1	1	1	1	3	3	1	3	2	1	1
	BH13	1	1	1	1	1	1	1	1	1	1	1	1	1	1	1	1	1	1	3	3	1	1	1	1	1
	LBU	3	1	.	1	.	1	.	.	.	1	1	2	1	1	1	1	2	1	3	3	3	2	1	1	.
Dw9 (DB10)	SI	1	1	1	2	2	3	2	.	1	1	1	1	1	1	1	1	1	1	1	1	3	3	1	1	1
	DJ	1	1	1	1	2	1	3	.	1	3	1	1	1	1	1	1	1	1	1	1	3	3	1	1	2
DR5	FPA	1	1	2	2	3	2	3	1	1	1	1	1	1	1	1	1	1	1	1	1	1	1	3	1	2
	JVM	1	1	1	2	2	1	2	1	1	1	1	1	1	1	1	1	1	1	1	1	1	1	1	3	3

Scores: 1, SSR > 65; 2, SRR 45 – 64.9; 3, SRR < 45; . , not tested

Conclusions

In addition to DB5, five tentative new specificities (DB6, DB7, DB8, DB9 and DB10) were suggested from panel and checkerboard studies in the first level. (DB8 has now been officially recognised and given the designation Dw16 by the Nomenclature Committee 1984.) All have to be confirmed by segregation studies in families, as well as typing of larger panels. DB1 was confirmed as a subtype of Dw7. Of the other HTC tested, only HAG showed a clear pattern of typing responses with the selected panel. Some of these responder cells still have undefined specificities.

Acknowledgment. We are grateful to Denny Williams for typing the manuscript.

References

1. Jaraquemada D, Ollier W, Okoye RC, Sachs JA, Festenstein H, Grosse-Wilde H (1983) Tissue Antigens 22:315
2. Sachs JA, Duquesnoy R, Hansen JA, et al (1980) In: Terasaki PI (ed) Histocompatibility testing 1980. UCLA, Los Angeles, p 268
3. Mickelson EM, Nisperos B, Thomas ED, Hansen JA (1982) Hum Immunol 4:79
4. Dupont B, Braun DW, Yunis EJ, Carpenter CB (1980) In: Terasaki PI (ed) Histocompatibility testing 1980. UCLA, Los Angeles, p 229

Table 3 see page 284 ff.

Table 3. Heterozygous panel typing and correlations of HLA-D blank HTC

	DB5	DB6	DB7	HAG	Dw16 (DB8)	DB9	AZH	DB1	Dw9 (DB10)	DR5	Dw6	BL	DR, DRw	Dw
1	11	.....	111	1	...	111	1	131	..	...	....	..	9 8	– 8
2	32	.....	113	1	...	111	1	111	..	...	....	..	9 –	– –
3	32	.....	111	2	...	111	1	333	..	...	....	..	9 5	– –
4	33	.....	113	2	...	122	1	223	..	...	....	..	9 5	– 5
5	31	.....	111	1	...	111	1	121	..	...	....	..	9 2	– 2
6	33	.....	112	1	...	132	1	213	..	...	....	..	9 3	– 3
7	33	.....	122	1	...	222	1	133	..	...	....	..	9 4	– 4
8	22	.....	111	1	...	111	1	131	..	...	....	..	9 4	– 4
9	..	331	...	.	111	...	.	...	..	111	1121	..	. . .	– 9
10	..	332	...	.	111	...	.	...	..	111	1211	..	w 12 7	– 11
11	..	232	...	.	122	...	.	...	..	111	1111	..	w 12 7	– 11
12	..	213	...	.	112	...	.	...	..	311	1111	..	w 12 –	– –
13	..	313	...	.	233	...	.	...	..	123	1323	..	w 12 –	– –
14	..	333	...	.	131	...	.	...	..	232	1113	..	w 12 1	– 1
15	11	.....	113	1	...	111	1	111	..	...	....	..	8 4	– 4
16	31	.....	332	1	...	133	1	113	..	...	....	..	8 –	– –
17	11	.....	331	1	...	121	1	111	..	...	....	..	8 4	– YT
18	11	.....	331	1	...	111	1	111	..	...	....	..	8 2	– 2
19	11	.....	331	1	...	111	1	111	..	...	....	..	8 8	– –
20	11	.....	333	1	...	112	1	111	..	...	....	..	8 –	– –
21	3.	...1.	133	1	.12	1.1	1	131	11	11.	....	11	8 7	– –
22	13	..1..	223	.	...	..2	2	.11	..	122	....	13	8 6	8 6
23	11	.....	111	1	...	121	1	121	..	...	....	..	8 1	8 1
24	11	.....	111	1	...	111	1	233	..	...	....	..	8 7	8 7
25	13	..1.1	111	.	...	..3	1	.33	..	231	....	11	8 –	8 –
26	1.	.1.1.	311	1	.11	..1	3	333	11	11.	....	12	8 –	8 –
27	1.	...1.	311	1	.11	3.2	1	331	33	12.	....	21	8 –	8 –
28	..	232	...	.	133	...	.	...	..	121	1313	..	6 2	– 2
29	..	233	...	.	333	...	.	...	..	113	1313	..	6 7	– 7
30	..	.113.	...	.	1333	...	.	...	..	121	3323	..	6 1	6 1
31	..	.111.	...	.	121	...	.	...	..	121	2311	..	6 4	6 4
32	..	.111.	...	.	111	...	.	...	..	113	1333	..	6 2	6 2
33	..	.211.	...	.	131	...	.	...	..	221	2331	..	6 1	6 1
34	..	.111.	...	.	311	...	.	...	..	111	3113	..	6 2	6 2
35	..	.311.	...	.	112	...	.	...	..	311	2131	..	6 3	6 3
36	..	.111.	...	.	111	...	.	...	..	111	3133	..	6 2	6 2
37	..	.112.	...	.	112	...	.	...	..	113	1323	..	6 4	6 4
38	..	.111.	...	.	111	...	.	...	..	121	2321	..	6 4	6 4
39	..	.111.	...	.	321	...	.	...	..	111	1113	..	6 4	6 4
40	2.	...1.	321	1	.13	1.3	3	111	22	11.	....	11	6 3	6 3
41	1.	...1.	111	1	.22	111	1	111	33	123	....	..	6 5	9 5
42	1.	..1.1	111	.	...	..1	1	.11	..	311	....	11	6 –	9 6
43	1.	.1.1.	111	1	.11	..1	2	111	11	11.	....	11	6 7	9 7
44	1.	.2.3.	311	1	.12	..1	2	111	12	31.	....	11	6 5	9 5

DB5

DKB	–	
KT14	.32	–
	DKB	KT14

DB6

PBR	–				
HERL	.49	–			
BM16	ns	.56	–		
2171A	ns	ns	ns	–	
BM24	ns	ns	.47	ns	–
	PBR	HERL	BM16	2171A	BM24

DB7

SAS	–		
HI-2	.36	–	
LUY	ns	.34	–
	SAS	HI-2	LUY

Dw16 (DB8)

BELU	–		
CRI	ns	–	
AMA	ns	.50	–
	BELU	CRI	AMA

45	11	. . . . .	111	1	. . .	231	1	111	. .	. . .	. . . .	. .	2	8	–	8
46	21	. . . . .	111	1	. . .	332	1	132	. .	. . .	. . . .	. .	2	4	–	4
47	11	. . . . .	111	2	. . .	121	1	322	. .	. . .	. . . .	. .	2	4	–	4
48	11	. . . . .	211	2	. . .	111	1	111	. .	. . .	. . . .	. .	2	5	–	5
49	11	. . . . .	111	1	. . .	111	1	111	. .	. . .	. . . .	. .	2	–	–	–
50	11	. . . . .	111	1	. . .	111	2	131	. .	. . .	. . . .	. .	2	–	–	–
51	1.	. . . 1.	112	2	. 22	111	1	111	11	131	. . . .	11	2	–	2	–
52	1.	. . 1. 1	121	.	. . .	. . 3	3	. 11	. .	111	. . . .	31	2	6	2	6
53	1.	. . 1. 1	211	.	. . .	. . 1	1	. 11	. .	111	. . . .	11	2	4	12	4
54	11	. . . . .	111	1	. . .	111	1	333	. .	. . .	. . . .	. .	7	2	7	–
55	11	. . . . .	111	1	. . .	131	1	331	. .	. . .	. . . .	. .	7	4	7	4
56	11	. . . . .	111	1	. . .	111	1	321	. .	. . .	. . . .	. .	7	5	–	5
57	11	. . . . .	131	1	. . .	111	1	133	. .	. . .	. . . .	. .	7	–	–	–
58	12	. . . . .	112	1	. . .	232	1	332	. .	. . .	. . . .	. .	7	–	–	–
59	11	. . . . .	111	1	. . .	111	1	231	. .	. . .	. . . .	. .	7	–	–	–
60	11	. . . . .	111	1	. . .	111	1	232	. .	. . .	. . . .	. .	7	3	7	3
61	11	. . . . .	111	1	. . .	131	1	133	. .	. . .	. . . .	. .	7	2	7	2
62	1.	. . . 1.	111	1	. 11	111	1	133	11	111	. . . .	11	7	1	7	1
63	3.	. . . 1.	111	1	. 11	111	1	123	31	311	. . . .	12	7	–	11	–
64	1.	. . . 1.	133	1	. 11	111	1	333	11	112	. . . .	11	7	–	11	–
65	1.	. . . 3.	211	1	. 13	1. 3	3	332	23	11.	. . . .	22	7	4	7	4
66	11	. . . 3.	111	1	. 13	212	1	323	33	21.	. . . .	12	7	2	7	–
67	1.	. . 1. 1	111	.	. . .	. . 1	2	. 33	. .	111	. . . .	11	7	–	11	–
68	1.	. 1. 3 .	311	1	. 11	. . 1	2	113	13	11.	. . . .	11	7	6	7	6
69	3.	. . 1. 1	323	.	. . .	. . 1	3	. 31	. .	121	. . . .	22	7	1	11	–
70	1.	. . 3. 3	121	.	. . .	. . 1	2	. 11	. .	131	. . . .	11	7	6	7	9
71	11	. . . . .	111	1	. . .	131	1	121	. .	. . .	. . . .	. .	7	–	–	–
72	1.	. . . 1.	112	1	. 11	111	1	111	11	232	. . . .	12	5	3	5	3
73	1.	. . 1. 1	111	.	. . .	. . 1	2	. 11	. .	321	. . . .	11	5	2	5	2
74	. .	. 113.	. . .	.	112	. . .	.	. . .	. .	212	1211	. .	5	2	5	2
75	. .	. 112.	. . .	.	111	. . .	.	. . .	. .	211	1111	. .	5	3	5	3
76	2.	. . . 3.	231	2	. 12	1. 3	1	331	31	13.	. . . .	31	5	1	5	1
77	1.	. . . 1.	111	1	. 11	1. 1	1	133	11	11.	. . . .	12	5	–	5	–
78	. .	. 111.	. . .	.	111	. . .	.	. . .	. .	311	1311	. .	5	–	–	–
79	. .	. 121.	. . .	.	111	. . .	.	. . .	. .	311	1111	. .	5	1	–	–
80	. .	. 113.	. . .	.	111	. . .	.	. . .	. .	211	1131	. .	5	8	–	8
81	. .	. 132.	. . .	.	112	. . .	.	. . .	. .	111	1111	. .	5	1	–	–
82	. .	. 112.	. . .	.	111	. . .	.	. . .	. .	111	1111	. .	5	1	–	–
83	1.	. . . 1.	311	3	. 13	2. 3	1	311	23	13.	. . . .	11	–	6	–	6
84	2.	. . . 1.	113	3	. 21	113	2	121	11	131	. . . .	12	–	–	–	–
85	3.	. . . 1.	313	3	. 12	211	2	112	11	123	. . . .	13	–	–	–	–
86	1.	. . . 1.	111	3	. 11	111	1	111	11	122	. . . .	11	–	4	–	4
87	3.	. 1. 2.	321	3	. 12	. . 1	1	113	31	31.	. . . .	13	–	7	–	11
88	1.	. . . 3.	311	3	. 13	3. 3	1	111	23	32.	. . . .	13	7	3	7	3
89	1.	. . . 1.	111	1	. 12	1. 1	1	111	33	11.	. . . .	11	–	4	–	B3
90	1.	. . . 3.	111	1	. 12	1. 2	1	223	13	11.	. . . .	21	–	1	–	1
91	3.	. . . 3.	131	2	. 13	1. 1	3	211	23	11.	. . . .	11	–	–	–	–
92	. .	. 112.	. . .	.	121	. . .	.	. . .	. .	221	3111	. .	–	4	–	4
93	. .	. 131.	. . .	.	122	. . .	.	. . .	. .	221	1121	. .	–	1	–	1
94	. .	. 113.	. . .	.	111	. . .	.	. . .	. .	311	1112	. .	–	3	–	3
95	. .	. 112.	. . .	.	121	. . .	.	. . .	. .	111	3111	. .	–	–	–	–

DB9

BAS	–		
REM	.59	–	
FJO	.46	.32	–
	BAS	REM	FJO

DB1

BIBA	–		
BH13	.44	–	
LBU	.21	.36	–
	BIBA	BH13	LBU

HAG

., not tested

DNA Restriction Fragment Length Polymorphism of Some Ninth Workshop Homozygous Typing Cells Using a cDNA Probe Specific for DRβ*

G. Paulsen[1], L. Rask[2], P.A. Peterson[2], J. Böhme[2], H. Grosse-Wilde[3], T. Moen[1], and E. Thorsby[1]

1 Institute of Transplantation Immunology, University of Oslo and The National Hospital, Oslo, Norway
2 Department of Cell Research, The Wallenberg Laboratory, University of Uppsala, Uppsala, Sweden
3 Department of Immunogenetics, University Hospital of Essen, 4300 Essen, Federal Republic of Germany

Introduction

During the mixed lymphocyte culture (MLC) testing of some of the homozygous typing cells (HTC) in the Ninth International Histocompatibility Workshop, it became apparent that not all HTC believed to detect the same HLA-D specificity behaved similarly in panel testing. To investigate this further, preliminary restriction fragment length polymorphism (RFLP) studies on some of the HTC submitted to detect Dw6, Dw8, or Dw10 were made with Southern blotting and a cDNA probe specific for DRβ. The results demonstrate a remarkable correspondence between the RFLP detected and the behavior of the HTC in MLC panel testing.

Material and Methods

Cells

Lymphoblastoid cell lines (LCLs) were established from some of the HTC submitted to the cellular part of the Ninth Workshop (Table 1). The T cells from one ampule of each HTC studied were first removed by rosetting with AET-treated sheep red blood cells and Lymphoprep flotation. The non-rosetting B cells were then washed in RPMI 1640 and resuspended in 1.5 ml tissue culture medium (RPMI 1640 with 10% fetal calf serum and antibiotics). Then 1.5 ml of sterile filtered tissue culture medium from an Epstein-Barr virus (EBV)-shedding marmoset B cell line (B95-8) were added. The human B cells were cultured until 2×10^8 lymphoblastoid cells were formed, replacing the medium with fresh medium when needed. Due to infected cultures or lack of cells, it was not possible to investigate all HTC believed to detect HLA-Dw6, Dw8, or Dw10.

Isolation of DNA

A cell pellet made from 2×10^8 lymphoblastoid cells was resuspended in a solution containing 0.5 M EDTA (pH 8.0), Proteinase K (Merck) (0.1 mg/ml) and 0.5% *N*-lauroylsarcosine (Sigma) at a concentration of 1×10^7 cells/ml, and incubated for 9 h at 37 °C. The following procedure was essentially as described elsewhere [1], with the exception that the samples were also digested with RNase (Sigma), 10 μg/ml, for 4 h at 37 °C.

Restriction Enzyme Cleavages

DNA samples were digested separately with *Eco*RI, *Bam*HI, or *Hind*III (2.5 units/μg DNA) for 20 h at 37 °C, as described elsewhere [1].

Genomic Hybridization

Ten micrograms of restriction-enzyme-digested DNA was separated electrophoretically in 0.7% agarose gels and hybridization performed as described elsewhere [2]. The cDNA probe specific for DR is also described elsewhere [3].

Results

Dw6

Three different HTC, SCL, SLE, and STEPH, could be tested; they were assumed to type for three different splits of Dw6 – 6.1, 6.2, and 6.3 respectively. The results from the Workshop MLC experiments (H. Grosse-Wilde et al., Definition of HLA-D with HTCs, this volume) suggest that SCL is homozygous for the Dw6 split Dw18, while SLE and STEPH are homozygous for Dw19, the complementary split of Dw6 (see Table 1). The restriction fragment patterns obtained are given in Figs. 1 – 3. Similarities between the three different HTC are seen. However, using *Bam*HI (Fig. 1), an additional 4.2-kb fragment was seen with SCL

* This study was supported in part by The Norwegian Cancer Society and the Deutsche Forschungsgemeinschaft SFB102 TP B4

Histocompatibility Testing 1984
Edited by E. D. Albert et al.

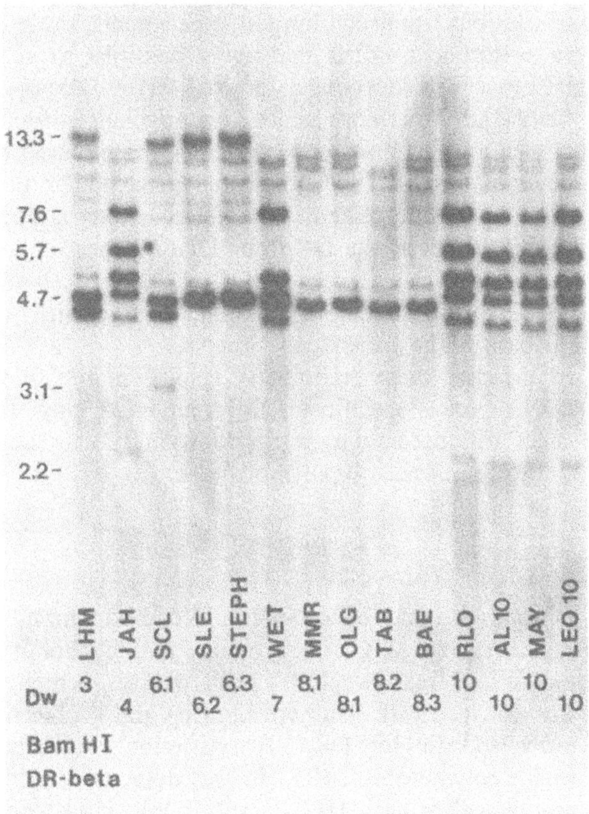

Fig. 1. Hybridization of a DRβ cDNA probe to DNA prepared by digestion with *Bam*HI of DNA from 14 different homozygous typing cells. Local designation and submitted specificity are given at *bottom* of figure (see also Table 1)

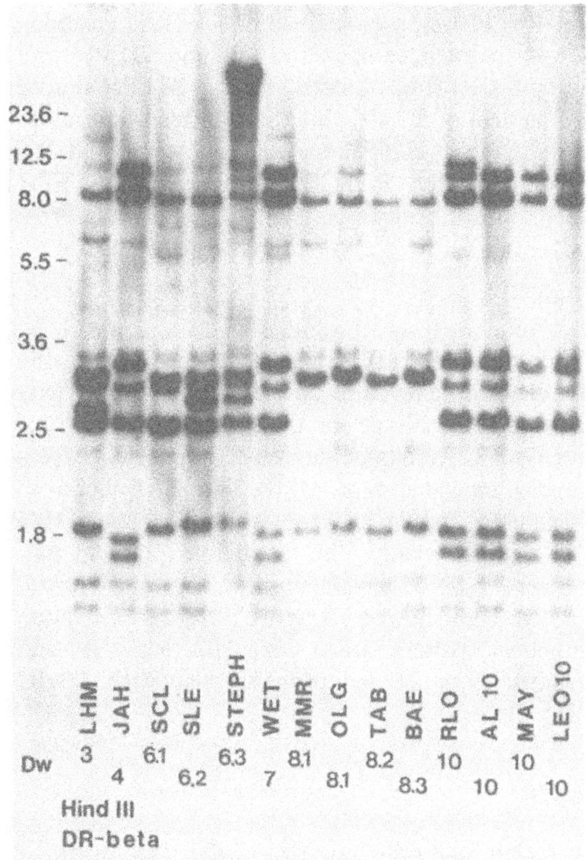

Fig. 2. As in Fig. 1, except that DNA digestion was performed with *Hin*dIII

Table 1. Homozygous typing cells investigated

Local id.	Origin	9w no.	HTC specificity[a]	
			Pre 9.ws.	Post 9.ws.
LHM	HAN	0305	Dw3	Dw3
JAH	HAN	0403	Dw4	Dw4
SCL	GSW	0604	Dw6.1	Dw18
SLE	HAN	0608	Dw6.2	Dw19
STEPH	HSU	0611	Dw6.3	Dw19
WET	WER	0705	Dw7	Dw17
MMR	ROO	0802	Dw8.1	Dw8
OLG	LAY	0803	Dw8.1	?
TAB	HAN	0806	Dw8.2	DB7
BAE	GSW	0807	Dw8.3	Dw8
RLO	STA	1004	Dw10	Dw10, w14
AL10	BAC	1001	Dw10	Dw10
MAY	BRA	1003	Dw10	Dw10
LEO 10	BAC	1002	Dw10	Dw10

HAN, J.H. Hansen, Seattle; GSW, H. Grosse-Wilde, Essen; HSU, H.S. Hsu, Baltimore; WER, P. Wernet, Tübingen; ROO, A. Termijtelen, Leiden; LAY, Z. Layrisse, Caracas; STA, P. Stastny, Dallas; BAC, N. Reinsmoen, Minneapolis; BRA, C. Brautbar, Jerusalem

[a] As ascertained in the final MLC data analysis

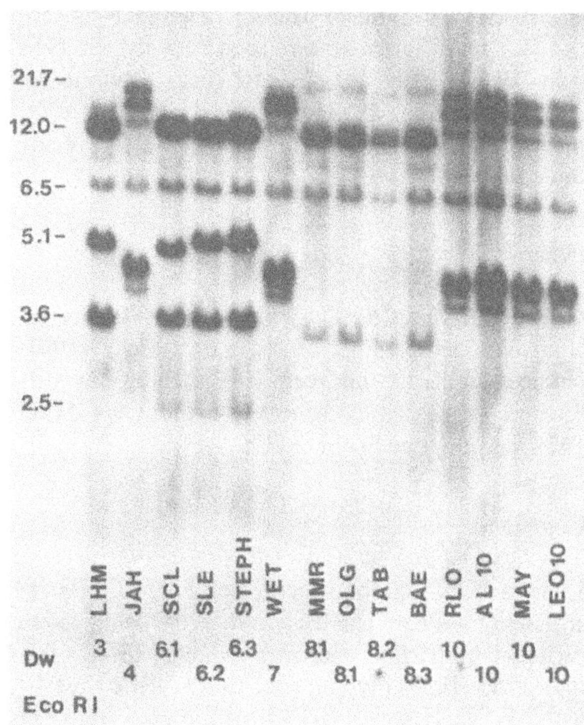

Fig. 3. As in Fig. 1, except that DNA digestion was performed with *Eco*RI

compared to SLE and STEPH, which gave identical RFLP. Using *Hind* III (Fig. 2), SCL lacked a 2.8-kb fragment compared to SLE and STEPH, and using *Eco* RI (Fig. 3), both SLE and STEPH shared a fragment of 5.1 kb, while SCL instead had a 4.8-kb fragment. STEPH showed an additional 9.6 band compared to SCL and SLE, but STEPH seems insufficiently digested.

Dw8

Four different HTC could be tested. MMR and OLG were believed to type for the subspecificity Dw8.1, TAB to type for Dw8.2, and BAE to type for Dw8.3. Results of the Workshop MLC experiments indicated that MMR and BAE behaved identically, typing for Dw8 while TAB and OLG behaved differently. The restriction fragment patterns of these cells were similar, but not identical, in that TAB showed a slightly different restriction fragment pattern using *Bam* HI (Fig. 1) and *Hind* III (Fig. 2), and probably also with *Eco* RI (Fig. 3).

Dw10

Four different HTC could be tested. The results of the Workshop MLC experiments indicated that the HTC AL10, MAY, and LEO 10 behaved identically, while RLO appeared HLA-D heterozygous (Dw10, w14). In the restriction fragment pattern analysis, no differences were seen between the cells using *Bam* HI (Fig. 1) or *Eco* RI (Fig. 3), while using *Hind* III (Fig. 2), RLO showed an extra fragment of approximately 12.5 kb not detected in the other three HTC.

Other HTC

Cells homozygous for Dw3, Dw4, or Dw7 were included as controls. Figs. 1 – 3 demonstrate clear differences in RFLP between HTC typing for different D specificities, except for the Dw4 HTC JAH and the three Dw10 HTC.

Comments

Using a cDNA probe specific for DRβ, DNA restriction fragment patterns were seen using three different restriction enzymes which closely followed the HLA-D typing specificity of the investigated HTC. However, RFLP differences between HTC assumed to type for the same HLA-D specificity were also seen, and were in accordance with the MLC results obtained at the Workshop. Even though caution must be exercised in drawing conclusions from such limited experiments, the results further confirm that it is possible to see RFLPs which are typical for each HLA-D specificity [2]. Furthermore, genetic heterogeneity which is seen in functional tests (i.e., MLC) may also be detected using a DRβ probe and a particular restriction enzyme. Whether the heterogeneity is due to differences at the DRβ1 or DRβ2 genes, or at other HLA class II genes (DQ, DP) because of cross-hybridization, is impossible to ascertain on the basis of the present experiments.
In any case, these preliminary results suggest that cDNA probes specific for different HLA class II genes will become powerful tools in the further study of HLA class II polymorphism.

Summary

DNA from some of the Ninth Workshop homozygous typing cells (HTC) believed to be homozygous for HLA-Dw6, Dw8, and Dw10 respectively was analyzed with Southern blotting and a cDNA probe specific for DRβ. A restriction fragment length polymorphism (RFLP) was detected which was typical of each HLA-D specificity. However, some differences in RFLP between the HTC belonging to the different groups were also detected, and the HTCs within each group which showed discrepant RFLP also behaved differently than typing cells in mixed lymphocyte culture (MLC) tests. Thus, the heterogeneity at HLA-D which is detected in functional tests (i.e., MLC) may also be seen using particular restriction enzymes and cDNA probes.

Acknowledgments. The marmoset B cell line (B95-8) was kindly donated by Dr. E. Klein, Department of Tumor Biology, Karolinska Institute, Stockholm. We are grateful to our colleagues (see Table 1) who submitted the HTC used in the present studies.

References

1. Böhme J, Owerbach D, Denaro M, Lernmark Å, Peterson PA, Rask L (1983) Human class-II major histocompatibility antigen beta-chains are derived from at least three loci. Nature 301:82 – 84
2. Andersson M, Böhme J, Andersson G, Möller E, Thorsby E, Rask L, Peterson PA (1984) Genomic hybridization with class II transplantation antigen cDNA probes as a complementary technique in tissue typing. Hum Immunol (in press)
3. Larhammar D, Andersson G, Andersson M, Bill P, Böhme J, Claesson L, Denaro M, Emmoth E, Gustafsson K, Hammerling U, Heldin E, Hyldig-Nielsen JJ, Lind P, Schenning L, Servenius B, Widmark E, Rask L, Peterson PA (1983) Molecular analysis of human class II transplantation antigens and their genes. Hum Immunol 8:95 – 103

Genetic Analysis of HLA-D Region Products Defined by PLT *

R. Wank and D.J. Schendel, on behalf of the participating laboratories

Institute of Immunology, University of Munich, Goethestraße 29, 8000 Munich 2, Federal Republic of Germany

Introduction

The finding that in vitro human primed lymphocytes (PLs) can function as memory cells allowed the analysis of genetic questions which had previously required in vivo immunizations [1]. It seemed it would be a simple task to clarify the polymorphic system of the HLA-D "locus" by priming against determinants encoded by a single haplotype [2], since the main responsibility of this locus for proliferation in primary mixed lymphocyte culture (MLC) [3] was demonstrated also in secondary MLC in an HLA-B : D recombinant family [4]. Despite the good correlation found between determinants defined by haplotype PLs and HLA-D homozygous typing cells (HTC), some evidence suggested that at least two antigenic systems encoded by one HLA haplotype were recognized by PLs [5, 6]. A considerable contribution to the strength of PL responses by products encoded by loci telomeric to HLA-DR/Dw was also shown in HLA-B : D recombinant families [7, 8].

In the PL exchange of the Seventh International Histocompatibility Workshop in Oxford, two PLs (7W704 and 7W709) were submitted which used phenotypically HLA-DR/Dw identical stimulating and responding cells for the priming combination [9]. Studies of such PLs, using families, HTC, and unrelated panels, led to the postulation of genetic systems encoded outside the HLA-DR/Dw segment [10–13]. A weak primary MLC reactivity observed between HLA-A, B, C, DR/Dw identical but GLO different siblings allowed separation of a locus encoding a stimulating determinant centromeric to HLA-DR [14]. Finally, a stringent approach was selected to define the secondary B cell (SB) system in which responding and stimulating cells for generating PLs were not only HLA-Dw, DR, and MB identical, but also HLA-A, B, and C identical. By this strategy, five alleles of a new HLA segregant series were defined in an elegant study [13].

The molecular analysis of the HLA-D region (see summary report in this volume) helps to clarify the complexities noted in PL studies of these HLA recombinant families. The findings that HLA-DR allospecificities are associated with a gene cluster comprised of one alpha and three beta chain sequences, that the DQ (formerly DC) gene cluster is composed of two alpha and two beta chain sequences, and that DP (formerly SB) belongs to yet another distinct gene cluster with two alpha and two beta chain sequences [15] indicate the degree of complexity that can be expected in lymphocyte responses measured between two individuals differing for the HLA-D region. This emphasizes the necessity of having methods that can be used to examine which of these DNA sequences are expressed and what functional roles their products play in lymphocyte activation. Primed lymphocyte typing (PLT) is such a method. The demonstration that PL analysis provided the first definition of a new segregant series of antigens encoded by the HLA-D region (i.e. the SB series), which was later confirmed by molecular mapping of the HLA-D region but has remained difficult to define with serological reagents (see report by S. Shaw et al., Analysis of SB Region Products by T Cells and Monoclonal Antibodies, this volume) reflects the importance of the PLT method for genetic analysis of the HLA-D region.

Goals of the Ninth Workshop PLT Study

1. A central goal of this workshop PLT study was to examine the DP (formerly SB) system in the frame of an international histocompatibility workshop. This was feasible because of the generous offer of S. Shaw to provide the original PL reagents by which he defined the SB specificities 1–5. These PLs and an additional pair of reagents provided by F. Robbins defining SB6 were expanded by R. Hartzman in interleukin-2 (IL-2)-containing medium to obtain adequate numbers of reagents for distribution to all participating laboratories. These reagents allowed 19 laboratories to study their local families and

* This project was supported in part by the Deutsche Forschungsgemeinschaft (A1 92/13-2).

panels and provided the data base for the central analysis of the DP system.

2. A special set of PL reagents was prepared to examine "classical" HLA-D region encoded determinants. These PLs were prepared in families with HTC donors: PLs primed to each of the single haplotypes of the HLA-D homozygous individual were made using responding cells obtained from the parents, and a third PL was primed to both haplotypes of the HTC, using responding cells from a two-haplotype different member of the family. Such sets were submitted for the specificities Dw1-Dw3 by R. Wank, M. Sasportes, and A. Termijtelen respectively.
3. It was hoped to distribute cloned PL reagents for fine-specificity analysis of HLA-D products, but few clones were available in adequate numbers. M. Sheehy and E. Yunis provided one cloned PL reagent to the workshop that was tragically lost by the shipping firm and thawed out before it could be retrieved.
4. Additional PL reagents having less well defined or unknown specificities were also submitted for analysis of HLA-D region encoded products.
5. The local families and unrelated individuals tested with the workshop PL reagents were also to be tested with the serological reagents of the Ninth Workshop, and where feasible also with the HTC reagents, thus allowing comparisons of HLA-encoded determinants defined by these three distinct methods.

Reagents and Participating Laboratories

A list of the 49 PL reagents distributed in the Ninth Workshop is given in Table 1. The reader is referred to R. Hartzmann et al. (Origin and Expansion of SB(DB)-Specific Reagents Characterized in the Ninth International Workshop, this volume) for detailed information on the DP set of PLs (PLs 20–31). All PL reagents were distributed to the participating laboratories, which are listed in Table 2. Some of these central laboratories did PLT analysis for "affiliated" laboratories in their regions.

Central Analysis of PL Responses

Data were submitted from 22 laboratories for central analysis, which was performed at the Institute of Immunology of the University of Munich. The methods for data analysis are summarized by K. Bickert et al. (Median Stabilization of Primed Lymphocyte Typing Data for the Central Workshop Analysis, this volume). The following information details the genetic analysis of PLT in the Ninth Workshop.

PLs 20–31 Defining DP Specificities

Sixteen laboratories submitted data testing PLs 20–31. The data selected for inclusion in the central analysis were divided into North American plus European files and Japanese files. The Japanese results are included in their separate report. The following analysis is based on the North American and European files, which included information from families and unrelated panel members. A subset of data including parents of the families and the additional unrelated individuals was made for the population analysis. Since not all PLs were tested in each experiment, the numbers of unrelated individuals analyzed with each PL varied from 132 to 208; 63% of all data was included in the analysis.

Distribution plots of the normalized values of the responses of each PL tested with the unrelated panel are presented in Figs. 1–12. From these diagrams, limits were selected to distinguish negative and positive reactions. These were numerically designated as follows: 0 = not tested; 2 = negative; 4 = questionably positive; 6 = positive; 8 = strongly positive. Relatively clear distinctions could be made for assigning scores of 6 and 8 for PLs 20–25, since the distributions showed a general bimodality. The distribution patterns for the remaining PLs were more complex. The limit of 6 for PLs 26 and 27 was set to include many more individuals, since previous studies had shown that the DPw4 specificity is very frequent. The distribution patterns with both PL26 and PL27 suggested that two groups of positive responses could be distinguished, and the limit of 8 was set particularly to distinguish the second positive group. Similarly complex patterns were found for PLs 28–31. Again, the 6 and 8 limits were chosen to include those responses that could be assigned as positive with the most confidence, while the 4 assignments were used to indicate broad clusters of responses that may have relationships to DPw5 or DPw6.

Two × two association analyses were made comparing PLs 20–31 with each other. The conservative limits of 6 or 8 were used to select the positive reactions. The correlation coefficients derived from this analysis are presented in Table 3. Pairwise sets of PLs (20 + 21, 22 + 23, 24 + 25, 26 + 27, 28 + 29, and 30 + 31) all showed significant positive associations and high r values for the first four pairs, with lower, yet still significant r values for the last two pairs. Weaker associations were found between PL 20 and PL 28, and between PL 29 and both PL 30

Table 1. List of submitted primed lymphocytes

Workshop listing	Local designation	HLA Antigens							Priming antigen	Lab. code
		A	Cw	B	DR	DQw	DPw	Dw		
PL 1 Priming cell	WAN-PL 1 Wi-V	2, 2 24, 2	3, – 3, 4	15, 18 15, 35	5, w8 1, 5	3, – 1, 3	2, 4 4, –	 1, –	Dw1	WAN
PL 2 Priming cell	WAN-PL 2 Wi-M	2, 2 2, 11	3, – 4, –	15, 18 18, 35, w6, w6	5, w8 1, w8	3, – 1, –	2, 4 2, 4	 1, –	Dw1	WAN
PL 3 Priming cell	WAN-PL 3 Wi-B	2, 2 11, 24	3, – 4, 4	15, 18 35, 35	5, w8 1, 1	3, – 1, –	2, 4 4, 4	 1, 1	Dw1	WAN
PL 4 Priming cell	SAS-CH 31 Gerard Chap	2, 19.2 19.2, 29	5, – 7, –	18, – 8, –	3, 5, w52 2, 3, w52	3			DR2	SAS/ DAU
PL 5 Priming cell	SAS-CH 32 Madeleine Chap	2, 19.2 2, 24	5, –	18, – 18, 18	3, 5, w52	3			DR2	SAS/ DAU
PL 6 Priming cell	SAS-CH 34 Hugues Chap	2, 19.2 24, 29	5, – 5, –	18, – 8, 18	3, 5, w52 2, 5, w52	3 3			DR2	SAS/ DAU
PL 7 Priming cell	AX* RT194 CAT	2, 28 1, 28	w2, – w2, –	51, 27 8, 27	5, w6 3, w6	1, 3 1, 2	3, 0 3, 4	5, 6 3, 6	Dw3	ROO
PL 8 Priming cell	AY* RT194 JAA	2, 28 1, 2	w2 –	51, 27 51, 8	5, w6 3, 5	1, 3 2, 3	3, 0 2, 0	5, 6 3, 5	Dw3	ROO
PL 9 Priming cell	AZ* RT194 CAA	2, 28 1, 1	w2 –	51, 27 8, 8	5, w6 3, 3	1, 3 2, 2	3, 0 1, 4	5, 6 3, 3	Dw3	ROO
PL 10 Priming cell	PT901 J. Latimer	29, 30 2, –	4, – –, –	13, 35 8, 18	1, 4 1, 4	1, –		1, 4 1, 4	Dw4	STA
PL 11 Priming cell	PT902 I. Flores	1, 11	6, –	37, w52	1, 4			1, 4 1, –	Dw14	STA
PL 12 Priming cell	PT903 T. Ball	1, 3 1, 2	–, – 5, 6	7, 8 37, 44	1, 3 1, w10			1, 3 1, –	DRw10	STA
PL 13 Priming cell	B* D* Emanuel	1, 2 1, 29	6, 6 3, 6	13, 17 13, 27	7, 7 3, 7	2, 3	4, 4 4, 4	11L, 11S 3, 11S	Dw3	HSU/ BIA
PL 14 Priming cell	FA* Stephen Sr.	2, 29 3, 29	3, 6 3, 6	17, 27 27, –	3, 7 3, 7	2, 3 2, 3	4, 4 4, 4	3, 11L 3, 7	Dw7, DPw2	HSU/ BIA

Table 1. (continued)

Workshop listing	Local designation	HLA Antigens							Priming antigen	Lab. code
		A	Cw	B	DR	DQw	DPw	Dw		
PL 15 Priming cell	FH Eli	2, 29 2, 3	3, 6 6, 6	17, 27 17, –	3, 7 7, 7	2, 3 2, 3	4, 4 2, 4	2, 11L 7, 11L	Dw7	HSU/ BIA
PL 16 Priming cell	AE* Naomi	3, 29 2, 3	3, 6 6, 6	27, – 17, –	3, 7 7, 7	2, 2 2, 3	4, 4 2, 2	3, 11S 7, 11L	Dw11L, DQ3	HSU/ BIA
PL 17 Priming cell	GF* David	1, 29 2, 29	3, 6 3, 6	13, 27 17, 27	3, 7 3, 7	2, 2 2, 3	4, 4 4, 4	3, 11S 3, 11L	Dw11L, DQ3	HSU/ BIA
PL 18 Priming cell	REI MN2 PLT Rei Pos	2, 3 2, 2	3, – 3, –	15, 44 15, 39	1, 1 1, 2			1, – 1, DMN2	DMN2	BAC
PL 19 Priming cell	Ebbe/Mad Madura								Dw/DRw8	SVE
PLs20 – 33: see Hartzman et al., PLT Joint Report										
PL 34 Priming cell	Mette/Maja* Maja								DP?	SVE
PL 35 Priming cell	Lone/Allan* Allan								DP?	SVE
PL 36 Priming cell	BRA-PZ ZED	3, 25 11, 25	–, – –, 2	7, 18 7, 40	2, 5 2, 5			2, 5 2, 5	?	BUC
PL 37 Priming cell	BRA-GN NYU	3, 23 1, 32	–, – 2, –	8, w52 27, 35, w4	3, 4 3, 4			3, 4 3, 4	?	BUC
PL 38 Priming cell	BRA1/2* BRA2	1, 2 1, 2	–, –	8, 44, w4, w6 8, 44, w4, w6	3, 7 3, 7				? ?	BRS
PL 39	BRA2/1	see PL 38: reverse priming combination								BRS
PL 40 Priming cell	PL 1 P 1	1, 3 1, 3		8, 35, w4 8, 35	3, 5 3				?	SIN
PL 41	PL 2	see PL 40: reverse priming combination							DR5	SIN
PL 42 Priming cell	SAS G 12 SAS G 2	2, 3 2, 19.2	–, – –, –	13, 15 13, 13	7, 7, w53, 53 7, 7, w53, 53				? ?	SAS/ DAU

PL 43 Priming cell	SAS P34 SAS P 4	2, 24 2, 25	2, 7 –, 7	40, 49 18, 49	4, 5 4, 5				?	SAS/ DAU
PL 44 Priming cell	SAS LS SAS S	1, 2 1, 2	5, 7 5, 7	8, 44 8, 44	3, 4 3, 4				?	SAS/ DAU
PL 45 Priming cell	SAS P 12 SAS P 2	2, 25 24, 25	7, – 2, –	18, 49 18, 40	4, 5 5, 5				?	SAS/ DAU
PL 46 Priming cell	SAS DB SAS B	2, 3 2, 30	4, 7 4, 6	35, 51 35, 51	1, 2 1, 2					SAS/ DAU
PL 47 Priming cell	BA* RT196 CB* RT190, QBL	1, 1 26, 26	7, 7 5, 5	8, 8 18, 8	3, 3 3, 3	2, 2 2, 2	4, 4 2, 2	3, 3 3, 3	LBQ1	ROO
PL 48 Priming cell	CB* 11RT192 CB* 6RT192, CA* RT190, BMJ	1, 1 1, 24	7, 7 5	8, 8 8, 8	3, 3 3, 3	2, 2 2, 2	4, 4 4, 4	3, 3 3, 3	LBQ1	ROO
PL 49 Priming cell	WAN-PL-6 WiR-1	2, 11 2, 11	3, 4 3, 4	15, 35 15, 35	1, 5 1, 1	1, – 1, –	4, – 4, 4	1, – 1, 1	?	WAN

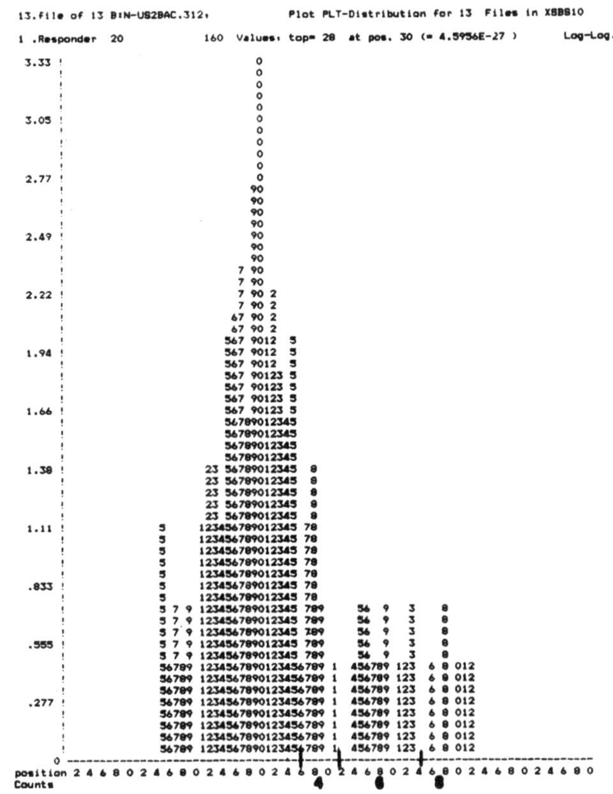

Fig. 1. Distribution plots of double normalized values (DNVs) of responses of PL 20. The number of responses (log scale) is given on the *y* axis and increasing DNVs are given from left to right on the *x* axis (log scale). The increments selected for assigning 4, 6, or 8 scores are shown below the *x* axis (4, questionably positive; 6, positive; 8, strongly positive)

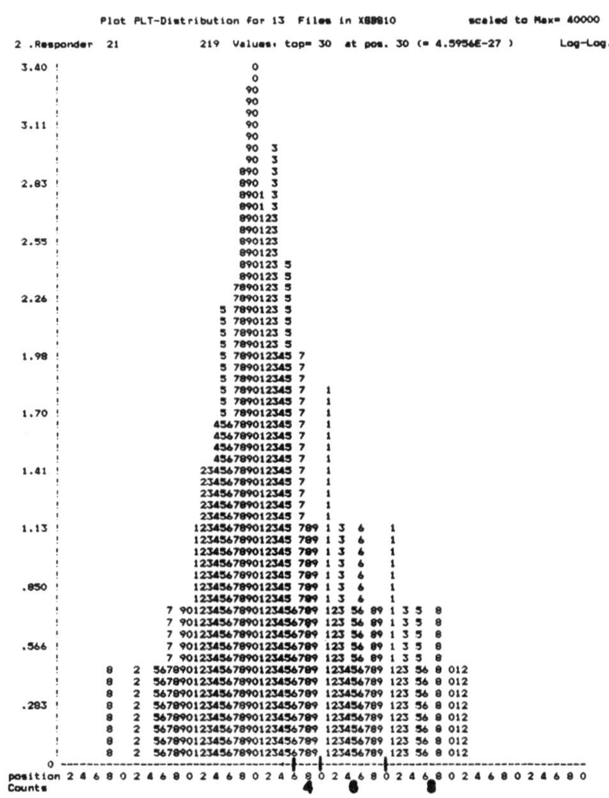

Fig. 2. Distribution plot for PL 21. Scales and scores as in Fig. 1

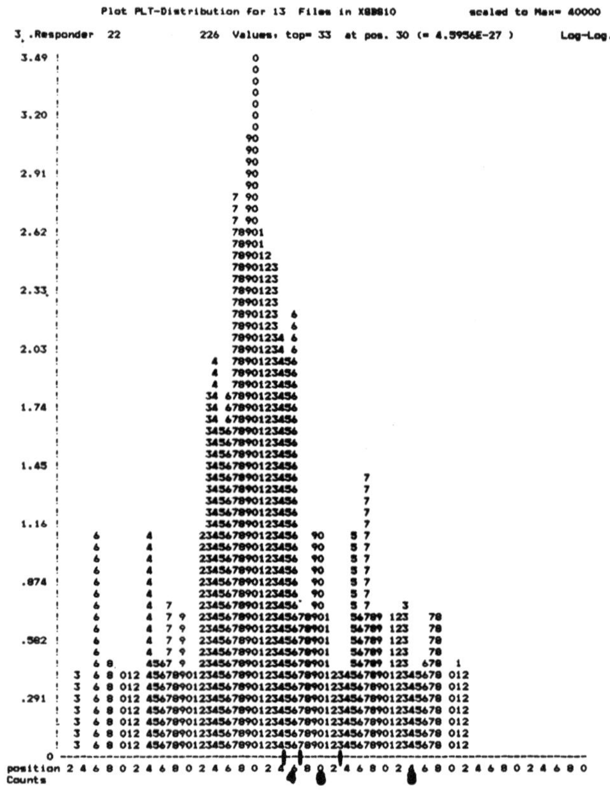

Fig. 3. Distribution plot for PL 22. Scales and scores as in Fig. 1

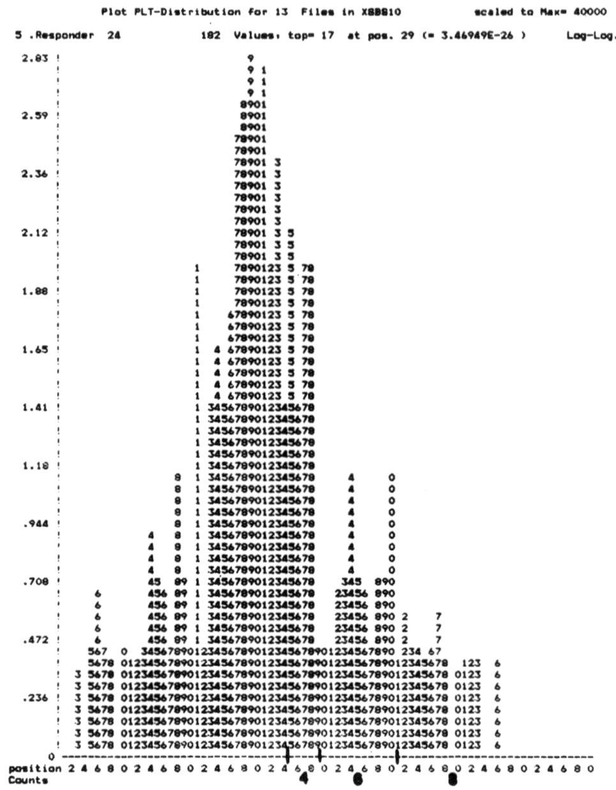

Fig. 5. Distribution plot for PL 24. Scales and scores as in Fig. 1

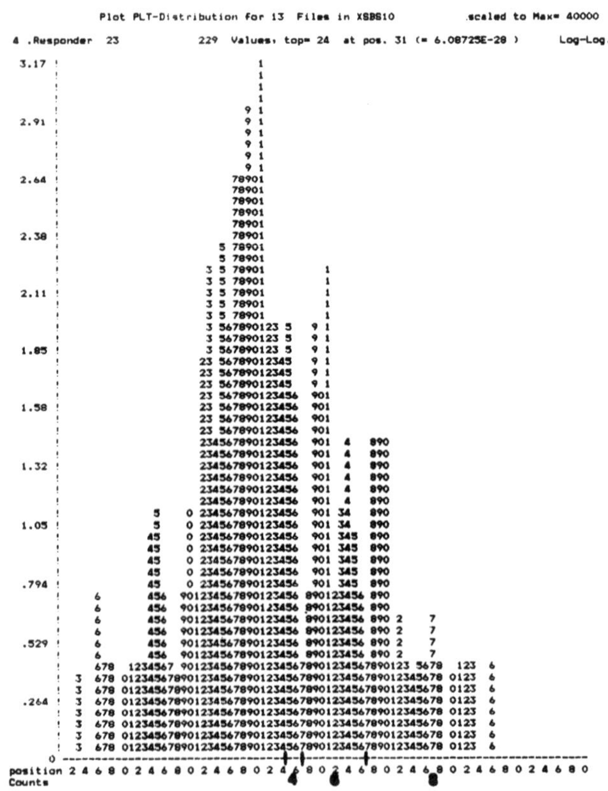

Fig. 4. Distribution plot for PL 23. Scales and scores as in Fig. 1

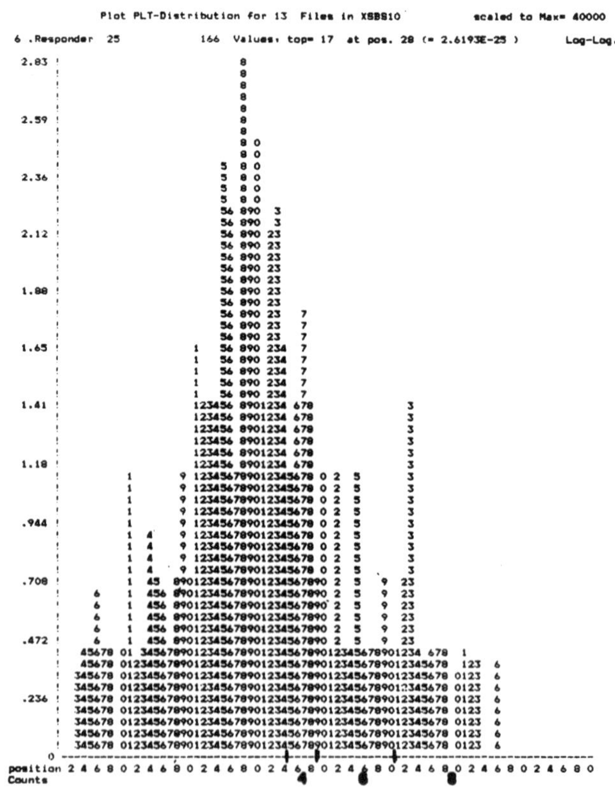

Fig. 6. Distribution plot for PL 25. Scales and scores as in Fig. 1

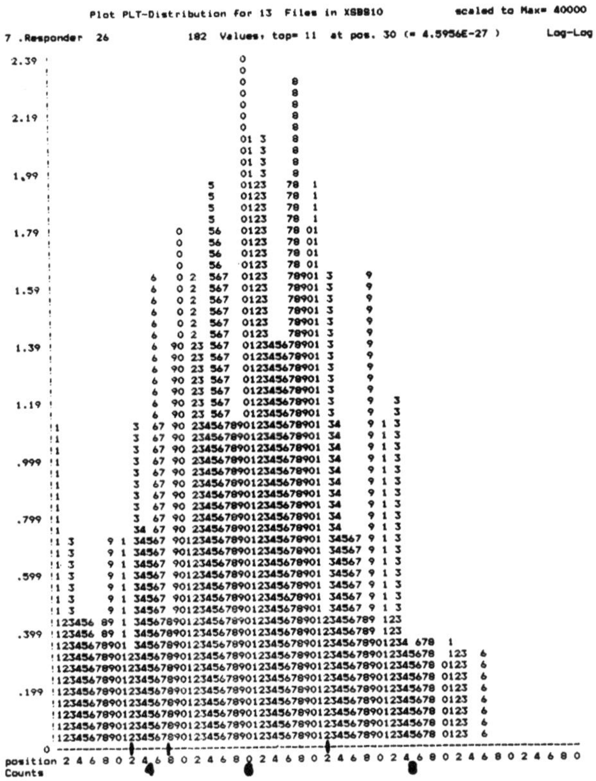

Fig. 7. Distribution plot for PL 26. Scales and scores as in Fig. 1

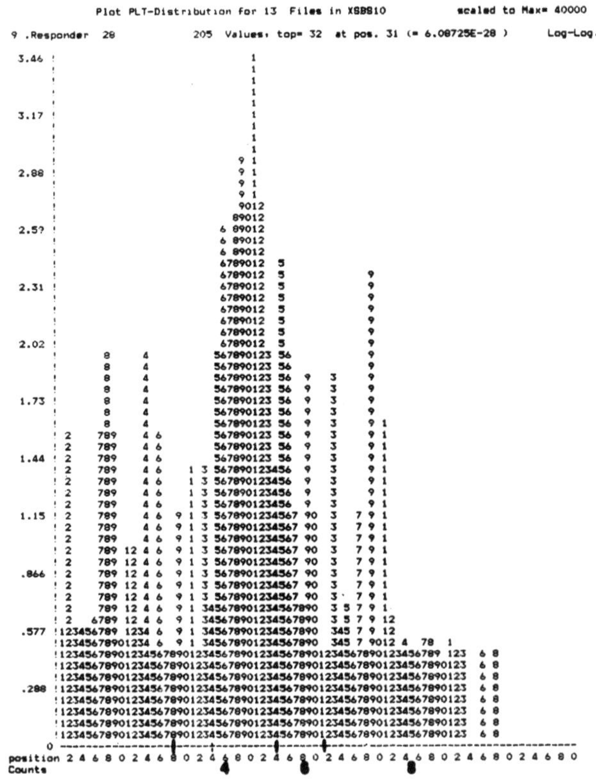

Fig. 9. Distribution plot for PL 28. Scales and scores as in Fig. 1

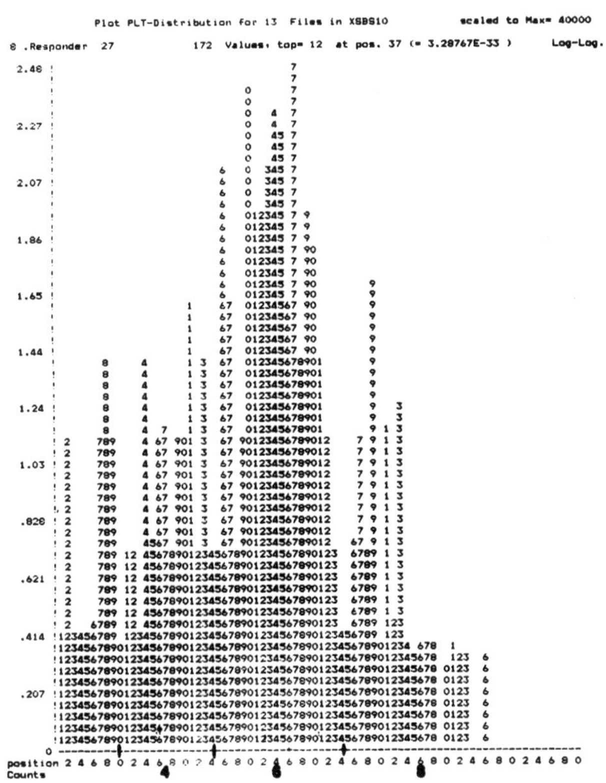

Fig. 8. Distribution plot for PL 27. Scales and scores as in Fig. 1

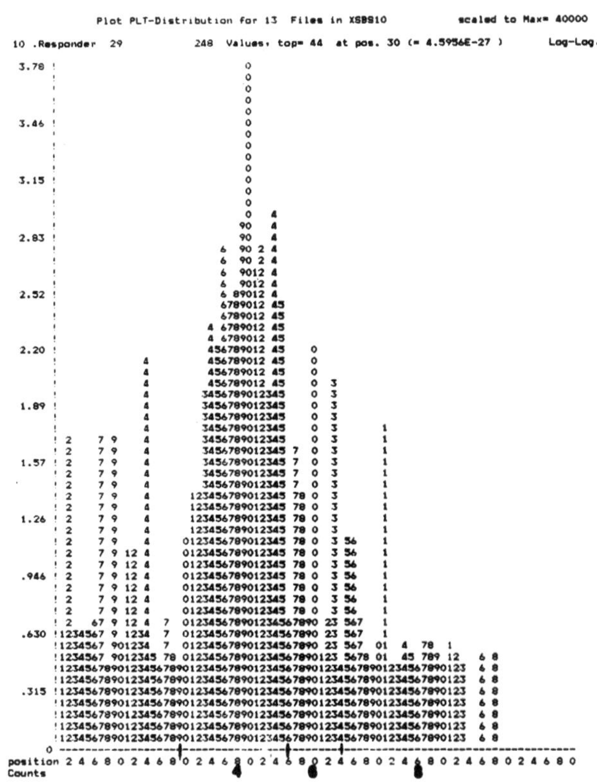

Fig. 10. Distribution plot for PL 29. Scales and scores as in Fig. 1

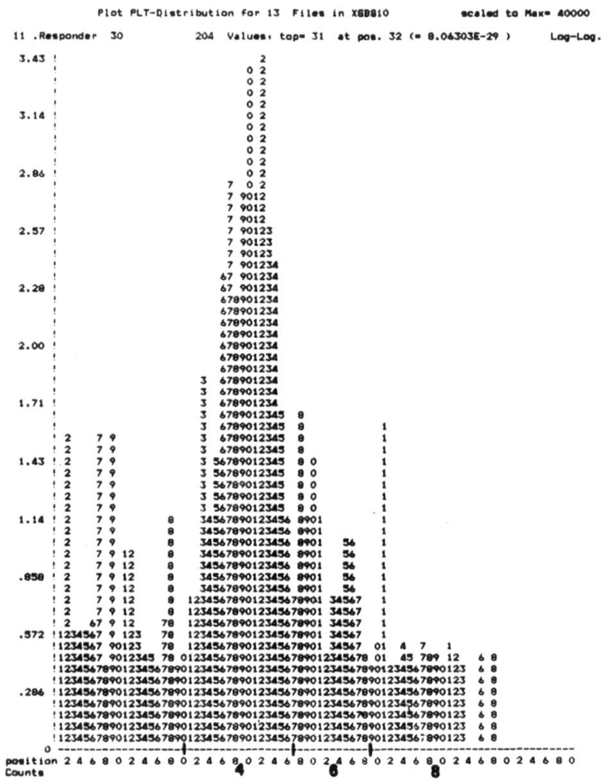

Fig. 11. Distribution plot for PL 30. Scales and scores as in Fig. 1

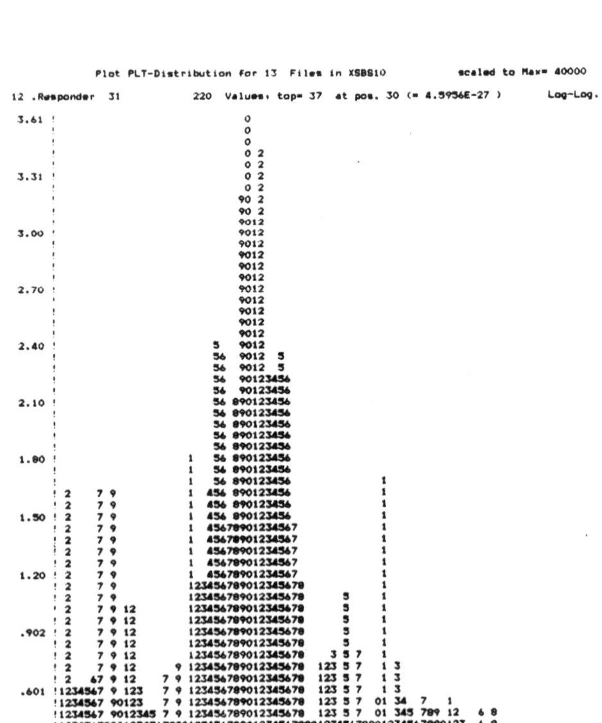

Fig. 12. Distribution plot for PL 31. Scales and scores as in Fig. 1

and PL 31. The strongly associated pairs of reagents were used to assign antigen specificities. Assignment of a DP specificity to any individual was made only when a 6 or 8 reaction was found with both reagents of the PL pair. The correlation coefficients comparing the workshop-assigned DP specificities with the individual PL reagents are shown in Table 4. For each specificity at least one member of the PL pair showed an excellent coefficient of correlation. Thus these PLs could be used to indicate a potential DP specificity although a workshop assignment was not made.

The antigen frequencies and gene frequencies for DP alleles in the unrelated panel are shown in Table 5. The central analysis antigen assignments were made only on the basis of positive reactions with both PL reagents identifying a given DP specificity, thus the percentages of positive individuals represent minimum estimates. The gene frequencies were calculated from these stringent antigen assignments. Antigen frequencies based on the assignment of a 6 or 8 reaction with the best member of the PL pair are also listed in Table 5 for comparison. No triplet antigen assignments were made in the unrelated panel using the stringent antigen assignment criteria (i.e., reactions of 6 or 8 with both PLs).

The selected subset of files used for central analysis of DP was recombined with the data on the remaining PL reagents, following normalization of both independently, to look for other reagents with potential DP reactivities (Table 6). Several associations were found, but the *r* values in general were quite low because of the few numbers of unrelated individuals that were tested with both sets of reagents. Only PL 48 showed significant associations to both members of the DPw4 PL pair. PLs 44 and 47 showed associations with the members of the PL pair showing higher associations with the workshop-defined specificities (Table 3), whereas PLs 40, 45, and 46 did not.

Analysis of "Classical" PLs (PLs 1–9)

Association analyses of the PL sets primed to one haplotype (PLs 1, 2, 4, 5, 7, 8) and two haplotypes (PLs 3, 6, 9), of HLA-DR/Dw homozygous donors is shown in Table 7. The correlations among the sets are lower than their correlations with the DR specificities associated with the priming haplotypes, except for the PL group 7–9, where both are comparable. Clearly, no better discrimination was found in reagents primed to single vs two haplotypes of the HTC donor. Interestingly, PLs 7–9 reacted as a set with non-DR3 cells of Japanese origin.

Table 2. Participating laboratories

REG/LAB	Research Center	Investigators	Affiliated Investigators
BENROO	University Hospital, Leiden, The Netherlands	A. Termijtelen, J.J. van Rood	
EAEBUC	Dept. of Medical Microbiology, Bratislava, Czechoslovakia	M. Buc, D. Busova	
FRADAU	Dept. of Immunology, Hôpital St. Louis, Paris, France	M. Sasportes, E. Villechenous-Pineda	
FRAJEA	Dept. of Immunology, Hôpital Cantonal, Geneva, Switzerland	F. Chardonnens, M. Jeannet	
GERBRA	Dept. of Immunohematology, Hadassah Hospital, Jerusalem, Israel	A. Amar, C. Brautbar	
GERGSW	Inst. of Virology and Immunology, Essen, Fed. Rep. of Germany	I. Doxiadis, H. Grosse-Wilde	
GERWAN	Inst. of Immunology, Munich, Fed. Rep. of Germany	D.J. Schendel, R. Wank	GERALB: E. Albert, Munich, Fed. Rep. of Germany EAEKAS: A. Kastelan, Zagreb, Yugoslavia
JAPKAS	University School of Medicine, Kitazato, Japan	N. Kashiwagi	
JAPTSU	Tokai Medical School, Kangawa, Japan	H. Inouye, K. Tsuji	
NCYBIA	Johns Hopkins School of Medicine, Baltimore, Maryland	W. Bias, S. Hsu	
NCYYUN	Sidney Farber Cancer Institute, Boston, Massachusetts	E. Yunis	
SCASVE	University Hospital, Copenhagen, Denmark	N. Morling, P. Platz, L. Ryder, A. Svejgaard	SCAKIS: T. Kristensen, P. Wendelboe Hansen Aarhus, Denmark
SCATSB	University Hospital, Oslo, Norway	T. Moen, E. Thorsby	
UKIBRS	Southwest Transfusion Centre, Bristol, England	B. Bradley	
UKIFES	London Hospital Medical School, London, England	H. Festenstein, D. Jaraquemada, T. Ollier	
US1HEJ	Naval Medical Research Institute, Bethesda, Maryland	R. Eckels, R. Hartzman, A. Johnson	NCYZIE: K. Zier Philadelphia, Pennsylvania
US2BAC	University of Minnesota, Minneapolis, Minnesota	F.H. Bach, N. Reinsmoen	
US4STA	Southwestern Medical School, Dallas, Texas	H. Ball, L. Dombravsky, P. Statsny	
US5SIN	McMaster University, Hamilton, Ontario, Canada	D. Singal	

Table 3. Correlation coefficients for DP reagents

21	.74**										
22	–.16	–.17*									
23	–.11	–.11	.68**								
24	–.03	–.11	–.08	–.15							
25	.13	–.03	–.15	–.19	.72**						
26	–.09	–.14	–.17	–.22	–.18	–.20**					
27	–.15	–.25	–.17	–.28	–.07	–.12	.69**				
28	.27*	.11	.00	–.05	–.15	–.07	–.07	–.07			
29	–.15	–.10	.04	.00	–.07	–.14	.02	.02	.28**		
30	–.12	–.12	.11	.03	–.04	–.06	–.28*	–.13	.01	.16*	
31	–.07	–.07	.01	.02	.01	–.07	–.16	–.02	.02	.20*	.39**
PL	20	21	22	23	24	25	26	27	28	29	30

* The coefficient of correlation (r) was calculated as follows: $\frac{a \cdot d - b \cdot c}{\sqrt{(a+b)(c+d)(a+c)(b+d)}}$

** The significance of r was determined using the χ^2 test with Yates' correction: * = χ^2 3.48 – 15; ** = $\chi^2 \geqq 15$

Table 4. Correlation coefficients between DP antigen assignments and individual DP primed lymphocytes

	PL (workshop no)											
	20	21	22	23	24	25	26	27	28	29	30	31
DP antigen												
DPw1	.78**	.95**	−.15	−.10	−.09	.06	.03	−.24	.21*	−.13	−.11	−.05
DPw2	−.14	−.16	.95**	.72**	−.12	−.14	−.22*	−.28*	−.03	.03	.10	−.09
DPw3	−.10	−.11	−.10	−.14	.94**	.78**	−.22**	−.11	−.13	−.09	.00	−.06
DPw4	−.18	−.30*	−.13	−.21*	−.07	−.14	.69**	1.00**	−.04	.10	−.22*	−.13
DPw5	−.11	−.11	.15	.10	−.11	−.14	−.01	−.14	.53*	.70**	−.05	.07
DPw6	−.07	−.06	.00	−.09	−.06	−.07	−.26*	−.10	.03	.17	.47**	.86**

** = $\chi^2 > 30.0$; * = $\chi^2 < 10.0$

Table 5. Frequencies of DP alleles in unrelated individuals

Allele	No. tested	Antigen frequency (+ve one PL)	Antigen frequency (+ve two PLs)	Gene frequency
DPw1	132	12.9	8.3	.07
DPw2	208	25.0	14.9	.07
DPw3	166	15.1	9.6	.12
DPw4	147	83.7	70.7	.35
DPw5	171	25.4	10.5	.05
DPw6	168	13.6	3.6	.02
Blank				.32

Antigen frequencies are calculated using assignments of positive responses with the PL reagent showing the highest coefficient of correlation with the defined specificity (Table 4). Gene frequencies are based on the stringent antigen assignment criteria of response values of 6 or 8 with both PLs defining a given DP specificity

Table 6. Other PL reagents showing associations with DP PLs 20 – 31

PL reagents	*r*	No. tested	*P*
46×25	0.45	25	0.04
48×26	0.36	56	0.01
48×27*	0.36	55	0.01
47×27*	0.25	80	0.05
45×28	0.62	26	0.01
40×28	0.43	26	0.06
44×31*	0.43	26	0.06

* The PL reagents marked with an asterisk represent those members of the PL pair that show the highest *r* values with the workshop-assigned DP specificities (see Table 4).
Significance was determined using Fisher's exact test for small samples

Table 7. Association analyses of classical PLs and DR specificities

PL reagents	No. tested	*r*	Specificities	No. tested	*r*
PL 1×2	209	0.35*	PL 1×DR 1	92	0.57*
PL 1×3	176	0.23*	PL 2×DR 1	95	0.39*
PL 2×3	197	0.39*	PL 3×DR 1	94	0.34*
PL 4×5	117	−0.6	PL 4×DR 2	40	0.69*
PL 4×6	115	0.44*	PL 5×DR 2	40	0.13
PL 5×6	115	0.02	PL 6×DR 2	40	0.62*
PL 7×8	225	0.45*	PL 7×DR 3	126	0.42*
PL 7×9	223	0.45*	PL 8×DR 3	124	0.53*
PL 8×9	223	0.45*	PL 9×DR 3	124	0.47*

* Significant *r* values ($p < 0.05$) are indicated with an asterisk

Conclusions

The emphasis of individual laboratories on typing families and panels for DP (SB) antigens limited the analysis of classical PL but provided an excellent data base for analyzing the genetics of the DP system in an international framework. The most striking points can be summarized as follows:

1. Cultured T cell lines established as paired reagents from six DP primed cell specificities (see R. Hartzman et al., Origin and Expansion of SB (DP)-Specific Reagents Characterized in the Ninth Histocompatibility Workshop, this volume) could be used very successfully for defining DP antigens. This advocates and opens new dimensions for collaboration with cellular reagents. Using such reagents, 19 laboratories were able to characterize their panels and families with reagents comparable to those originally reported by S. Shaw (13).
2. Population studies confirmed the existence of determinants behaving as products of a single genetic system.
3. Family studies which allowed segregation analysis of six DP specificities in 55 positive parents, including 341 tested family members, showed Mendelian segregation with HLA (for details see D. J. Schendel et al., Segregation Analysis of PLT Reagents in Families, this volume).

This fine specificity of DP PLs was not seen in the classical PLs despite the selection of homozygous donors and priming in restricted family combinations. The heterogeneity in these reagents probably reflects the complexity of the HLA-D region, whose functional diversity will be best defined with cloned PLs.

Acknowledgments. The support of Professor G. Riethmüller with the computer facilities of the Institute of Immunology is gratefully acknowledged. Particular thanks are due to A. Schreiter, C. Dalibor, M. Scheuerecker, J. Johnson, and N. Logothetis for assistance in the central data analysis.

References

1. Hayry P, Anderson L (1974) Generation of T memory cells in one-way mixed lymphocyte culture. II. Anamnestic responses of "secondary" lymphocytes. Scand J Immunol 3:823
2. Sheehy M, Sondel P, Bach M, Wank R, Bach F (1975) HLA typing: a rapid assay using primed lymphocytes. Science 188:1308
3. Yunis EJ, Amos DB (1971) Three closely linked genetic systems relevant to transplantation. Proc Natl Acad Sci USA 68:3031
4. Mawas C, Charmot D, Sasportes M (1975) Secondary response of in vitro primed human lymphocytes to allogeneic cells. I. Role of HLA-antigens and mixed lymphocyte reaction stimulating determinants in secondary in vitro proliferative response. Immunogenetics 2:449
5. Bach FH, Sondel PM, Sheehy MJ, Wank R, Alter B, Bach ML (1975) The complexity of the HLA LD system: a PLT analysis. In: Kissmeyer-Nielsen F (ed) Histocompatibility testing 1975. Munksgaard, Copenhagen, pp 576–580
6. Fradelizi D, Mawas C, Charmot D, Sasportes M (1975) In vitro primed cells: a probe for LD typing? In: Kissmeyer-Nielsen F (ed) Histocompatibility testing 1975. Munksgaard, Copenhagen, pp 584–587
7. Wank R, Schendel DJ, Hansen JA, Yunis EJ, Dupont B (1977) Two different HLA restimulating determinants separated by recombination and titration. Transplant Proc 9:1771–1775
8. Zier KS, Grosse-Wilde H, Huber C, Braunsteiner H, Albert ED (1978) Restimulation in secondary MLC by a non-D locus determinant within the MHC. Immunogenetics 6:451
9. Bradley B, Oliver RTD, Mendell N, Stevens A (1978) Joint report – the primed lymphocyte (PL) exchange. In: Bodmer WF, Batchelor JR, Bodmer JG, Festenstein H, Morris PJ (eds) Histocompatibility testing 1977. Munksgaard, Copenhagen, pp 142–148
10. Nunez-Roldan A, Sasportes M, Fradelizi D (1978) Analysis of products involved in primary and secondary allogeneic proliferation in man. II. Detection of products different from Ia-like, DRw antigens, activating secondary allogeneic proliferation in man. Immunogenetics 6:43
11. Wank R, Schendel DJ, Hansen JA, Dupont B (1978) The lymphocyte restimulation system: evaluation by intra-HLA-D group priming. Immunogenetics 6:107
12. Termijtelen A, Bradley BA, van Rood JJ (1980) A new determinant, defined by PLT, coded for in the HLA region and apparently independent of the HLA-D and DR loci. Tissue Antigens 15:267–274
13. Shaw S, Johnson AH, Shearer GM (1980) Evidence for a new segregant series of B cell antigens that are encoded in the HLA-D region and that stimulate secondary allogeneic proliferative and cytotoxic responses. J Exp Med 152:565
14. Mawas C, Charmot D, Sivy M, Mercier P, North ML, Hauptmann G (1978) A weak human MLR locus mapping at the right of a crossing over between HLA-D, Bf and GLO. J Immunogenet 5:583
15. Kaufmann JF, Auffray D, Korman AJ, Shackelford DA, Strominger J (1984) The class II molecules of the human and murine major histocompatibility complex. Cell 36:1

Segregation Analysis of PLT Reagents in Families

D. J. Schendel[1], R. J. Hartzman[2], D. Jaraquemada[3], T. Kristensen[4], N. Morling[5], W. Ollier[3], A. Termijtelen[6], and R. Wank[1]

1 Institute of Immunology, University of Munich, Goethestraße 29, 8000 Munich 2, Federal Republic of Germany
2 Naval Medical Research Institute, Bethesda, MD 20016, USA
3 Department of Immunology, London Hospital Medical College, London, U.K.
4 Tissue Typing Laboratory, University Hospital, Aarhus, Denmark
5 Tissue Typing Laboratory, University Hospital, Copenhagen, Denmark
6 Department of Immunohematology, University Hospital, Leiden, The Netherlands

Segregation of DP Alleles in Families as Defined with PLs 20 – 31

From the data included in the central analysis of DP, 36 families could be used for segregation analysis. The numbers of families informative for each DP allele are listed in Table 1. Only two families were informative for DPw1, since primed lymphocyte (PL) reagent 20 did not function well in several of the larger experiments. For the DPw2 specificity, nine informative families were analyzed. In one family, one child carried the DPw2 specificity who did not have the expected HLA haplotype carrying this specificity in the parent and three other children. Since data on GLO was not available, a recombination event could not be confirmed. For the specificities DPw2-DPw4, one child in each of several families was found to lack an antigen, although inheriting the given HLA haplotype with which the DP specificity was associated in at least two other children. Only in the case of DPw3 was information on GLO available

Table 1. Segregation analysis of DP alleles in 36 families using central workshop assignments

Allele	Positive parents	Children tested	Exceptions to HLA segregation	Comment
DPw1	2	8	0	
DPw2	9	36	1 extra, 2 missed	No outside markers
DPw3	6	27	1 missed	DR:GLO recombination; goes with DR
DPw4	23	96	1 missed	No outside markers
DPw5	4	16	3 missed	All in one family; 6 – 8 reaction seen with one PL
DPw6	3	14	0	
Total	47	197	8	

Table 2. Segregation analysis of "classical" PLs (PLs 1 – 9) in 21 families

No. of families	No. of haplotypes	PL reagent	No. +ve/no. expected	Exceptions
8	39	PL 1	6/15	9 misses; 1 extra
		PL 2	9/15	6 misses; 3 extra*
		PL 3	9/15	6 misses; 3 extra* *Segregates with DR2
6	38	PL 4	20/21	1 missed; 2 extra
		PL 5	16/21	5 missed; 2 extra
		PL 6	13/21	8 missed; 1 extra
7	40	PL 7	22/23	1 missed; 2 extra*
		PL 8	19/23	4 missed; 2 extra*
		PL 9	22/23	1 missed; 2 extra* * extra reactions occur in 2 identical siblings (DR7/DR–).

* Expected positives are based on the presence of the DR specificity to which the PLs were primed (i.e., DR1 for PLs 1 – 3; DR2 for PLs 4 – 6; DR3 for PLs 7 – 9)

Histocompatibility Testing 1984
Edited by E. D. Albert et al.

which could be used to confirm a recombinational event between DR and GLO; in this case the DPw3 antigen segregated with DR. The three missed assignments for DPw5 most likely represent false-negative assignments, since all three were found in one family in which the parent and one child showed reactions of 6 or 8 with both PL 28 and 29, while three children each showed a 6 or 8 reaction with only one of this PL pair.
No assignments of double specificities to an HLA haplotype were observed.

Segregation Analysis of PLs 1 – 9 in 21 Families

Although the coefficients of correlation among the three members of each "classical" PL group were very low, in general, their associations with the DR specificities DR1, 2, and 3, respectively, were better. Concordance was also seen between these PL specificities and DR in segregation in 21 families. Most exceptions were found in the PLs 1 – 3 group, but two DR1-positive families were not typed with these PLs and one family not having DR1 showed clear segregation with a DR2-bearing haplotype. For groups 4 – 6 and 7 – 9, no exceptions encompassing complete families were noted, and missed reactions were mostly lack of reactivity with one of the three members of the group. The most consistent patterns of all three reagents typing as a group were found for PLs 7 – 9, and 17 of 23 haplotypes with DR3 typed with all three PLs. Interestingly in one family, two HLA-identical but non-DR3 siblings were typed with all three reagents. In none of these exceptions was a Dw specificity of the predicted type present (Table 2).

Median Stabilization of PLT Data for the Central Workshop Analysis

K. Bickert[1], N. Morling[2], D.J. Schendel[1], W. Jennert[1], and R. Wank[1]

1 Institute of Immunology, University of Munich, Goethestraße 29, 8000 Munich 2, Federal Republic of Germany
2 Tissue Typing Laboratory, University Hospital, Copenhagen, Denmark

The data submitted for central primed lymphocyte typing (PLT) analysis encompassed 72 experiments from 22 laboratories, testing 49 workshop PL reagents and 12 "local" reagents. Stimulating cells were derived from 109 families and several hundred unrelated individuals, giving a total of 1057 different stimulating cells that were tested with some part of the workshop PL set. This resulted in 1.2 megabytes of information that was analyzed using a small system of two interconnected, 8-bit, CP/M microcomputers (PSI 80 and PSI 980, Kontron Electronics, Munich, Federal Republic of Germany). The PSI 980 was extended with a 20-megabyte hard disk in January, 1984 to complete the central analysis in Munich.
The data were submitted as counts per minute (cpm) of individual triplicates for each PL-stimulating cell combination. These data were assembled into experiment matrices, with PLs listed vertically and stimulating cells listed horizontally and included all replicate values. These data matrices were returned to the individual laboratories for correction. The *mean* values and their standard deviations and the *median* values were compared for the replicates of all test combinations. It was concluded that the median values provided an accurate representation of the data, and selection of this value resulted in elimination of the most extreme outliers. Reduced matrices containing only the median values were used for further analysis. A total mean value for each experimental matrix was calculated, and any row or column mean giving a value of < 10% of this total mean value was eliminated as technically deficient.
The wide range of median cpm (100 – 10 000) within individual experiments and among the 72 workshop experiments necessitated some form of data normalization to allow direct comparisons of data. To determine the appropriate method a subset of experiments was chosen, of which three showed clear negative and positive responses by simple visual inspection and the other three did not allow such distinctions, although the control values for the PLs showed discrimination. A computer program with a "menu" of methods was used to compare different parameters of stabilization in this subset, based on mean, median, or maximum values. Single normalization, either responder-wise (i.e., by row) or stimulator-wise (by column) was compared with double normalization, carried out

Histocompatibility Testing 1984
Edited by E. D. Albert et al.

first by row and then by column, or vice versa. These sets of "normalized" matrices were then evaluated by hand to determine which method would allow discriminative assignments for the different PLs and stimulating cells; would not give too many positive assignments to a single stimulating cell; and suggested patterns of segregation in families such that in general, responses in parents were found in some children. Segregation with HLA was not assumed at this stage.

All comparisons from the menu yielded disappointing results for defining a means of stabilization in the first round of analysis. Inspection of the raw data matrices suggested that the different nature of the PL reagents might account for some difficulties, since the levels of response with the cultured T cell lines (CTC), PLs 20–31, were normally much higher than those of the remaining PLs. In setting up their experiments, several laboratories had divided the PL reagents into two groups, one containing PLs 20–31, the other Pls 1–19 and 34–49. In such cases several of the stabilization methods looked promising. Therefore, each experiment containing a mixture of the two types of PL reagents was "split" into two experiments as described above. Since the total data submitted indicated that the majority of CTC reagents worked technically well for most labs, while the remaining PL were tested by fewer labs with many fewer stimulating cells, particular emphasis was placed on optimizing the analysis for PLs 20–31, comprising the standard DP set. Following this division of all experiments the menu was again utilized and double normalization using the median value was found to best fulfill the criteria listed above.

Median stabilization has been used successfully for normalization of PL data, as reported by Morling and colleagues [1, 2], and it was from these reports that this method was included in the workshop menu. Comparison of the method of median stabilization with other approaches, as well as its effect at each step of analysis for a single experiment, is well documented [1]. The reader is referred to this report for details. For the workshop analysis, one modification from the published procedure was made. The order of the double normalization was reversed: it was done first stimulatorwise (i.e., down the columns) and then responderwise (along the rows). This change presumably gave better results, because the dimensions of the DP data matrices generally had more stimulating cell values (up to 85) than PL values (maximum 12). The procedure for median normalization used in the workshop analysis was as follows:

Step 1. Copy the n elements of a column of experimental data (median values of triplicates) to a vector VE.

Step 2. Sort the vector according to increasing median cpm.

Step 3. Determine the "column" median of the vector as follows:

if n is odd: column median $= \mathrm{VE}\left(\frac{n+1}{2}\right)$

if n is even: column median

$$= 1/2 \times \left(\mathrm{VE}\left(\frac{n}{2}\right) + \mathrm{VE}\left(\frac{n}{2}+1\right)\right)$$

Step 4. Perform the first normalization by multiplying the column elements by

$$\frac{50}{\text{column median}}.$$

Step 5. Repeat steps 1–3 for the normalized data of a row to determine a "normalized row median".

Step 6. Perform the second normalization by multiplying the normalized row elements by

$$\frac{50}{\text{normalized row median}}.$$

Following median stabilization of all workshop experiments, a subset of data was selected for inclusion in the central genetic analysis of PLT. Three criteria were used for exclusion of experiments: (a) a minimum matrix size was not met (<5 PLs and <15 stimulating cells); (b) corrections of the data were not received from the submitting lab; (c) a minimum number of positive assignments could not be made ($<10\%$ positive assignments/experiment). The results of the genetic analysis are presented in the first two parts of this joint report (R. Wank and D. J. Schendel, Genetic Analysis of HLA-D Region Products by Primed Lymphocyte Typing, D. J. Schendel et al., Segregation Analysis of Primed Lymphocyte Typing Reagents in Families, both this volume).

References

1. Morling N, Platz P, Ryder LP, Svejgaard A, Thomsen M (1980) Data reduction in HLA-D typing with the primed lymphocyte typing (PLT) technique. The normalized median response (NMR). Tissue Antigens 15:123–136
2. Morling N, Jakobsen BK, Platz P, Ryder LP, Svejgaard A, Thomsen M (1981) Typing for human alloantigens with the primed lymphocyte (PLT) technique with notes on the interpretation of PLT data. Hum Immunol 2:333–340

Origin and Expansion of SB (DP)-Specific Reagents Characterized in the Ninth International Workshop

R.J. Hartzman[1], S. Shaw[2], and F.M. Robbins[3]

1 Naval Medical Research Institute, Bethesda, MD 20016, USA
2 Immunology Branch, NCI, NIH, Bethesda, MD, USA
3 Division of Immunologic Oncology, Georgetown University School of Medicine, Washington, D.C. 20007, USA

For definition of SB (DP) antigens, 12 sets of primed lymphocyte typing (PLT) reagents were submitted to the International Workshop. Two independent typing reagents were submitted for each of the 6 defined SB antigens. The antigens SB1, SB2, SB3, SB4, SB5 were defined originally [1, 2] and SB6 subsequently (F. M. Robbins). The typing reagents for SB1–5 are from the same donor combinations used in the original definition [1, 2]; phenotypes of the responding and stimulating donors are summarized in Table 1, and the donor combinations used to generate each reagent are indicated in Table 2. One of the criteria by which those donor combinations were originally chosen was that they should be completely matched for all known HLA antigens (except obviously SB); for SB6 the donor combinations were matched for HLA-DR, D, MB, MT but differ for some class I specificities as well as differing for SB. In the unrelated donors for SB1–5, matching was maximized by choosing haplotypes with strong linkage disequilibrium.

The procedure for the generation of the PL reagents is a routine MLC system described in detail previously [13, 18]. Responses in primary culture are dependent on optimization of the culture system, and even then are characterized by only weak proliferative responses and by low yield (100%). Responses during secondary (and subsequent) restimulation are very strong and characterized by about 500% yield per cycle of antigen stimulation. Other laboratories have tried to generate reagents of comparable specificity and strength of responsiveness; success has been variable. It is our impression that the most important parameters relate to choice of donors and optimization of primary culture. In particular: (1) careful choice of donors with maximal HLA identity; (2) optimal cryopreservation of the responding and stimulating cells; (3) good plasma/serum supplement for the culture (not heat inactivated, in the primary); (4) a good supplier of RPMI 1640 media (e.g. GIBCO; others have caused problems); (5) optimal CO_2 and humidity control during the incubation.

After priming and two rounds of specific stimulation with the priming antigen the primed cells were cryopreserved. They were subsequently thawed and expanded extensively using a method previously described [3–5].

One to 10×10^6 primed cells were cocultured with approximately fivefold irradiated (4500 R) stimulator cells in 80 ml tissue culture media (RPMI

Table 1. HLA phenotypes of donors used to generate SB-specific PLT reagents

Donor	SB	HLA-A	HLA-B	HLA-C	HLA-DR	HLA-Dw	DQw	DRw
Unrelated donors								
H9	1, 2	1, 2	7, 8	w7	2, 3	2, 3	1, 2	52
M14	3, 4	1, 2	7, 8	w7	2, 3	2, 3	1, 2	52
PM1	2, 4	1, 2	7, 8	w7	2, 3	2, 3	1, 2	52
S11	2, 5	1, 2	7, 8	w7	2, 3	2, 3	1, 2	52
W7	1, 4	1, 2	7, 8	w7	2, 3	2, 3	1, 2	52
B17	2, 4	1, 2	7, 8	w7	2, 4	2, 4	1, 3	53
F2	4, 5	1, 2	7, 8	w7	2, 4	2, 4	1, 3	53
Siblings identical except for recombinant SB								
FB6	4, 6	25, 31	15, 40	w3	4, 4	4	3, 3	53, 53
FB11	4, 1	25, 31	15, 40	w3	4, 4	4	3, 3	53, 53
Family members								
SUJA	4, 4	2, 2	27, 15	w3, w3	5, 4	5, 4	3, 3	52, –
SUGE	4, 6	2, 28	44, 15	w3, w5	5, 4	5, 4	3, 3	52, –
SUMK	4, (7)	2, 1	27, 37	w3, w6	5, 2	5, TB24	3, 1	52
SUMR	6, (7)	28, 1	44, 37	w5, w6	5, 2	5, TB24	3, 1	52

Histocompatibility Testing 1984
Edited by E. D. Albert et al.

Table 2. Combinations of donors used for generating reagents

Designation		Specificity	Comment	Responder	Stimulator[c]
Workshop	Local				
20	SB1A	DPw1		FB6	FB11
21	SB1B	DPw1		S11	H9
22	SB2A	DPw2		W7	H9
23	SB2B	DPw2		F2	B17
24	SB3A	DPw3		W7	M14
25	SB3B	DPw3		PM1	M14
26	SB4A	DPw4		S11	PM11
27	SB4B	DPw4	Broader[a] + minors[b]	H9	W7
28	SB5A	DPw5		B17	F2
29	SB5B	DPw5	Minors[b]	H9	S11
30	SB6A	DPw6		SUJA	SUGE
31	SB6B	DPw6		SUMK	SUMR

[a] Concordance between the pairs of reagents has proven to be good (0.85) for all reagents; however the discrepancies are greatest for 4A vs 4B where 4B is generally reactive with more donors

[b] Reagents 4B and 5B were both generated using donor H9 as responder. Analysis of these reagents by cell-mediated cytoxicity indicates that they include cytotoxic effector cells specific for human minor histocompatibility antigens [3]. However, responses to such minor antigens provide minimal background noise in proliferation assays

[c] The positive stimulator controls used in the workshop carried the following HLA antigens: cell Nr. 9 HLA-A1, B8, Cw7, DR3, 4, w52, Dw–, DQw2, 3, DPw1; cell Nr. 101 HLA-A2, 26, Bw41, w58, Cw6, DR5, w14, w52, Dw5, DQw1, 3, DPw2, 3; cell Nr. 695 HLA-A-2, 24, Bw46, 35, Cw1, 3, DRw8, w14, w52, Dw–, DQw1, DPw5; cell 1011 HLA-A28, 23, B18, 49, Cw7, DR1, 4, Dw1, DQw1, 3, DPw4, w6.

1640, L-glutamine, 25 mM HEPES, 10 µg/ml heparin and 10 µg/ml gentamycin) supplemented with 10% AB, Rh^+ plasma (heparin 5–20 µg/ml). The HEPES and heparin are not necessary and the gentamycin is usually omitted. The omission of gentamycin is important, as this permits staphylococci and streptococci to act as indicators of contamination for more subtle but functionally disruptive infections such as mycoplasma. The use of anticoagulants which function primarily by binding calcium, such as acid citrate dextrose, in the plasma must be avoided, as this can inhibit cell growth.

The stimulator cells also act as feeder cells in the expansion of the culture, so that a large excess is critical. The stimulator cells must have the appropriate DPw type, and no HLA-D or DR type which the responder cell does not express, as this can trigger an expansion of cells in the primed cell population which have been carried along but have not been previously stimulated. Large roller bottle flasks (Corning 490 cm^2) were used, but many types of tissue culture flasks can be used as long as the cells do not become crowded. In general there should be 1–10 times as much space between cells as space occupied by cells on the bottom of the flasks. Flasks are kept upright to decrease the risk of contamination. Cells are incubated for 2 days without interleukin-2 (IL-2) to permit conditions more favorable to the expansion of the intended cells and reduce the risk of expanding "non-specific" cells. On the 3rd day of culture, 20% of a crude preparation containing IL-2 is added. On the 4th day, at least 20% of the media is exchanged with fresh RPMI 1640 with 10% human plasma and 20% IL-2, adding an excess to be sure to keep the cell concentration well below 0.5×10^6/ml, and this exchange is repeated every 2 days. If growth is vigorous, as noted by cell crowding and/or slight media acidity, the culture is split into one or two additional flasks with a doubling or tripling of the media, plasma, and IL-2. The most likely reason for loss of an expanding culture at this stage is rapid cell growth outstripping the supply of IL-2 followed by massive cell death within a few hours. IL-2 is prepared from human peripheral blood leukocytes obtained at leukophoresis and has a high percentage of monocytes, diluted to 1×10^6 cells per ml in RPMI 1640 supplemented with 1% human plasma and 0.08% PHA-P and harvested at 48 h. IL-2 is produced from single donors. Several batches may be produced at one time and those which have high IL-2 as measured by growth of an IL-2-dependent cell pooled.

The most important single factor in obtaining large yields of functional cells is the relative number of feeder cells used (Table 3). A ratio of less than three feeder cells to one primed cell usually results in a low yield. Extremely vigorous expansion oc-

Table 3. Expansion using stimulator/feeder cells plus IL-2

	Number of cells × 10^6		
	Primed cells at start	Stimulator/ feeders	Primed cell yield
DPw1 (SB1A)	12.9	44	1165
DPw1 (SB1B)	8	25	872
DPw3 (SB3B)	30.8	60.5	638
DPw4 (SB4A)	13.6	75	971
DPw5 (SB5A)	22.8	104	624
DPw5 (SB5B)	10	80	2203
DPw6 (SB6A)	15	156	1036
DPw6 (SB6B)	12	156	1028

Data for cells expanded with single cycle of IL-2 and feeders

curs with ten feeder cells per primed cell, but these populations of expanded cells may lose the capacity for rapid proliferation in subsequent tests. These "non-functional" cells appear microscopically healthy and do not show a preponderance of any phenotype (e.g., T8) to suggest the cause. The use of five feeder cells per primed cell produces the most consistent result; 20–200-fold expansion with the maintenance of very high specific proliferative capacity.

Cells can be expanded through two to five cycles of stimulation/feeding and IL-2, producing extremely large numbers of cells. However after any one expansion, cells may perform well, may lose function, or may die. The risk of loss of function increases with each expansion. A cryopreserved aliquot from one expansion cycle may fail in a subsequent expansion, but a second vial from the same batch of cryopreserved cells may be successfully expanded with the maintenance of function. Thus the exact requirements for cell expansion are not fully understood. Finally, primed cells from some responder/stimulator pairs are easily expanded, such as the SB1A cell, and other primed cells, such as the SB4B set, require multiple attempts for successful expansion and are extremely difficult to re-expand with the maintenance of function.

The timing of cryopreservation is relatively important. If the cells are harvested too early, high background counts can be a problem from residual blast cells. If the cultures are harvested late, many of the cells may die. Thus cells are harvested after the cells reach a relative blast count of 5%–10% following the proliferation peak. Most cultures are harvested between days 7 and 8.

Cells are harvested being sure to perform any centrifugations in media that has 10–30 u/ml heparin to reduce the risk of clumping. Standard cryopreservation techniques using 10% fetal calf serum and 7.5% dimethyl sulfoxide are followed, and 0.5–50 × 10^6 cells can be frozen in a vial. A controlled rate freezer is used to reduce the sample temperature 1 °C/min to −30 °C, then 5 °C/min to −80 °C, and then the cells are stored in the vapor phase of liquid nitrogen. Extreme care is taken in the handling of cryopreserved cells, as the momentary increase in temperature to −30 °C can have deleterious effects on the function of the cells.

Cryopreserved, expanded cells are tested against a selected panel of previously SB-characterized cells for specificity and discrimination. In this workshop, several expanded cells did not produce results identical to the original primed cell and were discarded. A new batch of expanded cells was generated and these performed essentially identically with the unexpanded cell.

References

1. Shaw S, Johnson AH, Shearer GM (1980) Evidence for a new segregant series of B cell antigens that are encoded in the HLA-D region and that stimulate secondary allogeneic proliferative and cytotoxic responses. J Exp Med 152:565–580
2. Shaw S, Duquesnoy RJ, Smith PL (1981) Population studies of the HLA-linked SB antigens. Immunogenetics 14:153–162
3. Ruscetti FW, Morgan DA, Gallo RC (1977) Functional and morphologic characterization of human T-cells continuously grown in vitro. J Immunol 199:131–138
4. Pappas F, Bonnard GD, Hartzman RJ, Strong DM (1979) Human PL cells grown as continued T-cell cultures. Transplant Proc 11:1986–1989
5. Bach FH, Inouye H, Hank JA, Alter BJ (1979) Human T lymphocyte clones reactive in primed lymphocyte typing and cytotoxicity. Nature 281:307–309

CML: A Method for Cellular Typing *

D.J. Schendel, W. Jennert, K. Bickert, and R. Wank, on behalf of the participating laboratories

Institute for Immunology, University of Munich, Goethestraße 2, 8000 Munich 2, Federal Republic of Germany

Introduction

Cell-mediated lympholysis (CML) can be used as a cellular typing method to identify surface molecules that are recognized by cytotoxic T lymphocytes (CTLs). The target molecules recognized by CTLs in many cases correlated with HLA specificities (either class I or class II) that can be defined with serological reagents. On the other hand, several studies have clearly demonstrated that CTLs can detect HLA determinants that do not correspond to known serological specificities [1–9]. In several cases the CTL-defined specificities have been shown biochemically to represent distinct class I molecular variants, for example for HLA-A2, B27, and B44 [10–13]. Other CTLs have been described which show lysis of allogeneic target cells that share no serologically detectable HLA-A, B, C, or DR specificities with the sensitizing cells, and further investigation will be required to define the genetic and molecular basis of these anomalous CML reactions [14–16]. It is certainly clear that CTLs are unique reagents for identifying minor histocompatibility antigens in man and for defining the molecular epitopes important in HLA restriction [17–20].

The laboratories using CML typing for genetic analysis of HLA products have remained limited, but nevertheless several groups of investigators have collaborated, and these joint efforts provided a "preworkshop" basis, enabling CML to be included in the program of the Ninth International Histocompatibility Workshop (IHW) [21–23]. During the fifth meeting of the European CML Study Group, in fact, various proposals for the international CML study were designed.

Plans for the CML Study

Participating Laboratories

In 1981 a questionnaire was circulated through the Ninth IHW regional organization network to identify those laboratories interested in participating in a CML workshop study. This questionnaire was also designed to obtain information about the techniques used by the various labs and to ascertain whether CTL reagents would be available for exchange. Twenty laboratories expressed an interest in the CML study and 12 became active participants (Table 1).

Experimental Design

Responses to the questionnaire indicated that it would not be feasible to assemble an adequate set of CTL reagents for exchange on an international basis. Therefore, it was decided that each participating laboratory should prepare a specified set of CTLs to be tested on a standard target cell panel, that would be collected and distributed by the central organizing laboratory. The CTL reagents prepared locally were to include CTLs specific for HLA-A2, B7, and B8. In addition, data obtained from other locally derived CTLs tested on the standard panel could be submitted for central analysis. The standard target cell panel was composed of cells from members of five families in which the A2, B7, or B8 specificities were segregating. Where feasible, both parents and two children from each family were selected such that informative haplotypes for these specificities were present in one parent and one of the children (Table 2). The cryopreserved peripheral blood lymphocytes from one family each were provided by Aarhus, Amsterdam, Helsinki, Leiden, and Munich. Outside sets were shipped on dry ice to Munich, reassembled into complete workshop sets and distributed further to the participating laboratories.

CML Method

The participants agreed to adopt a standard method that had been used previously for combined analysis of CML results [22]. Each CTL was tested at varying effector to target cell ratios; the target cell panel, with one exception, was stimulat-

* This work was supported by the Deutsche Forschungsgemeinschaft (Al 92/13-2)

Histocompatibility Testing 1984
Edited by E. D. Albert et al.

Table 1. Participating laboratories

Laboratory designation	Research center	Investigators
BENIVA	Central Laboratory, Netherlands Red Cross Blood Center, Amsterdam, The Netherlands	B. Breur, P. Ivanyi
BENROO	Immunohematology Department, University Hospital, Leiden, The Netherlands	E. Blokland, E. Goulmy, J. van Rood
EAEKAS	Tissue Typing Center, Medical Faculty, Zagreb, Yugoslavia	M. Gerencer, A. Kastelan I. Durinovic-Bello
GERWAN	Institute of Immunology, University of Munich, Munich, F.R.G.	D. Schendel, R. Wank
NCYFUL	Blood Transfusion Service, Massachusetts General Hospital, Boston, Massachusetts	T. Fuller, C. Pinto
NCYYUN	Sidney Farber Cancer Institute, Boston, Massachusetts	P. Dubey, E. Yunis
NCYZIE	Children's Hospital of Philadelphia, Philadelphia, Pennsylvania	K. Zier
SCAKOS	Tissue Typing Laboratory, Finnish Red Cross Blood Transfusion Service, Helsinki, Finland	S. Koskimies
SCAJER	Blood Grouping and Tissue Typing Laboratory, Aalborg, Denmark	A. Elbaek, N. Grunnet
SCAKIS	Tissue Typing Laboratory, University Hospital, Aarhus, Denmark	T. Kristensen, J. Mossin, P. Wendelboe Hansen
UKIBRS	South West Regional Transfusion Centre, Bristol, England	B. Bradley, A. Doyle
UKIFES	The London Hospital Medical College, Department of Immunology, London, England	H. Festenstein, N. Yeatman

Table 2. Standard target cell panel

Target cell code	HLA haplotypes	Class I antigens	Class II antigens	Class III antigens
001	c/d	a: A1, B8, Cw7	DR5	C4AQO, C4B1, BFS, C2C
002	b/c	b: A2, B44, Cw5	DR2	C4A3, C4B1, BFS, C2C
003	a/d	c: A24, B15, Cw3	DR5	C4A3, C4BQO, BFF, C2C
004	a/b	d: A2, B18, Cw–	DR3	C4A3, C4B1, BFS, C2C
005	b/c	a: A3, Bw62, Cw3	DRw8	C4A3, C4B1, BFS, C2C
006	a/c	b: A32, B44, Cw5	DR–	C4A3, C4BQO, BFS, C2C
007	a/b	c: A2, B44, Cw–	DR7	C4A3, C4B1, BFF, C2C
008	c/d	d: A29, B44, Cw–	DR5	C4A3, C4B1, BFF, C2C
009	c/d	a: A32, B8, Cw–	DR3	C4AQO, C4B1, BFS, C2C
010	a/d	b: A32, B40, Cw2	DRw13	C4A3, C4B1, BFS, C2C
011	a/b	c: A31, B51, Cw4	DR1	C4A3, C4BQO, BFF, C2C
012	b/d	d: A2, B7, C–	DR4	C4A3, C4BQO, BFS, C2C
013	c/d	a: A24, Bw60, Cw3	DR2	C4A4, C4B2, BFS
014	a/b	b: A11, B7, Cw7	DRw6	C4A3, C4B1, BFS
015	a/d	c: A2, B8, Cw7	DR3	C4AQO, C4B1, BFS
016	b/c	d: A1, Bw57, Cw6	DR7	C4A6, C4B1, BFS
017	a/b	a: A2, Bw52, Cw–	DR2	C4A2, C4B1, BFS, C2C
018	c/d	b: A24, B35, Cw4	DRw6	C4A3, C4B1, BFS, C2C
019	a/c	c: A3, B7, Cw7	DR2	C4A3, C4B1, BFS, C2C
020	b/d	d: A1, Bw62, Cw3	DR4	C4A4, C4B2, BFS, C2C

ed with phytohemagglutinin for 48–72 h; and a ^{51}Cr release assay was used for measurement of cell lysis.

Workshop Goals

The primary goals of the CML study were to establish active collaboration among the different groups working with this specialized technique and to assess qualitatively and quantitatively the combined results obtained from multiple laboratories testing a standard target cell panel. Furthermore, the results from this exchange could be used to assess methods, reagents, and means of data analysis that would be applicable to collaborative studies involving numerous centers addressing more specific problems of the genetic basis of CTL recognition.

Central Analysis

Methods

Each laboratory submitted the raw data for each experiment, as well as a calculated percent CML (% CML) value determined according to the formula:

$$\frac{\text{experimental release (ER)} - \text{spontaneous release (SR)}}{\text{maximum release (MR)} - \text{spontaneous release (SR)}} \times 100$$

In addition, a local assignment of the reaction of each CTL with each target cell was submitted. A special set of cards was used to obtain information regarding technical parameters and comments on individual CTLs or target cells. The numerical data was assembled into a printout matrix (Fig. 1) which contained, in the first data block, the information on the maximum and spontaneous release values for each target cell, including the mean values of replicates (MM, SM) and their standard deviations (MV, SV). A percent SR (%SR) was calculated by dividing the mean SR by the mean MR (SM/MM × 100). This data was followed in sequence by the data for the CML responses of each CTL tested with each target cell. When the dilution of CTLs is transformed to $\log_{10}$ (L1–L6) in Fig. 1, and plotted against the %CML (C1–C6), a straight line should be obtained for each combination showing a positive reaction. The "best-fitting" line for the observed values was determined using the sum of least squares method (SS) and defined by its slope (SLO) and *y*-intercept (SEC). The significance of the linear correlation between the $\log_{10}$ (E/

C T L   D:M+GERWAN.001   26 Targets, 3 CTl's

Targets	1	2	3	4	5	6	7	8
.	1	2	3	4	5	6	7	8
Max./Spon.								
M1	2152	2500	4405	1677	2382	4133	2109	4599
M2	2084	2520	4507	1716	2586	4350	2158	4537
M3	2084	2425	4531	11840	2452	4254	2156	4602
MM	2106.7	2481.7	4481.0	5077.7	2473.3	4245.7	2141.0	4579.3
MV	39.3	50.1	66.9	5856.4	103.7	108.7	27.7	36.7
T/M	2	2	2	2	2	2	2	2
S1	377	419	525	174	231	381	172	413
S2	358	321	520	192	212	341	176	437
S3	336	372	537	187	211	356	169	433
SM	357.0	370.7	527.3	184.3	218.0	359.3	172.3	427.7
SV	20.5	49.0	8.7	9.3	11.3	20.2	3.5	12.9
%S	16.95	14.94	11.77	3.63	8.81	8.46	8.05	9.34
1 .CTL 10								
L1	1.699	1.699	1.699	1.699	1.699	1.699	1.699	1.699
L2	1.398	1.398	1.398	1.398	1.398	1.398	1.398	1.398
L3	1.097	1.097	1.097	1.097	1.097	1.097	1.097	1.097
L4	0.799	0.799	0.799	0.799	0.799	0.799	0.799	0.799
L5	0.491	0.491	0.491	0.491	0.491	0.491	0.491	0.491
L6	0.204	0.204	0.204	0.204	0.204	0.204	0.204	0.204
SS	24.5	9.3	53.3	134.3	109.5	49.6	9.9	36.9
REG	0.977	0.996	0.976	0.898	0.950	0.981	0.911	0.984
C1	29.0	46.0	51.0	45.0	45.0	49.0	13.0	54.0
C2	26.0	36.0	39.0	33.0	35.0	38.0	11.0	41.0
C3	15.0	29.0	30.0	25.0	18.0	23.0	6.0	30.0
C4	10.0	24.0	20.0	18.0	17.0	22.0	8.0	28.0
C5	8.0	13.0	15.0	13.0	8.0	13.0	6.0	19.0
C6	3.0	5.0	13.0	19.0	8.0	5.0	4.0	11.0
SEC	-1.913	0.286	3.399	7.653	-2.329	-1.756	2.757	4.921
SLO	18.015	26.594	25.947	18.824	25.485	28.220	5.530	26.979

Fig. 1. CML data matrix. Target cells, designated by sequential numbers and workshop numbers, are listed horizontally for each experiment. Replicate values for maximum release (*M1–M3*) with means (*MM*) and standard deviations (*MV*) are given, followed by the replicate values of spontaneous release (*S1–S3*) with their means (*SM*) and standard deviations (*SV*). The percentage spontaneous release (*%SR*) was calculated as SM/MM × 100. *CTLs* are listed vertically. The $\log_{10}$ E/T (L1–L6) are given, followed by the residual sum of squares (*SS*) and coefficient of correlation (*REG*) for the regression line obtained by plotting $\log_{10}$ E/T against the corresponding %CML (*C1–C6*). The regression line is defined by its *y*-intercept (*SEC*) and slope (*SLO*)

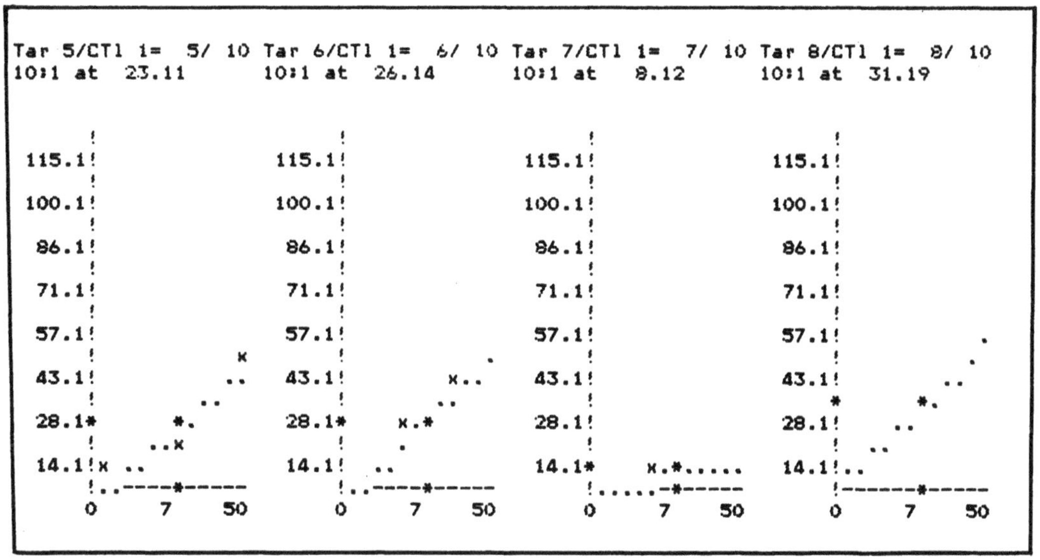

Fig. 2. Regression line plots. Each CTL-target cell combination is plotted with E/T (log scale) on the x axis and %CML on the y axis. The %CML, indicated by *, is determined for the selected E/T of 10 : 1. These four graphs represent the CML responses of CTL 10 (anti-A2) against target cells 05, 06, 07, and 08 of the standard target cell panel. Targets 05, 06, and 08 express A2, whereas 07 does not

3 Ctl's

CTL	Targets (1.. 26) 1 1	2 2	3 3	4 4	5 5	6 6	7 7	8 8	9 9	10 10
%S	16.95 *	14.94 *	11.77 *	3.63 *	8.81 *	8.46 *	8.05 *	9.34 *	10.80 *	11.76
1 .CTL 10										
SLOP	18.015 *	26.594 *	25.947 *	18.824 *	25.485 *	28.220 *	5.530 *	26.979 *	20.589 *	33.365
REGR	0.977 *	0.996 *	0.976 *	0.898 *	0.950 *	0.981 *	0.911 *	0.984 *	0.957 *	0.987
10:1	16.101 *	26.880 *	29.346 *	26.477 *	23.156 *	26.464 *	8.287	31.900 *	22.735 *	42.731
20:1	21.524	34.886	37.157	32.144	30.828	34.960	9.952	40.022	28.933	52.775
%RCR	55.570	90.065 *	95.930 *	82.986 *	79.588 *	90.256 *	25.692	103.325 *	74.697 *	136.251
2 .CTL 20										
SLOP	13.658 *	1.402 *	8.285 *	6.489 *	15.803 *	15.051 *	4.390 *	25.560 *	20.605 *	24.601
REGR	0.782	0.154	0.969 *	0.888 *	0.979 *	0.984 *	0.953 *	0.984 *	0.961 *	0.961
10:1	14.209 *	6.239	10.597 *	10.337 *	16.820 *	13.781 *	5.561	26.993 *	25.736 *	36.277
20:1	18.320	6.661	13.090	12.290	21.577	18.312	6.883	34.687	31.938	43.682
%RCR	48.045	17.470	34.330	32.231	56.587	48.023	18.050	90.968 *	83.759 *	114.557
3 .CTL 30										
SLOP	22.376 *	22.873 *	22.973 *	23.170 *	10.366 *	23.173 *	5.437 *	23.549 *	14.373 *	22.915
REGR	0.969 *	0.903 *	0.910 *	0.985 *	0.927 *	0.996 *	0.834	0.956 *	0.864 *	0.906
10:1	29.994 *	27.520 *	55.025 *	35.702 *	23.371 *	26.702 *	8.115	40.055 *	29.579 *	57.689
20:1	36.730	34.406	61.941	42.677	26.492	33.678	9.752	47.144	33.906	64.587
%RCR	61.985	58.062	104.529 *	72.021 *	44.707	56.834	16.457	79.559 *	57.218	108.995

Fig. 3. CML assignment matrix. Different criteria could be used for assignment of positive responses and selection of data for inclusion in the central analysis. These were marked in each case with *. In this example the following limits were set: %SR $\leq$ 25%; SLOP $\geq$ 1.0; REGR $\geq$ 0.9; %CML (E/T = 10 : 1) $\geq$ 10%; %RCR(E/T = 20 : 1) $\geq$ 67%

T) and %CML was expressed as a coefficient of correlation (REG) which is considered to be significant when $r \geq 0.9$. These values were calculated and included in the data matrix outprint. The results were also graphically presented for visual assessment (Fig. 2), which is important for identifying combinations in which a significant regression coefficient might not be obtained because a plateau of lysis occurs with several of the higher E/T values. From the regression line, the value of y (%CML) could be determined for any set value of x (E/T); these values were indicated with asterisks on the y and x axes respectively. To make central assignments, a program was designed that could evaluate the following parameters (Fig. 3): %SR, slope of the regression line and its coefficient of correlation. By extrapolation from this line the %CML was obtained for a selected E/T. In addition, a percent relative cytotoxic response (%RCR) was determined at a selected E/T if the specific control for the CTL was included in the same experiment. The %RCR was calculated by dividing the %CML of any given target cell at the selected E/T by the %CML for the specific target cell (i.e., the stimulating cell used for sensitizing the CTLs) obtained at the same E/T. This value was converted to a percentage by multiplication with 100. Variable limits could be selected for each of these parameters so that different criteria for assignment of positive responses could be assessed.

Results

Target Cells. To conserve on donation requirements for target cells, ampules with only $3-5 \times 10^6$ cells were submitted. Most laboratories reported difficulties in working with these minimal cell numbers, particularly since recoveries may have been further decreased through double shipments on dry ice. The labile nature of the target cell panel was reflected in the %SR values. The mean %SR for all target cells was 23.5%, but maximum values displayed a range of 28.7%–72.5%. No single target cell was consistently problematic, rather each cell gave difficulties in several experiments. The local negative and positive control target cells showed lower levels of %SR (mean 18.8%, range 4.8%–31.3%), indicating that the target cell problems were inherent in the exchanged panel. Using a conservative cutoff of 25% SR, the data from 60% of the tested combinations could be included in the central analysis.

CTL Reagents. Few problems were reported for CTLs, since these reagents were derived locally and pretested on local target cell panels. Data for at least three E/T were submitted for all CTL combinations, and the vast majority of CTLs showing lysis ≥ 10% at an E/T of 10 : 1 gave significant linear regression curves, demonstrating the discrete quantitative character of the CML response.

Assignment of Positive Reactions. Three criteria were compared centrally to define positive CML responses: (a) positive slope ≥ 10 for the regression line of a CTL-target cell combination, (b) %CML ≥ 25% at an E/T of 20 : 1, and (c) %RCR ≥ 67% at an E/T of 20 : 1. A combined assignment of positivity was made when two of these three criteria showed a positive assignment. The participating laboratories also scored each reaction using their local criteria for evaluating CML responses. Table 3 shows 2 × 2 association analyses comparing the local assignments with the three individual parameters, as well as the combined workshop assignments. Each individual method showed positive correlations with the local assignments, but the strongest correlation was obtained using the combined assignment.

Specificity of CTL Reactions. Positive reactions could be theoretically predicted on the basis of the "specificity" of the CTLs (i.e. anti-A2, -B7, or -B8) and the presence of this antigen in the target cell. These "specificities" were compared with the local and combined workshop reactions, based on the quantitative basis of a CTL-target cell interaction (Table 3). The strongest correlation was found with the local evaluation, and the combined workshop assignment showed a higher correlation than any of the individual methods of assignment. In general, however, the associations between CTL reaction patterns and the predicted "specificity" based on

Table 3. The 2×2 association analyses comparing local and workshop assignments and analyzing specificity of CTL reactions

Comparison	χ^2 [a]	r	n
Local vs slope	90.0	0.63	228
Local vs %CML	98.7	0.65	231
Local vs %RCR	123.7	0.71	247
Local vs combined assignment	133.7	0.74	243
Specificity vs local	114.3	0.69	243
Specificity vs combined assignment	95.3	0.56	307
Specificity vs slope	57.1	0.43	304
Specificity vs %CML	52.4	0.41	307
Specificity vs %RCR	66.7	0.47	300

[a] Chi-square calculated using Yates' correction

Table 4. Comparison of positive and negative CML reactions based on different parameters

Parameter	Local assignment		Combined assignment		Predicted specificity	
	+ve	−ve	+ve	−ve	+ve	−ve
Slope	22.0± 9.7	7.8± 7.2	24.4±9.6	7.2±6.8	20.5±10.3	10.2±11.0
%CML	30.7±13.3	10.2± 6.7	35.6±14.5	10.3± 6.4	29.2±15.4	15.8±15.0
%RCR	114.2±66.3	26.0±15.4	131.9±60.0	34.2±20.0	110.4±61.8	70.7±68.5

Data are presented as mean values ± standard deviations

sharing of classical serologically defined antigens indicated that the CTL responses were more heterogeneous. In all cases, more positive CTL reactions were assigned than could be accounted for by the presence of the HLA antigen in the target cell panel. Part of this heterogeneity certainly occurred because the CTL reagents were not cloned, but identity between serologically defined and CTL-defined epitopes or molecules need not be absolute, as discussed earlier.

Table 4 summarizes the mean values of the positive and negative groups of responses, comparing the division by local assignment, combined workshop assignment, or by predicted "specificity". The local and combined assignments show quite comparable values, and the discrimination between the positive and negative groups in all cases was greater than that seen for the division based on "specificity" assignments, demonstrating again that the CTL responses are more complex than or different from those predicted on the basis of the defined HLA antigens. In light of the complex organization of the HLA region, in particular of the HLA-D region, it is clearly difficult to obtain cell combinations that are identical for all products, except the desired HLA specificity. Therefore, such differences in reaction patterns are not unexpected.

Conclusions

The interest in development of CML as a cellular typing method and its application to problems of histocompatibility and immunogenetics is evidenced by the number of laboratories joining to collaborate in this international histocompatibility workshop. A conservative protocol was selected for this study that enabled participants to use target cell reagents supplied by other laboratories and to test these with locally derived CTLs. The precise quantitative nature of the CML response was clearly reflected in the results and provided an objective basis for central analysis. On the other hand, because the target cell panel was supplied in coded form the local assignments were valuable for evaluating "specificity" of CTL reactions. In fact, the local assignments could take into account a more multifaceted evaluation of reactions than could be made through computer assignments. In few cases were predicted reactions missed by the CTLs, showing the reliability of CTLs for detecting given class I antigens. More interestingly, however, were the extra reactions seen by CTLs. Some of these may be accounted for by technical difficulties or by heterogeneity in the CTL populations, but on the other hand, they also reflect the biological complexity of CTL recognition. Future collaborative efforts using cloned CTLs and transfected target cells expressing cloned HLA genes can be expected to yield exciting new information on the genetic basis of CTL recognition.

Acknowledgments. We gratefully acknowledge the enthusiastic support of Prof. Gert Riethmüller throughout the entire workshop activities. We thank C. Dalibor, M. Scheuerecker, and A. Schreiter for technical assistance and S. Förster for help in the preparation of this report. The members of the European CML Study Group are warmly thanked for their continual support with ideas and discussion. The members of the Tissue Typing Laboratory of the University Hospital, Aarhus, Denmark, kindly provided their computer programs.

References

1. Kristensen T, Grunnet N, Kissmeyer-Nielsen F (1974) Cell mediated lympholysis in man. Occurrence of unexpected, HLA ("LA" and "Four") irrelevant lympholysis. Tissue Antigens 4:378–382
2. Mawas C, Christen Y, Legrand L, Sasportes M, Dausset J (1974) Cellular and humoral response against determinants other than the classical HLA specificities. Transplant 18:256–266
3. Schapira M, Jeannet M (1974) Cell-mediated lympholysis in HLA identical unrelated individuals. Tissue Antigens 4:178–182
4. Kristensen T, Grunnet N (1975) Cell mediated lympholysis in man. Evidence of a separate CML locus within the major histocompatibility complex and an approach to CML typing. In: Kissmeyer-Nielsen F (ed)

Histocompatibility testing 1975. Munksgaard, Copenhagen, p 835
5. Goulmy E, Termijtelen A, Bradley B, van Rood JJ (1976) HLA restriction of non-HLA-A, -B, -C, and -D cell mediated lympholysis (CML). Tissue Antigens 8:317 – 326
6. Long MA, Handwerger BS, Amos DB, Yunis EJ (1976) The genetics of cell mediated lympholysis. J Immunol 177:2092 – 2099
7. Tekolf WA, Biddison WE, Aster RD, Shaw S (1982) Two subgroups of HLA Bw44 defined by cell-mediated lympholysis that differ in Bw44 expression on platelets and in patterns of genetic linkage disequilibrium. J Immunol 129:1474 – 1478
8. Kato S, Ivanyi P, Lacko E, Breur B, du Bois R, Eijsvoogel VP (1982) Identification of human CML targets. HLA-B locus (B12) antigen variants defined by CTL generated between B-locus-identical (B12) responder-stimulator pairs. J Immunol 128:949 – 955
9. Breuning MH, Lucas CJ, Breur BS, Engelsma MY, De-Lange GG, Dekker AJ, Biddison WE, Ivanyi P (1982) Subtypes of HLA-B27 detected by cytotoxic T lymphocytes and their role in self-recognition. Hum Immunol 5:259 – 268
10. Biddison WE, Kostyu DD, Strominger JL, Krangel MS (1982) Delineation of immunologically and biochemically distinct HLA-A2 antigens. J Immunol 129:730 – 734
11. van der Poel JJ, Mölders HH, Thompson A, Ploegh H (1983) Definition of four HLA-A2 subtypes by CML typing and biochemical analysis. Immunogenetics 17:603 – 608
12. Mölders HH, Breuning MH, Ivanyi P, Ploegh H (1983) Biochemical analysis of variant HLA-B27 antigens. Hum Immunol 6:111 – 117
13. Hahn AW, Schendel DJ, Wendelboe Hansen P, Ploegh H (1984) Biochemical and cellular identification of HLA-Bw44 subtypes. Hum Immunol (in press)
14. Ward MJ, Stiller CR, McGirr DA, Fung M, Cousins HK, Paty DW, Hawson WT, Sinclair NRSTC (1977) CML problems and possibilities defining specificities. Transplant Proc 9:1781 – 1784
15. Kristensen T (1978) Studies on the specificity of CML. Report from a CML workshop. Tissue Antigens 11:330 – 349
16. Schendel DJ, Wank R, Dupont B (1978) Cell-mediated lympholysis: examination of HLA genetic fine structure and complementation using cytotoxic lymphocytes. Eur J Immunol 8:634 – 640
17. Goulmy E, Termijtelen A, Bradley BA, van Rood JJ (1977) H-Y antigen killing by women is restricted by HLA. Nature 266:544 – 546
18. Dickmeiss E, Soeberg B, Svejgaard A (1977) Human cell-mediated cytotoxicity against modified target cells is restricted by HLA. Nature 270:526 – 528
19. McMichael AJ, Ting A, Zweerink HJ, Askonas BA (1977) HLA restriction of cell-mediated lysis of influenza virus-infected human cells. Nature 270:524 – 526
20. Elkins WL, Pierson G, Negendank W, Zier KS (1982) Recognition of minor lymphocyte alloantigen(s) on cells of HLA matched siblings and unrelated individuals by cytotoxic T lymphocytes in vitro. Immunogenetics 15:485 – 499
21. Bradley BA, Charmot D, Goulmy E, Johnson HE, Kristensen T, Mawas C, Pfeffer P, Schendel DJ, Wank R (1980) Histocompatibility typing by cell mediated lympholysis (CML): workshop II technical standardization. Tissue Antigens 16:73 – 90
22. European CML Study Group (1980) Human histocompatibility testing by T cell mediated lympholysis: a European standard CML technique. Tissue Antigens 16:335 – 367
23. Breuning MH, Tekolf WA, Kato S, Breur BS, Engelsma MY, Spits H, Ivanyi P (1983) High resolution HLA typing by cytotoxic T lymphocytes. Transplant Proc 15:118 – 122

The Second Complement Component, C2, in the Ninth Workshop*

W.H. Marshall[1], M. Neugebauer[2], M.P. Baur[2], and E.D. Albert[3]

With data provided by:
A. Arnaiz-Villena, C. Alper, H. Bashir, J. R. Batchelor, J. Bertrams, J. Bodmer, G. Bruun Petersen, C. B. Carpenter, C. Chandanayingyong, R. B. Chen, P. Chiewshilp, R. Cross, R. Dawkins, H. Dick, I. A. Dodi, E. Dupont, E. DuToit, E. Ferreira, H. Festenstein, A. Fielder, R. Fong, E. Giblett, C. Gorodezky, Chan So Ha, J. A. Hansen, G. Hauptmann, J. Hay, T. Juji, A. Kastelan, R. Kirk, F. Kissmeyer-Nielsen, S. Knight, L. U. Lamm, B. Larsen, P. Mackintosh, G. Mauff, S. Mayer, R. McLean, N. Mehra, T. Miyajima, J. R. Moraes, Ch. Mueller-Eckhardt, S. Naito, H. Neumeyer, B. Olaisen, G. O'Neill, Ch. Rittner, M. Robinson, J. J. van Rood, T. Rosales, D. Schendel, S. Serjeantson, A. Svejgaard, B. Tait, E. Thorsby, K. Tokunaga, L. Wells, G. Woodfield, J. Woodrow, Y. G. Yao, P. O. Yoshida, and E. Yunis

1 On sabbatical leave from the Memorial University of Newfoundland, St. John's, Newfoundland, Canada A1B 3V6
2 Biometrical Department, Diabetes Research Institute, Auf'm Hennekamp 65, 4000 Düsseldorf, Federal Republic of Germany
3 Laboratory for Immunogenetics, Children's Polyclinic, University of Munich, Pettenkoferstr. 8a, 8000 Munich 2, Federal Republic of Germany

Since the invention of the hemolytic overlay technique to reveal the presence of C2 in gels after isoelectric focusing [1, 4, 5], studies have been made in several populations [reviewed in 6], initially in Caucasoids and latterly in Mongoloids. In all groups studied, polymorphism of C2 has been shown. In Caucasoids there is one common allele, C2*1, which accounts for some 96% of C2 genes, and a less common allele, C2*2 (or C2*B), which accounts for about 4%. There are then a few much rarer variants.

The C2*2 allele has been shown to have allelic associations with HLA-B15 and HLA-Bw22, as well as with BF*S. It has been suggested, particularly because of differing C4 associations in these two cases (the common haplotypes being HLA-B15, BF*S, C2*2, C4*A4B2 on the one hand and HLA-Bw22, BF*S, C4*A4B4 on the other), that these haplotypes may represent independent founder haplotypes for the present European population and perhaps independent mutations. It was also suggested that other C2*2-bearing haplotypes might have been derived from these two putative founder haplotypes by ancestral recombination. These hypotheses lacked information on the splits of B15 and Bw22, lacked for the most part data on B cell antigens, and were generally insufficient for making broader generalizations on geographic distribution and allele age.

The Ninth Workshop has provided an important opportunity to examine in greater detail a further batch of data which is spread among several disparate populations.

Methods

There was no formal exchange of reference sera for C2 in this workshop, nor indeed has there ever been, but the C4 typing, which is of considerable importance, has been partly standardized by an international collaborating group of laboratories in separate workshops [7]. A C4 allele which was reported earlier as B4 came out as B5 in this workshop.

The family analysis program produced one or more haplotype interpretations for each family in the workshop, so far as the data allowed. Data that was incompatible with the genetic rules assumed by this program (M. Neugebauer et al., Analysis of Multilocus Pedigree Data by Computer, this volume) could not be included in the haplotypes. For this reason, a number of the haplotypes lack data on C4 alleles even though C4 typing was performed; in the same way some other data may have been lost.

The C2*2-bearing haplotypes listed in this paper are those which were assigned the highest probability by the computer.

Results

Two hundred and ninety-four families were found in the family analysis output with results for C2

* We acknowledge with gratitude the following financial support: a Visiting Scientist award from Health and Welfare Canada to W. H. M., and Deutsche Forschungsgemeinschaft grants Ba 660/5-1 to M. B. and Al 92-13-2 to E. A

Histocompatibility Testing 1984
Edited by E. D. Albert et al.

Table 1. Caucasoid haplotypes with C2*2

A	Cw	B	C2	BF	C4	DR	Country (lab)
The Bw62 haplotype and its fragments							
1	3	w62	2	S	A4B2	4	Canada (NCY MAR)
24	3	w62	2	S	??	4	Germany (MUE)
2	3	w62	2	S	A4B2	2	Australia (BSH)
2	3	w62	2	S	A4B2	?	UK (WOR)
3	–	w62	2	S	A4B2	4	Australia (HAY)
2	6	w62	2	S	??	4	Germany (BER)
2	–	w62	2	S	A4B2	2	Australia (DAW)
2	1	w62	2	S	A4B2	–	USA (HAN)[a]
2	3	w62	2	S	A6B3	5	Germany (BER)
2	–	51	2	S	A4B2	4	UK (KNT)
2	6	37	2	S	A4B2	4	Australia (YEG)
2	3	w60	2	S	A4B2	4	Australia (HAY)
3	2	w61	2	S	A4B2	1	Canada (NCY MRV)
29	4	35	2	S	A4B2	w6	Venezuela (BEN ROO)
Possible Bw62 fragments							
30	4	35	2	S	??	4	Germany (MUE)
32	?	12	2	S	??	4	Scandinavia (TSB)
24	–	35	2	S	??	4	USA (HAN)
2	3	27	2	S	??	4	S. Africa (DUT)
The Bw55 haplotype and its fragments							
26	3	w55	2	S	A4B5	w6	Australia (DAW)
1	3	w55	2	S	A4B5	w6	Canada (NCY MRV)
26	3	w55	2	S	A4B5	w6	France (MYE)
11	3	w55	2	S	A4B5	1	Australia (BSH)
2	–	w60	2	S	A4B5	4	Australia (DAW)
Possible Bw55 fragment							
29	4	35	2	S	??	w6	Venezuela (BEN ROO)
Unidentifiable "? equilibrium" fragments							
2	5	44	2	S	A3B1	5	Canada (NCY MRV)
2	6	50	2	OT[b]	A2B1	7	Canada (NCY MRV)
23	8	7	2	S	A3B1	5	Venezuela (BEN ROO)
29	–	44	2	F	A3B1	7	France (MYE)
3	6	13	2	S	A3B1	7	Germany (BER)
3	4	35	2	S	A3B2	7	Germany (BER)
1	7	8	2	S	A3B3	3	Germany (BER)
w33	–	14	2	S	A3B1	3	Germany (NEU)
1	–	–	2	S	A3B1	4	Spain (FRA ARN)

[a] Haplotype from North American Indian; [b] OT="other"

Table 2. C2*2 haplotypes from non-Caucasoid groups

A	Cw	B	C2	BF	C4	DR	Ethnic group (lab)
24	–	–	2	S	??	–	Japanese (US7 HAN)
2	–	–	2	S	??	–	Japanese (JUJ)
2	7	39	2	S	??	4	Japanese (JUJ)
26	3	w60	2	S	??	w9	Japanese (US7 HAN)
2	3	w60	2	S	??	5	Cape coloured (SAF DUT)
24	4	35	2	S	??	5	Cape coloured (SAF DUT)
2	–	35	2	S	A4B1	w6	Cape coloured (SAF DUT)
24	7	7	2	S	OTB2[a]	w6	Asian indian (ANZ MEH)
2	–	45	2	F	??	7	Negro (SAF DUT)

[a] OT=C4A "other"

typing, and in them were 671 unrelated individuals, the majority being Caucasoid. There were 42 haplotypes from unrelated people bearing a genetic variant of C2 which was coded as C2*2. All but 10 were found in Caucasoids. In the Caucasoid data several features were immediately apparent: (1) the two haplotypes noted in preworkshop data were easily recognised either as complete haplotypes or as fragments of the complete haplotypes; (2) these haplotypes were seen to comprise one split of B15 (Bw62), one split of Bw22 (Bw55), and two predominant DR types, DR4 and DR6. Thus the full haplotypes were A?, Cw3, Bw62, C2*2, BF*S, C4*A4B2, DR4 and A?, Cw3, Bw55, C2*2, BF*S, C4*A4B5, DR6. There was no particular A locus allele found on either of the haplotypes.

In Table 1 the Caucasoid haplotypes are sorted into (1) Bw62 haplotypes and putative fragments, (2) Bw55 haplotypes and putative fragments, and (3) miscellaneous haplotypes with no recognizable portions of either Bw62 or Bw55 haplotypes. The first two groups are listed with the more complete haplotypes at the top and the smaller fragments at the bottom.

In Table 2 are given 9 of the 10 non-Caucasoid C2*2-bearing haplotypes; the 10th was found in a North American Indian, and because it resembled a Bw62 haplotype it has been placed in Table 1. The most interesting of the non-Caucasoid haplotypes is the Japanese haplotype which carries C blank, B blank, and DR blank alleles. This was found in two Japanese subjects, one in Japan and one in the USA; a possible fragment of this haplotype, with C blank and B blank, was also found in a Spanish Caucasoid (see Table 1).

Discussion

If we postulate that the Caucasoid population had two founder haplotypes with C2*2, one with Bw62 and the other with Bw55, and if we disregard the effects of selection, which are sure to be there but cannot be estimated, then we can perhaps make some comments about these two founder haplotypes and some inferences from them on fine mapping of the complement loci.

The Bw62 haplotype is considerably more fragmented than the Bw55 haplotype and is also, in this material, more frequent. Both of these features suggest it is the older of the two. In earlier data [6], among the haplotypes with C2*2 in association with other HLA-B alleles, 13 were recognisable as fragments of Bw62 haplotypes by virtue of the associated A4B2, against only one with the C4 associated with Bw55-, viz A4B4 (or A4B5 as typed in this workshop); this is in agreement with the Ninth Workshop findings.

The putative ancestral recombinant haplotypes show that a total of six had recombined between the complement region and the HLA-B locus, whereas nine had recombined between the complement region and DR. This suggests that the complement loci are not far from the mid-point between HLA-B and DR, but nearer to B. In another chapter in this volume (M. Baur et al., Analysis of MHC Recombinant Families), the B/DR recombinants from the Ninth workshop families are analyzed and show a ratio of 1 : 2 between HLA-B/complement recombinants and HLA-DR/complement recombinants. This is in good agreement with the ancestral recombinant data and confirms the position (in recombination terms) of the complement loci nearer to B than to DR.

Analysis of the complement genes by gene cloning techniques [2] has shown the order of the genes to be C2, BF, C4, but the orientation of this stretch of DNA in relation to HLA-B and HLA-DR remains uncertain. Examination of the putative ancestral recombinant haplotypes in this material and in earlier work [6] shows three haplotypes where the familiar B locus allele is in association with C2*2 but the C4 alleles are not the familiar ones. Table 3 shows that if the order is B, C2, BF, C4, the unfamiliar C4 genes could have crossed over to those haplotypes by single recombinant events in each case; if, however, the order is B, C4, BF, C2, then the exchange of the C4 genes is now more complex, requiring either a double recombinant event or a specific recombination with a haplotype bearing

Table 3. Origins of ancestral recombinants with differing orientations of the complement region

If C2 is next to B							If C2 is next to DR							Source
A	Cw	B	C2	BF	C4	DR	A	Cw	B	C4	BF	C2	DR	
11	?	15	2	S*	A3B1	?	11	?	15*	A3B1*	S	2	?	[6]
10	?	w22	2	S*	A3B1	?	10	?	w22*	A3B1*	S	2	?	[6]
2	3	w62	2	S*	A6B3	5	2	3	w62*	A6B3*	S	2*	5	Ninth Workshop

* indicates break positions for recombination

the familiar HLA-B allele. Since double recombination or chance recombination with a familiar allele is less likely than single random recombinants, the most likely orientation of the loci is B, C2, BF, C4, DR. From this we conclude that a "chromosome walk" from the complement region will be shorter from the C2 locus than from the C4 locus and that the walk from C2 will terminate at HLA-B, not at HLA-DR.

Finally, a few remarks about ages of the C2*2-bearing haplotypes. Both haplotypes appear to have had so many recombinations between HLA-A and HLA-B that the founder A alleles can no longer be recognized. This would mean that two or more "half-lives" for that part of the haplotype have passed [6]. On the other hand, the maximum number of haplotypes which have lost both the B and the DR alleles by recombination is 11 out of 24 for the Bw62 haplotype (nine unidentified haplotypes plus two of the identified ones). Since some of the unidentified haplotypes are likely to have a Bw55 origin, this indicates that less than one half-life, for losing both B and DR alleles, has passed for that haplotype. If we take Edwards' calculation for haplotype half-life [3], based on recombination frequencies, we can state that the age of these haplotypes is more than 5000 years and less than 20 000 years (the latter assumes the C2 locus is about 0.25 cM from B and about 0.45 cM from DR, so that the combined recombination fraction for losing both B and DR alleles is 0.45×0.25). It should be noted that it is not possible to distinguish between haplotype "age" dating from an original C2 mutation and "age" dating from a population bottleneck through which only one example of a haplotype passed. It is presumably more likely that we are measuring the latter event. Because in both haplotypes C2*2 is found with only one of the splits of the B antigens, we can conclude that the mutations to C2*2 occurred after the mutations which split these antigens.

Some of these conclusions, reached from typing of C2 gene products in serum, can be confirmed at the level of the DNA. Apart from showing the orientation of the complement region, it will be interesting, for example, to see how many independent mutations the C2*2 genes on different haplotypes and in different ethnic groups represent.

Summary

Forty-two HLA haplotypes bearing C2*2 were found in the Ninth Workshop. Analysis suggests there were two founder haplotypes in the Caucasoid population which have become partially fragmented by ancestral recombination. Ancestral recombinants indicate that the C2 locus is nearer to B than to DR and that the gene order is B, C2, BF, C4, DR. The founder haplotypes appear to be more than 5000 and less than 20 000 years old, with the Bw62 haplotype being the older.

One interesting haplotype in the Japanese data may represent a founder haplotype for the oriental population.

Acknowledgments. Members of the participating laboratories are grateful to the many families who volunteered blood samples and to the many staff members and technologists who helped with the work.

References

1. Alper CA (1976) Inherited structural polymorphism in human C2: evidence for genetic linkage between C2 and Bf. J Exp Med 144:1111–1115
2. Carroll MC, Campbell RD, Bentley DR, Porter RR (1984) A molecular map of the human major histocompatibility complex class III region linking complement genes C4, C2 and factor B. Nature 307:237–241
3. Edwards JH (1978) Human Genetics. Chapman and Hall, London, p 42
4. Hobart MJ, Lachmann PJ (1976) Allotypes of complement components in man. Transplant Rev 32:26–42
5. Hobart MJ, Lachmann PJ, Alper CA (1975) Polymorphism of human C6. In: Peeters H (ed) Protides of the biological fluids. Pergamon, Oxford, p 575
6. Marshall WH, Barnard JM, Churchill D, Farid NR, Grandy R, Larsen B, Payne RH, Skanes VM, Ebers GC, Paty DW, Mervart H, Schroeder M (1984) Studies of alleles of the second complement component (C2) on Canadian HLA haplotypes. Tissue Antigens 23:229–239
7. Mauff G, Alper CA, Awdeh Z, Batchelor JR, Bertrams J, Bruun-Petersen G, Dawkins RL, Demant P, Edwards J, Grosse-Wilde H, Hauptmann G, Klouda P, Lamm L, Mollenhauer E, Nerl C, Olaisen B, O'Neill G, Rittner C, Roos MH, Skanes VM, Teisberg P, Wells L (1983) Statement on the nomenclature of human C4 allotypes. Immunobiol 164:184–191

Properdin Factor B

S. W. Serjeantson

John Curtin School of Medical Research, Australian National University, Canberra, Australia

The properdin factor B (BF) polymorphism comprises two common alleles, F and S; two less common alleles, F1 and SO.7 (previously termed S1); and several further rare alleles, described by Mauff et al. [1]. These electrophoretic variants have been used in traditional linkage analyses to map the structural gene coding for factor B between HLA-B and HLA-DR [2]. Molecular mapping [3] suggests a single factor B locus in this region, closely linked with the C2 locus and proximal to C4A and C4B loci.

Table 1. Frequencies of BF alleles in Caucasoid and Oriental populations (%)

BF	Caucasoid	Oriental
S	76.0	85.7
F	21.2	14.3
SO.7	1.3	0.0
Fl	1.3	0.0
Variants	0.2	0.0
Number of haplotypes	2304	182

Table 1 provides the percentage frequencies of BF alleles in healthy Caucasoid (ethnic codes 31 – 59) and Oriental (ethnic codes 11 – 29) populations. BF*SO.7 and BF*F1 were absent from Chinese, Thai, and Japanese groups.

BF alleles were found in significant positive linkage disequilibrium with MHC alleles, as shown in Table 2 for Caucasoid populations and in Table 3 for Oriental populations. For Orientals, however, the number of healthy haplotypes available for counting was small, and Japanese and Chinese populations, known to differ in HLA antigen profiles, were pooled. There was no significant linkage disequilibrium between BF and C2 or GLO alleles in either Caucasoids or Orientals.

Table 2. Caucasoid populations: MHC alleles in significant positive linkage disequilibrium with BF alleles

BF	HLA-A	HLA-C	HLA-B		C4A	C4B	HLA-DR
S	A2	Cw7	B7*	B38	A4	B2*	DR2*
	A11		B8*	Bw41	AQO	B3	DR3
			B13	Bw52	A6		DR4
			B27	Bw60*			DR5
F	A3	Cw4*	B35	Bw58*	A3*	BQO	DRw6*
	A29*		B37*	Bw62			DR7*
			B44*	Bw63			DRw10*
			Bw47*				
SO.7	–	Cw6*	Bw50*		A2*	B1*	DR7*
			B45				
F1	–	Cw5*	B18*		A3*	BQO*	DR3*

* $P < 0.001$

Table 3. Oriental populations: MHC alleles in significant positive linkage disequilibrium with BF alleles

BF	HLA-A	HLA-C	HLA-B	C4A	C4B	HLA-DR
S	A2*	Cw1*	–	C4A3	–	DR7*
	A11*	Cw6				DRw8
	A31					DRw9*
F	Al	Cw2	Bw41	–	C4B3	DR2*
	A3*	CwX*	B38			DR3
	A26*		B44			DRw10*
	Aw33					

* $P < 0.001$
(Tables 1 – 3 extracted from Baur et al. preliminary population analysis)

Several Ninth Workshop families demonstrated irregularities in BF segregation, apparently confirming the existence of a BF null allele, reported previously by Suciu-Foca et al. [4] on the haplotype A2,B15,Cw3,DR4. Some of these irregularities require confirmation before the frequency of the BF null allele can be estimated.

The Ninth Workshop family material has confirmed BF linkage disequilibrium relationships estimated from population data in the Eighth Workshop. It has provided additional information re-

Histocompatibility Testing 1984
Edited by E. D. Albert et al.

garding linkage disequilibrium between BF and C4A, C4B alleles.

References

1. Mauff G, Hauptmann G, Hitzeroth HW, Gauchel F, Scherz F (1978) The nomenclature of properdin factor B allotypes. Z Immunforsch 154:115
2. Weitkamp LR, Lamm LU (1982) Report of the committee on the genetic constitution of chromosome 6. Cytogenet Cell Genet 32:130
3. Carroll MC, Campbell RD, Bentley DR, Porter RR (1984) A molecular map of the human major histocompatibility complex class III region linking complement genes C4, C2 and factor B. Nature 307:237–241
4. Suciu-Foca N, O'Neill G, Rubenstein P (1980) Evidence for the existence of a possible Bf "null" allele. In: Terasaki PI (ed) Histocompatibility testing 1980. UCLA Tissue Typing Laboratory, Los Angeles, p 935

C4 Polymorphism *

C. Rittner [1] and G. Mauff [2]

1 Institute of Legal Medicine, University of Bonn, Stiftsplatz 12, 5300 Bonn, Federal Republic of Germany
2 Institute of Hygiene, University of Cologne, Goldenfelsstraße 21, 5000 Cologne, Federal Republic of Germany

On behalf of:
E. D. Albert, C. Alper, A. Arnaiz-Villena, H. Avakian, H. Bashir, J. R. Batchelor, J. Bertrams, H. Betuel, J. Bodmer, B. Bradley, D. Briggs, G. Bruun Petersen, A. Cambon-Thomsen, C. B. Carpenter, P. Chiewshilp, J. Dausset, R. Dawkins, P. Dewar, H. Dick, I. A. Dodi, I. Doxiadis, E. Dupont, E. du Toit, C. Evans, E. Ferreira, H. Festenstein, A. Fielder, K. Gelsthorpe, R. Giblett, R. C. Gorodezky, H. Grosse-Wilde, J. A. Hansen, G. Hauptmann, B. R. Hawkins, D. James, T. Juji, A. Kastelan, P. Kay, E. Keller, F. Kissmeyer-Nielsen, P. Klouda, S. Knight, L. U. Lamm, B. Lambert, J. Lee, P. Mackintosh, S. Mahadeo, A. Marcelli-Barge, W. H. Marshall, S. Mayer, R. McLean, N. Mehra, H. Mervart, T. Miyajima, C. Mueller-Eckhardt, S. Naito, H. Neumeyer, G. O'Neill, E. Ohayon, M. Robinson, S. Rodriguez de Cordoba, J. J. van Rood, T. Rosales, P. Rubinstein, B. Schacter, D. Schendel, M. L. Schroeder, V. M. Skanes, K. Tokunaga, N. Usher, R. Wank, K. Welsh, L. Wells, J. Woodrow, E. Yunis

Eighty laboratories have contributed data on class III gene products to the Ninth International Histocompatibility Workshop. Therefore, it can be concluded that these investigations of complement markers in studies on population genetics and disease associations reflect the increasing importance of the class III loci of the major histocompatibility complex. The study of the highly polymorphic C4 loci, in particular, poses a number of problems, only some of which can be addressed in this report. For a more detailed discussion the reader may consult some recent publications [6, 10, 12, 14]. The results of the association studies of C2, BF, C4A, and C4B in the workshop diseases will be found in the disease reports in this volume.

Only recently has the map order of human class III loci been established, by Carroll et al. [2], as shown in Fig. 1.

Whereas no reasonable doubt is cast on the position of these genes between HLA-DR and HLA-B on the short arm of chromosome 6 (see also M. Baur et al., Analysis of MHC Recombinant Families, this volume), the orientation of the genes within this region remains to be shown. Studies on C2 and BF have been summarized elsewhere in this volume (W. Marshall et al., C2 in the Ninth Workshop; S. Serjeantson, Properdin Factor B). Also, the identification of the genes named "C4z" and "C4y" as C4A and C4B respectively is under way. C4A- and C4B-specific cDNA probes are now available [3]. Yet, the definition of the human C4 polymorphism at the phenotypic level has to be completed. There is increasing evidence that more than 12 C4A and 20 C4B structural gene products seem to exist, as summarized recently [4]. Clearly, not all of these variants are equally well defined. As can be seen in Table 1, only four C4A and three C4B allotypes were included in the 1980 International Reference Typing and reached a more than 80% confidence level (G. Mauff, unpublished results). A second round of reference typing is currently under way (C. A. Alper and Z. L. Awdeh, manuscript in preparation). Subject to error are generally areas with variants needing a second digit for distinction. Obviously, some form of quality control has to be performed in future workshops to allow a comparison of data from individual laboratories.

* This work was supported in part by Deutsche Forschungsgemeinschaft Ri 164/16-1 and Ma 848/1

Histocompatibility Testing 1984
Edited by E. D. Albert et al.

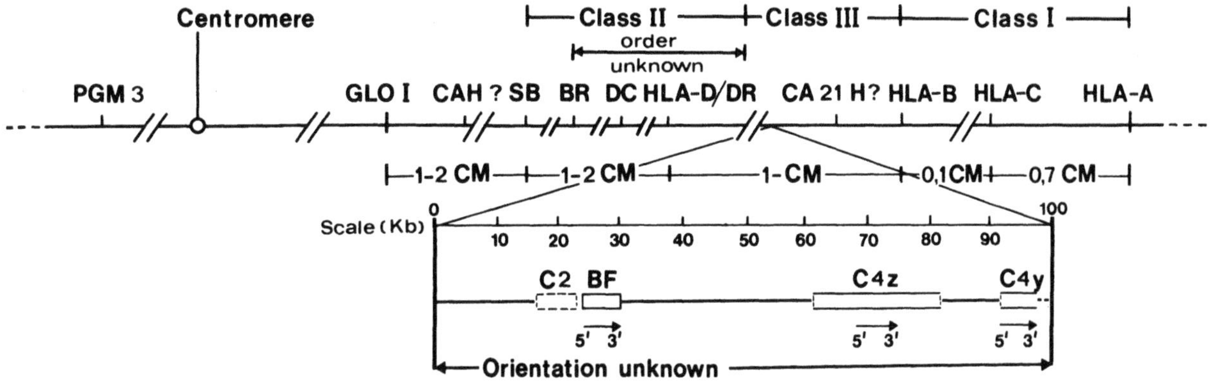

Fig. 1. Preworkshop state of human MHC on chromosome 6 (modified from reference 2). CM = Centimorgan

A second major problem of human C4 polymorphism lies in the frequent occurrence of so-called silent alleles which cannot easily be deduced from any typing method, as discussed in more detail elsewhere [6, 10]. In selecting the families from the Ninth Workshop Central Analysis the presence of silent alleles was assumed as safe only in cases of homozygosity for QO, in the absence of A 3, B 1, or if cosegregation with non-A 3, B 1 was seen. Only 50% of the families with locally assumed silent C4 alleles fulfilled these criteria. It is apparent that by this definition many families with silent alleles were not evaluated.

A third problem consisted in the difficulty of coding for duplicated C4 haplotypes, although the existence of duplications has in the meantime been well established [see, e.g., 6, 10, 13] (see B. Uring-Lambert et al., C4 Haplotypes with Duplicated C4A or C4B, this volume). In cases where more than two C4 genes were assigned locally to single haplotypes, the family could not be analyzed by the family analysis program. For this reason, of the 612 families submitted to the Workshop with class III gene data, 148 were excluded from haplotype analysis.

Table 1. C4 allotypes found in Ninth Workshop families

Well-defined[a]		Ill-defined	
A2	B1	A1	B92
A3	B2	$A12^{Cauc}$	B11
A4	B3	$A12^{Jap}$	B12
A6		A13	B21
		A5	B31
		A51	B4
		OT	B5
			B6
			B7
			OT
		AQO	BQO

[a] According to 1980 International C4 Reference Typing

Besides these more general problems, the level of the Ninth Workshop C4 data was determined by the typing techniques employed. Several established methods for the determination of C4 polymorphism are known [1, 4, 8], and new techniques are currently emerging for the recognition of the polymorphism on the protein level with monoclonal antibodies and on the DNA level with C4-cDNA [2, 13, 14], as listed in Table 2.

No specifications on the procedure for complement typing were made for the submission of data to the Ninth Workshop. As far as could be judged, family data for Central Analysis was based on two of the standard techniques accepted for C4 reference typing [4]: agarose-gel immunofixation electrophoresis and functional assignment of allotypes to C4A and C4B protein by hemolytic overlay after agarose gel electrophoresis. Some contributors used additional informations from Rodgers/Chido and C4α- and C4β-chain typings in assigning haplotypes [5, 9–12]. Since C4α- and β-chain typing techniques were not available at the time of planning, inclusion of this data was not provided for in the Central Analysis of complement typing results. As a consequence, discrepancies were observed between the results of Central Analysis and local analysis. Families submitted to the Ninth Workshop could therefore be classified according to their C4 data into three groups:

1. Pedigrees congruent by Central Analysis and by local analysis of the submitting laboratory
2. Pedigrees rejected by Central Analysis, but duplications of C4 loci assumed by local analysis on the basis of cosegregation or phenotypic patterns
3. Difficult or complex pedigrees rejected by Central analysis on the basis of conflicting rare variant attribution by the submitting laboratory and/or duplications of C4 loci

In the following, examples will be given which are considered as representative for the total C4 family

Table 2. Evidence for genetic polymorphism of human C4

Method	Information
1. Immunofixation agarose-gel electrophoresis	> 30 allelic banding patterns
2. Hemolytic detection on agarose-gel electrophoresis	C4B allotypes > C4A allotypes
3. Rodgers (Rg) and Chido (Ch) antigen determination	– complete – partial – aberrant – no } inhibition
4. C4α- and C4β-chain determination on SDS-gel electrophoresis	silent alleles by relative quantitation of: – C4αA- and C4αB-bands – C4βH- and C4βL-bands
5. Immunoblotting of C4 on SDS-gel electrophoresis with Rg and Ch antisera	– Rg epitope on C4αA-chain – Ch epitope on C4αB-chain – aberrant Rg/Ch epitopes
6. Immunoblotting of C4 on agarose-gel electrophoresis with C4B MOAB	– C4B epitopes on C4B allotypes – aberrant epitopes on "C4A" allotypes
7. DNA typing with C4 cDNA	– number of C4 genes – DNA polymorphism

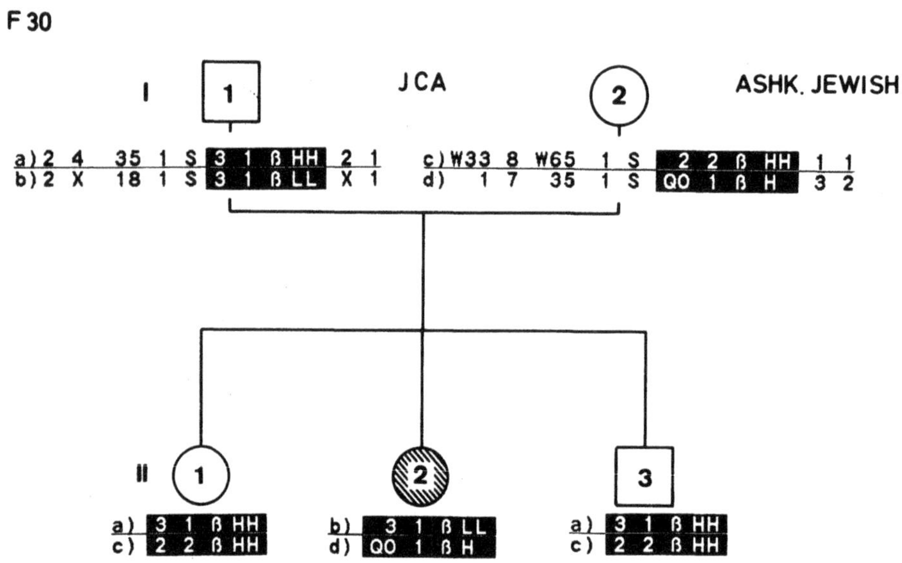

Fig. 2. Family 30 (SAF DUT 30). *Co-segregation* of C4A QO on haplotype d. Arbitrary sequence of typing data: HLA-A, C, B, C2, BF, C4A, C4B, C4β, HLA-DR, GLO. HLA, GLO typing results from Dr. Ernette du Toit, Cape Town.

data submitted to the Ninth Workshop. In family 30 (Fig. 2) identical haplotypes were assigned by Central Analysis and by local analysis on the basis of segregation. Proof for C4A 3 on haplotype b and for C4A QO on haplotype d was derived from child II,2. C4B 1 on haplotype b was assumed by Central Analysis but could be substantiated by the constellation of C4β H = L in individual I,1, C4β H in I,2, and foremost by C4β H < L in II,2, unequal distribution of C4β-chain banding pattern giving evidence for an unequal number of expressed C4 loci (C4A 3, B1/C4A QO, B 1 vs C4A 3, BQO/C4A QO, B 1 [4, 5]).

In family 29 (Fig. 3) duplication of C4A was observed in individual I,2 by expression of three allotypes. No allowance having been made for more than two C4 loci in the planning, the third C4A allotype *A2* in individual I,2 was not accepted by the family analysis program, and in consequence the children II,2 and 3 were excluded.

Duplication of *C4A 3, A 2* on haplotype d (in association with HLA-B35) as well as non-expression of C4A on haplotype a and C4B on haplotype b were presumed by local analysis to be the most likely interpretation on the basis of segregation patterns. Although not essential for the assumed constellation in this family, the findings were supported by the distribution of C4β-chain types.

Complex families with difficult C4 allotypes were in the minority of data submitted to the Ninth Workshop, but will be more often encountered in non-Caucasoid populations. They pose special problems due to unusual C4 allotypes and unexpected duplication, as seen in family 39 (Fig. 4).

In this family six rare C4 variants were observed (C4A 6; A 5; A '22'; A 1; B '28'; B 92), one of which, A '22', had not been described previously. Local analysis assumed duplication of C4B 2, B 92 on haplotypes g and h, phenotypically visible by three C4B allotypes in individuals III,6, 7, and 8. In individual II,2 the new allele A '22' was not recognizable due to its very close migration distance to C4A 3. The submitted data was therefore not accepted by the family program. Only on retyping individual II,2 with a new blood sample could the phenotype C4A 3, '22', B 92 successfully be as-

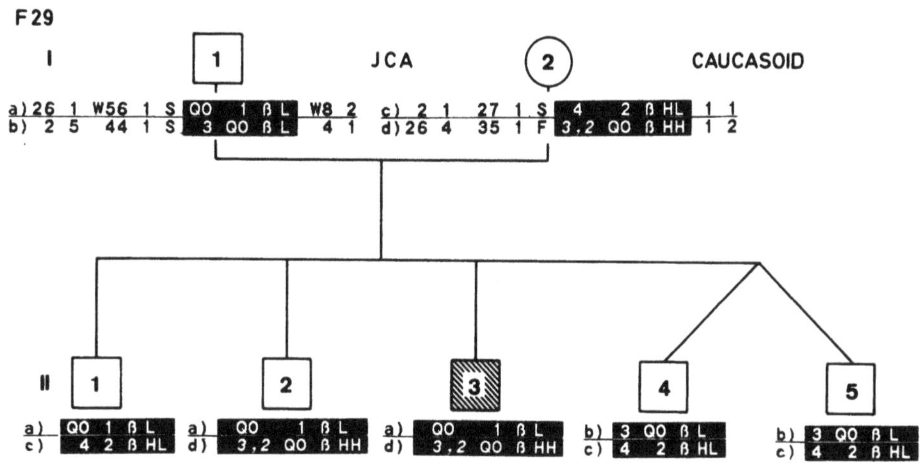

Fig. 3. Family 29 (SAF DUT 29). Individual I,2 with three C4A bands; *duplicated haplotype* C4A 3, A 2, B QO on d. Sequence of data and HLA typing results as in Figure 2.

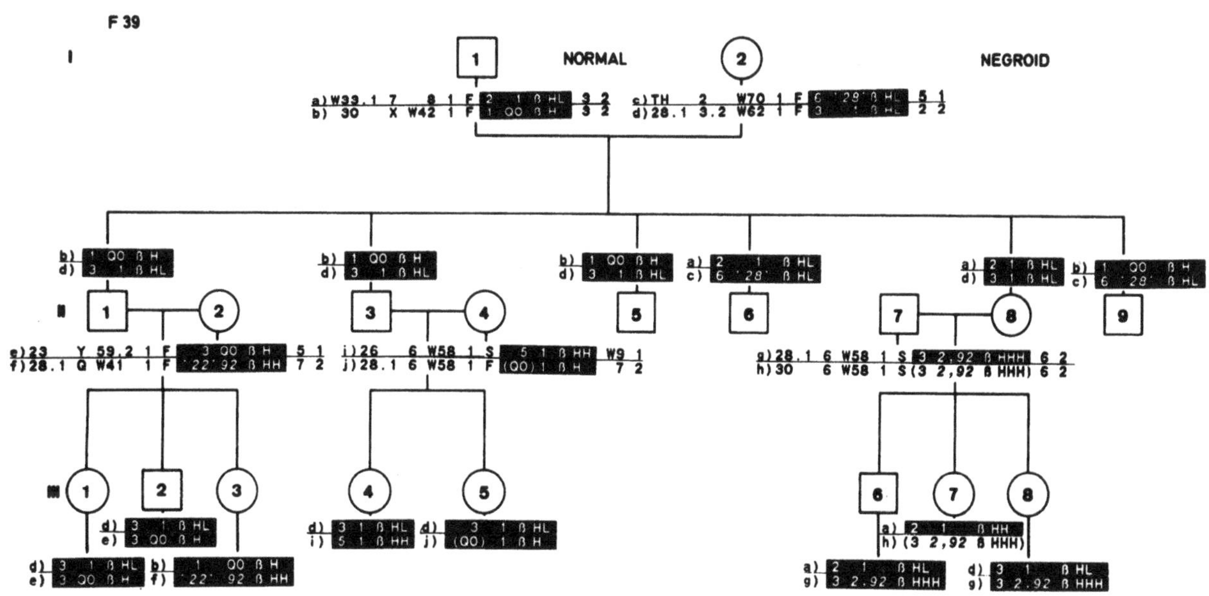

Fig. 4. Family 39 (SAF DUT 39). Apostrophes denote new Negroid C4 variant allotypes; *duplicated haplotype* C4A 3, B 2, B 92 on g and h. Sequence of data and HLA typing results as in Figure 2.

Table 3. Frequent Ninth Workshop haplotype associations of C4 alleles

Haplotype	HLA-Cw	HLA-B	C2	BF	C4A	C4B	HLA-DR
Healthy	8	w65	–	S	2	2	1/5
Healthy	6	w57	1	S	6	1	7
Healthy	3	w55	2	S	4	6	1/w6
Healthy	3	w60	2	S	4	5	1/w6
Healthy	7	8	1	S	QO	1	3
Healthy	4	35	1	S	3	QO	1/2/4
Healthy	5	44	1	F/S	3	QO	2/4/w6
IDDM/healthy	3	w62	1	S	3	3	4

certained. In addition, this pedigree contained three haplotypes unusual in Caucasoids but more often observed in Negroids:

1. b) C4A 1, B QO, BF F, C2 C(1) in five out of six haplotypes, also associated with HLA-Bw42 in three out of five haplotypes of all C4-typed Negroid Ninth Workshop families
2. c) C4A 6(resp. 5), B '28', BF F, C2 C(1) in five out of five haplotypes, also associated with HLA-Bw70 and DR5 in three out of six haplotypes
3. g) h) C4A 3, B 2, B 92, C4βHHH, BF S, C2 C(1) in five out of six haplotypes, also associated with HLA-Bw58, DRw6 in five out of five haplotypes

Furthermore, in this family the silent C4 alleles on haplotypes b, e, and j could be derived from the segregation patterns.

Neglecting most of these problems, all C4 typing results accepted by the computer analysis were used to calculate gene frequencies and haplotype frequencies as well as delta values for linkage disequilibria (cf. M. Baur et al., Population Analysis, this volume), which include certain HLA-B and HLA-DR alleles. Strongly positive delta values were found for the haplotypes in Table 3.

It may be mentioned that some laboratories apparently had difficulties in defining the C4A*4, B*6 haplotype in association with HLA-Bw55, C2*2, and DR1 which is also a subject of the present C4 reference typing. Recently it was observed [12] that the C4A*4, B*5 haplotype can be subdivided by Ch/Rg typing on blotted C4α chains. It could also been shown that the "A*QO" included in the haplotype with HLA-A1, Cw7, B8, and DR3 is a deleted gene of at least 22 kb [3], whereas in the cases of B*QO a non-expressed gene can be found. Finally, the C4A*3, B*3 haplotype in association with Bw62 and DR4 occurred relatively frequently not only among healthy Caucasoids, but also among Caucasoid IDDM patients of the Ninth Workshop (cf. J. Bertrams et al., IDDM joint disease report, this volume).

One of the aims of the Ninth Workshop was to establish a cross-over registry (cf. M. Baur et al., Analysis of MHC Recombinant Families, this volume). For the analysis of class III genes, 71 families with HLA-B/DR cross-overs were considered. Fifty-one families had to be rejected for the following reasons:

1. Ambiguous QO assignment
2. Intra-class III gene region cross-over (not yet unequivocally demonstrated in a single family)
3. B/DR double cross-over (extremely unlikely to detect)
4. Family not informative for class III genes

The list of 20 provisionally accepted HLA-B/DR cross-over families informative for one or more complement markers is given in Table 4. Not accounting for possible intra-class III gene cross-overs, the fragment carrying the complement genes travelled in 12 families with HLA-B and in eight families with HLA-DR. Excluding possible selection bias, this figure would support the data of Olaisen et al. [7] in as much as these authors place the class III gene cluster slightly more adjacent to HLA-B than to HLA-DR, although their complement gene map order has not been confirmed regarding C2 [2]. Also, it should be noted in Table 4 that only a restricted number of HLA-B alleles seems to be involved in the recombinational events. The typing results of these selected families should be confirmed and extended by a second laboratory to apply the whole C4 typing repertoire as outlined in Table 2 in close cooperation with the submitting laboratory in order to explore all informations provided by the Ninth Workshop.

The conclusions to be drawn from the Ninth Workshop C4 results for future comparison of accumulated data from different laboratories must include the requirement for standardized techniques allowing for the recognition of silent alleles and duplications, as well as reference samples for the classification of C4 allotypes.

No.	REG	LAB	No.	Original haplotypes HLA-A	Cw	B	C2	BF	C4A	C4B	DR	Recombinant haplotypes HLA-A	Cw	B	C2	BF	C4A	C4B	DR
1	ANZ	MEH	4	2	0	w61	1	F	3	1	2	24	7	7 #	1	F	3	1	2
				24	7	7	2	S	OT	2	w6								
2	ANZ	MEH	32	2	0	w61	1	S	3	1	2	2	0	w61 #	1	F	3	1	4
				3	4	35	1	F	3	1	4								
3	ANZ	DAW	2	26	3	w62	2	S	4	2	2	1 #	3	w62	2	S	4	2 #	3
				1	7	8	1	S	0	1	3								
4	EAE	KAS	85	26	0	38	1	S	2	1	w6	26	0	38	1	S	2	1 #	5
				24	0	51	1	S	3	1	5								
5	FRA	FAU	26	24	0	39		S	3	1	2	24	0	39		S	3	1 #	4
				33	3	w56		F	3	1	4								
6	FRA	MYE	17	24	0	51			3	1	w6	2	0	51			4	1 #	w6
				2	0	51			4	1	5								
7	NCY	MAR	3	3	4	35	1	S	3	1	2	3	4	35 #	2	S	4	2	4
				1	3	w62	2	S	4	2	4								
8	NCY	YUN	6	3		35		S	3	1	5	24		49 #		S	3	1	5
				24		49		F	3	11	7								
9	UKI	DEW	5	2	0	14	1	F	4	1	0	28	0	14	1	S	2	2 #	0
				28	0	14	1	S	2	2	5								
10	UKI	FES	6	26	4	35	1	S	3	1	w10	26	4	35	1	S	3	1 #	0
				2	8	14	1	S	3	2	0								
11	US7	HAN	4	24	1	w62	1	S	3	1	0	2	1	w62	2	S	4	2 #	0
				2	1	w62	2	S	4	2	6								
12	US7	HAN	5	11	1	27	1	S	3	0	w9	28	6	37	1	F	3	1 #	w9
				28	6	37	1	F	3	1	w10								
13	SCA	SVE	8	23	4	44	1	F	3	[0]	7	28	7	44	1	S	3	[0] #	7
				28	7	44	1	S	3	[1]	5								
14	GER	GSW	1	2	6	w57		S	6	1	7	2	6	w57 #		F	3	2	1
				3	0	39		F	3	2	1								
15	GER	NEU	2	1	7	8			0	1	3	1	7	8			0	1 #	7
				24	6	13			3	1	7								
16	FRA	OHA	10	2	5	w50		SO7			7	3	4	35 #		SO7			7
				3	4	35		F			1								
17	NCY	YUN	4	1	0	8	1	S			3	1 #	0	44	1	F		#	3
				23	4	44	1	F			7								
18	US3	GRU	10	25	0	39		S			2	25	0	39 #		F			7
				3	6	w47		F			7								
19	SCA	LIN	1	2	2	w62		S			4	2	2	w62 #		F			5
				29	0	44		F			5								
20	NCY	BIA	8	2	6	17		S			7	2	0	39		F		#	7
				2	0	39		F			1								

= assumed position of cross-over (possible intra-class III gene recombination not accounted for). In families 3 and 17, additional HLA-A/C cross-over

Acknowledgments. The authors acknowledge all discussion remarks from the submitting laboratories. We are especially grateful to Dr. Ernette du Toit, Cape Town, for making available the family material of families 29, 30, and 39.

References

1. Awdeh ZL, Alper CA (1980) Inherited structural polymorphism of the fourth component of human complement. Proc Natl Acad Sci USA 77:3576–3580
2. Carroll MC, Campbell RD, Bentley DR, Porter RR (1984) A molecular map of the human major histocompatibility complex class III region linking complement genes C4, C2 and factor B. Nature 307:237–241
3. Carroll MC, Belt KT, Palsdottir A, Yu CY, Porter RR (1984) Structural studies on the human fourth component of complement genes and their products. Third H-2, HLA Cloning Meeting, Strasbourg, 2–4 May
4. Mauff G, Alper CA, Awdeh ZL, Batchelor JR, Bertrams J, Bruun-Petersen G, Dawkins RL, Démant P, Edwards JH, Grosse-Wilde H, Hauptmann G, Klouda P, Lamm L, Mollenhauer E, Nerl C, Olaisen B, O'Neill G, Rittner C, Roos MH, Skanes V, Teisberg P, Wells L (1983) Statement on the nomenclature of human C4 allotypes. Immunobiol 164:184–191
5. Mauff G, Steuer M, Weck M, Bender K (1983) The C4β-chain: evidence for a genetically determined polymorphism. Hum Genet 64:186–188
6. Mauff G, Bender K, Giles CM, Goldmann S, Opferkuch W, Wachauf B (1984) Human C4 polymorphism: Pedigree analysis of qualitative, quantitative, and functional parameters as a basis for phenotype interpretations. Hum Genet 65:362–372
7. Olaisen B, Teisberg P, Jonassen R, Thorsby E, Gedde-Dahl T Jr (1983) Gene order and gene distance in the HLA region studied by the haplotype method. Ann Hum Genet 47:285–292
8. O'Neill GJ, Yang SY, Dupont B (1978) Two *HLA*-linked loci controlling the fourth component of human complement. Proc Natl Acad Sci USA 75:5165–5169
9. Rittner C, Tippett P, Giles CM, Mollenhauer E, Berger R, Nordhagen R, Buskjoer L, Bruun-Petersen G, Lamm L, Roos MH (1984) An international reference typing for Ch and Rg determinants on rare human C4 allotypes. Vox Sang. 46:224–234
10. Rittner C, Giles CM, Roos MH, Démant P, Mollenhauer E (1984) Genetics of human C4 polymorphism: detection and segregation of rare and duplicated haplotypes. Immunogenetics 19:321–333
11. Roos MH, Mollenhauer E, Démant P, Rittner C (1982) A molecular basis for the two-locus model of human complement component C4. Nature 298:854–856
12. Roos MH, Démant P, Giles CM, Mollenhauer E, Rittner C (1984) Polymorphism of human C4A and C4B-chains as detected by analysis of Rodgers and Chido determinants. J Immunol (in press)
13. Schendel DJ, Wank R, O'Neill GJ (1984) C4 phenotypic variation suggests an unusual class III gene organization. Vox Sang (in press)
14. Whitehead AS, Woods DE, Fleischnick E, Chin JE, Yunis EJ, Katz AJ, Gerald PS, Alper CA, Colten HR (1984) DNA polymorphism of the C4 genes. A new marker for analysis of the major histocompatibility complex. New Engl J Med 310:88–91

Genetics of HLA

Analysis of MHC Recombinant Families *

M.P. Baur [1], S. Sigmund [2], M. Sigmund [2], and C. Rittner [3]

1 Biometrical Department, Diabetes Research Institute, Auf'm Hennekamp 65, 4000 Düsseldorf 1, Federal Republic of Germany
2 Institute for Medical Statistics University of Bonn, 5300 Bonn, Federal Republic of Germany
3 Institute for Legal Medicine University of Bonn, Stiftsplatz 12, 5300 Bonn, Federal Republic of Germany

One of the aims of the Ninth Workshop was the collection of MHC recombinant families to gather confirmatory information about the known sequence of HLA-A, C, B, DR and to gather further information about sequence and orientation of the class III gene complex of C2, Bf, C4A, and C4B, which was postulated to be situated between HLA-B and HLA-DR without known orientation (Fig. 1) [1].

All families submitted to the Workshop masterfile were analysed by the Family Analysis Package (FAP) (M. Neugebauer et al., Analysis of Multilocus Pedigree Data by Computer, this volume) using the laboratory assignments for all loci as submitted on cards 2–7. In case of a family interpretation demanding at least one cross-over, FAP listed the solution with the highest likelihood, i.e., the so-

* Supported by Deutsche Forschungsgemeinschaft Ba 660/5-1, Ri 164/16-1

 Histocompatibility Testing 1984
Edited by E. D. Albert et al.

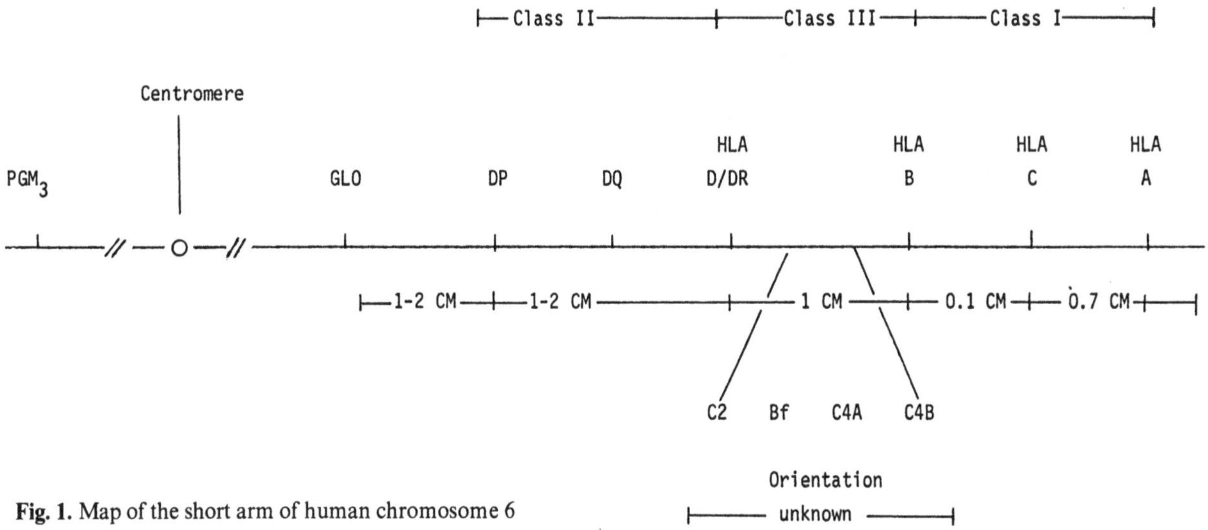

Fig. 1. Map of the short arm of human chromosome 6

lution with the smallest number of cross-overs, and, if possible, with the position of the cross-over between loci with a "large" recombination fraction. The results of FAP – position of cross-over and recombinant individual – were compared to the original coding for type of recombinant family and recombinant individual as given by the submitting laboratories on card 1. When there was agreement between laboratory coding and program interpretation, the family was accepted as correctly analyzed and added to the set of cross-over families.

In addition, all recombinant interpretations which did not correspond to the codes on card 1 were sent to the originating laboratories for checking. Finally, a list of discrepant "cross-over families" was presented during the Workshop for checking and confirmation of the results of FAP. In this way, a set of 217 confirmed and correctly analyzed recombinant families was available for analysis.

The position of the cross-over observed in this set is given in Table 1.

In the total set of 217 families, there was no single contradiction to the well-established order of the class I and class II loci as given in Fig. 1. Estimation of recombination fractions, though straight forward from the deduced recombinant haplotypes, was not possible due to the selection bias in the total Workshop masterfile, which favored recombinant families, especially the B/DR recombinant type. Map distances in Fig. 1 were therefore taken from the literature [2, 3]. From the large number of B/DR recombinant families, only 20 were accpeted for the complement markers. These families are discussed in detail in the C4 polymorphism report of this Workshop (C. Rittner and G. Mauff). In 12 cases the complement group travels with the B-locus; in eight cases it segregates with the DR-locus, confirming strongly the location of C2, Bf, C4A, C4B between HLA-B and HLA-DR. The question of orientation cannot be solved from these families, because no intracomplement recombination could be confirmed. To solve this question an attempt will be made to type the 62 further B/DR recombinant families available for the complement markers.

Table 1. Confirmed recombinations in the masterfile of the Ninth Workshop

Position	Number
A: C	42
A: B	15
C: B	4
C: DR	5
DR: GLO	50
B: DR (not informative for C2, Bf, C4A, C4B)	62
B: (Compl.)	8
DR: (Compl.)	12
Multiple (in different individuals)	23
Multiple (double cross-over)	0

References

1. Carroll MC, Campbell RD, Bentley DR, Porter RR (1984) A molecular map of the human major histocompatibility complex class III region linking complement genes C4, C2 and factor B. Nature 307:237–241
2. Olaisen B, Teisberg P, Jonassen R, Thorsby E, Gedde-Dahl T (1983) Gene order and gene distance in the HLA-region studied by the haplotype method. Ann Hum Genet 47:285–492
3. Robson EB, Lamm LU (1984) Report of the committee on the genetic constitution of chromosome 6. Human gene mapping 7. Cytogenet Cell Genet 37:47–70

Linkage Between HLA-A, C, B, Bf and DR Alleles: Haplotype Study of Healthy Families by Factorial Correspondence Analysis

D. Grange[1], M.M. Tongio[2], G. Hauptmann[2], B. Uring-Lambert[2], M.L. North[2], S. Mayer[2], M. Neugebauer[3], and M.P. Baur[3]

1 Unité Statistique, Centre de Calcul du CNRS, 23, rue du Loess, 67200 Strasbourg, France
2 Institut d'Hématologie, Centre de Transfusion Sanguine, 67200 Strasbourg, France
3 Biometrical Department, Diabetes Research Institute, Auf'm Hennekamp 65, 4000 Düsseldorf 1, Federal Republic of Germany

The most commonly used methods for the analysis of HLA linkage disequilibria allow two- or three-loci alleles to be investigated [1, 6]. In 1978, Dausset et al. [3] evolved a method to solve the problem to n loci; in 1981 [4], we suggested using factorial correspondence analysis (FCA), which is a method of multidimensional analysis worked out by Benzecri [2].

Material and Methods

Methods

The main stages of FCA and its aim are described briefly. First, a table showing the presence or absence of alleles of each haplotype is drawn up (Table 1): for example, haplotype 54, which is A2, Cw5, B44, BfS, DR4, is coded 1 in column A2 and 0 for other HLA-A alleles; 1 in column B44 and 0 for other B alleles, and so on for the other loci. This table is only composed of numbers 0 and 1, the sum of each row being equal to the number of loci to be studied. No missing data is allowed in this table. If an allele of a given locus commonly occurs concurrently with an allele of another locus, these alleles are said to have similar profiles. The method consists of representing all alleles in multidimensional space; it establishes a distance between alleles such that the alleles of similar profiles are very close together, whereas the alleles of very different profiles are very far apart. If there are linkage disequilibria between alleles of several loci, all these alleles will be found together in the same region in space. As it is very difficult to visualize data in multidimensional space, the method looks for subspaces, i.e., for planes (called factorial planes) which contain a maximum of information and on which the alleles will be projected and visualized. Because of distortions due to projection on a factorial plane, the method provides coefficients for estimating the quality of these projections on each of these planes. Calculations were done using the SPAD program [5].

Material

The haplotypes of 1887 families were available in the data files, but only 1098 haplotypes could be finally studied, for the following reasons: (1) FCA can be extended to study n loci, but it is essential that the alleles be determined for all the n loci of the haplotypes studied. Because C2, C4, and GLO had not been typed in many laboratories, only the families typed for HLA-A, C, B, Bf, and DR (a total of 579 families) were considered. (2) Only healthy families were selected (321 of the previous 579 families), and from these, individuals not genetically related were used. (3) Finally, only haplotypes whose genetic transmission was unquestionable were retained. Of the 1098 haplotypes selected, 851 were from Caucasoids, 183 from Mongoloids, 59 from Negroids, five were undefined.

Results

All the HLA-A, C, B, Bf and DR alleles as defined at the Los Angeles Workshop were investigated, with the exception of alleles with a count lower than 3. The new splits found in the 1984 Workshop could not be investigated since they had not been officially recognized at the time of this analysis. The allelic frequencies seen in each ethnic group in our sample were similar to those calculated from the total Workshop data (Baur et al., Population Analysis, in this volume). Figures 1 and 2 show the most striking factorial planes for the Caucasian and Mongoloid groups. For the Negroid population there was insufficient data for reliable results. Tables 2 and 3 show the linkage disequilibria found in the Caucasian and Mongoloid populations. The results are presented in the order given by the analysis. The strongest parts of the linkage disequilibria mainly involve the alleles of two or three loci, even if the linkages in some cases are extended to the whole haplotype. The number of the axis on which the haplotypes appear, and a

Histocompatibility Testing 1984
Edited by E. D. Albert et al.

Table 1. Presence/absence of alleles

Haplotype no. \ Locus	HLA-A (1 2 3 11 28 .)	HLA-Cw (1 2 3 4 5 6 7 8)	HLA-B (5 7 8 . 44 .)	Bf (S F F1 S07)	HLA-DR (1 2 3 4 .)
1	. .	. .	. .	.	. .
.	. .	. .	. .	.	. .
.	. .	. .	. .	.	. .
.	. .	. .	. .	.	. .
.	. .	. .	. .	.	. .
54	0 1 0 0 0 0	0 0 0 0 1 0 0 0	0 0 0 0 1 0	1 0 0 0	0 0 0 1 0
.	.	.	.	.	.
.	.	.	.	.	.
112	1 0 0 0 0 0	0 0 0 0 0 0 1 0	0 0 1 0 0 0	1 0 0 0	0 0 1 0 0
.					
.					
.					
851					

Haplotype no. 54 = A2, Cw5, B44, BfS, DR4; no. 112 = A1, Cw7, B8, BfS, DR3

Table 2. Linkage disequilibria found in Caucasians

Star rating		Linkage disequilibria			Axis no.	Star rating		Linkage disequilibria			Axis no.
++++	A1	Cw7 B8		DR3	1	+++	A2	Cw3 Bw60		DRw6	5
+++	A1	Cw7 B8	S	DR3	1	+++		Cw3 Bw55			5
+++		Cw7 B7			2	++++		Cw4 B35			6
+++		B7	S	DR2	2	++	A3	Cw4 B35			6
+++		Cw7 B7	S	DR2	2	++	A3	Cw4 B35	F		6
++	A3	Cw7 B7	S	DR2	2	++	A3	Cw4 B35	F	DR1	6
++++		Cw6 B13			2	+++	A11	Cw4 B35			4
+++		Cw6 B13		DR7	2	+++	A11	Cw4 B35	S		4
+++	A30	Cw6 B13		DR7	2	++	A11	Cw4 B35	S	DR1	4
++++		Cw6 Bw57			2	+		Cw4 B35		DR5	5
+++		Cw6 Bw57		DR7	2	++++		Cw2 B27			6
++	A1	Cw6 Bw57	S		4	+++		Cw2 B27	S		6
++++		Cw6 B37			1	++++		Cw2 Bw61			6
++	A1	Cw6 B37			1	++	A32	Cw2 Bw61			6
++		Cw6 B37	F		2	++		Cw2 Bw61		DR5	6
++		Cw6 B37	F	DRw10	2	+++		Cw1 B27			6
++++		Cw6 Bw50*	S0.7		2	++	A2	Cw1 B27			6
						+	A2	Cw1B27*		DR1	6
++++		Cw8 B14			3	+++		Cw1 Bw56*			6
+++	Aw33	Cw8 B14			3	+++		C– B44			4
++	Aw33	Cw8 B14		DR1	3	++		C– B44	F		4
+++	A28	Cw8 B14			3	+		C– B44		DR7	4
+++		Cw5 B44			4	+	A29	C– B44	F		4
++	A2	Cw5 B44			4	+	A29	C– B44	F	DR7	4
++	A2	Cw5 B44		DR4	4	++		C– B51			5
+++		Cw5 B18			4	+	A31	C– B51			5
+++		Cw5 B18	F1		4	+	A31*	C– B51	F	DR4	5
++		Cw5 B18**	F1	DR3	4	+++		C– Bw52			5
++++		Cw3 Bw62			5	+		C– Bw52*		DR2	5
++	A2	Cw3 Bw62			5	+++		C– B38			6
+++	A24	Cw3 Bw62			1	++		C– B38		DRw6	6
++	A24	Cw3 Bw62	F		1	++		C– B18			4
++		Cw3 Bw62	F	DRw6	1	++	A25	C– B18			4
++++		Cw3 Bw60			5	+++		C– Bw41*			6
+++	A2	Cw3 Bw60			5						

* low frequency haplotype; ** linkage disequilibrium with A30, frequently found in diabetic patients, was not found in this healthy population

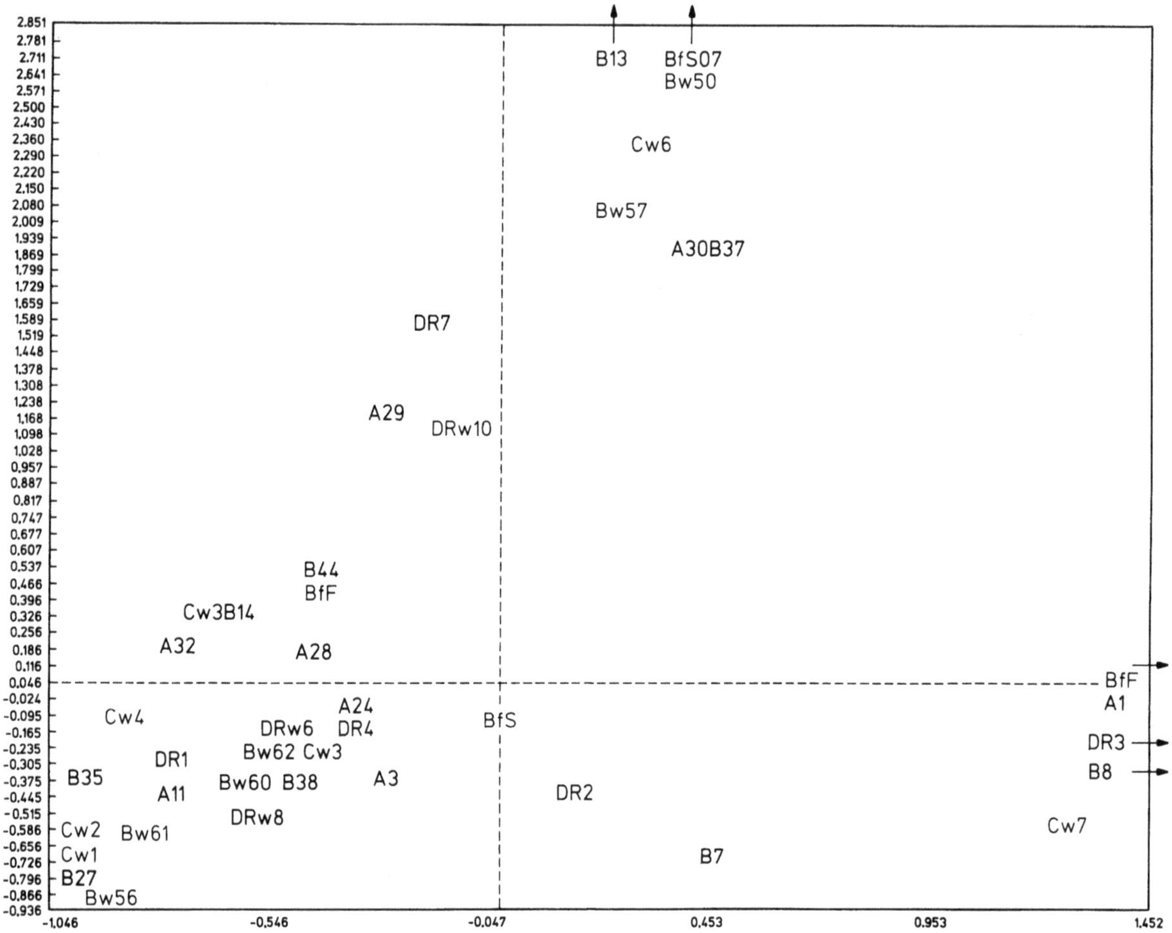

Fig. 1. FCA Plane (1, 2) Caucasians

Fig. 2. FCA Plane (1, 2) Mongoloids ▼

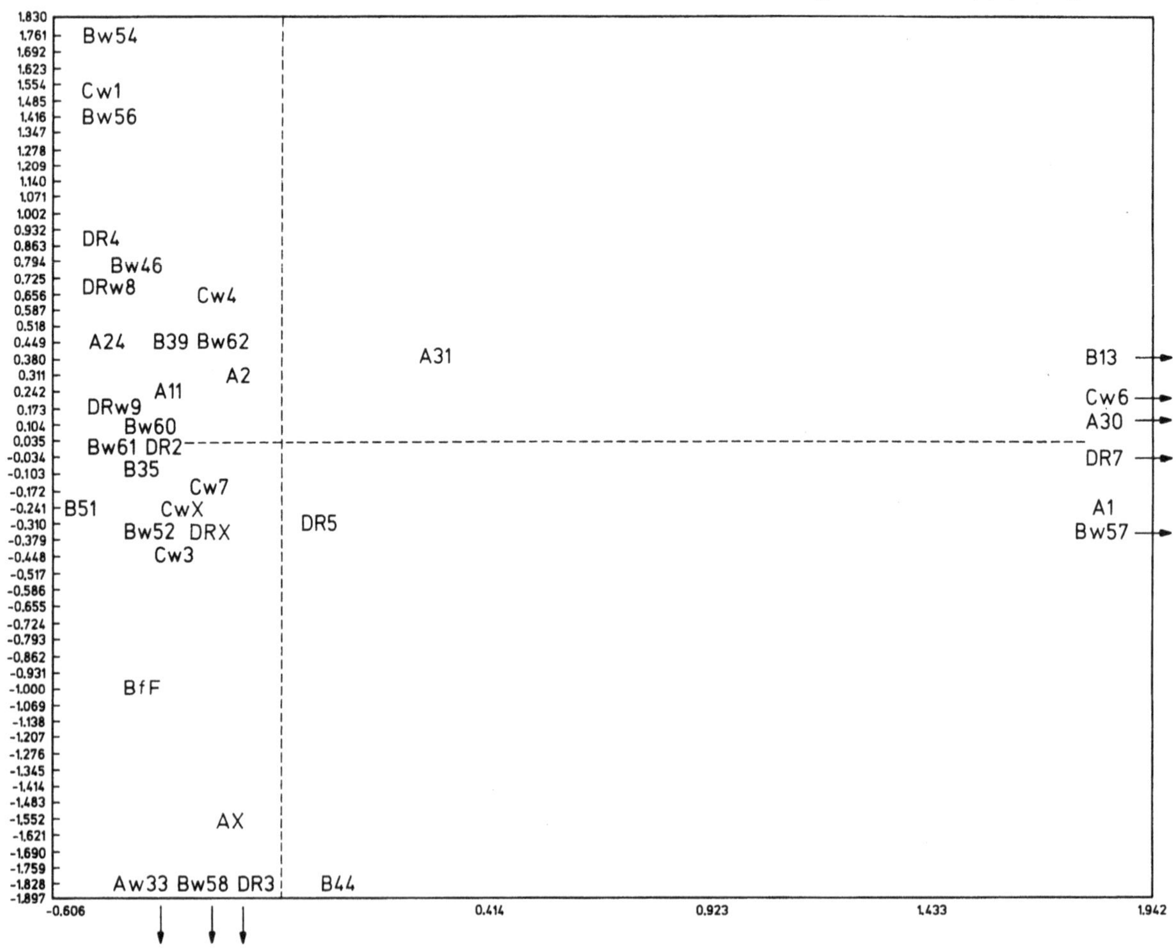

Table 3. Linkage disequilibria found in Mongoloids

Star rating		Linkage disequilibria		Axis no.	Star rating		Linkage disequilibria			Axis no.
+ + +	A30	Cw6 B13	DR7	1	+ +		Cw3 B35			6
	A1	Cw6 Bw57		1	+ + +		Cw7 B39			3
+ + +		Cw1 Bw54		2	+ +		Cw7 B39		DRw8	3
+		Cw1 Bw54	DR4	2	+ +		Cw7 B7		DR1	3
+ + +		Cw1 Bw56		2	+	A24	Cw7 B7		DR1	3
+ + + +		Cw3 Bw58		2	+		Cw7 Bw60			4
+	Aw33	Cw3 Bw58		2	+ +		C– B51			3
	A–	Cw3 Bw58		2	+ +	Aw33	C– B44	F		2
		Cw3 Bw58	DR3	2	+	Aw33	C– B44	F	DR–	2
+		Cw3 Bw60		1			Cw4 B35			6
+		Cw3 Bw60	DRw9	1						

star rating [4], which allows one to quantify the linkage disequilibria, are given in these two tables.

Discussion

FCA showed that the C alleles determined the factors around which linkage disequilibria appeared. The strongest linkages were between HLA-C and B alleles; this can be explained by the proximity of C and B loci and the low rate of recombinations between them. It was also confirmed that for broad HLA-B alleles with known splits, each split was linked to a different HLA-C allele. Linkages of HLA-C and B with the alleles of the HLA-A, Bf, and DR loci were less strong. Nevertheless, these alleles play an important role, as (1) they appear on some important haplotypes (e.g., A1, Cw7, B8, BfS, DR3; A3, Cw7, B7, BfS, DR2 in Caucasians), and (2) in some cases where the linkage disequilibrium between HLA-C and HLA-B concerns the same alleles, different haplotypes can appear, depending on the linked HLA-A, Bf, or DR alleles (e.g., linkage disequilibria involving Cw4, B35 can be either A3, Cw4, B35, BfF, DR1 or A11, Cw4, B35, BfS, DR1).

The linkage disequilibria found also depended upon the ethnic origins of the populations. This was because: (1) the gene frequencies of the alleles differed from one population to another, some of them being found exclusively in a given population, and (2) when the same alleles were present in different populations, the linkage disequilibria could either be the same in these populations (e.g., A30, Cw6, B13, DR7 found in both Caucasians and Mongoloids) or different (e.g., A3, Cw7, B7, BfS, DR2 in Caucasians and A24, Cw7, B7, DR1 in Mongoloids). Because of the relatively small size of the samples studied, the results given in this paper are probably incomplete. This is mainly true for the Mongoloids, where only 183 haplotypes were investigated. For example since Cw2, Cw5, and Cw8 were nearly absent in this small sample, linkage disequilibria involving these three alleles could not be studied.

In conclusion, FCA can be used to solve the problem of linkage disequilibria to n loci. Nevertheless, such a study can only be performed if all n loci are determined for each family. In this Workshop two-thirds of the data were unusable because they were incomplete for the five loci investigated.

For the future, it would be important to note that if a linkage disequilibrium study to n loci is planned, a protocol should be drawn up which specifies all the loci to be studied in each family.

References

1. Baur MP (1977) Errata corrigé; on some misprintings in the paper by Piazza "Haplotypes and linkage disequilibrium from the three-locus phenotypes" and a Fortran program to use its formulae. Tissue Antigens 9:181–186
2. Benzecri JP (1973) Analyse des données. Analyse des correspondances, tome II. Dunod, Paris
3. Dausset J, Legrand L, Lepage V, Contu L, Marcelli-Barge A, Widloecher I, Benajam A, Meo T, Degos L (1978) A haplotype study of HLA complex with special reference to the HLA-DR series and to Bf, C2 and glyoxalase I polymorphisms. Tissue Antigen 12:297–307
4. Grange D, Tongio MM, Mayer S, Hauptmann G, Klein J (1981) Haplotype study. Linkage between HLA-A, B, C and Bf alleles: results obtained by different statistical methods. Tissue Antigens 18:166–177
5. Lebart L, Morineau A (1982). SPAD. Système portable pour l'analyse des données. CESIA, Paris
6. Piazza A (1975) Haplotypes and linkage disequilibria from the three-locus phenotypes. In: Kissmeyer-Nielsen F (ed) Histocompatibility testing 1975. Munksgaard, Copenhagen, pp 923–927

The Nature of Selection in the HLA Region Based on Population Data From the Ninth Workshop*

W. Klitz[1], G. Thomson[1], and M.P. Baur[2]

1 Department of Genetics, University of California, Berkeley, California 94720, USA
2 Biometrical Department, Diabetes Research Institute, Auf'm Hennekamp 65, 4000 Düsseldorf, Federal Republic of Germany

The HLA region is a model system for the study of multilocus interactions. There are several well-defined, tightly linked, highly polymorphic loci. The physiology of the gene products is relatively well understood, information is available on the history of past generations, including disease and migration patterns, and comparative studies (e.g., H-2 in mice) supply useful background data. With the Ninth Workshop we have the additional asset of pedigree data which permits the accurate scoring of haplotypes and the testing of selection components.

Three separate approaches have been taken in the analysis of the population data from the Ninth Workshop: the level of homozygosity at each locus, an overall population measure of two-locus disequilibrium, and haplotype pattern analysis, which evaluates disequilibrium patterns to determine which haplotypes have been subject to selection.

In 1973, Ewens [1] determined the expected distribution of alleles in a population subject only to the effects of mutation rate and population size. More recently, Watterson [2] determined that this distribution is well characterized by the total homozygosity at a locus, measured by F, which is the sum of the squared allele frequencies. This assumes Hardy-Weinberg proportions of genotypes.

Figure 1 shows the homozygosity of the Caucasian population data for each of the HLA loci. The lines of neutrality expectation from Ewen's theory and the theoretical minimum (which occurs when all of the alleles at a locus are present in equal frequency) forms a basis for evaluating the observed values. All observed points differ from the neutrality expectation. The Histocompatibility loci A, B, C, and DR have allelic distributions more even than neutrality, while the three complement loci each demonstrate the dominance of a single allele even greater than that found under neutrality.

The three classes of HLA loci roughly comprise three discrete sets in terms of homozygosity. The class II locus, DR, departs furthest from neutrality expectation, and approaches the theoretical minimum for a locus with 11 alleles, suggesting the possible influence of strong stabilizing selection. The three class I loci are also far below the neutrality expectation. Similar results for the A, B, C, and DR loci hold for the Japanese sample (insufficient data was available for the class III loci). The class III or complement loci BF, C4A, and C4B show a striking departure in the other direction. Each of these loci is dominated by a single common allele. Directional selection is a possible explanation, but not really feasible, as we are looking at just one slice of time here and should not expect to observe the moment that allelic variation is disappearing. This leaves us with the possibility that allelic variation among these loci has not been completely defined. It is useful to emphasize that this evaluation of the HLA loci is made strictly on a population genetics basis, and is quite independent of any knowledge of the physiological function or history of definition of the various loci.

The linkage disequilibrium patterns observed among haplotypes of the tightly linked HLA loci can indicate the nature of evolutionary events, particularly selection events, since linkage disequilibria are retained and decay in time only as a function of recombination between loci. Tightly linked, highly polymorphic loci such as HLA retain evidence of distorted haplotype ratios for many generations.

A standard measure of disequilibrium is $D = x_{ij} - p_i q_j$, where x_{ij} is the observed frequency of a haplotype and $p_i q_j$ is the expected frequency based on the frequencies of the constituent alleles when there is no linkage equilibrium. If we square the observed number of haplotypes deviating from the expected value and divide by the expected value, we get the chi square distributed statistic Q, which is useful for testing whether the total disequilibrium of a population differs from zero (defined in Hedrick [3]). All the pairwise combinations among the loci A, B, C, and DR are highly significant, while none of the Q values of these loci in combination with the GLO locus, which is separated from the others by four or five map units, is significant. When adjusted for differing allele numbers and sample size, the total population

* This work was supported by the DFG Ba 660/5-1, and Al 92/13-2, West Germany; and by NIH Grant HD 12731 to G.T.

Histocompatibility Testing 1984
Edited by E. D. Albert et al.

disequilibria from the six pairs of HLA loci form a significant linear regression with map distance.

We have developed a method, haplotype pattern analysis, for examining the disequilibrium distribution of an entire population of two locus haplotypes. It is possible to plot all the haplotypes in the disequilibrium space, which is defined by D, the disequilibrium parameter, and $p_i q_j$, the haplotype frequency expected in the absence of linkage disequilibrium. Each point on such a graph then represents the position of a single haplotype in the population. There are from one hundred to several hundred such two-locus haplotypes among the major HLA loci. The points on such a graph form no particular pattern, limited only by the maximum D values, and showing an excess of negative over positive haplotypes.

If we look at only a single column or row of disequilibrium values in the ordered matrix of all possible haplotypes, i.e., those formed from combi-

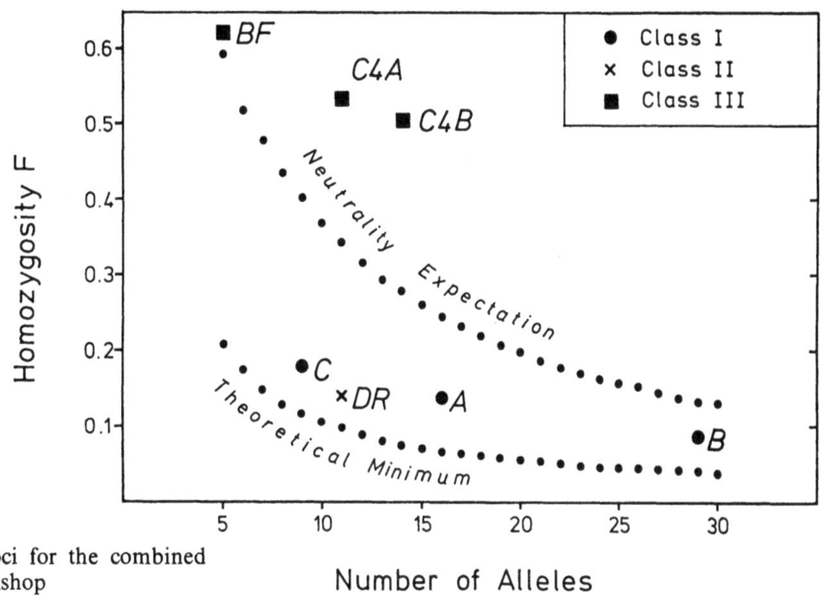

Fig. 1. Homozygosity among HLA loci for the combined Caucasian sample from the Ninth Workshop

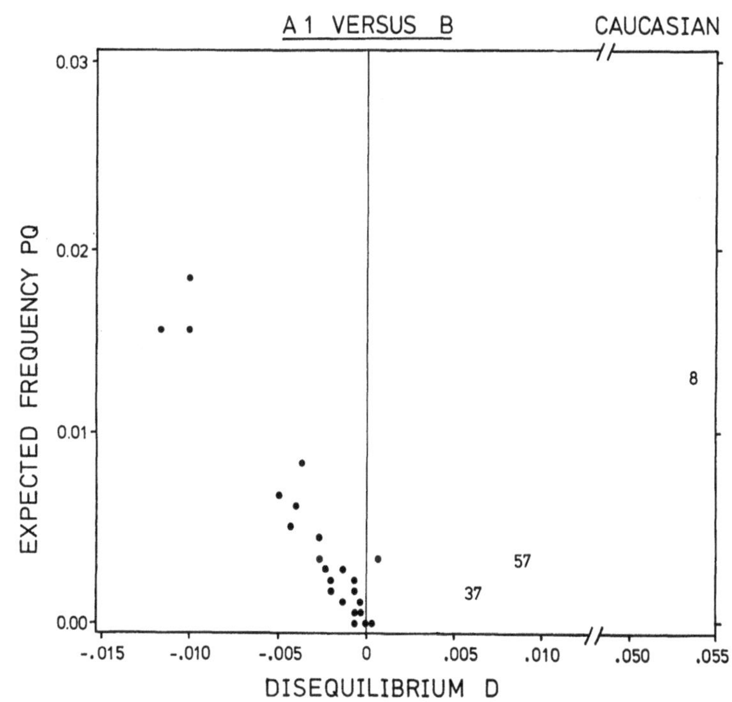

Fig. 2. The distribution of all HLA-B locus haplotypes formed from combination with the allele HLA-A1 based on the Ninth Workshop Caucasian population sample. The position of each haplotype is indicated by a dot, or, for the three haplotypes with strong positive disequilibria, by the B allele designation

nation with a single allele. For example A1 with all B locus alleles, we notice the algebraic constraint that the sum of these values must be zero. By subdividing and then plotting the disequilibrium values of the haplotypes in this way, we note that a few alleles form patterned arrangements of haplotypes, consisting of one haplotype with strongly positive disequilibrium and the remaining haplotypes all arrayed in a linear sequence in the negative D space. The disequilibria of the negative haplotypes, which share an allele with the favored haplotype, are proportional to the allele frequency of the unshared allele. All haplotypes in a population are assignable to one of three classes, depending on their relationship to the few favored haplotypes: favored haplotypes with high positive D values; those haplotypes related to the favored haplotypes by sharing one of their alleles (and which have negative D values); and those haplotypes which share neither allele with the favored haplotype and have low positive values. This scheme has been confirmed by deterministic models and by computer iterations of simple multiallelic systems.

Ramifications of this approach include a prediction of the minimum number of selection events in a population based on the ratio of the number of positive to negative haplotypes, the estimation of the order of appearance of the two alleles comprising a favored haplotype (based on a combination of their relative frequencies and the strength of the patterning observed in the disequilibrium space), possible prediction of splits, and finally association of diseases with the identified favored haplotypes.

The principles of haplotype pattern analysis are well demonstrated in the Ninth Workshop data. Figure 2 shows the plot of A1 versus all haplotypes formed with alleles of the B locus for the total Caucasian population sample. The haplotype A1, B8, having a disequilibrium value of 0.053 and normalized value of 0.65, is nearly alone in the positive space, sharing it with A1, B57 and A1, B37, which also have significant positive disequilibrium values. All of the other A1-associated B haplotypes are found in a linear array in the negative space. The plot of B8 with all A alleles is even more striking, as there are no other haplotypes in the positive space. Only a minority of single-allele haplotype plots show patterning.

The presence or absence of patterning is not a function of high or low allele frequencies of the constituent alleles. The two secondary positive haplotypes found in Fig. 2 can be explained as possibly having existed in the population before the appearance of A1, B8. This is supported by the fact that the allele frequency of B8 is lower than that of A1. Patterning is not restricted to A-B locus haplotypes, nor to only the Caucasian population sample.

Figure 2 can also be used to show the results of allelic splits. At the 1980 Workshop, B17 was divided into B57 and B58. The A1, B17 haplotype had a lower D value and higher expected value than shown for A1, B57 in Fig. 2. After the split, A1, B58 moved into alignment in the negative space and the A1, B57 haplotype had a higher D value than the old A1, B17.

The observation of disequilibrium patterns consistent with selective events bodes well for further dissection of the evolutionary forces acting in the HLA region.

References

1. Ewens WJ (1973) The sampling theory of selectively neutral alleles. Theor Popul Biol 3:87–112
2. Watterson GA (1973) The homozygosity test of neutrality. Genetics 88:405–417
3. Hedrick PW, Jain S, Holdren L (1978) Multilocus systems in evolution. Evol Biol 11:101–182

Population Analysis on the Basis of Deduced Haplotypes from Random Families *

M.P. Baur[1], M. Neugebauer[1], H. Deppe[1], M. Sigmund[2], T. Luton[1], W.R. Mayr[3], and E.D. Albert[4]

1 Biometrical Department, Diabetes Research Institute, Auf'm Hennekamp 65, 4000 Düsseldorf 1, Federal Republic of Germany
2 Institute for Medical Statistics, University of Bonn, 5300 Bonn, Federal Republic of Germany
3 Institut für Blutgruppenserologie der Universität Wien, 1090 Wien, Austria
4 Laboratory for Immunogenetics, University of Munich, 8000 München 2, Federal Republic of Germany

This report presents the results of the population analysis on the basis of the Masterfile [1] of the Ninth International Histocompatibility Workshop. The analysis was done for all the specificities – as newly defined by the WHO nomenclature committee [2] – of the loci HLA-A, B, C, DP, DQ, DR, D, as well as the complement loci C2, C4A, C4B, and Bf and the GLO polymorphism.

For reference purposes, Table 1 lists the gene frequency estimates for all loci within the ethnic (geographic) subgroups as defined by the ethnic code on card 1 columns 46–47. Due to the extremely small sample sizes for most of the groups (samples with less than 30 haplotypes were not included in Table 1), all other analyses were performed for the three major ethnic groups of Caucasians (CAU), Orientals (ORI), and Negroes (NEG) as defined on card 1 of the workshop coding sheet [1].

Besides the ethnic group code, the definition of the three samples was based on the family selection status (random healthy, not selected for specific antigen, no disease family). Whereas for C2, C4A, C4B, Bf, and GLO laboratory assignments were used, antigen assignments for HLA-A, B, C, DR, DQ were the results of the cell typing program [3] on the basis of the submitted serological reactions. In this way, all officially accepted specificities (new antigens, new splits) could be included. Furthermore, the data were based on an identical set of typing reagents and all antigen assignments were made according to the same algorithmic procedure, thus avoiding subjective bias. Assignments for HLA-D and HLA-DP were provided by the chairmen of the respective cellular technique working groups. The high quality of the data was guaranteed by the proven segregation of specificities due to the available family information. The basis for all parameter estimates were the deduced multilocus haplotypes (result of the family analysis package, FAP [4]) of unrelated individuals – individuals with parental codes "NPR" on card 1 – from families as described above.

As a consequence of this sample definition, which guaranteed the best quality of data attainable through confirmation of typing by segregation, the gain in sample size is rather small from families with a large number of offspring and few unrelated family members. Since for population NEG only about 100 deduced haplotypes were available from families as described above, we decided to include also healthy family members of disease families, being well aware of the possible bias thus introduced for this group (see justification in [5]).

Estimation Procedure

When dealing with a problem of several linked highly polymorphic loci – as in the MHC – the gametic distributions given by the frequencies of combinations of allelic expressions on each of the considered loci (frequencies of haplotypes) are generally described by a model including the gene frequencies for each locus and the association parameters between alleles of different loci in the same gamete. This association parameter, termed linkage disequilibrium or gametic association, was introduced for the two-locus problem by Jennings [6] and Robbins [7] as early as 1917 and extended to the three-locus problem by Greiringer [8]. A decomposition for the general n-locus case was given by Bennett [9] in 1954. Procedures to estimate the frequency of a specific haplotype or, as equivalent, its involved gene frequencies and linkage disequilibrium (delta) and their application to the HLA system were given for the two-locus problem by Mattiuz et al. [10] and for the three-locus problem by Piazza [11].

These procedures were extensions of the well-known "square root formula" and are useful as "point estimates" for specific haplotypes, but are of limited use when estimating a total frequency table. The optimal solution for an estimation problem including a large number of parameters is for all levels (gene frequencies, two-locus haplotype frequencies, ..., n-locus haplotype frequencies) the simultaneous maximum likelihood estimation of all parameters in the model. This can be done using the general expectation maximization (EM) procedure (iterative haplotype counting) of Smith [12] and Ceppellini et al. [13], which can be easily extended to the n-locus haplotype problem, as has

* Supported by Deutsche Forschungsgemeinschaft Ba 660/5-1, Al 92/13-2

Table 1. Gene frequencies for HLA, A, B, C, DR, DQ, Bf, GLO, C2, C4A, C4B by ethnic group code (see page 38; card 01)

Ethnic code:	2	11	12	13	21	31	33	34	36	39	40	41	42	44	48	54
A1	8.3	2.3	0.2	4.4	0.8	17.4	17.6	8.7	10.4	19.0	12.5	11.5	16.4	10.7	17.0	17.3
A2	17.4	34.8	26.2	36.9	25.6	27.1	9.5	29.4	32.8	31.9	24.2	29.2	28.4	29.3	36.6	23.1
A3	13.6	4.1	0.4	0	2.5	15.5	10.8	13.0	20.7	18.7	17.2	14.2	11.0	10.4	11.6	1.9
A11	4.6	19.8	10.3	0	5.0	3.9	17.0	9.8	10.4	4.8	6.3	6.9	4.1	4.9	4.9	15.4
A23	9.1	0	0	0	0	4.1	0	0	0	1.1	0.8	2.3	1.4	2.0	1.3	1.9
A24	4.6	11.1	36.1	33.5	46.9	10.5	12.2	9.8	6.9	3.2	11.7	9.2	11.6	14.2	10.3	9.6
A25	0	0	0	0	0	2.2	0	5.4	3.5	3.7	3.1	3.5	1.4	2.0	0.9	0
A26	4.6	3.5	10.4	4.4	1.7	2.8	2.7	2.2	3.5	3.2	3.9	3.8	5.5	2.0	1.8	7.7
A28	4.6	4.1	0.2	8.7	4.2	5.5	10.8	5.4	5.2	2.1	3.9	3.8	2.1	3.5	7.6	5.8
A29	2.3	0.6	0	2.2	0.8	2.8	0	7.6	1.7	1.6	2.3	3.1	3.4	3.2	2.2	0
A30	6.8	8.0	0.2	0	2.5	3.0	0	4.4	1.7	2.7	3.1	2.3	4.8	7.8	1.3	5.8
A31	0	2.3	6.2	8.7	4.2	3.9	5.4	2.2	1.7	2.1	5.5	3.1	2.7	1.5	1.8	9.6
A32	4.6	1.7	0	0	0	2.8	1.4	1.1	1.7	5.9	3.1	5.0	4.1	6.1	2.2	0
Aw33	0	6.4	7.1	0	1.7	1.1	6.8	0	0	0	2.3	1.2	2.7	2.3	0	0
Aw34	4.6	0	0	0	1.7	0	1.4	1.1	0	0	0	0	0	0	0	0
Aw36	10.5	0	0	0	0	0	0	0	0	0	0	0.4	0	0	0	0
Aw43	0	0	0	0	0	0	0	0	0	0	0	0	0	0	0	0
Aw66	0	0	0.9	0	0	0	0	0	0	0	0	0.4	0	0	0	0
A X	4.9	1.4	1.9	1.3	2.6	0.3	4.7	0	0	0	0	0.1	0.4	0	0.4	1.9
Sample size[a]	44	172	562	46	120	362	74	92	58	188	128	260	146	345	224	52
B7	18.4	2.9	5.9	0	4.3	12.2	5.6	12.0	15.5	14.4	13.3	14.3	11.2	6.6	15.3	4.2
B8	0	0.6	0	2.1	0	11.9	2.8	8.7	3.5	13.7	7.8	8.4	11.2	3.9	15.3	10.4
B13	2.6	11.6	0.9	0	3.5	2.2	1.4	1.1	3.5	1.1	2.3	3.4	3.7	4.2	2.7	0
B18	2.6	0	0	2.1	0.9	6.1	2.8	7.6	6.9	4.3	4.7	5.1	3.0	9.9	1.4	6.3
B27	2.6	2.3	0.2	6.3	5.2	2.8	1.4	1.1	6.9	6.0	1.6	2.9	1.5	0.3	8.1	8.3
B35	10.5	6.3	10.6	28.8	10.4	8.0	13.9	8.7	12.1	9.6	10.9	10.5	11.9	14.0	8.1	10.4
B37	0	2.9	0.2	0	0	1.1	7.0	0	1.7	0.5	2.3	2.9	2.2	1.2	1.8	0
B38	0	1.7	0.6	0	0	3.3	1.4	2.2	0	0.5	1.6	3.8	3.0	1.8	1.8	8.3
B39	0	4.1	4.2	8.3	0.9	2.8	0	2.2	0	2.1	0.8	1.3	3.0	2.4	1.4	0
Bw41	0	0.6	0	0	0	0.8	0	0	5.2	0.5	0.8	0.8	1.5	0.6	0.5	6.3
Bw42	2.6	1.2	0.6	0	0	0.8	0	0	0	0	0	0	0.8	0	0.5	0
B44	2.6	3.5	7.9	2.1	1.7	13.3	4.2	21.7	12.1	16.5	10.2	14.3	10.4	8.1	11.3	8.3
B45	5.3	0	0	0	0.9	0.3	0	1.1	0	0.5	0	0.8	1.5	0.3	0.5	0
Bw46	0	0.7	0.3	0	2.6	0	0	0	0	0	0	0.4	0	0	0	0
Bw47	0	0.6	0.2	2.1	0	0	1.4	0	0	0.5	0.8	0	0	0.6	0	0
Bw48	0	0.6	1.8	0	3.5	0	0	0	0	0	0	0	0	0	0	0
B49	2.6	0	0	0	1.7	0.8	0	0	0	2.1	3.1	1.7	3.0	3.6	1.8	0
Bw50	0	0	0	6.3	0	0.6	1.4	0	1.7	1.6	1.6	1.3	0	2.7	0.5	0
B51	2.6	3.5	9.0	16.7	7.8	4.2	7.0	5.4	8.6	3.2	7.0	5.5	7.5	12.2	3.2	2.1
Bw52	0	6.4	10.3	2.1	1.7	1.4	11.1	1.1	1.7	0	1.6	3.4	3.7	1.2	0.9	2.1
Bw53	10.3	0	0	2.1	0.9	0.3	1.4	1.1	0	0	0.8	0	1.5	0.9	0	0
Bw54	0	2.9	9.4	0	5.2	0.3	0	0	0	0	0	0	0	0	0	0
Bw55	0	1.7	2.2	0	4.3	0.6	1.4	0	5.2	1.1	3.1	1.3	1.5	2.4	0.5	2.1
Bw56	0	0	1.3	0	5.2	0	0	3.3	0	0.5	1.6	2.5	0.8	0.6	1.8	0
Bw57	5.3	1.2	0	2.1	0.9	3.3	7.0	5.4	3.5	2.7	1.6	1.7	1.5	4.5	2.3	4.2
Bw58	13.2	5.8	0.6	2.1	2.6	1.4	5.6	0	0	1.1	0.8	1.3	0	4.9	0	6.3
Bw59	0	0	1.8	0	0.9	0	0	0	0	0	0	0	0	0	0	0
Bw60	2.6	10.5	4.4	2.1	7.8	5.5	1.4	5.4	5.2	3.7	2.3	1.3	3.0	1.2	9.0	2.1
Bw61	2.6	7.6	13.9	12.5	12.9	1.1	11.1	1.1	0	1.6	3.1	1.7	3.7	1.8	9.0	6.3
Bw62	0	13.6	8.0	0	12.1	7.8	5.6	2.2	5.2	9.0	9.4	5.5	3.7	4.8	8.1	4.2
Bw63	0	0	0	0	0	1.1	2.8	0	1.7	0	0	0.4	0	1.5	0	0
Bw64	0	0	0	0	0	1.4	0	3.3	0	0.5	0	1.7	3.0	0.6	0.5	2.1
Bw65	0	0	0.2	0	0	4.2	0	4.4	0	2.7	6.3	0.4	1.5	2.1	1.8	6.3
Bw67	0	0	0.2	0	0	0	0	0	0	0	0	0	0	0	0	0
Bw71	2.6	0	0.6	0	0	0	1.4	0	0	0	0	0	0	0	0	0
Bw72	7.9	0.6	0.4	2.1	0	0	1.4	0	0	0	0	0.4	0.8	0.6	0.5	0
Bw73	0	0	0	0	1.7	0	0	0	0	0	0	0.8	0	0.3	0	0
B X	2.7	0.5	1.9	0.4	0.9	0.6	0	1.1	0	0	0.8	0.4	0.1	0.5	0	0
Sample size[a]	38	172	544	48	116	361	72	92	58	188	128	238	134	335	222	48
Cw1	2.4	12.8	19.8	0	14.5	2.2	5.7	2.2	1.7	1.1	2.4	5.1	5.1	1.8	5.4	5.6
Cw2	15.8	1.2	0.2	8.3	1.7	2.2	2.8	3.3	5.2	5.5	3.2	2.8	5.4	3.2	7.6	7.4
Cw3	4.7	28.3	26.4	26.5	34.0	15.1	5.6	10.0	15.5	16.0	12.7	11.4	8.0	9.5	18.2	13.0
Cw4	25.7	4.7	3.4	27.0	6.1	7.5	11.3	11.1	17.7	10.6	11.1	11.1	16.7	14.4	9.7	9.2

Table 1 (continued)

Ethnic code:	2	11	12	13	21	31	33	34	36	39	40	41	42	44	48	54
Cw5	0	0.6	0.2	2.1	0.9	7.3	0	13.3	8.6	10.4	4.0	6.3	5.8	5.9	7.3	0
Cw6	9.5	12.7	0	2.1	2.6	7.9	15.3	6.7	10.4	5.8	8.7	10.8	8.0	11.7	7.1	3.7
Cw7	14.2	18.2	11.1	6.6	8.6	30.4	13.1	18.9	20.6	30.1	20.8	25.6	26.8	18.6	28.2	16.7
Cw8	2.4	0	0.4	0	0	5.5	0	7.8	0	3.2	6.4	2.0	3.6	2.7	2.2	7.4
C X	25.4	21.6	38.5	27.5	31.6	21.8	46.4	26.7	20.3	17.3	30.8	24.9	20.7	32.3	14.2	37.1
Sample size[a]	42	172	556	48	116	358	72	90	58	189	126	254	138	340	224	54
DR1	8.6	1.1	6.2	2.4	2.5	10.6	1.5	2.3	12.0	14.5	8.9	9.7	9.9	7.0	11.1	13.1
DR2	19.6	15.8	15.5	2.4	21.8	12.0	20.2	10.5	24.0	17.3	16.6	18.9	12.6	16.4	17.8	10.9
DR3	12.8	4.6	0.6	7.5	0	10.8	14.2	13.6	3.7	13.3	6.5	8.0	17.4	11.4	16.3	15.2
DR4	5.7	8.7	24.3	47.0	17.5	15.8	2.2	21.7	7.4	19.9	11.3	15.7	10.4	8.2	13.5	17.4
DR7	11.5	13.3	0	2.4	0	11.9	16.5	17.4	14.8	13.3	9.7	11.8	11.9	12.2	7.5	10.9
DRw8	0	3.2	9.1	4.8	0	1.6	3.0	4.7	0	3.6	4.0	2.2	2.6	3.4	2.6	2.2
DRw9	1.1	16.1	12.7	0	7.5	1.2	0	1.2	0	0.6	0.8	2.2	0.9	0	1.1	0
DRw10	0	1.1	0.2	2.4	0	0.3	6.0	1.2	1.9	0	0	0.9	1.7	0.6	1.6	0
DRw11	12.8	6.3	2.3	4.8	17.5	10.3	4.5	10.4	14.5	4.8	11.5	11.6	15.5	21.2	9.5	17.4
DRw12	0	5.3	6.1	23.5	5.0	3.7	3.1	3.5	1.9	0.6	0	1.8	1.7	2.1	2.1	0
DRw13	5.7	0	3.9	0	2.5	4.5	3.0	2.5	1.9	4.8	11.3	5.3	4.4	5.5	7.4	4.4
DRw14	17.2	3.2	7.9	0	12.5	7.2	9.0	8.1	9.3	3.0	4.0	6.2	6.1	5.5	1.6	6.5
DR X	4.9	21.4	11.3	2.9	13.2	10.1	16.8	2.9	8.7	4.3	15.0	5.7	5.0	6.6	8.1	2.2
Sample size[a]	35	95	514	42	40	332	66	86	54	166	124	225	115	328	190	46
DQw1	48.4	20.3	33.2	6.6	41.2	32.5	30.8	24.9	43.7	34.0	29.7	35.7	26.6	33.1	28.4	33.7
DQw2	24.2	16.8	1.3	8.8	2.5	16.8	17.7	31.8	19.0	23.2	10.2	17.5	14.9	19.4	12.6	23.2
DQw3	15.6	16.4	34.4	59.9	31.5	29.5	13.5	31.6	20.2	24.6	13.3	24.0	22.8	24.6	18.9	34.7
DQ X	11.8	46.6	31.2	24.7	24.8	21.2	38.1	11.8	17.1	18.2	46.9	22.8	35.7	23.0	40.1	8.4
Sample size[a]	35	98	535	45	40	316	68	87	58	174	128	250	125	314	204	54

Table 1 (continued)

	11	34	39	40	41	44	48
Bf S	87.4	78.4	76.8	75.0	85.5	77.3	82.2
Bf F	12.6	18.2	21.2	23.8	10.7	18.2	16.4
BfS0.7	0	0	1.0	1.2	2.6	2.3	0
Bf F1	0	3.4	1.0	0	1.3	2.3	0.8
Bf V	0	0	0	0	0	0	0
Sample size[a]	87	88	99	84	77	44	128
GLO 1	24.0	45.5	50.5	47.6	45.2	46.8	47.7
GLO 2	76.0	54.5	49.5	52.4	50.7	53.2	52.3
GLO V	0	0	0	0	4.1	0	0
Sample size[a]	96	88	46	84	98	32	172

Table 1 (continued)

	34	39	41
C2 1	96.6	94.2	84.3
C2 2	2.3	5.8	15.7
C2 3	0	0	0
C2 V	1.1	0	0
Sample size[a]	88	52	38

Table 1 (continued)

	11	34	39	40	41	48
C4 A1	0	0	1.4	0	0	0
C4 A12	3.6	0	0	0	0	0
C4 A13	0	0	0	0	2.9	1.2
C4 A2	2.4	7.0	1.4	7.1	5.9	3.6
C4 A3	80.5	68.8	55.4	82.7	72.1	76.3
C4 A4	6.0	4.7	9.5	4.8	2.9	6.0
C4 A51	0	0	0	0	0	1.2
C4 A6	0	5.8	4.1	0	5.9	2.4
C4 AQO	7.5	13.7	28.4	5.4	10.3	9.5
Sample size[a]	83	86	74	84	68	84
C4 B1	59.0	73.6	71.0	74.4	68.0	64.5
C4 B11	0	0	0	0	0	1.2
C4 B12	1.2	0	0	0	0	0
C4 B2	22.6	9.3	10.6	7.1	10.2	10.1
C4 B3	1.2	0	1.3	1.2	13.1	6.0
C4 B4	0	0	0	1.2	0	1.2
C4 B5	0	1.2	0	1.2	0	0
C4 B51	0	0	0	0	0	1.2
C4 B6	0	0	0	1.2	0	0
C4 B7	0	0	0	0	0	0
C4 BQO	16.0	15.9	17.1	13.7	8.7	15.9
Sample size[a]	84	83	76	84	69	84

[a] Number of haplotypes counted

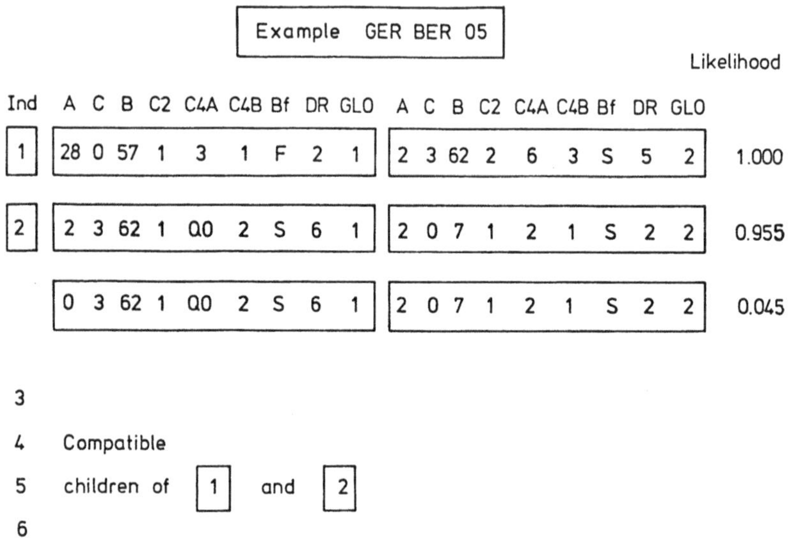

Fig. 1. Haplotypes and their relative likelihoods from FAP as basis of frequency estimates

been done by Baur and Danilovs [14] for three-locus HLA frequencies from the phenotypes of unrelated individuals.

Given the family material at hand from the Ninth Workshop even more information was available from the deduced haplotypes as a result of FAP [4]. Figure 1 shows as an example the deduced parental haplotypes of family GER BER 05. In this example both haplotypes of individual 1 are unique and can be directly counted in gene frequency estimates for all nine loci listed up to theoretically the nine-locus haplotype frequency estimate. Since both haplotypes of individual 2 are unique except for the HLA-A locus, they are counted for all estimation problems excluding the A locus. In case of an inclusion of the A locus, the first haplotype, carrying A2 with relative likelihood .955 and carrying AX with relative likelihood .045, is "counted" with the weight of this likelihood (expectation). Since these likelihoods are a function of the haplotype frequencies used for their calculation, this step has to be repeated (iterated), using for each cycle the estimates of the previous cycle and stopping the iteration after the change in frequencies has fallen below an arbitrarily set limit. Simple as it seems, this procedure needs a large computational effort and much computer time for each cycle (haplotyping of families, relative likelihood calculation for each haplotype explanation on the basis of given parameters, haplotype "counting" from these relative likelihoods, estimation of frequencies, linkage disequilibria, relative linkage disequilibria and chi-squares, improvement of the parameter set for the next cycle). Fortunately, though, it takes only a few cycles to convergence, due to the fact that most haplotypes are unique and their count is not influenced by the likelihood argument.

Results

Tables 2–13 present the gene frequency estimates for the three ethnic groups on the basis of the Workshop Masterfile [1] and the analysis as described above.

HLA-A, B, C

Generally there is good agreement to previously published frequency estimates [14, 15], especially for the well-defined specificities (Tables 2–4). The

Table 2. Gene frequencies for HLA-A

HLA-	Caucasians	Orientals	Negroids
A1	14.2	1.0	8.1
A2	28.9	28.1	17.5
A3	13.2	1.5	6.7
A11	6.3	11.7	1.9
A23	1.4	0.1	8.0
A24	10.3	31.4	4.8
A25	2.4	0	0
A26	3.2	7.2	4.5
A28	4.7	2.1	9.9
A29	2.9	0.4	4.9
A30	3.5	2.3	11.0
A31	2.9	5.2	1.6
A32	3.9	0.4	2.3
Aw33	1.4	6.0	3.9
Aw34	0.1	0.3	5.1
Aw36	0.1	0.1	3.2
Aw43	0	0	1.3
Aw66	0.2	0.5	0.3
A X	0.4	1.7	5.0
Sample size[a]	2163	976	311

[a] Number of haplotypes counted

Table 3. Gene frequencies for HLA-B

HLA-	Caucasians	Orientals	Negroids
B7	11.5	4.7	12.1
B8	9.6	0.2	5.5
B13	2.9	3.8	1.6
B18	5.5	0.3	4.2
B27	3.4	1.6	1.9
B35	10.5	10.2	7.1
B37	1.6	0.6	1.3
B38	2.5	0.7	1.6
B39	2.0	0.4	0
Bw41	0.9	0.1	2.3
Bw42	0.2	0.5	5.8
B44	12.3	6.0	7.7
B45	0.4	0.1	2.3
Bw46	0.1	3.6	0
Bw47	0.2	0.4	0
Bw48	0	1.6	0
B49	1.8	0.3	2.3
Bw50	1.1	0.3	0.6
B51	6.2	7.8	1.9
Bw52	2.0	7.3	0.6
Bw53	0.5	0.3	6.7
Bw54	0.1	6.7	0
Bw55	1.6	2.1	0
Bw56	1.1	1.5	0.3
Bw57	2.9	0.7	2.9
Bw58	0	1.2	0
Bw60	3.8	6.5	2.3
Bw61	2.1	11.7	1.5
Bw62	6.1	9.6	2.6
Bw63	0.7	0	1.9
Bw64	1.1	0	1.3
Bw65	2.6	0.2	1.6
Bw67	0	0.1	0
Bw71	0.1	0.4	0.8
Bw72	0.3	0.5	7.1
Bw73	0.1	0.2	0
B X	0.4	1.6	1.3
Sample size[a]	2132	968	311

[a] Number of haplotypes counted

following points are of special interest though:

1. The frequencies of AX and BX have dropped to about 1% in all populations (except for AX in NEG) as a result of the family information showing only in very rare cases the segregation of an AX or BX. Consequently there is little "room" left for the detection of the new specificities on these two loci unless they are rare variants.
2. The frequencies of CX were reduced to 24.9% (CAU), 33,3% (ORI), and 21.3% (NEG), not by definition of new C alleles but by improvement of the definition of Cw7, of which the frequencies increased – 24.3% (CAU), 12.1% (ORI), 24.1% (Neg) – by the same amount as the corresponding CX frequency decreased.
3. The new (provisional) specifities Aw66, Bw67, Bw71, Bw72, Bw73 have frequencies of less than 1%, except for Bw72, which in NEG has a frequency of 7.1%.
4. The splits Bw64, Bw65 of the broad specificity B14 have frequencies of 1.1%–2.6% in CAU, are almost equally frequent in NEG (1.3%–1.6%), and practically absent in ORI.

HLA-DR

For the DR locus, too, a notable decrease of the DRX frequency can be observed in all three populations which is compensated by an increase of the frequencies of all other specificities, especially those of DRw13, DRw14 – new splits of DRw6 (Table 5). These frequency changes are most likely caused by improved recognition of DRw6 and its splits and by better B lymphocyte typing.

Table 4. Gene frequencies for HLA-C

HLA-	Caucasians	Orientals	Negroids
Cw1	3.3	16.3	1.0
Cw2	4.1	1.0	11.9
Cw3	12.6	27.3	8.3
Cw4	11.6	5.3	14.0
Cw5	6.9	0.6	3.0
Cw6	8.6	3.8	12.9
Cw7	24.3	12.1	24.1
Cw8	3.7	0.3	3.5
C X	24.9	33.3	21.3
Sample size[a]	2106	968	316

[a] Number of haplotypes counted

Table 5. Gene frequencies for HLA-DR

HLA-	Caucasians	Orientals	Negroids
DR1	9.5	5.0	5.1
DR2	15.8	15.1	15.1
DR3	12.0	1.8	14.9
DR4	12.7	21.8	7.6
DR7	12.0	2.9	13.2
DRw8	3.0	7.3	0.8
DRw9	0.8	11.5	1.5
DRw10	0.8	0.5	2.3
DRw11	12.3	4.0	16.5
DRw12	2.0	7.2	3.4
DRw13	5.4	2.9	3.8
DRw14	5.8	6.8	10.7
DR X	7.9	13.2	5.3
Sample size[a]	1926	752	263

[a] Number of haplotypes counted

The newly defined splits DRw11, DRw12 of the broad specificity DR5, and DRw13, DRw14, of DRw6, have frequencies as follows:

	CAU	ORI	NEG
DRw11	12.3	4.0	16.5
DRw12	2.0	7.2	3.4
DRw13	5.4	2.9	3.8
DRw14	5.8	6.8	10.7

HLA-DQ

Frequencies of the newly recognized locus DQ are given in Table 6 for the three major ethnic groups. Comparison to previously published frequencies is not possible because results from a comparable sample are not available. The low frequency of DQw2 in ORI corresponds to the frequencies of DR3 and DR7 in Orientals.

HLA-DP and HLA-D

Gene frequency estimates for the DP and D polymorphisms were attempted only in population CAU due to the small sample sizes available. The typing results were provided by the chairmen of these cellular technique studies, entered into the family data, and thus confirmed by segregation (Tables 7, 8).

Table 6. Gene frequencies for HLA-DQ

HLA-	Caucasians	Orientals	Negroids
DQw1	32.3	30.2	40.1
DQw2	18.1	5.0	23.1
DQw3	23.3	32.7	24.6
DQ X	26.3	32.1	12.2
Sample size[a]	2016	776	256

[a] Number of haplotypes counted

Table 7. Gene frequencies for HLA-DP

HLA-	Caucasians
DPw1	4.3
DPw2	11.5
DPw3	4.0
DPw4	41.8
DPw5	4.4
DPw6	0
DPX	40.0
Sample size[a]	115

[a] Number of haplotypes counted

Table 8. Gene frequencies for HLA-D

HLA-	Caucasians
Dw1	12.8
Dw2	6.5
Dw3	8.2
Dw4	6.7
Dw5	14.4
Dw8	4.4
Dw9	5.7
Dw10	2.2
Dw11	3.2
Dw12	1.1
Dw13	1.1
Dw14	2.2
Dw15	0
Dw16	0
Dw17	6.6
Dw18	1.3
Dw19	5.3
DX	18.6
Sample size[a]	92

[a] Number of haplotypes counted

Table 9. Gene frequencies for C4A

	Caucasians	Orientals	Negroids
C4 A1	0.3	0	3.7
C4 A12	0	12.2	0
C4 A13	0.5	0	0
C4 A2	6.4	1.9	6.2
C4 A3	70.2	67.0	71.2
C4 A4	6.1	7.7	1.2
C4 A51	0.2	0	4.9
C4 A6	3.8	1.3	1.2
C4 AQO	12.5	9.9	11.6
Sample size[a]	558	156	81

[a] Number of haplotypes counted

Table 10. Gene frequencies for C4B

	Caucasians	Orientals	Negroids
C4 B1	71.4	65.4	68.5
C4 B11	0.2	0	0
C4 B12	0.2	0.7	0
C4 B2	9.1	22.1	8.4
C4 B3	3.2	0.7	3.6
C4 B4	0.7	0	0
C4 B5	0.7	0	0
C4 B51	0.2	0	0
C4 B6	0.4	0	0
C4 B7	0.2	0	0
C4 BQO	13.7	11.2	19.5
Sample size[a]	557	154	83

[a] Number of haplotypes counted

Table 11. Gene frequencies for C2

	Caucasians	Orientals	Negroids
C2 1	94.5	98.8	97.8
C2 2	5.2	1.2	2.2
C2 3	0	0	0
C2 V	0.3	0	0
Sample size[a]	361	86	91

[a] Number of haplotypes counted

Table 12. Gene frequencies for GLO

	Caucasians	Orientals	Negroids
GLO 1	47.6	16.9	26.5
GLO 2	51.8	83.1	73.5
GLO V	0.6	0	0
Sample size[a]	639	166	88

[a] Number of haplotypes counted

Table 13. Gene frequencies for Bf

	Caucasians	Orientals	Negroids
Bf S	77.1	87.3	47.0
Bf F	20.3	12.7	51.0
Bf SO.7	1.2	0	1.0
Bf F1	1.3	0	1.0
Bf V	0.1	0	0
Sample size[a]	691	173	100

[a] Number of haplotypes counted

C4A and C4B

Gene frequencies for the two loci coding for the fourth component of complement (C4) are given in Tables 9, 10. In spite of the problems in typing (difficult recognition, numerous rare variants, occasional reduplication [16]) frequency estimates for these loci, with one common allele each, three low-frequency alleles for C4A and two low-frequency alleles for C4B, and a number of rare variants, are reproducible [17, 18] and seem not to be influenced by the above-mentioned problems. The only completely deviating result is the frequency of C4A12 in ORI, which was most likely caused by a systematic coding error in these regional data. The good quality of the estimates is supported by the result of the Hardy-Weinberg fit for these loci, as given below.

C2, Bf, and GLO (Tables 11–13)

The frequency estimates for C2, Bf, and GLO as given in Tables 11–13 are in good accordance with previously published results.

Hardy-Weinberg Fit (Table 14)

The results of the Hardy-Weinberg test (Table 14) show a generally good fit to the expected distribution for all 12 loci analyzed. This is no surprise as significant deviations in this kind of analysis usually point out problems in the differentiation of certain phenotypes rather than true deviation from the equilibrium state in a population. This had been especially true in the case of previous analyses for HLA loci whenever newly defined specificities

Table 14. Hardy-Weinberg fit for the loci of the MHC

Locus	CAU			ORI			NEG		
	χ^2	df	*P*	χ^2	df	*P*	χ^2	df	*P*
A	107.6	149	≈0.5	64.7	129	≈0.55	108.9	143	≈0.5
B	360.9	571	≈0.5	184.0	543	≈0.7	184.7	385	≈0.5
C	38.4	36	0.36	35.8	32	0.29	24.4	35	0.91
DR	93.5	78	0.11	85.8	77	0.23	55.8	74	0.84
DQ	8.6	6	0.20	9.9	6	0.13	4.3	6	0.64
DP	9.6	15	0.84	–			–		
D	67.8	148	≈0.7	–			–		
Bf	6.5	10	0.77	0.2	1	0.65	6.1	6	0.41
C2	0.6	3	0.90	0.1	1	0.75	0.2	1	0.65
C4A	8.7	28	0.99	47.6	13	0.00001	5.4	19	0.99
C4B	17.2	54	0.99	9.8	10	0.46	4.5	6	0.61
GLO	0.7	1	0.40	0.8	1	0.37	0.5	1	0.48

had been included (see Hardy-Weinberg fit for the HLA-DR locus of the previous Workshop [14]). The good results of this analysis in spite of the inclusion of new complicated polymorphisms like C4; new loci like DP, DQ; and D, and new splits of DR-, B-, and A-locus specificities again shows the high quality of the data through confirmation of typing by segregation in families.

Some special points regarding Table 14 have to be made:

1. The highly significant deviation for the C4A locus in population ORI was caused only by an abnormal distribution of C4A12 homozygous and heterozygous individuals.
   This allele, which is usually very rare in all populations, had been coded as being present homozygously in a large number of individuals. Obviously, a systematic coding error in the regional data must have caused this distortion.
2. The comparatively low *P*-values for DR in CAU and ORI were due solely to distortions of the frequency of DRw11, DRw12 heterozygotes or homozygotes as well as phenotypes involving DRw13, DRw14. Obviously these splits of DR5, DRw6 are still difficult in their serological definition.

Linkage Disequilibrium

It is a well-known fact that strong associations termed linkage disequilibria exist between a multiplicity of the alleles at all loci within the MHC. The definition of this parameter (often called delta), its relative magnitude (relative delta), and its testing by chi-square have been given in numerous publications [e.g., 6–11, 14, 20, 21] and will not be repeated here. It should be again pointed out, though, that whereas two-way associations are straightforward, the definitions of higher order associations as given by Bennett [9] are problematic and not in correspondence to the higher order chi-square statistics [22, 23].

The multiplicity of chromosome 6 loci considered in the analysis has provided a large number of significant two-point associations which may be found in the haplotype reference tables for CAU, ORI, and NEG.

As in previous analyses, it can be noted that there are patterns of linkage disequilibria which are typical for certain populations, such as in the most simple case A1, B8 in Caucasians and A2, Bw46 in Chinese.

For some of the new splits we find characteristic associations involving one but not the other split partner, as is exemplified by the B14 splits [19]: Bw64 is associated with A32 and with DR7, while Bw65 is found predominantly on haplotypes with A28, Aw33, and DR1, as well as with C4A2, B2.

DR-DQ-Relationship

While haplotypes involving loci between which recombinations have been observed (such as HLA-A, B or HLA-B, DR) show a strong variation between populations, it can be observed that the known relationships between DR and DQ alleles are more or less constant (though at different levels of frequency) in the three major race groups, indicating that in evolution the DR-DQ block existed before the separation of these groups.

DP System

The DP alleles did not reveal significant associations with the alleles of the HLA-B, DR, and DQ-loci (sample sizes between 113 and 117). The weak association of DPw1 with A1 and Cw7 may well be due to chance.

The absence of associations between DP and Bf, C2, C4A, C4B, and GLO cannot be taken as strong evidence, due to the very small sample sizes (between 30 and 36).

Thus, these data place the DP locus outside the range of linkage disequilibrium of HLA-DR and DQ.

Relationship Between DR, DQ, and Dw Alleles

Analysis of the haplotype reference tables for DR-Dw and DQ-Dw shows again that with very few exceptions, which could well be technical in nature, the serologically defined specificities 'include' the corresponding Dw specificities. This finding is expected if one accepts that the HTC-defined Dw specificities represent not a single antigen but the haplotypic combination of antigens from two or more loci on chromosome 6. The fact that 'Dw' is for all practical purposes included in 'DR' indicates strongly that DR is one of the loci forming the Dw haplotype. The same must be assumed also for DQ, although the inclusion of Dw in DQ shows a few exceptions which may be due to the serological problems involved in the definition of the DQ-alleles.

Whether the simple formula DR + DQ = Dw, which was put forward during the workshop, is indeed correct will have to be shown by MLC experiments. At present, it is probably safer to change the formula to DR + DQ + X = Dw, where X stands for further splitting products of DR or DQ and/or an additional locus.

GLO System

The alleles of the GLO locus did not show any significant linkage disequilibrium with alleles of other MHC loci in any of the populations tested. Therefore the two-point haplotype frequencies involving GLO were not included in the reference tables. A sufficiently accurate frequency estimate of any two-point haplotype may be obtained by simple multiplication of the gene frequencies of the two alleles involved. For example, the HLA-B8, GLO-2 haplotype frequency in Caucasians is estimated as
$f(\text{GLO-2}) \times f(\text{B8}) = 0.518 \times 0.096 = 0.050$.

As a closing remark, we want to stress the point that the general use of frequencies and associations as given in this report and the reference tables is always problematic with respect to the sample sizes available for a highly polymorphic region like the MHC on the one hand, and the wish for subclassification of samples according to ethnic and/or geographic attributes on the other. Nevertheless, we are confident that the quality of the data which were available for this analysis is the best attainable and that, consequently, the results are reliable.

References

1. Baur MP, Albert ED, Mayr WR (this volume) The central data analysis of the Ninth Workshop
2. Bodmer W, Albert ED, et al (this volume) Nomenclature for factors of the HLA system 1984
3. Deppe H, Albert ED, Baur MP (this volume) Cell typing by computer
4. Neugebauer M, Willems J, Baur MP (this volume) Analysis of multilocus pedigree data by computer
5. Baur MP, Neugebauer M, Albert ED (this volume) Reference tables of two-locus haplotype frequencies for all MHC marker loci
6. Jennings HS (1917) The numerical result of diverse systems of breedings with respect to two pairs of characters. Genetics 2:97
7. Robbins RB (1918) Some applications of mathematics to breeding problems. Genetics 3:375
8. Greiringer H (1944) On the probability theory of linkage in Mendelian heredity. Ann Math Stat 15:25
9. Bennett JH (1954) On the theory of random mating. Ann Eugen 18:311
10. Mattiuz PL, Ihde D, Piazza A, et al (1970) New approaches to the population genetic and segregation analysis of the HLA system. In: Terasaki PI (ed) Histocompatibility testing 1970. Munksgaard, Copenhagen, 193
11. Piazza A (1975) Haplotypes and linkage disequilibrium from the three-locus phenotype. In: Kissmeyer-Nielsen F (ed) Histocompatibility testing 1975. Munksgaard, Copenhagen, 923
12. Smith CAB (1957) Counting methods in genetical statistics. Ann Hum Genet 21:254
13. Ceppellini R, Siniscalco M, Smith CAB (1955) The estimation of gene frequencies in a random mating population. Ann Hum Genet 20:97
14. Baur MP, Danilovs J (1980) Population analysis of HLA-A, B, C, DR and other genetic markers. In: Terasaki PI (ed) Histocompatibility testing 1980. University of California, Los Angeles, 955
15. Baur MP, Danilovs J (1980) Reference tables of two- and three-locus haplotype frequencies for HLA-A, B, C, DR, Bf and GLO. In: Terasaki PI (ed) Histocompatibility testing 1980, University of California, Los Angeles, 994
16. Rittner C, Mauff G (this volume) C4 polymorphism
17. Awdeh ZL, Alper CA (1980) Inherited structural polymorphism of the fourth component of complement. Proc Natl Acad Sci USA 77:3576
18. Bertrams J, Hintzen U, Schlicht V, Schoeps S, Louton TK, Baur MP (1984) Gene and haplotype frequencies of the fourth component of complement (C4) in type 1 diabetics and normal controls. Immunobiology 166:335
19. Mueller-Eckhardt G, Darke C, Fauchet R, Dewar PJ (this volume) HLA-B14: definite splitting into Bw64 (14.1) and Bw65 (14.2)
20. Baur MP, Grangé D (1983) Negative linkage disequilibria. Tissue antigens 21:262
21. Thomson G, Baur MP (1984) Third order linkage disequilibrium. Tissue Antigens (in press)
22. Bartlett MS (1935) Contingency table interactions. JR Statist Soc [Suppl] 2:248
23. Hill WG (1976) Non-random association of neutral genes in finite populations. In: Karlin S, Neno E (eds) Population genetics and ecology. Academic, New York, 339

Ninth International Histocompatibility Workshop Renal Transplant Study*

G. Opelz

Institute of Immunology, University of Heidelberg, Im Neuenheimer Feld 305, 6900 Heidelberg, Federal Republic of Germany

The Ninth International Histocompatibility Workshop Renal Transplant Study commenced in February 1983 with the distribution of Workshop HLA-typing reagents. A special set of reagents, including 113 sera recognizing HLA-A or B specificities and 58 sera recognizing HLA-DR specificities, was provided by the Workshop laboratories for the purpose of typing recipients and donors of kidney transplants. A mechanism of communication, data collection, and computerization was available through the Collaborative Transplant Study, a voluntary multicenter study initiated a year earlier. The centers participating in the Collaborative Transplant Study were invited to use the standard Workshop HLA-typing set for the duration of 1 year. The Workshop study's aim was to determine whether improvements in tissue typing would result in an improved correlation of HLA matching with kidney graft survival.

Reaction scores of typings performed with Workshop reagents were reported to the study center at the University of Heidelberg, West Germany. Information on the patients' background medical condition had to be submitted within 1 month of the transplant operation. Clinical follow-up data were requested at 3 months, 6 months, 9 months, and 12 months. Because of the short clinical follow-up in many patients at the time of this analysis, the results provided here must be considered preliminary.

Actuarial graft survival rates were computed by the method of Kaplan and Meier [1] and statistical significance was estimated be means of either Student's *t*-test or weighted regression analysis [2]. All types of failures were included. Patients who died with a functioning graft were counted as graft failures. An HLA antigen present in the donor and absent in the recipient was considered a mismatch. "Blanks" were not counted. Transplants were included in the analysis only if both donor and recipient had at least one antigen assigned on the HLA locus that was analyzed. If the quality of HLA typing had been rated "poor" for technical reasons by the submitting laboratory, the transplant was excluded.

A total of 2973 transplants that had been typed with Workshop reagents were reported by 160 transplant centers (Table 1). Because second grafts were not analyzed, and because some transplants had not yet been followed for 3 months at the time of analysis, the numbers of transplants contained in Figs. 1–8 are smaller than the total number given in Table 1.

The well-established correlation of graft survival with the number of HLA haplotypes shared between recipient and donor is confirmed by the data shown in Fig. 1. The 6-month survival rate for transplants from HLA-identical sibling donors (both HLA haplotypes shared) was 97% ± 2% (± SE). The corresponding rate for transplants from donors sharing one HLA haplotype with the recipient was 90% ± 2%. Grafts from unrelated cadaver donors had a much lower 6-month survival rate of 73% ± 1%. Nevertheless, this cadaver transplant survival rate is 10% higher than that observed in the 1980 Histocompatibility Workshop study [3].

The number of mismatched antigens on the HLA-A and B loci correlated to some extent with graft survival, although the difference between the survival rates of grafts with zero mismatches and those with four mismatches was a mere 11% at 6 months (79% ± 4% versus 68% ± 3%; $P = 0.04$) (Fig. 2). The correlation did not improve when the analysis was restricted to transplants in which all donors and recipients were Caucasians.

Analysis of the number of mismatches on the HLA-DR locus showed an effect approximately equal to that of HLA-A and B combined. Grafts with no DR mismatch survived at a rate of 78% ± 2% at 6 months, those with one mismatch at a rate of 73% ± 1%, and those with two DR mismatches at 67% ± 3% (P regression < 0.001) (Fig. 3.). This correlation improved when a subset of transplants was analyzed for which the submitting laboratories had indicated that the quality of DR typing was "good." That is, the serological typing reactions in both donor and recipient left no doubt about the DR antigen assignment. Figure 4 shows that in this patient subset, the graft survival curves separate more widely during the initial 3-month period.

* This work was supported in part by grants from the Deutsche Forschungsgemeinschaft and the Deutsche Krebshilfe eV

Histocompatibility Testing 1984
Edited by E. D. Albert et al.

Table 1. Participants in Ninth Histocompatibility Workshop transplant study

Center	No. of grafts	Center	No. of grafts	Center	No. of grafts
Basel	25	Iowa City	45	Paris (6)	33
Belfast	32	Israel Tx (2)	37	Perth	16
Berlin West	40	Japan Tx (13)	57	Phoenix	24
Birmingham, Ala	105	Kaiserslautern	17	Piraeus	9
Boston (9)	108	Kansas City (5)	68	Portland	44
Bristol	28	Leicester	17	Porto Alegre (5)	7
Brussels	36	Leningrad	5	Prague	41
Budapest	4	Leuven	46	Quebec	30
Buenos Aires (5)	22	Lisbon	25	Rennes	13
Cambridge	51	Louisville	14	Rochester, MN	12
Capetown (2)	51	Luebeck	10	Rome	2
Chicago (2)	23	Lyon	64	Rostock	8
Cincinnati (3)	53	Madrid (6)	56	San Antonio	39
Cleveland	34	Manchester	56	San Francisco	38
Cologne	21	Marburg	6	Seattle (4)	75
Dallas (2)	43	Melbourne	17	St. Etienne	24
Dublin	25	Mexico City	1	St. Louis	11
Essen	22	Milan (6)	45	Sydney (8)	68
Frankfurt	29	Minneapolis	38	Szeged	9
Freiburg	31	Montreal	8	Toledo, OH	12
Glasgow	54	Moscow	20	Torino	24
Gothenburg	101	Muenster	19	Toronto (2)	70
Groningen	34	Munich	14	Toulouse	33
Hamburg	34	Nancy	16	Tuebingen	6
Hannover	81	Nantes	59	Ulm	21
Hartford	25	Nashville	2	Uppsala	32
Heidelberg	58	New York (3)	19	Vancouver	14
Helsinki	60	Nijmegen	35	Vilnius	14
Hong Kong	7	Nürnberg	3	Winnipeg	10
Houston	63	Omaha	25	Zagreb	3
Innsbruck	29	Oxford	29	Zürich	29

Total number of transplants: 2973 (Numbers in parentheses denote cities with more than one transplant center)

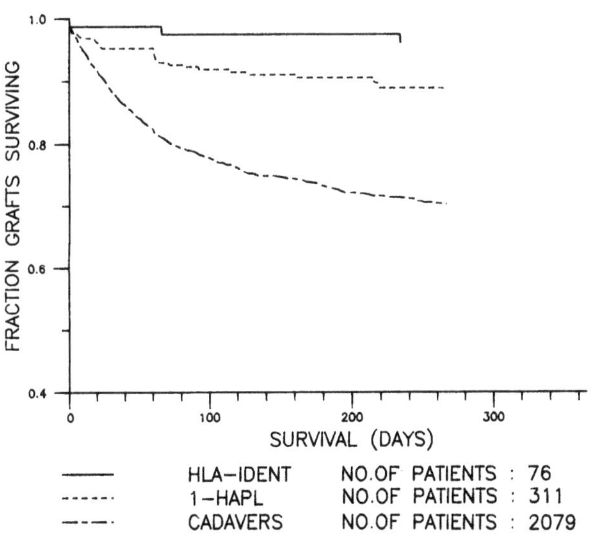

Fig. 1. Actuarial graft survival rates of first kidney transplants shown separately for the number of HLA haplotypes shared between recipient and donor. *HLA-IDENT,* transplants from HLA-identical sibling donors (both HLA haplotypes shared); *1-HAPL,* transplants from related donors who shared one HLA haplotype with the recipients (siblings, parents, or offsprings). *CADAVERS,* transplants from cadaveric donors

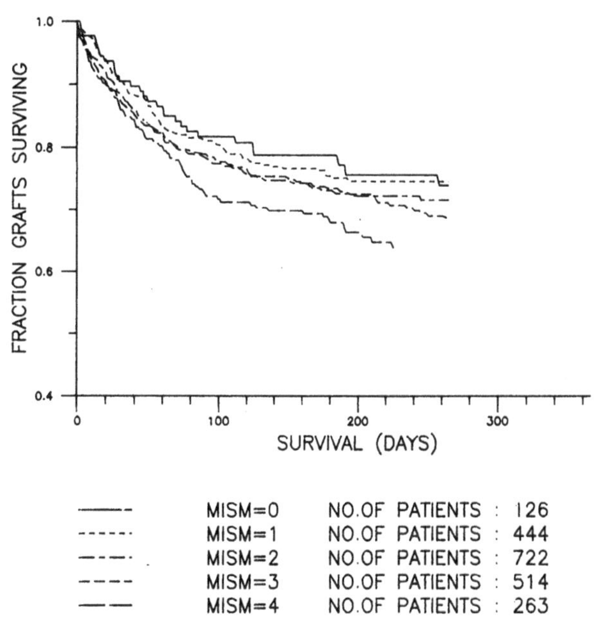

Fig. 2. Actuarial survival rates of first cadaver donor transplants shown separately for the number of incompatibilities at the HLA-A and B loci. The difference between grafts with no and four mismatched antigens is statistically significant at 6 months (P = 0.04)

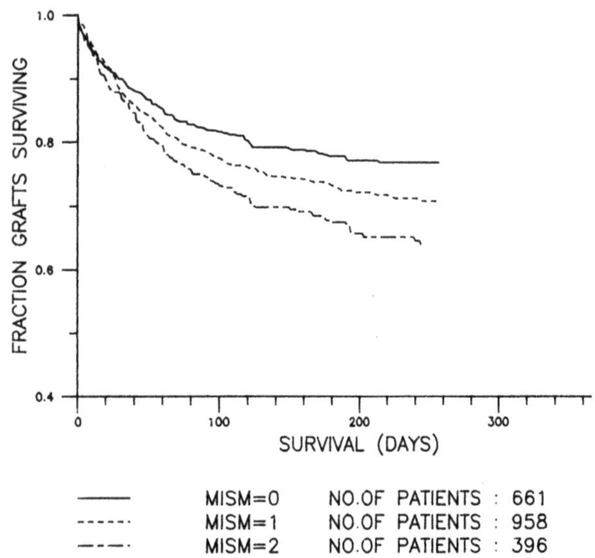

Fig. 3. Influence of incompatibilities at the HLA-DR locus on survival rate of first cadaver kidney transplants. The correlation of graft survival with the number of incompatibilities is statistically significant (P regression 0.001 at 6 months)

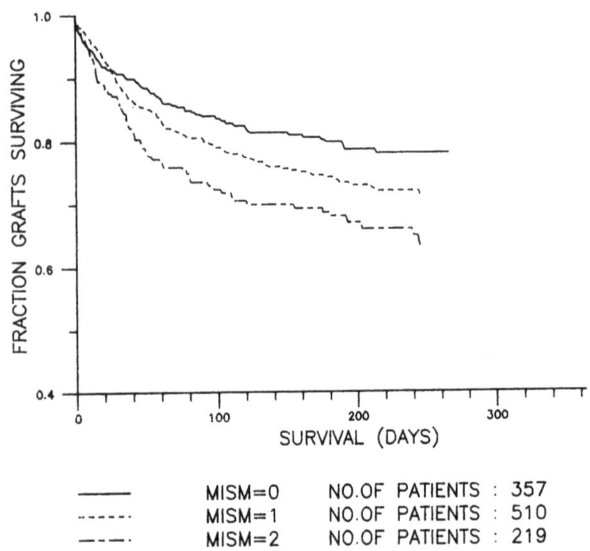

Fig. 4. Analysis of HLA-DR matching in subset of transplants with good-quality DR typing. The curves can be seen to separate better than those in Fig. 3

A much stronger correlation was obtained when the HLA-B and DR loci were analyzed together. There was a stepwise decline in graft survival with an increase in the number of mismatches. At 6 months, the graft survival rates were: 79% ± 4% for no mismatches, 77% ± 2% for one mismatch, 74% ± 2% for two mismatches, 69% ± 2% for three mismatches, and 63% ± 4% for four mismatches (P regression < 0.0001) (Fig. 5). A similar result was obtained when the number of HLA-B and DR antigens shared between recipient and donor was analyzed. The correlation was essentially the same as that obtained in the analysis of mismatches, except that grafts with four shared HLA-B and DR antigens survived at an exceptionally high rate (Fig. 6). Because only 47 transplants were "perfect matches" for HLA-B and DR, these results must await confirmation in a larger patient series. Nevertheless, the difference in graft survival between grafts with zero or four shared antigens was an impressive 21% at 6 months (87% ± 5% and 66% ± 3%, respectively, P < 0.001).

Combined consideration of the HLA-A, B, and DR loci improved the correlation even further. Whereas the difference between the best and the worst match grade was 16% when mismatching for HLA-B and DR was analyzed (Fig. 5), grafts with zero mismatches survived at a 22% higher rate than those with six mismatches in the combined analysis of HLA-A, B, and DR (85% ± 5% versus 63% ± 6% at 6 months; P < 0.01) (Fig. 7). Unfortunately, only seven transplants shared all six antigens at the three loci, too few for meaningful analysis.

Recipients who possessed the antigen HLA-DRw6 had a slightly lower graft survival rate than those negative for HLA-DRw6 (71% ± 2% versus 75% ± 1% at 6 months; difference not significant) (Fig. 8). However, DRw6-positive recipients who received kidneys from DRw6-positive donors enjoyed a much better graft outcome than DRw6-positive recipients who received DRw6-negative kidneys (graft survival rates at 6 months: 80% ± 3% and 64% ± 4%, respectively; P < 0.001) (Fig. 8). If the same type of analysis was carried out with DRw6 substituted by any other DR antigen the results were much less striking. Thus, the Workshop data confirm the finding of Hendriks et al. [4] that DRw6-positive recipients are at an increased risk of graft failure if they receive DRw6-negative kidneys. The Workshop data do not, however, support Hendriks' claim that DRw6-negative recipients do particularly well if they receive DRw6-positive kidneys. The 221 grafts analyzed in this series had a comparatively low (71% ± 3%) survival rate at 6 months (Fig. 8).

Furthermore, the effect of matching for HLA-DR was influenced greatly by the presence or absence of DRw6 in the recipient. In DRw6-negative recipients there was a small, although statistically significant, correlation of DR matching with graft outcome. Transplants with no, one, or two mismatches survived with 6-month rates of 77% ± 2%, 74% ± 2%, and 69% ± 3%, respectively (P regression < 0.03) (Fig. 9). In contrast, DR matching in DRw6-positive recipients revealed 6-month survival rates of 82% ± 3% for grafts with no mismatches,

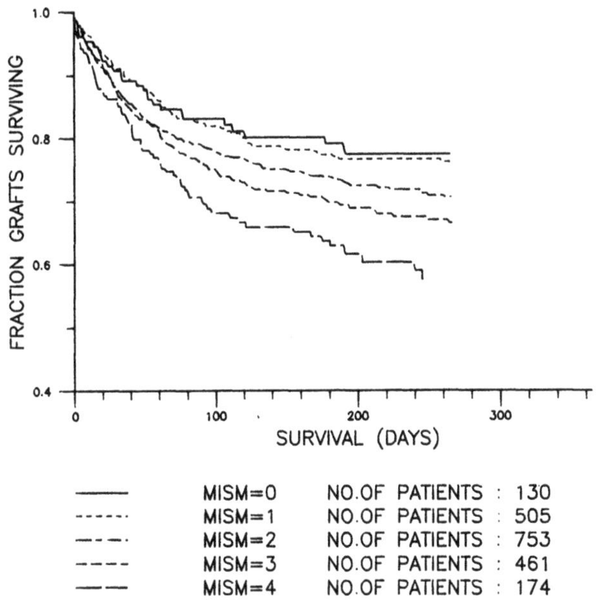

Fig. 5. Combined analysis of HLA-B and HLA-DR incompatibilities on survival rate of first cadaver kidney transplants. *MISM*, number of mismatched or incompatible antigens. The correlation of graft survival with the number of mismatches is highly significant (P regression 0.0001 at 6 months)

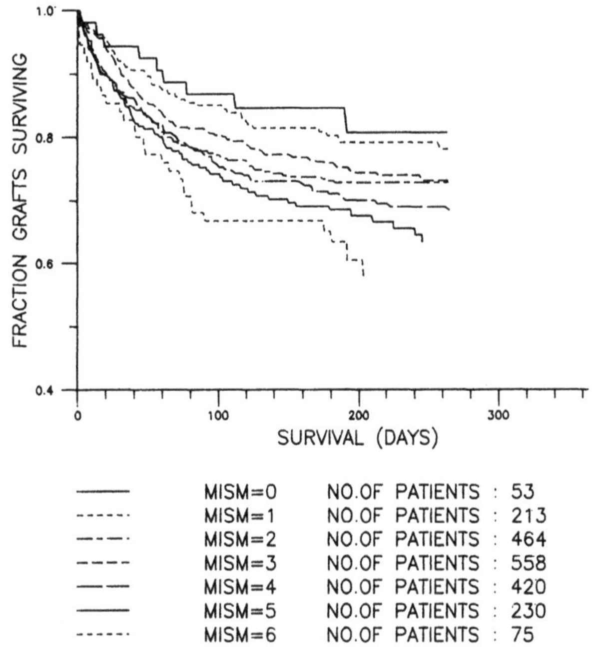

Fig. 7. Combined analysis of HLA-A, B, and DR incompatibilities in first cadaver transplants. The difference between grafts with no (*top curve*) or six mismatches (*bottom curve*) is an impressive 22% at 6 months

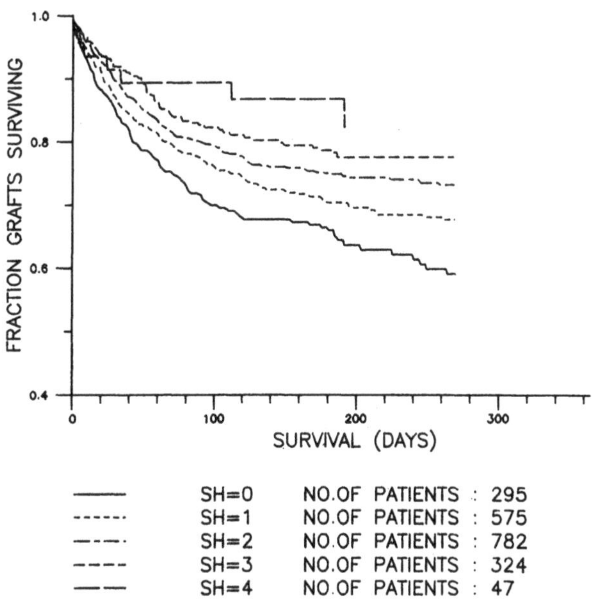

Fig. 6. Combined analysis of HLA-B and DR according to the number of antigens shared between recipient and donor. Graft survival is particularly good with four antigens shared, but the number of transplants analyzed is small

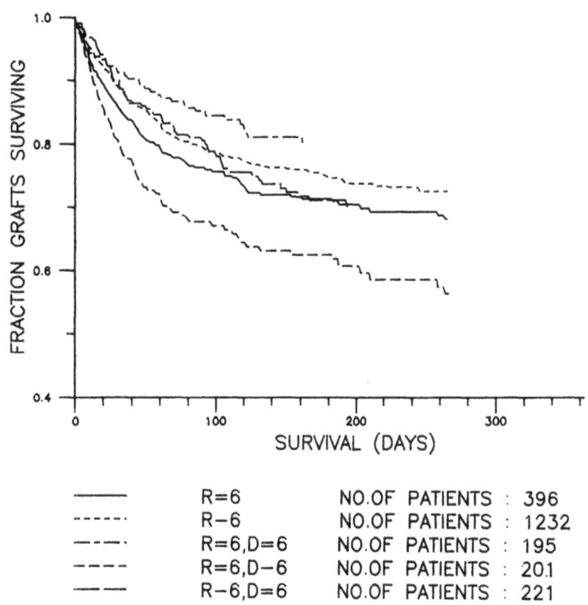

Fig. 8. Actuarial survival rates of first cadaver transplants plotted according to whether donors and recipients were positive or negative for the HLA antigen HLA-DRw6. *R* indicates recipients, *D* indicates donors. Whether the recipients or donors possessed the DRw6 antigen is indicated by = or –. DRw6-positive recipients did significantly better with DRw6-positive kidneys (*top curve*) than with DRw6-negative ones (*bottom curve*) (P 0.001 at 6 months)

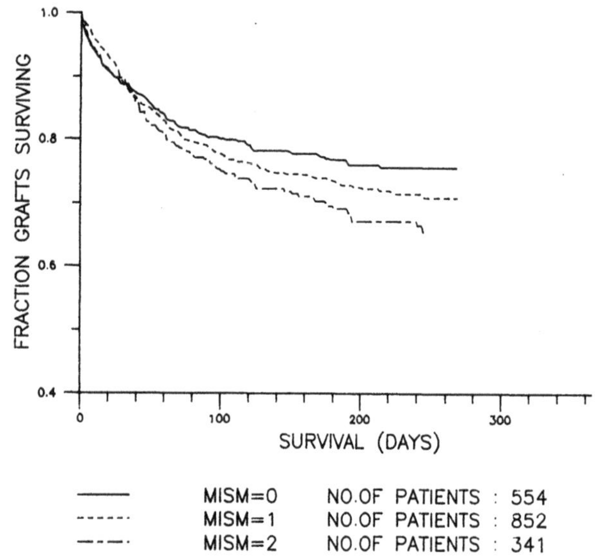

Fig. 9. Analysis of HLA-DR incompatibilities in DRw6-negative recipients

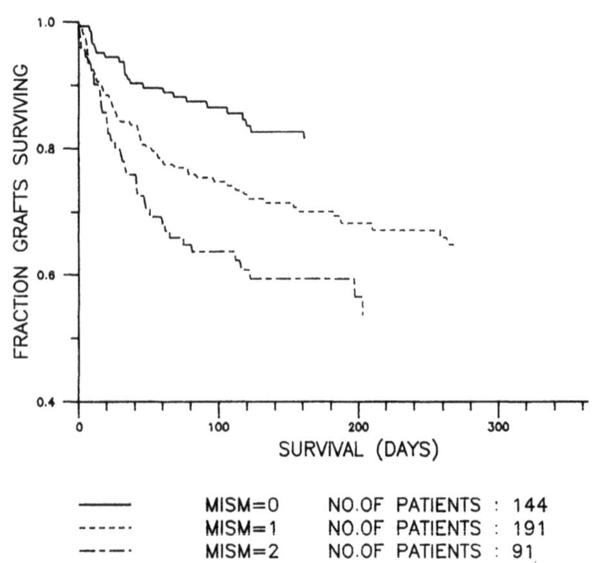

Fig. 10. Analysis of HLA-DR incompatibilities in DRw6-positive recipients. The correlation is much stronger than that in the DRw6-negative recipients shown in Fig. 9

70% ± 3% for grafts with one mismatch, and 59% ± 5% for grafts with two mismatches (P regression < 0.001) (Fig. 10).

Discussion

Compared with the Eighth International Histocompatibility Workshop Study in 1980, the current report provides a much more positive outlook for HLA matching in renal transplantation. It was difficult to show any effect of matching in the 1980 study [3]. Now, 4 years later, a highly significant effect of HLA matching on graft survival has been found. Although some had felt that a renewed collaborative effort would not serve any useful purpose, especially if, as in the 1980 Workshop, no significant effect of HLA matching were demonstrated, many more centers participated in the current study than in the 1980 Workshop. The question whether HLA matching matters or not is not only of scientific interest. With increasing cost pressures in most countries, the relevance of expensive laboratory tests is being scrutinized. The centers participating voluntarily in this effort demonstrated courage and a high degree of responsibility toward the community of renal transplant patients.

Although the results must still be considered preliminary, they show fairly convincingly that HLA typing and matching have a definitive place in clinical kidney transplantation. Why is the correlation of matching with graft survival better this time than in the 1980 Workshop study? A number of possible reasons can be thought of: The number of transplants is more than double that in the 1980 study. The quality of HLA typing reagents has improved. Technical skill in the performance of typing has improved, especially in smaller laboratories, which 4 years ago were not familiar with the then new DR-typing technique. There was a 1-month deadline on reporting in the current study, and the centers had been instructed to report consecutive cases.

The current results provide a first, preliminary answer to the frequently asked question as to whether matching for HLA-DR is all that is required, or whether the HLA-A and B loci must also be considered. Certainly, it is less difficult to find a good match if only DR compatibility is desired. The results shown in this report provide evidence that while matching for DR alone does improve graft survival, the improvement is about the same as that achievable with HLA-A, B matching. Most importantly, combination of HLA-B and DR, or of HLA-A, B, and DR provides significant further advantages.

It must be pointed out that the data provided in this report are preliminary overview results on the effect of HLA matching on graft survival. They do not take into account various factors that were shown previously to influence transplant outcome, such as pretransplant blood transfusions, the presence of preformed lymphocytotoxic antibodies, and the type of immunosuppression. There is an obvious need for more detailed analyses that consider HLA matching in the context of these other variables. Nevertheless, that clear correlations were found in the overall data, without selection, is most encouraging and rewarding.

An example of a differential HLA matching effect in certain patient subsets is shown in the analysis of

HLA-DR matching in DRw6-positive or DRw6-negative recipients. We would expect to see similar effects if transfused and nontransfused patients were analyzed separately, or if patients with and without preformed lymphocytotoxic antibodies were separated, etc. To identify additional categories of potential transplant recipients that benefit especially from improved HLA compatibility is an important research task. Because it is logistically impossible to provide all patients with HLA-A-, B-, and DR-compatible kidneys, it is important to concentrate efforts on those for whom the benefit is greatest.

The Ninth International Histocompatibility Workshop Renal Transplant Study can be considered a success. It demonstrated that, provided high quality reagents are used, HLA typing has reached a degree of reliability that can be used to improve clinical transplant results. That significant correlations were obtained even though the typings were carried out in many different laboratories, the transplants were performed in many different hospitals, the patient material was heterogenous, and the clinical treatment regimen were not standardized, is an impressive demonstration of useful international scientific cooperation.

Acknowledgment. It is impossible to acknowledge individually all persons who contributed to this study. Countless hours were invested by doctors, laboratory technicians, nurses, transplant coordinators, clerical personnel, and secretaries. The following is a list of individuals who were responsible for coordinating the work at the individual centers and who reported the data to the study center at the University of Heidelberg:

Dr. Thiel (Basel); Dr. Middleton (Belfast); Dr. Molzahn, Ms. Müller (Berlin-West); Dr. Barger (Birmingham, AL); Dr. Carpenter, Ms. Goguen (Boston); Dr. Bradley (Bristol); Dr. Dupont (Brussels); Dr. Petranyi (Budapest); Dr. Prigoshin de Godelman, Dr. Suarez (Buenos Aires); Dr. Joysey (Cambridge); Dr. Du Toit, Dr. Oudshoorn (Capetown); Dr. Lazda, Dr. Radvany (Chicago); Dr. Balakrishnan (Cincinnati); Dr. Braun (Cleveland); Dr. Meider (Cologne); Dr. Stastny (Dallas); Ms. Spencer (Dublin); Dr. Jakubowski, Dr. Grosse-Wilde (Essen); Dr. Fassbinder, Dr. Kühnl (Frankfurt); Dr. Tanzi-Fetta, Dr. Wilms (Freiburg); Dr. Dick (Glasgow); Dr. Brynger, Dr. Sandberg (Gothenburg); Dr. Beelen (Groningen); Dr. Hiller, Mr. Clausen (Hamburg); Dr. Robin-Winn (Hannover); Ms. Bow (Hartford); Dr. Schäfer, Dr. Dreikorn (Heidelberg); Dr. Koskimies (Helsinki); Dr. Hawkins (Hong Kong); Dr. Kerman (Houston); Dr. Margreiter, Mr. Fetz (Innsbruck); Dr. Goeken (Iowa City); Dr. Gazit, Ms. Efter (Israel Transplant); Dr. Amemiya (Japan Transplant); Dr. Albert, Dr. Gumbel (Kaiserslautern); Dr. Cross, Ms. Weaver (Kansas City); Dr. Veitch (Leicester); Dr. Shabalin (Leningrad); Dr. Vanrenterghem, Dr. Vermylen (Leuven); Dr. Caetano (Lisbon); Mr. Richardson (Louisville); Dr. Hoyer (Lübeck); Dr. Betuel (Lyon); Dr. Kreisler, Dr. Moreno (Madrid Transplant); Dr. Dyer (Manchester); Dr. Lange (Marburg); Dr. d'Apice (Melbourne); Dr. Lehne (Mexico); Dr. Sirchia, Dr. Mercuriali (Milan); Dr. Andersen (Minneapolis); Dr. Guttmann (Montreal); Dr. Zaretskaya (Moscow); Dr. Lison (Münster); Dr. Albert, Dr. Land (Munich); Dr. Perrier (Nancy); Dr. Soulillou (Nantes); Dr. Johnson, Ms. Candler (Nashville); Dr. Fotino, Dr. Nehlsen-Cannarella (New York); Dr. Reekers (Nijmegen); Dr. Leibold (Nürnberg); Dr. Larsen (Omaha); Dr. Ting (Oxford); Dr. Frantz, Dr. Thibault, Dr. Raffoux (Paris); Dr. Dawkins, Dr. Christiansen (Perth); Dr. Vanderwerf (Phoenix); Dr. Hadjiyannakis (Piraeus); Dr. Norman (Portland); Dr. Kraemer (Porto Alegre); Dr. Kocandrle, Dr. Ivaskova (Prague); Dr. Lachance, Dr. Roy (Quebec); Dr. Fauchet (Rennes); Dr. Moore (Rochester, MN); Dr. Casciani (Rome); Dr. Hudemann (Rostock); Dr. Saunders, Ms. Anderson (San Antonio); Dr. Garovoy (San Francisco); Dr. Hansen, Ms. Nisperos (Seattle); Dr. Le Petit (Saint Etienne); Dr. Anderson (St. Louis); Dr. Bashir (Sydney); Dr. Csajbok (Szeged); Dr. Senitzer (Toledo, OH); Dr. Curtoni, Dr. Amoroso (Torino); Dr. Falk, Dr. Cardella (Toronto); Dr. Calot (Toulouse); Dr. Bockhorn (Tübingen); Dr. Franz, Dr. Goldmann (Ulm); Dr. Säfwenberg (Uppsala); Dr. Reeve (Vancouver); Dr. Seksteliene (Vilnius); Dr. Jeffery (Winnipeg); Dr. Kastelan (Zagreb); Dr. Largiader (Zürich).

Thanks are due Dr. C. Koehler of the German Cancer Research Center, Heidelberg, and his staff for providing computer support for the study, Mr. M. Henninge for writing the computer programs, and Ms. E. Feisthammel and Ms. U. Mülker for handling the countless report forms and maintaining the data files.

References

1. Kaplan EL, Meier P (1958) Non-parametric estimation from incomplete observations. J Am Stat Assoc 53:457–81
2. Dunn OJ, Clark VA (eds) (1974) Applied statistics: Analysis of variance and regression. Wiley, New York
3. Opelz G, Terasaki PI (1980) International Histocompatibility Workshop study on renal transplantation. In: Terasaki PI (ed) Histocompatibility Testing 1980. UCLA Tissue Typing Laboratory, Los Angeles, California, pp 592–624
4. Hendriks GFJ, Schreuder GMT, Class FHJ, D'Amaro J, Persijn GG, Cohen B, van Rood JJ (1983) HLA-DRw6 and renal allograft rejection. Br Med J 286:85–87

Disease Reports:

Insulin-Dependent Diabetes Mellitus*

J. Bertrams[1] and M.P. Baur[2]

In collaboration with: F. Clerget-Darpoux[3], M.-C. King[4], C. Kollmar[1], M. Neugebauer[2], and H. Payami[5]

1 Department of Laboratory Medicine, St. Elisabeth Hospital, 4300 Essen, Federal Republic of Germany
2 Biometrical Department, Diabetes Research Institute, Auf'm Hennekamp 65, 4000 Düsseldorf, Federal Republic of Germany
3 INSERM U 155, Chateau de Longchamp, Paris, France
4 School of Public Health, University of California, Berkeley, CA, USA
5 Genetics Department, University of California, Berkeley, CA, USA

Purpose of the Study

Different autoimmune diseases often occur together in the same individual or family. Among the clustering autoimmune diseases, those mainly observed are insulin-dependent (type 1) diabetes mellitus (IDDM), diseases of the thyrogastric group [autoimmune thyroid disease (ATD); Graves' disease, Hashimoto's disease], and rheumatoid arthritis (RA). This clinical observation suggests a shared etiology due to genetic predisposition which is supported by the fact that these clustering autoimmune diseases are associated with the same HLA antigens: DR3 and DR4. For example, IDDM and ATD are significantly associated with DR3, while DR4-associated diseases include IDDM and RA.
Accordingly, one of the purpose of this study was to investigate the hypothesis of a shared genetic predisposition within the HLA region. For this purpose we proposed to type multiplex families with IDDM and other DR3 and/or DR4 associated diseases. In collaboration with Drs. Doniach (London) and Farid (Newfoundland) a detailed definition and diagnostic criteria were produced for the following DR3- and DR4-associated diseases: ATD (Graves' disease, Hashimoto's atrophic autoimmune thyroiditis, goitrous autoimmune thyroiditis), idiopathic Addison's disease, pernicious anemia, celiac disease, and RA. Part of the diagnostic criteria and clinical information for all patients was given on the disease card no. 52 (Table 1).
Another purpose of this study was to investigate different aspects of the still open question of the mode of inheritance of IDDM susceptibility (and the susceptibility of the other DR3- and DR4-associated diseases) by analyzing the family data using different genetic models.

Participating Laboratories and Case Material

A total of 28 laboratories submitted family data. The names and institutions of the participating groups and the numbers of investigated families are given in Table 2. Of the total data submitted, 167 families (41 of them of Japanese origin) were included in the analysis. According to the diseases involved, the submitted families were divided into three groups:
Group I: 70 families with only one IDDM patient
Group II: 45 families with more than one IDDM patient
Group III: 49 families with at least one IDDM patient and at least one patient with a DR3- or DR4-associated disease other than IDDM
The results obtained within these three groups of families are given in the following tables under the symbols I, II and III.

Results

HLA-B, DR Gene Frequencies

Table 3 presents the frequencies of selected HLA-B alleles and of all tested HLA-DR alleles, as counted from the genes of Caucasian IDDM patients and controls. From multiplex families, the first-born IDDM child was taken for this analysis as well as the analyses given in Tables 4, 5, and 9. Control frequencies are those obtained by the population analysis of this workshop (M. P. Baur et al. Population Analysis, this volume).

* The study was supported by the Deutsche Forschungsgemeinschaft, SFB 113, projects B3 and B8

Histocompatibility Testing 1984
Edited by E. D. Albert et al.

CARD 52

Type I diabetes study
Submit this card in addition to the WS card set for every individual of a family included in the type I diabetes study

Item	Column	Code
Card Number	1–2	52
Region Code	3–5	
Typing Lab Code	6–8	
Family ID Number	9–10	
Individual ID Number	11–13	
	14	X
Type I diabetes	15	0=no inf., 1=no, 2=yes
Age at onset (years)	16–17	01-99
Month at onset	18–19	01=January,....,12=December
Retinopathy	20	0=no inf., 1=no, 2=yes
ICA	21	0=no inf., 1=never defected, 2=present, 3=earlier
ICA first investigated (years after diagnosis)	22–23	01-99
ICA persisted (years after diagnosis)	24–25	(still present=99)
Thyroglobulin antibodies	26	0=not tested, 1=neg, 2=low, 3=high
Microsomal antibodies	27	0=not tested, 1=neg, 2=low, 3=high
Gastric antibodies	28	0=not tested, 1=neg, 2=low, 3=high
Adrenal antibodies	29	0=not tested, 1=neg, 2=low, 3=high
	30	X
Graves disease	31	0=no inf., 1=no, 2=yes
Age at onset (years)	32–33	01-99
Incr. 24hr radio-iodine uptake	34	0=not tested, 1=no, 2=yes
Absence of nodularity	35	0=not tested, 1=no, 2=yes
Thyroid hormone level	36	0=not tested, 1=normal, 2=increased
Thyroid stimulating antibodies	37	0=not tested, 1=neg, 2=low, 3=high
Microsomal antibodies	38	0=not tested, 1=neg, 2=low, 3=high
Thyroglobulin antibodies	39	0=not tested, 1=neg, 2=low, 3=high
	40	X
Atrophic autoimmune thyroiditis	41	0=no inf., 1=no, 2=yes
Age at onset (years)	42–43	01-99
Thyroid hormone level	44	0=not tested, 1=normal, 2=low
Serum thyrotropin level	45	0=not tested, 1=normal, 2=high
Microsomal antibodies	46	0=not tested, 1=neg, 2=low, 3=high
Thyroglobulin antibodies	47	0=not tested, 1=neg, 2=low, 3=high
	48	X
Goitrous autoimmune thyroiditis	49	0=no inf., 1=no, 2=yes
Age at onset (years)	50–51	01-99
Thyroid hormone level	52	0=not tested, 1=normal, 2=low
Serum thyroglobulin	53	0=not tested, 1=normal, 2=high
Lymphocytic infiltration	54	0=not tested, 1=no, 2=yes
	55	X
Idiopathic Addison's disease	56	0=no inf., 1=no, 2=yes
Age at onset (years)	57–58	01-99
Serum cortisol	59	0=not tested, 1=normal, 2=low
Abs. diurnal var. of cortison secr.	60	0=not tested, 1=no, 2=yes
Serum ACTH	61	0=not tested, 1=normal, 2=high
Adrenal antibodies	62	0=not tested, 1=neg, 2=pos
	63	X
Pernicious anemia	64	0=no inf., 1=no, 2=yes
Age at onset (years)	65–66	01-99
B12 absorption test typical	67	0=not tested, 1=no, 2=yes
Parietal cell antibodies	68	0=not tested, 1=neg, 2=pos
Intrinsic factor antibodies	69	0=not tested, 1=neg, 2=pos
	70	X
Celiac disease	71	0=no inf., 1=no, 2=yes
Age at onset (years)	72–73	01-99
Dermatitis herpetiformis	74	0=no inf., 1=no, 2=yes
	75	X
Rheumatoid arthritis	76	0=no inf., 1=no, 2=yes
Age at onset (years)	77–78	01-99
RF average titre	79	0=not tested, 1=low, 2=medium, 3=high
	80	X

Table 1. Patient coding form

Table 2. Participating laboratories and number of families investigated

Lab. code	No. of families	Investigators	Institutions
ALB	1	E. Albert[1], E. Rossipal[2]	[1] Labor für Gewebetypisierung, München, FRG [2] Universitätsklinik Graz, Austria
ARN	5	A. Arnaiz-Villena[1] I.L. Vicario, R. Barrio[2]	[1] Centro Especial Ramon Y Cajal, Immunologia, Madrid, Spain [2] Centro Especial Ramon Y Cajal, Pediatria, Madrid, Spain
BER	30	J. Bertrams[1], C. Kollmar[1], F.A. Gries[2], A. Wittenborg[3]	[1] Elisabeth Hospital, Essen, FRG [2] Diabetes-Research Institute, Düsseldorf, FRG [3] Rheumaklinik, Herne, FRG
BLA	11	J. Blank	Histocomp. Lab. University of Wisconsin Hosp., Madison, USA
BRG	1	B. Barger, D. Bell, R. Acton	Univ. of Alabama, Dept. of Microbiology, Birmingham, USA
BRN	1	W.E. Braun	Histocomp. & Immunogen. Lab., Cleveland Clinic Foundation, USA
BRU	2	M. de Bruyere	Université Catholique de Louvain, Bruxelles, Belgium
BSH	2	H. Bashir	Tissue Typing Lab., Red Cross Blood Transf. Serv., Sidney, Australia
CRB	3	A. Carbonara, E.S. Curtoni[1], A. Amoroso[2]	[1] Inst. di Genetica Medica di Università, Torino, Italy [2] CNR Immunogenetica ed Istocompatibilita, Torino, Italy
DAW	1	R. Dawkins	Tissue Typing Lab., Royal Perth Hosp., Perth, Australia
DPT	2	E. Dupont	Dept. of Immunology, Erasme, Hospital, Bruxelles, Belgium
DUT	12	E. du Toit, M. Stein[1], F. Bonnici[2]	[1] Provincial Lab. for Tissue Immunology, Cape Town, South Africa [2] Div. of Pediatrics and Child Health, Univ. of Cape Town, South Africa
FAU	2	R. Fauchet[1], H. Allanic[2]	[1] Lab. d'Histocompatibilite, Centre de Transfusion, Rennes, France [2] Clinique Medicale F, Rennes, France
JLE	5	J. Lee	American Red Cross National Headquarters, Bethesda, USA
JUJ	2	T. Juji[1], H. Maruyama, S. Ishiba[2]	[1] Blood. Transf. Service, Womens Medical College Tokyo, Japan [2] Dept. of Pediatrics, Women's Medical College, Tokyo, Japan
KAS	5	A. Kastelan[1], M. Bello[1], M. Kadrnka[2]	[1] Tissue Typing Ctr., Faculty of Medicine, Zagreb, Yugoslavia [2] Dept. of Pediatrics, M. Stojanovic Hospital, Zagreb, Yugoslavia
KAT	17	M.-C. King[1], C. Torfs[1], W. Epstein[2], J. Karam[2], G. Friedmann[3], P. Singleton[4]	[1] School of Public Health Univ. of California, Berkeley, USA [2] Univ. of California, San Francisco, USA [3] Kaiser Permanente Medical Group, Oakland, USA [4] Lettermann Hospital, San Francisco, USA
MEH	1	N.K. Mehra, M.C. Vaidya[1], E. Bhatia, M.M.S. Ahuja[2]	[1] Cellular Immunol. Lab., All-India Inst. of Med. Sci., New Delhi, India [2] Dept. of Endocrinology, All-India Inst. of Med. Sci., New Delhi, India
MIY	6	T. Miyajima	Dept. of Surgical Research, National Cardiovasc Center, Osaka, Japan
MOL	12	E. Moller[1], R. Persson[2]	[1] Dept. of Clinical Immunol., Huddinge Univ. Hosp. Stockholm, Sweden [2] Dept. of Pediatrics, St. Göraus Hospital, Stockholm, Sweden
NEU	2	H. Neumeyer	Zentraler Blutspendedienst, Göttingen, FRG
RAD	4	R. Radvany[1], H. Traismann[2]	[1] Dept. of Surgery, Northwestern Medical School, Chicago, USA [2] Dept. of Pediatrics, Northwestern Medical School, Chicago, USA
RUB	8	P. Rubinstein[1], F. Ginsberg[2]	[1] Lindsley F. Kimball Research Inst., New York Blood Center, USA [2] Mt. Sinai Hospital, New York, USA
STA	2	P. Stastny[1], J.F. Marks[2]	[1] Health Science Center, Univ. of Texas, Dallas, USA [2] Dept. of Pediatrics, Univ. of Texas, Southwestern Med. School, Dallas, USA
THP	1	J. Thompson[1], G. Sperling[2]	[1] Hoxworth Blood Center, University of Cincinnati, USA [2] Childrens Hospital, Cincinnati, USA
TSU	41	K. Tsuji, Y. Yamashita, K. Sato, M. Kusama, Y. Nose, T. Sukegawa, T. Nakatsuji[1], G. Mimura[2], K. Kida[3], T. Kobayashi[4], K. Nakamura[5], S. Sonoda[6], H. Inouye[7]	[1] Tokai University School of Medicine, Isehara, Japan [2] University of the Ryukjus, Naha, Japan [3] Ehime University School of Medicine, Ehime, Japan [4] Toranomon Hospital, Tokyo, Japan [5] Osaka Prefectural Hospital, Osaka, Japan [6] Ehime Prefectural Institute of Public Health, Matsuyama, Japan [7] Osaka Prefectural Hospital, Osaka, Japan
WAL	2	R.L. Walford	Dept. of Pathology, Univ. of California, Los Angeles, USA
ZAR	4	Y. Zaretskaya, R. Voylokova, V. Abramov, S. Ignatenko[1], M. Balabolkin, Shaginova[2]	[1] Lab. of Immunogenetics, Inst. of Transplantation, Moskau, USSR [2] The 3rd. Moscow Medical Inst., Moskau, USSR

Table 3. HLA-B and -DR gene frequencies in Caucasian IDDM patients and controls

Gene	Controls $n = 1152$	IDDM				χ^2
		I $n = 43$	II $n = 21$	III $n = 45$	Total $n = 109$	
HLA-B8	0.10	0.15	0.21	0.30	0.22	31.60
HLA-B18	0.05	0.05	0.12	0.04	0.06	2.24
HLA-Bw62	0.06	0.08	0.02	0.13	0.09	7.71
HLA-DR1	0.09	0.09	0.10	0.08	0.09	
DR2	0.15	0.06	0.05	0.01	0.04	22.57
DR3	0.12	0.30	0.31	0.34	0.32	66.49
DR4	0.13	0.35	0.35	0.38	0.36	76.14
DR5	0.14	0.01	0	0.03	0.02	27.26
DRw6	0.12	0.03	0.05	0.05	0.05	10.56
DR7	0.12	0.07	0.14	0.07	0.08	3.83
DRw8	0.03	0.05	0	0.02	0.01	
DRw9	0.01	0.01	0	0.01	0.01	
DRw10	0.01	0	0	0	0	
DRX	0.08	0.03	0	0.01	0.02	

I = Single case IDDM
II = Multiplex IDDM
III = Multiplex IDDM + other DR3- or DR4-associated disease

As expected, HLA-B8 is significantly increased among all diabetics ($\chi^2 = 31.6$), whereas the increase in B18 and Bw62 is insignificant. Looking at the IDDM subgroups, the increasing B8 frequency in groups I, II, and III and the significant increase of Bw62 only in group III ($\chi^2 = 7.7$), not in groups I and II, is remarkable. The deviations observed for HLA-DR alleles among Caucasian IDDM patients are in good agreement with previous findings [14]. DR3 and DR4 are significantly increased; DR2, DRw6, and also DR7 are significantly decreased in the total IDDM patient group (Fig. 1). The frequency of DR1 was not decreased but insignificantly increased, a result also described previously [4]. It is of special interest that all DR alleles exhibit nearly identical frequencies when analyzed in the IDDM subgroups. Accordingly, differences found among IDDM subgroups for B8 and Bw62 are not paralleled by DR3 and DR4, respectively. This could be the result of a stronger linkage disequilibrium between B8 and DR3 alleles and between Bw62 and DR4 alleles in multiplex families of group III IDDM patients.

C2, C4, BF Allele Frequencies

Among the C2, C4, BF complement alleles, BF*F1, C2*2, and C4B*3 showed significant increases; the C4B*2 allele was nonsignificantly increased; and

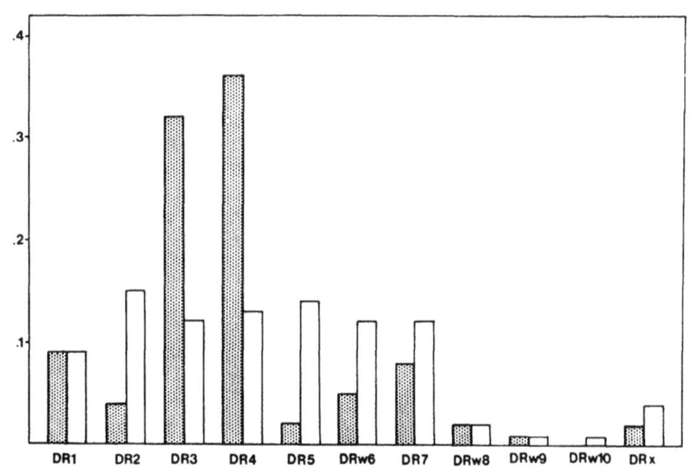

Fig. 1. HLA-DR allele frequencies in Caucasian IDDM patients (▨) and normal controls (□)

Table 4. BF, C2, and C4 gene frequencies in Caucasian IDDM patients and controls

Gene	Controls	IDDM				χ^2
		I	II	III	Total	
BF*F1	0.013 (420)	0.06 (16)	0.08 (13)	0.03 (45)	0.05 (74)	6.44
BF*SO.7	0.013	0.09	0.04	0.01	0.03	
C2*2	0.053 (141)	0.00 (7)	0.12 (4)	0.15 (36)	0.13 (47)	4.80
C4A*QO	0.108 (323)	0.08 (13)	0.08 (6)	0.14 (33)	0.11 (52)	
C4B*QO	0.126	0.15	0.08	0.03	0.07	2.48
C4B*2	0.071	0.19	0.17	0.09	0.12	2.89
C4B*3	0.032	0.04	0.00	0.15	0.11	10.07

Numbers in parenthesis = numbers of individuals tested

Table 5. HLA-DR gene frequencies in Oriental IDDM patients and controls

Gene	Controls $n = 381$	IDDM				χ^2
		I $n = 26$	II $n = 24$	III $n = 4$	Total $n = 54$	
HLA-DR1	0.04	0.04	0.08	0.12	0.07	
DR2	0.149	0.04	0.00	0.00	0.02	12.97
DR3	0.02	0.02	0.00	0.00	0.01	
DR4	0.236	0.33	0.29	0.62	0.33	4.25
DR5	0.076	0.04	0.04	0.00	0.03	
DRw6	0.036	0.00	0.00	0.00	0.00	
DR7	0.028	0.03	0.02	0.00	0.03	
DRw8	0.103	0.19	0.12	0.00	0.15	1.62
DRw9	0.128	0.27	0.35	0.26	0.30	22.19
DRw10	0.008	0.00	0.00	0.00	0.00	
DRX	0.17	0.04	0.10	0.00	0.06	7.01

the frequency of the silent alleles C4A*QO and C4B*QO did not deviate from the control frequencies (Table 4). While the deviation of the structural C2, C4, BF alleles is similar to that found in previous published results [1, 2], the lack of increase in C4A*QO and C4B*QO is surprising. It may be caused by the pooling of data of different laboratories for a system with technical typing problems affecting especially the frequency of the silent alleles (see also C. Rittner and G. Mauff, C4 Polymorphism, this volume).

HLA-DR and C2, C4, BF Frequencies in Oriental Patients

HLA-DR allele frequencies of 54 Oriental families (mainly Japanese) are given in Table 5. As in the last workshop, DR4 is significantly increased and DR2 significantly decreased. DRw8, which was significantly increased in the Japanese IDDM patients of the last workshop, shows a nearly normal frequency, whereas the HLA-DRw9 allele is strongly increased (30% vs 12.8%; $\chi^2 = 22.19$). Another interesting finding is the significant decrease of the DRX allele among the Oriental diabetic patients. C2, C4, BF alleles have been determined in so small a number of Oriental families that reliable gene frequencies cannot be given.

DR3 and DR4 in RA and ATD

DR3 and DR4 genes have been counted in multiplex families for patients with RA or ATD (Graves' disease or Hashimoto's thyroiditis). The number of patients with other DR3- and/or DR4-associated diseases was too small for an analysis of DR allele frequencies. As shown in Table 6, DR3 is significantly increased among ATD and IDDM patients, while DR4 occurs significantly more often among RA and IDDM patients.

Table 6. Gene frequencies of DR3 and DR4 among patients with RA, ATD, and IDDM in Caucasian multiplex families

Gene	a RA $n = 18$	b TD $n = 43$	c IDDM $n = 109$	d Controls $n = 1152$	χ^2
HLA-DR3	0.22	0.43	0.32	0.12	a-d: n.s. b-d: 67.50 c-d: 66.49
HLA-DR4	0.39	0.15	0.36	0.13	a-d: 16.83 b-d: n.s. c-d: 76.14

Table 7. HLA-DR allelic combinations in Caucasian IDDM patients

	IDDM $n = 167$	Eighth Workshop	Controls $n = 1147$	Relative risk
DR3/X[a]	25 (15.0%)	7.1%	219 (19.1%)	0.75
DR3/3	12 (7.2%)	10.7%	15 (1.3%)	5.84
DR3/4	56 (33.6%)	41.1%	28 (2.4%)	20.16
DR4/4	13 (7.9%)	9.8%	23 (2.0%)	4.13
DR4/X[a]	43 (25.8%)	25.9%	239 (20.8%)	1.32
DRX/X[a]	17 (10.2%)	5.4%	623 (54.3%)	0.10

[a] DRX: all DR except DR3, 4

Table 8. HLA-DR allelic combinations in Oriental IDDM patients

	IDDM $n = 89$	Controls $n = 391$	Relative risk
DRw9/X[a]	26 (29.9%)	71 (18.2%)	1.86
DRw9/9	5 (5.7%)	6 (1.5%)	3.82
DRw9/4	16 (18.4%)	18 (4.6%)	4.54
DR4/4	25 (28.7%)	108 (27.7%)	1.02
DR4/X[a]	8 (9.2%)	28 (7.2%)	1.28
DRX/X[a]	9 (10.3%)	160 (41.0%)	0.16

[a] DRX: all DR except DR4, w9

HLA-DR Allelic Combinations

HLA-DR3, 4 allelic combinations among 167 Caucasian IDDM patients and 1147 Caucasian controls are given in Table 7. Analogous frequencies obtained from the diabetes study of the Eighth Workshop [14] are added for comparison. The most interesting finding in relation to the discussion of the genetic models of IDDM susceptibility is that the relative risk for the DR3, 4 heterozygotes is much higher than the sum of the risk values of both the DR3 and DR4 homozygotes. Accordingly, the effect of the DR3- and DR4-associated IDDM genes cannot be only additive. As also pointed out by Svejgaard et al. [14], the relative risk values for DR3 and DR4 homozygotes are both considerably higher than those for DR3,X and DR4,X heterozygotes, indicating a dose effect for both the DR3-associated and the DR4-associated IDDM genes.
Analysis of DR4,w9 allelic combinations among Japanese IDDM patients yielded rather different results (Table 8). Although DR4,w9 heterozygotes have the highest relative risk, the sum of the risk values of DR4 and DRw9 homozygotes is nearly equal to the risk value of the DR4,w9 heterozygotes. In addition, the risk value for DRw9 homozygotes is in fact considerably higher than the relative risk for DRw9,X heterozygotes, but the risk for DR4 homozygotes is even lower than that for DR4,X heterozygotes. Accordingly, the genetics of IDDM among Orientals seems to be even more difficult to interpret than among Caucasians.
In an additional analysis, we compared the DR3, 4 allelic combination in the IDDM patients of the three subgroups (Table 9). The occurrence of RA in several families of group III may be the reason for the highest frequency of DR4 among diabetics of this group. Also included in the table are frequencies obtained from all IDDM patients of all investigated families (sibs and parents included). Frequencies of the different DR allelic combinations of all diabetics are not different from frequencies obtained by counting only the first-born diabetic child in multiplex families of groups II and III.

IDDM "High-Risk Haplotypes"

When HLA haplotypes including HLA-A, B, C, DR and C2, C4, BF alleles were arranged according to positivity for DR3 and DR4, it became obvious that the following three "super-haplotypes" occurred frequently among IDDM patients:
a) A1, Cw7, B8, C2*1, BF*S, C4A*QO, B*1, DR3;
b) A30, Cw5, B18, C2*1, BF*F1, C4A*3, B*QO, DR3;
c) A2, Cw3, Bw62, C2*1, (C2*2), BF*S, C4A*1, B*3, DR4.

These super-haplotypes have also been found in other previously published studies of IDDM pa-

Table 9. HLA-DR allelic combinations in Caucasian IDDM patients

	IDDM			Total	All IDDM
	I (n = 43)	II (n = 21)	III (n = 45)	(n = 109)	(n = 167)
DR3/X[a]	7 (16.3%)	4 (19.0%)	6 (13.3%)	17 (15.6%)	15.0%
DR3/3	3 (7.0%)	0	6 (13.3%)	9 (8.3%)	7.2%
DR3/4	13 (30.2%)	9 (24.9%)	13 (28.9%)	35 (32.1%)	33.6%
DR4/4	3 (7.0%)	1 (4.8%)	4 (8.9%)	8 (7.3%)	7.9%
DR4/X[a]	11 (25.5%)	4 (19.0%)	13 (28.9%)	28 (25.7%)	25.8%
DRX/X[a]	6 (14.0%)	3 (14.3%)	3 (6.7%)	12 (11.0%)	10.2%

[a] DRX: all DR except DR3, 4

tients [4, 5]. Patients with DR3-associated diseases other than IDDM often carry haplotype a, while haplotype c shows an increased frequency among patients with RA.

Haplotype Sharing Among Sib Pairs Affected by IDDM

Results of the haplotype-sharing analysis among Caucasian and Oriental sib pairs affected by IDDM are given in Table 10. In the combined material, 51.1% share both, 37.8% share one, and 11.1% share no haplotype. This distribution differs significantly from the expected distribution of 25%, 50%, and 25% in independent segregation ($p < 0.025$). The data of the haplotype-sharing analysis of the Eighth Workshop diabetes study [14], also given in the table, are in relatively good agreement with the data of the present study. The results can be considered independently because the amount of overlap between the two family samples of the Eighth and Ninth Workshop diabetes studies is less than 5%.

Genetic Interrelationship and Mode of Inheritance of DR3- and DR4-Associated Diseases in Multiplex Families

The clustering of different DR3- and/or DR4-associated diseases in one individual or one family suggests a common HLA-associated genetic interrelationship between these diseases. To test this hypothesis, the HLA haplotype-sharing distributions among sib pairs with different affectional status combinations were calculated under two hypotheses. In the first model, a common allelele predisposes for both diseases, each disease being expressed according to its specific mode of inheritance and penetrance. In the second model, different alleles exist at the same locus predisposing for the two diseases, which again have their own mode of inheritance and penetrance. Both hypotheses assume single-locus models. The multiplex family data of the Ninth Workshop (including the data given by C. Torfs et al., Inheritance and Possible Coinheritance of HLA-Linked Susceptibilities to Insulin-Dependent Diabetes Mellitus, Autoimmune Thyroid Diseases, and Rheumatoid Arthritis, this volume) were pooled with family data from the literature [6, 7] to get a sample large enough for the genetic analysis. A total of 89 sib pairs with two diseases in different combinations were analyzed for their HLA haplotype sharing; the results are given in Table 11. According to the observed disease combinations in sib pairs, the ex-

Table 10. Haplotype sharing among IDDM-affected sib pairs

	Number of shared haplotypes		
	0	1	2
Caucasians n = 26	3 (11.5%)	8 (30.7%)	15 (57.7%)
Orientals n = 19	2 (10.5%)	9 (47.4%)	8 (42.1%)
Total n = 45	5 (11.1%)	17 (37.8%)	23 (51.1%)
Expected	25%	50%	25%
Eighth Workshop	4.6%	36.9%	58.6%

Significance for the deviation from the expected distribution: total χ^2 (2 d.f.) = 8.43; $p < 0.025$

Table 11. HLA haplotype sharing among sib pairs of multiplex families

Affectional status combination	Shared HLA haplotypes			
	2	1	0	Total
IDDM, ATD -ATD	.22	.71	.07	27
IDDM, ATD -IDDM	.71	.29	0	7
IDDM, ATD -IDDM, ATD	.67	.22	.11	9
IDDM -ATD	.40	.40	.20	10
IDDM -RA	.29	.57	.14	7
RA, ATD -ATD	.29	.64	.07	14
RA, ATD -RA	0	.75	.25	4
RA -ATD	.18	.55	.27	11

pected haplotype sharing was calculated for three possible cases: (a) one sib affected with two diseases, the other with only one (AB-A), (b) both sibs affected with two diseases (AB-AB), and (c) each sib affected with one (different) disease (A-B). The expected haplotype-sharing distribution for these three affectional status combinations under model I (common allele) and model II (different alleles) were plotted on trinomial plotting paper (Figs. 2–4). The shaded areas in the figures represent the expected outcomes on the basis of the postulated model and varying penetrance parameters.

IDDM-ATD: Since IDDM and ATD are both associated with DR3, the two diseases may have a common genetic susceptibility allele. The observed haplotype sharing values are in agreement with this hypothesis. A predisposition by different alleles, however, cannot be ruled out (Figs. 2, 3). The observed sharing distribution among sibs with different diseases (IDDM-ATD, Fig. 4) is incompatible with both models. Due to the small sample size, however, neither model can be rejected.

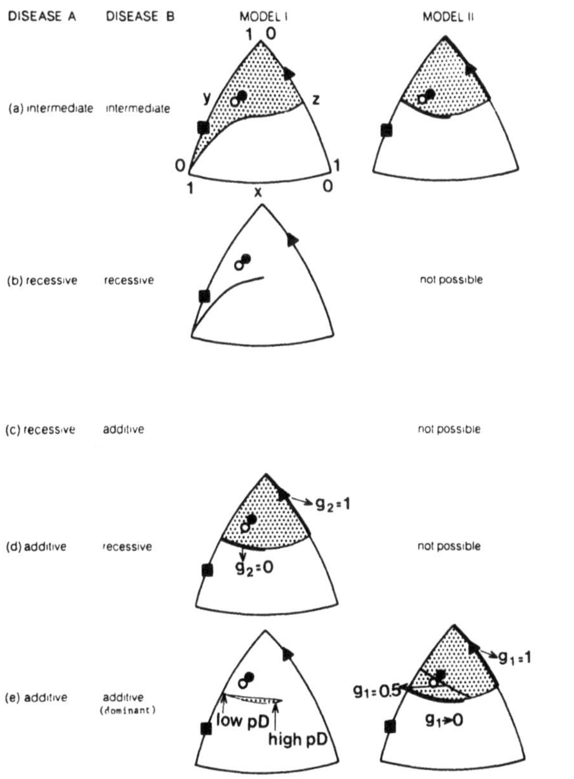

Fig. 2. Expected and observed HLA haplotype sharing (x, y, z) in sib pairs with one sib affected with two diseases, the other with only one of them (AB-A) under model I (common allele) and model II (different alleles) for various modes of inheritance and penetrances of each disease, *g1*, penetrance of B in heterozygotes; *g2* penetrance of the recessive disease; ●, IDDM, ATD – ATD; ■, IDDM, ATD – IDDM; ○, RA, ATD – ATD; x, RA, ATD – RA

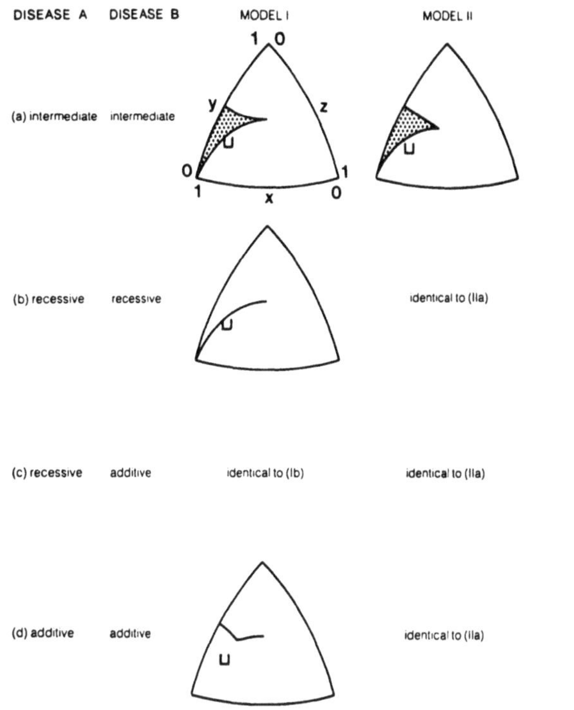

Fig. 3. Expected and observed HLA haplotype sharing (x, y, z) in sib pairs with both sibs affected with two diseases (AB-AB) under model I (common allele) and model II (different alleles) for various possible modes of inheritance of each disease. ⊔, IDDM, ATD – IDDM, ATD

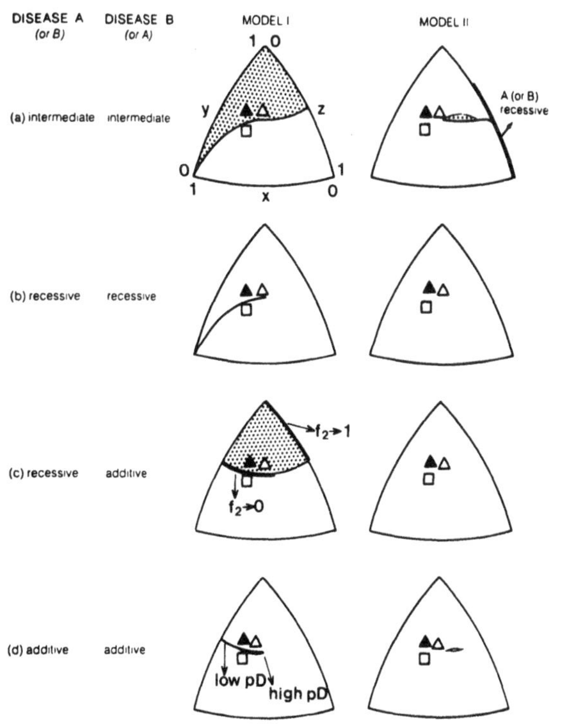

Fig. 4. Expected and observed HLA haplotype sharing (x, y, z) in sib pairs with both sibs affected with one but different diseases (A-B) under model I (common allele) and model II (different alleles) for various possible modes of inheritance of each disease. □, IDDM – ATD; ▲, IDDM – RA; △, RA – ATD

Preliminary results indicate that the observed values are more compatible with a model which assumes one allele predisposing for both diseases and another predisposing for one, allowing for negative complementation for IDDM.

IDDM-RA: Similarly, IDDM and RA are associated with the same HLA antigen, this time DR4, again suggesting a common genetic susceptibility. The IDDM-RA data point (Fig. 4) fits the expectation under model I (common allele), but not under model II (different alleles). The different-allele hypothesis can be rejected if IDDM, RA, or both are recessive.

ATD-RA: The third disease combination is that of ATD and RA, which are associated with different HLA antigens (ATD-DR3/RA-DR4), suggesting the existence of different susceptibility alleles (model II). The data favors the different-allele hypothesis and is in agreement with the suggested near-dominant, high-penetrance model for ATD and near-dominant, low-penetrance model for RA. The common-allele model can be ruled out if either RA or ATD is recessive, additive, dominant, or close to any of these (Fig. 2).

Figure 5 summarizes the possible relationship between IDDM, RA, and ATD on the basis of the observed haplotype sharing in multiplex families. Whereas the disease susceptibility alleles for RA (S_{RA}) and for ATD (S_{ATD}) are most likely not identical, they both occur on the same haplotypes predisposing for IDDM. The model of inheritance for both RA and ATD is indicated to be close to dominant, whereas IDDM is transmitted according to a near-recessive model or a model involving at least two susceptibility alleles (negative complementation).

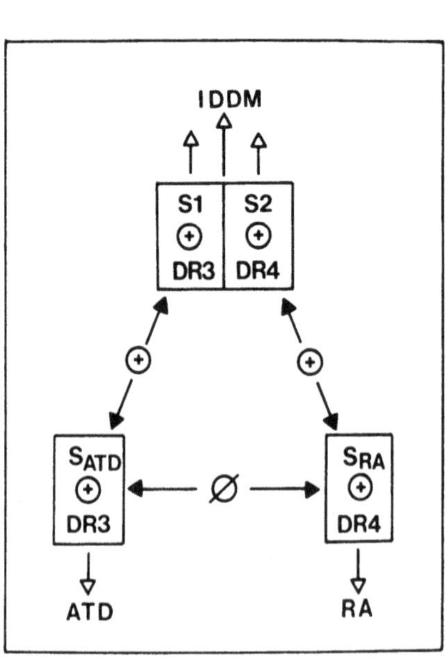

Fig. 5. Genetic interrelationship between susceptibility (*S*) to IDDM, ATD, and RA. ⊕, positive linkage disequilibrium

IDDM Susceptibility Gene Frequency and Its Penetrance in the Population and Families

An analysis for the underlying genetic model for IDDM was performed on the following three (partly overlapping) samples:

a) Families with IDDM only: 77 families, 132 affected members;
b) Families with IDDM and other DR3/DR4-associated diseases: 159 families, 234 affected members (affected status: individuals with at least IDDM);
c) Families with IDDM and other DR3/DR4 associated diseases: 159 families, 322 affected family members (affected status: individuals with IDDM *or* other DR3/DR4-associated diseases);

The model for transmission of IDDM was given by a single locus in the HLA region with a susceptibility allele g (alleles $s_1, \ldots s_n$) with frequency $q = \sum_{i=1-n} q_i$. The penetrance of s/s genotypes *in families* is termed f_1, that of heterozygous s/non-s genotypes λf_1. It is important to realize that the penetrance parameter is defined as *intra*familial (probability for an individual to be affected knowing one relative has the disease) and differs from the population penetrance, which is denoted as f_0.

The aim of the analysis was the estimation of q, λ, f_1, f_0 by:

1. Maximization of the conditional likelihood for marker genotypes given trait phenotypes
2. Using the recurrence risk in sibs as well as the prevalence in the population

In order to calculate the conditional likelihoods of marker genotypes (observed HLA haplotypes) given trait phenotypes (disease status), it was assumed that recombination between disease locus and HLA-DR is negligible, i.e., $\theta = 0$. On the basis of a recurrence risk of $r = 0.05$ [9] and an estimated 95% confidence interval for λ with $0 \leq \lambda \leq 0.12$ [10] the frequency q, the intrafamilial penetrance f_1, and the population penetrance f_0 were estimated in the three family samples listed above (Table 12).

Due to a rather "flat" likelihood curve, the estimate of λ has a large variance. The estimate of q, though, is not strongly affected, and is high under all conditions. This observation of a high gene frequency estimate has been described before [14], but was always disputed on the basis of population prevalence and recurrence risk in sibs. Given the

Table 12. Frequency (q), intrafamilial penetrance (f_1), and population penetrance (f_0) in the three family samples

$\lambda=0$				$\lambda=0.12$		
Sample	q	f_1	f_0	q	f_1	f_0
a)	0.39	0.10	0.01	0.30	0.13	0.011
b)	0.43	0.10	0.01	0.33	0.13	0.011
c)	0.49	0.09	0.008	0.42	0.11	0.010

well-supported assumption of different penetrance values within families, and on the population level as expressed in a factor of $f_1/f_0 \approx 10$, a rather high gene frequency q with a low population penetrance f_0 and a higher intrafamilial penetrance f_1 is acceptable with the observed data. In conclusion, it can be stated that the total familial correlation is by no means explained by the MHC; additional environmental and/or genetic components have a major role in the development of IDDM.

One or Two Susceptibility Alleles for IDDM?

The so-called intermediate or gene-dose model [3, 13], with one susceptibility gene causing a higher penetrance when present in double dose (homozygotes) than when present in single dose (heterozygotes), cannot be rejected completely on the basis of the existing information. Nevertheless, the existence of two IDDM genes, one in association with DR3 and the other with DR4, seems very likely. There is accumulated evidence for immunogenetic heterogeneity within IDDM. This heterogeneity suggests that more than one type of IDDM may exist. The separation of IDDM according to immunogenetic markers into a DR3-associated autoimmune type and a DR4-associated insulin antibody responder type is still difficult. The ability of mathematical models based on the heterogeneity arguments to make accurate population predictions seems to be additional evidence in the favor of different IDDM types [12].

It was attempted by another mathematical analysis to compare two models for IDDM on the basis of marker as well as disease information in 130 diabetes families, using the family analysis package FAP (M. Neugebauer et al., Analysis of Multilocus Pedigree Data by Computer, this volume). The two models were defined by the two loci HLA-B and HLA-DR and a postulated disease susceptibility ("DS") locus between HLA-B and HLA-DR. Recombination between these three loci was assumed to be negligible. The two models differed only by the number of postulated alleles at the disease susceptibility locus: two (one susceptibility allele S and one normal allele s) for model 1 and three (two susceptibility alleles S1 and S2 and one normal allele s) for model 2 [see also 8]. Consequently, the models contained the following parameters:

Model 1: Two alleles at the "DS" locus with the parameters:

Gene frequencies for disease locus:	f(S), f(s)
Penetrances:	p(S,S), p(S,s), p(s,s)
HLA gene frequencies:	f(DR1)... f(B5)...
Linkage disequilibria:	B-DR, B-"DS", DR-"DS"

Model 2: Three alleles at the "DS" locus with the parameters:

Gene frequencies for disease locus:	f(S1), f(S2), f(s)
Penetrances:	p(S1,S1), p(S1,S2), p(S2,S2), p(S1,s), p(S2,s), p(s,s)
HLA gene frequencies:	f(DR1)... f(B5)...
Linkage disequilibria:	B-DR, B-"DS", DR-"DS"

On the basis of estimates taken from the literature [8], FAP was used to iteratively improve all included parameter estimates simultaneously and to finally calculate the likelihood of the observed family sample conditional to the two alternative models.

The results of the maximum likelihood estimates are obviously biased due to the sampling procedure, and consequently are not given as estimates here. The qualitative results, though, show especially for model 2 that the genotype S1/S2 at the disease locus has the highest penetrance, and that the S1 allele in Caucasians is in high linkage disequilibrium with DR3 as well as B8, whereas S2 is positively associated with DR4 and Bw62.

To test model 1 vs model 2, the negative logarithms of the likelihoods for all 130 families were summated [see also 11], which resulted in 3034.6 for model 1 and 3019.6 for model 2. The difference on the log scale of d = 15.0 is equivalent to a likelihood ratio of 1 : 3 000 000 in favor of model 2. The corresponding likelihood ratio test yields a chi square of 30, which on the basis of an additional number of 15 degrees of freedom in model 2 has a p value of < 0.01, showing that the model of a disease locus with two different susceptibility alleles is significantly superior in explaining the observed family data to a model with only one susceptibility allele.

Accordingly, we believe that at least two IDDM genes exist and should be considered for all susceptibility models. In relation to the difficulty in understanding the risk value of DR3,4 heterozygotes, which is much higher than the sum of the risks of DR3 and DR4 homozygotes, the suggestion made by Svejgaard et al. [15] should be mentioned. They discussed the possibility that so-called "hybrid" or "combinatorial" factors exist in DR3,4 heterozygotes, increasing the susceptibility to IDDM. Combinatorial antigens with alpha and beta chains controlled by different haplotypes may exist in DR3,4 heterozygotes, resulting in a strongly increased IDDM risk.

Summary

Data from 70 families with only one IDDM patient, 45 families with more than one IDDM patient, and 49 families with at least one IDDM patient and at least one patient with a DR3- or DR4-associated disease other than IDDM were analyzed for the international IDDM study. The main results are:

1. The positive association between IDDM and HLA antigens DR3 and DR4 in Caucasians is confirmed, as is the excess of DR3, DR4 heterozygotes among the patients.
2. Among Japanese, IDDM is associated with DR4 and DRw9 (rather than DRw8).
3. The frequency of the IDDM gene seems to be high in the population as well as in families. The penetrance, however, is about 10 times higher in families.
4. The three-allele model with two common IDDM genes, being associated with DR3 and DR4, fits the family data significantly better than the two-allele model.
5. In multiplex families with IDDM, autoimmune thyroid disease (ATD), and rheumatoid arthritis (RA), the inheritance of IDDM susceptibility is close to recessive, that of susceptibility to ATD and RA close to dominant. IDDM and ATD, as well as IDDM and RA, may have a common disease allele. ATD and RA have no genetic susceptibility in common.

Acknowledgments. The authors acknowledge the excellent technical assistance by Fe Barberan, Christine Bienek, Christina Erlenkämper, Ute Hintzen, Susanne Raml, and Kristin Quinkert, and the expert assistance in preparing the manuscript by Anne Frankenstein.

References

1. Bertrams J, Dewald G, Spitznas M, Rittner C (1980) HLA-A, B, C, DR, Bf, and C2 alleles in insulin-dependent diabetes mellitus with proliferative retinopathy. Immunobiology 158:113–118
2. Bertrams J, Hintzen U, Schlicht V, Schoeps S, Gries FA, Louton TK, Baur MP (1984) Gene and haplotype frequencies of the fourth component of complement (C4) in type 1 diabetics and normal controls. Immunobiology 166:335–344
3. Bodmer WF (1980) The HLA system and disease. Oliver Sharpey Lecture 1979. J R Coll Physicians London 14:43–50
4. Contu L, Deschamps J, Lestradet H, Hors J, Schmid M, Busson M, Benjamin A, Marcelli-Barge A, Dausset J (1982) HLA haplotype study of 53 juvenile insulin-dependent diabetic (I.D.D.) families. Tissue Antigens 20:123–140
5. De Jongh BM, Burining GJ, Schreuder GNT, Schuurmann RKB, Radder JK, van Loghem E, Meera Khan P, Hauptmann G, van Rood JJ (1984) HLA and Gm in insulin-dependent diabetes in the Netherlands: report on a combined multiplex family and population study. Hum Immunol 10:5–21
6. Farid NR, Larson B, Payne R, Noel EP, Sampson L (1980) Polyglandular autoimmune disease and HLA. Tissue Antigens 16:23–29
7. Grennan DM, Dyer PA, Clague R, Dodds W, Smeaton I, Harris R (1983) Family studies in RA – the importance of HLA-DR4 and of a gene for autoimmune thyroid disease. J Rheumatol 10:584–589
8. Hodge SE, Rotter JI, Lange KL (1980) A three allele model for heterogeneity of juvenile onset insulin dependent diabetes. Ann Hum Genet 43:399–412
9. Lestradet H, Besse J (1975) Prévalence et incidence du diabète juvénile insulin-dépendent en France. Diabete Metab 3:44–53
10. Louis EJ, Thomson G, Payami H (1984) Affected sib method to the intermediate model. Ann Hum Genet 47:225–243
11. Risch N (1984) Segregation analysis incorporating linkage markers. I. Single locus models with an application to type I diabetes. Am J Hum Genet 36:363–386
12. Rotter JI (1981) The modes of inheritance of insulin dependent diabetes mellitus. Am J Hum Genet 33:835–851
13. Spielmann RS, Baker L, Smijewski CM (1980) Gene dosage and susceptibility to insulin-dependent diabetes. Ann Hum Genet, London 44:135–150
14. Svejgaard A, Platz P, Ryder L (1980) Joint report: insulin dependent diabetes mellitus. In: Terasaki PI (ed) Histocompatibility testing 1980. Regents of University of California, Los Angeles, p 638
15. Svejgaard A, Platz P, Ryder L (1983) HLA and disease 1982 – a survey. Immunological Rev. 70:193

HLA-DR3 and DR7-Negative Celiac Disease*

M. DeMarchi and A.O. Carbonara, with the collaboration of N. Ansaldi, P.A.S. Hetzel, S. Koskimies, M. Werkasalo, and J.C. Woodrow

Istituto di Genetica Medica e CNR, Centro di Studio Immunogenetica e d'Istocompatibilità, Via Santena 19, 10226 Torino, Italy

Introduction

HLA studies of celiac disease (CD) have shown an association with DR3 and a weaker one with DR7, with a particularly increased risk for DR3/7 heterozygotes [1, 3–6, 9, 13]. This situation, in several respects, mirrors that found in insulin-dependent diabetes mellitus (IDDM), where DR3 and DR4 are involved [12]. The two main models put forward to explain this dual association are (1) that there are two separate disease susceptibility genes for CD, either DR3 and DR7 themselves or genes in linkage disequilibrium with them, and (2) that there is one susceptibility gene in linkage disequilibrium with both DR antigens, e.g., possible candidates would be the genes underlying the cross-reacting specificity DQw2 [7], as recently proposed on the basis of radioimmunological typing of CD patients' cells [16].

Moreover, in all studies some cases lacking both DR3 and DR7 have been reported, ranging from 1.6% to 13.6% (Table 1). This group might be explained in two main ways: (a) the serological markers are associated by linkage disequilibrium with the unknown responsible gene, which is actually present in both the "positive" and the "negative" patients; (b) the disease is heterogeneous and only one subtype is associated with HLA. In the "negative" patients, the disease might be due to other vicarious genetic factors, or to exposure to overwhelming environmental risks (sometimes these patients are called "phenocopies" or "sporadics" [15]). In CD the association with HLA-B8, before typing for DR3 was possible, was clearly an example of (a). However, the difficulties of serological definition of Class II specificities leave the choice between the two explanations open.

* Work supported in part by CNR P.F. Basi molecolari delle malattie genetiche

Aims of the Study

According to the above framework, two main lines of investigation were proposed to the interested laboratories: (1) to collect DR3- and DR7-negative cases of CD and analyze their HLA genotype with the aim of clarifying whether DR3 and DR7 are directly or only secondarily associated with CD, possibly as a consequence of their known linkage disequilibrium with DQw2; and (2) to compare the clinical and immunological features of this rare group of patients with those of the common DR3 and/or DR7 positives, in order to detect possible heterogeneity between the two groups.

Participating Laboratories

After excluding a few DR7-positive patients, the sample was represented by the families of nine DR3- and DR7-negative probands, contributed by the laboratories of Dr. Hay in Australia, Dr. Koskimies in Finland, Prof. Woodrow in England, and our laboratory in Italy (Table 2). The results

Table 1. Proportion of DR3- and DR7-negative genotypes in Caucasian celiac disease patients

Population	No. negatives	Total	% negatives	Reference
Ireland	4	58	6.9	cited in [13]
England	3	126	2.4	[8]
Australia	4	54	7.4	[9]
Germany – Austria	9	91	9.9	[13]
France	3	22	13.6	[3]
Italy	4	140	2.9	[6]
	1	63	1.6	[16]
Spain	9	163	5.5	[10]
Total	37	717	5.2	

Histocompatibility Testing 1984
Edited by E. D. Albert et al.

Table 2. Main features of the DR3- and DR7-negative patients

Reg.	Lab.	Fam	HLA genotype								Sex	Age at onset[a]
			A	C	B	DR /	A	C	B	DR		
SKA	KOS	11	24	w3	w60	w10 /	2	w3	w62	4	M	6.0
UK1	WOR	10	26	w2	27	4 /	2	–	44	4	M	34.0
	WOR	11	11	–	7	2 /	2	w7	7	4	F	61.0
	WOR	12	11	–	51	1 /	2	w3	w63	4	F	27.0
ANZ	HAY	7	28	w3	w60	w8 /	2	w3	w60	4	F	12.6
	HAY	8	3	w1	51	5 /	3	–	7	4	F	28.4
IT1	CRB	15	1	w7	51	5 /	2	–	w73	4	M	1.8
	CRB	19	30	w5	18	4 /	28	w6	13	4	F	0.7
	CRB	20	3	–	49	2 /	3	–	38	4	M	0.8

[a] Years, months

obtained by cytotoxicity, using WS reagents, are reported here; a parallel study, performed by Dr. Tosi in Rome with radioimmunoassay for selected DR and DQ specificities, is reported elsewhere. Furthermore, a group of five IDDM families where CD is also present, although separately reported [2], will be referred to briefly here because of their special relevance to the present study.

Clinical Features and Patient Selection

It was mandatory that all submitted patients should fulfill the strict diagnostic criteria established by E.S.P.G.A.N. [11]. However, we decided to include four adult cases, though the data on all three specified biopsies were lacking. The overall symptom frequency in the nine patients was quite typical for CD: 78% anemia; 66% anorexia; 55% mood disturbances; 55% failure to thrive; 22% dwarfism; 12% stypsis; 11% edema; 35% other symptoms. In all the patients, clinical improvement occurred within 1 month of gluten-free diet, and in 66% relapse of malabsorption took place within 3 months after gluten challenge. The age of onset ranged from childhood to adulthood, suggesting that this genotype is not preferentially represented in any special age group as suggested for DR7 by some authors [8] but not by all [3, 4]. According to the overall clinical judgement, in 25% of patients the onset of disease showed atypical features: a proportion which corresponds to that usually reported for the whole group of CD patients [5]. In two cases, CD was accompanied by other disease (ulcerative colitis in one case, an unidentified disorder in the other). Thus, within the limitations of the small sample, no obvious evidence of clinical heterogeneity was found between this selected group of DR3- and DR7-negative patients and the overall CD population.

Serology

All the patients were confirmed as negative for DR3 and DR7 with WS reagents. In agreement with our previous report [5], all the patients were DR4 positive; note that two of them were shown to be DR4 homozygous on the basis of family studies, and that in the heterozygotes all other DR specificities were also found (Table 2). Complement polymorphism was performed by only one laboratory (WOR), and will not be discussed here. The serological patterns of the relevant DR4s, both in the probands and in their DR4-positive relatives, encompassed both the long DR4.1 and the DR4.2 pattern, and in the Finnish patient (KOS 11) even the short DR4.3, so that no clear correlation of the CD-associated DR4 gene to one of the "splits" could be substantiated. DQw3 as defined by sera 748, 746, and 744 was present in all patients. It must be noted that two of the present cases had previously been typed in Torino as Dw4 positive. Further studies are needed to establish whether the Dw4-associated split of DR4 is directly associated with CD, or secondarily involved because of association with one of the new DR or DQ (DC) specificities, e.g., DQw3 or DC5.

Family Studies

CD Families. Only two of the families featured multiple cases of CD. In family CRB 19, one HLA-identical sister had just completed the diagnostic series of three jejunal biopsies, as had her older brother. In family HAY 8, the DR3- and DR7-negative proband married a healthy DR3/7 man, and two children, one DR3- and one DR7-positive, developed CD, suggesting a common familial background favoring CD in any of the DR risk genotypes. This single family might indicate that DR4 can act in a similar manner to DR3 or DR7.

Families with IDDM + CD. Five families are included in this group. In two of them the proband suffers from both diseases, a well-known clinical association [14]. In one, a grandfather suffered from IDDM and a granddaughter from CD; he was DR3/4 and she DR3/7, having inherited the same DR3 gene from him. In another family, two HLA-identical children were affected, one with IDDM + CD and the other with IDDM. All probands in this groups were DR3 and DQw3 positive, but their number is too low to make the absence of DR3 positive, DQw3 negative haplotypes significant.

Genetics

As shown in Table 1, only a few cases of "negative" CD patients have been reported, and only nine of them could be included in this collaborative study. Therefore, some caution is appropriate in considering the available sample as representative for all DR3- and DR7-negative CD patients. For example, among nine Spanish DR3 and 7 negatives, five were DR5, but no special mention is made of DR4 [10], which might indicate that no special association was seen. Taking this limitation into account, the finding that DR4 is present in 100% of this group can be discussed in relation to the genetics of CD. Firstly, the frequency of DR antigens in the DR3- and DR7-negative CD patients must be compared with that in DR3- and DR7-negative controls. Otherwise, an apparent negative association of DR4 would result, since the frequency of this antigen in the general population is higher than the entire category of "negatives" in CD. Based on the Eighth Workshop data, the Caucasian DR4 antigen frequency ranges from 18% in Europe to 31% in Australia; after subtraction of DR3 and DR7 these values become 32.6% and 75.3% respectively, with RR estimates between 39 and 6.3. When this value is compared with those of DR3- and DR7-positive genotypes, against the same X/X genotype (X = alleles other than 3, 7, and 4), the result is a weaker association: RR = 1800 – 1400 for DR3/3 and DR3/7, 400 – 300 for DR3/X and 7/X [6]. Unfortunately, this cannot be computed in the selected sample of this study.
Secondly, the hypothesis that DQw2 is the class II antigen primarily associated with all CD patients, and responsible for the increased frequency of DR3 and DR7 [16], is apparently rejected. It could only be maintained with the ad hoc assumption that CD encompasses two separate entities, one associated with DQw2 (+DR3 and/or DR7), and one negative for these antigens. However, this is not substantiated by any evidence of clinical heterogeneity between the "positive" and "negative" cases, and would in any case render ineffective the formal genetic approach to discriminate primary from secondary associations through the "negatives". Other in vitro experiments are required to analyze which of the DR, DQ alpha, DQ beta, or other loci, or shared determinants between their products, are involved in recognition of the gluten protein. This latter hypothesis might be favored, in order to explain how the response to a single protein is common to as many as three different alleles.
Finally, if these data are confirmed in larger samples, CD becomes the only example of 100% association with HLA, thus excluding, or making very rare, the "phenocopies".

References

1. Albert ED, Harms K, Bertele R, Andreas A, McNicholas A, Kuntz B, Scholz S, Schiessl B, Wetzmüller H, Reissinger P, Weeser-Krell C (1978) B-cell alloantigens in coeliac disease. In: McNicholl B, McCarthy C, Fottrell PF (eds) Perspectives in coeliac disease. MTP, Lancaster, p 123
2. Bertrams J, Baur MP (1984) Joint report: insulin-dependent diabetes mellitus (this volume)
3. Betuel H, Gebuhrer L, Percebois H, Descos L, Minaire Y, Bertrand J (1979) Association de la maladie coeliaque de l'adulte avec HLA-DRw3 et DRw7. Gastroenterol Clin Biol 3:605 – 606
4. Betuel H, Gebuhrer L, Descos L, Bertrand J, Freycon F, Lepetit JC (1980) Celiac disease and its association with HLA markers. In: Terasaki PI (ed) Histocompatibility testing 1980. UCLA Tissue Typing Laboratory, Los Angeles, p 668
5. DeMarchi M, Carbonara AO, Ansaldi N, Santini B, Barbera C, Borelli I, Rossino P, Rendine S (1983) HLA-DR3 and DR7 in coeliac disease: immunogenetic and clinical aspects. Gut 24:706 – 712
6. DeMarchi M, Carbonara AO, Mayr W, van Loghem E, de Lange G, Ansaldi N, Curtoni ES (1984) HLA-DR, Gm allotypes and sex as risk factors for coeliac disease (this volume)
7. Duquesnoy RJ (1981) Immunogenetic aspects of the relationship between HLA-DR and the MB and MT system. Transplant Proc 13:1804 – 1807
8. Ellis A, Taylor CJ, Dillon-Remmy M, Woodrow JC, McConnell RB (1984) HLA-DR typing in coeliac disease. Evidence for genetic heterogeneity. Br Med J (in press)
9. Hetzel PAS, Propert DN, Brown RJ, Schanfiels MS, Hay J, Davidson GP, LaBrooy JT, Shearman DJC (1984) HLA and Gm allotype association with coeliac disease in Australian subjects. Abstract, Ninth Histocompatibility Workshop
10. Mearin ML, Biemond I, Pena S, Polanco I, Vazquez C, Schreuder GTHM, DeVries RRP, van Rood JJ (1983) HLA-DR phenotypes in Spanish coeliac children: their contribution to the understanding of the genetics of the disease. Gut 24:532 – 537

11. Meeuwisse GW (1970) Diagnostic criteria in coeliac disease. Acta Paediatr Scand 59:461 – 465
12. Rotter J (1981) The modes of inheritance of insulin-dependent diabetes mellitus. Am J Hum Genet 33:835 – 851
13. Scholz S, Rossipal E, Brautbar C, Ashkenazi A, Harms K, Betuel H, Freycon F, Shmerling DH, McKenna R, Stevens FM, McNicholl B, McCarthy CF, Albert ED (1981) HLA-DR antigens in coeliac disease. A population and multiple case family study. In: McConnell RB (ed) The genetics of coeliac disease. MTP, Lancaster, p 143
14. Scott BB, Losowsky MS (1975) Coeliac disease: a cause of various associated diseases? Lancet i:956 – 957
15. Thomson G (1983) Investigation of the mode of inheritance of the HLA associated diseases by the method of antigen genotype frequency among diseased individuals. Tissue Antigens 21:81 – 104
16. Tosi R, Vismara D, Tanigaki N, Ferrara GB, Cicimarra F, Buffolano W, Follo D, Auricchio S (1983) Evidence that coeliac disease is primarily associated with a DC locus allelic specificity. Clin Immunol Immunopathol 28:395 – 404

Leprosy*

R.R.P. de Vries[1], S.W. Serjeantson[2], and Z. Layrisse[3]

1 Dept. of Immunohematology and Blood Bank, University Hospital, 2333 AA Leiden, The Netherlands
2 Dept. of Human Biology, Johan Curtin School of Medical Research, P.O. Box 334, Canberra 2601, Australia
3 Instituto Venezuelano de Investigaciones Cientificas (IVIC), Apartado 1827, Caracas 1010a, Venezuela

Participants

Alvarez, I., Perez-Campos, H., Vila, V., Rosen, V. Laboratorio de Histocompatibilidad. Banco Nacional de Organos Tejidos, Montevideo, Uruguay

De Vries, R. R. P., van Eden, W., Schreuder, G. M. T., Convit, J., Gonzalez, N. M.: Dept of Immunohematology and Blood Bank, University Hospital, Leiden, The Netherlands; Instituto de Dermatologia, Caracas 101, Venezuela

du Toit, E. D., Hitzeroth, H. W., Kleeberg, H. H., Kok, S.: Provincial Laboratory for Tissue Immunology, Cape Town; Genetic Services, Dept. of Health Welfare and Pensions, Tuberculosis Research Institute of the SAMRC; Westford Hospital, Pretoria, South Africa

Gerbase-de Lima, M., Persoli, L. B., Stilmann R. F., Gerbase, A. C., Mendes, N. F.: Disciplina de Imunologia, Escola Paulista de Medicina São Paulo, Brazil; Secretaria da Saude, Rio Grande do Sul, Brazil

Giraudo, C., Tello, E., Gomez, V.: Laboratorio de Histocompatibilidad, Hospital Privado, Cordoba, Argentina

Gorodezky, C., Alvarenga, M. V., Flores, J., Castro, L. E., Erosa, G., Debaz, H., Castro Bernal, E., Hernandez, O., Rodriguez, O.: Laboratorio de Investigaciones Immunologicas, ISET, S.S.A. Centro Dermatologica Pascua (CPD), S.S.A., Mexico

Jobim, L. F.: Laboratorio de Imunogenetica, Hospital de Clinicas, Universidade Federal Rio Grande do Sul, Porto Alegre, Brazil

Ferreira, E., Catanio, R. I. I. S., Pereira, N. F., Guilherme, L., Niedfeld, M. F., Miranda, R. N.: Laboratorio de Imunogenetica, Hospital de Clinicas, Universidade Federal Do Parana, Curitiba, Parana, Brazil

Hansen, J. A., Kim, S. J.: Puget Sound Blood Center, University of Washington, Seattle, USA; Dept. of Microbiology, Yosei University, Seoul, Korea

Mauff, G.: Hygiene Institut, University of Cologne, West Germany

Mehra, N. K., Vaidya, M. C., Sharma, A. K., Shastri, S.: All India Institute of Medical Sciences and Safdarjang Hospital, New Delhi; Gandhi Memorial Leprosy Foundation, Wardha, India

Moraes, M. E., Ricart, J., Gallo, M. E. N., Almeida, S. M., Salatiel, I. S., Zamolyi, G., Zamolyi, M., Faria, L., Rutowitsch, M., Moraes, J. R.: Hospital Servidores do Estado, Universidad Estado do Rio de Janeiro, Centro de Saude C. Antonio da Silva, AMB. Souza Araujo Fiocruz, Rio de Janeiro, Brazil

Pollack, M. Ching, C., Reinhardt, E., Levis, W.: Memorial Sloan-Kettering Cancer Center, 1275 York Avenue, New York 10021, USA

Prigoshin de Godelman, N., Uccello, C. M., Schnurmajer, D., Gatti, R.: Laboratorio de Histocompatibilidad, Instituto Medico Antartida, Hospital Privado; Servicio de Dermatologia, Hospital Muniz, Buenos Aires, Argentina

Rosales, T., Oliveira de Paula, D., Xavier, M. A., Cossermeli, W.: Laboratorio de Investigacoes em Reumatologia, Hospital das Clinicas, Facultade de Medicina, Sao Paulo, Brazil

Sasazuki, T., Kikuchi, I., Ozawa, T.: Dept of Human Genetics, Medical Research Institute, Tokyo Medical and Dental University, Japan

Sekiguchi S.: National Defense Medical College, 3-2 Namiki, Tokorozaura, Saitama 359, Japan

* Material and financial support was provided via the Immunology of Leprosy (IMMLEP) component of the UNDP/World Bank/WHO special programme for Research and Training in Tropical Diseases

Histocompatibility Testing 1984
Edited by E. D. Albert et al.

Introduction

Clinical and Immunological Aspects of Leprosy

Leprosy is a chronic infectious disease which presently affects more than 15 million individuals. The disease is the result of the interaction between *Mycobacterium leprae* and the immune system of the infected host, *M. leprae* by itself being a virtually harmless bacillus. Apparently the majority of individuals exposed to or infected with *M. leprae* develops effective immunity to *M. leprae* without disease. A minority, however, may develop a wide range of clinical symptoms, which show striking interindividual variability. This clinical spectrum closely parallels the immunological spectrum of responsiveness displayed by the host [1, 2].

The two extremes of the leprosy spectrum are polar tuberculoid (TT) and polar lepromatous (LL) leprosy. TT leprosy is characterized clinically by one or a few well-demonstrated skin lesions with anesthesia due to nerve involvement which may subsequently lead to deformities. There are few bacteria and the process is self-healing. Immunologically, there is obvious cellular immune reactivity toward *M. leprae:* lymphocyte (mainly OKT4-positive T cells) infiltration with epitheloid cell granulomata in the lesions, and strongly positive skin test (Mitsuda reaction) and in vitro (lymphocyte transformation test) immune reactivity. Untreated LL leprosy patients, on the other hand, have nodules or skin lesions containing large numbers of macrophages loaded with *M. leprae* and a striking absence of cellular immune reactivity toward *M. leprae:* no or only slight lymphocyte infiltration (mainly OKT8-positive T cells), no granuloma formation, negative skin test and in vitro reactivity. An inverse relationship exists between cellular and humoral immune reactivity toward *M. leprae:* antibody titers are low or absent in TT and high among LL leprosy patients, the latter probably being secondary to the defective cellular immunity leading to persistent bacterial load. The absence of cellular immune reactivity in lepromatous leprosy is specific for *M. leprae.*

Between the two extremes (TT and LL leprosy) there is a range of clinical, histopathological, and immunological symptoms. For research purposes, the most widely used classification is the five-group scale according to Ridley and Jopling [2]: polar tuberculoid (TT), borderline tuberculoid (BT), borderline (BB), borderline lepromatous (BL), and polar lepromatous (LL). From TT to LL there is a gradual decrease of cellular immunity and an increase in bacterial load. The nature of the immune defect underlying the *M. leprae*-specific anergy in lepromatous leprosy is still unknown, although most evidence has been presented for *M. leprae*-specific suppressor T cells. Even less is known about the defect leading to tuberculoid leprosy as opposed to effective immunity without disease.

HLA and Leprosy

Soon after the demonstration of MHC-linked immune response genes and the first associations between HLA and disease, a number of population studies were performed comparing the HLA-A and B antigen frequencies between different categories of leprosy patients and controls [reviewed in 3, 4]. The associations reported were either weak or not confirmed in other populations, and different associations were reported among different populations.

Because these data might be compatible with HLA-linked disease susceptibility genes showing different linkage disequilibria in different populations, family studies were performed to demonstrate such genes. Until recently, sufficient data were available only for TT leprosy, which was shown to be controlled by an HLA-linked gene, most probably recessive [4, 5]. Recently, two studies have been performed which indicate that the development of lepromatous leprosy is controlled by another HLA-linked gene [5]. These family studies also provided evidence against susceptibility to leprosy per se being controlled by HLA-linked genes [5]. In search for genetic markers for HLA-linked control of the development of these leprosy types, HLA-DR and other class II HLA antigens were studied. Stronger and more consistent associations were found for these HLA class II antigens than for the HLA class I antigens. Thus HLA-DQw1 was found to be associated with lepromatous leprosy in several populations [3–5]. However, the associations reported are still rather weak and therefore of little or no practical value. There still exists considerable interpopulation heterogeneity which indicates that the associated HLA antigens are not directly responsible. Therefore we may expect to discover better markers in the future. This not only has practical implications but is also important for studies on the mechanism of HLA-linked control of leprosy type.

A direct role for HLA class II molecules in the interaction between antigen-presenting cells and T cells in *M. leprae*-specific cellular immune responsiveness has been shown [6]. Furthermore, an in vitro correlate for an in vivo association between a particular HLA-DR type (DR3) and TT leprosy has been demonstrated [5, 6]. Thus the nature and role of HLA class II immune response gene products in leprosy may be unraveled in the future. This immunogenetic approach may answer how effective vs defective immune responsiveness to *M.*

leprae is established and thus provide tools for prevention and therapy of leprosy.

Aim of this Study

The evidence for a role of HLA-linked genes controlling the differential host response to *M. leprae* is derived from a limited number of family studies performed by only a few investigators [3–5]. Therefore, this Ninth International Histocompatibility Workshop study on HLA and leprosy was planned to document in a collaborative effort the relationship between HLA and leprosy, in particular the TT and LL types. To this purpose, the families to be included in the study were selected according to uniform criteria in order to obtain as homogeneous a data set as possible. Apart from the use of the same set of HLA typing sera, uniformity was further realized by using the same criteria for leprosy classification and the same lepromin (lepromin-A, provided via WHO) to measure in vivo cellular immune reactivity toward *M. leprae.*

Materials and Methods

Families Tested

In order to be maximally informative and to avoid ascertainment bias, the participants were asked to select families according to the following four criteria:

1. Not previously typed for HLA
2. At least two siblings affected (presently or in the past) with TT leprosy, or at least two siblings affected with BL or LL leprosy
3. At least one healthy sibling older than the youngest affected sibling
4. Both parents available for examination

Data were sent from 75 families containing 434 individuals. They belonged to at least ten different ethnic groups and originated from 11 different countries. The majority, however, were from Latin America and of mestizo or Caucasian descent.

Leprosy Classification and Lepromin Testing

Every member of a family included in this workshop study had to be examined by an experienced leprologist, and a detailed history had to be taken in order not to miss a cured case of leprosy. In the genetic analysis, cured patients were considered as susceptible or affected.

For every active or cured leprosy patient, the following information had to be available:

1. Leprosy classification according to the Ridley and Jopling [2] five-group system: TT, BT, BB, BL, LL.
2. A biopsy specimen taken before treatment.

Every participant was urged to perform a lepromin skin test on every individual tested. To this purpose, lepromin-A, all derived from the same batch of *M. leprae*-infected armadillo tissue and prepared in the National Hansen Disease Centre (Carville, USA), was made available through the Immunology of Leprosy section (IMMLEP) of the World Health Organisation. Lepromin results were scored in millimeters duration. Results of > 3 mm were considered positive.

HLA and Complement Typing

Both parents, affected siblings, and at least one healthy sibling older than the youngest affected sibling had to be typed for HLA-A, B, C, DR, and non-DR class II antigens using the workshop serum set. Every participant was requested to type or refer material for typing for GLO and the Bf, C2, and C4 polymorphisms. Bf, C2 and C4 typing was performed for most of the Latin American families and the South African family by Dr. G. Mauff (Cologne, West Germany).

Data Analysis

Cosegregation of Leprosy Status and Lepromin Responsiveness with HLA. Using the original selection criteria only a limited number of families would have been acceptable for analysis. Therefore, we decided to use somewhat less strict criteria which we considered not to induce an ascertainment bias. We included all families in which HLA haplotypes could be reliably assigned, also those where the leprosy status of both parents was not completely known. Some families were included that contained no healthy sibling older than the youngest patient, but at least one sibling affected with TT and one with BL or LL leprosy. Thus 50 families were available for analysis.

The method used to analyze deviations from randomness of the observed HLA haplotype segregation in relation to leprosy status and lepromin responsiveness indicating the involvement of HLA-linked genes was developed by Nijenhuis and has been described previously [7]. Briefly, the observed difference between the number of siblings that inherited one haplotype from a parent and those that inherited the other haplotype (D) is compared with the expected difference (d) assuming random segregation. The method allows for pooling of data from sibships of different sizes. The test statistic is:

$$\chi^2 = \frac{\{|\sum D - \sum d| - 0.5\}^2}{\sum \sigma_d^2}$$

where σ_d^2 is the variance of d.

Because of the nature of the material, no systematic search for associations with particular HLA types was performed. However, we did look particularly for the possible preferential segregation of two HLA antigens, namely DQw1 and DR3 toward children affected with lepromatous or lepromin-negative leprosy [4, 5]. To this purpose the one-sided p value from the binomial distribution with $P = 0.50$ was approximated with the one-sided p of the standard normal distribution $T = x_i - ½ - ½N$ divided by $½\sqrt{N}$, where N is the number of segregations studied and x_i the highest of the two values obtained for inheritance or not of the particular HLA type.

Linkage Analysis. Formal linkage analyses of HLA haplotypes and several clinical parameters were undertaken in multiple-case families. These parameters included presence or absence of leprosy, in vivo response to lepromin, and clinical type of leprosy. Linkage was measured by maximum likelihood estimation of the recombination fraction (θ), based on the relative probability (P_R) of having generated the observed family distribution. The probability of obtaining the observed combinations of HLA haplotypes and leprosy status when recombination values varied between 0.0 and 0.5 was compared with the probability of no linkage ($\theta = 0.5$). $Log_{10} P_R$, defined as the lod score, was estimated for each family. Since lod scores are additive, they were summated for all families irrespective of ethnic group.

Lod scores were calculated using the computer program LIPED [8]. Conventionally, a lod score less than −2 is sufficient to exclude linkage. A lod score greater than +3 confirms linkage of two loci, and one of between +2 and +3 is suggestive of linkage. In the initial exploratory analyses of multiple-case leprosy families, the recombination fraction was considered equal in males and females. For families where one or neither parent had been examined for leprosy it was necessary to provide an estimate of the population frequency of the putative susceptibility allele to accommodate the possibility that the untested parent carried the allele. The population prevalence of genetic predisposition to leprosy was assumed to be 1%, so that the gene frequency was given as 0.1 under models where leprosy susceptibility was recessive and as 0.005 under dominant models.

Results

Cosegregation Analyses

The most important results are summarized in Table 1. We first analyzed the possible cosegregation of leprosy or leprosy type with HLA. No significantly increased sharing of HLA haplotypes was observed among siblings affected with leprosy but including those with different leprosy types. The same was true for siblings affected with TT leprosy, but only a few sibships were available for this analysis. In contrast, siblings affected with lepromatous (BL or LL) leprosy shared an HLA haplotype significantly more often than expected ($p < 0.025$). The latter was only true for haplotypes from parents not affected with lepromatous leprosy. Next, we analyzed lepromin responsiveness irrespective of leprosy status. We observed significantly ($p < 0.05$) decreased sharing of haplotypes inherited from lepromin-positive parents among sibships containing both lepromin-positive and -negative siblings. This indicated HLA-linked genetic heterogeneity of lepromin responsiveness. Whereas lepromin-positive siblings still tended to show decreased haplotype sharing and thus heterogeneity, lepromin-negative siblings seemed to show an excess sharing of haplotypes from lepromin-positive parents. However, these data failed to reach significance.

Finally, we combined the lepromin data with leprosy status. Among lepromin-positive siblings, healthy or affected, no significant deviation from random segregation was observed. In contrast, lepromin-negative leprosy patients shared HLA haplotypes significantly more often than expected, but only from their lepromin-positive affected parents. There was only one family containing more than two lepromin-negative healthy siblings.

A preferential segregation of DQw1 from DQw1 heterozygous healthy parent to children affected with lepromin-negative leprosy was observed: of 35 informative segregations, DQw1 was inherited 25 times ($p < 0.01$). No significantly non-random segregation was observed for HLA-DR3.

Linkage Analysis

Linkage analysis showed that presence or absence of leprosy was not closely linked with HLA (Table 2). Both dominant and recessive models with varying degrees of penetrance were explored. When penetrance was low, lod scores uninformatively actively tended to zero, and these data are not shown. However, since the chance of a monozygotic twin with an affected twin developing leprosy has been

Table. 1. Cosegregation of leprosy status and lepromin responsiveness with HLA

Sibs		Parents		ΣD	Σd	$\Sigma \sigma_d^2$	χ^2	P
Leprosy	Lepromin	Leprosy	Lepromin					
T+L				62	59.8	41	0.07	n.s.
TT				16	17	14	0.02	n.s.
L				59	45	39.5	4.61	< 0.025
	pos. + neg.		pos.	32	46.3	41.9	4.55	< 0.05
	pos. + neg.		neg.	48	47.1	42.2	0.00	n.s.
	pos.			36	47.8	47.2	2.71	n.s.
	neg.		pos.	27	19.5	16.25	3.02	n.s.
	neg.		neg.	33	32.5	27.25	0.00	n.s.
pos.	pos.			28	25	23.5	0.27	n.s.
neg.	pos.			36	41.2	44.7	0.50	n.s.
	neg.	pos.	pos.	12	6	4.50	6.72	< 0.01
pos.	neg.	other		54	49.5	40.25	0.40	n.s.

estimated as 60%−85% in different studies, a penetrance value of 70% may not be unrealistic. When susceptibility to *M. leprae* was considered to be under the control of a dominant gene, linkage with HLA could be excluded at recombination fractions less than 20%. When leprosy susceptibility was considered recessive, close linkage with HLA could also be excluded, with significantly negative lod scores at $\theta = 0.10$. Under the recessive hypothesis, lod scores obtain a maximum value at $\theta = 0.3$, although they do not reach statistical significance. When the lod score of 0.81 observed in the 65 Ninth Workshop families at a penetrance value of 70% is added to that observed in 109 previously published families, the total lod score of 2.93 suggests that HLA haplotype sharing may be a significant determinant of leprosy status in some families. This possibility was explored further in the Ninth Workshop families. Clinical type of leprosy was taken into account by estimating lod scores separately in families concordant for lepromatous leprosy, families concordant for tuberculoid leprosy, and discordant families.

Analyses were repeated with healthy sibs excluded, to allow for the possibility that healthy sibs had not been sufficiently exposed to *M. leprae* to permit clinical infection. In addition, three-allele genetic models that incorporated leprosy clinical type were tested to examine the hypothesis that more than one HLA-linked susceptibility allele is involved in determining clinical status. None of these analyses could unequivocally implicate or exclude linkage between HLA and leprosy type, although the highest lod scores occurred in families with at least two lepromatous sibs and an affected parent, as demonstrated in the cosegregation analysis.

Convincing evidence was obtained for linkage between HLA and in vivo response to lepromin in 43 families tested with standardized WHO lepromin-A (Table 3). When positive response to lepromin-A was considered dominant, with penetrance of 90%, there was strong evidence for close linkage with HLA, with the lod score attaining a maximum value of 2.84 at a recombination value tending to zero. Nonresponders included LL, BL, and BB patients, as well as some healthy family members.

There was no clear evidence for linkage of complement haplotypes or any single complement allotype to leprosy in general or to the clinical types of leprosy in those Ninth Workshop families in which segregation of complement types could be deduced.

Table 2. Lod scores for HLA haplotypes and leprosy in 65 families, ignoring clinical type

Genetic model	Recombinant fraction (θ)				
	$\theta = 0.0$	$\theta = 0.1$	$\theta = 0.2$	$\theta = 0.3$	$\theta = 0.4$
Leprosy recessive					
Penetrance: 100%	−57.96	− 8.96	−0.50	0.59	0.52
90%	−32.92	− 6.82	−0.37	1.05	0.54
70%	−21.22	− 4.52	−0.11	0.81	0.39
Leprosy dominant					
Penetrance: 100%	−71.29	−13.52	−4.36	−1.06	−0.17
90%	−31.45	− 9.67	−3.12	−0.68	−0.10
70%	−18.61	− 5.13	−1.29	−0.10	−0.01

Table 3. Lod scores for HLA haplotypes and lepromin-A positive responses in 43 families

Genetic model	Recombination fraction (θ)				
	$\theta = 0.0$	$\theta = 0.1$	$\theta = 0.2$	$\theta = 0.3$	$\theta = 0.4$
Dominant	2.84	2.26	1.45	0.72	0.20
Recessive	−11.91	−3.60	−0.93	−0.02	0.07

For C4, this may be attributed in part to the difficulties in defining duplicated and silent alleles (see C. Rittner and G. Mauff, C4 Polymorphism, this volume), and in part to the relative lack of unusual allotypes.

Discussion

Analysis of Ninth Workshop families has shown that susceptibility to leprosy per se is not controlled by MHC-linked factors. This should provide greater impetus for identifying non-HLA genetic factors. In the mouse, a single non-H2 locus codes for resistance or susceptibility to a number of intra-cellular parasites, including *Mycobacteria* [9], and mouse strain differences in susceptibility to intracellular parasites can be attributed to differences in bacteriostatic or bacteriocidal activity of macrophages. A similar locus may well exist in man.

The most significant role for HLA-linked factors in leprosy related to control of in vivo response to lepromin, evidenced in both the cosegregation and linkage analyses. There are two possible interpretations of this observation. First, classification of leprosy type according to lepromin response may have defined a more homogeneous group of patients than was otherwise possible. In addition, some healthy sibs who failed to respond to lepromin may have preclinical leprosy infection, but in the absence of antibody studies, this is conjectural. Definition of this homogeneous group then permitted classification of the role of MHC factors in determining clinical type of leprosy. The second interpretation is that MHC-linked factors control immune response to lepromin, in healthy individuals as well as in those with leprosy. Because we were only able to study a few lepromin-negative healthy individuals, it is not possible to discriminate between these two possibilities.

Within clinical subcategories of leprosy, there is often wide variation in individual immune response. The testing of families with lepromin-A successfully identified one such immune response category, predominantly lepromatous in clinical type, and HLA distributions strongly suggest that HLA-related mechanisms are involved in determining this clinical group. Within the category of tuberculoid leprosy there is great variation in lymphocyte transformation test responses to *M. leprae*, but these were not determined in Ninth Workshop families. Also, the number of tuberculoid patients submitted to the Workshop was comparatively small. Thus we were unable to demonstrate a role for HLA in determining susceptibility to tuberculoid leprosy.

A few comments regarding the suggested mode of inheritance and ascertainment bias are warranted. In determining the genetic model for susceptibility to *M. leprae*, the method of ascertainment of leprosy families on the basis of two affected offspring levels tends to bias the model in favor of an recessive model of transmission. In many families neither parent was affected, so that comparatively low penetrance rates would need to be invoked to accommodate a dominant model. Clearly, if selection had been based on families with one parent affected, a dominant mode of inheritance would have been favored. A similar bias has not affected the analysis of lepromin-A responses. In this analysis, the informative families were those where one parent was a heterozygote for the putative "lepromin response" locus and the other parent was a homozygous responder or a nonresponder.

We conclude that susceptibility to leprosy is determined by non-HLA factors, which may be genetic as well as environmental, but that in the presence of infection, HLA-related mechanisms determine host response and thus clinical type of leprosy. HLA-DQw1 might be a universal genetic marker for lepromin unresponsiveness, i.e., for lepromin-negative leprosy.

References

1. Godal T (1978) Immunological aspects of leprosy: present status. Prog Allergy 25:211–242
2. Ridley DS, Jopling WH (1966) Classification of leprosy according to immunity. A five group system. Int J Lepr 34:225–273
3. De Vries RRP, van Eden W, Van Rood JJ (1981) HLA-linked control of the course of *M. leprae* infections. Lepr Rev 52 suppl 1:109–119
4. Serjeantson SW (1983) HLA and susceptibility to leprosy. Immunol Rev 70:24–47
5. Van Eden W, de Vries RRP (1984) HLA and leprosy: a re-evaluation. Lepr Rev 55:89–104
6. De Vries RRP, van Eden W, Ottenhoff THM (1984) HLA class II immune response genes and products in leprosy. Prog Allergy (in press)
7. De Vries RRP, Lai A Fat RFM, Nijenhuis LE, Van Rood JJ (1976) HLA-linked genetic control of host response to *Mycobacterium leprae*. Lancet 2:1328–1330
8. Ott J (1974) Estimation of the recombination fraction in human pedigrees: efficient computation of the likelihood for human linkage studies. Am J Hum Genet 26:588–597
9. Skamene E, Gros P, Forget A, Kongshavn PAL, St Charles C, Taylor BA (1982) Genetic regulation of resistance to intracellular pathogens. Nature 297:506–509

Juvenile Chronic Arthritis, Pauciarticular Type

B.M. Ansell and E.D. Albert

1 Division of Rheumatology, Clinical Research Centre Northwick Park Hospital, Harrow, Middlesex, U.K.
2 Immunogenetics Laboratory München, Pettenkoferstraße 8 a, 8000 München 2, Federal Republic of Germany

On behalf of: A. Arnaiz Villena, V. Balog, S. Barocci, E. Bhettay, W. Braun, L. Brkljacic, D. Bucin, C. B. Carpenter, F. Celada, F. Eawood, H. Dick, E. duToit, D. Glass, J. Gomez-Reino, P. J. Hall, K. G. Heide, A. Kastelan, S. Knight, M. Kreisler, R. M. Küster, M. Larson, A. Leak, B. Löw, R. Madhok, D. J. Mazanec, F. Mercuriali, T. Moore, M. Moreno, J. Mulero, L. Muylle, K. G. Oen, J. W. Oldfather, L. Pachmann, R. E. Petty, N. Prigoshin, R. Radvanyi, P. Reekers, K. Rich, G. Rodey, F. Rre, S. Scholz, E. Schretlen, M. L. Schroeder, E. Schuchmann, R. Sturrock, N. Suciu- Foca, H. Svantesson, B. Taskesi, E. Thorsby, H. Truckenbrodt, L. van de Putte, H. Venning, J. L. Vicario, L. Wells, E. Westphal, A. A. Zachary
The following laboratories contributed families to the study: BEN MUY, BEN REE, EAE KAS, FRA ARN, FRA KRE, GER ALB, GER WES, IT1 MRC, IT2 CEL, LAT PRZ, NCY CAR, SAF DUT, SCA LOW, SCA TSB, UKI DIC, UKI KNT, US1 STL, US4 RAD, US5 MLS, US6 BRN, US8 NSF

Aims of Study

The early onset pauciarticular form of juvenile chronic arthritis (JCA) was chosen because it provides a relatively well established clinical entity within the heterogeneous group of disease defined as JCA. The aim of the study was to confirm and extend the observations on the association of this subgroup with HLA-DR5 and DRw8 [2–6]. Due to the high degree of serological cross-reactivity between DR5 and DRw8 it has been asked whether the high frequency of DRw8 observed in JCA patients might not be due to an artefact caused by serological cross-reactivity. Furthermore, it was intended to investigate whether other HLA-linked alleles or haplotypic combinations of alleles are involved in coding for disease susceptibility or correlate with other features, such as the age at onset, the presence of antinuclear antibodies and iridocyclitis. Families with double cases were sought to increase the knowledge on the distribution of HLA haplotypes among sib pairs.

Exclusions

Of a total of 153 families submitted for which there was adequate information, 11 families were excluded because the patients had a clinically different form of JCA i.e. a polyarticular onset, or the typical symptoms of juvenile spondylitis. Among the excluded were patients in whom psoriasis was found or in whose family members psoriasis was known.

Controls

Since the patients in this study originate from many different ethnically quite heterogeneous areas of North America, South Africa and Europe, two types of controls were used throughout:

1. A control panel of haplotypes from unrelated healthy Caucasian individuals ($n = 2134$ haplotypes for the HLA-A, B haplotype frequencies and $n = 2032$ for the HLA-B, DR haplotypes). This panel represents the total Caucasian frequencies.
2. A control panel selected from healthy individuals belonging to the same ethnic groups from which the patients had originated. If, for example, one laboratory submitted 10 patients and their families, 10 healthy Caucasian individuals also tested by this laboratory were included in the control panel. Thus a heterogeneous control panel was established which contained the same type of ethnic variation as the panel of patients.

Variations in antigen frequencies were only considered significant if they could be shown in comparison with both control populations.

HLA Allele Frequencies

Since all patients were genotyped, the analysis of HLA antigen frequencies is done on the genotypic level.

The HLA-A, B and C gene frequencies of 141 patients with JCA and the two types of controls are listed in Table 1. The gene frequencies of HLA-A2, DR5 and DRw8 are increased, while HLA-DR2 and DR4 show a decreased frequency. There are no significant deviations among the alleles of the B locus or the C locus.

The supertypic specificities DRw52 and DRw53 show significant deviations in frequency among patients. The increase for DRw52, however, does not go beyond that expected on the basis of the known

Histocompatibility Testing 1984
Edited by E. D. Albert et al.

Table 1. Gene frequencies of HLA alleles in 141 patients with juvenile chronic arthritis

	Patients $n = 282$	Matched controls (a) $n = 284$	Caucasian controls (b) $n = 2134$	Chi-square a	Chi-square b
HLA-A1	0.123 (38)	0.106 (30)	0.143		
HLA-A2	0.418 (118)	0.324 (92)	0.278	5.6*	11.9**
HLA-A3	0.085 (24)	0.116 (33)	0.131		
HLA-A11	0.046 (13)	0.106 (30)	0.065		
HLA-A23	0.011 (3)	0.032 (9)	0.017		
HLA-A24	0.099 (28)	0.070 (20)	0.102		
HLA-A25	0.018 (5)	0.018 (5)	0.025		
HLA-A26	0.046 (13)	0.021 (6)	0.029		
HLA-A28	0.035 (10)	0.035 (10)	0.046		
HLA-A29	0.018 (5)	0.021 (6)	0.034		
HLA-A30	0.025 (7)	0.035 (10)	0.032		
HLA-A31	0.025 (7)	0.032 (9)	0.032		
HLA-A32	0.018 (5)	0.063 (18)	0.041	6.3*	2.2
HLA-Aw33	0.011 (3)	0.018 (5)	0.017		
HLA-Aw34	0.007 (2)	– (0)	0.001		
HLA-Aw66	0.004 (1)	0.004 (1)	–		
HLA-AX	– (0)	– (0)	0.007		
* $p = 0.02$; ** $p = 0.0006$					
HLA-B7	0.089 (25)	0.123 (35)	0.115		
HLA-B8	0.103 (29)	0.099 (28)	0.100		
HLA-B13	0.025 (7)	0.035 (10)	0.027		
HLA-B14	0.014 (4)	0.032 (9)	0.037		
HLA-B18	0.057 (16)	0.039 (11)	0.056		
HLA-B27	0.074 (21)	0.042 (12)	0.038	2.3	2.7
HLA-B35	0.135 (38)	0.095 (27)	0.107		
HLA-B37	0.004 (1)	0.014 (4)	0.014		
HLA-B38	0.043 (12)	0.021 (6)	0.024		
HLA-B39	0.046 (13)	0.014 (4)	0.025	4.1	1.3
HLA-Bw41	0.004 (1)	0.011 (3)	0.009		
HLA-B44	0.142 (40)	0.165 (47)	0.138		
HLA-B45	– (0)	0.007 (2)	0.005		
HLA-Bw47	– (0)	– (0)	0.004		
HLA-Bw48	– (0)	– (0)	0.001		
HLA-B49	0.011 (3)	0.028 (8)	0.023		
HLA-Bw50	0.007 (2)	0.004 (1)	0.012		
HLA-B51	0.071 (20)	0.025 (7)	0.047	5.2	1.2
HLA-Bw52	0.007 (2)	0.021 (6)	0.016		
HLA-Bw53	– (0)	0.011 (3)	0.005		
HLA-Bw54	– (0)	– (0)	–		
HLA-Bw55	0.011 (3)	0.014 (4)	0.017		
HLA-Bw56	0.007 (2)	0.004 (1)	0.007		
HLA-Bw57	0.014 (4)	0.046 (13)	0.028	3.7	
HLA-Bw58	0.011 (3)	0.007 (2)	0.018		
HLA-Bw59	– (0)	– (0)	–		
HLA-Bw60	0.064 (18)	0.046 (13)	0.037		
HLA-Bw61	0.004 (1)	0.018 (5)	0.013		
HLA-Bw62	0.053 (15)	0.060 (17)	0.059		
HLA-Bw63	0.004 (1)	0.004 (1)	0.005		
HLA-BX	0.007 (2)	0.018 (5)	0.013		
HLA-Cw1	0.039 (11)	0.018 (5)	0.037		
HLA-Cw2	0.088 (25)	0.063 (18)	0.089		
HLA-Cw3	0.116 (33)	0.120 (34)	0.134		
HLA-Cw4	0.127 (36)	0.120 (34)	0.115		
HLA-Cw5	0.078 (22)	0.074 (21)	0.068		
HLA-Cw6	0.046 (13)	0.099 (20)	0.043		
HLA-Cw7	0.236 (67)	0.222 (63)	0.267		
HLA-Cw8	0.014 (4)	0.025 (7)	0.014		
HLA-CwX	0.257 (73)	0.261 (74)	0.232		

Table 1. (continued)

	Patients $n = 278$	Matched controls (a) $n = 284$	Caucasian controls (b) $n = 2032$	Chi-square a	b
HLA-DR1	0.054 (15)	0.098 (28)	0.096	3.4	3.1
HLA-DR2	0.093 (26)	0.172 (49)	0.163	6.9*	5.2*
HLA-DR3	0.139 (38)	0.133 (32)	0.128		
HLA-DR4	0.054 (15)	0.134 (38)	0.136	9.6**	10.1**
HLA-DR5	0.221 (62)	0.148 (42)	0.152	4.8*	4.3*
HLA-DRw6	0.146 (41)	0.113 (32)	0.114		
HLA-DR7	0.075 (21)	0.144 (41)	0.120	6.1*	2.5
HLA-DRw8	0.139 (39)	0.028 (8)	0.027	21.6***	20.9***
HLA-DRw9	0.021 (6)	0.004 (1)	0.010		
HLA-DRw10	– (0)	0.004 (1)	0.008		
HLA-DRX	0.054 (15)	0.042 (12)	0.049		

	Patients $n = 282$	Matched controls (a) $n = 284$	Caucasian controls (b) $n = 2134$	Chi-square a	b
HLA-DRw52	0.550 (153)	0.401 (114)	0.400	11.9**	12.5**
HLA-DRw53	0.151 (42)	0.292 (83)	0.290	15.4**	14.7**
HLA-DQw1	0.309 (86)	0.370 (105)	0.370	2.0	1.8
HLA-DQw2	0.169 (47)	0.190 (54)	0.190	0.3	0.3
HLA-DQw3	0.281 (78)	0.239 (68)	0.240	1.0	0.9

Absolute numbers of haplotypes given in parentheses
* p 0.05 – 0.005; ** p 0.005 – 0.001; *** $p < 10^{-5}$

inclusion of DR5 and DRw8 into DRw52. Likewise, the decrease for DRw53 is in complete agreement with the low frequencies of DR4, 7 and w9. The DQ alleles DQw1, DQw2 and DQw3 do not exhibit any significant deviation.

Compensation of the Frequency Increase

If some alleles of a gene locus show an increased frequency, the other alleles of the same locus must show a compensatory decrease in frequency. If the other HLA alleles are neutral with respect to disease susceptibility, it can be expected that this compensatory frequency decrease should be distributed evenly, so that a frequent allele should show a more prominent decrease than an infrequent allele. Thus the expected degree of decrease can be calculated for the alleles of each locus on the genotypic level. These calculations are shown for the HLA-A locus and the DR locus in Tables 2 and 3. From Table 2 it is seen that the antigen A26 is found more commonly than one would expect on the basis of an evenly distributed decrease. All other alleles do not differ significantly from the frequency which is expected under the assumption of neutrality with respect to disease susceptibility. In the DR locus, it appears that DR4 is less frequently found and DRw6 more frequently found than expected on the basis of neutrality with respect to disease susceptibility. We also observed a relative increase in frequency for the allele DR3, although this does not quite reach statistical significance compared with the control population.

Bf Polymorphism

The Bf alleles were tested in 77 patients and their relatives. The results are listed in Table 4. The allele Bf S appears to have a slightly although not significantly higher frequency in patients than in the controls.

C4 Polymorphism

C4 polymorphism was tested in 52 of the patients and their families. The frequencies of the C4-A and C4-B alleles as well as of some C4-A, B haplotypes in patients and controls are listed in Table 5. There is a slight increase in frequency for the C4-haplotype A3, B1; however, this deviation is not significant after correction for the large number of comparisons. It has been reported [7] that the C4 allele B2 is frequent among patients with JCA. In the

Table 2. Compensation for the frequency increase of HLA-A2 among the other HLA-A alleles

HLA allele	Gene frequencies			Chi-square	
	Observed	Expected (matched controls; a) $n = 284$	Expected (Caucasian controls; b) $n = 2134$	a	b
A1	0.137 (38)	0.091 (26)	0.115 (32)	5.5	1.1
A3	0.085 (24)	0.100 (28)		0.6	
A11	0.046 (13)	0.091 (26)	0.034 (10)	5.3	0.9
A23	0.011 (3)	0.027 (8)	0.013 (4)	3.1	0.2
A24	0.099 (28)	0.060 (17)	0.082 (23)	7.1	1.1
A25	0.018 (5)	0.015 (4)			
A26	0.046 (13)	0.018 (5)	0.023 (7)	12.8*	7.2*
A28	0.035 (10)	0.030 (8)		0.5	
A29	0.018 (5)	0.018 (5)			
A30	0.025 (7)	0.030 (8)			
A31	0.025 (7)	0.028 (8)			
A32	0.018 (5)	0.054 (15)	0.033 (9)	6.7	1.8
Aw33	0.011 (3)	0.015 (4)			
Aw34	0.007 (2)	– (0)			
Aw66	0.004 (1)	– (0)			
AX	– (0)	0.003 (1)			

* $p < 0.01$

Table 3. Compensation for the frequency increase of HLA-DR5 and DRw8 among the DR alleles

HLA allele	Gene frequencies			Chi-square	
	Observed	Expected (matched controls; a) $n = 284$	Expected (Caucausian controls; b) $n = 2032$	a	b
DR1	0.054 (15)	0.076 (21)		1.7	
DR2	0.093 (26)	0.133 (37)	0.130 (36)	3.3	2.8
DR3	0.139 (38)	0.088 (24)	0.101 (28)	8.2*	3.6*
DR4	0.054 (15)	0.104 (29)	0.109 (30)	6.8*	7.5*
DRw6	0.146 (41)	0.088 (24)	0.091 (25)	12.0*	10.2*
DR7	0.075 (21)	0.118 (33)	0.096 (27)	4.4	1.3
DRw9	0.021 (6)	0.003 (1)			
DRw10	– (0)	0.003 (1)			
DRX	0.057 (15)	0.033 (9)	0.039 (11)	4.0	1.5

* $p < 0.01$

present sample the frequency of C4 B2 is greater, although not statistically significantly so, than in controls.

Ig Allotyping

Seventeen families submitted by UKI KNT were typed for 12 Gm allotypes, A2m and K2m by Dr. G. de Lange (Amsterdam). There were no deviations from Caucasian controls.

Table 4. Gene frequencies of Bf alleles in 77 patients with JCA

	BfS	BfF	BfS1	BfF1
Patients $n = 154$ haplotypes	0.85	0.11	0.01	0.03
Matched controls $n = 162$ haplotypes	0.80	0.18	0.01	0.01
Caucasian controls $n = 841$ haplotypes	0.76	0.21	0.01	0.01

Table 5. Gene frequencies of C4A and C4B alleles and of C4A, B haplotypes in 54 patients with JCA

Allele	Patients (104 haplotypes)	Controls (648 haplotypes)	Allele	Patients (104 haplotypes)	Controls (648 haplotypes)
C4A1	–	0.004	C4B1	0.770	0.688
C4A2	0.050	0.057	C4B2	0.130	0.071
C4A3	0.800	0.690	C4B3	0.020	0.032
C4A4	0.040	0.056	C4BQO	0.080	0.168
C4A5	–	0.003			
C4A6	–	0.028			
C4AQO	0.110	0.143			
A3B1	0.660*	0.500	A4B2	0.040	0.040
A3BQO	0.080	0.130	A2B1	0.020	0.040
AQOB1	0.090	0.110	AQOB2	0.020	0.010
A2B2	0.030	0.003	A3B2	0.040	0.020
A3B3	0.020	0.020	AQOBQO	0.010	0.020

* Chi-square = 5.1

HLA-DR5-Positive Haplotypes of JCA Patients

When the 62 DR5-positive haplotypes of JCA patients were analyzed as to the frequencies of the B locus alleles on DR5-positive haplotypes, four different HLA-B alleles were observed to appear in relative high frequency: B35 (18 of 62 = 29%); B44 (12 of 62 = 19%); B51 (7 of 62 = 11%); and B18 (7 of 62 = 11%). When these frequencies were compared with those of a normal control population, it was seen that B35 is found on a significantly higher proportion of the DR5-positive haplotypes in patients than in controls (29% vs 15%; chi-square = 8.2). The relative frequency of B44, B51 or B18 on DR5 haplotypes in patients was not different from that observed in the normal controls.

The number of B35-positive, DR5-positive haplotypes was greater in patients than in normal controls (chi-square = 5.3), whereas the DR5-negative, B35-positive haplotypes were not more frequent in patients than in controls. The DR5-positive, B35-negative haplotypes were only slightly more frequent in patients (0.158) than in controls (0.129). From this it may be concluded that the presence of B35 is only correlated with JCA in the presence of DR5. The high frequency of B35 is probably due to linkage disequilibrium between DR5 and B35.

The frequency increase for HLA-A2 was seen both on the DR5- and DRw8-positive haplotypes [47 of 101 haplotypes (47%) carried HLA-A2] and in the DR5- and DRw8-negative haplotypes [71 of 181 DR5- and DRw8-negative haplotypes (39%) carried A2]. If one compares the proportion of A2-positive haplotypes among the DR5- or DRw8-positive and -negative haplotypes in patients and in controls, one can observe that A2-positive, DR5- or DRw8-positive haplotypes are significantly more common in patients than in controls (chi-square = 3.86), and that A2-positive, DR5- or DRw8-negative haplotypes are more common in patients than in controls. These figures are interpreted as indicating that the increase of HLA-A2 is independent of the increase of HLA-DR5 and DRw8.

HLA-DRw8-Positive Haplotypes of JCA Patients

Among the 39 DRw8-positive haplotypes, the HLA-B alleles HLA-Bw60 and B39 were found in relatively high frequency. The proportions of Bw60 and B39 on DRw8-positive haplotypes are not significantly different from the control population.

In the analysis of Bf and C4 polymorphism, it has been noted that the DR5-positive haplotypes very frequently carry Bf-S and the C4 haplotype A3, B1. However, both C4-A3, B1 and Bf-S are also associated with DR5 in the normal control population. Therefore, there appear no particular haplotypic combinations which, in connection with DR5 or DRw8, would be involved in coding for disease susceptibility for JCA.

Antinuclear Antibodies

The relationship between the presence of antinuclear antibodies and HLA allele frequencies is shown for 132 patients. Table 6 shows the frequency for A2 and DRw8 could be lower in patients without antinuclear antibodies than in pa-

Table 6. Antinuclear antibodies (ANA) and HLA gene frequencies in 132 patients with JCA

	HLA-A2	HLA-B27	HLA-DR5	HLA-DRw8
ANA-positive female patients $n = 132$ haplotypes	0.48	0.09	0.23	0.18
ANA-positive male patients $n = 22$ haplotypes	0.50	0.00	0.27	0.18
All ANA-positive patients $n = 154$ haplotypes	0.48	0.08	0.24	0.18
ANA-negative patients $n = 110$ haplotypes	0.36	0.07	0.22	0.09*

* Chi-square = 4.3

Table 7. Chronic iridocyclitis (CIC) and HLA gene frequencies in 132 patients with JCA

	HLA-A2	HLA-B27	HLA-DR5	HLA-DRw8
Female patients with CIC $n = 80$ haplotypes	0.58	0.05	0.18	0.21
Male patients with CIC $n = 24$ haplotypes	0.46	0.08	0.25	0.08
All patients with CIC $n = 104$ haplotypes	0.55	0.06	0.19	0.18
All patients without CIC $n = 160$ haplotypes	0.36	0.09	0.26	0.12

* Chi-square = 9.4

Table 8. HLA gene frequencies in relation to age at onset and sex of 141 patients with JCA

	Age at onset (years)	HLA-			
		A2	B27	DR5	DRw8
Female patients $n = 166$ haplotypes	1 – 5	0.46	0.07	0.20	0.15
Male patients $n = 36$ haplotypes	1 – 5	0.53	0.08	0.33	0.14
Subtotal	1 – 5	0.47	0.07	0.22	0.15
Female patients $n = 62$ haplotypes	6 – 14	0.27	0.09	0.27	0.14
Male patients $n = 18$ haplotypes	6 – 14	0.33	0.00	0.09	0.00
All patients	1 – 14	0.42	0.07	0.22	0.14
Matched controls	–	0.32	0.04	0.15	0.03
Caucasian controls	–	0.28	0.04	0.15	0.03

tients with antinuclear antibodies. This difference is, however, not significant for A2 and shows a borderline significance for HLA-DRw8.

Chronic Iridocyclitis

The relationship of chronic iridocyclitis (CIC) with HLA frequencies is listed in Table 7. The patients without CIC do not seem to have as high a gene frequency of A2 as is observed for patients with CIC. There is, however, no appreciable difference in the frequency of HLA-DR5 and DRw8 between patients with and without CIC.

Age at Onset

Analysis related to the age at onset and sex of the patient, shows (Table 8) that at low age of onset (between 1 and 5 years) there is no appreciable difference between the frequencies for selected HLA alleles in female and male patients. In the group of patients with age at onset of 6 years and older, the female patients show a pattern of HLA association similar to that in the younger patients, while the male patients appear to have no increase in frequency for the alleles A2, DR5 and DRw8. From this it might be concluded that the subgroup of pauciarticular JCA includes male and female patients with typical joint involvement and age of onset between 1 and 5 years and also female patients with age at onset of 6 – 14 years. Male patients with an age at onset of greater than 6 years do not appear to have the same genetic markers.

Double-Case Families

The present study includes seven sib pairs with JCA. Three of these sib pairs share both HLA haplotypes, two share one, and two share none. If these results are added to those reported by Clemens et al. in 1984 [1], there is a total of 13 sib pairs sharing two haplotypes, four sharing one, and two sharing none. These data represent an excess of sib pairs sharing both HLA haplotypes, which indicates that both HLA haplotypes contribute to disease susceptibility in the majority of cases.

Discussion

Allele and Haplotype Frequencies

The present study has clearly confirmed earlier reports that the antigens DR5 and DRw8 are associated with pauciarticular JCA. Since all patients were investigated with the same serum set and all patients were genotyped, it is now clear that cross-reactivity between DR5 and DRw8 does not play a major role in the increased frequency observed for both DR5 and DRw8.
A new feature is the significant increase of the frequency of HLA-A2, which is unrelated to the increase of DR5 and DRw8. The analysis of the DRw8- and DR5-positive haplotypes of patients has provided no clear evidence for the existence of a particular "extended haplotype" in connection with susceptibility for JCA. The high frequencies for the Bf S allele and the C4 A3, B1 haplotype appear possibly to be due to linkage disequilibrium with DR5.

Clinical Parameters

The analysis of clinical parameters revealed some indications for heterogeneity of the HLA associations with JCA. Concerning the age at onset, there appears to be a difference between male and female patients aged 6 years and older; pauciarticular JCA with onset at age 6 and later is associated with A2, DR5 and DRw8 in females, but not in males.
Patients with CIC have a high frequency of HLA-A2, while patients without this complication have a normal frequency of A2. On the other hand, it is somewhat surprising that antinuclear antibodies in the serum of patients do not show any clear correlation with the HLA antigens. It must be stressed, however, that there was no standardisation of the assay methods for antinuclear antibodies.

Mode of Inheritance of Disease Susceptibility

Of the 139 patients, 11 were found to be heterozygous DR5/DRw8, compared to 8.5 expected on the basis of the significantly increased gene frequencies for DR5 and DRw8. Thus, the observation is not significantly different from expectation. There is no evidence for an increased frequency of DR5 homozygous patients (8 observed, 6.8 expected). None of the patients were found to be homozygous for DRw8. The latter findings do not support the hypothesis of a recessive mode of inheritance for HLA-linked susceptibility for JCA. The excess of sib pairs sharing two HLA haplotypes, and the above population data, can be explained by the assumption of several different HLA-linked susceptibility genes (be they identical with certain HLA antigens or not): one associated with A2, one with DR5 and one with DRw8. The analysis of allele frequencies taking into account the deviations expected as compensation for the frequency increases of A2, DR5 and DRw8 shows that there must be several more DR alleles which contribute in a positive way (= susceptibility; DR3, DRw6) or in a negative way (= protection; DR4) to disease susceptibility. Thus at least five of the ten DR alleles are not neutral with respect to susceptibility to JCA.
In this context, it seems worth noting that the alleles of the DQ locus, which is very closely linked with the DR locus, do not show any significant association with pauciarticular JCA.

References

1. Clemens LE, Albert E, Ansell BM (1984) J Rheumatol (in press)
2. Glass D, Litvin D, Wallace K, et al (1980) J Clin Invest 66:426–429
3. Stastny P, Fink CW (1979) J Clin Invest 63:124–130
4. Glass D, Litvin DA (1980) Arthritis Rheum 23:796–799
5. Miller ML, Glass DN (1981) Bull Rheum Dis 31:21–25
6. Hall PJ, Burmann SJ, Laurent MP, Briggs D, Venning H, Leak A, Ansell BM (1984) 9th Workshop Abstracts, p 53

A Family Study of Gold-Induced Nephropathy in Patients with Rheumatoid Arthritis

J.R. Batchelor[1], I.A. Dodi[1], P. Woo[2], G.S. Panayi[2], B.M. Ansell[3], and P.L. Williams[3]

1 Department of Immunology, Royal Postgraduate Medical School, Hammersmith Hospital, Ducane Road, London W12 OHS, U.K.
2 Department of Rheumatology, Guy's Hospital, Guy's Tower, London Bridge, London U.K.
3 Division of Rheumatology, MRC Clinical Research Centre, Northwick Park, Harrow, Middlesex, U.K.

Introduction

Membranous glomerulonephritis is a serious toxic complication which may affect subjects treated parenterally with gold. The gold is commonly administered as a therapeutic agent for rheumatoid arthritis (RA). Two earlier studies have suggested that the nephropathic complications of gold occur with significantly higher frequency in RA patients with HLA-B8 and/or DR3 [2, 5]. This study was undertaken to confirm or refute the earlier ones, and if possible to extend the analyses to include alleles of the HLA region complement polymorphisms (C4A, C4B, Bf, and C2).

Patients and Methods

Patients

The objective was to compare antigen frequencies in two groups of RA patients, namely those parenterally treated with gold who developed nephropathy and those treated with gold who did not develop nephropathy. The gold preparation used in all patients was sodium aurothiomalate. In order to be admitted to the study, the patients had to conform to the criteria for definite or classical RA laid down by the American Rheumatism Association (see Table 3-2 in [3]). The laboratories contributing patients who fulfilled the diagnostic criteria for RA, and for whom there was complete data on gold treatment and proteinuria are listed in Table 1. Full data on very few non-Caucasoid patients were submitted, and therefore the analyses have been confined to Caucasoids.

Gold is normally administered, after preliminary test doses, in 50-mg amounts at appropriate intervals (usually 1 week) until a total of 1 g has been given. If there is evidence of toxicity before 1 g has been given, treatment with gold is halted. Therefore many patients who developed gold nephropathy received less than 1 g of gold, but all pa-

Table 1. Rheumatoid arthritis patients in gold-induced nephropathy workshop study

Submitting lab. (region)		Investigators	No. of patients with nephropathy	No. of patients without nephropathy	Race
BAT	(UK-1)	J.R. Batchelor, I.A. Dodi, P. Woo, G.S. Panayi, A.H. Fielder	10	10	Caucasoid
BIA	(NCY)	W. Bias, C. Arnett	0	1	Caucasoid
CXH	(UK-1)	R.N. Maini, C. Evans, D. McCluskey, J. Markwick	2	0	Caucasoid
EWA	(GER)	D. Ewald	0	1	Caucasoid
HAR	(UK-1)	R. Harris, P. Dyer, R. Cleague	2	1	Caucasoid
JOY	(UK-1)	V. Joysey, J. Herriott, B. Hazelman	2	0	Caucasoid
KNT	(UK-1)	B. Ansell, P. Hall, P. Bedford, P.L. Williams	8	0	Caucasoid
REE	(BEN)	P. Reekers, L. Vanderpuppe	1	0	Caucasoid
RVE	(US-5)	C.E. Reeve	4	5	Caucaosid
SIN	(US-5)	D.P. Singal, W.G. Benson	5	5	Caucasoid
DUT	(SAF)	E. Dutoit, M. Stein	1	2	Cape coloured
NAI	(JAP)	S. Naito	1	0	Oriental

Histocompatibility Testing 1984
Edited by E. D. Albert et al.

tients included in our analyses of the gold without nephropathy received a full course of treatment of 1 g of gold and showed no proteinuria during or at completion of the treatment. If proteinuria was detected by dipstick, the total amount excreted in a 24-h urine sample was measured.
There were 34 patients with gold nephropathy, 23 of whom had 1 g or more proteinuria/24 h. Eight patients showed 0.5 – 0.99 g proteinuria/24 h, and three had levels below 0.5 g/24 h.
For comparison, there were 23 RA patients who received a full course of 1 g of gold, but did not develop proteinuria.

Serology

The HLA typing was carried out in accordance with the Workshop rules. All but two of the subjects included were genotyped by family studies. Methods for allotyping for C4A, C4B, Bf, and C2 were as previously described [1]. Only 17 of the patients with gold nephropathy and nine of the group without nephropathy were fully allotyped for all the HLA region complement polymorphisms.

Results

HLA Antigen Frequencies

The subjects were analyzed for differences in frequency of HLA-A, B, C, and DR antigens between the nephropathic and non-nephropathic patient groups. Only four antigens (Table 2) showed marked differences in frequency, and these reached statistically significant.
It is relevant that the antigens B8, Cw7 and DR3, are in positive linkage disequilibrium in Caucasoid populations. No correction factor need be applied to the probability values, because the null hypothesis was that there would be no difference between the patient groups specifically in B8 and DR3.
A significantly lower frequency of HLA-DR7 was observed in the group of patients with gold nephropathy, a finding which confirms the data of Repice et al. [4]. Of the three patients with DR7 who developed gold nephropathy, two also expressed DR3.
HLA-DR4 was, as expected, of high frequency in both the group of patients with nephropathy and the group without nephropathy (59% and 65% respectively). There was no significant difference between the groups.

Sex Distribution

A significantly higher proportion of males was seen in the group of patients developing gold nephropathy than in the group without nephropathy (Table 3). Consistent with this observation is that idiopathic membranous nephropathy, which has many similarities with gold-induced nephropathy, is commoner in males than females. It is also of interest that in the sample studied, none of the males with HLA-DR3 escaped the development of nephropathy.

HLA Haplotypes

The data presented in Table 2 showed that there was a raised frequency of B8, Cw7, and DR3 in the patients with gold nephropathy. Because these antigens are in positive linkage disequilibrium, analysis of all haplotypes with DR3 was carried out. Table 4 shows that all the DR3-positive haplotypes in the patients with nephropathy also carried B8 (haplotype assignment was not possible in one patient because of lack of family data). Twelve of the 16 DR3-positive haplotypes also carried Cw7, and four showed no Cw antigen, suggesting that Cw7 may have been missed.
In contrast, there was only one example of B8+, Cw7+, DR3+ haplotype observed in the gold-treated patients without nephropathy.

Table 2. Significant differences in frequency of HLA-antigens between patients with and without gold nephropathy

Antigen	Patients with nephropathy	Patients without nephropathy	χ^2	Probability
HLA-B8	21 (62%)	4 (17%)	10.97	$p<0.001$
HLA-Cw7	22 (65%)	8 (35%)	4.92	$0.05>P>0.01$
HLA-DR3	16 (47%)	3 (13%)	7.14	$0.01>P>0.001$
HLA-DR7	3 (9%)	8 (35%)	5.93	$0.05>P>0.01$

Only Caucasoid patients were included in the analysis; there were 34 patients with nephropathy, and 23 without nephropathy

Table 3. Sex distribution in patients with and without gold nephropathy

Sex	Patients with nephropathy	Patients without nephropathy
Male	14 (5)	3 (0)
Female	20 (11)	20 (3)

The frequency of males is significantly higher in the group of patients with nephropathy than in the group without nephropathy. The figures in brackets denote the number of subjects with DR3
$\chi^2 = 5.19$; $0.05 > p > 0.01$

Table 4. Frequency of haplotypes with DR3

DR3-positive patients with gold nephropathy	A	B	C	DR	No. of times haplotypes observed
	1 or 2	8	w7	3	11
	11	8	w7	3	1
	3	8	–	3	2
	2	8	–	3	1
	No haplotype assigned				1
				Total	16
DR3-positive patients without gold nephropathy	1	8	w7	3	1
	30	13	w6	3	1
	No haplotype assigned				1
				Total	3

Complement Allotypes

Unfortunately, too few of the patients were allotyped for complement polymorphisms to allow a productive analysis. A high frequency of null alleles was observed in both the patients with nephropathy and those without. *C4A*QO is known to be in positive linkage disequilibrium with the A1, B8, Cw7, DR3-positive haplotype, so the high frequency (10/17) of *C4A*QO in the group of patients with nephropathy is not unexpected. However, three of nine patients allotyped in the group without nephropathy also had the *C4A*QO allele.

Discussion

This study confirms the results of the two previous ones [2,5] in which strict criteria for patient selection were applied and RA patients developing gold nephropathy were compared with non-nephropathic RA patients who received a full course of 1 g of intramuscular sodium aurothiomalate. In both these previous papers an excess of B8 and/or DR3 was observed in the nephropathy patient group. A point which may be of importance is that the gold preparation used in these studies was sodium aurothiomalate. However, aurothiopropanol sulphate-induced nephropathy has also been observed in association with the same antigens [6]. In addition to confirming an excess of both these antigens, the present study demonstrated a non-significant increase of Cw7. Because of the known disequilibrium between these antigens in Caucasoids, it was thought likely that the haplotype coding for these antigens was present in high frequency. Analysis of the haplotypes from the family material confirms that gold-induced nephropathy is strongly associated with haplotypes encoding B8, Cw7, and DR3; commonly, the same haplotype includes A1, but may instead include A2, 11, or 3. Due to the small number of cases in the study in which HLA complement allotypes were identified, it is not possible to make any definite statements regarding the effects of these polymorphic loci. However, the possibility that they may have some relevance should not be overlooked. The *C4A*QO allele is in very strong positive linkage disequilibrium with A1, B8, Cw7, DR3.

This study also confirms a brief report by Repice et al. [4], who observed a significant deficit of DR7 in a group of 14 RA patients with gold-induced renal or skin toxicity. We have observed only three patients with DR7 who subsequently developed gold nephropathy, and two of these also expressed DR3 and B8.

Lastly, the present study shows that a significantly higher proportion of males than females treated with gold go on to develop nephropathy (82% vs 50%).

In conclusion, it appears that both HLA haplotype and sex affect the patient's susceptibility to gold-induced nephropathy.

Summary

Thirty-four rheumatoid arthritis (RA) patients who developed proteinuria during treatment with intramuscular gold and 23 gold-treated RA patients who did not develop nephropathy were studied. Family material permitted haplotype analyses in all but two patients. The results showed a significant excess of HLA-B8, Cw7 and DR3 in the group of patients with nephropathy. Haplotype analyses showed that these antigens were present on the same haplotypes; of 33 patients with nephropathy whose haplotypes could be analyzed, 15 inherited an haplotype carrying B8, Cw7 or Cw–, and DR3.

Amongst 22 gold-treated RA patients without nephropathy, this haplotype was observed once. Another observation was that HLA-DR7 was significantly reduced in the group of patients with nephropathy. Lastly, it was found that a higher proportion of males than females treated with gold develop nephropathy.

Addendum. During the discussions, two groups presented further data which was in agreement with the results of the Ninth Workshop analysis. Dr. Ewald (Mannheim, Germany), in a study of 198 patients with definite RA, found the antigens HLA-A1, Cw7, B8 and DR3 in seven of eight patients with gold-induced nephropathy. Dr. Leibold (Erlangen, Germany), in a similar study of 74 patients, found A1, B8 and DR3 present together in six of 17 subjects with gold-induced nephropathy.

References

1. Fielder AH, Walport MJ, Batchelor JR, Rynes RI, Black CM, Dodi IA, Hughes GRV (1983) Family study of the major histocompatibility complex in patients with systemic lupus erythematosus: importance of null alleles of C4A and C4B in determining disease susceptibility. Br Med J 286:425
2. Gran JT, Husby G, Thorsby E (1983) HLA-DR antigens and gold toxicity. Ann Rheum Dis 42:63
3. Masi AT, Medsger TA (1979) In: McCarty DJ Jr (ed) Arthritis and allied conditions, 9th edn. Lea and Febiger, Philadelphia, p 11
4. Repice MM, Radvany RM, Schmid FR (1979) HLA-A-B-C-DR locus antigens and gold toxicity in rheumatoid arthritis. Clin Res 27:647a
5. Wooley PH, Griffin J, Panayi GS, Batchelor JR, Welsh KI, Gibson TJ (1980) HLA-DR antigens and toxic reaction to sodium aurothiomalate and D-penicillamine in patients with rheumatoid arthritis. New Engl J Med 303:300
6. Bardin T, Dryll A, Debeyre N, Ryckewaert A, Legrand L, Marcelli A, Dausset J (1982) HLA system and side effects of gold salts and D-penicillamine treatment of rheumatoid arthritis. Rheum Dis 41:599

Rheumatoid Arthritis*

F.T. Christiansen, H. Kelly, and R.L. Dawkins

Publication 8435 of the Departments of Clinical Immunology, Royal Perth Hospital and The Queen Elizabeth II Medical Centre, Perth, Western Australia

Background

Since the association of rheumatoid arthritis (RA) with Dw4 [1] and DR4 [2] was shown for Caucasian patients, a number of hypotheses have been advanced to account for the immunogenetic basis of the disease. It has been variously suggested that DR4 itself is important in conferring disease [3], that the D-DR region is important in coding for possible Ir genes [4] and that DR4 or supratypes including DR4 mark a "disease allele" that is necessary but not sufficient to confer susceptibility to RA [5]. DR4 is not associated with RA in all populations studied. In samples of Asian Indians [6] and Israeli Jews [7] DR1 was increased, though supratypes were not identified. Moreover, in Caucasoids approximately one-third of patients are DR4 negative. No theory to date has been able to satisfactorily explain differences in racial associations with disease, DR4-negative RA in Caucasoid patients and the apparent increase in the frequency of DR4 in familial versus non-familial RA [8].

The current study addresses some of these questions:

1. Is there a degree of haplotype sharing between sibs with RA that is different from that expected by chance?
2. Are supratypes that are associated with non-familial RA implicated in familial RA?
3. Are certain supratypes associated with DR4-negative RA?

Methods

A supratype refers to a particular combination of alleles at certain loci within the MHC [5]. Supratypes were identified from the phenotypes of unrelated healthy subjects submitted to the Australasian and New Zealand (ANZ) region of the Ninth Workshop. A large number of apparently stable supratypes occurring relatively frequently were identified.

The frequency of these supratypes was compared in healthy subjects and patients with RA (tested as part of the Second Asian and Oceanic Histocompatibility Workshop; 2AOHWS), and a number of supratypes which were increased in fre-

* Support for this study was provided by the West Australian Arthritis and Rheumatism Foundation.

quency in patients with RA were identified. In the present study these supratypes are compared to the haplotypes shared between sibs in families with multiple affected sibs.

Supratypes are written in the shorthand form HLA-B, C4A, C4B, Bf, HLA-DR, since recombinant families suggest that C4A, C4B and Bf lie between B and DR and this has recently been confirmed by mapping with overlapping cosmid clones [9].

Clinical details, whenever possible, were collected on all patients included in the study. With very few exceptions, all had classical or definite RA, with erosions visible on radiography.

Haplotype Sharing Between Sibs with RA

Table 2 gives the data for haplotype sharing between affected sibs for the families submitted to the Ninth Workshop and adds data of other published families. The combined data indicate there is no significant deviation from chance in haplotype sharing among sibs with RA.

The lack of haplotype sharing between affected sibs is in contrast to the report by Stastny in the previous workshop [13] and in contrast to a number of other MHC-associated diseases, e.g. IDDM, coeliac disease and Graves disease [reviewed in 14].

Table 1. Source and composition of data contributed

Lab/clinician	Data contributed	Race
Dawkins	4 multi-sib families	Aust. Cauc.
Highton	8 multi-sib families[a]	N. Z. Cauc.
Mehra/Vaidya	2 families with single case of RA 2 multi-sib families	Asian Indian Asian Indian
Bertrams	1 multi-sib family (also with IDDM) 7 families with single case of RA + IDDM	German Cauc. German Cauc.
Ewald	2 families with single case of RA	German Cauc.
Tsuji	2 families with single case of RA	Japanese
Bias	1 family with single case of RA	Amer. Cauc.
Batchelor	9 families with single case of RA	English Cauc.
Barger, Acton/ Alarcoa, Koopman	1 family with single case of RA	Amer. Cauc.
Bodmer	1 family with single case of RA	English Cauc.
Dutoit	4 families with single case of RA	Cape Coloured
Parsa	50 cases of DR4-negative RA	Amer. black; other negroids; Amer. Cauc.; Hispanic

[a] Families were C4 typed as part of the Ninth Workshop but HLA A, B, C, antigen assignment was local

Table 2. Haplotype sharing in familial RA

Lab/Published data	No. of families	No. of sib pairs	No. of haplotypes shared with proband		
			0	1	2
Ninth Workshop data					
BER	1	1	0	0	1
DAW	12	16	4	9	3
MEH	3	3	1	2	0
Literature review					
Ström and Möller 1981 [110]	5	8	1	4	3
Khan et al. 1981 [11]	4	5	0	4	1
Zilko and Dawkins 1982 [12]	3	3	2	1	0
Grennan et al. 1983 [3]	9	12	1	8	3
Total observed	37	48	9	28	11
Expected by chance			12	24	12

$\chi^2 = 1.7$ (not significant)

The lack of haplotype sharing suggests that either there is an extremely common MHC-associated susceptibility factor allowing the development of RA, or that alleles at another independently segregating locus are as important as "disease alleles" associated with the MHC. In any event, twin studies indicate that the penetrance of the disease is low [15].

Haplotype Sharing Between Sibs with RA and Sibs with IDDM

A number of families were submitted which included one sib with RA and at least one other with IDDM. The data on haplotype sharing between these sib pairs is presented in Table 3. Although there were no sibs who shared zero haplotypes, the deviation in haplotype sharing did not reach statistical significance.

Although the numbers are small, the haplotype sharing between sibs with RA and those with IDDM is more like that observed between sibs with IDDM than that between sibs with RA. In the family BER35, the shared haplotype is A2, Cw3, Bw62, C4A3, B3, BfS, DR4, which has been previously identified as increased in frequency in patients with RA as well as IDDM [16].

DR4 in Familial RA

The frequency of DR4 was examined in the eight families of the Ninth Workshop and 22 suitable families from the literature with familial RA. A total of 69 siblings had RA, and DR4 was present in 53 (76.8%), of whom seven (10.1%) were homozygous. The DR4 genotypes of the propositi in these 30 families were determined and analyzed by the method of antigen genotype frequencies described by Thomson [17]. A summary of the data is presented in Table 4. This analysis has been based simply on the DR4 genotypes and relates simply to a MHC susceptibility gene marked by DR4. However, as shown in the next section, only some DR4 bearing supratypes may be relevant, and additional non-DR4-associated supratypes are probably relevant. Further analyses and model testing based on the presence of the relevant "RA-associated" supratypes are required.

Table 3. Number of haplotypes shared between one sib with IDDM and another with RA

Family		No. of haplotypes		
		0	1	2
BER	12	0	1	0
	15	0	0	1
	16	0	2	0
	19	0	1	0
	35	0	0	1
	44	0	1	0
KAT	08	0	1	0
	19	0	0	1
Observed		0	6	3

Table 4. DR4 genotype frequencies amongst propositi in familial RA

	Genotype			
	DR4/DR4	DR4/DRX	DRX/DRX	
Observed	2	22	6	Total 30
Recessive	5.6[a]	14.7	9.6	$\chi^2 = 7.8$; $p<0.01$
Additive	3.1[a]	20.8	6.0	$\chi^2 = 1.48$; p n.s.

DRX indicates any non-DR4 antigen.
[a] Numbers predicted under recessive or additive models as described by Thomson [17]

Table 5. Important supratypes in non-familial RA

	Supratype		CPR
B8	3, 0, S	DR4	22.3
Bw62	3, 2.9, S[a]	DR4	9.3
Bw60	3, 1, S	DR4	5.5
B51	3, 0, F	DR4	5.4
Bw60	4, 2, S	DR4	2.7
Bw62	3, 1, S	DR4	2.7

[a] C4B2.9 (Perth) has been coded for the workshop as C4B3

Familial and Non-Familial RA

Five local patients and 112 patients typed for the 2AOHWS were examined and supratypes were assigned from the phenotypes. Two reference groups were used for comparison: a core group of 189 subjects from the population of Busselton in Western Australia, and 136 unrelated healthy Caucasian subjects submitted from the ANZ region to the Ninth Workshop.

Certain supratypes were found to occur in increased frequency in the patient group (Table 5). Although all listed supratypes had a cross-product ratio (CPR) of greater than 2, only the first three were increased in frequency at the 5% level of significance, after correcting for the number of DR4 supratypes. Several DR4 bearing supratypes, including the one found most commonly in the reference population, had CPRs of about 1.0.

Table 6. Shared haplotypes in familial RA

Lab	Family reference	Shared haplotype					Comments
DAW	11	A2	Cw–	B44	4, 2, S	DR4	Common to all three sibs
DAW	11	A32	Cw3	Bw60	3v, 1, S	DR4	Shared by two sibs only
DAW	05	A2	Cw3	Bw62	3, 2.9, S	DR4	Common to all three sibs
DAW	05	A24	Cw2	Bw65	2, 1, S	DR1	Shared by two sibs only
DAW	12	A2	Cw6	Bw50	3, 0, S	DR4	Common to all three sibs
DAW	12	A1	Cw–	B51	3, 2, F	DR4	Shared by two sibs only
BER	23	A31	Cw3	Bw62	3, 1, S	DR4	Two haploidentical sibs
BER	23	A24	Cw3	Bw60	3, 1, F	DRw6	Two haploidentical sibs
Rosen et al. [18]		A1	Cw–	B8	3, 0, S	DR4	Another recombinant haplotype is also shared between two affected sibs

Table 7. Frequency of RA supratypes in familial and non-familial RA

		Familial RA	Non-familial RA
RA supratype identified	Yes	11	3
	No	4	16

Fisher's exact $p = 0.001$

Haplotypes shared between Caucasian sibs with RA are listed in Table 6. This list only includes those haplotypes with C4 and DR data necessary for the complete identification of a supratype.

Four supratypes occur in both these lists. They are (a) Bw62, 3,1,S,DR4; (b) B8, 3,0,S,DR4; (c) B51, 3,0/2,F,DR4; (d) Bw62, 3,2.9,S,DR4. It is likely that Cw3, Bw60, 3,1,S,DR4 should also be included in this list, since the haplotype B40-DR4 is shared in three of the families reported in the literature and Cw3, B40, DR4 was reported in association with RA in the previous workshop [19].

These supratypes may be considered as marking a disease allele. The frequency of these supratypes in familial and non-familial RA is shown in Table 7. Both are associated with these particular DR4-bearing supratypes, though they are more common in familial RA. The data for non-familial RA is consistent with the data from the 2AOHWS where "RA supratypes" as defined above could be definitely identified from the phenotypes of 31/117 (26.5%) of patients.

RA and DR4 Serology

The DR4 report (this volume) indicates that three serological patterns of DR4 may be recognized, and these patterns correspond closely to the Dw associations with DR4. DR4.1 is the most common in Caucasoids, being found in approximately 70%. Amongst 20 unrelated Caucasian patients with RA studied in this workshop, 18 had a DR4 antigen that was of the longest pattern (4.1), while two had 4.1 or 4.2 in one laboratory where the critical sera separating these two patterns reacted only weakly. None had the shortest pattern (4.3).

The B locus antigens and supratypes (where they could be identified) associated with each DR4 pattern were examined in both healthy and diseased individuals. Many B locus antigens are associated with the longest pattern, including at least B7, B18, B37, B38, Bw41, B44, B49, Bw60 and Bw62. Two of the supratypes associated with RA, namely Bw62,3,2.9,S,DR4 and Bw60,3,1,S,DR4, are included in this group. With the 4.2 pattern, the B locus antigens include B7, B35, B44, B51, Bw60 and Bw62. However, among the shortest pattern, 4.3, there are only a limited number of associations to date, including B35 the A26, B38, 2, 1, S, DR4 supratype.

In conclusion, most, if not all, patients with RA have the longest DR4 pattern (4.1), and this pattern includes a large number of supratypes which contain DR4, including some of those associated with RA.

DR4-Negative RA

Given that DR4 itself is unlikely to be important in RA, a study of HLA antigens in DR4-negative RA was undertaken. From the material submitted, two racial groups, Caucasoid and Negroid, could be studied.

Fifty-four DR4-negative Caucasoids with RA were suitable for study. These included 18 from a number of North American and European laboratories and an additional 38 Australian Caucasoids studied previously in the 2AOHWS. The control group consisted of the 74 DR4-negative individuals out of 100 healthy unrelated individuals selected from the various regions submitting the disease cases. Thirty

Negroid cases were available, the majority being submitted from one laboratory (Parsa). Two reference populations were selected. The first consisted of 34 unrelated healthy DR4-negative Negroids submitted to the Ninth Workshop, the second consisted of the Negroid population included in the Eighth Workshop with appropriate correction to antigen frequencies to take account of the absence of DR4.

There were no notable differences in the HLA-A or B locus antigen frequencies in either racial group. The frequencies of the DR alleles are given in Tables 8 and 9. In the Caucasoid group there is a significant increase in the frequency of DR1, with a CPR of 3.4. Though the significance does not withstand correction for the number of alleles tested, it is nonetheless relevant that DR1 has been the only other DR antigen found increased in RA in at least some racial groups [5, 6, 13]. Similarly, in the Negroid group there is an increase in the frequency of DR1, though this was not significant at the 5% level (Table 9).

Table 8. DR antigen frequencies in Caucasoid DR4-negative patients with RA

	RA			Controls
	N. Amer. and Eur.	Aust.	Total (%)	Ninth Workshop
Antigen	$n = 16$	$n = 38$	$n = 54$	$n = 74$
DR1[a]	5	15	20 (39.4)	11 (14.9)
DR2	2	11	13 (24.1)	29 (39.2)
DR3	9	9	18 (33.3)	24 (32.4)
DR5	7	7	14 (20.0)	17 (23.0)
DRw6	2	7	9 (16.7)	17 (23.0)
DR7	4	10	14 (25.9)	30 (40.5)
DRw8	0	3	3 (5.6)	4 (5.4)
DRw9	0	2	2 (3.7)	2 (2.7)

[a] CPR = 3.4; $\chi^2 = 7.2$; $p < 0.01$

Table 9. DR antigen frequencies in Negroid DR4-negative patients with RA

	RA (%)	Controls	
		Eighth Workshop	Ninth Workshop
Antigen	$n = 30$	$n = 292$	$n = 34$
DR1[a]	8 (26.7)	(10.5)	2 (5.9)
DR2	7 (23.3)	(31.1)	13 (38.2)
DR3	8 (26.7)	(34.6)	10 (29.4)
DR5	8 (26.7)	(27.2)	8 (23.5)
DRw6	9 (30.0)	(34.9)	9 (26.4)
DR7	10 (33.3)	(20.4)	6 (17.6)
DRw8	1 (3.3)	(12.2)	1 (2.9)
DRw9	5 (16.7)	(5.9)	1 (2.9)
DRw10	1 (3.3)	(4.1)	2 (5.9)

[a] CPR = 5.8; $\chi^2 = 3.76$; $0.10 > p > 0.05$

Taken together and in view of the previous reports in the literature, these data suggest that in addition to DR4, DR1 may be important in marking susceptibility to RA. Unfortunately, there were insufficient numbers of cases with additional complement allotyping to determine whether, as with DR4, only some particular DR1-bearing supratypes are important. There did not appear to be any obvious association of DR1 with any one B locus product, suggesting the likelihood of several supratypes. However, further studies are required to confirm the DR1 association and characterize the relevant DR1-bearing supratypes.

Conclusion

Markers of Disease Susceptibility

Although the association with Dw4 and DR4 established that the MHC controls – at least in part – susceptibility to RA, the present results suggest that these alleles must be indirect markers of other relevant alleles within or close to the MHC. Only some DR4-containing supratypes are associated with RA. Further, there are other MHC alleles associated as shown clearly by the results in DR4-negative RA and in studies of patients from different races.

Examination of the alleles at many loci may reveal better disease markers than DR or D. To date, this aspect has been disappointing; however, it is unlikely that class I or class III alleles are important.

Comparison with IDDM

There is undoubtedly a common genetic background shared by RA and IDDM, and this is illustrated in part by the co-occurrence of these two diseases and by the increased frequency of the same supratype in both diseases, as well as by the sharing of this supratype (Bw62, 3, 2.9, S, DR4) between a sib with RA and another with IDDM. However, RA is different from IDDM in so far as there is a lack of haplotype sharing between sibs with RA, and DR3-bearing supratypes are not important except in relationship to the development of complications of therapy (J. R. Batchelor et al., A Family Study of Gold-Induced Nephropathy in Patients with Rheumatoid Arthritis, this volume).

Familial Vs Non-Familial RA

From the data given above it is clear that familial and non-familial RA are at least similar in their

MHC association. A number of DR4-bearing supratypes appear important in both, and these are likely to identify the presence of a relevant disease gene(s) which is the same in both. This would argue that at least from this aspect, familial and non-familial RA are similar. However, these supratypes appear to be particularly common in familial RA, suggesting the presence of more of these relevant disease genes.

Mode of Inheritance

Any attempt to devise a model of the inheritance of RA must take account of the following observations:

1. MHC markers are likely to be only an indirect indication of other relevant MHC alleles yet to be identified.
2. There is no evidence of increased haplotype sharing between affected siblings. These data are consistent with either a recessive or a dominant model for the MHC-linked gene.
3. There is no evidence of a qualitative difference between familial and non-familial RA; rather, families with multiple cases may have more relevant genes than families with a single case.
4. There are similarities and differences when RA and IDDM are compared. Some DR4-containing supratypes are relevant to both diseases, but other supratypes are involved in only one, whilst there is no evidence of excess haplotype sharing in familial RA.
5. The MHC gene must be common.
6. Penetrance is low.
7. Other factors must be important. There is some evidence that environmental as well as other genetic (e.g. Gm) and hormonal factors might be relevant, whilst additional genetic factors seem important in disease manifestations and complications of therapy.

Acknowledgements. We are grateful to the many laboratories and clinicians who were involved in this study for their efforts, without which this study would not have been possible, and to Dr Glenys Thomson for the sib pair and antigen genotype frequency analyses.

References

1. Stastny P (1976) Mixed lymphocyte cultures in patients with rheumatoid arthritis. J Clin Invest 5:1148–1164
2. Stastny P (1978) Association of the B cell alloantigen DRw4 with rheumatoid arthritis. New Engl J Med 298:869–873
3. Grennan DM, Dyer PA, Clague R, Dodds W, Smeaton I, Harris R (1983) Family studies in RA – the importance of HLA DR4 and of genes for autoimmune thyroid disease. J Rheumatol 10:584–589
4. Stastny P (1977) Immunogenetic factors in rheumatoid arthritis. Clin Rheum Dis 3:315
5. Dawkins RL, Christiansen FT, Kay PH, Garlepp M, McCluskey J, Hollingsworth PN, Zilko PJ (1983) Disease associations with complotypes, supratypes and haplotypes. Immunol Rev 70:5–22
6. Woodrow JC, Nichol FE, Zaphiropoulos G (1981) DR antigens and rheumatoid arthritis: a study of two populations. Br Med J 283:1287–1288
7. Schiff B, Mizrachi Y, Ograd S, Yaron M, Gazit E (1982) Association of HLA Aw31 and HLA DR1 with adult rheumatoid arthritis. Ann Rheum Dis 41:403–404
8. Khan MA, Kammer G, Dejelo CL, Kushner I, Braun WE, Ballou SP (1983) Study of HLA antigens in familial and sporadic rheumatoid arthritis. Tissue Antigens 21:35–38
9. Carrol MC, Campbell RD, Bentley DR, Porter RR (1984) A molecular map of the human major histocompatibility complex class III region linking complement genes C4, C2 and factor B. Nature 307:237–241
10. Ström H, Möller E (1981) HLA and rheumatoid arthritis: a study of five families. Tissue Antigens 18:92–100
11. Khan MA, Kushner I, Braun WE, Dejels CL, Ballou SP (1981) Clinical and HLA studies in multiple case families with rheumatoid arthritis. Tissue Antigens 18:136–138
12. Zilko P, Dawkins RL (1982) Family Studies. In: Dawkins RL, Christiansen FT, Zilko PJ (eds) Immunogenetics in Rheumatology. Excerpta Medica, Amsterdam, pp 142–174
13. Stastny P (1980) Rheumatoid arthritis. In: Terasaki PI (ed) Histocompatibility testing 1980. UCLA Tissue Typing Laboratory, Los Angeles, pp 681–686
14. Louis EJ, Thomson G, Payami H (1983) The affected sib method. II. The intermediate model. Ann Hum Genet 47:225–243
15. Lawrence JS (1970) Rheumatoid arthritis: nature or nurture. Ann Rheum Dis 29:357–379
16. McCluskey J, Kay PH, Dawkins RL, Komori K, Christiansen FT, McCann VJ (1983) Association of specific MHC supratypes with rheumatoid arthritis and insulin dependent diabetes mellitus. Disease Markers 1:197–212
17. Thomson G (1983) Investigation of the mode of inheritance of the HLA associated diseases by the method of antigen genotype frequencies among diseased individuals. Tissue Antigens 21:81–104
18. Rosen RD, Brewer EJ, Sharp RM, Yunis EJ, Schangfield MS, Birdsall HH, Ferrell RE, Templeton JW (1983) Familial rheumatoid arthritis: a kindred identified through a proband with seronegative juvenile arthritis includes members with seropositive, adult onset disease. Hum Immunol 4:183–196
19. Perez-Rojas G, Ppenchaszadeh G, Rodriguez M, Armas P, Bianco N (1980) HLA DR4 antigens and B40-Cw3-DRw4 haplotype in rheumatoid arthritis. In: Terasaki PI (ed) Histocompatibility testing 1980. UCLA Tissue Typing Laboratory, Los Angeles, pp 952–953

D-Penicillamine-Induced Myasthenia Gravis *

M.J. Garlepp and R.L. Dawkins

Departments of Clinical Immunology, Royal Perth Hospital and The Queen Elizabeth II Medical Centre, Perth, Western Australia

Background

D-Penicillamine (D-P) is used for the treatment of rheumatoid arthritis (RA), but is a potent inducer of autoimmune phenomena [5]. Approximately 1% of treated patients develop myasthenia gravis (MG) [4]. Since D-P-induced MG is clinically indistinguishable from spontaneous MG, it has been difficult to exclude the possibility that MG has occurred fortuitously.

Two recent studies [6, 7] have indicated that MG occurring after D-P given for RA is associated with B35 and DR1, in contrast to DR4 (RA) and the supratype A1, Cw7, B8, C4AQO, C4B1, BfS, DR3 (spontaneous MG) [3].

The present study was aimed at answering the following questions:

1. Is the MHC association specific for D-P? That is, will patients with RA plus MG (but no prior D-P) be similar to RA (DR4) or MG (A1, Cw7, B8, C4AQO, C4B1, BfS, DR3) or D-P MG (B35, DR1)?
2. What is the detailed supratype associated with D-P MG – including B35 and DR1? Will alleles elsewhere within the MHC show any similarities with RA or MG (e.g. C4)? Is there one particular locus which might provide a receptor for D-P?
3. Do the supratypes found in either RA or MG inhibit or preclude the development of the other diseases?

Patient Material

Typing data was submitted from seven laboratories: DAW, TAI (ANZ); MAC, WOR, KNT, DEW (UK1); RVE (US5). Patients and their families were contributed by the following clinicians: Dr. B. Ansell (Northwick Park), Dr. J. Delamere (Birmingham), Dr. W. Essigman (Lister Hospital), Dr. P. Fawcett (Newcastle), Dr. J. Hassall (Sydney), Dr. P. Keary (Townsville), Dr. K. Muirden (Melbourne), Dr. A. Nicholls (Suffolk), Dr. C. Reeve (Vancouver), Dr. M. Webley (Oxford) and Dr. J. Woodrow (Liverpool).

Data were received on 27 patients. Of these, 18 were accompanied by sufficient family data to allow genotyping, seven had phenotype data only, and three were typed without using Ninth Workshop trays. Twenty-two patients had received D-P for treatment of RA, two for primary biliary cirrhosis and one for Wilson's disease. Two patients had RA and MG without D-P therapy.

The primary criterion for classification as MG was the demonstration of antibodies to the acetylcholine receptor (anti-AChR). Four of the submitted patients were not shown to have anti-AChR. All patients were Caucasian.

Results

Table 1 provides a summary of selected antigen frequencies in D-P MG derived from those patients typed using Ninth Workshop reagents who were anti-AChR positive (see Tables 2 and 3).

Both DR1 (78%) and DR7 (59%) were increased compared to their frequencies in controls or RA patients in the Eighth Workshop [10]. DR1 and

Table 1. Selected phenotype frequencies in D-P MG

Antigen	Frequency (%)
B8	7 (37)
B27	4 (21)
B35	4 (21)
B44	6 (32)
DR1	13 (76)
DR2	1 (6)
DR3	2 (12)
DR4	4 (24)
DR5	1 (6)
DR7	10 (59)
B35, DR1	4 (24)
B27, DR1	4 (24)
B8, DR3	2 (12)
DR1 and DR7	7 (39)
DR1 and/or DR7	16 (94)

Only anti-AChR-positive, Ninth-Workshop-typed patients have been included. Nineteen patients were typed for HLA-A, B and C, and 17 for DR

* Publication 8425 of the Departments of Clinical Immunology, Royal Perth Hospital and The Queen Elizabeth II Medical Centre, Perth, Western Australia

Histocompatibility Testing 1984
Edited by E. D. Albert et al.

Table 2. Haplotypes of patients with D-P MG or coincident MG and RA

Patient	HLA				Complement			
	A	Cw	B	DR	C4A	C4B	Bf	C2
KNT 131	2	4	35	1	3	0	S	1
	1	6	w57	7	6	1	S	1
TAI 061	3	4	35	1	2	0	F	1
	24	–	18	5	3	1	S	1
DAW 039	3	7	7	1	3	1	S	1
	11	–	7	–	4	2	S	1
DAW 935[a]	w33	8	14	1	2	2	S	1
	1	6	37	1	4	2	S	2
WOR 115[b]	2	6	17	1	3	0 or 1	S	ND
	2	6	w50	7	2	0 or 1	S1	ND
WOR 112	11	4	35	1	2	1 or 0	F	ND
	1	7	8	3	0	0 or 1	S	ND
MAC 152	26	–	38	1	2	0 or 1	S	ND
	2	6	13	7	3	0 or 1	S	1
MAC 133	1	7	8	1	3	1	S	1
	29	–	44	7	0	1	F	1
MAC 122	2	3	w62	1	3	0	F	1
	3	–	–	7	2	1	F	1
MAC 104	26	1	27	1	3	1	S	1
	1	–	8	w6	4	51	S	2
KNT 128	2	4	44	7	–	–	F	1
	1	7	8	4	–	–	S	1
TAI 056	1	7	8	7	0	1	S1	1
	2	–	w61	2	5	0	S	1
DEW 105	1	–	8	7	0 or 3	1	S	ND
	26	–	7	3	0 or 3	1	S	ND
MAC 114	2	5	44	–	3	0	S	1
	1	2	w61	–	3	1	S	1
MAC 164	2	5	44	–	0	1	S	1
	1	–	8	–	0	1	S	1
MAC 144[c]	11	–	7	4	3	1	S	1
	1	–	8	3	0	1	S	1
DAW 137[c]	2	–	8	3	0	1	S	1
	2	2	40	4	3	1	F	1
WEB[d]	2	–	27	1	ND	ND	ND	ND
	3	–	7	4	ND	ND	ND	ND

– = blank or unassignable; ND = not done
[a] D-P given for Wilson's disease
[b] D-P given for primary biliary cirrhosis
[c] MG and RA: not treated with D-P
[d] Not Ninth Workshop typed

Table 3. Phenotypes of patients with D-P MG

Patient	HLA				Complement		
	A	Cw	B	DR	C4A	C4B	Bf
DAW 793	1, 11	2, 4	35, w61	1, 4	2, 3	1	F
DEW 101	2, 29	1	27, 44	1, 7	3	1, 2	SF
DEW 103	1, 2	1, 6	27, 44	1, 7	4	1, 2	S
DEW 108[a]	1, 3	4, 7	7, 44	4	3	1	F
DEW 107[b]	1, 29	7	8	3	0	1	S
RVE 001[b]	2, 24	1, 3	27, w62	1	3	1, 2	SF
RVE 002[b]	2, 3	7	7, 51	1, 4	3	1, 2	SF
KEA[c]	2	2	18, 27	1, 4	4	1, 2	S
NIC[c]	2, 3	–	15, 27	1, 5	ND	ND	ND

No family data was available
[a] D-P given for primary biliary cirrhosis
[b] Anti-AChR not demonstrated
[c] Not Ninth Workshop typed

Table 4. DR1-bearing haplotypes in D-P MG

A	Cw	B	C4A	C4B	Bf	C2	DR
2	4	35	3	0	S	1	1
3	4	35	2	0	F	1	1
11	4	35	2	0 or 1	F	ND	1
3	7	7	3	1	S	1	1
2	6	17	3	0 or 1	S	ND	1
26	–	38	2	0 or 1	S	1	1
1	7	8	3	1	S	1	1
2	3	w62	3	0	F	1	1
26	1	27	3	1	S	1	1
w33	8	14	2	2	S	1	1[a]
1	6	37	4	2	S	2	1[a]

[a] Both haplotypes from patient DAW 935

Table 5. DR7-bearing haplotypes in D-P MG

A	Cw	B	C4A	C4B	Bf	C2	DR
1	6	w57	6	1	S	1	7
2	6	w50	2	0 or 1	S1	ND	7
1	7	8	0	0 or 1	S	ND	7
2	6	13	3	0 or 1	S	1	7
1	–	8	0 or 3	1	S	ND	7
29	–	44	0	1	F	1	7
2	4	44	–	–	F	1	7

Table 6. HLA-B8-bearing haplotypes in D-P MG

A	Cw	B	C4A	C4B	Bf	C2	DR
1	7	8	–	–	S	1	4
1	7	8	0	1	S1	1	7
1	7	8	0	0 or 1	S	ND	3
1	7	8	0 or 3	1	S	ND	7
1	7	8	3	1	S	1	1
1	–	8	4	51	S	2	w6
1	–	8	0	1	S	1	–

DR7 occurred together in 39% of patients, while 94% had either DR1, DR7 or both.

The DR data on eight of these patients (DAW 039, DAW 793, TAI 061, TAI 056, WOR 112, MAC 133, MAC 104, MAC 152) have been published previously [6, 7]. Of the previously unreported cases, 67% (6/9) had DR1, 56% (5/9) DR7 and 89% (8/9) either DR1 or DR7. Notably the three non-Workshop-typed patients (KEA, NIC, WEB) had DR1.

The genotypes of those patients with family data are shown in Table 2. No B locus antigen was universally found on the DR1- or the DR7-bearing haplotypes. Similarly, no particular complotype was found in all cases (Tables 4 and 5). Consideration of the phenotypic data (Table 3) and the data from non-Workshop typed patients suggests that a supratype bearing A2, B27, DR1 may prove to be important.

Both patients with MG and RA who had not been treated with D-P (Table 2) had B8, C4AQO, B1, BfS, C2 1, DR3, the supratype associated with idiopathic MG [3]. This contrasts with the B8-bearing haplotypes in D-P MG (Table 6). Only one was shown to have C4AQO,B1, BfS, DR3, and this patient (WOR 112) also had a DR1-bearing haplotype.

Discussion

The present data confirm and extend the DR1 association with D-P MG. This iatrogenic disease clearly differs immunogenetically from idiopathic generalized MG (see below) [3] and restricted ocular MG (increased DR5) [2]. The present data also indicate an increase in DR7. This antigen was marginally increased in the study by Delamere et al. [6].

No single DR1- or DR7-bearing supratype can be designated as being primarily responsible for conferring susceptibility to D-P MG. This contrasts with idiopathic generalized MG, where the A1, Cw7, B8, C4AQO, C4B1, BfS, DR3 supratype is of primary importance in the development of early onset disease, particularly in females [3]. These data are, however, reminiscent of RA, where several DR4-bearing supratypes confer susceptibility to disease [8].

In the present data DR4 was demonstrated in only six patients with D-P MG; in four of these it was accompanied by DR1, in one by DR7, and the remaining patient (DEW 108) had received D-P for the treatment of primary biliary cirrhosis. Thus it seems unlikely that DR4-bearing supratypes preclude the development of either D-P MG or idiopathic MG, since both patients with RA and idiopathic MG (MAC 144, DAW 137) had DR4. It seems that DR1-bearing supratypes do predispose to development of both RA and D-P MG, since a proportion of DR4-negative RA patients have DR1-bearing supratypes and DR1 has been shown to be increased in RA in at least two racial groups [9, 11].

Whether the A1, B8, C4AQO, C4B1, BfS, DR3 supratype precludes the development of D-P MG is less clear. The anti-AChR-positive patient (WOR 112) in whom this supratype could not be excluded also had DR1. This supratype occurs relatively rarely in RA but clearly does not prevent its development, at least in the presence of DR4 (e.g. patients MAC 144, DAW 137).

In D-P MG a striking feature of those haplotypes with B8 was the absence of DR3 and the frequent disturbance of the complotype C4AQO, C4B1, BfS, C21 usually seen with A1, Cw7, B8 [1, 8]. Whether this observation is unique to D-P MG or rather to RA remains to be determined. In RA, HLA-B8 is associated with DR4 more frequently than expected [3].

The absence of a predominant supratype bearing DR1 or DR7 might suggest a direct role for these antigens in susceptibility to D-P MG. This remains a possibility, but important aspects which need to be clarified are:

1. The importance of the supratypes bearing A2, B27, DR1
2. The complotypes associated with each of these alleles in D-P MG
3. The alleles of other class II loci (e.g. Dw, DP) which are associated with DR1 and DR7

References

1. Awdeh ZL, Raum D, Yunis EJ, Alper CA (1983) Evidence for T/t-like complex in man. Proc Natl Acad Sci USA 80:259–263
2. Dawkins RL, Garlepp MJ (1984) Autoimmune muscle disease. In: Rose NR, Mackay I (eds) The autoimmune diseases. Academic, New York (in press)
3. Dawkins RL, Christiansen FT, Kay PH, Garlepp MJ, McCluskey J, Hollingsworth PN, Zilko PJ (1983) Disease associations with complotypes, supratypes and haplotypes. Immunol Rev 70:5–22
4. Dawkins RL, Garlepp MJ, McDonald BL, Williamson J, Zilko PJ, Carrano J (1981) Myasthenia gravis and D-penicillamine. J Rheum 8 [Suppl 7]:169–172
5. Dawkins RL, Zilko PJ, Carrano J, Garlepp M, McDonald BL (1981) Immunobiology of D-penicillamine. J Rheum 8 [Suppl 7]:56–61
6. Delamere JB, Jobson S, Mackintosh LP, Wells L, Walton KW (1983) Penicillamine-induced myasthenia in rheumatoid arthritis: its clinical and genetic features. Ann Rheum Dis 42:500–504
7. Garlepp MJ, Dawkins RL, Christiansen FT (1983) HLA antigens and acetylcholine receptor antibodies in D-penicillamine induced myasthenia gravis. Br Med J 286:338–340
8. McCluskey J, Kay PH, Dawkins RL, Komori K, Christiansen FT, McCann VJ (1983) Association of specific MHC supratypes with rheumatoid arthritis and insulin-dependent diabetes mellitus. Disease Markers 1:197–212
9. Schiff B, Mizrachi Y, Orgad S, Yaron M, Gazit E (1982) Association of HLA Aw31 and HLA-DR1 with adult rheumatoid arthritis. Ann Rheum Dis 41:403–404
10. Terasaki PI (ed) (1980) Histocompatibility testing 1980. UCLA Tissue Typing Laboratory, Los Angeles
11. Woodrow JC, Nichol FE, Zaphiropoulos G (1981) DR antigens and rheumatoid arthritis: a study of two populations. Br Med J 283:1287–1288

HLA-B27-Negative Ankylosing Spondylitis

J. Edmonds[1], H. Bashir[2], G. Thomson[3], and A.O. Carbonara[4]

1 St. George Hospital, Dept. of Rheumatology, Sydney, NSW 2217, Australia
2 Blood Transfusion Service, 153 Clarence Street, Sydney, N.S.W. 2000 Australia
3 University of California, Berkeley, CA, USA
4 Instituto di Genetica Medica, Torino, Italy

On behalf of: F. Barboni, W. Bias, A. Cambon, R. L. Dawkins, R. W. Ewald, R. Fauchet, K. Gelsthorpe, D. C. O. James, A. Kastelan, J. M. Kreisler, J. C. Lepetit, W. Marshall, M. Matsuyama, S. Mayer, H. Mervart, H. Neumeyer, E. Ohayon, E. Thorsby, M. M. Tongio, S. Wegener

Since the description, in 1973, by Caffrey and James [1] and Schlosstein et al. [2] of the association of HLA-B27 with ankylosing spondylitis, evidence has continued to accumulate of the universality of the association. The association is strongest amongst Caucasians, Japanese and certain North American Indians, and considerably less so in American Blacks, Jews and Pima [3]. In no ethnic group is the association an absolute one, and even in Caucasians a small group of HLA-B27-negative ankylosing spondylitis patients can be recognised.
Two major hypotheses are advanced to explain the strong association between HLA-B27 and ankylosing spondylitis:

1. The linked gene hypothesis, which proposes that the gene for HLA-B27 is in linkage disequilibrium with a second gene, which is more directly responsible for susceptibility to disease. This theory would explain HLA-B27-negative ankylosing spondylitis by postulating dissociation of the disease susceptibility gene from the gene for HLA-B27. One would, on this basis, expect a similar frequency of ankylosing spondylitis or associated seronegative arthropathies among the family members of HLA-B27-negative propositi as among the HLA-B27-positive ankylosing spondylitis families [4]. However, on the contrary, to date there are no reports of families with more than one affected HLA-B27-negative individuals in the absence of psoriasis or inflammatory bowel disease.
2. HLA-B27 itself may be involved in the pathogenesis of ankylosing spondylitis, either by cross-reacting with, or acting as a receptor for, an environmental agent [5]. This theory does not easily accommodate HLA-B27-negative disease either, except by the proposition that either such patients possess the HLA-B27 CREG alloantigens (B7, Bw22, Bw42, Bw47) which may substitute for B27 because of shared functionally important epitopes, or the ankylosing spondylitis is associated with the presence of other genes such as those for psoriasis or inflammatory bowel disease.

Thus the aims of the study were to clarify these issues:

1. By characterising the entity "B27-negative ankylosing spondylitis" by the clinical features of the disease and its immunogenetic and other markers, using rigid criteria for patient selection
2. By examining its degree of independence from (a) B27 CREG antigens [6], (b) psoriasis or inflammatory bowel disease [7], and (c) antigens associated with psoriasis [8], both in the patients themselves and in their first-degree relatives.

Patient Data

Clinical Data

Participants were asked to provide the following clinical data on each patient: number of years since diagnosis of ankylosing spondylitis; age at onset; duration of characteristic pelvic, lumbar or dorsal pain in years; presence of iritis; presence of thoracic or thoracolumbar junction pain; limitation of motion of the lumbar spine in all three planes; limitation of chest expansion to 2.5 cm or less measured at the level of the fourth intercostal space; presence of other diseases: Reiter's disease, reactive arthritis, chronic inflammatory bowel disease, psoriasis, rheumatoid arthritis, urethritis, persistent diarrhoea, acute anterior uveitis, inflammatory arthritis in limb joints other than hips or shoulders.

X-Ray Data and Evaluation

For each patient, participating centres were asked to state the radiological grade of sacroiliitis (0 – 5) using the New York criteria [9] and specify whether syndesmophytes were present.
One to twelve X-ray films on each of 31 patients were also made available for independent review by three rheumatologists and one radiologist, each of whom examined the films on one occasion. In 17 patients, grading was concordant or differed by one

Histocompatibility Testing 1984
Edited by E. D. Albert et al.

grade in only one of the four assessments. In seven patients, grading differed by one grade in more than one of the four assessments but did not affect the classification. In three patients, grading differed by more than one grade and the majority grading was accepted. In four patients, the films were considered unsuitable for interpretation and the grade stated by the participating centre was accepted. These patients were classified together with those in whom the X-rays were unavailable.

Patient Classification

To reduce as far as possible the effects of heterogeneity amongst the patients included in the study, rigid diagnostic criteria were devised for patient inclusion. These have been entitled the Ninth International Histocompatibility Workshop (IHW) criteria for ankylosing spondylitis, and are as follows:

1. Grade 3–4 bilateral radiological sacroiliitis
2. Two of the following four conditions: iritis; thoracic or thoracolumbar junction pain; limitation of chest expansion to 2.5 cm or less measured at the level of the fourth intercostal space; radiological syndesmophytes; limitation of motion of the lumbar spine in all three planes.

Patient Classification for Study

For the purposes of this study three sets of criteria were applied to each patient, viz the above IHW criteria, the New York criteria [9] and the Rome criteria [10]. On this basis they could be divided into the following groups:

Group A: Patients who fulfilled the IHW criteria.

a) Those in whom X-rays were graded by independent evaluation
b) Those in whom X-rays were graded by the participating centre
c) Those in whom family studies were not available

Group B: Patients who failed to fulfill the IHW criteria but fulfilled the New York criteria.

a) Those in whom X-rays were available for independent evaluation
b) Those in whom X-rays were graded only by the participating centre
c) Those reported to have only unilateral sacroiliac joint changes

Group C: Patients who failed to fulfil either the IHW criteria or the New York criteria.

a) Those fulfilling the New York criteria for probably ankylosing spondylitis only
b) Those fulfilling the Rome criteria only
c) Those fulfilling the Rome criteria for whom family studies were not available

Results

In all, 49 families and five unrelated individuals were submitted by the 19 laboratories shown in Table 1. On the basis of the classification outlined above, 48 patients were admitted to the study and were distributed as shown in Table 2. Thirty-one patients were assigned to group A, 13 to group B, and four to group C. In each group there was a predominance of males (77% overall) and of subjects whose age at onset was 30 years or less (65%). The mean duration of illness was similar in all three groups.

Table 3 shows for each subject the presence or absence of B27 CREG, of psoriasis-associated antigens (Cw6; DR7; B37, 38, 39, w57; B13) and of concomitant disease (psoriasis, inflammatory bowel disease or other arthropathy). The same data is shown for family members where available. In all, 181 first-degree relatives of 43 of the subjects were included in the study.

B27 CREG

Fifteen (31%) individuals were positive for B27 CREG antigens: 9/31 in group A, 4/13 in group B and 2/4 in group C. HLA B7 was present in 10, Bw22 in four, and one individual was positive for both antigens. The B27 CREG-positive group showed no special features and was derived from virtually all the ethnic groups in the sample.

At least one first-degree relative of a further four individuals was B27 positive. With the exception of one family with multiple diseased individuals (family of individual #11), these families were free of concomitant disease, and apart from the propositi were free of ankylosing spondylitis. None of the propositi in these families showed evidence of recombination.

Psoriatic Antigens

One or more psoriasis-associated antigens were defined in 18 subjects: 11 from group A, five from group B and two from group C. In 12 of these subjects two or more of the antigens were defined, and in five of them the haplotype B37 or 38 or39 or w57/Cw6/DR7 was present. In six individuals, themselves lacking these antigens, a single psoriasis-associated antigen was present in one or more

Table 1. Contributing laboratories

Region	Laboratory	Contributors	No. of families	No. of unrelated individuals
ANZ	BSH	Dr. H. Bashir, Dr. J. Edmonds, Sydney	4	
	DAW	Professor R.L. Dawkins, Dr. E. Owen, Perth	1	
EAE	KAS	Professor A. Kastelan, Dr. V. Kerhin, Dr. J. Jajic, Zagreb	3	4
	RIC	Dr. S. Wegener, Rostock	2	
France	FAU	Dr. R. Fauchet, Dr. Y. Pawlowsky, Dr. P. Charles, Rennes	3	
	KRE	Dr. J.M. Kreisler, Dr. M.E. Moreno, Dr. J. Mulero, Madrid	5	1
	LEP	Dr. J.C. Lepetit, Prof. G. Riffat, St Etienne	1	
	MYE	Professor S. Mayer, Dr. M.M. Tongio, Professor L. Asch, Strasbourg	2	
	OHA	Professor E. Ohayon, Dr. A. Cambon, Dr. B. Mazières, Dr. B. Fournier, Central Immunology, Toulouse	2	
Germany	EWE	Dr. R.W. Ewald, Mannheim		
	NEU	Dr. Hans Neumeyer, Dr. G. Janning, Göttingen	1	
Italy	BAR	Professor F. Barboni, Dr. P. Tabacchi, Professor L. Frizziero, Bologna	4	
Japan	MAT	Dr. M. Matsuyama, Osaka	1	1
NCY	BIA	Professor W. Bias, Dr. F. Arnett, Baltimore	3	
	MAR	Dr. W. Marshall, Newfoundland	1	
	MRV	Dr. H. Mervart, Dr. D. Gladman, Toronto	2	
SCA	TSB	Professor E. Throsby, Dr. O. Förre, Oslo	6	
UK	GEL	Dr. K. Gelsthorpe, Dr. J. Lawrence, Sheffield, Manchester	2	
	JAM	Dr. D. James, Professor D. Brewerton, Dr. A. Ebringer, London	5	

Table 2. Classification of subjects by sex and age at onset

Classification	Number of subjects (48)	Sex: Male (37)	Sex: Female (11)	Age at onset: < 30 (31)	Age at onset: > 30 (17)
Group A					
a)	14	10	4	10	4
b)	13	12	1	8	5
c)	4	4	0	1	3
Total	31	26	5	19	12
Group B					
a)	2	1	1	1	1
b)	8	5	3	6	2
c)	3	1	2	3	0
Total	13	7	6	10	3
Group C					
a)	2	2	0	1	1
b)	1	1	0	0	1
c)	1	1	0	1	0
Total	4	4	0	2	2

first-degree relatives, again without evidence of recombination in the propositi. Thus in 50% of subjects, psoriasis-associated antigens were present in the individuals and/or their first-degree relatives.
It is of interest that in only two subjects did B27 CREG and psoriasis-associated antigens co-occur ($p < 0.05$).

Concomitant Disease

Concomitant disease was present in 19 of 48 individuals: nine from group A, seven from group B and three from group C. The diseases comprised psoriasis alone in three cases, other arthropathy in 11, psoriasis + other arthropathy in three, inflammatory bowel disease in one, and acute anterior uveitis in one. The presence or absence of concomitant disease could not be correlated with any antigen or group of antigens.
In eight of the individuals, the same concomitant disease was present in at least one first-degree relative. Three other individuals, themselves lacking concomitant disease, had a first-degree relative with psoriasis, psoriasis + inflammatory bowel disease or rheumatoid arthritis. Thus, 22 of the 48 individuals in the study (46%) demonstrated concomitant disease in themselves and/or at least one first-degree relative.

Multiple-Case Families

In all, seven families in which more than one individual was suspected of having B27-negative ankylosing spondylitis were submitted for study. In six of these families, two individuals were thought to have the disease, but in four of them, the disease in the second individual failed to fulfil any of the three sets of criteria. In a fifth family, the second

Table 3. Characteristics of subjects and families

Series number	Patient	Patient characteristics: B27 CREG	Other disease	Psoriatic alleles: Cw6	DR7	B37, 38 39, w57	B13	Family characteristics: B27 CREG	Other disease	Psoriatic alleles: Cw6	DR7	B37, 38 39, w57	B13
Group A a)													
1	M.M.	+	–	–	–	–	–	+	–	•	•	•	•
2	J.P.	+	PS	–	–	–	–	+	–	–	–	–	–
3	R.Q.	+	IBD	–	–	–	–	+	–	–	–	–	–
4	H.B.	–	AAU	+	+	+	+	•	–	•	•	•	•
5	A.W.	–	–	+	•	+	+	•	–	+	•	+	+
6	P.W. (F)	–	–	+	+	+	–	–	PS	+	+	+ +	–
7	C.D.	–	–	+	•	+	–	–	–	+	•	+	–
8	K.B.	–	PS	+	+	+	–	–	PS	+	+	+	–
9	S.S. (F)	–	–	+	–	–	–	–	–	+	–	–	–
10	R.P.	–	–	–	+	–	–	•	RA	•	•	•	•
11	D.C.	–	–	–	–	–	–	B27	PS, IBD	–	–	–	–
12	J.P. (F)	–	–	–	–	–	–	B27	–	–	–	+	–
13	P.K.	–	–	–	–	–	–	–	–	–	+	–	–
14	K.C. (F)	–	–	–	–	–	–	–	–	+	–	–	–
Group A b)													
15	J.J.G.	+	OA	–	–	–	–	+	OA	–	–	–	–
16	T.B.	+	OA	–	–	–	–	+	–	–	–	–	–
17	W.G.	+	OA	–	–	–	–	+	OA	–	–	–	–
18	A.C.	+	–	–	–	–	–	+	–	–	–	–	–
19	M.A.	+	–	–	–	–	–	+	–	–	–	+	–
20	N.B.	+	–	–	–	–	–	+	–	–	–	–	–
21	L.K. (F)	–	OA	–	–	–	–	•	–	•	•	•	•
22	H.B.	–	–	+	–	+	–	B27	–	+	–	+	–
23	G.B.	–	–	+	–	+ +	–	–	–	+	–	+ +	–
24	#51	–	–	–	–	+ +	–	–	–	–	–	+ +	–
25	S.B.	–	–	–	–	–	–	–	–	–	+	–	–
26	C.O.S.	–	–	–	–	–	–	–	–	–	–	–	–
27	R.C.	–	–	–	–	–	–	–	–	–	–	–	–
Group A c)													
28	E.M.	–	OA, RD	–	–	–	–						
29	H.G.	–	–	–	+	–	+						
30	A.P.	–	–	–	–	–	–						
31	H.E.	–	–	–	–	–	–						
Group B a)													
32	M.C. (F)	–	OA	–	–	–	–	–	OA	–	–	+	–
33	A.W.	–	–	–	–	–	–	–	–	–	–	–	–
Group B b)													
34	J.F. (F)	+	–	–	–	–	–	+	–	–	–	–	–
35	C.L. (F)	+	OA	–	–	–	–	+	–	–	–	–	–
36	P.J.	+	OA	–	–	+	–	•	•	•	•	•	•
37	A.P.	–	PS	–	–	–	–	•	•	•	•	•	•
38	E.N.	–	PS, OA	–	+	+	–	+	OA, RA	–	+	–	–
39	H.I.	–	OA	–	+	–	–	•	•	•	•	•	•
40	U.S.	–	PS, OA	–	–	+	–	–	PS	–	–	+	–
41	L.L. (F)	–	–	–	+	+ +	–	–	–	–	+	+ +	–
Group B c)													
42	A.F. (F)	+	–	–	–	–	–	+	–	–	–	–	–
43	M.S. (F)	–	–	–	–	–	–	B27	–	–	–	–	–
44	A.M.	–	–	–	–	–	–	–	–	–	–	–	–
Group C a)													
45	W.S.	+	OA	–	–	–	–	+	–	–	–	–	–
46	L.E.	–	PS, OA	–	–	–	–	–	PS, OA	–	–	–	–
Group C b)													
47	#52	+	–	+	+	–	+	+	–	+	+	+	+
Group C c)													
48	R.R.	–	OA	–	–	+	–						

PS, psoriasis; IBD, inflammatory bowel disease; AAU, acute anterior uveitis; RA, rheumatoid arthritis; OA, other arthropathy; RD, Reiter's disease; (F), female; •, not tested

individual failed to fulfil the minimal criteria and the propositus suffered from pure psoriasis.

Two families submitted by Dr. Mervart included five and two diseased individuals respectively. In family MRV # 20 (family of individual # 11), three of the affected individuals were B27 positive and suffered from inflammatory bowel disease + psoriasis + ankylosing spondylitis, pure ankylosing spondylitis and psoriasis + ankylosing spondylitis respectively. Two individuals were B27 negative. One suffered from psoriasis + ankylosing spondylitis and one from ankylosing spondylitis alone. The latter patient was included in the study. In family MRV # 21 (family of individual # 8), the two HLA-identical B27-negative male sibs both suffered from psoriasis, but one suffered from ankylosing spondylitis as well and is included among the 48 subjects for analysis. These were the only two families in the study in which more than one B27-negative individual suffered from ankylosing spondylitis. However, as is indicated, both these families were complicated by concomitant disease and/or B27 in the family.

Table 4. B27-negative ankylosing spondylitis: B27-CREG antigens and psoriasis-associated antigens in Caucasian patients and controls

HLA antigen	Frequency		Odds ratio
	Patients ($n = 47$)	Controls ($n = 2035$)	
B7	0.234	0.222	1.07
Bw22	0.085	0.053	1.66
B13	0.085	0.054	1.63
B38	0.085	0.052	1.69
B39	0.106	0.051	2.21
Bw57	0.128	0.055	2.52*
Cw6	0.191	0.166	1.19
DR7	0.205	0.237	0.83

* $p < 0.05$

B27-Negative AS Without Complicating Factors

One of the aims of the study was to determine whether individuals with disease independent of the contributing factors defined above were common amongst patients with B27-negative ankylosing spondylitis. Only two of the 31 individuals of group A (# 26 and # 27) satisfied these conditions. A further two for whom family data were lacking (# 30 and # 31) were also themselves free of recognised contributing factors. Two of the 13 individuals of group B (# 33 and # 44) lacked contributing factors in themselves and their families, but there were no such individuals in group C.

Thus in the entire series of 48 subjects only four individuals who were negative for B27 CREG and/or psoriatic antigens, lacked concomitant disease and had first-degree relatives known to be free of disease and free of these antigens could be identified. A further two individuals whose families were not included in the study could in their own right be considered to have uncomplicated B27-negative anyklosing spondylitis.

HLA Antigens

Because of the small numbers of subjects from each of a variety of ethnic backgrounds, no control group could be deemed entirely satisfactory for comparison of HLA antigen frequencies with the study group. The HLA-ABC DR antigen frequencies of the 47 Caucasian subjects were compared with a control Caucasian group of subjects of appropriate ethnic backgrounds studied in the Ninth IHW. The single Negro subject was excluded. The B locus allele frequencies were appropriately adjusted for the exclusion of B27. (The effect of removal of B27 from the control population on the A, C and DR allele frequencies in linkage disequilibrium could not be adjusted for at this time.) No A, B, C or DR antigens showed significant differences between patients and controls when the

Table 5. Caucasian haplotypes in B27-negative ankylosing spondylitis

Haplotypes	Observed (42 families)	Expected (42 families)	Haplotypes	Observed (42 families)	Expected (42 families)
B35, Cw4	7	8.064	B13, Cw6	3	2.074
Bw57, Cw6	5	1.738*	Bw62, Cw3, DR4	3	1.034[a]
Bw57, DR7	4	1.512	B45, Cw6	2	0.268*
Cw6, DR7	4	3.990	B45, Cw6, DR2	2	0[a]
Bw57, Cw6, DR7	3	1.260[a]	B18, Cw5, DR3	2	0.622[a]

* $p < 0.05$

[a] Eighth IHW Caucasian data

probabilities were corrected for the number of comparisons made. The patient and control frequencies are shown in Table 4. Slight increases in frequencies of B13, B38, B39, Bw57 and Cw6 and a decrease of DR7 could be shown, but were not significant.

No differences could be shown in the frequency of any antigen or antigen group in relation to age at onset, sex or the occurrence of concomitant disease.

Haplotypes

The haplotypes observed more than once in the 42 Caucasian families are shown in Table 5. With the exception of B35, Cw4; Bw62, Cw3, DR4; and B18, Cw5, DR3, all are psoriasis associated. The haplotypes Bw57, Cw6 (p =0.032) and Bw45, Cw6 (p = 0.030) were significantly increased in frequency in the patients; however, the corrected p values are not significant.

Discussion

The heterogeneity of B27-negative ankylosing spondylitis has been emphasised in a number of reports [6, 7, 11–14] and is amply demonstrated in this workshop study. It was as apparent in the group of subjects classified by the most stringent criteria (Ninth IHW) as in the groups defined by New York and Rome criteria. In age at onset and mean duration of disease, the three groups were comparable and were similar to an unrelated group of B27-positive ankylosing spondylitis patients.

The notable characteristics of the condition [15] – a high incidence of concomitant disease such as peripheral arthritis, psoriasis or chronic inflammatory bowel disease in the patients or their first-degree relatives and psoriasis-associated antigens or haplotypes in the patients or their first-degree relatives – were spread fairly evenly over the three groups of patients and over all ethnic groups. Whilst each of these factors alone was barely statistically significant, just nine individuals of the 43 whose families were available for study lacked all of these characteristics. Of the five whose families were not evaluated, two could be said in their own right to have "pure" B27-negative ankylosing spondylitis.

In a number of studies, especially of American blacks, it had been suggested that B27 CREG antigens may substitute for B27 in the disease. However, this study could give no support to this contention, since the frequencies of these antigens were not increased.

Although seven families with more than one individual suffering from disease were submitted to the study, in only two of these families did a second individual fulfil the criteria for inclusion, and both of these families were complicated by psoriasis.

Thus, in the absence of HLA-B27, ankylosing spondylitis occurred sporadically on a heterogeneous genetic background. As demonstrated in this study, the disorder does not appear to have any distinguishing *clinical* features and is not of significantly later onset than B27-positive ankylosing spondylitis. In the absence of psoriasis, psoriatic alleles or haplotypes in the patient or his family, and B27 CREG, the disease is rare in Caucasians, and no family has yet been described with more than one confirmed case (this study) [15].

B27-negative ankylosing spondylitis appears to occupy a niche in the spectrum of spondylarthritides [16] in which a number of different diseases with spondylitis as one manifestation interact or overlap. It is well known that in psoriasis or inflammatory bowel disease, the development of ankylosing spondylitis is much less dependent on the presence of B27 or its associated genes. Thus, other disease susceptibility genes may in certain circumstances be responsible. Many of the patients in the study and their families possessed antigens known to be associated with susceptibility to psoriasis, but displayed no psoriatic disease. It seems likely that in some subjects the underlying disease has not been or may not be expressed, as Woodrow [7] has suggested. Nevertheless, further follow-up studies on the families will be of interest.

Acknowledgments. The contribution of all participants and the co-operation of the patients, their families and the rheumatologists involved in the study is most gratefully acknowledged. We are grateful for the advice of Professor J. C. Woodrow in the preparation of this report.

References

1. Caffrey MFP, James DCO (1973) Human lymphocyte antigen association in ankylosing spondylitis. Nature 242:121
2. Schlosstein L, Terasaki PI, Bluestone R (1973) High association of an HL-A antigen, W27, with ankylosing spondylitis. N Engl J Med 288:704
3. Thomson G (1983) The human histocompatibility system: anthropological considerations. Am J Phys Anthropol 62:81
4. Woodrow JC, Nichol FE, Whitehouse GH (1983) Genetic studies in ankylosing spondylitis. Br J Rheumatol 22 [suppl 2]:12
5. Edmonds J, Geczy A, Bashir H (1983) Ankylosing spondylitis and HLA B27: possible mechanisms. In: Dawkins RL, Christiansen FT, Zilko PJ (eds) Immunogenetics in rheumatology. Excerpta Medica, Amsterdam

6. Khan MA, Kushner I, Braun WE (1980) Genetic heterogeneity in primary ankylosing spondylitis. J Rheumatol 7:383
7. Woodrow JC (1977) Histocompatibility antigens and rheumatic diseases. Sem Arthritis Rheum 6:257
8. Hawkins BR, Tiwari JL, Lowe N, Wolfish P, Pollack CA, Cho YW, Terasaki PI (1980) HLA and psoriasis. In: Terasaki PI (ed) Histocompatibility testing 1980. UCLA, Los Angeles, p 711
9. Bennett PH, Wood PHN (eds) (1968) Population studies of the Rheumatic diseases. Proceedings of Third International Symposium. Excerpta Medica, New York, p 445
10. Kellgren JH, Jeffery MR, Ball J (eds) (1963) The epidemiology of chronic rheumatism, vol 1. Blackwell, Oxford
11. Van Den Berg-Loonen E, Dekker-Saeys B, Meuwissen SGM, Nijenhuis LE, Engelfreit P (1977) Histocompatibility antigens and other genetic markers in ankylosing spondylitis and inflammatory bowel disease. J Immunogenet 4:167
12. Wagener P, Zeidler H, Eckert G, Deicher H (1983) Increased frequency of HLA-Bw35 CREG antigens in HLA-B27 negative ankylosing spondylitis. Br J Rheumatol 22 [suppl 2] 134
13. Jajic I, Kerhin V, Kastelan A (1983) Ankylosing spondylitis syndrome in patients without HLA-B27. Br J Rheumatol 22 [suppl 2]:136
14. Armstrong RD, Panayi GS, Welsh KI (1983) Histocompatibility antigens in psoriasis, psoriatic arthropathy and ankylosing spondylitis. Ann Rheum Dis 42:142
15. Woodrow JC (1983) Genetics of anklyosing spondylitis. In: Dawkins RL, Christiansen FT, Zilko PT (eds) Immunogenetics in rheumatology. Excerpta Medica, Amsterdam
16. Moll JMH (1983) Pathogenetic mechanisms in B27 associated diseases. Br J Rheumatol 22 [suppl 2] 93

Scleroderma: Possible Association with the C4 System – A Progress Report*

C. Rittner[1], P. Kühnl[2], C.M. Black[3], S. Pereira[3], and K.I. Welsh[4]

1 Institute of Legal Medicine, University of Bonn, Stiftsplatz 12, 5300 Bonn, Federal Republic of Germany
2 Institute of Immunohematology, University of Frankfurt, 6000 Frankfurt, Federal Republic of Germany
3 Rheumatology Unit, West Middlesex Hospital, Isleworth, Middlesex, U.K.
4 Tissue Typing Laboratory, Guy's Hospital, London, U.K.

Introduction

Scleroderma (progressive systemic sclerosis; PSS) is a systemic connective tissue disorder characterized by proliferative vascular lesions, obliterative microvascular lesions, and residual atrophy with fibrosis of multiple organs, e.g., skin, gastrointestinal tract, heart, lung, and kidney. The etiology is unknown. Immune mechanisms such as hyperimmunoglobulinemia, circulating immune complexes, anti-nuclear antibodies, mononuclear cell infiltrates in the skin, aberrant T cell subpopulations, and decreased lymphocyte transformation by nonspecific mitogens, though unspecific findings, have been described. Also, a scleroderma-like disease may occur in graft-versus-host reactions. Yet association studies of PSS with HLA region markers have revealed heterogeneous results. Associations with A9, B8, B27, B35, Dw1, and DR5 have been reported. In two investigations, no associations were found. Most recently, three C4B*QO,QO individuals were found among 17 patients with PSS, compared with three C4B*QO,QO individuals among 144 normal controls ($P = 0.016$ in Fisher's test). The aim of the Workshop scleroderma study was to see whether this previous finding [3] could be confirmed.

Material and Methods

A total of 11 patients (all female) and their families were studied with the Ninth Workshop HLA-A, B, C, DR typing sets (see Table 1) using the NIH technique. Eight of these 11 patients were investigated in the C4 system with high-voltage agarose gel electrophoresis (HVAGE) with anti-C4 fixation and C4-dependent lysis, SDS-gel electrophoresis of immunoprecipitated and reduced C4 for detection and quantitation of α chains, and immune blotting with anti-Chido and anti-Rodgers as described recently by Rittner et al. [6]. In addition, the β chains of C4 were studied as described by Mauff et al. [2]. BF typing was performed according to Alper et al. [1].

* This study was supported in part by a grant from Deutsche Forschungsgemeinschaft (Ri 164/16-1)

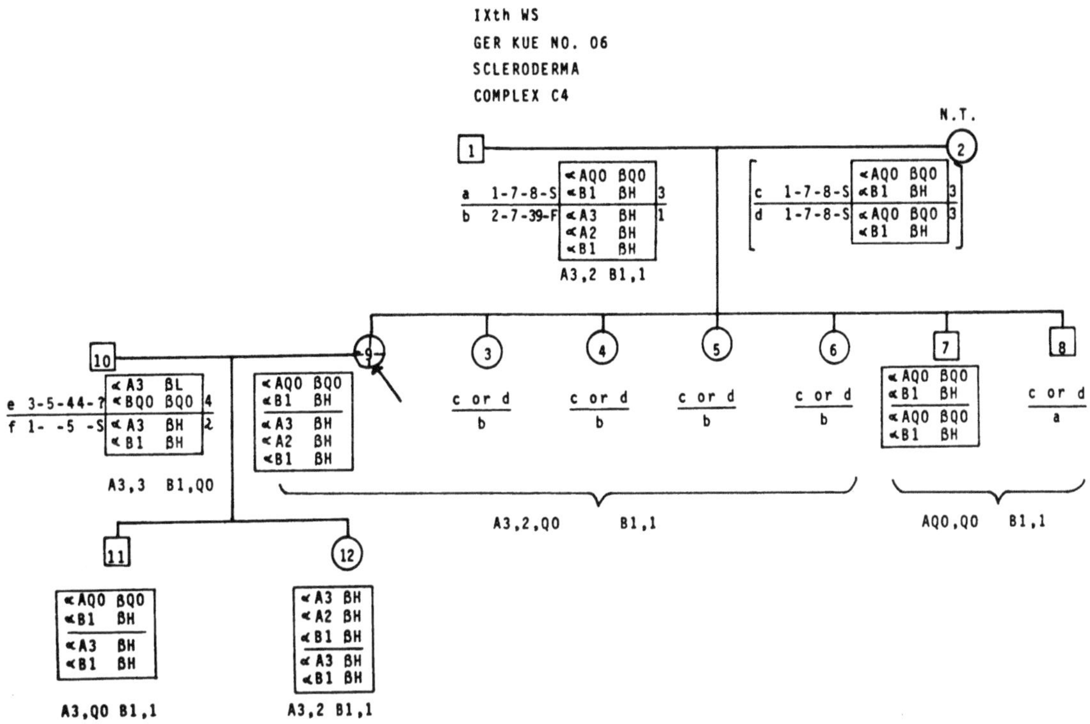

Fig. 1. Pedigree of family GER KUE 06: duplicated C4 haplotype

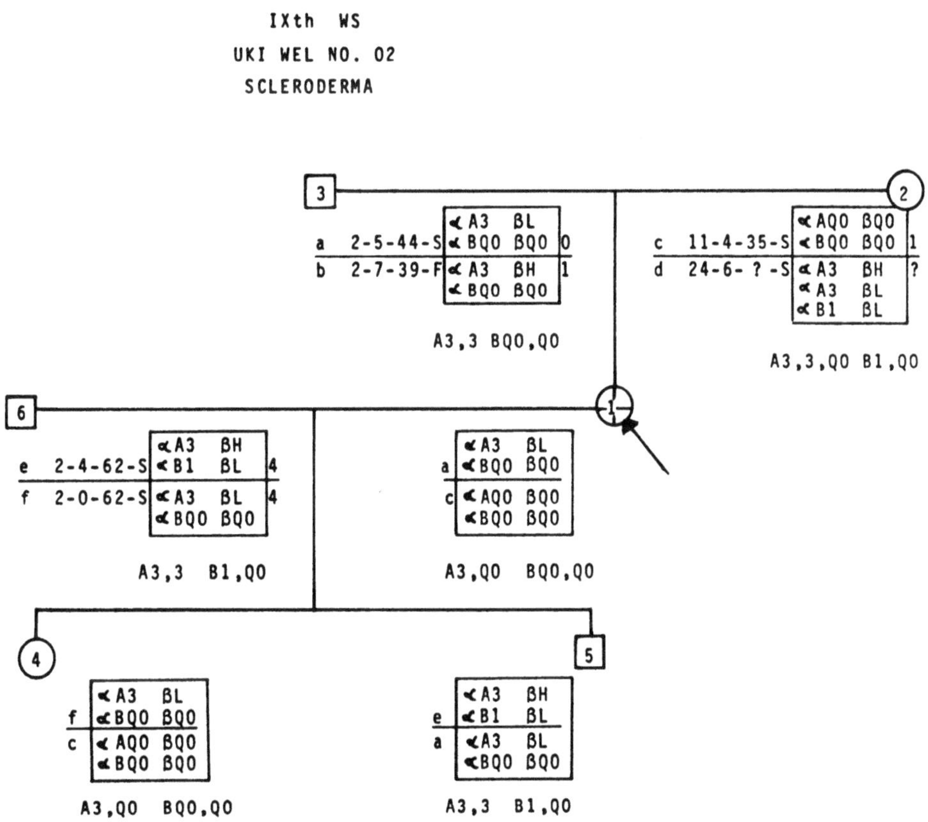

Fig. 2. Pedigree of family UKI WEL 02: assignment of silent C4 alleles in the patient and her relatives

Table 1. Ninth Workshop patients with diffuse scleroderma

Pat. no.	REG	LAB	Fam. no.	HLA-A	C	B	BF	C4A	C4B	DR
1	GER	KUE	05	1	w7	8	S	0	1	3
				2	w6	17	S	6	1	7
2	GER	KUE	06	1	w7	8	S	0	1	3
				2	w7	39	F	3, 2	1	1
3	GER	KUE	07	3	?	51	S	3	1	1
				11	w3	w55	S	3	1	2
4	GER	KUE	08	28	w5	w55	S	4	5	1
									Rg-	
				29		44	F	3	1	4
5	UKI	WEL	01	1	w7	8	F	0	1	3
				28	0	51	S	3	1	w6
6	UKI	WEL	02	2	w5	44	S	3	0	0
				11	w4	35	S	0	0	1
									Ch-	
7	UKI	WEL	03	24	w7	18	S	3	1	4
				1	w7	8	S	0	1	3
8	UKI	WEL	04	3		18		A3, QO	B1, 2	
				23		14				
9	US6	BRN	21	24	w7	18				1
				32	w4	35				5
10	US6	BRN	24	2	w5	44				7
				3	0	51				w8
11	US6	BRN	25	2	w2	27				w6
				1	w7	8				3

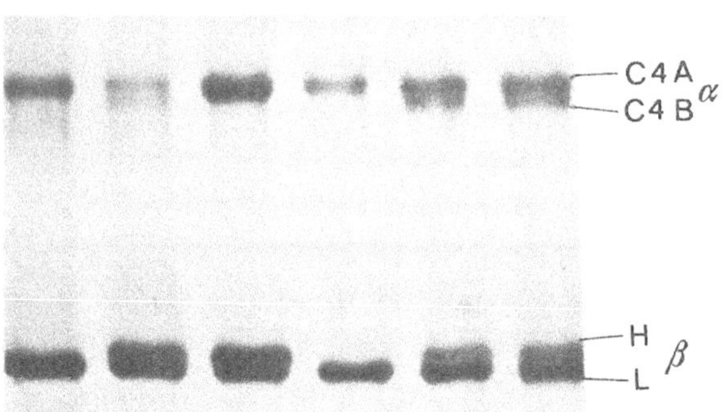

Fig. 3. SDS gel electrophoresis of immunoprecipitated and reduced C4 protein of members of family UKI WEL 02 (see Fig. 2). Origin at top. From left to right: nos. 1 to 6

Results

The results of our study are summarized in Table 1. Five of the 11 patients with diffuse scleroderma carry the haplotype HLA-A1, Cw7, B8, BFS(F), C4A*QO-B*1, DR3, compared to about one in ten in a normal Caucasoid population. The frequencies of all other HLA-A, B, C, DR, and BF allotypes do not differ from those in a normal population.

Interesting results, however, were noted in the C4 system: six of eight patients carry C4A*QO, assigned by quantitation of the α chains. The C4A*QO allele frequency is 0.2941 compared to 0.1472 in the previous study [3]. In patient no. 6, A*QO is associated with B*QO on the same haplotype. Patient no. 2 carries a duplicated C4A*3A*2 haplotype, as seen in Fig. 1. She shares this haplotype b with her father, four sisters, and her daughter. The existence of this haplotype in family KUE 06 is proven by cosegregation with C4A*QO (see also C. Rittner and G. Mauff, C4 Polymorphism, this volume).

Patient no. 6 of family WEL 02 possesses only one expressed C4 gene (A*3,QO B*QO,QO) as does her daughter (no. 4 in Fig. 2). Both have only C4A α and βL chains on the SDS-gel (Fig. 3). The patient, her mother, and her daughter have in addition a very weak expression of the C4 α chains, sharing the C4A*QOB*QO haplotype. The patient's mother may carry a homoduplicated haplotype, but this cannot be proven at the phenotypic level [6].

Discussion

Though resting on a very limited number of scleroderma patients and their families studied, this investigation seems to support our previous findings on a possible association of scleroderma and the C4 system. It is known that the disease manifestation can be induced by acute viral and bacterial infections. We have put forward the hypothesis [4, 5] that "impaired" or deficient C4 molecules may have an insufficient capacity to clear immune complexes. Therefore, C4 may be directly involved in the pathogenesis of scleroderma.

Summary

To test the hypothesis of a possible association of the C4 system with scleroderma [3, 4], eight patients with diffuse scleroderma and their families were investigated for the HLA linkage group (HLA-A, C, B, BF, C4A, C4B, DR) within the Ninth Workshop. C4 typing included HVAGE with immune fixation with anti-C4, C4-dependent lysis, SDS-PAGE of immunoprecipitated and reduced C4 for α and β chain typing and quantitation, and Ch/Rg precipitation of blotted α and β chains. This advanced C4 technology revealed silent C4A*QO alleles in six of eight patients and one duplicated C4A*3A*2 haplotype. A C4A*QO haplotype also carried C4B*QO. Although no statistical evaluation can be performed, in view of the limited number of patients studied, these results seem to support our previous findings that the C4 system could be involved in the pathogenesis of scleroderma.

Acknowledgment. The excellent technical assistance of Ms. Beate Stradmann is gratefully acknowledged.

References

1. Alper CA, Boenisch T, Watson L (1972) Genetic polymorphism in human glycine-rich beta- glycoprotein. J Exp Med 135:68–80
2. Mauff G, Steuer M, Weck M, Bender K (1983) The C4 β-chain: evidence for a genetically determined polymorphism. Hum Genet 64:186–188
3. Mollenhauer E, Schmidt R, Heinrichs M, Rittner C (1984) Scleroderma: possible significance of silent alleles at the C4B locus. Arthritis Rheum 27:711–712
4. Rittner C (1983) Chromosomes and complement in scleroderma. In: Black CM (ed) Proceedings of the Scleroderma Symposium, London, May 12–13. Smith Kline & French Laboratories Ltd, pp 23–28
5. Rittner C, Bertrams J (1981) On the significance of C2, C4, and Factor B polymorphisms in disease. Hum Genet 56:235–247
6. Rittner C, Giles CM, Roos MH, Demant P, Mollenhauer E (1984) Genetics of human C4 polymorphism: detection and segregation of rare and duplicated haplotypes. Immunogenetics 19:321–333

Behçet's Disease *

T. Okuyama [1], H. Kunikane [1], M. Kasahara [1], S. Ohno [1], M. Aizawa [1], C. Conighi [2], S. Perrone [3], and P.L. Mattiuz [2]

1 Department of Pathology and Department of Ophthalmology, Hokkaido University School of Medicine, Sapporo, 060 Japan
2 Istituo Genetica Medica, University of Ferrara, Italy
3 Clinica Oculistica, University of Padova, Italy

Introduction

Since Ohno et al. reported a strong association of HLA-B5 with Behçet's disease in 1973 [1], this observation has been confirmed in various ethnic groups [2, 3, 4]. After HLA-B5 was subdivided into two specificities, B51 and Bw52, B51 was shown to be increased in the patients [5].

However, associations of HLA-D region antigens with Behçet's disease have not been studied enough. In the Japanese patients, an increase of DRw52 (MT2) was reported [6, 7], while Lehner postulated that HLA-B5 and DR7 were increased in Caucasian patients with ocular lesions [8].
Thus, the aims of the present study were:
1. To confirm an association with HLA-B51,
2. To investigate whether any HLA-D region serologically defined antigens are associated with Behçet's disease, and whether any special haplotype including HLA-B51 exists in the patients,
3. To document the relationship between sex, clinical features, and associated HLA antigens.

* The Italian investigation was supported in part by CNR "Pregetto finalizzato Ingegneria Genetica e Basi Molecolari delle Malattie Ereditarie" and by the Fondo Ministeriale per la Ricerca Scientifica (40□) 1981–82

Materials and Methods

A total of 47 patients from two laboratories, 37 from AIZ (Japan) and 10 from MTT (Italy), were typed for HLA-A, B, C, DR (+DRw52, 53), and DQ antigens. The patients were diagnosed and classified into two groups, complete and incomplete types, on the basis of their clinical manifestations according to the guidelines for diagnosis of Behçet's disease proposed by the Behçet's Disease Research Committee of the Japanese Ministry of Health and Welfare [9]. All patients were examined as to clinical symptoms and laboratory findings. Table 1 shows the number of patients and family members included in this study.

Statistical significance was evaluated using chi-square tests with Yates' correction; *P* values were corrected by multiplying them with the number of antigens tested, except for HLA-B51, a well-established antigen associated with Behçet's disease.

Table 1. Number of patients and family members tested

	Japanese (AIZ)	Italian (MTT)	Total
Patients	37	10	47
Fathers	22	10	32
Mothers	27	10	37
Siblings	25	38	63

Table 2. HLA-A, B, C antigen frequencies (%) in patients with Behçet's disease

Antigen	Japanese				Italian	
	Control	Complete	Incomplete	Total	Control	Patients
A1	0.0	0.0	0.0	0.0	29.7	10.0
A2	36.7	50.0	38.5	45.9	40.5	40.0
A3	0.0	0.0	0.0	0.0	16.2	10.0
A24	57.1	41.7	61.5	48.6	29.7	40.0
A26	24.5	45.8	23.1	37.8	8.1	10.0
A11	14.3	16.7	7.7	13.5	9.5	30.0
A29	0.0	0.0	0.0	0.0	5.4	10.0
A30	0.0	0.0	0.0	0.0	20.3	10.0
A31	24.5	20.8	23.1	21.6	4.1	10.0
Aw33	10.2	4.2	0.0	2.7	4.1	0.0
B51	12.2	58.3*	53.8*	56.8*	10.8	80.0*
Bw52	22.4	12.5	7.7	10.8	6.8	0.0
Bw53	0.0	0.0	0.0	0.0	5.4	10.0
B7	10.2	0.0	0.0	0.0	16.2	0.0
B8	0.0	0.0	0.0	0.0	13.5	10.0
B14	0.0	0.0	0.0	0.0	4.1	0.0
B18	0.0	0.0	0.0	0.0	12.2	0.0
B44	14.3	4.2	7.7	5.4	13.5	20.0
B45	0.0	0.0	0.0	0.0	0.0	10.0
Bw54	16.3	0.0	15.4	5.4	0.0	0.0
Bw55	4.1	0.0	7.7	2.7	2.7	10.0
Bw56	0.0	0.0	7.7	2.7	0.0	0.0
B39	12.2	8.3	7.7	8.1	5.4	10.0
Bw46	2.0	20.8***	7.7	16.2***	0.0	0.0
B49	0.0	0.0	0.0	0.0	6.8	10.0
B35	12.2	25.0	23.1	24.3	28.4	0.0
Bw62	18.4	4.2	0.0	2.7	13.5	0.0
B27	0.0	0.0	0.0	0.0	0.0	0.0
B37	0.0	0.0	0.0	0.0	2.7	10.0
Bw60	18.4	8.3	7.7	8.1	4.1	0.0
Bw61	34.7	20.8	38.5	27.0	1.4	0.0
Cw1	22.4	16.7	23.1	18.9	2.7	0.0
Cw2	0.0	0.0	0.0	0.0	1.4	10.0
Cw3	57.1	54.2	46.2	51.4	21.6	10.0
Cw4	6.1	4.2	7.7	5.4	32.4	20.0
Cw5	0.0	0.0	0.0	0.0	9.5	10.0
Cw6	0.0	0.0	0.0	0.0	27.0	10.0
Cw7	20.4	12.5	0.0	8.1	39.2	0.0
Number	49	24	13	37	74	10

* $P<0.0001$; ** $P<0.004$; *** $P<0.05$, Pc n.s.

Results

HLA-A, B and C Antigen Frequencies

The disease was classified as complete or incomplete type according to the clinical manifestations (Table 2). Twenty-four of the Japanese patients were classified as complete, 13 as incomplete types. The 10 Italian patients, eight complete and two incomplete types, were analyzed together because subgrouping made the number of patients too small for any statistical comparison.

Japanese. A significant increase of B51 was observed in both complete type patients (58.3% vs 12.2% controls, χ^2 c = 14.96; $P < 0.0001$; relative risk = 10.0) and incomplete type patients (53.8% χ^2 c = 8.37; $P < 0.004$; relative risk = 8.4). This increase was also significant when the patients of both types were taken into account (χ^2 c = 17.38; $P < 0.0001$; relative risk = 9.4). Although Bw46 was also increased in the complete type (20.8% vs 2.0% controls; χ^2 c = 5.26; $P < 0.05$; *Pc* n.s.), this increase was not significant.

Italians. Eight of the 10 patients possessed B51 (80.0% vs 10.8% controls; χ^2 c = 23.05; $P \ll 0.0001$; relative risk = 33.0). No significant deviation was noted for other HLA-A, B, and C antigens.

HLA-D Region Antigen Frequencies

Japanese (Table 3). DRw52 was increased in the patients (86.1% vs 52.1% controls; χ^2 c = 9.24; $P < 0.003$; $Pc < 0.05$). Furthermore, a decrease of DQw1 (38.9% vs 64.6% controls) and a high frequency of positive reactions with the monoclonal antibody 9w925 (61.1% vs 25.5% controls; χ^2 c = 9.25; $P < 0.003$; $Pc < 0.05$; relative risk = 4.6) were observed.

Italians (Table 4). Slight increases of DRw6 and DRw8 were observed (30.0% and 20.0% vs 19.1% and 4.4% controls respectively). DRw52 was also slightly increased (80.0% vs 69.1% controls). However, these increases were not statistically significant. The frequency of 9w925-positive reactions was not shown because the reactivity was too weak to define the antigen.

Relationship Between B51 and DRw52

In order to determine whether the increase of DRw52 was secondary to or independent of the increase of B51, the frequencies of DRw52 were compared between B51-positive and B51-negative patients (Table 5).

Table 3. Frequencies of HLA-D region antigens (%) in patients with Behçet's disease in Japan

Antigen	Control	Patients		
		Complete	Incomplete	Total
DR1	14.6	0.0	0.0	0.0
DR2	31.3	13.0	7.7	11.1
DR3	0.0	0.0	0.0	0.0
DR4	54.2	39.1	30.8	36.1
DR5	10.9	26.1	30.8	27.8
DRw6	10.9	4.3	15.4	8.3
DRw6.2	9.1	9.1	12.5	10.0
DR7	0.0	0.0	0.0	0.0
DRw8	15.2	34.8	30.8	33.3*
DRw9	29.2	34.8	7.7	25.0
DRw52 (MT2)	52.1	87.0**	84.6	86.1***
DRw53 (MT3)	68.8	65.2	38.5	55.6
DQw1 (MB1)	64.6	43.5	30.8	38.9*
DQw2 (MB2)	0.0	0.0	0.0	0.0
DQw3 (MB3)	63.0	82.6	76.9	80.6
9w925	25.5	65.2***	53.8	61.1***
Number	48	23	13	36

* $P < 0.05$, *Pc* n.s.; ** $P < 0.01$, *Pc* n.s.; *** $P < 0.003$, $Pc < 0.05$

Table 4. Frequencies of HLA-D region antigens (%) in Italian patients with Behçets disease

Antigen	Control	Patients
DR1	17.6	10.0
DR2	27.9	30.0
DR3	16.2	10.0
DR4	18.9	10.0
DR5	36.8	40.0
DRw6	19.1	30.0
DR7	25.0	20.0
DRw8	4.4	20.0
DRw9	0.0	0.0
DRw10	2.9	0.0
DRw52	69.1	80.0
DRw53	33.3	30.0
DQw1	60.3	70.0
DQw2	36.8	20.0
DQw3	41.9	40.0
Number	68	10

Table 5. Comparison of the frequency of DRw52 between B51-positive and B51-negative patients

	Japanese DRw52 positive		Italian DRw52 positive	
	n	%	*n*	%
B51 positive	17/20	85.0	7/8	87.5
B51 negative	14/16	87.5	1/2	50.0
Total	31/36	86.1	8/10	80.0

Table 6. Correlation of B51, DRw52 assignments, and clinical features

		Japanese			Italian		
		No.	B51 (%)	DRw52 (%)	No.	B51 (%)	DRw52 (%)
Sex	male	22	54.5	86.4	8	87.5	87.5
	female	15	60.0	85.7	2	50.0	50.0
Age (years)	male	34.0	[20 – 42]		37.9	[23 – 61]	
	female	40.2	[20 – 57]		39.0	[31 – 47]	
Age at onset (years)							
	< 30	19	73.7*	84.2	8	75.0	87.5
	male	14	71.4	78.6	7	85.7	100.0
	female	5	80.0	100.0	1	0.0	0.0
	≧ 30	18	38.9*	83.3	2	100.0	50.0
	male	8	25.0	100.0	1	100.0	0.0
	female	10	50.0	70.0	1	100.0	100.0
Aphthae	(+)	34	58.8	87.9	9	77.8	77.8
	(–)	2			1		
Erythema	(+)	25	60.0	87.5	7	85.7	85.7
	(–)	10			3		
Folliculitis	(+)	14	57.1	92.3	6	100.0	100.0
	(–)	12			2		
Iridocyclitis	(+)	34	61.8	84.8	9	77.8	77.8
	(–)	3			1		
Uveoretinitis	(+)	30	60.0	82.8	10	80.0	80.0
	(–)	7			0		
Optic nerve	(+)	5	80.0	80.0	3	100.0	66.7
atrophy	(–)	30	63.3		7	71.4	
Cataracts	(+)	7	71.4	85.7	3	100.0	66.7
	(–)	28	60.7		7	71.4	
Genital ulcer	(+)	26	53.8	84.6	7	85.7	85.7
	(–)	10			3		
Arthritis	(+)	20	65.0	85.0	7	85.7	85.7
	(–)	15			3		
Intestinal	(+)	5	60.0	85.0	3	33.3	33.3
Symptoms	(–)	26			7	100.0	100.0
Prick test	(+)	8	75.0	80.0	6	100.0	83.3
	(–)	11	36.4		4	50.0	
Leukocytosis	(+)	13	38.5	92.3	2	100.0	100.0
	(–)	19	68.4	88.9	6	83.3	83.3
Patients		37	56.8	86.1	10	80.0	80.0

* $\chi^2 c = 4.56$, $P < 0.05$

Table 7. Frequencies (%) of HLA antigens of the parents and unaffected siblings of the patients

Antigen	Japanese					Italian				
	Controls ($n = 49$)	Patients ($n = 37$)	Fathers ($n = 22$)	Mothers ($n = 27$)	Unaffected siblings ($n = 25$)	Controls ($n = 74$)	Patients ($n = 10$)	Fathers ($n = 10$)	Mothers ($n = 10$)	Unaffected siblings ($n = 38$)
B51	12.2	56.8	31.2	44.4*	44.0	10.8	80.0	40.0	50.0	44.7
Bw46	2.0	16.2	9.1	7.4	8.0	–	–	–	–	–
DR5	10.9	27.8	9.1	23.1	24.0	36.8	40.0	10.0	60.0	26.3
DRw6	10.9	8.3	9.1	7.7	24.0	19.1	30.0	20.0	20.0	18.4
DRw8	15.2	33.3	27.3	30.8	28.0	4.4	20.0	20.0	20.0	7.9
DRw52	52.1	86.1	68.2	76.9	80.0	69.1	80.0	50.0	80.0	68.4
DQw1	64.6	38.9	59.1	61.5	72.0	60.3	70.0	50.0	50.0	57.9
9w925	25.5	61.1	42.9	53.8**	32.0	–	–	–	–	–

* $P < 0.01$ compared with controls; ** $P < 0.05$ compared with controls
–, not defined

Japanese. DRw52 was increased in both B51-positive and B51-negative patients. Haplotype frequency of B51-DRw52 was increased in the patients (0.185 vs 0.034 controls; $P < 0.001$; relative risk = 7.5), though no significant linkage disequilibrium was observed ($\Delta = -0.013$; $t = -0.22$).

Italians. There were only two B51-negative individuals; one had DRw52, the other did not. Haplotype frequency of B51-DRw52 was increased in the patients (0.30 vs 0.043 controls; $P < 0.001$; relative risk = 11.6). In the seven B51 DRw52-positive patients, two had DRw52 in cis position, one in trans position, and four in both cis and trans positions. Thus six out of the seven patients had B51 and DRw52 in the same haplotype.

Clinical Features and HLA Antigens

Japanese. The average present age and age at onset were lower in the male patients (34.0 and 28.0 years respectively) than in the females (40.2 and 33.9 years respectively). Concerning the association with B51, 73.7% of the patients who were under 30 years old at onset were B51-positive, whereas only 38.9% of the patients who were over 30 at onset were B51-positive ($\chi^2 c = 4.56$; $P < 0.05$). Other findings of interest were that B51 appeared to be associated with prick test positivity and to have a negative association with leukocytosis (Table 6).

Italians. An association between age at onset and B51 was not observed in Italians. Here also, B51 appeared to be associated with prick test positivity. Furthermore, intestinal symptoms were more frequent in the B51-negative patients.

Family

No families were available for linkage analysis between disease susceptibility genes and HLA haplotypes because no affected siblings were present. Thus, only the frequencies of the antigens that showed increases or decreases in the patients are given (Table 7).

Japanese. B51 and DRw52 were also increased in parents and siblings. Although simple comparison was impossible because of the sampling bias, the frequencies of DQw1 and 9w925 antigen in the unaffected siblings were 72.0% and 32.0% respectively, about the same as in the controls.

Italians. A slight increase of B51 was observed in parents and siblings. DRw8 was increased in the parents, DR5 and DRw52 only in the mothers. In the 10 families with a total of 48 offspring, we observed four recombinants (two A/C and two B/DR), three of which were of maternal origin. Two of the four were observed in patients and two in healthy brothers. Although there were no definite patients, some symptoms associated with Behçet's disease were present in five out of the 20 parents and 12 of the 38 siblings. Unexpectedly, B51 was only 20.0% in the five parents and 25.0% in the 12 siblings. In the 12 siblings, there were only two who were two-haploidentical with the patients, and four shared no haplotype with the patients. There was no evidence that B51 or the HLA complex contributed to the appearance of symptoms associated with Behçet's disease.

Conclusions

A strong association between B51 and Behçet's disease was confirmed in the Japanese and Italian populations. A slight but not statistically significant increase of Bw46 was observed in the Japanese patients.

In HLA-D region antigens, the frequency of DRw52 was increased in the Japanese patients. A decrease of DQw1 and an increase of the unknown antigen detected with 9w925 were observed in the Japanese patients. 9w925 was reported to react with DRw6.2-positive cells and DRw8-positive cells in this Workshop. More serological and immunochemical characterization of 9w925 will be needed to determine the relationship between Behçet's disease and this antigen. Slight increases of DRw6 and DRw8 were observed in the Italian patients. These results suggest that HLA-D region antigens also play a part in the pathogenesis of Behçet's disease.

B51 and DRw52 appeared to be increased independently in the Japanese patients. They may have complementary roles in the pathogenesis of this disease. In the Italian patients, B51 and DRw52 had a tendency to exist in the same haplotype; that is, there may be linkage disequilibrium between B51 and DRw52 in the patients. However, the sample number examined was too small to be sure of this.

B51 was associated with earlier onset in the Japanese patients, and also appeared to be associated with prick test positivity in both ethnic groups. Intestinal symptoms were more frequent in the B51-negative Italian patients.

References

1. Ohno S, Aoki K, Sugiura S, Nakayama E, Itakura K, Aizawa M (1973) HLA-A5 and Behçet's disease. Lancet 2:1383–1384
2. Dausset J, Hors J (1975) HL-A and genetics of human diseases. Transplant Rev 22:44–74
3. Brautbar C, Chajek T, Ben-Turia S, Lamm L, Cohen T (1978) A genetic study of Behçet's disease in Israel. Tissue Antigens 11:113–120
4. Adorno D, Pezzi PP, Bonini S, Masala C, Bonini S, Amendolea MA, Casciani CU (1979) HLA-B5 and Behçet's disease. Tissue Antigens 14:444–448
5. Ohno S, Asanuma T, Sugiura S, Wakisaka A, Aizawa M (1978) HLA-Bw51 and Behçet's disease. JAMA 240:529
6. Ohno S, Ohguchi M, Matsuda H, Wakisaka A, Aizawa M (1982) Close association of HLA-Bw51, MT2 and Behçet's disease. In: Inaba G (ed) Behçet's disease. University of Tokyo Press, Tokyo, p 73
7. Sasazuki T, Nishimura YK, Mineshita S, Miyashita H, Inaba G (1982) Genetic analysis of Behçet's disease. In: Inaba G (ed) Behçet's disease, University of Tokyo Press, Tokyo, p 33
8. Lehner T (1982) Cellular and humoral immunity in Behçet's syndrome. In: Inaba G (ed) Behçet's disease. University of Tokyo Press, Tokyo, p 357
9. Shimizu T (1974) Editorial: Behçet's disease. Jpn J Ophthalmol 18:291–294

Kawasaki Disease (Mucocutaneous Lymph Node Syndrome)

T. Sasazuki[1], F. Harada[1], M. Sada[2], T. Kamiya[2], Y. Yanase[3], and T. Kawasaki[3]

1 Department of Human Genetics, Medical Research Institute, Tokyo Medical and Dental University, Tokyo 113, Japan
2 National Cardiovascular Center, Research Institute, Osaka 565, Japan
3 Department of Pediatrics, Japanese Red Cross Center, Tokyo 150, Japan

Since mucocutaneous lymph node syndrome (MCLS) was first described by Kawasaki in 1967 [1], several environmental agents have been reported to be involved in the disease. However, nothing has been widely accepted, and the involvement of genetic factors in the pathogenesis of MCLS is obscure.

MCLS is an acute febrile eruptive disease commonly occuring in infants and young children. It is most frequent in Japan, although several cases have been reported from all over the world. Although at first the prognosis was believed to be favorable, further study revealed that mortality was not negligible (0.5%–1.0%), mainly due to the unique pathological changes of the coronary arteries, such as aneurysms.

According to six nationwide Japanese epidemiological surveys conducted by the MCLS Research Committee, more than 47 000 cases of MCLS had been reported as of October 1982 and more than 270 patients had died, mainly of myocardial infarction or mitral insufficiency. Because the numbers tend to increase year by year, it is extremely important to discover the etiology.

To clarify the immunogenetic factors involved in the pathogenesis of MCLS, multiplex families were studied in which at least two siblings were affected. Diagnosis was based on the diagnosis guideline of MCLS published by the MCLS Research Committee (3rd edn, August 1978). Data were received from two Japanese laboratories (SAS and SAD). Twenty-three multiplex families with 63 members were studied.

Table 1. HLA-A, B antigen frequencies in patients with MCLS

HLA	MCLS ($n = 24$) %	Controls ($n = 50$) %	Relative risk[a] %
A 1	4.0	1.0	4.30
2	21.0	43.2	0.35
11	21.0	17.2	1.28
24	71.0	58.5	1.69
26	21.0	18.7	1.12
31	4.0	15.3	0.25
w33	8.0	13.1	0.61
B 7	25.0	11.4	2.70
13	4.0	4.0	1.04
35	8.0	14.0	0.56
37	4.0	1.1	4.30
40	21.0	29.5	0.61
44	13.0	12.5	0.97
51	13.0	15.9	0.75
w52	17.0	20.5	0.75
w54	21.0	14.1	1.62
w58	4.0	1.7	2.13
w59	8.0	4.2	2.18
w60	13.0	12.7	1.13
w61	4.0	16.8	0.19
w62	4.0	16.7	0.21

[a] Statistically not significant at 5% level

Histocompatibility Testing 1984
Edited by E. D. Albert et al.

Table 2. HLA-C, DR antigen frequencies in patients with MCLS

HLA	MCLS (n = 24)	Controls (n = 50)	Relative risk[a]
Cw1	29.0%	32.1%	0.88
w3	42.0	46.5	0.81
w4	4.0	9.3	0.44
w6	4.0	1.4	4.30
w7	13.0	–	–
DR1	21.0	12.4	1.86
2	25.0	29.0	0.82
4	58.0	37.4	2.34
w6	not assigned		
w8	13.0	23.9	0.45
w9	21.0	27.2	0.70
w10	4.0	0.3	2.13

[a] Statistically not significant at 5% level

Table 3. Distribution of shared HLA haplotypes in affected sib pairs with MCLS

Number of shared HLA haplotypes	Observed number	Random number	χ^2
Two	4	5.75	0.532
One	12	11.50	0.217
None	7	5.75	0.271
Total	23	23.00	1.020

(D.F. = 2, $P > 0.60$)

Antigen frequencies of HLA of propositi with MCLS are summarized in Tables 1 and 2. There is no association between MCLS and any HLA specificities.

We analyzed multiplex families with MCLS by the affected sib pair method [2]. Out of 23 affected sib pairs with MCLS, four shared two HLA haplotypes identical by descent, 12 shared one HLA haplotype identical by descent, and seven shared no HLA haplotype identical by descent (Table 3). This HLA haplotype distribution did not differ from the random distribution ($\chi^2 = 1.09$, D.F. = 2, $P > 0.60$). Thus this method could not detect a major gene linked to HLA controlling the susceptibility to the disease.

Similary, there was no association between MCLS and any Gm allotype, and the affected sib pair method using Gm allotype marker did not reveal any significant distortion in the distributuion of shared Gm allotypes between affected sib pairs.

References

1. Kawasaki T (1967) Febrile oculo-oro-cutaneo-acro-desquamatous syndrome with or without acute non-suppurative cervical lymphadenitis in infancy and childhood. Clinical observations of fifty cases (in Japanese). Jpn J Allerg 16:178
2. Cudworth AG, Woodrow JC (1975) Evidence for HL-A-linked genes in juvenile diabetes mellitus. Br Med J 3:133

Classical and AIDS Kaposi's Sarcoma *

M.S. Pollack[1], J. Falk[2], E. Gazit[3], D. Lawrence[4], B. Safai[6], P. Rubinstein[5], and B. Dupont[6]

1 Baylor College of Medicine, Houston, TX 77030, USA
2 Toronto Western Hospital, Toronto M5T258, Ontario, Canada
3 Sheba Medical Center, Tel-Hashomer, Israel
4 Centers for Disease Control, Atlanta, Georgia, U.S.A.
5 New York Blood Center, New York, NY, USA
6 Sloan Kettering Institute for Cancer Research, New York, NY, USA

Introduction

Acquired immunodeficiency syndrome (AIDS) is a relatively new syndrome of high mortality and morbidity that has been seen in large cities since 1979, predominantly among homosexuals, intravenous drug users, Haitians, and patients with hemophilia. AIDS patients always have evidence of defective cellular immunity, including lymphopenia and grossly decreased ratios of helper to suppressor T cells. Cutaneous anergy and diminished proliferative responses to mitogens and specific antigens are also often observed. Neutrophil function appears normal, and immunoglobulin levels are usually normal or elevated. Epidemiological studies have recently suggested that one or another variant form of human T4 lymphotropic retrovirus

* This study was supported in part by NIH grants CA-08748, CA-22507, CA-34995, and CA-37888

(e.g., LAV or HTLV-III) may be responsible for the secondary, very severe immunodeficiency seen at least among the homosexual AIDS patients [6].
The AIDS syndrome is manifested by the occurrence of unusual, severe opportunistic infections (OIs) and/or malignancies not seen in individuals with normal immune systems. More than a third of the homosexual AIDS patients develop the particular malignancy Kaposi's sarcoma (KS). An HLA-DR5 association has been established among unrelated patients with AIDS-KS in New York [4, 7], and a similar association was also recently reported for a smaller group of AIDS-KS patients in Los Angeles [9]. DR5 has also been reported to be significantly increased among patients with the "classical" form of KS which generally occurs at a much later age and progresses much less rapidly than AIDS-KS. Such an association was reported for classical KS patients in New York [4, 7], Sardinia [3], and Greece (A. Kaloterakis, personal communication).
Other similarities in previous reports relating to both AIDS-KS and classical KS include decreases in frequencies for the antigens B8 and DR3 [4, 7–9]. Additional associations reported for small groups of patients include an increased frequency of Aw19 complex antigens in classical KS [2] and increased frequencies of A23 [9], A29 [5, 9], B44 [5, 8, 9], B49 [9], and DR2 [8] in AIDS-KS.
The purpose of the Workshop study was to clarify and confirm the previously reported HLA associations and to determine whether the same or different HLA associations would be found in other patient populations. Although the "family study" requirement for Workshop disease studies discouraged the submission of family data from AIDS-KS *or* AIDS-OI patients (who in most cases are homosexuals), sufficient Workshop family HLA data for classical KS patients and sufficient new (non-workshop) AIDS-KS data are available to confirm that a significant HLA association may indeed exist for both forms of this malignancy.

Patient Material

For purposes of classification, classical KS is a slowly progressive disease occurring in otherwise healthy, heterosexual individuals above the age of 60. In contrast, the U.S. Centers for Disease Control define a case of AIDS-KS as "a disease, at least moderately predictive of a defect in cell-mediated immunity, occurring in a (younger) person with *no known cause* of diminished resistance to that disease." Because there are no previously published data relating to AIDS-OI, and because no patients with this disease were reported in the workshop, the present report summarizes Workshop and other new data relating only to KS in either the classical or AIDS form. Unfortunately, too few family studies were included to warrant haplotype frequency analysis even for the classical KS patients. The laboratories that were the primary sources of the data are shown in Table 1.
Data analysis found no new significant deviations in HLA-A, B antigen frequencies. Tables 2 and 3 therefore summarize the combined Workshop and previously unpublished (Pollack, Safai, Dupont) antigen frequencies for selected (previously reported) HLA-A and B locus antigens and for all DR locus antigens for both classical and AIDS-KS patients.
The results of the new data summarized in this report are consistent with previous reports: decreases in B8 and DR3 among AIDS-KS patients [4, 7–9], an increase in B44 in AIDS-KS [5, 8, 9], and a DR5 increase in Italian patients with either classical or AIDS-KS [4, 7, 8]. (No clear increase in DR5 was seen in the present group of Ashkenazi patients with classical KS, and no clear decrease in either

Table 1. Sources of data

Laboratory and collaboratina clinicians	Patient classification	Ethnic subgroup(s)	
Pollack/Dupont (Safai, Myskowski)	Classical KS AIDS-KS (previously unreported)	Italian Other Caucasian	1 20
Falk (Cummings, Harwood)	Classical KS (Workshop data)	Italian Ashkenazi Other Caucasian	6 13 8
Gazit (Brenner)	Classical KS (Workshop data)	Ashkenazi Non-Ashkenazi Jewish	2 5
US6 BLA	AIDS-KS (Workshop data)	Other Caucasian	2

Table 2. Selected HLA antigen frequencies in ethnic subpopulations of patients with classical Kaposi's sarcoma

HLA antigen	Ethnic subpopulation					
	Italian		Ashkenazi		Other Caucasian	
	Patients # (%)	Controls (522/455)%	Patients # (%)	Controls (127/133)%	Patients # (%)	Controls (867/979)%
B8	0 (0)	12	1 (7)	9	1 (13)	18
B35	3 (43)	31	4 (29)	28	1 (13)	15
B44	0 (0)	15	2 (14)	9	2 (25)	26
DR1	1 (14)	17	6 (40)[a]	16	5 (63)[a]	20
DR2	0 (0)	23	2 (33)	17	2 (25)	26
DR3	2 (29)	17	1 (7)	14	4 (50)	23
DR4	0 (0)	12	5 (33)	24	1 (13)	28
DR5	6 (86)[a]	36	5 (33)	39	0 (0)	19
DRw6	2 (29)	25	5 (33)	20	1 (13)	22
DR7	0 (0)	24	2 (13)	27	2 (25)	23

The patients included in this table are from the sources listed in Table 1 (seven Italians, 15 Ashkenazim, and eight other Caucasians). Control antigen frequencies are taken from [1], with numbers in parentheses representing the number of individuals tested for HLA B locus antigens/the number tested for DR antigens.

[a] These antigen frequencies show significant deviations from those found in the appropriate control group ($P < 0.05$)

Table 3. Selected HLA antigen frequencies in ethnic subpopulations of patients with AIDS Kaposi's sarcoma

HLA antigen	Ethnic subpopulation					
	Italian		Other Caucasian		Black	
	Patients # (%)	Controls (522/455)%	Patients # (%)	Controls (867/979)%	Patients # (%)	Controls (186/168)%
A23	0 (0)	4	1 (5)	5	1 (25)	24
A29	1 (25)	5	1 (5)	7	0 (0)	12
B8	0 (0)	12	0 (0)[a]	18	0 (0)	4
B35	2 (50)	31	5 (23)	15	2 (50)	14
B44	1 (25)	15	8 (36)[b]	26	0 (0)	14
B49	0 (0)	8	2 (9)	5	0 (0)	1
DR1	0 (0)	17	7 (32)	20	1 (25)	14
DR2	1 (25)	23	5 (27)	26	2 (50)	34
DR3	0 (0)	17	1 (5)[b]	23	1 (25)	28
DR4	1 (25)	12	8 (36)	28	0 (0)	8
DR5	3 (75)	36	13 (59)[a]	19	2 (50)	29
DRw6	2 (50)	25	3 (14)	22	1 (25)	28
DR7	0 (0)	24	3 (14)	23	0 (0)	22

The patients included in this table are from the sources listed in Table 1 (four Italians, 22 other Caucasians, and four blacks). Control antigen frequencies are taken from [1], with the numbers in parentheses representing the number of individuals tested for HLA-A, B antigens/the number tested for DR antigens.

[a] These antigen frequencies show significant deviations from those found in the appropriate control group ($P < 0.05$)

[b] These antigen frequencies show strong trends towards deviations from those found in the appropriate control group ($P < 0.075$)

B8 or DR3 was seen in any of the classical KS groups in this study.) Interestingly, there was a complete absence of DR5 among the eight non-Italian, non-Ashkenazi patients (Table 2) reported by Falk (Canada) with classical KS, but this must be considered a very small patient sample size. One of five non-Ashkenazi Jewish patients with classical KS reported by Gazit (data not shown) did have DR5, and the non-Italian, non-Ashkenazi "other Caucasian" patients with AIDS-KS included in this study had a significant increase in DR5 in comparison with controls.

Although one previous study of AIDS-KS suggested that the increase in DR5 might not exist in all ethnic subpopulations [8], and although new data from one New York group suggest that the magnitude of the increase in DR5 among AIDS-KS patients has decreased since the epidemic first started [10], the present report suggests that DR5 continues to mark a susceptibility factor for AIDS-KS in all ethnic groups, especially in patients of Italian descent. Since the specific ethnic backgrounds of the patients in some of the previous studies, e.g., [9], were not specified, it is possible that these included an excess of individuals of Italian descent. The question of the ethnic distribution of the still prominent association of DR5 with both AIDS-KS and classical KS thus remains to be clarified.

The relative decrease in B8 and DR3 among KS patients found in this and previous [3, 4, 7, 9] studies has led to the suggestion [9] that the B8, DR3 haplotype might protect against the malignant manifestations of the primary disease. (However, Rubinstein et al. [10] no longer find this trend in New York.) Additional new findings in the present report include the suggestion that HLA-DR5 may also be increased among black patients with AIDS-KS (Table 3) and that HLA-DR1 may be increased among non-Italian (Ashkenazi Jews and "other") Caucasians with classical KS (Table 2). These findings should be confirmed by repeat studies. It is also noteworthy that previous reports of increases in A23 [9], A29 [5, 9], B34 [4, 7], and B49 [9] were not confirmed; this serves as a reminder that "significant" HLA associations will occur by chance and must always be verified by studies of new samples of patients.

In addition to the HLA data described above, Workshop participants and others report additional observations: Dr. E. Gazit (Tel-Hashomer, Israel) reports that patients with the classical form of KS do *not* show grossly abnormal T4 : T8 lymphocyte subclass ratios, and Dr. D. Lawrence (CDC, Atlanta) reports that there are no HLA antigen associations with AIDS patients' levels of antibodies to HTLV antigens. These observations, together with HLA antigen frequency data reported here and previously, support the hypothesis that the etiology of classical and AIDS-KS involves different initiation step's but that HLA-associated immune response factors may determine which *already susceptible* individuals develop manifest malignant disease.

Acknowledgment. The authors wish to thank Brenda Connelly for typing and editing the manuscript.

References

1. Baur MP, Danilovs JA (1980) Reference tables of two and three locus haplotype frequencies for HLA-A, B, C, DR, Bf and GLO. In: Terasaki PI (ed) Histocompatibility testing 1980. UCLA, Los Angeles, pp 994–1210
2. Brenner S, Krakowski A, Schewach-Millet M, et al (1982) Increased frequency of Aw19 in Kaposi's sarcoma. Tissue Antigens 19:392–394
3. Contu L, Cerimele D, Pintus A, et al (1984) Genetic and immunologic studies on Kaposi's sarcoma in Sardinia. Abstracts of Ninth International Histocompatibility Workshop and Conference, München Wien 1984, p 61
4. Friedman-Kien AE, Laubenstein LJ, Rubenstein P, et al (1982) Disseminated Kaposi's sarcoma syndrome in young homosexual men. Ann Int Med 96:693–700
5. Lawrence D, Bias W, Pollard K, et al (1982) HLA studies in an epidemic of Kaposi's sarcoma and opportunistic infections (KS/0I) among homosexual males. Abstracts of 8th Annual Meeting, American Association for Clinical Histocompatibility Testing, San Francisco, p A-30
6. Marx JL (1984) Research news. Strong new candidate for AIDS agent. Science 224:475–477
7. Pollack MS, Safai B, Myskowski PL, et al (1983) Frequencies of HLA and Gm immunogenetic markers in Kaposi's sarcoma. Tissue Antigens 21:1–8
8. Pollack MS, Safai B, Dupont B, et al (1983) HLA-DR5 and DR2 are susceptibility factors for acquired immunodeficiency syndrome with Kaposi's sarcoma in different ethnic subpopulations. Disease Markers 1:135–139
9. Prince HE, Schroff RW, Ayoub G et al (1984) HLA studies in acquired immune deficiency syndrome patients with Kaposi's sarcoma. J Clin Immunol 4:242–245
10. Rubinstein P, Walker M, Carpenter C, et al (1984) HLA in patients with disseminated, epidemic, Kaposi's sarcoma (EKS). A different type of disease association. Abstracts of Ninth International Histocompatibility Workshop and Conference, München Wien 1984, p 61

HLA and Familial Malignant Melanoma

J. Hors[1], F. Demenais[2], J.P. Cesarini[3], O. Verola[4], M. Prade[5], G. Mueller-Eckhardt[6], E. Gazit[7], L. Gebuhrer[8], M. Busson[1], and R.L. Dawkins[9]

With the collaboration of: H. Betuel, C. Bouillenne, C. Dehay, R. Ewald, P. Kühnl, S. Mayer, H. Neumeyer, G. Pellegris, F. Riedel, M. M. Tongio, and L. P. de Waal

1 INSERM, U93, Hôpital St. Louis, 2, Place du Dr. Fournier, 75010 Paris, France
2 INSERM, U155, Chateau de Longchamp, Paris, France
3 Hopital Fondation Rothschild, Paris, France
4 Departement Anatomopathologie, Hôpital St. Louis, Paris, France
5 Departement Anatomopathologie, Centre G. Roussy, Villejuif, France
6 Institute of Clinical Immunology and Blood Transfusion, Giessen, Federal Republic of Germany
7 Chaim Sheba Medical Center, Tel Hashomer, Israel
8 Centre Transfusion Sanguine, Lyon, France
9 Department of Clinical Immunology, Royal Perth Hospital, Perth, Australia

The aim of this work was to study a possible linkage between susceptibility to familial malignant melanoma (FMM) and the HLA region by genotyping multiplex-case families.

Genetic Background

The incidence rate of MM is about 4/100 000/year [12] and its familial occurrence has been widely reported in the literature [7]. Dysplastic nevi (DN) have been described both in association with melanoma [5] and not in association with melanoma [17].

Recently, a new clinical entity associated with precursor lesions has been isolated among FMM cases [2, 11, 18]. This new syndrome is known as "BK mole" [2, 18] or "FAMM syndrome" [11, 12], since these DN have been observed in FMM patients and their relatives. The reported frequency of FMM among all occurrences of the disease varies from 4% to 12%.

Although irregular transmission patterns have suggested reduced penetrance of a dominant gene or a polygenic mechanism [4, 19], the familial vertical transmission of FMM is probably consistent with autosomal dominant inheritance [7].

Previous Linkage Studies

The first observation of a possible linkage between FMM and HLA was made by Dawkins, who found a maximum lod score of 1.25 at a recombination distance of 10 units in a unique large multiplex-case family [9]. In a series of six multiplex families published by Pellegris et al. [15], five pairs of patients shared at least one HLA haplotype. In an independent series of seven pedigrees, Demenais et al. [3] observed a maximum lod score of 1.64 at a recombination fraction of 5% assuming low penetrance values, suggesting a possible linkage between HLA and FMM. No observed association between MM and any HLA allele has been proved, except for A9 in the case of metastatic or relapsing forms [1].

Criteria and Methods

There were three criteria for selection of the families studied. First, the family had to include at least two cases of MM.

Second, the diagnosis had to be established on the basis of histopathological data. Slides of melanoma tissue from each patient were required for submission to a panel of pathologists (JPC, MP, OV, Paris) for independent readings. For the review of pathological material, the following criteria were applied:

1. The MM was classified according to the International Nomenclature (UICC 1972, Sydney) [6].
2. Borderline and/or precursor lesions in which the melanocytic proliferation were evaluated were classified into three categories of atypia: high, moderate, and severe [16].
3. Particular attention was paid to the association of a nevocytic component with either malignant or precursor lesions. All patients and relatives had to be carefully examined by a dermatologist experienced in pigmented lesions. FMM may be (a) observed in patients with no other pigmented lesions; (b) associated with a DN; or (c) associated with multiple nevi (MN; ≥ 20), some of which may be pleiomorphic.

Third, HLA geno- and haplotype determination had to be clearly established.

Histocompatibility Testing 1984
Edited by E. D. Albert et al.

Linkage analysis was performed using the computer program LIPED [14] with age correction [10]. Homogeneity of the lod scores was tested using the Morton method [13]. Three successive linkage analyses were performed considering each of the following patterns as a single trait: (1) only individuals displaying an MM; (2) only individuals with precursor lesions (DN and/or MN) with or without FMM; (3) all individuals affected. Each of these traits was assumed to be determined by a single autosomal dominant gene. The lod scores were computed for a large range of gene frequencies (10^{-4}, 10^{-3}, 10^{-2}, 10^{-1}, 0.2, 0.3) and penetrance values (0.01, 0.05, 0.1, 0.3, 0.5 and 0.7).

Families and Patients

A total of 22 families (Table 1) were submitted for analysis to the Ninth Workshop, including 61 patients with FMM; 23 patients belonging to 10 families displayed DN lesions, and 50 members from 17 families had MN. They were all new families being studied for the first time except for two: family 1 [3] and family 4 [9]. In most of the families (12/16 with a disease status documented for the parents), FMM is vertically transmitted over two or three generations, fitting with a dominant pattern of inheritance with incomplete penetrance.

Results

The age at onset of the 61 FMM patients (29 M, 32 F) varied from 18 to 71 years with an average of 37 years. Thirty-nine FMM patients had a superficial spreading melanoma, eight had a nodular form, and 14 were unclassified. Haplotypes shared by at least two patients with FMM are listed in Table 2. Lod scores for the three patterns studied (see above) are displayed in Tables 3–5, and are given for the extreme values of gene frequency (10^{-4} and 0.30) and two different penetrances (0.05 and 0.50). As far as FMM is concerned, the maximum lod score observed is 0.94 at a recombination fraction of 20% (Table 3), which is far from the significance level (+ 3). A very tight linkage at a recombination fraction) of (θ) value $\leq$ 2% can be excluded when the gene frequency is low $\leq 10^{-1}$. When precursor lesions (DN with or without MN) are considered alone, or together with MM, the lod scores are even lower: a close linkage can be firmly excluded at a distance of $\leq$ 5% or 10% recombination, especially when the gene frequency is $\leq 10^{-1}$.

Linkage homogeneity was tested within the Ninth Workshop material (Table 6) and also by compari-

Table 1. Distribution of the clinical pattern in the 22 families

Family	Total subjects tested	Lesions found		
		FMM	DN	MN
1 ANZDAW04	38	12	5	5
2 BENBOU01	4	2	0	3
3 BENENG06	7	3	2	2
4 FRABET11	21	3	2	1
5 FRADAU58	4	2	2	2
6 FRADAU59	8	2	1	4
7 FRADAU60	11	2	0	0
8 FRAMYE23	11	2	4	7
9 FRABET04	23	4	2	3
10 GEREWA03	10	2	2	4
11 GERKUE12	4	2	1	2
12 GERMUE16	23	3	0	4
13 GERMUE17	7	2	2	2
14 GERMUE18	15	3	0	2
15 GERMUE19	19	2	0	4
16 GERMUE20	18	2	0	3
17 GERNEU07	13	2	0	1
18 IT2PEL01	4	2	0	0
19 GERGAZ07	4	2	0	0
20 GERGAZ08	4	2	0	0
21 GERGAZ09	4	3	0	1
22 GERGAZ10	3	2	0	0

Table 2. HLA haplotypes shared by patients with MM

Family	A	C	B	DR	No. of patients
ANZDAW04	2	w1	27	2	9
	24	w3	w55	w6	6
BENBOU01	11	w4	44	7	2
BENENG06	28	w7	44	5	3
FRABET11	3	–	7	2	2
	1	w2	w61	w6	2
FRADAU58	28	–	51	4	2
FRADAU59	31	w7	18	5	3
FRADAU60	30	w5	18	3	2
FRAMYE23	2	w5	44	4	2
FRABET04	26	5	51	5	3
GEREWA03	2	w7	49	w6	2
GERKUE12	2	w7	7	2	2
GERMUE16	2	–	38	2	2
	25	–	44	4	2
GERMUE17	26	–	18	2	2
GERMUE18	24	–	38	2	2
GERMUE19	2	w7	39	2	2
	24	–	w61	w6	2
GERMUE20	29	w3	w55	4	2
GERNEU07	1	w7	8	–	2
GERGAZ07	23	–	w41	5	2
GERGAZ08	24	–	38	5	2
GERGAZ09	3	–	8	3	3
GERGAZ10	30	–	38	5	2

Table 3. Lod scores for linkage between a dominant gene for MM and HLA

Gene frequency	Maximal penetrance at 40 years	Recombination fraction θ 0.00	0.05	0.10	0.20	0.30	0.40
10^{-4}	0.05	−15.43	−0.81	0.38	0.94	0.75	0.34
	0.50	−18.59	−1.35	−0.04	0.69	0.61	0.28
0.30	0.05	0.41	0.42	0.39	0.29	0.17	0.07
	0.50	−0.60	−0.21	0.00	0.16	0.14	0.07

Table 4. Lod scores for linkage between a dominant gene for precursor lesions and HLA

Gene frequency	Maximal penetrance at 30 years	Recombination fraction θ 0.00	0.05	0.10	0.20	0.30	0.40
10^{-4}	0.05	−14.51	−3.18	−1.67	−0.48	−0.07	0.04
	0.50	−17.69	−4.43	−2.61	−0.99	−0.30	−0.02
0.30	0.05	0.39	−0.28	−0.20	−0.09	−0.03	0.00
	0.50	−1.51	−1.05	−0.73	−0.33	−0.11	−0.02

Table 5. Lod scores for linkage between a dominant gene for precursor lesions and/or MM and HLA

Gene frequency	Maximal penetrance	Recombination fraction θ 0.00	0.05	0.10	0.20	0.30	0.40
10^{-4}	0.05	−23.80	−4.74	−1.97	−0.02	0.40	0.27
	0.50	−27.57	−5.54	−2.57	−0.36	0.22	0.20
0.30	0.05	0.22	0.27	0.28	0.24	0.15	0.07
	0.50	−0.78	−0.37	−0.12	0.12	0.14	0.08

Table 6. Test of linkage homogeneity according to clinical and geographical criteria (HLA and FMM)

Families without DN (n = 12)		Families with DN (n = 10)	
Max. lod score	0	+ 1.23	
θ	0.45	0.15	NS
European families (n = 17)		Others (n = 5)	
Max lod score	0	+ 1.71	NS
θ	0.45	0.07	

The differences are not significant

son to the data already published [3, 9, 15]. There were no significant differences, and therefore we performed linkage analysis of pooled data including other published cases [3]; the maximum lod scores then reached 1.78 ($\theta = 0.20$) and 0.72 ($\theta = 0.05$) with gene frequencies of 10^{-4} and 0.30 respectively.

Discussion

The results of this study enable us to definitely rule out a close linkage between HLA and a single gene assumed to determine precursor lesions of any type occurring alone or together with FMM. However, when FMM is studied alone, such firm exclusion cannot be asserted; only very tight linkage is excluded when the low gene frequencies are considered.

The fact that different results were obtained in the exclusion of linkage in FMM alone and precursor lesions alone suggests the possible existence of different genetic mechanisms controlling these two entities, including genes possibly linked to the Rh locus [8].

In conclusion, further studies are needed in order to determine whether HLA plays a role in the genetic determination of MM, with special attention paid to a possible heterogeneity of the disease, which requires larger series of multiplex families. When considering heterogeneity, it would be important to examine the genetic contribution to the sequential steps in the development of FMM: non-HLA genes may be involved in the development of precursor lesions, while HLA may influence the progress to malignancy.

Acknowledgments. We are greatly indebted to the following clinicians who kindly referred their patients to us and provided the pathological slides: M. F. Avril, C. Brocheriou (Paris), A. Azizi, S. Brenner (Tel Aviv), A. Castermans (Liège), M. Hundeiker (Gießen), V. Voigtländer (Mannheim), P. Altmeyer, H. Holzmann (Frankfurt), E. Großhans (Strasbourg), G. Moulin, J. Bouchet (Lyon)

References

1. Cavelier B, Daveau M, Gilbert D, et al (1980) Augmentation de l'antigène HLA-A9 dans les mélanomes malins principalement dans les formes métastatiques ou les récidives. A propos de 105 mélanomes dont 34 formes graves. C R Acad Sci 291:241–243
2. Clark WH, Reimer RR, Greene M et al (1978) Origin of familial malignant melanomas from heritable melanocytic lesions. Arch Dermatol 114:732–738
3. Demenais F, Cesarini JP, Daveau M, Cavelier B, Gony J, Feingold N, Hors J (1984) A linkage study between HLA and cutaneous malignant melanoma and/or precursor lesions. J Med Genet (in press)
4. Duggleby WF, Stoll H, Priore R (1981) A genetic analysis of melanoma: polygenic inheritance as a threshold trait. Am J Epidemiol 114:63–72
5. Elder DE, Goldman LI, Goldman SC, et al (1980) Dysplastic nevus syndrome: a phenotypic association of sporadic cutaneous melanoma. Cancer 46:1787–1794
6. McGovern VJ, Mihm MC, Bailly C et al (1973) The classification of malignant melanoma and its histologic reporting. Cancer 32:1446–1457
7. Greene MH, Fraumeni JF (1979) The hereditary variant of malignant melanoma. In: Clark WH, Goldman MJ, Mastrangelo (eds) Human malignant melanoma. Grune and Stratton, New York, pp 139–166
8. Greene MH, Goldin LR, Clark WH, et al (1983) Familial cutaneous malignant melanoma: autosomal dominant trait possibly linked to the Rh locus. Proc Nat Acad Sci USA 80:6071–6075
9. Hawkins BR, Dawkins RL, Hockey A, et al (1981) Evidence for linkage between HLA and malignant melanoma. Tissue Antigens 17:540–541
10. Hodge SE, Morton LA, Tiderman S, Kidd KK, Spence MA (1979) Age of onset correction available for linkage analysis (LIPED) Am J Hum Genet 31:761–762
11. Lynch HT, Frichot BC, Lynch JF (1978) Familial atypical multiple mole-melanoma syndrome. J Med Genet 15:352–356
12. Lynch HT, Fusaro RM, Danes BS, et al (1983) A review of hereditary malignant melanoma including biomarkers in familial atypical multiple mole melanoma syndrome. Cancer Genet and Cytogenet 8:325–358
13. Morton NE (1963) Segregation and linkage. In: Burdette WJ (ed) Methodology in human genetics. Holden Day, San Francisco, pp 17–52
14. Ott J (1974) Estimation of the recombination fraction in human pedigrees: efficient computation of the likelihood for human linkage studies. Am J Hum Genet 26:588–597
15. Pellegris G, Illeni MT, Rovini D, et al (1982) HLA complex and familial malignant melanoma. Int J Cancer 29:621–623
16. Prade M, Levene A, Cesarini JP, Bailly C, Van der Esch E, Smith N, Suurkula CM, Verhest A (1984) Intraepidermal melanocytic proliferation: a practical guide to the histological classification of some possible precursors of malignant melanoma. Br J Dermatol (in press)
17. Rahbari H, Mehregan AH (1981) Sporadic atypical mole syndrome. Arch Dermatol 117:329–331
18. Reimer RR, Clark WH, Greene MH, et al (1978) Precursor lesions in familial melanoma. A new genetic preneoplastic syndrome. JAMA 239:744–746
19. Wallace DG, Exton LA, McLeod GRC (1971) Genetic factor in malignant melanoma. Cancer 27:1262–1266

Hodgkin's Disease

J. Hors[1], C. Bonaïti-Pellie[2], M.F. D'Agay[3], H. Rappaport[4], J.M. Andrieux[5], L.P. de Waal[6], G.G. de Lange[6], and N. Feingold[2]

With the collaboration of W. Braun, A. Cambon-Thomsen, M. de Bruyere, P. A. Dyer, P. Engelfriet, R. Fauchet, H. Festenstein, M. Gueguen, S. Lawler, S. Mayer, M. Muylle, P. Perrier, and M. M. Tongio

1 INSERM, U93, Hôpital St. Louis, 2, Place du Dr. Fournier, 75010 Paris, France
2 INSERM, U155, Chateau de Longchamp, Paris, France
3 Departement d'Anatomopathologie, Hôpital St. Louis, Paris, France
4 Department of Anatomopathology, City of Hope Medical Center, Duarte, CA, USA
5 Departement de Hemato-Oncology, Hopital Laennec, Paris, France
6 Central Laboratory Transfusion Service, Amsterdam, The Netherlands

The aim of this work was to study a possible linkage between susceptibility to Hodgkin's disease and the HLA region by genotyping multiplex case families. Because familial incidence of the disease is low, international cooperation is a unique opportunity for providing sufficient cases for a linkage study.

Epidemiological and Genetic Background

The average incidence rate of the disease is known to be about 4/100 000 [4, 6]. Siblings of Hodgkin's patients have a 7 times higher risk of contracting the disease [4]. This estimate leads to an approximate recurrence risk among siblings of 0.5% (eight of 1569 siblings). Little information exists concerning the mode of transmission of the disease. On account of the time intervals between diagnoses being shorter than the age differences between family members, Vianna et al. [14] concluded that shared environmental factors played an important role in familial incidence. Gruffermann et al. [4], noting an excess of sex concordance, reached the same conclusions.

HLA and Hodgkin's Disease Susceptibility

From numerous studies made on the relationship between HLA and Hodgkin's disease, two main conclusions emerge:

1. From the review of population data, there are converging arguments in favor of the prevalence of A1 – particularly in the case of mixed cellularity – and, to a lesser degree, of B5, B8, and B18 [12] among Hodgkin's patients.
2. From a total series of 21 pairs of affected siblings published in the literature, an excess of HLA-identical pairs was observed to be significant [8]: 12 shared two haplotypes, seven shared one, and two none. These results suggest the possible existence of a disease susceptibility gene inside or near HLA.

Methods

The only *criteria for selection* of the cases submitted to the workshop were that they should belong to multiplex families, that HLA genotyping could be clearly established, and that the diagnosis of the disease be proven on the basis of histological data (Luke's classification [9]). Slides of an enlarged lymph node from each patient were required to be submitted to a panel of two pathologists (M. F. d'A, Paris, and H. R., Los Angeles), for two independent readings.

The *histopathological* study was important in order to differentiate Hodgkin's from non-Hodgkin's lymphomas and to place each case histologically into one of five main categories: mixed cellularity, nodular sclerosis, lymphopredominant, lymphodepletion, and others. It was recommended that all patients and relatives be carefully examined and that *clinical pathological staging* [2, 3] and course of development be quoted (card 69). However, staging has not been considered as a critical point of the study, since follow-up is very short and the cases have been selected nonrandomly.

The *linkage analysis* was made using the LIPED program [11] with age correction [7] for the lod score calculation. When the genetic model and parameters are unknown, the lod score method does not permit to estimate the recombination fraction, but remains a powerful method to detect linkage. Moreover it permits to take into account all types of affected relatives and not only affected siblings. The computations were performed under extreme single-locus models, recessive and dominant, for various gene frequencies and an average level of penetrance of 1%, deduced from the recurrence risk in sibs. Homogeneity of the lod scores was tested using the method proposed by Morton [10].

Histocompatibility Testing 1984
Edited by E. D. Albert et al.

Table 1. Haplotypes shared by pairs of affected siblings

Pair	Family	HLA haplotype				Shared haplotypes
1	FRA DAU 61	A3	C–	B7	DR4	2
		A2	Cw7	B18	DR5	
2	FRA FAU 20	A29	C–	B7	DR–	2
		A1	Cw3	Bw62	DRw6	
3	US6 BRN 18	A2	Cw7	B7	DR2	2
		A28	C–	B35	DR–	
4	FRA DAU 62	A2	Cw2	B27	DRw6	2
		A3	Cw7	B7	DR7	
5	FRA OHA 8	A11	Cw4	B35	DRw6	2
		A11	Cw7	B7	DR5	
6	FRA MYE 24	A1	C–	B35	NT	2
		A1	C–	B–	NT	
7	BEN ENG 4	A2	Cw7	B7	DR2	2
		A28	Cw3	Bw60	DR2	
8	BEN MUY 2	A2	Cw3	Bw60	DRw6	1
9	BEN BRU 1	A2	Cw7	B7	DR2	1
10	BEN ENG 2	A2	C–	B51	DR5	1

Table 2. Haplotypes shared by parent/child pairs

Pair	Family	HLA haplotype			
11	FRA MYE 24	A11	C–	B35	DR1
12	UKI HAR 3	A1	C–	B35	DR1
13	FRA OHA 8	A11	Cw4	B35	DRw6
14	UKI LAW 13	A11	Cw6	B45	DR4
15	FRA MYE 25	A2	Cw7	B18	DR2

Table 3. Haplotypes not shared by related patients

Pair	Family					Relationship
16	BEN ENG 3	A31	C–	B51	DR5	S/S
		A24	Cw5	B44	DR5	
		A24	C–	B44	DRw6	
		A30	Cw4	B35	DR1	
17	BEN MUY 1	A2	Cw7	B7	DR2	S/S
		A2	Cw7	B27	DR4	
		A28	C–	B51	DRw6	
		A29	C–	B51	DR5	
18	FRA PRR 20	A3	C–	B8	DR4	S/S
		A11	Cw3	Bw60	DR2	
		A2	C–	Bw60	DR–	
		A3	C–	B35	DR5	
19	BEN ENG 1	A1	Cw6	Bw57	DR3	C/C
		A1	Cw7	B7	DR2	
		A2	Cw3	Bw62	DRw6	
		A28	Cw3	Bw60	DRw6	
20	BEN ENG 5	A1	Cw7	B8	DR3	C/C
		A1	Cw7	B8	DR2	
		A2	C–	B18	DR5	
		A3	Cw4	B35	DR1	
21	FRA FAU 20	A2	Cw3	B15	DRw6	C/C
		A29	Cw4	B35	DR5	
22	UKI FES 27	A3	Cw7	B7	DR7	U/N
		A–	Cw7	B51	DR–	
		A2	Cw5	B44	DR1	
		A28	Cw7	B44	DR2	

S/S, pairs of siblings; C/C, first cousins; U/N, uncle and nephrew

Families and Patients

A total of 19 multiplex families were submitted: they included four parent/child(ren) situations, ten families in whom only siblings were affected, two families with only first cousins, and three other situations: one uncle/nephew pair, one with two sibs and a first cousin, and one with two sibs, an uncle, and a first cousin.

Haplotype comparisons were carried out after subdividing families into 22 pairs of patients with reference to one index case per family (Tables 1–3), except for families FRA MYE 24 and FRA FAU 20 where two nuclear families were considered for simplification. All the families were new, being studied for the first time, except three who had already been analyzed previously and retyped for the workshop (FRA OHA 8, FRA FAU 20, FRA DAU 62) (family "SOU", no. 17 "GUI" and no. 5 respectively from [8]).

Table 4. Linkage analysis on workshop data (19 families)

Recessive model				Dominant model			
q	θ_{max}	Z_{max}	Z_0	q	θ_{max}	Z_{max}	Z_0
0.01	0.37	0.036	−17.290	0.01	0.34	0.046	−5.322
0.35	0.25	0.091	−0.830	0.10	0.20	0.150	−0.431
0.78	0.00	0.103	0.103	0.26	0.00	0.254	0.254

q, gene frequency; θ_{max}, value of recombination fraction for which maximum lod score (Z_{max}) is obtained; Z_0, value of lod score for $\theta = 0$

Results

Patients. A total of 42 patients, 21 male and 21 female, were studied. The age at onset varied from 2 to 53 years, with an average of 27 years.

Genotype. Seven pairs of affected siblings shared two haplotypes, three pairs shared only one, and three pairs none. This distribution is not significantly different from the expected Mendelian pattern of 3.25, 6.5, and 3.25 pairs respectively ($\chi^2 = 4.63$ after Yates correction; df 2). None of the three pairs of first cousins shared any haplotypes.

Haplotypes. The list of shared haplotypes is given in Table 1 (siblings) and Table 2 (parent/child). The list of unshared haplotypes in the other pairs of patients (three siblings, three first cousins) is shown in Table 3. It can be noted that the haplotype A2, Cw7, B7, DR2 is present in three families (pairs 3, 7, and 9) and A1, C–, B35, DR1 in two (pairs 11 and 12). It can be seen that three patients are A1 homozygotes (pairs 6, 19, and 20; Tables 1, 3) and that two antigens are shared by two pairs: A24, B44 (pair 16) and A3, Bw60 (pair 18)

Table 5. Concordance in time, histology, and sex

Pair	Time intervals (years)	Age intervals (years)	Histological type		Sex		Shared haplotypes
1	28	19	NS	NS	F	F	2
2	0	1	NS	NS	F	F	2
3	1	5	NS	NS	F	F	2
4	11	3	UN	NS	F	M	2
5	4	6	NS	NS	M	M	2
6	1	6	MC	MC	M	F	2
7	8	6	MC	MC	M	F	2
8	4	12	MC	NS	F	M	1
9	1	4	NS	NS	M	F	1
10	5	1	NS	NS	F	F	1
11	7	22	NS	LD	M	M	1
12	9	24	NS	NS	F	M	1
13	4	21	NS	NS	M	M	1
14	0	24	LP	LP	M	F	1
15	1	15	LP	LP	M	M	1
16	6	8	NS	NS	F	F	0
17	6	1	MC	MC	M	F	0
18	7	10	NS	NS	M	M	0
19	5	12	NS	NS	M	F	0
20	1	1	LP	NS	M	M	0
21	1	7	NS	MC	F	F	0
22	3	20	UN	UN	M	M	0

NS, nodular sclerosis; UN, unclassified; MC, mixed cellularity; LD, lymphodominant; LP, lymphodepletion

Lod Scores. Under recessive mode of inheritance, the lod scores never exceeded the value of 0.11, whatever the postulated gene frequencies. When a dominant model was considered, the maximum score obtained was 0.28. The results are shown in detail in Table 4.

Antigen Frequencies. The proportion of individuals bearing the antigen HLA-A1 was 26% (11 : 42).
The *time intervals* ranged from 0 to 28 years and the *age intervals* at onset from 1 to 24 years, as shown in Table 5.
The *histological subtypes* are concordant in 17 pairs and discordant in 5 pairs.

Discussion

The very low, nearly null, value of the maximum lod scores obtained in the present study is far from the +3 value necessary to assume a linkage between HLA and a putative gene of susceptibility to Hodgkin's disease. For low gene frequencies, lod scores are less than −2 for small values of θ, permitting rejection of close linkage under those particular hypotheses. This seems in contradiction with the results obtained from previous studies published in the literature. The revised lod score calculations in this material after withdrawing the cases resubmitted in this workshop are shown in Table 6. Heterogeneity between the two series is almost significant (χ^2 varying from 2.30 to 3.96, df 1, according to the parameters used).
Hypotheses can be formulated in order to explain such a discrepancy:
1. The selection of family pedigrees published in the literature could be biased by the over-representation of concordant pairs, i.e., those in favor of a linkage, while the observed discordant pairs may not have reached publication. This possible bias has been discussed by F. C. Grumet [5].
2. Different histological features, and also clinical involvement [13], may support the possible heterogeneity of Hodgkin's disease. However, it can be noted that in the present series the three HLA-different pairs of affected siblings are histologically concordant (Table 5).

Table 6. Linkage analysis on data from the literature (26 families)

Recessive model				Dominant model			
q	θ_{max}	Z_{max}	Z_0	q	θ_{max}	Z_{max}	Z_0
0.01	0.16	3.121	−11.276	0.01	0.08	3.349	1.425
0.15	0.10	2.601	1.225	0.05	0.03	2.926	2.819
0.37	0.00	2.293	2.293	0.08	0.00	2.757	2.757

Abbreviations: see Table 4

Besides postulated immune response genes responsible for resistance to the disease, allowing a higher survival rate – for example A1, B8, which could partly explain the association with A1 observed mainly in the retrospective studies [8] – the existence of a susceptibility gene within the HLA region, particularly near the A locus [1], is still questionable.
However, the fact that previous results exhibited significant lod scores makes further studies necessary before any definite conclusion can be reached on the possibility of a genetic linkage between HLA and susceptibility to Hodgkin's disease. It is hoped that further publication of all the multiplex families observed prospectively will be continued, on the basis of an international registry.

Acknowledgments. We are greatly indebted to the following clinicians who kindly referred their patients to us and provided the pathological slides: C. Brocheriou, F. Teillet (Paris), J. K. Weick, R. E. Hermann (Cleveland), N. Buyssens (Antwerpen), F. Oberling (Strasbourg), J. Pris, A. Robert (Toulouse), I. E. Smith, G. S. Tobis (London), J. Garbet (Angers).

References

1. Bodmer WF (1973) Genetic factors in Hodgkin's disease: association with a disease-susceptibility locus (DSA) in the HL-A region. Natl Cancer Inst Monogr 36:127–134
2. Carbone PP, Kaplan HS, Musshof K, Smithers DW, Tubiana M (1971) Report of the committee on Hodgkin's disease staging classification. Cancer Res 31:1860–1861
3. De Vita TV, Heilman S, Rosenberg SA (1982) Hodgkin's disease and the non-Hodgkin's lymphoma. In: Cancer principles and practice of oncology. Lippincott, Philadelphia, p 1331–1401
4. Grufferman S, Cole P, Smith PG, Lukes RJ (1977) Hodgkin's disease in siblings. N Engl J Med 296:248–253
5. Grumet FC Personal communication
6. Gutensohn N, Cole P (1977) Epidemiology of Hodgkin's disease in the young. Int J Cancer 19:595–604
7. Hodge SE, Morton LA, Tideman S, Kidd KK, Spence MA (1979) Age of onset correction available for linkage analysis (LIPED). Am J Hum Genet 31:761–762
8. Hors J, Dausset J (1983) HLA and susceptibility to Hodgkin's disease. Immunol Rev 70:167–192
9. Lukes RJ, Butler JJ (1966) The pathology and nomenclature of Hodgkin's disease. Cancer Res 26:1063–1081
10. Morton NE (1962) Segregation and linkage. In: Burdette WJ (ed) Methodology in human genetics. Holden-Day, San Francisco, pp 17–52
11. Ott J (1974) Estimation of the recombination fraction in human pedigrees: efficient computation of the likelihood for human linkage studies. Am J Hum Genet 26:588–597
12. Ryder LP, Anderson E, Svejgaard A (eds) (1979) HLA and disease registry. Munksgaard, Copenhagen
13. Teillet F, Boiron M, Bernard J (1971) A reappraisal of clinical and biological signs in staging of Hodgkin's disease. Cancer Res 31:1723–1729
14. Vianna NJ, Davies JNP, Polan AK, Wolfgang P (1974) Familial Hodgkin's disease: an environmental and genetic disorder. Lancet ii:854–857

Original Contributions

Human Histocompatibility Antigens in Malignant Tumors of Nonlymphoid Origin

P.G. Natali[1], A. Bigotti[2], and S. Ferrone[3]

1 Departments of Immunology, Regina Elena Cancer Institute, Rome, Italy
2 Department of Pathology, Regina Elena Cancer Institute, Rome, Italy
3 Department of Microbiology and Immunology, New York Medical College, Valhalla, NY 10595, USA

The availability of monoclonal antibodies has facilitated the analysis of the distribution of histocompatibility antigens in surgically removed tissues.

Staining of surgically removed normal tissues of nonlymphoid origin has provided surprising data on the tissue distribution of histocompatibility antigens: class I antigens have a more restricted tissue distribution than originally assumed, since they were not detected in brain cortex, cerebellum, sympathetic ganglia, hypophysis, parathyroid gland, thyroid, exocrine pancreas, hepatocytes, spermatozoa, seminiferous tubules, or skeletal or smooth muscles. The distribution of HLA-DR antigens is broader than that of DQw1 antigens, since the latter were not detected in epithelia of stomach, small intestine, colon, or breast. The tissue distribution of both class I and class II HLA antigens is different from that of their counterparts in mice, since H-2 antigens have not been found in adrenal glands, esophagus, ovarian follicles, or pancreatic islet cells, and the murine analogs of DQ antigens are expressed by epithelial cells of small intestine and colon.

Malignant transformation of cells may be associated with changes in the expression of HLA antigens. Class I antigens became detectable in 5 of 20 brain tumors, in 7 of 8 liver carcinomas, and 2 of 7 thyroid carcinomas. On the other hand, loss of class I antigens occurred in 14 of 37 breast carcinomas, in 21 of 97 melanomas, in 7 of 14 lung carcinomas, and in 14 of 30 breast carcinomas. Breast carcinomas frequently display discrepancies in the reactivity with antibodies to the two subunits of class I antigens, since the lack or decrease in staining with antibodies to the heavy chain is not paralleled by a comparable reduction in the staining with antibodies to β_2 microglobulin.

Class II antigens can be acquired by a variety of tumors and especially by melanomas. HLA-DR antigens appear more frequently than DQ antigens; staining of 58 tumors of different origins detected HLA-DR antigens and DQ antigens in 33 and in 17 tumors, respectively. No tumor was found to express DQ antigens and to lack DR antigens. This finding and the differential susceptibility to modulation by interferons combine to suggest that HLA-DR and DQ antigens are controlled by different regulatory mechanisms.

Class I and class II antigens are heterogeneous in their expression among cells within a lesion, among primary lesions and autologous metastasis removed from different anatomical sites, and among lesions removed from different patients. Both class I and class II HLA antigens may become detectable in cytoplasms of tumor cells. This localization is not unique for tumor cells, since it also occurs in normal cells, both in man and in other animal species. In view of the role of HLA antigens in cell–cell interactions and of the relationship in animal model systems between abnormalities in the expression of histocompatibility antigens and metastatic spread of tumors, the abnormalities we have described may play a significant role in the aberrant behavior of tumor cells.

Histocompatibility Testing 1984
Edited by E. D. Albert et al.

B27 Subtypes

L.P. de Waal, J. Lieder, G.G. de Lange, B. Huis, C.J.M. Melief, C.P. Engelfriet, and P. Ivanyi

Central Laboratory, Netherlands Red Cross Blood Transfusion Service, The Laboratory for Experimental and Clinical Immunology, University of Amsterdam, Amsterdam, The Netherlands

Cytotoxic T lymphocytes (CTL) generated between HLA-A, B, C (B27-positive) full-house identical responder stimulator pairs recognized three B27 subtypes. These were provisionally designated as B27W, B27K, and B27C. B27W and B27K antigens behaved as HLA-B locus alleles in population and family studies, functioned as virus restriction elements, and were found to be biochemically different [1–3]. A CTL clone was obtained, which typed for B27K [4]. In the Caucasian population 8% of B27-positive cells are of B27K type and 1% of the B27C type. We examined the possibility of finding sera that could be used for typing in the routine two-step microlymphocytotoxicity test for these subtypes; we selected 50 pregnancy and polytransfused patient sera because of their known (albeit imperfect) association with B27. The sera were tested against a panel of cells previously typed by CTL for the B27W and B27K and B27C subtypes. Four sera were found that are almost specific for these B27 subtypes (Table 1).

Furthermore, two monoclonal antibodies, M1 and M2 (a kind gift from Dr. Grumet), were tested against the same cell panel (Table 2). The results indicate that M2 is almost specific for B27W + C. In addition, M2 also recognizes Bw47 [5]. Since B27W-specific CTL fail to lyse Bw47 target cells, the results with the M2 monoclonal antibody indicate that the epitopes recognized by CTCs differ from those recognized by M2.

Thus the combined data indicate that (1) B27 CTL-defined subtypes can also be recognized by

Table 1. Recognition of CTL-defined HLA-B27 subtypes by pregnancy sera

CTL-defined B27 subtype		Pregnancy sera			
		0567/1:2	BROK/1:1	Cassel/1:1	KCJR/1:4
B27-W	1	8	8	1	1
	2	8	8	1	1
	3	8	8	2	1
	4	6	8	1	1
	5	8	8	1	1
	6	8	8	1	1
	7	8	8	1	1
	8	8	8	1	4
	9	8	8	2	1
	10	8	6	1	1
	11	8	8	1	1
	12	8	8	1	1
	13	8	6	1	1
	14	8	8	1	4
	15	6	8	1	1
B27-K	1	1	1	8	8
	2	1	1	8	6
	3	1	1	8	6
	4	1	1	8	4
	5	1	1	8	8
	6	1	1	8	6
	7	1	2	8	6
	8	1	1	4	8
B27-C	1	8	4	1	1
	2	8	8	1	1
	3	8	8	1	1
	4	8	8	1	1
	5	8	2	1	1

Table 2. Recognition of CTL-defined HLA-B27 subtypes by monoclonal antibodies

CTL-defined B27 subtype		Monoclonal antibody	
		Grumet M-1/1:200	Grumet M-2/1:10
B27-W	1	8	8
	2	8	6
	3	8	8
	4	8	1
	5	8	8
	6	8	8
	7	6	8
	8	8	8
	9	8	8
	10	8	8
	11	8	8
	12	8	8
	13	8	1
	14	8	8
	15	8	8
B27-K	1	8	4
	2	8	1
	3	8	1
	4	8	1
	5	8	1
	6	8	1
	7	8	1
	8	8	1
B27-C	1	8	0
	2	8	2
	3	8	8
	4	8	2
	5	8	4

Histocompatibility Testing 1984
Edited by E. D. Albert et al.

alloimmunesera and monoclonal antibody; and (2) epitopes recognized by CTL differ from those recognized by antibody.

Reference

1. Breuning et al (1982) Subtypes of HLA-B27 detected by cytotoxic T lymphocytes and their role in self-recognition. Hum Immunol 5:259 – 268
2. Breuning et al (1983) Specificity of anti-HLA-B27 cytotoxic T lymphocytes. Tissue Antigens 22:267 – 282
3. Mölders et al (1983) Biochemical analysis of variant HLA-B27 antigens. Hum Immunol 6:111 – 117
4. Breuning et al (to be published) A cloned cytotoxic T-lymphocyte line recognizing a subtype of HLA-B27. Hum Immunol
5 Grumet et al (1982) Monoclonal antibody (B27M2) subdividing HLA-B27. Hum Immunol 5:61

Segregation of DQ and DR: "Exceptions to the Rule"

M. Oudshoorn[1], G.M.T. Schreuder[2], E.M. Campbell[1], and E.D. du Toit[1]

1 Provincial Laboratory for Tissue Immunology, Private Bag 4, Observatory, 7935 Cape Town, South Africa
2 Dep. of Immunohematology and Blood Bank, University Hospital, Rijnsburgerweg 10, 2333 AA Leiden, The Netherlands

The strong associations of DQw1 with DR1, 2, w6, and w10, of DQw2 with DR3 and 7, and of DQw3 with DR4 and 5 have been defined in studies with cells of Caucasoid origin. The use of monoclonal antibodies and carefully selected alloantisera made it clear that these associations are in fact a reflection of strong linkage disequilibrium between HLA-DR and DQ in Caucasoid populations, but that exceptions can occur when other populations are studied.

In Cape Town we typed 42 families for HLA-A, B, C, and DR with Ninth Workshop sera. The DR serology was analysed in Cape Town and Leiden and no problems were encountered with the definition of the DR specificities, but some of the DQ alleles appeared to segregate in a rather unexpected way. Of the 16 DR3-positive haplotypes found among 34 unrelated South African Negroes, nine segregated with DQw2, five with DQ blank, and two with DQw3. The 14 DR3-positive haplotypes found among unrelated Caucasoids and the six found among unrelated Cape Coloureds all segregated with DQw2. Of the 11 DR5-positive haplotypes found in unrelated Cape Coloureds, nine segregated with DQw3 and two with DQw1. Amongst the 15 DR5-positive haplotypes found in the unrelated South African Negroes, nine segregated with DQw3 and six with DQw1. The serological reaction patterns of DR3, 5 and 7 positive haplotypes with different DQ alleles are shown in Table 1.

Although the DQw1 sera sometimes reacted weakly, the patterns were as expected. Of the so-called

Table 1. Serological reaction patterns of DR3-, 5-, and 7-positive haplotypes with the different DQ alleles

9W[a] sera: DR3, DR5, DR7

DR	DQ	DR3 564	DR3 565	DR3 570	DR5 608	DR5 610	DR7 629	DR7 630
3	w2	+	+	+	–	–	–	–
3	w3	+	+	+	–	–	–	–
3	–	+	+	+	–	–	–	–
5	w3	–	–	–	+	+	–	–
5	w1	–	–	–	+	+	–	–
7	w2	–	–	–	–	–	+	+
7	w3	–	–	–	–	–	+	+

9W[a] sera: DQw1

DR	DQ	653	654	655	657	661	662	664	667	668	669	664	701	793	794	672
3	w2	–	–	–	–	–	–	–	–	–	–	–	–	–	–	–
3	w3	–	–	–	–	–	–	–	–	–	–	–	–	–	–	–
3	–	–	–	–	–	–	–	–	–	–	–	–	–	–	–	–
5	w3	–	–	–	–	–	–	–	–	–	–	–	–	–	–	–
5	w1	+	+	+	+	+	+	+	+	+	+	+	+	+	+	+
7	w2	–	–	–	–	–	–	–	–	–	–	–	–	–	–	–
7	w3	–	–	–	–	–	–	–	–	–	–	–	–	–	–	–

9W[a] sera: DQw2

DR	DQ	726	792	+5 775	+7 723	+7 727	+3 +7 720	+3 +7 721	+5 +3 722	+7 719	+7 724
3	w2	+	+	+	+	+	+	+	+	+	+
3	w3	–	–	–	–	–	+	+	+	–	–
3	–	–	–	–	–	–	+	+	+	–	–
5	w3	–	–	+	–	–	–	–	+	–	–
5	w1	–	–	+	–	–	–	–	+	–	–
7	w2	+	+	+	+	+	+	+	+	+	+
7	w3	–	–	–	+	+	+	+	–	+	+

9W[a] sera: DQw3

DR	DQ	761	744	745	746	774	787	748	+5 741	+5 794	+6 +5 756	+3 760
3	w2	–	–	–	–	–	–	–	–	–	–	+
3	w3	+	+	+	+	+	+	+	+	+	+	+
3	–	–	–	–	–	–	–	–	–	–	–	+
5	w3	+	+	+	+	+	+	+	+	+	+	+
5	w1	–	–	–	–	–	–	–	+	+	+	–
7	w2	–	–	–	–	–	–	–	–	–	–	–
7	w3	–	+	–	+	+	+	+	+	+	+	+

[a] 9W, Ninth Workshop

Histocompatibility Testing 1984
Edited by E. D. Albert et al.

DQw2 or DR3 + 7 sera only 9w726 and 792 were monospecific; all other sera reacted with DQw2-negative DR5, DR3, and/or DR7-positive cells [1]. Of the 11 DQw3 sera, three reacted with DR5-positive, DQw3-negative cells and one with DR3-positive, DQw3-negative cells.

Conclusion. Our family data clearly showed that DQ is a series of specificities different from DR and that strong associations between DQ and DR as described in Caucasoid populations can be different in other populations. The study of families with DR-DQ combinations different from the usual ones is very helpful in defining DR antibodies in supposedly monospecific DQ alloantisera, thus proving that they are not monospecific.

Reference

1. Schreuder I, Parlevliet J (1983) HLA-DR, LB, MB, MT and 8W13 with 9 HTCs. In: Ninth International Workshop Newsletter V, pp 41 – 51

Characterization of a New Subset of B Cell Alloantigens

A.H. Johnson[1], D.B. Amos[2], M. Woodbury[2], R.J. Hartzman[3]

1 Georgetown University School of Medicine, Washington, DC 20007, USA
2 University Medical Center, Durham, NC 27710, USA
3 Naval Medical Research Institute, Bethesda, MD 20014, USA

The complexity of the human class II molecules is well established. A minimum of four distinct serologically defined molecular subunits have been identified (DR, BR, DQ, DP). We report here a new serologically defined B cell specificity designated MA4. The absorption data is consistent with the interpretation that the MA4 specificity is located on a molecule or chain distinct from DR, BR, DQ, DP.

The defining antiserum (MAX) was raised by planned immunization of a father with lymphocytes from his son (immunizing haplotype = A31, Cw–, B14, Dw7, DR7, BR4, DQw2, DPw2). ABC activity was removed with specific platelet absorption. Antiserum MAX absorbed with cell line JEDA (DR7, w6/DRw52, w53/DQw1/DPw2, w4) reacted with only DQw2 cells and with DR4+ cells in a panel ($n = 180$). All activity segregated with HLA in families. Absorption experiments were performed to characterize the DR4-associated serological activity. The HLA types of the LCL used for absorption are as follows: JEDA (see above), 90 = DR4, 4/BR4/DQw3/DPw2, 94 = DR5, 5/DRw52, 52/DQw3, w3/ DPw2, w4; LOST = DR3, 3/DRw52, w52/DQw2/ DPw4, w4. Absorption which characterizes the new specificity MA4 is given in Table 1.

Table 1. Specific absorption of alloantiserum MAX/P1

Absorbing cell(s)	Remaining specificity		Specificity of B cell panel[a]								
			DR7+ DQw2+ BR4+	DR7+ DQw2+ BR4–	DR7+ DQw2– BR4+	DR4+ DQw3+ BR4+	DR4+ DQw3+ BR4–	DR4+ DQw3– BR4–	DR5+ DQw3+	DR3+ DQw2+	DR3+ DQw2–
	DQw2	MA4									
JEDA	+	+	6/11	1/1	0/2	2/3	6/8	1/1	0/5	4/4	0/3
JEDA/90	+	–	6/11	1/1	0/2	0/3	0/8	1/1	0/5	4/4	0/3
JEDA/94	+	+	6/11	1/1	0/2	2/3	6/8	1/1	0/5	4/4	0/3
JEDA/LOST	–	+	6/11	0/1	0/2	2/3	6/8	1/1	0/5	0/4	0/3
JEDA/LOST/90	–	–	0/11	0/1	0/2	0/3	0/8	1/1	0/5	0/4	0/3
JEDA/LOST/94	–	+	6/11	0/1	0/2	2/3	6/8	1/1	0/5	0/4	0/3

[a] Number of positive reactions over number of cells tested

Histocompatibility Testing 1984
Edited by E. D. Albert et al.

Thus an antiserum raised against a DR7 haplotype contains alloantibody activity against DR4+ individuals. This activity (designated MA4) cannot be BR4 or DPw2, since the absorbing cell, JEDA, is BR4+, DPw2+. MA4 has been shown to segregate with HLA in families and is associated with DR4 and with DR7 in panel studies. Since this antibody was raised against a single haplotype, we feel that the most likely interpretation of the data is the existence of a new subset of B cell alloantigen. MA4 may be identical to the DQ-like activity in antiserum HON7, which has been shown to be distinct from the BR4 activity. If so, then MA4 could be located on the DQ alpha chain or on a second DQ/I-A-like molecule. The presence of similar, as yet undefined allospecificities on class II polypeptide chains could explain the reported findings of alloreactive T cell clones which react with a specificity apparently different from the immunizing specificity (i.e., a DR7 stimulator giving rise to DR4-related allospecific T cell clones). Likewise it could explain the immunochemical differences observed between two "serologically identical" phenotypes.

Serologic Detection of New Polymorphisms on DQ Molecules Distinct from the DQw1, 2, and 3 Specificities

G. Nunez, M.J. Latimer, E.J. Ball, L.K. Myers, and P. Stastny

Dept. of Internal Medicine, The University of Texas Health Science Center at Dallas, Southwestern Medical School, 5323 Harry Hines Blvd., Dallas, TX 75235, USA

Recent structural studies have suggested that DQ molecules are more polymorphic than presently defined by conventional serology [1–3]. We have analyzed 9W reagents for the presence of sera that might detect new polymorphisms on DQ molecules. To do this, we have utilized the following criteria: (1) expression on B cells but not on most monocytes; (2) specific inhibition of cytotoxicity by monoclonal anti-DQ but not by anti-DR antibodies; (3) panel distribution distinct from the known DQw1, 2, and 3 specificities.

Table 1. Inhibition of cytotoxicity of selected DR, DQ, and DSP sera by monoclonal antibodies

Blocking antibody[a]	Specificity	Serum dilution	9W Alloantisera				
			613 DR5	747 DQw3	607 DSP	712 DSP	773 DSP
			cytotoxicity scores				
L368	ß2-microglobulin	1	8	8	8	8	8
		1:2	8	8	8	8	8
		1:4	8	8	4	8	8
		1:8	8	8	1	1	8
		1:16	1	1	1	1	1
L203	DR	1	2	8	8	8	8
		1:2	1	8	8	8	8
		1:4	1	8	1	8	8
		1:8	1	8	1	8	8
		1:16	1	1	1	1	1
TU22	DQ	1	8	1	1	1	1
		1:2	8	1	1	1	1
		1:4	8	1	1	1	1
		1:8	8	1	1	1	1
		1:16	1	1	1	1	1

[a] B cells from a DR3, 5; DQw2, w3 donor were incubated with mouse monoclonal antibody, washed, and incubated with $F(ab')_2$ goat antimouse IgG before cytotoxicity testing

These determinants appear to represent private or short epitopes of DQ molecules that also carry antigens DQw1, w2, and w3 and have been tentatively named DSP. The specificity DSP5 × 4 was defined by two sera (9w601 and 9w607) which react with most DR5 and a small percentage of DR4 cells. Other sera reacting with DSP determinants were 9w712 and 9w773 associated with DR5 and 9w705 associated with DRw6. Sera 9w759 and 9w761 were similar but distinct from DQw2 and DQw3 respectively. DSP antigens appear to stimulate allogeneic T cells and serve as restriction elements for antigen-specific T cell responses (see E. J. Ball et al., Private Specificities of Human IA-Like Molecules Detected by T Cell Lines, this volume). The relation of DSP antigens with recently described polymorphisms of DQ alpha chains [4] remains to be explored.

References

1. Giles R, Hurley CK, Capra JD (1984) Primary structural variation among serologically indistinguishable DS antigens: the MB3 bearing molecule in DR4 cells differs from the MB3 bearing molecule in DR5 cells. J Immunol (in press)
2. Goyert SM, Moriuchi J, Winchester R, Silver J (1983) HLA-DS molecules and their relation to supertypic specificities. Hum Immunol 70:53–63
3. Shackelford DA, Eibl B, Strominger JL (1983) Structural polymorphism of the DC light chains from DR1-, DR2-, and DRw6-positive cell lines. Immunogenetics 18:625–637
4. Tosi R, Tanigaki N, Sorrentino R, Centis D, Ferrara GB (1984) Serologically detectable polymorphism of the HLA-DC α-subunit. J Immunol 132:277–282

Analysis of 9W Antisera Detecting DR4- and DR2-Associated Epitopes by Use of Anti-idiotypic Antibodies *

E. Reed, C. Rohowsky-Kochan, and N. Suciu-Foca

Columbia University, College of Physicians and Surgeons, 630 W. 168th Street, New York, NY 10032, USA

Idiotypes are phenotypic markers of immunoglobulins which are defined by anti-idiotypic antibodies present in antisera directed against the variable region of Ig molecules. The library of idiotypes (Id) includes individual Id (Id I) and cross-reactive Id (Idx) which are shared by different individuals of the same species. Recently, we have shown that pregnancy sera contain both idiotypic and anti-idiotypic (anti-Id) antibodies to class I and class II HLA antigens [1, 2]. We have postulated that human anti-Id antibodies to HLA recognize, in alloantisera, public Id (Idx) that are products of highly conserved germ-line genes. This hypothesis was tested in the present study by determining the capacity of two anti-Id reagents to block the corresponding Id of relevant Ninth International Histocompatibility Workshop (9W) antisera.

Anti-Id (Ab2) Reagents. The selection and characterization of the anti-Id antisera FH (anti-anti-DR4) and ES (anti-anti-DR2) has been previously described [2]. Serum FH was obtained from a woman immunized to the HLA-DR4, Dw10, DRw53, DQw3 haplotype of her child. Serum ES derives from a parous woman immunized to DR2, Dw9 (HTC 8W205) DQw1 haplotype. Following absorption on lymphoblastoid cell lines, the $F(ab')_2$ of these sera was obtained and tested for its capacity to block idiotypic antibodies to various HLA-DR specificities.

Idiotypic (Ab1) Antibodies to HLA-DR2 and DR4. The HLA-DR antibody specificity of the 9W sera was determined by analyzing the pattern of reactions displayed by each serum on a panel of 20 families and 100 unrelated individuals including a minimum of two homozygous cells for each HLA-D/DR specificity [3]. 9W antisera defining the HLA antigens DR2, DR4, DQw1 (associated with DR1 + 2 + w6 + w10), DRw53 (associated with DR4 + 7 + w9), and DQw3 (associated with DR4 + 5 + w8 + w9) were selected for study if they showed an internal correlation of $r \geqq 0.7$ at a 1 : 2 dilution when tested on an informative panel of $DR2^+$ and $DR4^+$ cells.

Determination of FH (Anti-DR4) and ES (Anti-DR2) Idiotypic Antibodies in 9W Sera. The $F(ab')_2$ of serum FH and ES was tested at a concentration of 2 mg/ml for its capacity to block the cytotoxic activity of various dilutions of Ab1 contained by workshop antisera.

* This work was supported by grant NO1-AI-32505-01

Histocompatibility Testing 1984
Edited by E. D. Albert et al.

As previously shown by us, the DR4 specificity is associated with at least three distinct HLA-D/DR antigens: Dw4, Dw10, and SFNI (Dw14) [4]. 9w sera 575, 576, 580, 585, 587, 589, 592, 594, and 595 react indiscriminatively with cells expressing these specificities. Sera 576, 594 and 595 were blocked by Ab2 of FH, while sera 575, 580, and 585 were not. Two sera, 578 and 590, react with DR4^{+} or SFN1^{+} targets but not with Dw10. Serum 590 was not blocked by Ab2 of FH. The titer of sera reacting exclusively with SFN1+ cells (582 and 593) was not sufficient for inhibition studies. Since FH was immunized to the Dw10-associated DR4 specificity, it is possible that the failure of her Ab2 to inhibit serum 9W590, which recognizes another (not Dw10- associated) DR4 variant, is due to idiotypic differences between the paratopes of Ab1 binding to epitopes of Dw10 and Dw4 targets. Recent molecular studies indeed confirm our former contention that although serologically similar, the Dw4, Dw10, and SFN1 (Dw14) antigens are structurally distinct [4], since they differ with respect to the patterns of migrations of the DR beta chains [5].

The FH serum also contains anti-Id antibodies which inhibit the cytotoxic activity of some but not all anti-DRw53 and anti-DQw3 9w antisera (Table 1).

Table 2 summarizes the results obtained by studying the anti-idiotypic activity of serum ES. The haplotype to which ES was immunized carried the DR2, DQw1-associated Dw9 specificity defined by the 8W205 HTC. Serum ES inhibits three 9W sera (534, 552, 542) which react with cells expressing the Dw2 or the Dw9 specificity, yet fails to block another seven sera from the same cluster (530, 533, 535, 538, 545, 550, 555). Only one of these seven sera (555) fails to react with 8W205 HTC or with cells typing with it. Therefore, it seems that, as in the previous case, the anti-Id antibody discriminates between two different types of idiotypic antibodies, one that reacts with an epitope shared

Table 1. Anti-idiotypic inhibition of 9W sera by serum FH

HLA-DR/DQ	Associated HLA-Dw	9W sera	9W sera sharing the Idx detected by F(ab')$_2$ from serum FH	
			Idx^{+}	Idx^{-}
4	4, 10, SFN1	575, 576, 580, 585, 587, 589, 592, 594, 595	576, 594, 595	575, 580, 585
4	4, SFN1	578, 590		590
4	SFN1	582, 593		
DRw53 (4+7+w9)	4, 10, SFN1, 7, 11	729, 734, 736, 743	729	736, 743
DQw3 (4+5+w8+w9)	4, 10, SFN1, 5, 8	584, 744, 746, 747, 748, 750, 754, 779, 786, 915, 969	744, 747, 750	748, 754, 786

Underlined numbers represent sera with sufficient titer (≧ 1/2) for anti-Id testing

Table 2. Anti-idiotypic inhibition of 9W sera by serum ES

HLA-DR/DQ	Associated HLA-Dw	9W sera	9W sera sharing the Idx detected by F(ab')$_2$ from ES	
			Idx^{+}	Idx^{-}
2	2, 9 (8W 205 HTC)	530, 531, 533, 534, 535, 538 541, 542, 543, 545, 547, 549 550, 552, 553, 554, 555, 540, 546	534, 542, 552	530, 533, 535, 538 545, 550, 555
DQw1 (1+2+w6+w10)	1, 2, 6, 9 (8W 205 HTC)	652,653, 654, 655, 656, 657 661, 662, 663, 664, 667, 668, 669, 670, 671, 672, 674, 700, 701, 703, 706, 793, 794, 660, 667	664, 667, 669	657, 661, 668, 674 794

Underlined numbers represent sera with sufficient titer (≧ 1/2) for anti-Id testing

by Dw9- and Dw2-positive cells and a private epitope that is expressed by Dw2-carrying cells exclusively. Serum ES also contains anti-Id antibodies which block certain DQw1 antisera (9w664, 667, 669), although the other sera (9w657, 661, 668, 674, 794) were not inhibited.

Since the internal correlation between sera containing antibodies with the FH or ES Id was not higher than their correlation with sera that do not contain these antibodies, it appears that the reactivity of anti-DR alloantisera reflects the cumulative effect of a whole spectrum of idiotypic antibodies recognizing various determinants of HLA-DR molecules.

The fact, however, that anti-Id antibody (Ab2) present in anti-HLA sera inhibit not only autologous idiotypic antibodies (Ab1) to HLA but also antibodies formed by unrelated women, indicates that these are germ-line-encoded regulatory Id. This suggests that the spontaneous development of anti-Id antibodies to HLA plays an important role in down-regulating the maternal reactions against the fetus and that such anti-Id antibodies might become of therapeutic interest in transplantation.

References

1. Suciu-Foca N, Reed E, Rohowsky C, Kung P, King DW (1983) Anti-idiotypic antibodies to anti-HLA receptors induced by pregnancy. Proc Natl Acad Sci USA 80:830–834
2. Reed E, Bonagura V, Kung P, King DW, Suciu-Foca N (1983) Anti-idiotypic antibodies to HLA-DR4 and DR2. J Immunol 131:2890–2894
3. Suciu-Foca N, Rohowsky C, Godfrey M, Khan R, Malavet J, Woodward K, Hardy M (1980) HLA-D-DR relationships. 1. Patterns of reactions of HTCs with the genetic set of 8th workshop sera. In: Terasaki PI (ed) Histocompatibility Testing 1980. UCLA Tissue Typing Laboratory, Los Angeles, pp 287–288
4. Suciu-Foca N, Rubinstein P, Nicholson JF, Susinno E, Weiner J, Godfrey M, Hardy M, Rayfield E, Reemtsma K (1979) Juvenile diabetes mellitus and the HLA system. Transplant Proc 11:1309–1313
5. Bach FH, Anichini A, Reinsmoen N, Groner J, Watson A, Segall M (1983) Genetic and molecular analyses of lymphocyte-defined HLA-D regions specificities. Hum Immunol 8 [1]:25–32

The HLA-D Region: Serology, Structure, Tissue Distribution, and Function of Human Class II Molecules and Their Antigenic Determinants

P. Stastny[1], J.D. Capra[2], C.K. Hurley[2], R. Giles[2], R. DeMars[3], G. Nunez[1], L.K. Myers[1], and E.J. Ball[1]

1 Department of Internal Medicine, The University of Texas Health Science Center at Dallas, Southwestern Medical School, 5323 Harry Hines Boulevard, Dallas, TX 75235, USA
2 Department of Microbiology, The University of Texas Health Science Center at Dallas, Southwestern Medical School, 5323 Harry Hines Boulevard, Dallas, TX 75235, USA
3 Laboratory of Genetics, University of Wisconsin, Madison, WS, USA

DR, DQ, and DP Molecules are Structurally Distinct by N-terminal Amino Acid Sequence Analysis. Amino acid sequences for alpha chains of the three types of molecules are shown in Table 1. The major populations of molecules that carry the DRw52-like determinants recognized by monoclonal antibodies I-LR2 (Nadler) or 7.3.19.4 (Koning) and also those that bear DRw53 epitopes reactive with 109d6 (Winchester) are indistinguishable from DR molecules [1].

Lysostrip Testing of Ninth Workshop Sera with Anti-DR and Anti-DQ Monoclonal Antibodies Demonstrated that Some Sera Contain Antibodies against Class II Antigens Other Than DR. Sera 9w601 and 9w607 which correlate well with DR5 ($r = 0.7$) were completely inhibited by anti-DQ monoclonal antibodies (Table 2). They define the new specificity DSP5X4. Additional anti-DSP sera are described in another paper from our group. Thus in addition to the broad antigens DQw1, DQw2, and DQw3, the DQ molecules carry the narrow DSP specificities. These antigens are not expressed in type I monocytes. They therefore give weak or negative cytotoxicity reactions when B cell preparations containing large numbers of monocytes are used.

A Model of the HLA-D Region Products Based on Biochemical Data, Mutant Cell Lines, Fluorescence Inhibition with Monoclonal Antibodies, and Lysostrip Experiments with Ninth Workshop Sera. To explain our results we postulate at least two, possibly three, DR-like, and two DQ-like molecules

Histocompatibility Testing 1984
Edited by E. D. Albert et al.

Table 1. N-terminal amino acid sequence data for DR, DQ, and DP antigens

Class II antigen	Monoclonal antibody	Alpha chain Amino acid sequencce										
Position no.		9	11	12	13	16	19	22	24	25	26	29
DR	L203	–	–	F	Y	–	–	F	F	–	F	–
DQw3	IVD12	–	Y	–	–	Y	Y	–	–	Y	–	F
DP	I-LR1	Y	–	Y	–	–	–	F	F	–	F	–

Table 2. Lysostrip testing of Ninth Workshop sera with various monoclonal antibodies

Monoclonal antibody	Specificity	Reactivity remaining after lysostrip[a]			
		DR5 597	DRw52 688	DQw3 747	DSP4X5 601, 607
L368	β_2-M	+	+	+	+
L203	DR	–	–	+	+
TU22	DQ	+	+	–	–
IVD12	DQw3[b]	+	+	–	–

[a] On DR5, DRw52, DQw3-positive peripheral blood B cells.
[b] IVD12 defines a specificity that resembles DQw3 defined by alloantisera

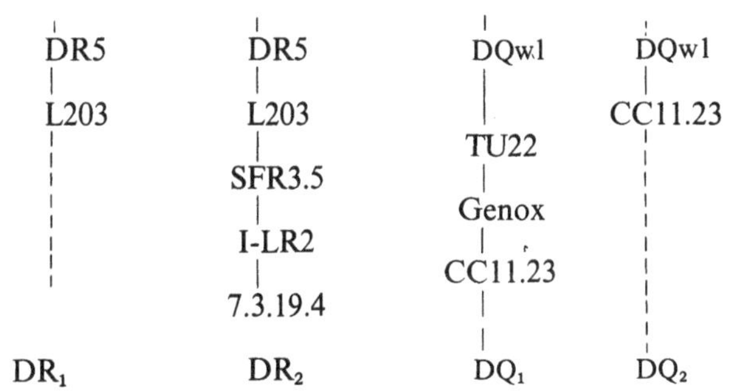

Fig. 1. Interpretation of data obtained by fluorescence inhibition and lysostrip with monoclonal antibodies

(Fig. 1). The DR5 allodeterminants appear to be on both sets of DR molecules. DQw1 defined with alloantisera appears to be present on a subset of DQ molecules which also carry epitopes recognized by TU22 and Genox 3.53.

Summary

The genes encoding human class II molecules are clustered closely together in the HLA-D region. Linkage disequilibrium has made it difficult to separate their serologic reactions. Monoclonal antibodies have been used to identify DR, DQ, and DP molecules which are structurally distinct by N-terminal amino acid analysis. Fluorescence inhibition in the FACS and lysostrip testing of Ninth Workshop sera with anti-DR and anti-DQ monoclonal antibodies demonstrated that some sera contain antibodies against class II antigens other than DR. DSP antigens corresponding to "private" specificities on the DQ molecules have been described. A model of HLA-D region products showing the location of epitopes recognized by monoclonal antibodies and allodeterminants is presented.

Reference

1. Hurley CK, Giles RC, Nunez G, DeMars R, Nadler L, Winchester R, Stastny P, Capra JD (1984) Molecular localization of human class II MT2 and MT3 determinants.

Definition of MC1, a Novel HLA Determinant Associated with DR1 and DR4*

R.J. Duquesnoy[1], M. Marrari[2], S. Hackbarth[3], and A. Zeevi[1]

1 The Department of Pathology, University of Pittsburgh, School of Medicine, Room 406 Scaife Hall, Pittsburgh, PA 15261, USA
2 Central Blood Bank of Pittsburgh, HLA Laboratory, 812 Fifth Avenue, Pittsburgh, PA 15219, USA
3 The Blood Center of Southeastern Wisconsin, 1701 W-Wisconsin Avenue, Milwaukee, WI 53233, USA

We have recently identified a new HLA-D encoded determinant defined by a cluster of six B cell alloantisera, none of which have been tested in the Ninth Workshop [1]. This determinant, designated as MC1, is associated with DR1 and DR4 and has an antigen frequency of 47% in North American Caucasians and 43% in North American Blacks. The following sera were used to define MC1: Hol (from K. Gelsthrope, Regional Blood Transfusion Center, Sheffield, England), McL (from R. Payne, Stanford University, Palo Alto, CA), Coc (from J. Hay, Red Cross Blood Transfusion Service, Adelaide, Australia), Bon and Dia (from R. Fauchet, Regional Blood Bank, Rennes, France), and Lin (from C. Raffoux, Nancy, France). The reactivity patterns of these sera were highly significantly correlated, and their mean r values were 0.56 in Caucasoid panels and 0.46 in Black panels.

Family studies have shown that MC1 largely segregates with DR1- and DR4-containing haplotypes. However, DR1 and DR4 are not completely included within MC1 because several DR1- and DR4-containing phenotypes have been found to be negative for MC1 while other DR1 and DR4 negative phenotypes are positive for MC1. Absorption studies with CLL cells and B lymphoblastoid cell lines showed that both DR1 and DR4 cells remove MC1-specific antibody activity. However, most anti-MC1 sera also contained DR1-specific antibodies, while others had extra DR4 antibody activity. The extra DR antibody activity presents a problem regarding the serological assignment of MC1, and better MC1-specific antisera need to be identified.

Additional support for the existence of the MC1 determinant was obtained through the identification of an alloreactive T cell clone with PLT specificity strongly associated with MC1 ($r = 0.86$). Clone HJ6 was generated from an MLR culture of a DR2,−; DQw1,−; and MC1-negative responder and a DR4,−; DQw3,−; DRw53,−; and MC1-positive stimulator and showed PLT reactivity with both DR1, MC1 and DR4, MC1 cells. These data show that an MC1-associated cellular determinant can induce T lymphocyte alloactivation.

Serological studies on alloreactive T cell clones have also demonstrated that certain clones generated from MC1-negative responders and maintained in long-term culture may preferentially acquire the expression of MC1 but not DR4 in the presence of DR4, MC1 irradiated feeder cells and IL2. These findings suggest that MC1 and DR4 may reside on different molecular entities. However, biochemical studies with properly selected antisera need to be conducted in order to define a molecular basis for the association between MC1 and DR1 and DR4.

Finally, a disease association study has suggested a role of MC1 in rheumatoid arthritis. In a population of 31 patients with adult rheumatoid arthritis, 29 (93.5%) typed for MC1, a significant increase over the 47.4% frequency of MC1 in normal Caucasoids. In this group of patients, the frequency of DR4 was 74.1% (vs 29.0% in controls). The relative risks for DR4 and MC1 were 7.0 and 16.1 respectively.

The above findings suggest that MC1 may be a novel HLA-DR associated determinant which can be detected both in serological and cellular assays and which may serve as a useful disease association marker. MC1 may be similar to the "second locus" specificity Te23 which was described by Park and Terasaki in the Eighth Histocompatibility Workshop [2]. This determinant was defined by a single alloantiserum (8W1211) and was associated with DR1 and DR4 in Caucasoids but only with DR1 in Blacks. Also it was suggested that Te23 was allelic to Te21 (analogous to DQw1), Te22 (or DQw3) and Te24 (or DQw2). However, our studies have ruled out allelism of MC1 with DQ antigens and family studies have shown that many DR1, DQw1 and DR4, DQw3 haplotypes also express MC1. Thus, it is possible that MC1 might be different from Te23. This determinant appears also unrelated to DQw1, DRw52 and DRw53 and DP. (In this workshop Richiardi has described a monoclonal antibody apparently specific for MCI. Also, Lepage has identified a class II antigen similar to MCI).

References

1. Duquesnoy RJ, Marrari M, Hackbarth SA, Zeevi A (1984) Hum Immunol (in press)
2. Park MS, Terasaki PI (eds) (1980) Histocompatibility Testing 1980. UCLA Tissue Typing Laboratory, Los Angeles, p 578

* Supported by AI 21410, AI 18923, and grant IM373 from the American Cancer Society

A Monoclonal Antibody (GH-3): "Non-orthodox" Anti HLA-A3 or A11 Induced by a Lymph Node Extract from a Hodgkin's Disease Patient

J. Gony, M. Garcia, F. Teillet, J. Kadouche, and J. Hors

Sce Pr Dausset, Centre Hayem, INSERM U 93, Hôpital Saint-Louis, 75475 Paris Cedex 10, France

A monoclonal antibody GH-3 (IgG produced by a hybridoma rat × mouse; SP20 myeloma) derived from an immunization against cells from a patient with Hodgkin's disease and acute myeloid leukemia, can be considered as nonorthodox since:
It reacts serologically against lymphocytes of HLA A3 or A11 individuals ($r = 0.87$) (Fig. 1)
It segregates in families with HLA-A3 or A11 ($r = 0.94$)
It precipitates solubilized cell surface antigen of healthy subjects A3 or A11 only although the immunizer was neither A3 nor A11, but A29, Aw19.2.
GH-3 reacts against the circulating blast cells of the immunizer but is negative against the lymphocytes of his HLA-identical sister.
GH-3 antibody is weakly absorbed by A3 and A11 lymphocytes.
With the blotting technique GH-3 recognizes a 50-kd−45-kd structure in reduced extracts of pathologic lymph node from a Hodgkin's disease patient neither A3 nor A11 (Fig. 2).
Capping experiments show that the recognized antigen does not co-cap with HLA
These data suggest that monoclonal antibody GH-3 recognizes an epitope shared by HLA antigen and a differentiation antigen in Sternberg cells.

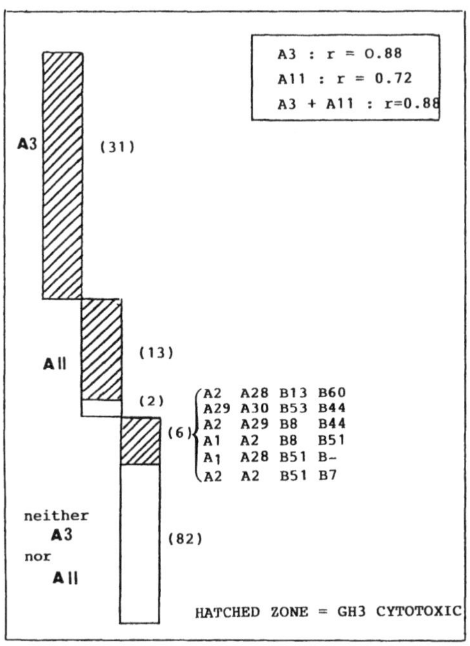

Fig. 1. Pattern of the reactivity of GH-3 on 132 normal PBL

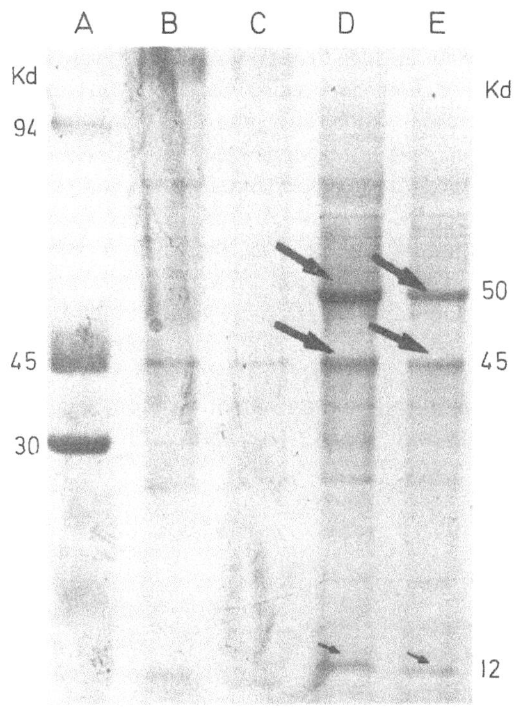

Fig. 2. Blotting of GH-3 with NP40 extract antigen from a lymph node of a Hodgkin's patient neither A3 nor A11. *A* Molecular weight control; *B* Nonreduced extract Dose 40 µl; *C* Nonreduced extract Dose 20 µl; *D* Reduced extract Dose 40 µl; *E* Reduced extract Dose 20 µl

Histocompatibility Testing 1984
Edited by E. D. Albert et al.

Enhancing Monoclonal Antibodies Against HLA-Bw4 Molecules

B. Uchańska-Ziegler, D. Martin, C. Müller, P. Wernet, and A. Ziegler

Immunology Laboratory, Medical University Clinic, 7400 Tübingen, Federal Republic of Germany

The relationship of antigenic determinants on HLA-Bw4-bearing molecules has been analyzed by means of the monoclonal antibodies (MOABs) TÜ48 (IgM), TÜ109 (IgG) and TÜ110 (IgG). TÜ48 [1] and TÜ109 [C. Müller et al., in preparation] recognize HLA-Bw4 molecules, but TÜ48 also reacts with certain HLA-A antigens. Inhibition studies carried out with the human monocytoid cell line U937 (HLA-A3, Aw19, B18, Bw53, Bw4, Bw6, Cw1, Cw3) and the B cell line BJAB-B95.8.6 (HLA-A1, A2, B13, B35, Bw4, Bw6, Cw4) showed that TÜ48 and TÜ109 recognize two different epitopes on molecules bearing the "supertypic" specificity Bw4; neither MOAB was able to compete for binding with the other (max. level of inhibition ~ 15%). Although both MOABs react very reliably in serological assays, they are problematic reagents for immunoprecipitations. The MOAB TÜ48 does not precipitate its antigen from ^{125}I-labeled lysates of Bw4/Bw6 or Bw4/Bw4 cells. Precipitations with TÜ109 were only successful, and then not with all Bw4-bearing cells tested, when the MOAB was directly coupled to *Staphylococcus aureus* bacteria. Nevertheless, the amount of radioactivity specifically precipitated was very low. However, a combination of TÜ48 and TÜ109 proved very effective for the precipitation of HLA-Bw4 molecules from all cells tested. Even in the few cases where TÜ109 alone precipitated the HLA-Bw4 molecule, there was a several-fold enhancement in cpm bound when TÜ48 was added. The ability of both reagents to cooperate with antibodies directed against "private" HLA-B specificities was investigated using TÜ110, which reacts with HLA-B13 molecules on the cell surface [2], but only very poorly in cell lysates. Only the TÜ48/110 pair precipitated HLA-B13/Bw4 molecules; no cooperation was observed when TÜ109 and TÜ110 were used simultaneously. Inhibition studies showed that TÜ109 inhibited the binding of TÜ110 completely, but TÜ48 did not compete with this MOAB at all. However, TÜ110 could not prevent the subsequent binding of TÜ109. These results lead to the following conclusions: (1) The Bw4 "supertypic" specificity consists of at least two spatially separate epitopes (TÜ48, Tü109); (2) the TÜ48 determinant is spatially separate from the B13 private specificity (TÜ110); (3) binding of TÜ109 prevents detection of the B13 specificity (TÜ110); and (4) TÜ48/TÜ109 and TÜ48/TÜ110 are pairs of MOABs enhancing the recognition of certain HLA-B molecules.

References

1. Müller C, Ziegler A, Müller G, Schunter F, Wernet P (1982) Monoclonal antibody (TÜ48) defining alloantigenic class I determinants specific for HLA-Bw4 and HLA-Aw23, -Aw24 as well as -Aw32. Hum Immunol 5:269–281
2. Müller C, Herbst H, Löffler G, Ziegler A, Wernet P (1983) A cytotoxic monoclonal antibody specific for the private alloantigenic determinant of the HLA-B13 molecule. Hum Immunol 7:229–237

Histocompatibility Testing 1984
Edited by E. D. Albert et al.

Spatial Localization of Allospecific HLA Class I Epitopes by Antibody Blocking Studies

P. Gladstone, P. Antonelli, and J.A. Hansen

Genetic Systems Corporation, 3005 First Avenue, Seattle, WA 98121, USA

A series of polymorphic and monomorphic monoclonal HLA class I antibodies was used in competitive blocking studies to explore the spatial relationships of the epitope sites recognized. This study asks whether four different polymorphic determinants present on A- and B-locus alleles have the same spatial position with respect to the epitopes recognized by the monomorphic antibodies (60.5, 71D9, H1DE, BB5). Cells (a B lymphoid cell line) were incubated with saturating quantities (approximately 2.0 μg/2 × 10^5 cells) of "blocking" antibody (at 4 °C). In the second step, a limiting amount of a fluorescein-isothiocyanate (FITC)-conjugated monoclonal was added without washing. Staining intensity was quantitated on an FACS, and percent blocking was calculated from the change in modal fluorescence in the presence and absence of blocking antibody. Maximal blocking was assessed by blocking each FITC-conjugated antibody by itself. Each antibody was tested as an FITC-conjugated probe and as a blocking antibody (unconjugated) on a single B-lymphoblastoid cell line (B-LCL) which reacted with all four polymorphic antibodies. The four polymorphic antibodies were P8.1, anti-B8; P5.3 and P7.1, anti-B27+; and P5.1, anti-A2+. None of the polymorphic antibodies except P5.3 and P7.1 blocked one another.

The blocking of polymorphic by monomorphic antibodies can be due either to steric hindrance or to alteration of conformation. The results show that each of the four polymorphic antibodies is unique with relation to the monomorphic antibodies (mAbs).

Table 1 shows a partial matrix of results in terms of percent blocking. The results, taken together, cannot be due to differences in affinity. Other features of the data include: (1) One monomorphic antibody, H1DE, causes a uniform reduction of binding of most of the other antibodies (both mono- and polymorphic) and may cause a change in conformation of the entire molecule. This hypothetical conformational change leads to increased binding of one antibody, BB5, and occurs regardless of which of these two antibodies is used as an FITC-labeled probe. (2) The two B27-related epitopes (P5.3 and P7.1) are differentially affected by H1DE, BB5, and P10.1. This suggests that although both epitopes are present on identical series of B-locus alleles (B27, 7, 17, w22, w63, 14, w46) and strongly block each other, they are different antibodies. Both may possibly see the same primary sequence but have distinct conformational dependencies. (3) Two instances in which no blocking was seen (P5.3 and P7.1 with 60.5) were actually due to nonreaction of 60.5, an alleged monomorphic, with the B27 allele in isoelectric focusing gel analysis (Choo Y, personal communication). In interpreting these data, we postulate that the monomorphic mAbs define a series of fixed sites on HLA class I molecules of any allele. The blocking studies thus permit localization of the allospecific epitopes defined by the antibodies with respect to the epitopes recognized by fixed monomorphic determinants. By this analysis, the A2+, B27+, and B8 allospecific epitopes appear to be four distinguishable sites on the class I molecule.

Table 1. Competitive blocking of anti-class I mAbs (unconjugated): percent blocking

		blockers							
		60.5	71D9	H1DE	BB5	H8G1	P10.1	P5.3	P7.1
	60.5	98	90	61	nd[a]	nd	nd		
	71D9	86	99	58	−16	99	0		
FITC	H1DE	2	30	99	−25	39	−12		
2nd	BB5	nd	nd	−28	89	12	0		
Ab	H8G1	nd	nd	12	4	99	39		
	P5.3	0	87	61	0	92	48	94	83
	P7.1	0	90	0	−41	77	−16	99	96
	P5.1	25	50	70	48	54	99		
	P8.1	71	50	52	−16	99	28		

[a] nd, not done

Histocompatibility Testing 1984
Edited by E. D. Albert et al.

Analysis of Homozygous Typing Cells with Primed Lymphocytes and Monoclonal Antibodies Directed Against Polymorphic Ia Antigen Epitopes

R. Wank, D.J. Schendel, and J.P. Johnson

Institute for Immunology, Goethestraße 29, 8000 Munich 2, Federal Republic of Germany

LCL were derived from homozygous typing cells of the Ninth Histocompatibility Workshop. A panel of eight murine monoclonal antibodies (moabs) directed against distinct polymorphic Ia epitopes expressed on Dw6 cells [1, 2] was analyzed for binding on cells expressing the specificities Dw1–Dw12 and other new groups. Although the eight moabs are directed against DR- or DQ-like molecules on Dw6 cells, seven also reacted with cells of other specificities (Fig. 1 a). Distinction between cells with the same DR antigen but with different Dw specificities (i.e., Dw6 vs Dw9; Dw7 vs Dw11; Dw4 vs Dw10) was seen in the expression of epitopes residing on both DR- and DQ-like molecules. Interestingly, the Dw7 group failed to react with any of the moabs. The dichotomy of Dw7 and the other Dw specificity groups was examined with two mutually primed HTCs in primed lymphocyte (PL) testing. The PL responses showed that the priming of the Dw7 HTC against Dw6 did not lead to increased cross-reactivity against other HTC groups, though this might have been expected because of sharing of multiple Ia-like epitopes between Dw6 and the other Dw specificity groups (Fig. 1 b).

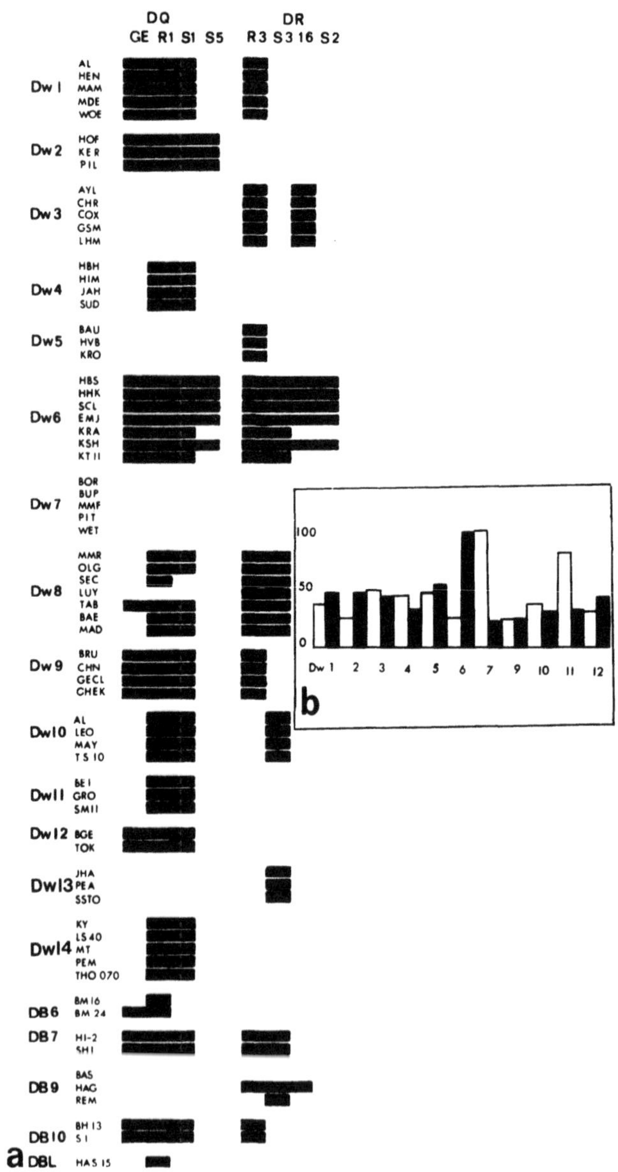

Fig. 1. **a** Binding of monoclonal antibodies with Workshop HTC. Moabs Ge, R1, S1, and S5 are directed to polymorphic epitopes on DQ molecules and R3, S3, 16, and S2 to polymorphic epitopes on DR molecules (determined by biochemical criteria). Reactivity was assessed using a single-cell ELISA. *Black bars,* positive; *blank spaces,* negative; **b** responses of two reciprocally primed HTC (Dw6, SCL and Dw7, BOR) restimulated by HTC from the specificity groups Dw1, 2, 3, 4, 5, 6, 7, 9, 10, 11, and 12 (depicted in **1 a**). The mean in each group was derived from the median cpm of each HTC and divided by the median cpm of the specific priming cell. The resulting precentages represent relative responses compared with the reference response (% RR). *Solid bars,* Dw7 primed against Dw6; *open bars,* Dw6 primed against Dw7

References

1. Johnson JP, Meo T, Riethmüller G, Schendel DJ, Wank R (1982) Direct demonstration of an HLA-DR allotypic determinant on the low molecular weight (beta) subunit using a mouse monoclonal antibody specific for DR3. J Exp Med 156:104–111
2. Johnson JP, Wank R (1984) Monoclonal antibodies to polymorphic epitopes on Ia antigens: three independent groups of determinants expressed on DRw6 homozygous cells. Eur J Immunol 14:739–744

 Histocompatibility Testing 1984
Edited by E. D. Albert et al.

A Monoclonal Antibody Detects a New Antigenic Determinant Shared by DR1 and DR4/Dw4 Molecules *

P. Richiardi, T. Crepaldi, I. Borelli, F. Malavasi, and A.O. Carbonara

Istituto di Genetica Medica, Università di Torino, Via Santena 19, 10126 Torino, Italy

A cytotoxic murine monoclonal antibody (MoAb), AC1.59, detects a new DR specificity coded by HLA haplotypes carrying DR1, DR4, DRw6, DRw8, or DRw9 alleles, thus defining a new group of cross-reacting DR specificities. Moreover, AC1.59 allows the serological definition of two genetically determined subtypes of DR4, one correlated with Dw4 and one with Dw10.

These conclusions come from the following results:

1. AC1.59 was produced after primary immunization with a DR1 homozygous human lymphoblastoid cell line (IBw4). From the immunizing cell line it precipitates a glycoprotein complex of 28–35 kd.
2. Tests of complement-dependent lymphocytotoxicity show that it is negative against a panel of peripheral T cells, while against B-enriched suspensions it has a polymorphic pattern significantly correlated with DR1 + DR4 ($P < 10^{-7}$). DR1 is completely included, while only some DR4-positive individuals react with this MoAb. The few extra-reactions concern DRw6-, DRw8-, DRw9-, and DR5-positive individuals. Family studies confirm these results: AC1.59 consistently segregates with HLA haplotypes carrying DR1 ($n = 5$), DR4 ($n = 10$), DRw6 ($n = 2$), or DRw8 ($n = 1$) specificities. AC1.59 specificity is carried only by DR4/Dw4 and not by DR4/Dw10 haplotypes. Analogously, only some DRw6 + haplotypes (2 of 6) code for the AC1.59 epitope. These DRw6+ haplotypes type as DRw14 with Workshop sera. As far as DR5 is concerned, the reactivity of AC1.59 is weak and not reproducible.
3. Competition experiments performed on the immunizing cells with cold MoAbs and alloantisera and AC1.59 labelled with ^{125}I show that: (a) binding of AC1.59 is inhibited by three out of three anti-DR1 alloantisera, by an anti-DR1+4 alloantiserum, by monomorphic anti-DR MoAbs TÜ35 (gift from Dr. Müller) and by HOT 214 (from Dr. Ferrone); (b) binding of AC1.59 is not inhibited by 3 out of 3 anti-DQw1 alloantisera, by the monomorphic anti-DR AA3.84 [1], or by the monomorphic anti-DQ MoAb TÜ22 (from Dr. Müller). These results indicate that the AC1.59 epitope is likely to be carried on DR molecules spatially close to the DR1 epitope defined by some typing alloantisera.
4. Sequential immunoprecipitation experiments were performed with AC1.59 and the monomorphic anti-DR MoAb AA3.84, using a IBw4-^{125}I lysate. Precipitation with AA3.84 produces complete depletion of AC1.59 molecules, while precipitation with AC1.59 does not remove all AA3.84 molecules.

These results suggest that AC1.59 recognizes a subset of DR molecules, though this should be confirmed with different DR1 and DR4 homozygous cells.

Reference

1. Malavasi F, Milanese C, Fabbi M, Richiardi P, Caligaris-Cappio F, Ferrero E, Roggero S, Dellabona P (1984) Generation and characterization of murine monoclonal antibodies against HLA class II molecules. Diagnostic Immunology 2:53–62

* Work supported in part by "Progetto Finalizzato Tecnologie Biomediche e Sanitarie" Contratto CNR 830052557

Serological Analysis of Two Monoclonal Antibodies: One Detecting an DRw53 Supertypic Determinant and One Detecting a New Supertypic Determinant Related to HLA-DR7

K. Horibe, R.W. Knowles, M.S. Pollack, and B. Dupont

Sloan-Kettering Memorial Cancer Center, Box 41, 1275 York Avenue, New York, NY 10021, USA

Two cytotoxic monoclonal antibodies (MoAbs), PL3 (IgG3) and PL2 (IgG2a), were produced by immunization with an HLA-DR7 homozygous cell line, PLH. Their serological specificities were determined by binding assays and by complement-dependent microcytotoxicity on an extensive cell panel.

MoAb PL3 reacts with all HLA-DR7-, DR4-, and DRw9-positive cells tested. This specificity is in complete concordance with the DRw53 allospecificity. In blocking studies, $F(ab')_2$ fragments of PL3 were found to block the cytotoxic reactivity of anti-DRw53 alloantisera. Although PL3 bound to each of the DRw53-positive cell lines, it showed significantly weaker binding to HLA-DR4 and DRw9 cells than to DR7 cells, both in titration and in quantitative absorption assays. This differential pattern of binding was not found for the polyclonal DRw53 alloantisera, suggesting that the PL3 determinant may be one of several closely related determinants which comprise the DRw53 allospecificity. $F(ab')_2$ fragments of PL3 were also tested with anti-DQw2 and anti-DR7 alloantisera. Binding of the PL3 $F(ab')^2$ fragments to DR7 homozygous target cells had no effect on the anti-DQw2 sera, but significantly enhanced the cytotoxic reactivity of some anti-DR7 sera. This suggested that the PL3 determinant is distinct from the DR7 determinant, but may be carried on the same molecule.

MoAb PL2 strongly reacts with HLA-DR7-positive B cell lines and more weakly with DR5-, DRw6-, DR3-, and DR2-positive B cell lines. The strength of PL2 binding was found to be in the order DR7 > DR5 > DRw6 > DR3 > DR2, both in titration and in quantitative absorption assays. PL2 bound to the B cell-enriched fraction isolated from the peripheral blood of HLA-DR7- or DR5-positive individuals using nylon wool columns, but did not react with the T cell-enriched fraction. In families including HLA-DR7- or DR5-positive individuals, expression of the PL2 determinant was found to segregate with the major histocompatibility antigens (lod score = 3.051). Therefore, PL2 appears to recognize a new supertypic determinant on HLA class II molecules.

Study of Monoclonal Antibodies to the HLA-D Region Products DQw1 and DRw52

J.G. Bodmer, J.M. Heyes, and J. Lindsay

Imperial Cancer Research Fund, Lincoln's Inn Fields, London WC2A 3PX, U.K.

Abbreviations

ELISA enzyme-linked immunosorbent assay; FCS foetal calf serum; IP intraperitoneally; IV intravenously; MLC mixed lymphocyte culture; NEPHGE non-equilibrium pH-gradient electrophoresis; NP40 Nonidet P40; PAP peroxidase anti-peroxidase; PAS protein A on Sepharose CL-4B; PBS phosphate-buffered saline; PLT primed lymphocyte typing; RAM rabbit anti-mouse; SaCI *Staphylococcus aureus* Cowan I strain; SDS PAGE sodium dodecyl sulphate polyacrylamide gel electrophoresis.

Introduction

Monoclonal antibodies are proving to be very powerful tools for the analysis of the HLA-D region products. Serological studies of the Seventh Workshop identified a series of antigens which showed a close but not perfect relationship with the D locus antigens defined by MLC (1). Even at this stage the lack of complete agreement between the two types of assay indicated that the region would prove complex, with more than one locus involved. This was supported by serological studies by Tosi et al. which indicated the presence of another locus

Histocompatibility Testing 1984
Edited by E. D. Albert et al.

they called DC [2]. At present, three D region loci are clearly defined by MLC, PLT and serology, while DNA studies, which have to date identified six D region α chains and seven β chains, indicate even greater complexity, as discussed by W. F. Bodmer in this volume (The HLA System 1984).

The aim of this study was to produce antibodies to HLA-D region products which could be used in both serological and immunochemical studies to help to unravel the complexity of the region. In particular, the intention was to define clearly the components contributing to the DRw6 specificity and to identify the subregion in which each of these components was coded. In the previous studies carried out in this laboratory Brodsky et al. and de Kretser et al. [3, 4] had produced DQw1 antibodies, but so far no DRw6-specific monoclonal antibody has been reported in this or any other laboratory. It was also of interest that the majority of polymorphic antibodies produced were directed to the DQ product, indicating either greater immunogenicity or easier accessibility of DQ than DR products. In the two fusion experiments described here, one produced an antibody to a DQ subregion product DQw1. The other was a deliberate attempt to produce a DR- rather than a DQ-specific antibody, if possible to the DRw6 antigen, by coating the DRw6, DQw1 immunising cells with anti-DQw1 mouse antiserum.

Materials and Methods

Cell Lines and Media

Details of the cell lines used are given in Table 1. B-lymphoblastoid cell lines were grown in RPMI 1640 culture medium (Gibco Biocult Ltd., Paisley, Scotland) supplemented with 10% FCS (Flow Labs, Irvine, Scotland), penicillin (100 U/ml) and streptomycin (100 µg/ml).

Table 1. Cell lines

Name	Cell type	Original source of cells or cell line
WT46	B line	Trucco/Cepellini, Basel
IGR3	Melanoma line	Carrel, Ludwig Institute, Switzerland
MAJA	B line	Thomsen/Svejgaard, Copenhagen
MAPP	C-ALL	Greaves, ICRF/London
B85	B line	Minowada, RPMI, USA
NALM 6	C-ALL	Minowada, RPMI, USA
WT46	B line	Trucco/Cepellini, Basel
WVB	B line	Bradley/Van Rood, Leiden
KT11	B line	Kashiwagi, Japan
ARNT	B line	Thomsen/Svejgaard, Copenhagen

The hybrids 4.1 and 8.1 were grown initially in the same medium with the HAT constituents hypoxanthine (10^{-4} mol), methotrexate (10^{-5} mol) and thymidine (1.6×10^{-5} mol) and 20% FCS. After cloning the cells were weaned over a period of a month on to RPMI 1640, antibiotics and 10% FCS:

Immunisation and Fusion

The antibodies were produced using the following protocols.

4.1

An A strong mouse was immunised as follows:
Day 1 IP 5×10^6 WT46 whole cells in PBS
Day 7 IV 5×10^6 WT46 whole cells in PBS
Day 10 Fused with P3/NS1/1-AS4-1 mouse myeloma [5]

8.1

A BALB/c mouse was immunised as follows:
Day 1 IP 5×10^6 WVB whole cells "coated" with mouse antiserum
Day 38 IP 5×10^6 WVB whole cells "coated" with mouse antiserum
Day 98 IV 50 µg WVB class II antigen
Day 99 IV 50 µg WVB class II antigen
Day 100 IV 50 µg WVB class II antigen
Day 102 Fused as above

Method for "Coating" Cells. 5×10^6 WVB whole cells were incubated for 15 min at 37 °C with serum from a mouse which had previously been immunised with MST Class II product. The spleen from this mouse had been used for an earlier fusion producing an anti-DQw1 (DC1) antibody (5).

Purification of WVB-Class II Product. This product was prepared according to the method described by Snary and Crumpton [6]. The cell fusion for both hybrids was performed using the procedure described by Galfrè et al. [7] with a slight modification of the technique involving the use of polyethylene glycol 4,000 (Merck) instead of PEG 1,500.

4.1 Fusion Plating. The suspension of fused cells was plated into 4 x 24-well and 2 x 96-well tissue culture plates at a density of 4×10^7 spleen cells/plate. Conditioned medium (from NSI cultures) was used in the 96-well plates.

8.1 Fusion Plating. After fusion the hybrids were plated in HAT-containing medium into nine 96-well tissue culture plates at varying dilutions from 3×10^7 spleen cells/plate down to 7.5×10^6 spleen cells/plate. Mouse spleen were used as a feeder layer.

Screening

The supernatants from wells with actively growing hybrids were screened using an ELISA PAP complex technique [8] against a panel of homozygous B cell lines which were attached to 96-well plates for this purpose. Extensive cytotoxicity screens were also performed on the hybrid supernatants.
4.1 and 8.1 were double-cloned using a single-cell cloning technique. Ascites tumours were produced in pristane-primed Balb/c mice in the case of 8.1. For 4.1, F1 hybrids of A strong x Balb/c mice were used. The mice were inoculated with $1-3 \times 10^6$ cloned hybrid cells in serum free RPMI 1640.

Characterization and Purification of the Ig Secreted by Hybridomas

The subclass characterisation of 4.1 and 8.1 was performed using immunodiffusion analysis [9]. RAM subclass-specific antisera were obtained from Miles Labs.
The monoclonal antibodies were purified from the ascites fluid on a protein A-Sepharose 4B column (Pharmacia) [10].

Preparation of [^{35}S]Methionine-Labelled Cell Lysates

Cells were grown in RPMI 1640 medium supplemented with 10% FCS, penicillin (100 U/ml) and streptomycin (100 μg/ml) maintained at $5 \times 10^5 - 10^6$ cells/ml. Prior to labelling, the cells were washed three times in RPMI 1640 lacking methionine, resuspended at 5×10^7/ml in methionine-free medium supplemented with 1 mCi [^{35}S]methionine (Radiochemical Centre, Amersham) and incubated at 37 °C in CO_2 for 4 h.
The cells were then harvested and washed three times in ice-cold PBS, suspended in 900 μl NP40 lysis buffer (1% NP40, 10 m*M* Tris pH 7.4, 1 m*M* phenylmethylsulphonyl fluoride, 20 m*M* iodoacetamide) [11] and incubated on ice for 30 min. The nuclear debris was pelleted using a Beckman Microfuge B centrifuge and the lysate passed through a 0.22-μm MILLEX GS Millipore filter [12]. The lysate was then precleared using protein A bearing SaCI prepared according to Kessler [13]. After preclearing for 30 minutes the lysate was used immediately for precipitation. Immunoprecipitation was done using PAS [14] obtained from Pharmacia. Radiolabelled proteins were precipitated from the precleared lysate using 20 μg purified Ig or 20 μl ascites of all the antibodies used. After incubation overnight at 4 °C with the antibodies, 30 μl of a 10% suspension of PAS in NP40 lysis buffer was added and further incubated for 1 h. The immune complexes attached to the PAS beads were washed three times [11] and dissociated by heating at 50 °C for 30 min in NEPHGE sample buffer and separated on 13-cm tube gels containing ampholines of a 3.5 – 10 pH range (LKB Instruments, Croydon) as described by O'Farrell et al. [15]. After separation on 12.5% SDS PAGE, the labelled proteins were visualised by autoradiography using KODAK SB5 film.

Western Blot Procedures: Preparation of Glycoprotein Fractions

10^8 cells grown routinely in RPMI 1640 medium were harvested and washed 3 times in PBS. They were then suspended in 2 ml NP40 lysis buffer as previously described and incubated on ice for 30 min. The nuclear debris was removed by centrifugation in a Microfuge B and the lysate passed through a 2-ml column of Lentil Lectin on Sepharose-4B (Pharmacia). The column was then washed with 40 ml lysis buffer and the bound glycoproteins eluted with 10% α-methyl-D-mannoside (Sigma) in lysis buffer.
The glycoproteins were separated on a 12.5% polyacrylamide slab gel. Electrophoretic transfer was performed essentially as described by Towbin et al. [16], using nitrocellulose with a pore size of 0.1 μm (Schleicher and Schüll) and transferred at 400 mA for 1 h. After transfer the membranes were washed in PBS Tween [17], cut into strips, and incubated with the test antibodies at a concentration of 10 – 20 μg/ml in PBS Tween overnight at 4 °C. The strips were then washed extensively with PBS Tween, incubated for 2 h with ^{125}I-labelled RAM [18], which was used as the second antibody, then further washed in PBS Tween. Autoradiography was performed on the dried nitrocellulose strips using SB5 film.

Results

Characterisation of the Antibodies Using Normal and Tumour Cell Lines by ELISA and Cytotoxicity Assays

After initial screening of the antibodies 4.1 and 8.1, both were double-cloned using the single-cell cloning method and their immunoglobulin class established as IgG2 by immunodiffusion. Although the two antibodies were originally screened using the ELISA method, because they were both IgG2 and therefore complement-fixing, they were also extensively screened in cytotoxicity assays and gave

Table 2. Reactivity of antibodies on normal B-lymphoblastoid and tumour cell lines

				Antibody					
				31.1	CA2	IB5	1.2	4.1	8.1
Specificity				DR, DQ(DC) DP(SB) (mono)	DR, DQ(DC) (mono)	α chain (mono)	DQw1 (DCI) (poly)	DQw1 (DCI) (poly)	DRw52 (MT2) (poly)
Cell line	DR	DQ	Cell type						
WT46	w6, w6	+	B line	+	+	+	+	+	+
IGR3	1, 7	–	Melanoma line	+	+	–	–	–	–
MAJA	1, 1	+	B line	+	+	+	+	+	–
MAPP	1, –	–	C-ALL	+	+	–	–	–	–
B85	3, 7	+	B line (Same donor)	+	+	+	–	–	+
NALM 6	3, 7	–	C-ALL (Same donor)	+	+	–	–	–	+

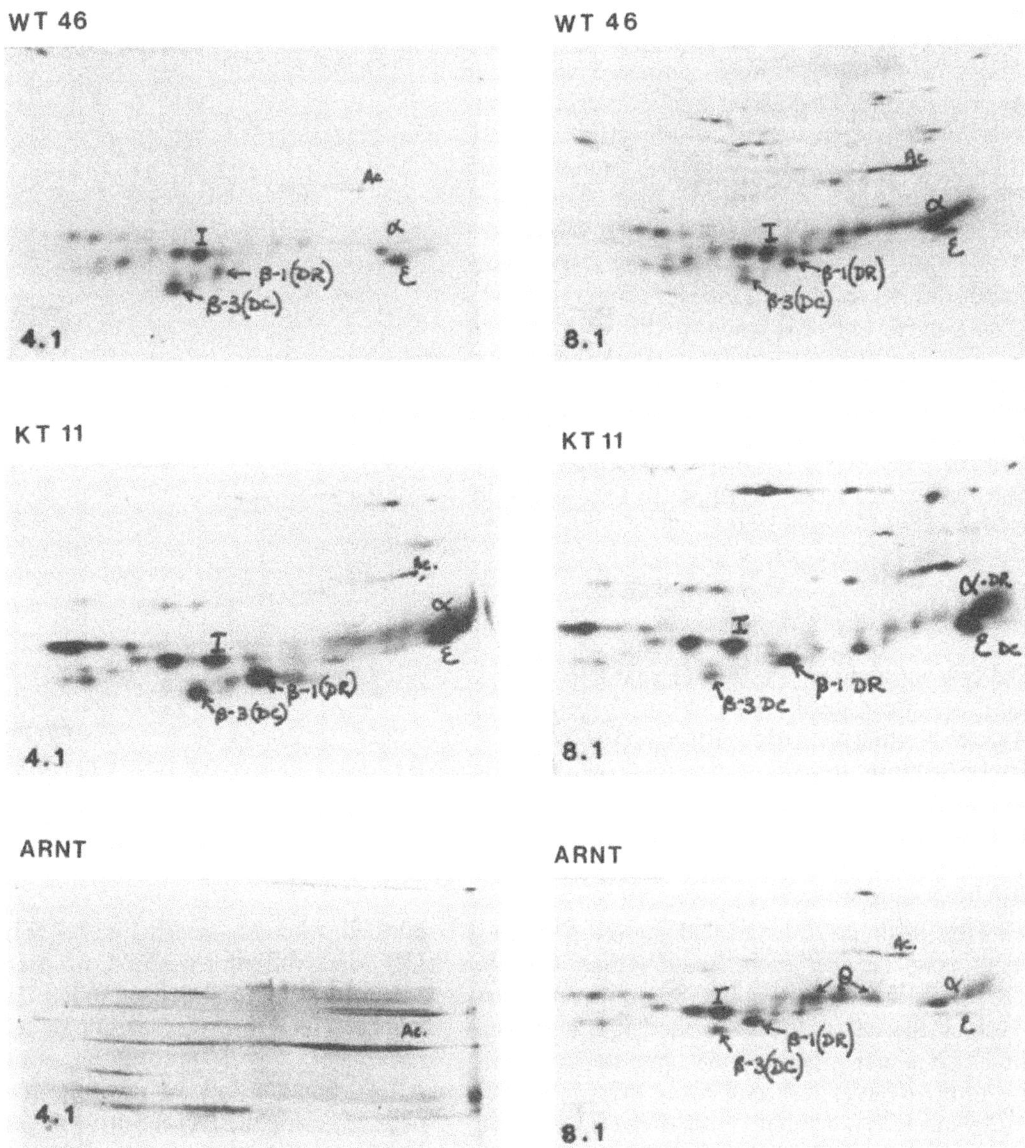

Fig. 1. NEPHGE/SDS PAGE analyses of the DRw6 cell lines WT46, KT11 and ARNT using antibodies 4.1 and 8.1 (DC in the figure is DQ with the new nomenclature)

identical results with the two methods. Further results on their specificity can be found elsewhere in this volume (J.G. Bodmer et al., HLA-D Region Monoclonal Antibodies) as they were included in the Ninth Workshop monoclonal study. 4.1 was numbers 945 and 660 in the Workshop, and 8.1 at different concentrations was numbers 946, 947 and 948. It was shown, as previously established in our laboratory, that 4.1 reacted with all DR1, DR2 and DRw6 cells. 8.1 reacted with DR3, DR5 and DRw6 but failed to react with DRw12 (Herluf) and DRw8. Thus it shows a specificity shorter than the previously defined DRw52 (MT2) antigen.

In order to determine whether the antibodies were reacting with DR or DQ products, they were further tested on a series of tumour cell lines known to express the DR product but lacking the DQ product, as shown by Newman et al. [19], Carrel et al. [20] and independently in this laboratory. A selection of the data are shown in Table 2. The reactions of 4.1 and 8.1 were compared with four other antibodies. CA2 [21] is a monomorphic antibody presumed to react with all D region products, 31.1 [12] reacts primarily with DR products. 1B5 [22] reacts mainly with α chains, particularly DR α, and SDR1.2 [4] is a DQw1 antibody. It was shown by this study that 4.1 and SDR1.2, the DQw1 antibodies, did not react when the DQ product was absent, as on cell lines IGR3 and MAPP. This showed that these antibodies were primarily DQ directed and did not cross-react with DR specificities in the absence of DQ. On the other hand, 8.1, the DRw52 antibody, did react when the DQ product was absent, as is shown by its reactivity with NALM6, the C-ALL cell like lacking DQ.

Immunochemical Studies

The two antibodies were further characterised using two-dimensional gel electrophoresis and Western blotting methods as described above.

Figure 1 shows the two-dimensional gel patterns produced by the antibodies on three DRw6 cell lines: WT46, the line used to produce 4.1; KT11, a Japanese DRw6 cell line; and ARNT. Clear precipitation patterns are seen using 8.1 on all three cell lines. It should be noted that the DR β chain is in all cases labelled more heavily than the DQ (DC) β chain, suggesting that 8.1 is directed primarily at the DR product. Further, it is clear that the DQ β is precipitated in the same position relative to the I (invariant) spot in the top two panels, WT46 and KT11, while it is in a different position, directly below the I spot, in the bottom panel, ARNT. Looking at the precipitations with 4.1 in WT46 and KT11, the DQ β spot is more heavily labelled, whereas for cell line ARNT, which has a DQ β in a different position, no precipitation was seen with 4.1. This lack of precipitation with 4.1 has been seen in the other DRw6 cell lines which have their DQ β spot in the same position as ARNT. Similar lack of precipitation using 4.1 is observed using the DQ-negative melanoma cell line IGR3 (Fig. 2).

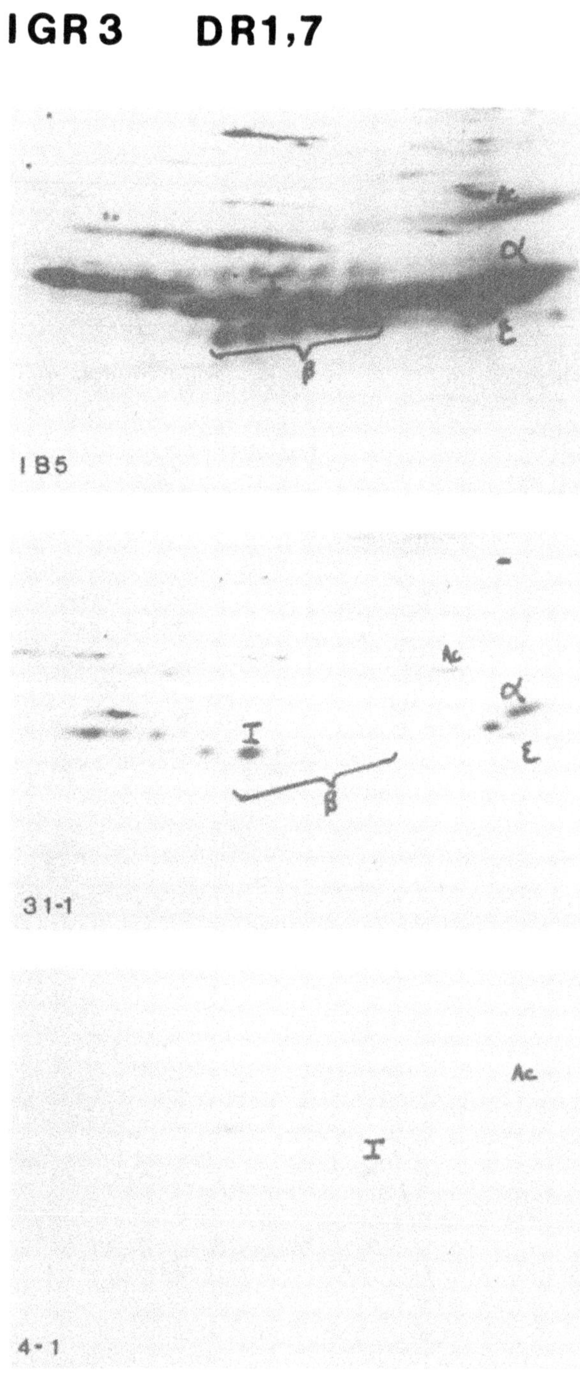

Fig. 2. NEPHGE/SDS PAGE analyses of DQ-negative melanoma cell line IGR3 using IB5, 31.1 and 4.1

In order to determine whether the DQw1 specificity was coded on the α or the β chain and to con-

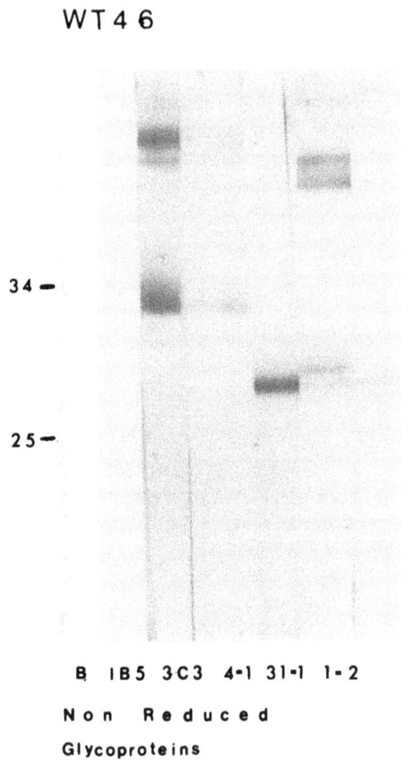

Fig. 3. Western blot analysis of WT46 using antibodies 1B5, 3C3, 4.1, 31.1 and 1.2

firm that it was coded in the DQ subregion, an analysis using Western blotting procedures was carried out. Five antibodies were used in a one-dimensional Western blot analysis, and the results are shown in Fig. 3. Here the two α chain antibodies IB5 and 3C3 are shown clearly to label the 33K α band of the WT46 preparation, while the DR monomorphic antibody 31.1 labels two β bands, the higher molecular weight DR β and the lower DQ β. The two DQw1 antibodies label only the lower molecular weight β band which corresponds to the DQ product.

Conclusions

For the antibody 4.1, the serological studies suggest, and the immunochemical studies confirm, that the product identified is coded for in the DQ subregion of HLA, as it neither reacts nor precipitates in the absence of DQ. Further, the polymorphism seen, as shown by the Western blots, resides on the DQ β chain. The antibody SDR1.2 has been shown to precipitate DQw1 β products in both WT46 and ARNT, indicating that it is in some sense supertypic, recognising more than one split of DQw1. 4.1, on the other hand, precipitates only those DQw1 products of a specific subset. It is of great interest to note that the two cell lines whose DQw1 products are recognised by 4.1 have been identified as having the MLC-defined specificity Dw18 (6A), whereas the cell lines not recognised have the specificity DRw19 (6b). Thus this antibody is capable of recognising, in biochemical analysis, a specificity previously only seen by cellular assays. Another monoclonal antibody in the Workshop, 929 [23], previously identified as a DR3 antibody, also seems to define this subset of DRw6, as is discussed elsewhere in this volume (J. G. Bodmer et al., HLA-D Region Monoclonal Antibodies).

The antibody 8.1, in contrast to 4.1, shows, both by serology and by biochemical techniques, the now clearly recognised fact that the DRw52 product it identifies is from the DR rather than the DQ subregion. As there are at least three DR β chains coded for, and probably usually at least two expressed (see W. F. Bodmer, The HLA System 1984, this volume), this DRw52 product is probably not usually, possibly never, coded for by the same β chain gene as the so-called DR specificities. However, the complexity of this region, the possibility that different numbers of DR β chains are expressed in different haplotypes and, as suggested by Nepom et al. [24] and others, the possibility that the same antibody can recognise products of different subregions in different DR types makes any firm identification of the specific DR β chain coding for DRw52 premature. Studies with this antibody and other DRw52 antibodies, for example 930 in this workshop, show that the DRw52 specificity will be further divided. Whereas 8.1 reacts only with cells which are DR3, DR5 and DRw6, 930 reacts with DRw12 as well, and yet other DRw12 antibodies appear to react also with DRw8. The study of the two antibodies discussed here underlines the exquisite specificity of monoclonal antibodies for the fine analysis of the HLA system.

Acknowledgments. We should like to thank Dr. Walter Bodmer for helpful discussion and Carol Figg for technical assistance.

Summary

Two monoclonal antibodies 4.1 and 8.1, specific for DQw1 and DRw52 respectively, have been produced. 4.1, made by immunisation with whole cells from a DRw6 cell line WT46, identifies the DQw1 product but immunoprecipitates only a specific subset of DQw1 molecules, indicating that it may define a narrower specificity than the presently defined DQw1. 8.1 was produced by immunising a mouse with whole cells from another DRw6 cell line which had been coated with mouse DQw1 antiserum in order to block DQ sites and produce a DR antibody. This antibody identifies the DRw52 antigen in DRw6, DR3 and DR5, but not in DRw8 and DRw12. This indicates that the antibody is defining a split of DRw52. These antibodies also detect variation in DQ as compared to DR expression in certain melanoma and lymphoma cell lines.

References

1. Bodmer J, Richards S, Bodmer WF (1977) The definition of Ia antigens using 7th Workshop sera. Tissue Antigens 10:140
2. Tosi R, Tanigaki N, Centis D, Ferrara GB, Pressman D (1978) Immunological dissection of human 1A molecules. J Exp Med 148:1592–1611
3. Brodsky FM, Parham P, Barnstable CJ, Crumpton MJ, Bodmer WF (1979) Monoclonal antibodies for analysis of the HLA system. Immunol Rev 47:3–61
4. de Kretser TA, Crumpton MJ, Bodmer JG, Bodmer WF (1982) 2-Dimensional gel analysis of the polypeptides precipitated by a polymorphic HLA-DRI,2,W6 monoclonal antibody – evidence for a 3rd locus. Eur J Immunol 12:600–606
5. Kohler G, Howe GS, Milstein C (1976) Fusion between immunoglobulin-secreting and nonsecreting myeloma cell lines. Eur J Immunol 6:292
6. Snary D, Crumpton MJ (1974) Preparation and properties of lymphocyte plasma membrane. Contemp Top Mol Immunol 3:27–56
7. Galfrè G, Howe SC, Milstein C, Butcher GW, Howard JC (1977) Antibodies to major histocompatability antigens produced by hybrid cell lines. Nature 266:550
8. Lansdorp PM, Astaldi GCB, Oosterhof F, Janssen MC, Zeijlemaker WP (1980) Immunoperoxidase procedures to detect monoclonal antibodies against cell surface antigens. Quantitation of binding and staining of individual cells. J Immunol Methods 39:393–405
9. Ouchterlony O, Nilsson LA (1978) In Handbook of Experimental Immunology (ed. Weir DM). Vol 1, Chapter 19, p 16. Blackwell Scientific Publications, London
10. Ey PL, Prowse SJ, Jenkins CR (1978) Isolate of pure IGG1, IGG2A and IGG2B immunoglobulins from mouse serum using protein A-sepharose. Immunochem 15:429
11. Owen MJ, Kissonerghis AM, Lodish HF, Crumpton MJ (1981) Biosynthesis and maturation of HLA-DR antigens in vivo. J Biol Chem 256:8987–8993
12. Dekretser TA, Crumpton MJ, Bodmer JG, Bodmer WF (1982) Demonstration of 2 distinct light chains in HLA-DR-associated antigens by 2-dimensional gel-electrophoresis. Eur J Immun 12:214–221
13. Kessler WW (1975) Rapid isolation of antigens from cells with a staphylococcal protein A-antibody absorbent: parameters of the interaction of antibody-antigen complexes with protein A. J Immunol 115:1617–1624
14. McSween JM, Eastwood SL (1981) Recovery of antigen from staphylococcal protein A-antibody adsorbents. Methods Enzymol 73:459–471
15. O'Farrell PZ, Goodman HM, O'Farrell PH (1977) High resolution two-dimensional electrophoresis of basic as well as acidic proteins. Cell 12:1133
16. Towbin H, Staehelin T, Gordon J (1978) Electrophoretic transfer of proteins from polyacrylamide gels to nitrocellulose sheets: procedure and some applications. Proc Natl Acad Sci USA 76:4350–4354
17. Batteiger B, Newhall WJ, Jones V, Jones RB (1982) The use of Tween 20 as a blocking agent in the immunological detection of proteins transferred to nitrocellulose membranes. J Immunol Methods 55:297–307
18. McConahey PJ, Dixon FJ (1980) Radioiodination of proteins by the use of the chloramine-T method. Meth Enz Vol 70:210–225
19. Newman RA, Delia D, Greaves MF, Navarrete C, Fainboim L, Festenstein H (1983) Differential expression of HLA-DR and DR-linked determinants of human leukemia and lymphoid cells. Eur J Immunol 13:172
20. Carrel S, Tosi R, Gross N, Tanigaki N, Carmagnola AL, Accolla RS (1981) Subsets of human Ia-like molecules defined by monoclonal antibodies. Mol Immunol 18:403–411
21. Charron DJ, McDevitt HO (1979) Analysis of HLA-D region-associated molecules with monoclonal antibody. Proc Natl Acad Sci USA 76:6567–6571
22. Adams TE, Bodmer JG, Bodmer WF (1983) Production and characterization of monoclonal-antibodies recognizing the alpha-chain subunits of human A1 alloantigens. Immunology 50:613–624
23. Johnson JP, Meo T, Riethmüller G, Schendel DJ, Wank R (1982) Direct demonstration of an HLA-DR allotypic determinant on the low-molecular weight (Beta) subunit using a mouse monoclonal antibody specific for DR3. J Exp Med 156:104–111
24. Nepom GT, Nepom BS, Antonelli P, Mickelson E, Silver J, Goyert SM, Hansen JA (1984) The HLA-DR4 family of haplotypes consists of a series of distinct DR and DS molecules. J Exp Med 159:394

Characterisation of the HLA-D Region DQw3 Specificity Using the Monoclonal Antibodies 2HB6 and IVD12

A.D. Shannon, C.E. Rudd, J.G. Bodmer, W.F. Bodmer, and M.J. Crumpton

Imperial Cancer Research Fund, P.O. Box 123, Lincoln's Inn Fields, London WC2A 3PX, UK

Introduction

Human class II histocompatibility antigens are expressed mainly on B cells, activated T cells, monocytes and macrophages. They comprise two non-covalently associated, glycosylated polypeptides of molecular weights 32–34 kd (α) and 27–29 kd (β). A combination of serological, cellular and biochemical techniques has shown that these antigens are the products of at least three distinct genetic subregions, namely HLA-DP (SB), HLA-DQ (DC) and HLA-DR [1]. They are the analogues of the I-A and I-E subregion products of the mouse H-2 region and control immune responses by regulating interactions between T and B cells and antigen-presenting cells.

In addition to the defined HLA-DR specificities, several series of supertypic specificities, including DQ, have been reported [2, 3]. It appears likely that the DQ supertypic specificities are carried by molecules other than those expressing the DR specificities [4–6]. The present study involves the characterisation of the DQw3 supertypic specificity, associated primarily with HLA-DR4, 5 and w9, using the monoclonal antibodies 2HB6 and IVD12.

Materials and Methods

Cell Lines. The B cell lines used were derived either from Burkitt lymphomas or by in vitro transformation of peripheral blood cells with Epstein-Barr virus (EBV) and included a previously described panel of homozygous typing cells [4, 7]. HPB-ALL, J6 and HUT-78 are T lymphoma cell lines which, on the basis of expressing T3 antigen, are derived from mature T cells. The cell lines MOLT-4 and HSB2 were derived from T-ALL and correspond to immature T cells. All lines were grown in RPMI-1640 medium supplemented with foetal calf serum [10% (v/v)], penicillin (100 units/ml) and streptomycin (50 µg/ml).

Human peripheral blood lymphocytes (PBLs) were prepared by defibrination and separation using standard Ficoll-Hypaque flotation techniques.

Monoclonal Antibodies. Hybridoma CSB-2HB6 was derived from an ATH mouse which had been primed by the intraperitoneal injection of 5×10^6 ATL mouse spleen cells at monthly intervals for a period of 5 months prior to intravenous boosting with 10^7 PRIESS (HLA-DR4) cells. Four days later the ATH spleen cells were fused with P3/NS1/1-Ag4-1 mouse myeloma cells [8] according to methods described by van Heyningen et al. [9]. Hybridoma culture supernatants were initially screened against the cell lines PRIESS and MOLT-4. PRIESS-specific supernatants were then screened against a panel of homozygous typing cells to identify polymorphic anti-class II antibodies.

Hybridoma 2HB6 was single-cell cloned and ascites tumours were propagated by inoculation of cells into pristane-primed ATH × Balb/c F_1 mice. The class and subclass of the 2HB6 antibody were determined using the Ouchterlony technique and standard antisera.

Antibody IVD12 was a gift of Giles et al. [5] in the form of an ascitic fluid. The corresponding hybridoma had been obtained from a Balb/c mouse immunised with PRIESS cells. Antibody 17.15 was obtained from Hansen et al. [13].

Binding Assays. Solid-phase radioimmunoassays (RIA) and enzyme-linked immunosorbent assays (ELISA) were used to detect the binding of monoclonal antibodies to cell surface determinants. The assays were performed as previously described [10, 11] using cells of > 90% viability that had been fixed with 0.25% glutaraldehyde. Titrations confirmed that saturating levels of antibody were used.

Cytotoxic Assays. Although an IgG_1 antibody, 2HB6 proved to be cytotoxic when equal amounts of 10× concentrated hybridoma culture supernatant and rabbit anti-(mouse Ig) serum were incubated at room temperature for 15 min (Anne Atkinson and Julia Bodmer, unpublished observations). Complement-dependent microcytotoxicity tests were performed according to the standard method adopted at the Eighth Histocompatibility Workshop (1980).

Biochemical Analyses. Immunoprecipitates were prepared from [^{35}S]methionine-labelled cells as described by Owen et al. [12]. Routinely, 200 µl 10×

Histocompatibility Testing 1984
Edited by E. D. Albert et al.

concentrated hybridoma culture supernatant or 5–10 µl ascitic fluid were added to 5×10^6 cell equivalents. As both 2HB6 and IVD12 bind weakly to *Staphylococcus aureus* (Cowan I strain) bacteria, 5–10 µg of rabbit anti-(mouse Ig) serum (DAKO Laboratories, Denmark) was added prior to the addition of fixed *S. aureus* bacteria.

One-dimensional SDS-PAGE and 2-D NEPHGE/SDS-PAGE analyses of immunoprecipitates were performed using previously described techniques [4, 7, 15].

Results

Reactivity with Lymphoblastoid Cell Lines. The reactivities of 2HB6 with various homozygous B lymphoblastoid cell lines are shown in Table 1. Antibodies 2HB6 and IVD12 had identical reactivities in all RIA and ELISA tests. Unlike 2HB6, however, IVD12 was refractory to treatment with rabbit anti-(mouse Ig) serum and thus could not be used in microcytotoxicity assays. In this case, the monoclonal antibody 17.15 was used as a positive control. The results obtained showed that 2HB6 and 17.15 have similar reactivities except on some DR7 lines which were positive for 17.15 and negative for 2HB6.

The combined results (Table 1) show that although the DQw3 specificity is classically associated with the HLA-DR4, 5 and w9 specificities, antibody 2HB6 reacted positively with a number of B cell lines outside this association (namely, some HLA-DR2, w6, 7 and w8 cells). Additional RIA testing using five T cell lines (Table 1) showed a strong positive reaction of 2HB6 and IVD12 with HUT-78 cells. This line was shown to be HLA-DR4 and DQw3 positive by alloantisera. All remaining T cell lines were negative to both antibodies. Limited microcytotoxicity testing on PBLs confirmed the preferential reactivity of antibody 2HB6 with HLA-DR4 and 5 cells, the strongest reactivity being with DR5 cells.

Analyses of Immunoprecipitates. Immunoprecipitates prepared from cell lysates of [^{35}S]methionine-labelled PRIESS cells were analysed by 1-D SDS-PAGE (Fig. 1). Comparisons of the polypeptides precipitated by the monomorphic anti-HLA-DR antibody TAL-1B5 (track *a*) with those of the two anti-DQw3 antibodies 2HB6 and IVD12 (tracks *b* and *c* respectively) showed that 2HB6 and IVD12 precipitated similar complexes comprising a 33- to 34-kd (α) chain (faintly labelled), a 32-kd invariant (Ii) chain (heavily labelled) and a 27- to 28-kd (*β*) chain. Notably, the *β* chain precipitated by the anti-DQw3 antibodies has an apparently smaller

Table 1. Reactivity[a] of monoclonal antibody 2HB6 with human B and T cell lines

DR type	No. lines	Positive[b, c]	Negative
B cell lines			
1	2	–	MAJA, METTE
2	4	RML[d]	PGF, MST, BRI-8
3	2	–	WT20, WT49
4	5	PRIESS, KT2[d] WT51, LEIF-T	SJAH[d]
5	5	IDF, DHF, WT48 WT50	FPF[d]
w6	7	AZL[d], RPB, WPB	WT46, DAUDI[d] WVB, ARNT
7	3	SCCA	IBW9, MANN
w8	3	JOM-TC	MADURA-T, 231
w9	2	KOZ[d], KT14[d]	–
T cell lines			
–	5	HUT78[e]	MOLT-4, HSB2, J6 HPB-ALL

[a] Based on combined results of RIA, ELISA and microcytotoxicity assays
[b] Binding on RIA ≧ 4 times background; ELISA ≧ 3 times background; microcytotoxicity ≧ 50% lysis
[c] All cell lines positive for 2HB6 were shown to express the DQw3 specificity by microcytotoxicity assays using alloantisera and the monoclonal antibody 17.15
[d] Non-Caucasoid origin
[e] Typed by alloantisera as HLA-DR4, DQw3

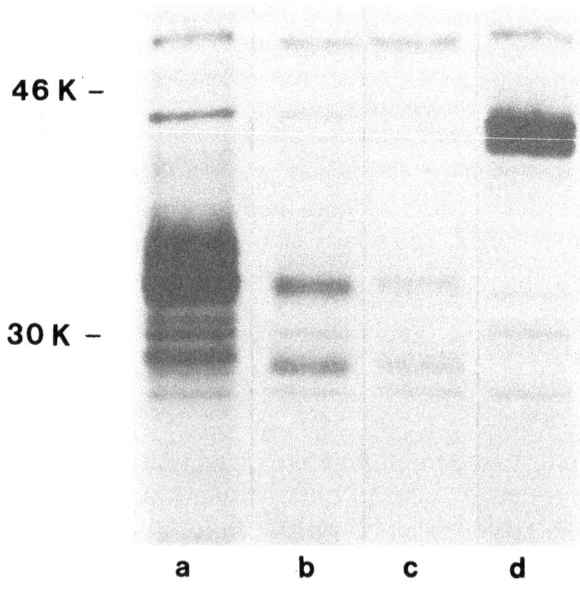

Fig. 1. SDS-PAGE analysis under reducing conditions of immunoprecipitates prepared from lysates of [^{35}S]methionine-labelled PRIESS cells using the monoclonal antibodies *a* TAL-1B5; *b* 2HB6; *c* IVD12; *d* W6/32 (monomorphic anti-HLA-A, B, C control antibody)

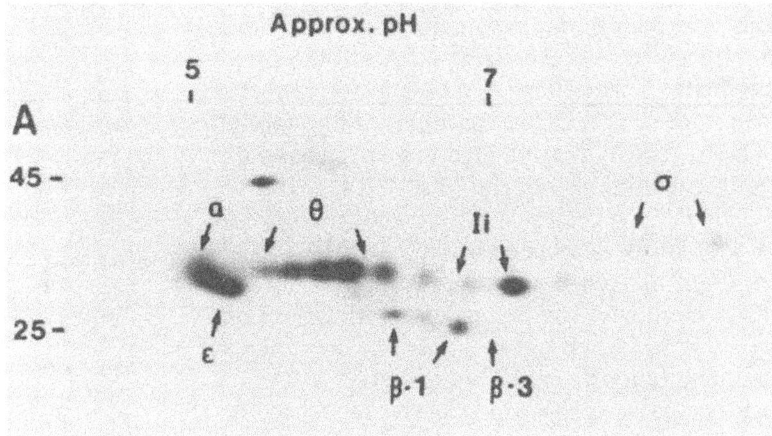

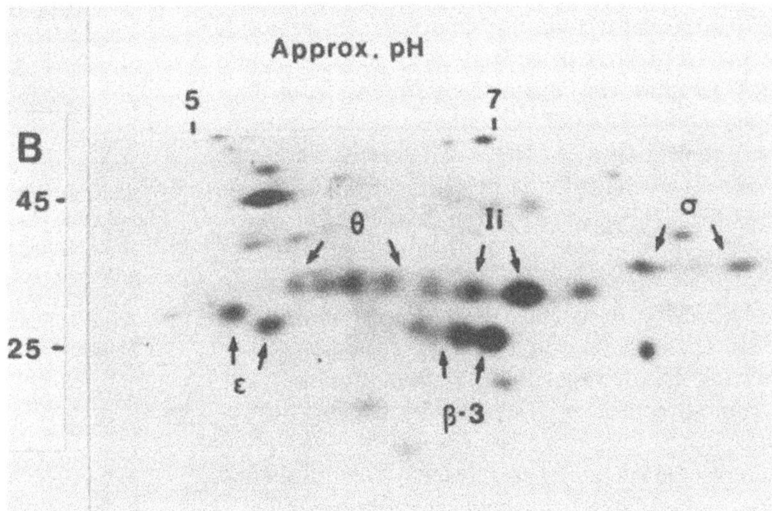

Fig. 2. A, B. 2-D NEPHGE/SDS-PAGE analysis of immunoprecipitates obtained by reacting the monoclonal antibodies TAL-1B5 **(A)** and 2HB6 **(B)** with lysates of [^{35}S]methionine-labelled LEIF-T (HLA-DR4, 4) cells. The designation of polypeptide spots is as previously described [4, 7]

molecular size than the major β chain precipitated by TAL-1B5 (DRβ chain approximately 29 kd). Track *d* of Fig. 1 shows the pattern for the positive control antibody, W6/32, which recognises class I antigens [14]. Similar one-dimensional results were obtained from cell lysates of [^{35}S]methionine-labelled LEIF-T cells (not shown).

Immunoprecipitates obtained from [^{35}S]methionine-labelled LEIF-T cells using the antibodies TAL-1B5 and 2HB6 were also analysed by 2-D NEPHGE/SDS-PAGE (Fig. 2). As can be seen (Fig. 2A), TAL-1B5 precipitated a complex pattern of polypeptides. These included DRα and DQα (labelled ε in Fig. 2) polypeptides, at least two DRβ (β-1) polypeptides and one faint DQβ polypeptide (β-3). A series of invariant polypeptides (θ, Ii and σ) was also precipitated as previously described [7, 15]. By contrast, antibody 2HB6 (Fig. 2B) failed to precipitate polypeptides with pI values in the region of DRα and DRβ. Instead, this antibody gave a pattern which clearly comprised two polypeptide spots in the DQα (ε) region (molecular weight approx. 31 – 32 kd) and at least two major polypeptides in the DQβ (β-3) region that characteristically are more basic than the DRβ (β-1) spots. As before, a series of invariant polypeptides (θ, Ii and σ) were precipitated. Although similar results were obtained for the IVD12 antibody (not shown), the polypeptide pattern was considerably less intensely labelled than that obtained with 2HB6.

Discussion

The results of RIA and ELISA binding assays and of microcytotoxicity tests indicate that the antibodies 2HB6 and IVD12 have identical patterns of reactivity. Both show a polymorphic pattern, binding strongly to cells expressing HLA-DR4, 5 or w9 specificities, indicating that they are directed against the class II DQw3 specificity. Although the DQw3 specificity is considered to be in strong linkage disequilibrium with the HLA-DR4, 5 and w9 specificities, the present study has shown DQw3 to be additionally associated with some HLA-DR2, w6, 7 and w8 cell lines that are negative for the DQw1 specificity. This is consistent with DQw3 being allelic to DQw1 and indicates that the linkage disequilibrium between DQw3 and HLA-DR4 or 5 may not be as high as previously supposed, especially in non-Caucasoid populations.

One-dimensional SDS-PAGE analyses of immunoprecipitates demonstrated that 2HB6 and IVD12 recognise a similar complex comprising a 32- to 33-kd α chain and a 27- to 28-kd β chain. This complex was distinctly different from that carrying the HLA-DR specificity, as precipitated by TAL-1B5 (Fig. 1). These differences were emphasised by the 2-D NEPHGE/SDS-PAGE analyses (Fig. 2), which demonstrated that the polypeptides precipitated by 2HB6 possessed pI and molecular weight values indistinguishable from those previously assigned to products of the DQ locus. These analyses thus confirm previous studies showing that this specificity is most probably carried on glycoproteins coded for by the DQ subregion [5, 16].

Comparison of the present results with published data on anti-DQw3 monoclonal antibodies [5, 13, 17] highlights the similarity in binding patterns of 2HB6, IVD12 and HU-18. All three antibodies are positive on cells expressing the DKT2 and Dw4 specificities but negative on cells expressing Dw15 [cf. 17]. Unlike antibody 17.15, 2HB6 does not bind to a large number of cell lines carrying the HLA-DR7 specificity, and these two antibodies therefore have somewhat different patterns of reactivity. A notable feature is that 2HB6 appears to be specific for DQ products as judged by two-dimensional gel analyses of immunoprecipitates. In contrast, anti-DQw1 monoclonal antibodies cross-react with DR products [1, 4].

The results also demonstrate the value of novel approaches to immunisation in the derivation of polymorphic anti-HLA-D region monoclonal antibodies. In this case advantage was taken of the cross-reactivity between particular polymorphic types of mouse and human class II antigens.

References

1. Bodmer JG, Bodmer WF (1984) Monoclonal antibodies to HLA determinants. Br Med Bull 40/3:276–282
2. Tosi R, Tanigaki N, Centis D, Ferrara GB, Pressman D (1978) Immunological dissection of human Ia molecules. J Exp Med 148:1592–1611
3. Duquesnoy RJ, Marrari M, Annen K (1979) Identification of an HLA-DR associated system of B cell alloantigens. Transplant Proc 11:1757–1760
4. DeKretser TA, Crumpton MJ, Bodmer JG, Bodmer WF (1982) Two-dimensional gel analysis of the polypeptides precipitated by a polymorphic HLA-DR1, 2, w6 monoclonal antibody:evidence for a third locus. Eur J Immunol 12:600–606
5. Giles RC, Nuñez G, Hurley CK, Nuñez-Roldan A, Winchester R, Stastny P, Capra JD (1983) Structural analysis of a human I-A homologue using a monoclonal antibody that recognizes an MB3-like specificity. J Exp Med 157:1461–1470
6. Beckman I (1984) Monoclonal antibodies to HLA-DR antigens. Immunol Today 5:29–32
7. Adams TE, Bodmer JG, Bodmer WF (1983) Production and characterization of monoclonal antibodies recognizing the α-chain subunits of human Ia alloantigens. Immunology 50:613–624
8. Köhler G, Howe CS, Milstein C (1976) Fusion between immunoglobulin-secreting and nonsecreting myeloma cell lines. Eur J Immunol 6:292–295
9. van Heyningen V, Barron L, Brock DJH, Crichton D, Lawrie S (1982) Monoclonal antibodies to human α-fetoprotein: analysis of the behaviour of three different antibodies. J Immunol Methods 50:123–131
10. Stocker JW, Heusser CH (1979) Methods for binding cells to plastic: application to a solid-phase radioimmunoassay for cell surface antigens. J Immunol Methods 26:87–95
11. Lansdorp PM, Astaldi GCB, Oosterhof F, Janssen MC, Zeijlemaker WP (1980) Immunoperoxidase procedures to detect monoclonal antibodies against cell surface antigens. Quantitation of binding and staining of individual cells. J Immunol Methods 39:393–405
12. Owen MJ, Kissonerghis AM, Lodish HF (1980) Biosynthesis of HLA-A and HLA-B antigens in vivo. J Biol Chem 255:9678–9684
13. Hansen JA, Martin PJ, Kamoun M, Nisperos B, Thomas ED (1981) A supertypic HLA-DR specificity (DR4 + 5) defined by murine monoclonal antibody. Hum Immunol 2:103–111
14. Barnstable CJ, Bodmer WJ, Brown G, Galfre G, Milstein C, Williams AF, Zeigler A (1978) Production of monoclonal antibodies to group A erythrocytes, HLA and other human cell surface antigens – new tools for genetic analysis. Cell 14:9–20
15. Rudd CE, Bodmer JG, Bodmer WF, Crumpton MJ (1985) HLA-D region antigen associated invariant polypeptides as revealed by 2-D gel analysis: glycosylation and structural inter-relationships. J Biol Chem (in press)
16. Tanigaki N, Tosi R, Sagawa K, Minowada J, Ferrara GB (1983) The distribution of DR5, MT2 and MB3 specificities on human Ia subsets. Immunogentics 17:371–386
17. Kasahara M, Takenouchi T, Ogasawara K, Ikeda H, Okuyama T, Ishikawa N, Moriuchi J, Wakisaka A, Kikuchi Y, Aizawa M, Kaneko T, Kashiwagi N, Nishimura Y, Sasazuki T (1983) Serologic dissection of HLA-D specificities by the use of monoclonal antibodies. Immunogentics 17:485–495

Idiotypic Analysis of Anti-Human MHC Class II Monoclonal Antibodies by Syngeneic Anti-Idiotypes

D. Piatier-Tonneau, M. Viguier, P. Debré, and D.J. Charron

Laboratoire d'Immunogénétique, CNRS 500, CHU Pitié-Salpêtrière, 91 boulevard de l'Hôpital, 75013, Paris, France

Further definition of the reactivity of 43 monoclonal antibodies to human MHC class II antigens (anti-DR mAbs) was attempted at the idiotype level. Idiotypic analysis was performed with four syngeneic BALB/c anti-idiotypic sera (anti-Ids) raised against four anti-DR mAbs: D1.12, 206, 135, BM50 [1]. A large number of anti-DR mAbs (29/43) were shown to inhibit the binding of the four Ids to their homologous anti-Ids, indicating a large idiotypic recurrence. Analysis of the cross-reactions (Table 1) led to the distinction of two different sets of anti-Ids. The first set (anti-135 and anti-BM50 Ids) exhibited a large number of cross-reactions. Anti-135 Ids recognised idiotope(s) on 25 of 29 cross-reactive anti-DR mAbs, anti-BM50 Id, on 24 of 29. No relationship between idiotypy and specificity could be detected among these mAbs. In contrast, the second anti-Id set exhibited a more restricted number of cross-reactions: anti-206 Id recognized idiotope(s) on 13 of 29 cross-reactive anti-DR mAbs, 7 of which were specific for the DRβ chain and the NG2 epitope [2], as was the 206 immunizing mAb. Similarly, anti-Ids directed to D1.12, an anti-DR mAb specific for the DR complex and the NG1 epitope, recognised idiotope(s) on 11 of 29 mAbs, none of which recognised the NG2 epitope and only 2 the DRβ chain. The results suggest that anti-D1.12 and -206 Ids might recognise idiotypic determinants more or less closely associated with anti-DR mAb fine specificity.

The high idiotypic recurrence may suggest that mouse antibody response to human Ia antigens is restricted and possibly reflects the presence of immunodominant determinants on DR molecules. Anti-Ids from set I might alternatively constitute a "mirror image" of such a common determinant or a heterogeneous antibody population directed to idiotopes more or less closely associated with anti-DR mAb antigenic specificity.

Table 1. Cross-reactions of 43 anti-DR mAbs with the four anti-Ids

1. *Anti-135 and -BM50 Ids, anti-135 Id only°, anti-BM50 Id only°°*
   SG157, SG171, SG520 (J. Silver); TU34, TU35, TU36, TU37, TU39, TU43, TU22°, TU58° (A. Ziegler); Q2/80, LC12/9 (V. Quaranta); Leu10 (F. Brodsky); F5C9, 26.1 (I. McKenzie); 135, 141, 206, BMMag8, BM50 (D. Charron); SFR3.DR5, SFR.P1.1 (S. Radka); SC2 (R. Fox); DA6.147° (K. Guy); D1.12°° (R. Accolla); 21R.5°° (M. Letarte)
2. *Anti-206 Ids*
   SG171, SG520 (J. Silver); TU34, TU35, TU39 (A. Ziegler); Q5/13, 506AF (V. Quaranta); F5C9, 26.1 (I. McKenzie); 206, BM50 (D. Charron); SFR3.DR5 (S. Radka); SC2 (R. Fox)
3. *Anti-D1.12 Ids*
   DA6.147 (K. Guy); SG157 (J. Silver); TU34, TU35, TU39; TU58 (A. Ziegler); F5C9, 26.1 (I. McKenzie); DI.12 (R. Accolla); BM50 (D. Charron); SC2 (R. Fox)
4. *Non-cross-reactive anti-DR mAbs*
   DA5.164, DA6.231, HIG48, HIG78 (K. Guy); YD1/63.HLK (A. Ziegler); Q2/70, LC12/3, LC20/353 (V. Quaranta); L03 (F. Brodsky); D4.22 (R. Accolla); SG465 (J. Silver); XD5.H7 (S. Radka); SC3, SC4 (R. Fox)

References

1. Piatier-Tonneau D, et al (1983) J Immunol 131:1339
2. Accolla R, et al (1982) J Immunol 128:166

Comparison of Human–Human and Human–Mouse Hybridoma Systems for the Production of Alloreactive Human Monoclonal Antibodies

A. Cambon-Thomsen, A. Blancher, D. Clement, D. Fathallah, M. Calot, and M. Thomsen

INSERM U.100, CHU Purpan, F-31052 Toulouse Cedex, France

Introduction

Compared with monoclonal antibodies of rodent origin, human monoclonal antibodies (HuMAbs) have the theoretical advantage of a better correlation with reaction patterns observed with alloantibodies, and in addition might have therapeutic application. A number of HuMAbs have been produced [3], but none to the major histocompatibility complex products have so far been described. The aim of our work was to evaluate the human–human and the human–mouse hybridoma systems for the production of alloreactive HuMAbs by performing parallel fusions between peripheral blood lymphocytes (PBLs) from women HLA-immunized by pregnancy and four 8-azaguanine-resistant mouse and human cell lines.

Materials and Methods

PBLs from ten women HLA-immunized by pregnancy were obtained during the week after delivery and fused with various cell lines [1, 2, 4]: a mouse cell line, X63 Ag8.653, and three human cell lines: J3JH22 from Kaplan, RH-L4 from Olsson, and LICR-LON-HMy2 from Edwards. Hybrids were selected by azaserine or aminopterin. Ig screening was performed by a sandwich ELISA method. Antibody activity was tested by cell-binding ELISA and by two-colour fluorescence towards the father's and/or panel members' PBLs.

Results

Human–human fusions resulted in low hybrid growth in fewer than 25% of the wells, except in one case (65% of the wells with RH-L4). Hybrid growth was dependent on the feeder cells, which can vary in quality according to the individuals. Only IgG were detected and no antibody activity was demonstrated. More hybrids (repeatedly in more than 85% of the wells) were obtained from the human–mouse fusions. They grew earlier and faster. Ig-producing human–mouse hybrids were found in 7%–50% of the wells. The numbers of IgM- and IgG-secreting hybrids were about the same. IgG and IgM were simultaneously present in eight supernatants (10%). The amount of Ig was generally 1–10 μg/ml. Two fusions were performed with parallel hybrid selection by aminopterin and azaserine: more Ig-producing hybrids were observed with azaserine. Numerous Ig-producing human–mouse hybrids spontaneously lost their Ig production if they were not cloned very early. From four fusions, strong reactivity towards the father's lymphocytes was found by cell-binding ELISA in 1/5, 1/15, 6/50, and 5/22 supernatants, respectively. Positive supernatants underwent further testing: five of them, all containing IgM, were cytotoxic to B cells. They did not react with erythrocytes.

Conclusion

In our test conditions the human–mouse hybridoma system with hybrid selection by azaserine seems more valuable than the human–human hybridoma system for generating HuMAbs using PBLs from in vivo HLA-alloimmunized individuals. We obtained several alloreactive IgM antibodies. No HLA specificity could be defined. In spite of chromosomal instability the human–mouse hybridomas have some advantages over the human–human hybridomas at present: more hybrids are obtained and they grow rapidly; it is possible to kill the nonfused human cells with ouabain; no feeder cells are required; no Ig is produced by the malignant cell line; and the production of ascites in nude mice is possible.

References

1. Cambon-de Mouzon A, Olsson L (1983) Human monoclonal antibodies (HuMAbs) against cell membrane antigens. Transplant Proc 15:220–224
2. Garchon HJ, Blancher A, Champommier F, Blanchard de Vaucouleurs A, Bach JF, Hainaut J (1983) Production d'anticorps antitétaniques humains par des hybridomes. Rev Fr Transfus Immuno-Hématol 26:147–151
3. Kozbor D, Roder JC (1981) The production of monoclonal antibodies from human lymphocytes. Immunol Today 4:72–79
4. Olsson L, Kronstrøm H, Cambon-de Mouzon A, Honsik C, Brodin T, Jakobsen B (1983) Antibody-producing human–human hybridomas. I. Technical aspects. J Immunol Methods 61:17–32

Histocompatibility Testing 1984
Edited by E. D. Albert et al.

Crossreactivity of Monoclonal Anti-HLA Antibodies with Rhesus Monkey Lymphocytes

R. van Lambalgen, and M. Jonker

REP Institutes, Division for Health Research TNO, 151 Lange Kleiweg, P.O. Box 5815, 2280 HV Rijswijk, The Netherlands

Monoclonal anti-HLA class I and class II antibodies (MCAs) submitted to the Ninth Histocompatibility workshop were screened for crossreactivity with rhesus monkey lymphocytes with known RhLA antigens.

Anti-HLA Class I MCAs. Fifty-three anti-class I MCAs were screened against a panel of 76 rhesus monkey lymphocytes. Limited and often weak reactivity was found. The data showed that without exception the reactions segregated with the RhLA locus in families. Four MCAs showed an association with RhLA antigens (Table 1).

This is the first time that anti-HLA reagents have shown a good correlation with RhLA antigens, with the exception of the supertypic HLA-Bw4 and Bw6 antisera.

Anti-HLA Class II MCAs. Ninety anti-class II MCAs were screened against a panel of 50 AET-SRBC-separated B cells, using an NIH technique with shortened incubation times (15 min and 30 min). In total, 48 MCAs were positive and 16 were negative with all monkeys tested; 11 MCAs showed a limited reactivity with no apparent association and 15 MCAs recognised possible supertypic RhLA-DR determinants. Analysis of RhLA-identical siblings showed that it is likely that these determinants segregated with RhLA. Figure 1 shows the associations of these 15 MCAs with the known RhLA-DR specificities. A shaded box in-

Table 1. MCAs showing an association with RhLA antigens

Serum-RhLA	+ +	+ −	− +	− −	χ^2	r	P
9w1105-A2	11	0	1	64	68.6	0.95	0.001
9w1106-A13+A24	32	4	1	37	55.7	0.87	0.001
9w1124-A11+A26	24	1	20	31	22.2	0.54	0.001
9w1133-A11+A26	23	2	24	27	14.4	0.43	0.001

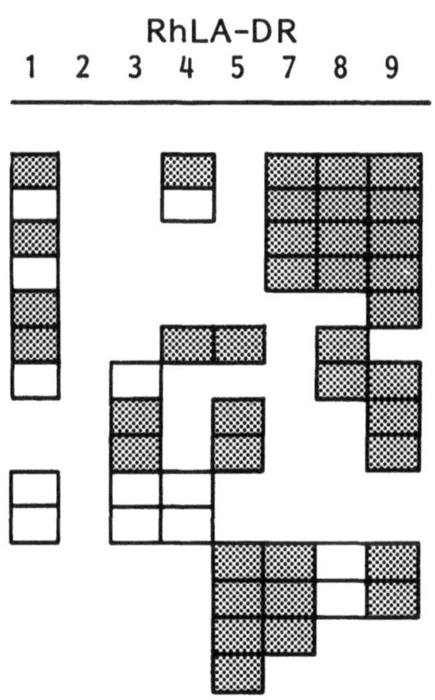

MCA	++	+−	−+	−−	X^2	r	P
9w956	25	4	6	15	14.8	0.54	0.0001
40	18	3	13	16	7.0	0.37	0.008
28	22	6	3	19	18.3	0.61	0.00002
33	17	3	8	22	14.1	0.53	0.0002
18	15	3	3	28	23.5	0.69	$<$ 0.00001
32	26	4	3	17	22.5	0.67	$<$ 0.00001
42	22	1	7	10	11.9	0.49	0.0006
30	24	7	2	17	18.5	0.61	0.00002
04	19	10	7	14	3.9	0.28	0.05
46	14	0	20	16	7.2	0.38	0.007
47	11	0	20	19	6.7	0.37	0.01
05	10	1	5	34	21.0	0.65	$<$ 0.00001
65	10	2	5	33	18.2	0.60	0.00002
77	4	12	0	33	9.0	0.43	0.005
43	3	5	0	42	16.8	0.58	0.0001

Fig. 1. Reaction patterns identified in 15 MCAs associated with RhLA-DR specificities

Histocompatibility Testing 1984
Edited by E. D. Albert et al.

dicates a strong, an open box a partial, and an open space no association with a particular RhLA-DR antigen. Good interpretation of the results is difficult, because 60% of the monkeys came from two harems, so there is a high incidence of haplotype sharing. Further research is needed to investigate whether these possible supertypic DR determinants are analogous to the human DRw52,53 and/or DQ specificities.

Conclusion

Both anti-HLA class I and anti-HLA class II MCAs showed meaningful cross-reactivity with rhesus monkey lymphocytes. An extended study with these MCAs is useful for further analysis of the RhLA system and a comparison of the results with the HLA system may provide insight into the conservation of MHC determinants in evolution.

A Simple and Rapid Procedure for Purification of Human Dendritic Cells from Peripheral Blood

G. Gaudernack, S. Bjercke, and E. Thorsby

Institute of Transplantation Immunology, The National Hospital, 0027 Oslo 1, Norway

Until recently it was believed that the principal antigen-presenting cell among peripheral blood mononuclear cells (PBMC) was the monocyte (MO). Recent evidence, however, indicates that the accessory function of the adherent cell population is due to contaminating dendritic cells (DCs) [1]. To compare the antigen-presenting capacity of MOs and DCs, we have developed a simple and rapid procedure for purification of human DCs from peripheral blood. Concentrated leukocyte fractions (buffy coat) were used as a source of MOs and DCs. The first step involves adherence of cells bearing receptors for fibronectin to plastic petri dishes coated with gelatin and fibronectin [2]. Since this binding is Ca^{2+}-dependent, adherent cells are easily eluted by 10 m*M* EDTA. Subsequently Fc receptor (FcR)-positive cells (MOs and contaminating B cells) are removed by adherence to plastic petri dishes coated with IgG. An alternative procedure involves selective absorption of monocytes after prior incubation with a monoclonal anti-monocyte/macrophage antibody (ID5), on plastic petri dishes coated with $F(ab')_2$ anti-mouse Ig. Both procedures yield a highly enriched dendritic cell population, depleted of MOs and highly purified MOs. The distribution of surface markers on purified dendritic cells and monocytes is summarized in Table 1.

Table 1. Distribution of surface markers on purified dendritic cells and monocytes

Surface marker		Dendritic cells	Monocytes
Mabs	Cellular specificity		
E 12.14	β-2 Microglobulin	+	+
D1C	pan-Leukocyte	+	+
ID5	Monocytes	−	+
C10.6a	Monocytes	−	+
IBC 12	Monocytes	−	+
Leu M2	Monocytes (some)	+/−	+/−
63D3	Monocytes and granulocytes	−	+
Leu M1	Monocytes and granulocytes	−	+
Leu M3	Monocytes	−	+
DRC1	Germinal center DRC	−	−
OKT6	Thymocytes and Langerhans DRC	−	−
Receptors			
FibR		+	+
FcR		−	+

When testing the capacity of these cell populations to present the soluble antigen PPD to purified T cells, we made the following observations: (1) Purified monocytes (> 95% pure) were weakly stimulatory or devoid of antigen-presenting capacity over a wide MO-to-T cell ratio; (2) highly enriched DCs were potent accessory cells; and (3) the yield of DCs was approximately 1% of the starting material (PBMC). On the basis of these findings we conclude that dendritic cells having receptors for fibronectin but lacking FcR and several monocyte/macrophage differentiation antigens are the active accessory cells in human blood.

References

1. van Voorhis WC, et al (1983) Relative efficiency of human monocytes and dendritic cells as accessory cells for T cell replication. J Exp Med 158:174–191
2. Freundlich B, Avdalovic N (1983) Use of gelatin/plasma-coated flasks for isolating human purified blood monocytes. J Immunol Methods 62:31–37

Histocompatibility Testing 1984
Edited by E. D. Albert et al.

HLA-A, B, C Typing Using Serum

C. Russo [1], M. Fotino [2], P. Antonelli [3], A.O. Carbonara [3], and S. Ferrone [4]

1 Department of Medicine, Cornell University Medical College, 1300 York Avenue, New York, NY 10021, USA
2 New York Blood Center, New York, NY, USA
3 Istituto di Genetica Medica, Torino, Italy
4 Department of Microbiology and Immunology, New York Medical College, Valhalla, NY, USA

We have applied a double determinant immunoassay (DDIA) [1] to HLA-A2, A28 and B13 typing, using serum as an antigen source. The results obtained show a correlation of 96% (B13) and 89.1% (A2, A28) with the results obtained by conventional HLA typing. In the DDIA, polyvinylchloride microtiter plates were coated with the anti-HLA-A2, A28 monoclonal antibody CR11-351 (MoAb) [2] and/or with the anti-HLA-B13 MoAb SYI [3]. Then 25 µl serum from HLA-typed donors was added to the well, and incubated for 2 h at room temperature. After the plates had been washed three times, ^{125}I-labeled anti-human B_2m MoAb NAMB I [2] (2×10^5 cpm/well) was added and incubation continued for 2 h. Then the microtiter plates were washed five times and bound radioactivity was counted. The results obtained (see Table 1) were highly reproducible, since testing of 28 sera (16 positive and 12 negative) on two occasions gave concordant results with 27 of the 28 samples tested. The variation in the content of HLA-A2 antigens in sera taken from a given donor was less than 5%. On the other hand, a seven-fold variation in the level of HLA-A2, A28 antigens was found in the sera from the 55 positive donors analyzed; the highest values were found in the HLA-A2, A28 phenotype, followed in decreasing order by those in A2 homozygotes, A28 homozygotes, A2 heterozygotes, and A28 heterozygotes. No relationship between the serum level of HLA-A2, A28 antigens and the total HLA-A, B, C serum level was found. Family studies suggest that the level of HLA-A2 and A28 antigens in the serum is subject to genetic control, which does not appear to be linked to the MHC region. The results indicated that the DDIA is a simple, rapid, and reproducible procedure for HLA-A, B, C typing with serum. The following points are noteworthy: (a) The DDIA provides qualitative and quantitative information; (b) it does not require viable cells, which facilitates retrospective studies; and (c) it eliminates spurious results caused by abnormal susceptibility of target cells to complement-dependent lysis. Since monoclonal antibodies to an increasing number of HLA-A, B, C allospecificities have become available, the DDIA may become a viable alternative to the complement dependent lymphocytotoxic assay.

Table 1. Results of HLA-A, B, and C typing with serum

DDIA					+	−
Sera tested	+	−	Total no.			
A2+	41	2	43	+	55	3
A28+	14	1	15			
A2, A28−	8	35	43	−	8	35
($\chi^2 = 60.5$)			101			
					+	−
Sera tested	+	−	Total no.			
B13+	7	2	9	+	7	2
B13−	2	113	115			
($\chi^2 = 71.1$)			124	−	2	113

References

1. Russo C, Pellegrino MA, Ferrone S (1983) Transplant Proc 1:66
2. Russo C, Ng AK, Pellegrino MA, Ferrone S (1983) Immunogenetics 18:25
3. Lepage V, Raffoux C, Dove C, Mallet C, Degos L (1983) Ninth International Histocompatibility Workshop, Newsletter no. 1, July 15

Histocompatibility Testing 1984
Edited by E. D. Albert et al.

Definition of Two Monocyte-Specific Antigens, One of Which Correlates with the 9a Antigen*

M.J. Jager[1], A. van Leeuwen[1], F.H.J. Claas[1], W.M. Baldwin[2], and J.J. van Rood[1]

1 Dept. of Immunohematology and Blood Bank, University Hospital, Leiden, The Netherlands
2 Dept. of Nephrology, University Hospital, Rijnsburgerweg 10, 2333 Leiden, The Netherlands

Anti-monocyte antibodies are negative factors in bone marrow and renal transplantation [1]. If the monocyte antigens themselves can be recognized, typing and perhaps matching for these antigens will be possible, which may further improve the results of transplantation.

For the detection of monocyte-specific antibodies we used the two-color fluorescence test on total post-Ficoll leukocytes [3]. The advantage of this assay is that antibodies against T cells, B cells, and monocytes can be detected separately, while extra manipulations to obtain the different cell types can be avoided. To circumvent known anti-HLA reactions, sera from parous women and kidney transplant patients were first screened on cells that were HLA-A-, B-, C-, and DR-compatible with the serum donors. Out of a total of 106 sera tested 6 were shown to be monocyte specific, identifying two main monocyte antigens, HMA-1 and HMA-2 (human monocyte antigen). With platelet-absorbed sera, the phenotype frequencies in a random panel were 0.54 and 0.66, respectively. Every cell tested had at least one of these two antigens, suggesting a di-allelic system for the HMA antigens. One of the anti-HMA-1 sera was also positive in the immunofluorescence test on peritubular endothelial cells, but because of the much lower phenotype frequency we think that another antigen than HMA-1 is involved.

Both in panel and in family studies a perfect correlation was observed between the presence of the HMA-1 antigen and the non-HLA agglutination antigen 9a [2].

Inhibition experiments showed that the anti-HMA-1 sera can completely block the agglutinating anti-9a sera: anti-HMA-1 sera probably recognize the same molecule as the anti-9a sera. These results indicate that it may be relevant to study the influence of HMA-1 and HMA-2 or of 9a on renal and bone marrow transplantation.

Acknowledgement. We would like to thank Marian Witvliet for her excellent technical assistance.

References

1. Claas FHJ, Van Rood JJ, Warren RP, Weiden PL, Su PJ, Storb R (1979) The detection of non-HLA antibodies and their possible role in bone marrow graft rejection. Transplant Proc 11:423–426
2. Van Rood JJ, Van Leeuwen A, Schippers AMJ, Pearce R, Van Blankenstein M, Volkers W (1967) Immunogenetics of the group four, five and nine systems. In: Curtoni ES, Mattiuz PL, Tosi RM (eds) Histocompatibility testing. Williams and Wilkins, Baltimore, pp 203–219
3. Van Rood JJ, Van Leeuwen A, Ploem JS (1976) Simultaneous detection of two cell populations by two-colour fluorescence and application to the recognition of B cell determinants. Nature 262:795

* This work was supported in part by the Dutch Foundation for Medical Research (FUNGO), which is subsidized by the Dutch Organization for the Advancement of Pure Research (ZWO) and the J. A. Cohen Institute for Radiopathology and Radiation Protection (IRS)

 Histocompatibility Testing 1984
Edited by E. D. Albert et al.

Anti-Idiotypic Antibodies in Women with Successful Pregnancy*

D.P. Singal, L. Butler, S.-K. Liao, and S. Joseph

Department of Pathology, McMaster University Hamilton, Ontario, Canada L8N 3Z5

We have recently shown that anti-idiotypic antibodies capable of inhibiting responses in MLC and CML can be induced by transplantation and transfusion [1–3]. Based on these observations, we reasoned that such antibodies may also be induced in women alloimmunized by pregnancy. To test this hypothesis, we tested sera from women for anti-idiotypic antibodies directed against husband-specific idiotypes on wife's lymphocytes.

Serum samples from 20 women were tested for inhibition in the MLC test. Nine sera were from parous women, eight from women with no children, and three from women with abortion(s). The MLC inhibition experiments were performed as described by us previously [3]. Responder lymphocytes were from the wife and stimulator cells were from the husband. The sera that showed inhibition by 17% or more (99% confidence limit) were considered as having MLC-inhibiting activity. The inhibition was 2.4% ± 1.52% (range 0%–12%) for sera considered noninhibiting as compared with inhibition of 47.0% ± 5.23% (range 32%–82%) for sera having inhibitory activity.

Serum from one primiparous woman did not inhibit responses in MLC. Sera from the remaining eight parous women inhibited responses of wife's lymphocytes to husband's cells in MLC. The results from one such experiment are shown in Fig. 1. It can be seen that treatment of wife's lymphocytes with autologous serum caused 48% inhibition of responses in MLC. Similar data were observed with the remaining seven sera. The inhibition in these experiments was 48.9% ± 5.53% (range 35%–82%).

Of the sera from women with no children, that from one woman caused 32% inhibition of responses of wife's lymphocytes to husband's cells in MLC. Sera from the remaining seven women did not cause any inhibition (mean 3.43% ± 2.09%, range 0%–12%). Also, no inhibition (0%) was observed with sera from all three women with recurrent abortion(s).

The specificity of the inhibitory factor in sera from parous women was investigated by absorption studies. Serum (1 ml) from a woman (A) was absorbed with either lymphocytes (10 × 10⁶) from the husband (B) or with wife-antihusband (ABx)

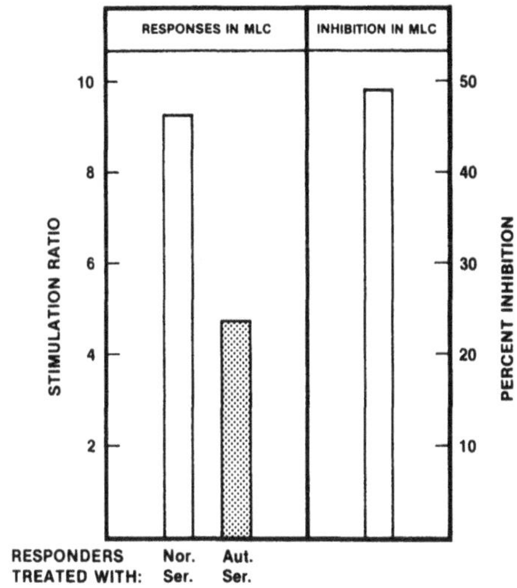

Fig. 1. Responses of lymphocytes from wife against stimulator cells from husband. Responder cells were treated with normal AB (*Nor. Ser.*) or autologous (*Aut. Ser.*) serum before setting up MLC cultures. Data are given as stimulation ratio and as percent inhibition

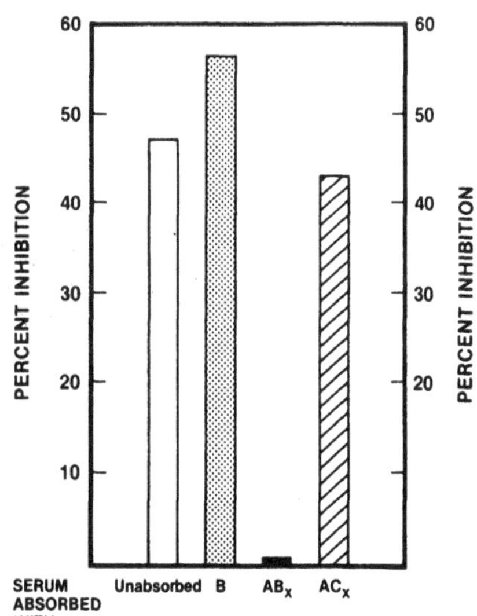

Fig. 2. Responses of lymphocytes from wife against stimulator cells from husband. Responder cells were treated with autologous serum [unabsorbed or absorbed with husband's cells (*B*), wife-anti-husband lymphoblasts (*ABx*), or wife-anti-third party lymphoblasts (*ACx*)] before MLC cultures were set up

* This work was supported by a grant from the Medical Research Council of Canada

orwife-anti-thirdparty(ACx)lymphoblasts(10×10^6). Responder (A) lymphocytes were treated with either unabsorbed or absorbed serum and then tested for responses against husband's stimulator cells. The results from an experiment are shown in Fig. 2. It is evident that absorption of serum with husband's lymphocytes or with ACx lymphoblasts did not remove the inhibitory activity. On the other hand, absorption of serum with ABx lymphoblasts removed the inhibitory activity. Similar results were obtained with serum from another woman.

Sera and IgG fractions from two parous women were tested for antibodies against ABx lymphoblasts by the indirect immunofluorescence technique. Sera and IgG fractions stained 35%, 43% and 25%, 31% ABx lymphoblasts. Antibodies directed against ABx lymphoblasts could not be demonstrated in serum from a woman with recurrent abortions.

Factors that block MLC reaction have been demonstrated in plasma and sera from pregnant women. These factors have been shown to be directed against stimulator as well as responder lymphocytes. The data in the present study confirm and extend these observations in that antibodies capable of inhibiting responses of wife's lymphocytes to husband's cells in MLC are present in sera from parous women, but not in women with no children or in women with abortions. The results also suggest that the inhibitory activity of the sera was due to the presence of anti-idiotypic antibodies directed against husband-specific idiotypes present on wife's lymphocytes. The data suggest that maternal tolerance to the fetus may be attributable to a similar mechanism occurring in vivo.

References

1. Nagarkatti PS, Singal DP (1983) Blood-transfusion-induced suppression of cytotoxic T lymphocyte responses in mice. Transplantation 36:520–525
2. Nagarkatti PS, Joseph S, Singal DP (1983) Induction of antibodies by blood transfusions capable of inhibiting responses in MLC. Transplantation 36:695–699
3. Singal DP, Joseph S (1982) Role of blood transfusions on the induction of antibodies directed against recognition sites on T lymphocytes in renal transplant patients. Hum Immunol 4:93–108

T-Cell Alloantigens

Class I MHC-Linked Determinants Expressed on Activated T Cells

R. Fauchet[1], D.J. Charron[2], O. Bouhallier[1], N. Genetet[1], G. Merdrignac[1], P. Turmel[2], D. Bourel[1], and B. Genetet[1]

1 Laboratoire d'Histocompatibilité – Centre Régional de Transfusion Sanguine et Groupe Universitaire de Recherche en Immunologie Fondamentale et Appliquée, Rue Pierre Jean Gineste, 35000-Rennes, France
2 Laboratoire d'Immuno-génétique Hôpital Pitié-Salpétrière, Paris, France

Introduction

Sensitized T-cells in mixed leukocyte culture possess HLA-D like antigens absent from nonactivated resting T cells. These antigens are synthesized by allostimulated T cells [1]. T cell expression of HLA-DR antigens has been demonstrated by several investigators using a variety of methods [2–6]. On activated T cells, specific anti-HLA-DR antisera showed unexplained reactivity, distinguishable from HLA-DR reactivity [7]. This antiblast activity had also been found in sera from multiparous women in which no anti-HLA-A, B, or DR antibodies were detectable [8]. Gazit and co-workers postulated the existence of a genetic system specific to activated T cells, in close linkage disequilibrium with the HLA system. They named this the HT system and suggested that it might be a human correlate of the mouse TLa region. Two possible alleles of the postulated HT locus (HT1 or K, HT3 or SF48) were identified [9, 10]. The genetic polymorphism of the HT locus has recently been confirmed [11]. The present study was undertaken to determine if sera from multiparous women clearly detected new determinants on blast cells different from the classical HLA-A, B, C antigens and similar to HTs. We also carried out this study to investigate the specificity of such determinants and their correlation with the HLA system.

Histocompatibility Testing 1984
Edited by E. D. Albert et al.

Material and Methods

Sera. A total of 536 sera were studied. All sera were initially screened for HLA-A, B, C, DR activity on the selected panel and absorbed twice with pooled platelets to remove any HLA-ABC activity. Absorption assay was performed on this sera. 100 µl serum was incubated at room temperature for 2 h with 2×10^9 mature platelets and/or with 2×10^6 lymphocytes.

Panel Cells. T, B [12], and PHA-T cells were isolated from the same subjects: 58 healthy unrelated donors and 60 members of 12 different families. PHA-T cells were obtained from peripheral blood cells (1×10^6 cells/ml) incubated in tissue flasks (37 °C in 5% CO_2) with PHA at a final concentration of 1 : 2000. The culture medium was changed on day 3. On day 5 of culture PHA cells were harvested and frozen (3×10^6 cells/ml). The microlymphocytotoxicity test was used on the different targets.

Antigen Blocking Test. Blocking experiments were carried out using PHA-T cells pretreated with turkey anti-β2m or anti-P29-34 sera (at 37 °C for 60 min), and all the tests were performed by microlymphocytotoxicity.

Cytofluorometric Analysis. This was used to compare patterns of detected determinants by specific antiblast and by anti-HLA specific sera. Determination was based on the analysis of 10^4 PHA-T cells scanned in the cell sorter (ORTH 50H). Dead cells were excluded on the basis of their characteristic low forward scatter profiles. As for the controls, the alloserum was replaced by an identical quantity of incubation medium (HBSS added 5% FCS).

*Immunoprecipitation and Polyacrylamide Gel Electrophoresis.*PHA blasts were labeled on day 5 with [^{35}S]methionine ($\geq$ 600 Ci/mmol, Amersham, UK) at day 5 of culture and the membranes extracted. Immunoprecipitates were prepared by reacting 100 µl 0.5% Nonidet P-40 (NP-40) extract (obtained from 10^7 cells) with 30–50 µl of antiserum 101 RE followed by 200 µl of a 10% solution of heat-killed, formalin-fixed *S. aureus* (Cowan). Unabsorbed and platelet absorbed sera were used. Normal human serum was used as control. Immunoprecipitated samples were reduced, dissociated, and electrophoresed on 12% polyacrylamide gel slabs (Fig. 1). Kodak NS-2T X-ray film with no screens was used for autoradiography. Two-dimensional gel electrophoresis was performed as previously described [13], except that IEF was used for the first dimension and 8.5% acrylamide for the second dimension in order to maximize separation in the 40–45K range.

Results

Of 536 multiparous women tested, 52 had defined anti-HLA-A, B, C but not DR activity (group 1) and 484 lacked defined anti-HLA-A, B, C and DR activity (group 2). All the sera were absorbed with pooled platelets and tested against PHA-activated T cells, as well as T peripheral blood lymphocytes and B cells from the same donors. Of the 536 sera tested, 39 (7.27%) reacted specifically in duplicate with PHA-activated T cells: Four of these 39 sera belonged to group 1 (7.6%) and 35 belonged to group 2 (7.23%). Out of the 39 selected sera, 21 were submitted to antigen-blocking test using anti-β2 microglobulin and/or anti-p29–34 turkey sera and to family segregation analysis.

These 21 sera fell into two groups: the first group with nine antisera reacting with neither with β2 microglobulin nor with p29-34 molecules on PHA-activated T cells; and the second group with 12 antisera whose anti-PHA-activated T-cell activity disappeared with blocking of the reaction by anti-β2 microglobulin antibodies but not by anti-p29-34 antibodies. These 12 sera may, therefore, contain antibodies against β2m-associated determinants (Table 1).

Five of these 12 sera reacted with determinants in linkage disequilibrium with HLA-A antigens: 101 RE with HLA-A3, 102 RE with HLA-A1, 106 RE with HLA-A9, 107 RE with HLA-A2, 111 RE with HLA-A10. Linkage appeared weaker for the other seven sera. One sera, 101 RE, detected a structure in close disequilibrium with HLA-A3 and can be similar to HT3 sera studied by Gazit. The following is a more detailed analysis of 101 RE.

Absorption Tests. On screening, serum 101 RE showed no anti-HLA-A, B, C, or DR activity. After absorption with pooled platelets, activity was found against A3 blasts but not against A3 B cells or resting A3 T cells. After three successive absorptions with A3 positive lymphocytes (20×10^6/ml), residual reactivity with blasts was seen. After sequential absorption with pooled platelets followed by absorption with A3 lymphocytes, the serum consistently showed activity against mitogen-activated A3 lymphocytes. After absorption with A3 blasts this activity disappeared, but was restored by elution. Absorption with A3-specific platelets reduced but did not remove PHA-T antibody activity.

Population Studies. Serum 101 RE was tested against a panel of 58 activated T cells from unrelated donors. Activity was seen against 17 A3 positive cells, among which only one showed a weakly positive result. 101 RE and HT3 were also tested

Table 1. Blocking test with turkey anti-β_2 microglobulin and anti-p29-34

PHA-T cells	Blocked with	101 RE	102 RE	104 RE	105 RE	106 RE	107 RE	121 RE	155 RE
A2, Bw62, DRw6, DRw8		1	1	6	6	1	8	1	1
	Turkey anti-β_2m	1	1	1	1	1	1	1	1
	Turkey anti-p29-34	1	1	6	6	1	8	1	1
A24, B8, Bw62, DR3, DR7		1	1	8	1	6	1	1	6
	Turkey anti-β_2m	1	1	1	1	1	1	1	1
	Turkey anti-p29-34	1	1	8	1	6	1	1	6
A1, A2, B44, Bw57, DR4, DR7		1	8	1	1	1	8	8	1
	Turkey anti-β_2m	1	1	1	1	1	1	1	1
	Turkey anti-p29-34	1	8	1	1	1	8	8	1
A2, A25, B18, Bw62, DR5, DR7		1	1	1	1	6	6	1	1
	Turkey anti-β_2m	1	1	1	1	1	1	1	1
	Turkey anti-p29-34	1	1	1	1	6	6	1	1
A1, A3, B7, B8, DR2, DR3		8	1	8	1	1	8	1	1
	Turkey anti-β_2m	1	1	1	1	1	1	1	1
	Turkey anti-p29-34	8	1	8	1	1	8	1	1

8: 75% – 100% reactivity; 6: 50% – 75% reactivity; 1: 0 – 10% reactivity

Table 2. Segregation of 101, 102 and 107 RE reactivity in four families

Family	Paternal haplotypes		Maternal haplotyes		Sibling reactions with 101 RE and 102 RE – 107 RE
	a	A2, B7, DR4	c	A11, B5, DRw6	b→ 101 RE+ a a
BIL	–		–		c d c
	b→	101 RE+A3, B7, DR1	d	Aw19.2, B5, DRw6	
	a	A2, B15, DR4	c	A1, B8, DR3	b→ 101 RE+ b→ 101 RE+ a
BLE	–		–		d→ 101 RE+ c c
	b→	101 RE+A3, B14, DR–	d→	101 RE+A3, B7, DR2	
	a→	102 RE+A1, B17, DR7	c	Aw19, B18, DR7	b→ 101 RE+ a→ 102 RE+
LEG	–		–		d→ 101 RE+ c
	b→	101 RE+A3, B27, DR1	d→	101 RE+A3, B5, DR1	
	a→	107 RE+A2, B35, DR4	c	A29, B12, DR7	a→ 107 RE+ b→ 101 RE+
ORA	–		–		d c
	b→	101 RE+A3, B35, DR1	d	A28, B18, DR5	

against the 58 cells; there was no reactivity pattern for the cells lacking A3 whether 101 RE or HT3 was used.

Family Studies. Table 2 shows the pattern of inheritance of HLA haplotypes and reactivities of activated lymphocytes with sera 101 RE and 102 RE in four families: in family BIL, 101 RE was positive with the father by haplotype b and sibling b/c, who inherited the paternal b haplotype A3, B7, DR1. In family BLE, both parents were positive and had haplotypes b and d including A3. Only A3-negative sibs having inherited a/c haplotypes were negative with this serum. The same was observed in families LEG and ORA. The families previously studied showed a significant genetic segregation concerning the inheritance of PHA-T determinants.

Cytofluorometric Analysis. This was initially performed on T cells from day 0 to day 5 of culture in the presence of PHA. The same percentage of cells was stained with A3 alloserum regardless of the day of culture with a great intensification of the fluorescence observed. On the other hand, 101 RE alloserum, negative on T cells at day 0, stained a high percentage of activated T cells strongly on day 5. The analysis showed a different profile for the determinants detected by A3 and 101 RE allosera. When the PHA-cells (day 5) were labeled by both A3 and 101 RE alloantisera (tests in quadruplicate), an increase in the intensity of fluorescence (without any modification in the number of labeled cells) was observed. This additional effect suggested that the A3 and the 101 RE antibodies were detecting different antigenic determinants expressed on the surface of the same cell.

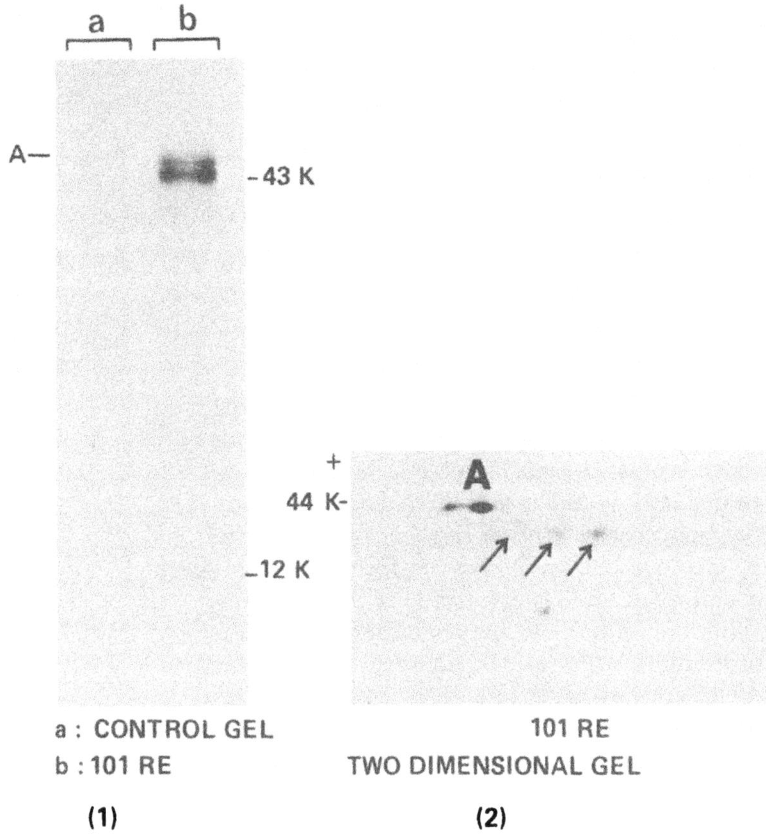

Fig. 1. Analysis of the specificity of 101 RE by immunoprecipitation. *1* One-dimensional gel electrophoresis. *2* Two-dimensional gel electrophoresis

Biochemical Studies. Absorbed and unabsorbed 101 RE serum specifically precipitated a 42K-12K molecular complex on PHA-activated T cells. Only a faint band was seen at 44K in the control gel, corresponding to actin and distinguishable from the main 42-43K band. Two-dimensional gel electrophoresis of serum 101 RE showed a class I molecule with a 42K heavy chain and a 12K light chain (Fig. 1).

Discussion

These data confirm the widely reported finding that sera obtained from multiparous women contain activity that cannot be explained on the basis of known anti-HLA-A, B, C, or DR activity against surface antigens expressed by activated lymphocytes. This is consistent with biochemical evidence of a rearrangement of glycoprotein structures and the formation of new protein structures during T cell stimulation [14, 15]. An HTA1 antigen expressed on the human lymphoblastoid T cell line MOLT4 was suggested to be the human correlate of a murine Tl determinants, structurally similar to HLA antigens and associated with $\beta 2$ microglobulin [16]. It had also been demonstrated that the membrane structures of the cells were impaired in culture activated human T cells [17]. Our own study deals with antigens associated with $\beta 2$m. These data support the hypothesis that the activities of some of the sera correlated with particular HLA antigens (A1, A2, A3, A9, A10), show inheritance in family studies and demonstrate that the detected determinants belong to a specific genetic system. Blocking by turkey anti-$\beta 2$ microglobulin and biochemical data added to demonstrate that the antigens detected are indeed associated with $\beta 2$ microglobulin and detect a molecular complex corresponding to a class I HLA structure. It should be pointed out that a significant increase in the intensity of fluorescence occurred with both A3 and 101 RE antibodies, suggesting that these antibodies were detecting two different antigen determinants on the surface of the same cells.

Three hypotheses could be put forward to explain the reactivity of these sera: (a) a second A locus could explain the correlation with known and frequent HLA antigens, (b) it could be a reaction against an epitope unveiled following the activation process of the cells, (c) it could be the human counterpart of the murine Qa system. Experiments are in progress (study of the thymocyte cells, cell lines, sequential immunoprecipitation) to analyze the difference between the differentiation T cell antigens and the classical class I products. The similarity of our findings to those of Gazit is striking and suggests that 101 RE and HT3 could detect the same structure, belonging to the "HT system."

Summary

About 7% of allosensitized or non-allosensitized HLA-A, B, C sera obtained from 536 multiparous women possessed anti-PHA T cell antibodies. Blocking tests by turkey anti-$\beta 2$ microglobulin and turkey anti-P29-34 antisera showed, in some sera, the presence of antibodies against $\beta 2$-microglobulin-associated determinants in linkage disequilibrium with HLA antigens. Immunoprecipitation studies with 101 RE detected a molecular complex corresponding to a class I molecule. Dependent fluorescence intensity tends to prove that different class I antigenic determinants are expressed on the surface of the same PHA-activated T cells.

References

1. Evans RL, Faldetta TJ, Humphreys RE, Pratt DM, Yunis EJ, Schlossman SF (1978) Peripheral human T cells sensitized in mixed leukocyte culture synthesize and express Ia-like antigens. J Exp Med 148:1140–1448
2. Greaves M, Verbi W, Festenstein H, Papaesteriadies C, Jaraquemada D, Hayward A (1979) "Ia-like" antigens on human T cells. Eur J Immunol 9:356–362
3. Metzgar RS, Bertoglio J, Anderson JK, Bonnard GD, Ruscetti FW (1979) Detection of HLA DRw (Ia-like) antigens on human T lymphocytes grown in tissue culture. Immunol 122:949–953
4. De Wolf WC, Schlossman SF, Yunis EJ (1979) DRw antisera react with activated T cells. J Immunol 122:1780–1784
5. Zimmerman R, Ozer H, DeWolf WC, Evans RL, Yunis EJ, Schlossman SF (1979) The detection of Ia like and DRw antigens on activated T cells. Transplant Proc 11:1770–1773
6. Reinherz EL, Kung PC, Pesando JM, Ritz J, Goldstein G, Schlossman SF (1979) Ia determinants on human T-cell subsets defined by monoclonal antibody. J Exp Med 150:1472–1482
7. Lima G, Wollman E, Lepage V, Degos L, Dausset J (1981) Alloantigens expressed on activated human T cells different from HLA-A, -B, -C and -DR antigens. Immunogenetics 13:529–537
8. Kim SJ, Christiansen FT, Gosar I, Silver DM, Pollack M, Dupont B (1980) Frequency of alloantibodies reacting with PHA-activated T lymphocytes unexplainable by known HLA activities. Hum Immunol 4:347–355
9. Gazit E, Terhorst C, Yunis EJ (1980a) The human "T" genetic region of the HLA-linkage group is a polymorphism detected on lectin activated lymphocytes. Nature 284:275–277
10. Gazit E, Terhorst C, Mahoney RJ, Yunis EJ (1980b) Alloantigens on the human T (HT) genetic region of the HLA linkage group. Hum Immunol 1:97–109
11. Gazit E, Gothelf Y, Gil R, Orgad S, Pitman TB, Watson ALM, Yang Young S, Yunis EJ (1984) Alloantibodies to PHA-activated lymphocytes detect human Qa-like antigens. J Immunol 132 [1]:165–169
12. Fauchet R, Bouhallier O, Genetet B (1980) B-cell typing by rosetting with treated sheep red blood cells. In: Terasaki PI (ed) Histocompatibility testing 1980. UCLA, Los Angeles, p 289
13. Charron D, Engleman EG, Benike CJ, McDevitt HO (1980) Ia antigens on alloreactive T cells in man detected by monoclonal antibodies: evidence for synthesis of HLA-D/DR molecules of the responder type. J Exp Med 152[2]:127–136
14. Anderson LC, Gahmberg CG, Kimura AK, Wigzell (1978) Activated human T lymphocytes display new surface glycoproteins. Medical Sciences 75:3455–3458
15. Boto WO, Humphreys RE (1981) Variation in the synthesis of membrane proteins of human T lymphocytes during mitogenic activation, recognition of a 70 000 dalton protein with anti-p23,30 heteroantiserum and a novel 42 000 dalton protein anti-44,12 heteroantiserum. J Immunol 126[2]:759–760
16. Ziegler A, Milstein C (1979) A small polypeptide different from $\beta 2$ microglobulin associated with a human cell surface. Nature 279:243–244
17. Burns GF, Battye FL, Goldstein G (1982) Surface antigen changes occurring in short-term cultures of activated T lymphocytes: analysis by flow cytometry. Cell Immunol 71:12–26

Alloantibodies to PHA-Activated Lymphocytes Detect Human Qa-Like Antigens*

E. Gazit[1], Y. Gothelf[1], R. Gil[1], S. Orgad[1], T.B. Pitman[2], A.L.M. Watson[2], S. Young Yung[2], and E.J. Yunis[2]

1 Chaim Sheba Medical Center, Tel-Hashomer, Israel 52621
2 The Dana-Farber Cancer Institute, Boston, MA, and Harvard Medical School, Boston, MA, USA

Introduction

At the Eighth Histocompatibility Workshop in 1980 and in several reports published thereafter [5–7], we provided evidence of the existence of class I non-HLA β_2-microglobulin (β_2m)-associated molecules on lectin-activated lymphocytes. This was shown by using PHA-activated lymphocytes as a cellular probe to screen platelet-absorbed alloantisera. In the initial study, two alloantisera, K and SF48, were shown to contain antibodies which reacted with PHA-activated lymphocytes but not with resting T or B lymphocytes separated from the same individual [5–7]. This reactivity was not absorbed either by pooled platelets or by platelets isolated from the individual donors of the activated lymphocytes. Turkey anti-β_2-microglobulin blocked the reactivity to the corresponding HT antibodies, but turkey anti-Ia-like did not. Thus, it appeared that the molecule recognized by SF48 and K is β_2m-associated. It was shown by family studies that the same reactivity segregated dominantly with HLA haplotypes and more specifically, in one recombinant family, with HLA-A locus [5, 6]. Here we described three new HT determinants (non-HLA class I MHC antigens) that are recognized by eight antisera. One of these (HT-2) is found to segregate with HLA in four families which were studied. Our experiments indicate that the products of the HT polymorphism are not expressed on thymocytes, a fact which suggest that these alloantigens may represent either the human counterpart of murine Qa system or else a new polymorphism of class I alloantigens.

Materials and Methods

Procurement of Alloantisera. Alloantisera from pregnant women were obtained as previously described [4].

* Supported in part by Grant # 3283 from the United States-Israel Binational Science Foundation (BSF), Jerusalem, Israel, and National Institutes of Health Grants AI-17120, CA-19589, and CA-06516

PHA Activation of Lymphocytes. PHA activation of peripheral blood lymphocytes (PBL) was carried out in Costar trays (Costar 3512; Costar, Cambridge, MA). PBL (2×10^6 Ficoll-Hypaque-separated) were placed in each well in 2 ml of 10% pooled human serum (PHS) in RPMI 1640 medium supplemented with glutamine, penicillin, and streptomycin and containing 1.0 µg/ml PHA (HA-17, Wellcome Laboratories, England). After 72 h at 37 °C, the cells were harvested and adjusted to a concentration of 1.5×10^5 living cells/ml. Ten-milliliter samples of the suspension, in RPMI 1640 medium containing 10% interleukin 2(IL 2) and 10% PHS, were incubated in plastic flasks in a CO_2 incubator at 37 °C. After 4 days, the cultures were harvested and frozen in dimethyl sulfoxide in samples of $2-4 \times 10^6$ cells/vial. The activated cell panels were kept frozen in liquid nitrogen until used. The average viability of the thawed and fresh activated lymphocytes was greater than 80%.

Preparation of IL 2. IL 2 was prepared according to published methods [3] from PBL from one or two 1000-rad-irradiated donors, or from T cell chronic lymphatic leukemia cells (T-CLL). The IL 2 was used at optimal concentrations of 10%, giving cultures of PHA-activated lymphocytes with 10–15 times the preactivation count (80%–90% viability).

Cytotoxicity Testing. Cytotoxicity testing was performed by the standard two-stage National Institutes of Health method utilizing the long incubation time [11].

Platelet Absorptions. Platelet absorptions were carried out with pooled, outdated, packed platelets or freshly isolated platelets from single donors in a ratio of 1 : 1 serum to packed platelets. The absorptions were carried out twice (at room temperature and at 4 °C), for 60 min each time.

Blocking with Turkey Antibodies. The preparation and assay of the turkey antisera were as reported previously [5]. Lymphocytes used in the blocking assay were centrifuged and resuspended in an appropriate volume of turkey antiserum and incubated at 37 °C for 60 min, after which they were plat-

Histocompatibility Testing 1984
Edited by E. D. Albert et al.

ed on the typing trays and tested in the cytotoxicity assay.

Preparation of Thymocytes. Thymuses were obtained from children undergoing cardiac surgery. Thymus fragments were teased into single-cell suspensions and applied to a Ficoll-Hypaque density gradient. The thymocytes were washed three times with RPMI 1640 medium and used for the cytotoxicity test or cryopreserved in ethylene glycol and minimal essential medium with Spinner salts, as previously described [11].

Correlation Coefficient. Reactions of the alloantisera with B lymphocytes and PHA-activated lymphocytes were analyzed by two-by-two comparisons with a well-defined HLA panel. Cluster analysis was performed comparing the pattern of reactivity of pairs of antisera with that of PHA-activated lymphocytes of the screening panel.

Lod Score. Lod scores in calculation of linkage of the new determinants of HT with HLA were calculated using the method described by Morton [13].

Results

HT Antibodies

Of 1100 sera tested, 69 were found to contain antibodies to HT antigens as revealed by reactions with a panel of PHA-activated lymphocytes obtained from 28 individuals. Cytotoxicity reactions of these sera were negative in tests against resting T lymphocytes obtained from the peripheral blood of the same donors or from a random panel of 60 individuals. The sera displayed three types of positive cytotoxicity pattern: (a) Positive reactions to PHA-activated lymphocytes only, with blocking of the reaction by turkey β_2m antibody but not by turkey Ia antibody. These reactions were classified as HT. (b) Positive reactions with B and PHA-activated lymphocytes, with blocking of the latter by both turkey antibodies (i.e., anti-β_2m and anti-Ia). These reactions were classified as due to antibodies against HLA-DR and HT. (c) Positive reactions with B and PHA-activated lymphocytes, with blocking of the latter by turkey anti-β_2m (Table 1). This pattern is illustrated by serum 1667; the reactivity against PHA-activated lymphocytes (Y-3 and Y-4) could be blocked by anti-β_2m, but not anti-Ia, despite the fact that the serum reacted with the B lymphocytes of these individuals. These reactions, however, indicate the anti-HT reactivity in this serum. It is conceivable that the absence of blocking of the PHA-activated lymphocytes by anti-Ia was due to the greater sensitivity of B lymphocytes compared with PHA-activated lymphocytes to C-mediated lymphocytotoxicity (unpublished experiments). The same cytotoxicity patterns were produced with the use of antibodies absorbed by platelets obtained from the individuals from whom the PHA blasts had been produced (Table 2). The reproducibility of these reactions, as tested in three independent assays with a panel of 30 individuals, was 89% (Fig. 1). Final HT assignments were made on the basis of at least two positive assays; of the 69 sera found to contain HT antibodies, 23 gave between five and 12 positive reactions per serum. The reactions of eight of these sera appeared to cluster in three groups, as detected by significant values of the coefficient of correlation, r. The r values indicate that sera 965 and 1032, sera SF48 and 1642, and sera 1136, 1605, 1014, and 1227 detect three

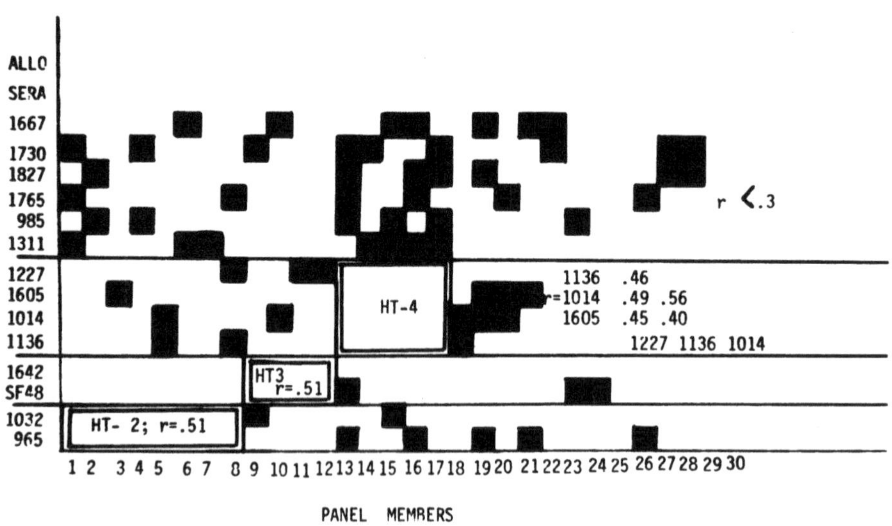

Fig. 1. Reactivities of selected "HT" alloantisera with a panel of PHA-activated lymphocytes ($n = 30$)

Table 1. HT and HLA-DR lymphocytotoxicity reaction patterns with the use of pooled platelet-absorbed alloantibodies

Sera	Y-1					Y-2				
	B	Act	Blocked a-β_2m	Blocked a-IA	Interpret[b]	B	Act	Blocked a-β_2m	Blocked a-Ia	Interpret[b]
SF48	1	6	1	4	HT	1	1	1	1	
693	1	1	1	1		1	1	1	1	
965	6	6	4 – 6	2	DR	2	4	1	1	HT + DR
1136	6	4	1	1	HT + DR	2	2	1	2	HT?
1188	1	1	1	1		1	1	1	1	
1605	1	6	1	4	HT	1	4	1	4	HT
1667	1	1	1	1		1	1	1	1	
	Y-3					Y-4				
SF48	1	2	1	2	HT?	1	1	1	1	
693	2	6	1	4	HT	1	1	1	1	
965	6	1	1	1	DR	4	4	4	1	DR
1136	1	1	1	1		4	4	4	1	DR
1188	1	1	1	1		1	1	1	1	
1605	1	1	1	1		2	4	1	1	HT + DR
1667	4	8	1	8	HT	4	8	2	8	HT

The numbers in the table represent cytotoxicity scores as follows: 1, less than 10% dead cells; 2, 10% – 25% dead cells; 4, 25% – 50% dead cells; 6, 50% – 75% dead cells; 8, 75% – 100% dead cells.
B, B lymphocytes; Act, PHA-activated T lymphocytes; Blocked a-β_2m, blocking by antibody against β_2m; Blocked a-Ia, blocking by antibody against human Ia-like; Interpret, interpretation of the serological reactions.

[a] The antibodies were absorbed with a platelet pool obtained from 200 individuals. The reactions with enriched T lymphocytes in all cases were also scored

[b] Blocking done on PHA-activated lymphocytes only

Table 2. HT and HLA-DR lymphocytotoxicity reaction patterns of PHA-activated lymphocytes by sera absorbed with platelets of each individual tested[a]

Sera	Y-1 PHA-activated					Y-2 PHA-activated				
	B	Alone	Plus a-β_2m	Plus a-Ia	Interpretation	B	Alone	Plus a-β_2m	Plus a-Ia	Interpretation
1605	1	6	1	4	HT	1	6	2	6	HT
1667	1	1	1	1		1	1	1	1	
1188	1	1	1	1		1	1	1	1	
	Y-3 PHA-activated					Y-4 PHA-activated				
1605	1	1	1	1		1	8	1	6	HT
1667	2	8	1	6	HT	4	8	2	6	HT
1188	1	1	1	1		1	1	1	1	

[a] The antibodies were absorbed with platelets obtained from the individuals listed from 1 – 4. The reactions with T lymphocytes are not listed but were negative. The scores given are explained in Table 1

different determinants, designated as HT-2, HT-3, and HT-4 respectively. The determinant detected by HT-3 was found to be associated with HLA-A3 ($r = 0.70$ for SF48; $r = 0.31$ for 1642). However, HT-2 and HT-4 were not found to be associated with any HLA specificity.

Inheritance of HT Determinants with HLA

Four families, comprising eight parents and 16 siblings, were studied. Twenty-seven sera gave informative cytotoxic reactions consistent with inheritance of antigens in linkage with the HLA

Table 3. Reactivities of thymocytes and PHA-activated lymphocytes with selected HT alloantisera

Thymus				Serum SF48	1079	1199	1311	1605	1709	1827
# 1	Peripheral blood lymphocytes	B		1	1	1	1	1	1	1
		PHA-activated	Untreated	6 – 8	1	1	4	4	1	1
			blocked by turkey anti β_2m	1	1	1	1	1	1	1
			Blocked by turkey anti-Ia	8	1	1	2 – 4	2 – 4	4 – 6	1
	Thymocytes			1	1	1	1	1	1	1
# 2	Peripheral blood lymphocytes	B		1	1	1	1	1	1	1
		PHA-activated	untreated	1	2 – 4	4	1	1	2 – 4	2 – 4
			blocked by turkey anti β_2m	1	1	1	1	1	1	1
			Blocked by turkey anti-Ia	1	4	2	1	1	4	2
	Thymocytes			1	1	1	1	1	1	1

Scores explained in Table 1

haplotypes. Two sera (the 965 and 1032 or HT-2 cluster) were informative in the four families and showed inheritance in 11 siblings. Linkage analysis indicated dominant inheritance in linkage with HLA (lod score value Z = 4.46). Other sera gave informative results for codominant inheritance in linkage with HLA in one to 12 children, with rare examples of missed or extra reactions. Some sera gave segregation patterns in five to 12 of the siblings: sera 1311, 1405, 1730, and 1827 in five; serum 1199 in six; serum 1014 in seven; and serum 985 in 12 siblings.

Reactivity in HT Antibodies with Thymocytes

The sera were tested against a panel of thymocytes and PHA-activated lymphocytes obtained from children undergoing cardiac surgery (Table 3). Invariably, the thymocytes and the PHA-activated lymphocytes obtained from the same donors did not react with the same sera.

Discussion

The present experiments demonstrate that human lymphocytes activated by lectins express class I histocompatibility alloantigens that are different from those encoded by the conventional HLA loci (A, B, C). Similar observations have been recently made by several investigators [8, 9] (R. Fauchet, personal communication; S. Mayer and M. M. Tongio, personal communication). Wollman et al [17] described very recently the presence of non-HLA antigenic determinants which were expressed on activated T and B lymphocytes but did not segregate with HLA.

Because the determinants we described, which were recognized on lectin-activated lymphocytes, were not shared by thymocytes, they are probably not the human equivalent of murine TLa locus gene products. (This possibility cannot be excluded, however, because a small subset of thymocytes not detected by the methods used here may indeed express the HT antigenic determinants.) If, in fact, the HT determinants are not analogous to murine TLa, it would appear that these antibodies are directed against Qa-like determinants.

We have been able to characterize 23 antisera containing antibodies to HT (non-HLA class I antigens) or to HT and HLA-DR, and have successfully used the ability of turkey anti-Ia to block cytotoxic reactions to HLA-DR alloantibodies. Reactions to HT antigens can be blocked by turkey anti-β_2m, but not by anti-Ia-like antibodies. Because the sera do not contain anti-HLA (A, B, C) antibodies, the blocking studies (anti-β_2m) are not due to steric hindrance to HLA (class I) molecules. Previously, we described two antibodies, SF48 and K, similar to those identified here. The present results identifies a second serum that appears to react to the same determinant as SF48 (HT-3), which is found in association with HLA-A3. Although the remaining sera and/or the other two clusters of reactivities (HT-2 and HT-4) could not be significantly associated with any known HLA (A, B, C or DR) alloantigens, our family studies suggest that the reactions of the anti-HT-like antibodies fit quite well with the inheritance patterns of HLA haplotypes. One of the clusters (HT-2), composed of two antisera, was in fact inherited in linkage with HLA. Because more than one kind of HT antibody may be present in each serum or cluster of sera, cross-reactivity between sera or clusters is possible, and would explain many of the combinations of reactivities observed in individuals and families.

Thus, the random-population and family-study results can be explained in at least two ways: sera may identify Qa-like gene products of a polymorphic locus in which each cluster of reactivity represents the product of an allele encoded by that locus, or alternatively, sera may recognize products, allelic monomorphic, that belong to several genetic loci closely linked to HLA in chromosome 6.

In mice, the Qa-1-like and Qa-2 phenotypes have been found to be expressed on activated lymphocytes and on a variety of nucleated blood cells, including T and B lymphocytes, hematopoietic stem cells, and granulocytic-macrophage precursors [1, 2, 10, 16]. It is anticipated that enriched PHA-activated lymphocytes would quantitatively express more of the HT antigen than would resting T or B lymphocytes. The murine Qa antigens are markers of differentiation that show quantitative variation in relation to specific cell types (or tissue types) and to the age of the animal. Because the Qa-2-like quantity differs in a strain-specific manner, detectability by different antisera may vary [12, 14, 15]. It is conceivable, therefore, that if HT antibodies do indeed behave like Qa-2 antibodies, they may react variably with hematopoietic cells in relation to the state of differentiation of the cells and/ or of the individual studied. Cell-surface molecules identified serologically as HT, as characterized here, and the thymocyte antigens previously described by us are restricted to specific cell types and therefore exemplify selective gene expression during development.

References

1. Flaherty L (1976) The TLa region of the mouse: identification of a new serologically defined locus, Qa-2. Immunogenetics 3:533–539
2. Flaherty L, Zimmerman O, Sullivan A (1978) Qa-2 and Qa-3 antigens on lymphocyte subpopulations: I. Mitogen responsiveness. J Immunol 121:1640–1643
3. Friedman SM, Thompson G, Halper JR, Knowles DM (1982) OT-CLL: A human T-cell chronic lymphatic leukemia that produces IL 2 in high titer. J Immunol 128:935–940
4. Gazit E, Mizrachi Y, Mashiach I, Serr D (1977) Acquisition of typing serum from post partum blood clot. Tissue Antigens 9:66–69
5. Gazit E, Terhorst C, Yunis E (1980) The human "T" genetic region of the HLA linkage group is a polymorphism detected on lectin-activated lymphocytes. Nature 284:275–277
6. Gazit E, Terhorst C, Mahoney RJ, Yunis E (1980) Alloantigens of the human T (HT) genetic region of HLA linkage group. Hum Immunol 1:97–109
7. Gazit E, Gothelf Y, Gil R, Orgad S, Pitman TB, Watson ALM, Yang SY, Yunis EJ (1984) Alloantibodies to PHA activated lymphocytes detect human Qa-like antigens. J Immunol 132:165–169
8. Gerbase de lima M, Wollman EE, Lepage V, Degos L, Dausset J (1981) Alloantigens expressed on activated human T cells different from HLA-A, B, C and DR antigens. Immunogenetics 13:529–537
9. Kim SJ, Christiansen FT, Gosar I, Sliver DM, Pollack MS, Dupont B (1981) Frequency of alloantibodies reacting with PHA-activated T lymphocytes unexplained by known HLA activities. Hum Immunol 1:341–348
10. Kinkade PW, Flaherty L, Lee G, Watanabe T, Michelson J (1980) Qa antigen expression on functional lymphoid myeloid and stem cells in adult mice. J Immunol 124:2879–2885
11. Mahoney RJ, Gazit E, MacCarthy-Shanley K, et al (1982) Alloantisera detect HLA-A, B, C and non HLA-differentiation antigens on human thymocytes. J Immunol 129:2630–2635
12. Michelson J, Flaherty L, Hutchinson B, Yudkouitz H (1982) Qa-2 does not display structural genetic polymorphism detectable on isoelectric focussing gels. Immunogenetics 16:363–366
13. Morton NE (1955) Sequential tests for detection of linkage. Ann J Hum Genet 9:55–74
14. Oudsshoorn-Snoek M, Ivauji D, Demant P (1981) Qualitative and Quantitative aspects of anti-H-2L^d sera. Transplantation 32:128–136
15. Rucker J, Horwitz M, Lerner EA, Murphy DB (1983) Monoclonal antibody reveals H-2 linked quantitative and qualitative variation in the expression of a Qa-2 region determinant. Immunogenetics 17:303–316
16. Stanton TH (1979) Expression of Qa-1 on mitogen-stimulated cells. Immunogenetics 9:597–600
17. Wollman EE, Guilherme I, Lepage V, Dausset J (1984) Non-HLA antigenic determinants expressed on activated T and B lymphocytes. Tissue Antigens 23:1–11

T Cell System A in Humans is Probably Equivalent to Qa or Tla in Mice

A. van Leeuwen[1], M.J. Giphart[1], G. de Groot[1], H. Festenstein[2], and J.J. van Rood[1]

1 Department of Immunohematology and Blood Bank, University Hospital Leiden, 2333 AA, Leiden, The Netherlands
2 Department of Immunology, London Hospital Medical College, London, UK

Introduction

Using the HLA-CAP approach [1] positive alloantisera which react with T cell subset alloantigens were found. With these highly selected alloantisera a diallelic antigenic system was recognized on T_G lymphocytes, designated T cell system A (TCA) with alleles TCA*1 and TCA*2 [2]. The gene frequencies of TCA*1 and TCA*2 are 0.44 and 0.56 respectively. No population association is found with any of the HLA antigens. This observation contrasts with the data of Ferrara et al. [3, 4] and Gazit et al. [5, 6], who also described alloantibodies that react with human T cells. These antibodies, however, identify antigens that segregate together with HLA antigens.
In this report we present evidence for linkage of TCA and HLA based on family data. The TCA antigens are dimers of peptides with molecular weights of $\approx 42\,000$ daltons and 12 000 daltons respectively. Furthermore, we presume that the TCA system might be the human equivalent of *Qa* or *Tla* in the mouse.

Materials and Methods

All families were typed using the NIH standard technique for the HLA-A, B, and C antigens and the TCF technique for the DR and DQ antigens [7]. To select antisera for typing for the TCA antigens, the HLA-CAP approach [1] was used, in which sera from HLA-A1, B8, DR3-positive parous women who had formed multiple leukocyte antibodies were tested on lymphocytes from HLA-A1, B8, DR3 homozygous individuals. In this manner interference with anti-HLA class I or class II antigens is minimized.
A T_G-enriched suspension was prepared from T cells using theophylline, as previously described [8]. In short, blood was layered over a Ficoll-Isopaque gradient. After centrifugation the T cells were isolated from the interphase by rosetting with papainized or AET-treated sheep red blood cells. To enrich the T_G population, the E rosettes were incubated with 3–10 m*M* theophylline. In this manner one can get up to 50%–60% enriched T_G cells.

The most promising sera were selected and absorbed with Epstein-Barr virus (EBV)-transformed B cell lines from the husband of the serum producer to remove all anti HLA-A, B, C, and DR antibodies. The absorbed sera were tested with the prolonged complement-dependent cytotoxicity test (1 h incubation with serum at 10 ° and 2 h with complement at 20 °) followed by the addition of ethidium bromide as a dye. To test the segregation of the TCA specificity, 15 two-generation families with 64 children were analyzed. Fourteen families were volunteers, and in one (family D.), two of the five children suffered from celiac disease. Only 12 families were informative for linkage computation between TCA and HLA. Linkage computation was performed as described by Race and Sanger [9]. Linkage is considered to be established when the sum of the lod scores is equal to or greater than 3. The blocking assay with turkey anti-β_2 microglobulin was carried out as described previously [10]. Lymphocytes used in the blocking assay were sedimented and resuspended in an appropriate volume of turkey anti-β_2 microglobulin (kindly donated by Dr. M. D. Poulik) and incubated at 20 ° for 60 min. They were then used, without washing, in the cytotoxicity assay.
The lod scores are used to test the weight of the accumulated evidence for or against linkage.
For characterization of TCA antigens, enriched populations of T_G cells were radiolabeled with ^{125}I and further processed for immunoprecipitation. Analysis by immunoprecipitation and subsequent polyacrylamide gel electrophoresis was done as described before [11].

Results

Using alloantisera from parous women absorbed with EBV-transformed B cell lines from the husband of the serum producer, 15 two-generation families were tested for the TCA antigens. Twelve families were informative for the computation of the lod score. Table 1 shows the segregation in the families.
Table 2 shows that linkage between TCA and HLA possibly exists. In previous population studies [2] no association was found with any of the HLA anti-

Histocompatibility Testing 1984
Edited by E. D. Albert et al.

Table 1. Segregation of TCA phenotypes in the families studied

Mating	*n*	Children					
		TCA1.1		TCA1.2		TCA2.2	
		observed	expected	observed	expected	observed	expected
TCA1.1×TCA1.1	0	–	–	–	–	–	–
TCA1.1×TCA1.2	5	11	12	13	12	0	0
TCA1.2×TCA1.2	3	1	3	6	6	5	3
TCA1.1×TCA2.2	0	–	–	–	–	–	–
TCA1.2×TCA2.2	7	0	0	18	14	10	14
TCA2.2×TCA2.2	0	–	–	–	–	–	–
	15	12	15	37	32	15	17

$\chi^2_6 = 5.1188$ $p = 0.530$

Table 2. Lod (z1) scores for 12 informative families tested for T-cell system TCA and HLA haplotypes

F[b]	ratio[a]	Recombination fraction 0.00	0.05	0.10	0.15	0.20	0.25	0.30
A	6:1	–	+0.371	+0.532	+0.559	+0.526	+0.456	+0.360
B	3:0	+0.602	+0.533	+0.465	+0.393	+0.318	+0.243	+0.170
D	3:2	–	–1.442	–0.887	–0.585	–0.388	–0.250	–0.151
G	3:1	–	–0.464	–0.229	–0.119	–0.060	–0.028	–0.011
K	3:0	+0.602	+0.533	+0.465	+0.393	+0.318	+0.243	+0.170
Pr	6:0	+1.505	+1.371	+1.231	+1.082	+0.924	+0.756	+0.578
Po	5:0	+1.204	+1.093	+0.975	+0.851	+0.720	+0.581	+0.436
vR	2:1	–	–0.721	–0.444	–0.292	–0.194	–0.125	–0.076
S	3:1	–	–0.464	–0.229	–0.119	–0.060	–0.028	–0.011
Si	3:1	–	–0.464	–0.229	–0.119	–0.060	–0.028	–0.011
W	5:0	+1.204	+1.093	+0.975	+0.851	+0.720	+0.581	+0.436
dV	3:0	+0.602	+0.533	+0.465	+0.393	+0.318	+0.243	+0.170
			+1.972	+3.090	+3.288	+3.082	+2.644	+2.060
Family D. excluded			+3.414	+3.977	+3.873	+3.470	+2.894	+2.211

[a] Nonrecombinant : recombinant
[b] F = family

gens. When the segregation of HLA haplotypes of the various families was analyzed for possible linkage to TCA, however, the sum of the lod scores at $\theta = 0.15$ was +3.288. Family D., the family with two children with celiac disease, is the only family with two recombinants who are precisely the two affected children. If this family is excluded from the study the total lod scores at a recombination fraction of 10% are +3.977. In the family material, three HLA-GLO cross-overs were discovered (data not shown). This is not unexpected from the known distance between these loci. Together with the knowledge that the order of loci on chromosome 6 is centromere-GLO-HLA (DR-B-C-A) and that the distance between HLA and TCA is bigger than between HLA and GLO (about 4%) [12], these three HLA/GLO recombinants might be useful for mapping TCA. They show that TCA should be on the HLA-A side of the chromosome. Table 3 shows two different cross-overs in one family (A.): one between TCA2 and HLA-A28 in child number 1 and one between GLO2 and HLA-DRw6 in child number 3.

No suggestions of linkage with other blood group or enzyme markers are found for TCA.

Blocking tests carried out for anti-TCA sera with turkey anti-β_2 microglobulin indicate that the anti-TCA sera can be blocked by anti-β_2 microglobulin,

Table 3. Family A. with two recombinant children, one TCA-HLA-A cross-over and one GLO-HLA-DR cross-over

Sex		Haplotypes
Father		TCA1, A1, B8, DR3, GLO2/TCA1, B51, DR5, GLO2
Mother		TCA1, A28, B27, Cw2, DRw6, GLO1/TCA2, A1, B8, DR3, GLO2
Ch. 1[a]	f	TCA1, A1, B8, DR3, GLO2/TCA2 [c] A28, B27, Cw2, DRw6, GLO1
Ch. 2	f	TCA1, A2, B51, DR5, GLO2/TCA2, A1, B8, DR3, GLO2
Ch. 3[b]	m	TCA1, A2, B51, DR5, GLO2/TCA1, A28, B27, Cw2, DRw6 GLO2
Ch. 4	m	TCA1, A2, B51, DR5, GLO2/TCA2, A1, B8, DR3, GLO2
Ch. 5	m	TCA1, A2, B51, DR5, GLO2/TCA2, A1, B8, DR3, GLO2
Ch. 6	f	TCA1, A2, B51, DR5, GLO2/TCA1, A28, B27, Cw2, DRw6, GLO1
Ch. 7	f	TCA1, A1, B8, DR3, GLO2/TCA2, A1, B8, DR3, GLO2

[a] TCA-HLA-A cross-over
[b] GLO-HLA-DR cross-over
[c] indicates cross-over

which suggests association with class I molecules. Because anti-TCA sera do not contain anti-HLA-A, B, or C antibodies (the sera are intensively absorbed with B cell lines from the husband) the blocking can only be due to nonreactivity of TCA molecules. The TCA alloantisera are in general too weak to allow straightforward immunoprecipitation of the antigens. Furthermore the cell populations used as antigen source are not pure, but only enriched for a given subtype. Thus, other cell populations are present which may express antigens which are not yet defined but are detectable by immunoprecipitation. We therefore screened a number of TCA alloantisera for their capacity to precipitate antigens in a "specific" way, i.e., more intense bands in a given area than with antisera on SDS-PAGE. In this way we were able to select an anti-TCA2 alloantiserum precipitating molecular species with molecular weights of ≈ 42 000 daltons, significantly more than with anti-TCA1 alloantiserum, using TCA2,2 homozygous cells as antigen source.

Further characterization was done by analyzing the relationship of the TCA2 antigenic species with molecules carrying the W6/32 determinant and with β_2 microglobulin. The results are summarized in Table 4. It can be seen that the TCA2 antigenic species on T_G cells does not carry the W6/32 determinant, but is associated with β_2 microglobulin. Antilymphocyte serum serving as a positive technical control (ALS) shows that the pretreatment of T_G cell extracts does not lead to a severe loss of precipitable molecular species.

The demonstration of a 42 000-dalton band after pretreatment with W6/32 followed by treatment with anti-β_2 microglobulin indicates that more class I products may be recognized in this way than with W6/32 alone (data not shown).

Table 4. Analysis of the relationship of TCA2 antigenic species with molecules carrying the W6/32 determinant and with β_2 microglobulin

Pretreatment	Treatment	T_G suspension
W6/32	Anti-TCA2	40 000–42 000
W6/32	Anti-β_2m	42 000
	W6/32	44 000
Anti-β_2m	Anti-TCA2	–
Anti-β_2m	ALS	Many, but none of 44 000

Discussion

The data obtained from 12 families informative for the segregation of TCA alleles were consistent with the hypothesis that the alleles are codominant. Further analysis of the linkage data suggests the possibility that TCA may be loosely linked to HLA at a fairly large map distance (maximum lod score at about θ 0.10 to 0.15). Because of the distance it should not be surprising that no evidence of population association has been found [2]. If indications for linkage to HLA are confirmed, the mapping position of TCA could be deduced from the existence of three HLA-GLO recombinants to be on the HLA-A side. DNA analysis has revealed that the mapping position of HLA non-ABC class I genes is telomeric from HLA-A [13]. Ideally, however, this should be confirmed in families also typed for PGM-3 and perhaps for PG-5, so that both telomeric and centromeric markers may be utilized. Characterization of the TCA antigens was done by immunoprecipitation. Due to the technical difficulties of these types of analysis using alloantisera and to the possibly weak expression of TCA antigen on the cell surface, firm conclusions cannot yet be drawn. However, based on the results so far obtained, we favor the interpretation that the TCA antigenic system is class I-like. Further and more refined techniques are needed to confirm this possibility. Thus, our data suggest that TCA antigens are dimers of peptides with molecular weights of $\approx 42\,000$ and 12 000 respectively, like Qa or Tla in the mouse [14]. However, the TCA antigens are only expressed on a subpopulation of T cells (T_G), whereas class I antigens are expressed on all nucleated cells. Therefore, the TCA antigens are referred to as class IV antigens [15].

The biochemical properties of the class IV and class I products in the mouse were originally thought to be identical; recently, however, slight differences in the biochemical features have been observed [14]. For Qa-2 the molecular weights are 40 000 and 12 000 respectively. There are more differences between the two classes, such as the wide tissue distribution of K, D, and L antigens (class I) versus the restricted distribution of Tla and its related antigens (class IV).

The location of TCA on chromosome 6 telomeric to the HLA-A side of the chromosome may be related to the possible existence of associations between diseases and HLA-A, such as those described between Hodgkin's disease and HLA-A1 and between acute lymphoblastic leukemia and HLA-A2 [16, 17]. If TCA is the equivalent of Qa or Tla, then one would expect to find an anomalous strong expression on some tumor cells. Preliminary data suggest that this is indeed the case (A. van Leeuwen, submitted for publication). Linkage of T cell alloantigens to HLA has been suggested by both Gazit et al. [6], for the activated T cell differentiation markers designated as HT, and by Ferrara et al. [4]. The relationships, if any, between these antigens and those described here remain to be determined.

References

1. Van Leeuwen A, Festenstein H, Van Rood JJ (1980) Human alloimmune sera against T cell subsets. J Exp Med 152:235s
2. Van Leeuwen A, Festenstein H, Van Rood JJ (1982) Diallelic alloantigenic systems on subsets of T cells. Human Immunol 4:109
3. Ferrara GB, Strelkauskas AJ, Longo A, McDowell J, Yunis EJ, Schlossman SF (1979) Markers of human T cell subsets identified by alloantisera. J Immunol 123:1272
4. Ferrara GB, Longo A, Tosi R, Biagini A, Mennucci M, Carminati G (1981) HLA segregation of human T-cell subpopulation markers. Human Immunol 2:213
5. Gazit E, Terhorst C, Yunis EJ (1980) The human "T" genetic region of the HLA linkage group is a polymorphism detected on lectin-activated lymphocytes. Nature 284:275
6. Gazit E, Terhorst C, Mahoney RJ, Yunis EJ (1980) Alloantigens of the human T (HT) genetic region of the HLA linkage group. Human Immunol 1:97
7. Van Rood JJ, Van Leeuwen A, Ploem JS (1976) Simultaneous detection of two cell populations by two-colour fluorescence and application to the recognition of B-cell determinants. Nature 262:795
8. Van Leeuwen A (1979) Alloantibodies that react with subsets of human T cells. Tissue Antigens 14:437
9. Race RR, Sanger R (1976) Blood groups in man. Blackwell, Oxford
10. Bernoco D, Bernoco M, Ceppellini R, Poulik MD, Van Leeuwen A, Rood JJ (1976) B cell antigens of the HLA system: A simple serotyping technique based on noncytotoxic anti-β_2 microglobulin reagents. Tissue Antigens 8:253
11. Giphart MJ, Morolli B, Van Vreeswijk W, Gerrits R, Balner H (1983) The major histocompatibility complex of rhesus monkeys. XV. Chemical characterization of DR locus antigens and antigen 48. J Immunogenet 10:45
12. Weitkamp LR, Lamm L (1982) Report of the committee on the genetic constitution of chromosome 6. Human gene mapping 6. Cytogenet Cell Genet 32:130
13. Orr HT, Bach FH, Ploegh HL, Strominger JL, Kavathas P, DeMars R (1982) Use of HLA loss mutants to analyse the structure of the human major histocompatibility complex. Nature 296:454
14. Michaelson J, Flaherty L, Bushkin Y, Yudkowitz H (1981) Further biochemical data on Qa-2. Immunogenetics 14:129
15. Snell GD (1981) Studies in histocompatibility. Science 213:172
16. Kourilsky FM, Dausset J, Feingold N, Dupuy JM, Bernard J (1967) Etude de la repartition des antigènes leucocytaires chez des malades attients de leucémie aique en remission. In: Advances in Transplantation. First Int. Congress of the Transplantation Society, Paris, 1967. Munksgaard, Copenhagen, p 515. Dausset J, Hamburger J and Mathé G (eds)
17. Ryder LP, Andersen E, Svejgaard A (1979) HLA and disease registry. Third report. Munksgaard, Copenhagen

New Determinants Expressed on Activated Lymphocytes and on Human Acute Lymphoblastic Leukemia Cells Closely Linked to Conventional HLA-A Antigens

Y. Mitsuishi, A. Falkenrodt, M.M. Tongio, and S. Mayer

Institut d'Hématologie, Centre de Transfusion Sanguine de Strasbourg, 10, Rue Spielmann, 67085 Strasbourg Cedex, France

Three antisera (GO, TM, PE) which, after intensive platelet absorption, reacted with microcytotoxicity to PHA-activated lymphocytes (PHA-L) but not to peripheral blood lymphocytes (PBL) or B lymphocytes (BL) were selected for further study. GO was positive with all HLA-A24 PHA-L; TM with all HLA-A9 PHA-L; PE with all HLA-A2, A28 PHA-L. Family segregation studies showed that the serum reactivity followed the HLA haplotype transmission. These antibodies could be absorbed by PHA-L carrying the corresponding antigen, but not by PBL from the same donors. In addition, kinetic studies showed that the antigen recognized by these antibodies appeared only after several hours of mitogenic stimulation of lymphocytes. Because PE was exhausted, further investigations could only be carried out with GO and TM. Chromatographic analysis showed that the cytotoxic activities of GO and TM were in the IgM fraction.

In 1980, Gazit et al. [1] described two analogous antisera, which were putatively called anti-HT1 and anti-HT3 and characterized as similar to human anti-TL-Qa antibodies.

Since TL antigens can be detected on murine leukemia cells, our sera were tested with 19 cases of acute lymphoblastic leukemia (ALL), 1 case of leukemic lymphosarcoma (LLS) and 25 cases of chronic lymphocytic leukemia (CLL). GO and TM were negative with CLL cells and the HLA-A9 LLS variety (markers: OKT3$^-$, 4$^-$, 8$^-$, 6$^+$, 9$^+$, 10$^+$; T11$^+$; E rosette$^+$; J5$^-$; TdT$^+$; DR$^-$).

When tested with ALL cells, GO reacted with all the A24 common ALL (cALL) (markers: OKT3$^-$, 4$^-$, 8$^-$, 6$^-$, 9$^-$, 10$^+$; T11$^-$; E rosette$^-$; J5$^+$; TdT$^+$; DR$^+$) but not with an A24 early T-ALL (eT-ALL) (markers: OKT3$^-$, 4$^-$, 8$^-$, 6$^-$, 9$^+$, 10$^+$; T11$^-$; E rosette$^-$; J5$^+$, TdT$^+$; DR$^-$; thymic mass$^+$). Absorption tests confirmed that the antibody could be absorbed by the A24 PHA-L and A24 cALL cells but not by an Aw24 eT-ALL variety. Anti-cALL reactivity was absorbed by PHA-Ls, and PHA-L reactivity was absorbed by cALL cells.

TM reacted with all the A9 cALL cells and also with the A24 eT-ALL variety. Absorption tests showed that this serum contained two different antibodies: one designated TM1, which could be absorbed by A9 PHA-Ls and by cALL cells but not by eT-ALL cells, and the other, TM2, which was only absorbed by the eT-ALL cells. Reactivity of GO and TM1 was blocked by a turkey anti-β_2 microglobulin serum (gift from Dr. Gazit), but TM2 was not blocked. These results showed that GO and TM1 recognized an unconventional class I antigen which was expressed on both PHA-Ls and cALL cells but not on PBL, BL or CLL and eT-ALL cells. TM2 recognized a non-class I antigen. Further work will be needed.

Reference

1. Gazit E, Terhorst C, Mahoney RJ, Yunis EJ (1980) Alloantigens of the human T (HT) genetic region of the HLA linkage group. Hum Immunol 1:97–109

Histocompatibility Testing 1984
Edited by E. D. Albert et al.

Analysis of DP Region Products by T Cells and Monoclonal Antibodies: Blocking of DP-Specific Proliferation and Cell-Mediated Cytotoxicity*

S. Shaw[1], M. Sanchez-Perez[1], and R. DeMars[2]

1 National Institutes of Health, Bethesda, MD 20205, USA
2 Laboratory of Genetics and Department of Human Oncology, University of Wisconsin, Madison, WI 53706, USA

Introduction

Three families of class II ("Ia") genes/molecules (DR, DQ, DP) have been defined within the human HLA region, each of which can stimulate allogeneic T cell responses and restrict T cell recognition of foreign antigen. We have explored the relationship between serologically defined epitopes on class II HLA molecules and T-cell-mediated responses to the DP antigens. Our approach has combined the use of (1) DP-specific primed T cells, (2) HLA-deletion mutant cell lines, and (3) 70 monoclonal antibodies (moabs) specific for class II molecules. The most informative analysis has been possible for DPw2-specific responses, since mutant lymphoblastoid cell lines (LCLs) have been derived which are positive for DPw2, but have lost expression of DR and DQ determinants. Analysis of moab inhibition of T cell proliferation [but not cell-mediated cytotoxicity (CML)] was complicated by the fact that many moabs which failed to bind to the stimulator (or target) cell inhibited the response. In CML, enhancement rather than inhibition was observed with a number of moabs. Three moabs inhibited CML specific for all DP alleles tested, while other moabs gave allele-specific inhibition. Overall patterns of inhibition suggested that DPw2 and DPw3 are more similar to each other than to DPw1.

Materials and Methods

Cell Lines. Derivation of HLA-deletion mutant LCL has been described in detail previously [1, 2]. The line 721.82 used in these studies (henceforth referred to as .82) retains expression of DPw2, but has lost expression of all other defined DR, DQ, and DP antigens present on its parental line [2, 3]. LCLs from normal donors H9 (DPw1, 2) and M19 (DPw3, 4) were also used as targets.

Moabs. 70 moabs specific for class II MHC molecules (18 mouse alloinduced and 52 rodent anti-human) were generously provided by 17 different laboratories (see [4] for sources and further references). These moabs have been characterized previously by flow microfluorometry (FMF) to measure binding to products of three distinct genetic subregions of HLA discriminated by the HLA-deletion mutants [2−6] and have been assigned, as a working hypothesis, to seven clusters differing in specificity of binding to this DR1, DQw1, DPw2 haplotype (see Table 1).

Functional Inhibition. Proliferation and CML were performed as described previously using extensively characterized DP-specific primed T cell reagents [7, 8]. Moabs tested for inhibition were present during the assay (3 days for proliferation, 1.5−4 h for CML) at a dilution of 1/5 for proliferation and 1/3 for CML. The stock concentrations (a) varied according to the preparation supplied to us; (b) were generally culture supernatant, ascites fluid (1/25), or purified antibody (200 μg/ml); and (c) are exactly as tabulated in studies of moab binding [4].

Results and Discussion

We analyzed the ability of 70 monoclonal anti-Ia antibodies to inhibit DPw2-specific proliferation and CML (Fig. 1). The response was assured to be DPw2-specific in two distinct ways − the known specificity of the responding population, and the restricted Ia expression of LCL .82 used as stimulating cell (for proliferation) or target cell (for cytotoxicity) (.82 expresses DPw2 but not DQ or DR; see [2, 3]). In both the assays, some moabs fell in the shaded region, designating no effect, some fell below that region, indicating an inhibitory effect, and some fell above that region, suggesting an enhancing effect. To elucidate the origins of these differences, the functional effect of each moab is plotted in each panel together with the magnitude of binding of that moab to the stimulating/target LCL .82.

* This work was supported in part by NIH grants AI 15486 and P30 CA 14520

Histocompatibility Testing 1984
Edited by E. D. Albert et al.

Table 1. Moab number and name listed by pattern of binding specificity on DR1, DQw1, DPw2 haplotype

Weak to negative				
1) ILR2	2) YD1/63	3) DA6.147	4) 40J	5) 391
6) K13	7) 41A	8) 39B	9) 40M	10) 40G
DR1-related				
11) 39D	12) 62.74	13) TU36	14) 10A	15) I2
16) 40K	17) TU34	18) IIIE3	19) L1.1.12	20) 62.3.34
21) L1.1.6	22) B3.15	23) OKIA2	24) MHM36	25) B8.13.6
26) IVG1	27) Q2/70	28) B8.11.2	29) IVF7	30) L203
31) OKIA1	32) DA6.164	33) D4-22	34) SG157	35) D1-12
DQw1-related				
40) 30	41) SDR1.2	42) 40I	43) TU22	44) 33.1
DPw2-related				
50) W63	51) 39H	52) MHM4	53) ILR1	
Cross-reactive DR + DPw2 + DQw1				
60) 39E	61) 7A	62) TU37	63) TU58	64) TU43
65) 40B	66) L03	67) DA2	68) B8.12.2	69) HIG48
70) L227	71) MHM21	72) TU39	73) 40D	74) DA6.231
75) SG520	76) Q5/13	77) TU35	78) DA6.121	79) IVAI2
80) 1641	81) SG171			
Cross-reactive DR1 + DQw1				
95) 39G	96) 8A	97) 39A		
Cross-reactive DR1 + DQw1 + DPw2				
90) SG465				

Specificity assigned by FMF studies of binding to HLA mutant cell lines (see [4] for details including sources of moabs and relevant citations on each)

It is apparent that there are marked differences in the patterns between the two different functional responses. Seven to ten moabs inhibit CML, while perhaps 21–34 inhibit proliferation. The most striking feature of this difference is that many preparations of moab which do not bind significantly (as measured by FMF) to the simulator LCL nevertheless inhibited proliferation. Such inhibition has many possible explanations: (1) anti-Ia antibody may inhibit by some effect independent of the stimulator cell [9]; (2) the moab may bind to the stimulator with such low affinity that it is not detected in an assay like FMF which involves extensive washing; (3) the moab preparation may contain other substances which account for the inhibition (only those preparations which were designated as containing azide were dialyzed in our laboratory so some preparations could have had azide; however, azide-independent effects must be invoked to explain inhibition observed by some preparations even after dialysis, e.g. # 20, 21).

For our purposes, CML constituted a more specific (although perhaps less sensitive) assay system, since: (1) CML results divide the moabs rather clearly into two groups: those which cause marked inhibition and those which do not; and (2) only moabs which bound the target markedly inhibited CML. Among moabs which bound well to the target, seven strongly inhibited CML, while 13 did not. It is not surprising that many moabs which bind to target Ia fail to inhibit DPw2-specific CML. Three different effects could be involved: (1) the moab binds DPw2 but has inadequate affinity or concentration to "cover" all the antigenic sites; (2) the moab binds to part of the DPw2 molecule which is distinct from those "seen" by the CML effectors; (3) the moab does not bind to DPw2, but to other Ia molecules (non-DR, non-DQ, non-DPw2) present on this LCL [in fact, studies of # 52 (MHM4, [10]) suggest that it binds an additional molecule on .82 which is retained by the DPw2-null mutant .174 [11] (De Mars and McMichaels, unpublished work)].

However, the high frequency of moabs whose presence apparently enhanced CML was somewhat surprising. At least two explanations need to be considered. First, since enhancement is also seen with moabs with minimal binding to the target (by FMF), it is possible that such an effect can be mediated at the level of the CML effector cell. Second, it is plausible that moabs can bind to the DPw2 molecule at a site which is distinct from that seen by T cells and thereby result in a conformational change [12] in the molecule which facilitates T cell recognition.

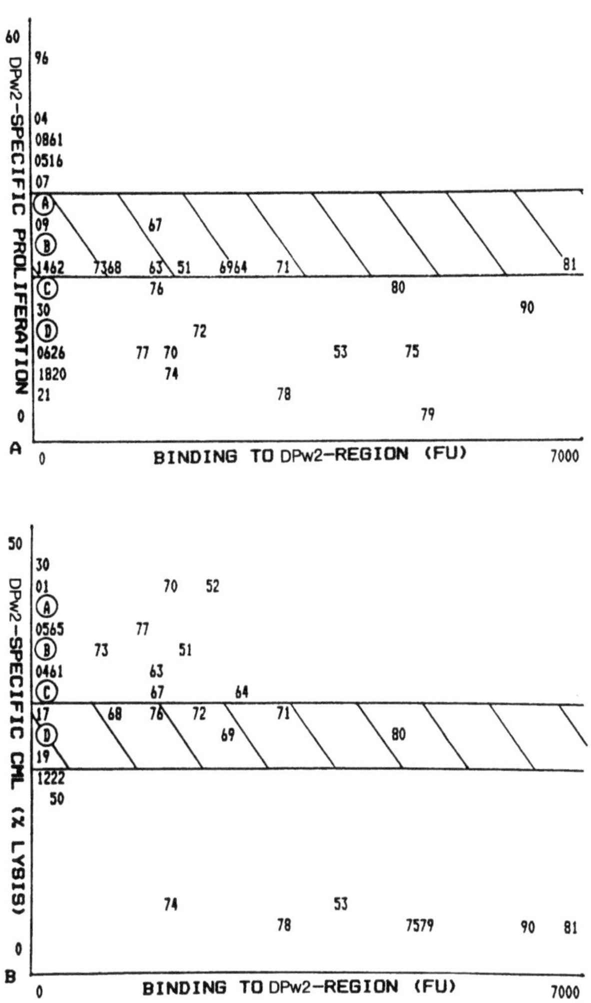

Fig. 1A, B. Correlations between moab binding to the DPw2 subregion and moab inhibition of DPw2-specific T cell responses. Binding to the DPw2 region of mutant LCL 721.82 was determined by FMF and results plotted on the *x* axis (as fluorescent units). This LCL was used as stimulator for DPw2-specific proliferation (*A*) and as a target for DPw2-specific CML (*B*) by the same bulk population of primed T cells (W7/H9; see [7, 8]). The *shaded region* represents the range of responses observed in five control groups (without added moab). Proliferative responses are given as cpm × 10^{-3} (*A*) and cytotoxicity as % lysis (*B*). Each *two-digit number* represents the data for a single moab (see Table 1). In areas where many moabs overlay each other, points have been displaced one unit laterally or vertically and the excess moabs combined into clusters designated by an encircled letter. Moabs included in such clusters are: *A* Ⓐ 02, 10, 15, 43, 60, 97; ○ 01, 11, 12, 13, 17, 19, 32, 41, 42; © 03, 22, 23, 24, 25, 27, 28, 33, 44, 50, 65, 95; Ⓓ 29, 31, 34, 35, 40. *B* Ⓐ 15, 23, 31, 32, 40; Ⓑ 03, 14, 16, 24, 27, 42, 44, 62; © 02, 06, 07, 08, 09, 10, 11, 13, 26, 34, 43, 60, 96, 97; Ⓓ 17, 20, 21, 25, 28, 29, 33, 35, 41, 95

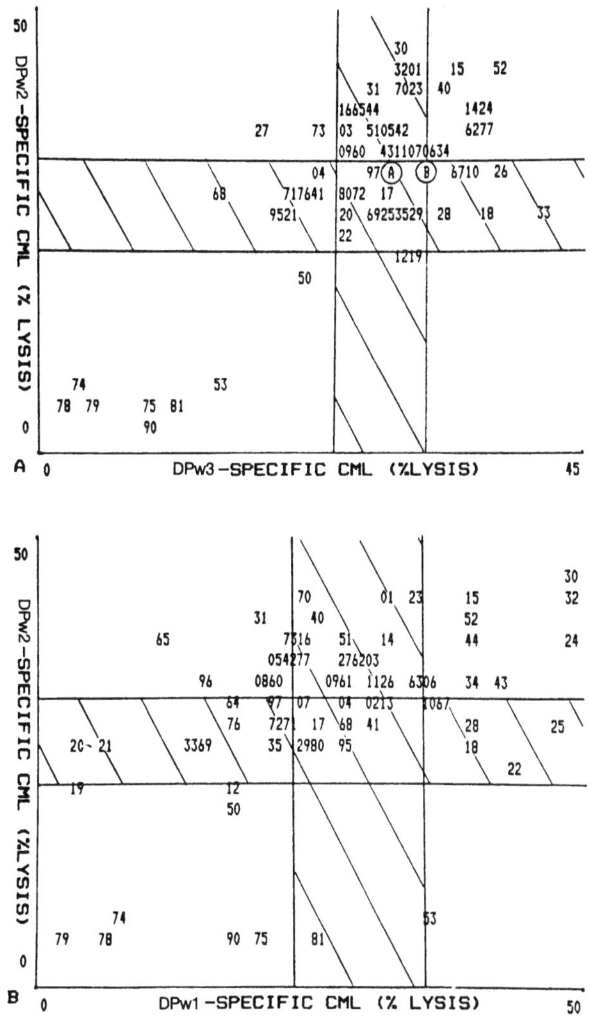

Fig. 2A, B. Correlations between moab inhibition of CML specific for different DP alleles. DPw1 CML is by FB6/11 effectors on H9 LCL, and DPw3 CML by W7/M14 effectors on M19 LCL (see [7, 8]). Conventions of data representation are identical to those in Fig. 1. Moabs included in lettered clusters in **A** are: Ⓐ 63, 64, 96; Ⓑ 02, 08, 13, 61

Although DPw2-specific CML is ideal for the foregoing analysis (because LCL .82 allows analysis of DPw2 in isolation from DR, DQ, and other DP), moab inhibition of CML has also been studied for other DP alleles, e.g., DPw3-specific and DPw1-specific CML (shown in Fig. 2). In each panel the pattern of inhibition is compared with the inhibition of DPw2-specific CML. Panel A illustrates that inhibition of DPw3-specific CML is rather similar to DPw2-specific CML. The same seven moabs strongly inhibit both responses. No moab inhibits either response markedly without also inhibiting the other (except perhaps # 68). This similarity suggests that: (1) the moabs which bind DPw2 strongly also bind DPw3 strongly; (2) on the DPw2 and DPw3 molecules there is a similar spatial relationship between the moab epitopes and the site seen by T cells; and (3) the assay system has inherent reproducibility (to find the same inhibition in two different responses).

It is interesting that the moabs which result in enhancement of the DPw2-specific CML are generally different from those that enhance DPw3-specific CML. Since the effector cells for DPw2 and DPw3 CML are derived from the same donor (W7), this discrepancy suggests that the effect may be at the stimulator cell. Since this effect can be mediated by antibodies which do not bind to the stimulator by FMF analysis, very low affinity interactions may be sufficient to give this enhancement.

A different pattern is seen with DPw1-specific CML. Although three moabs inhibit both responses strongly, several moabs inhibit DPw2-specific CML but not DPw1-specific and vice versa. These data suggest that there are marked differences between DPw1 and DPw2 as seen by these moabs. It is striking that the three DPw2-preferential moabs are from Goyert (# 75, 81, 90) and the DPw1-preferential moabs from Kalil (# 19, 20, 21). Perhaps the immunizing antigen (perhaps its DP allele) conferred an DP allospecificity on the moabs derived from that immunization even though the moabs are not exclusively DP-specific. Such "allospecific" binding of a moab to one family of Ia molecules plus "alloindifferent" binding on another family of Ia molecules has been observed for DR plus DS7 with moab # 81 [13].

It is noteworthy that DPw2 and DPw3 appear so similar in pattern of inhibition and that DPw1 is so easily distinguishable. This correlates with the pattern of binding of the one moab which is closest to being "DP specific" (# 53, ILR1), which binds to DPw2 and DPw3 but not DPw1. Thus, the pattern of CML inhibition by 70 moabs tends to support the impression that DPw2 and DPw3 may be more similar to each other (at least in some immunogenic epitope) than to DPw1. If DPw1 is quite different structurally, that might explain why many laboratories find DPw1-specific primed T cell reagents are easier to generate than DPw2-, DPw3-, etc. specific reagents.

The three moabs which inhibited DPw1-, DPw2-, and DPw3-specific CML (Fig. 2; 74, 78, 79) also inhibited DPw4-specific and DPw5-specific CML, but did not inhibit lectin-mediated killing (unpublished). Such antibodies appear to bind determinants present on all defined DP alleles and to inhibit T cell recognition of those molecules. It is tempting to postulate that such moabs bind to determinants that are highly conserved because they are of particular functional importance in T cell recognition.

Acknowledgments. We thank all the contributors of monoclonal antibodies, without whose generous contributions this analysis would have been impossible. We thank Ms P. Smith for excellent technical assistance.

References

1. Kavathas P, Bach FH, DeMars R (1980) Gamma ray-induced loss of expression of HLA and glyoxylase I alleles in lymphoblastoid cells. Proc Natl Acad Sci USA 77:4251–4255
2. DeMars R, Chang CC, Rudersdorf RA (1983) Dissection of the D-region of the human major histocompatibility complex by means of induced mutations in a lymphoblastoid cell line. Hum Immunol 8:123–129
3. Shaw S, DeMars R, Schlossman SF, Smith PL, Lampson LA, Nadler LM (1982) Serologic identification of the human secondary B cell (SB) antigens: correlations between function, genetics and structure. J Exp Med 156:731–741
4. Shaw S, Ziegler A, DeMars R (1985) Specificity of monoclonal antibodies directed against human and murine class II histocompatibility antigens as analyzed by binding to HLA-deletion mutant cell lines. Human Immun (in press)
5. Kavathas P, DeMars R, Bach FH, Shaw S (1981) SB: A new HLA-linked human histocompatibility gene defined using HLA-mutant cell lines. Nature 293:747–749
6. DeMars R, Chang CC, Marrari M, Duquesnoy RJ, Noreen H, Segall M, Bach FH (1983) Dissociation in expression of MB1/MT1 and DR1 alloantigens in mutants of a lymphoblastoid cell line. J Immunol 131:1318–1321
7. Shaw S, Duquesnoy RJ, Smith PL (1981) Population studies of the HLA-linked SB antigens. Immunogenetics 14:153–162
8. Shaw S, Johnson AH, Shearer GM (1980) Evidence for a new segregant series of B cell antigens that are encoded in the HLA-D region and that stimulate secondary allogeneic proliferative and cytotoxic responses. J Exp Med 152:565–580
9. Accolla RS, Moretta A, Cerottini JC (1981) Allogeneic mixed lymphocyte reactions in humans: pretreatment of either the stimulator or the responder cell with monoclonal anti-Ia antibodies leads to an inhibition of proliferation. J Immunol 127:2438–2442
10. Makgoba MW, Hildreth JEK, McMichael AJ (1983) Identification of a human Ia antigen that is different from HLA DR and DC antigens. Immunogenetics 17:623–635
11. DeMars R, Chang CC, Shaw S, Reitnauer PJ, Sondel PM (1984) Homozygous deletions that simultaneously eliminate in expressions of class I and class II antigens of EBV-transformed B-lymphoblastoid cells. I. Reduced proliferative responses of autologous and allogeneic T cells to mutant cells that have decreased expression of class II antigens. Hum Immunol (in press)
12. Tosi R, Tanigaki N, Sorrentino R, Accolla R, Corte G (1981) Binding of one monoclonal antibody to human Ia molecules can be enhanced by a second monoclonal antibody. Eur J Immunol 11:721–726
13. Goyert SM, Silver J (1983) Further characterization of HLA-DS molecules: implications for studies assessing the role of human Ia molecules in cell interactions and disease susceptibility. Proc Natl Acad Sci USA 80: 5719–5723

Typing for DP-like Determinants

N. Morling[1], R.J. Hartzman[2], B.K. Jakobsen[1], N. Oedum[1], P. Platz[1], L.P. Ryder[1], S. Shaw[3], and A. Svejgaard[1]

1 Tissue Typing Laboratory, State University Hospital (Rigshospitalet), Tagensvej 20, 2200 Copenhagen, Denmark
2 Transplantation and Immunology Branch, Naval Medical Research Institute, Bethesda, MD 20205, USA
3 Immunology Branch, National Cancer Institute, National Institutes of Health, Bethesda, MD 20205, USA

Primed lymphocyte typing (PLT) cells recognizing non-HLA-D/DR antigens were generated in Copenhagen in both family and unrelated combinations compatible for HLA-D/DR [1]. A number of determinants were defined, including six DP-like antigens. Each DP-like specificity was defined by repeated testings with from two to eight different PLT cell combinations. The correlation (r) between these antigens and DPw1-DPw6 each defined by two highly discriminating PLT cells developed in Bethesda by bulk expansion were investigated in 53 individuals, and the frequencies of the DP-like antigens were estimated in 71 healthy, unrelated randomly selected Danes (Table 1).

A "split" of DPw2 was detected by means of PLT cells from Bethesda. In a panel of 41 individuals, the reactions of the bulk-expanded PLT cells indicated that DPw2 could be split based on the following reactions of DPw2A and DPw2B: ++: 7; +−: 0; −+: 4; −−: 30 ($P < 10^{-4}$). The family of one of the DPw2A-negative/DPw2B-positive individuals was investigated, and the specific reactivity towards DPw2 followed one of the HLA haplotypes. In this family, however, there seemed to be cross-reactivity between DPw2B and DPw6.

The bulk-expanded DP reagents had a very high discriminatory power and allowed detection in one family of a clear-cut recombination between DR, DQ on the one hand and DPw6 on the other in a child known to be an HLA-DR/GLO recombinant [2]. This confirms the mapping of DPw6 centromeric to DR and DQ. DNA studies of this family are in progress. Three "new" determinants different from HLA-D/DR, DP and DQ were recognized by PLT cells primed in HLA-D/DR-compatible combinations. The determinants RA, HA, and MA seemed to be associated with DR2, DR3, and DRw6, respectively (Table 2).

These determinants behave as if controlled by a "new" segregant series, but more studies (particularly with bulk-expanded reagents) are needed to clarify the situation.

References

1. Morling N, Platz P, Ryder LP, Svejgaard A, Thomsen M (1981) Technical aspects of the Primed Lymphocyte Typing (PLT) technique. Tissue Antigens 17:162–173
2. Svejgaard A, Henningsen K, Jakobsen BK, Morling N, Platz P, Ryder LP (1983) Another DR/SB recombinant. Ninth International Histocompatibility Workshop and Conference, Newsletter no. II, September 15, 1983

Table 1. Sb antigens in Danes

	AL/DPw1	MOU/DPw2	EP1/DPw3	EP2/DPw4	MET/DPw5	BJA/DPw6
Correlation (r)	0.86	0.76	1.00	0.92	1.00	1.00
Frequency (%)	19.6	17.5	27.6	65.3	12.1	8.6

Correlations between local DP-like determinants and DPw1-DPw6, and frequencies of locally defined DP-like determinants

Table 2. "New" non-D/DR, DP, DQ determinants

Priming (D/DR)	Determinants	+ +	+ −	− +	− −	P
5, 7+ 5, 5×	RA-1 vs DR2	4	2	0	23	10^{-3}
5, 7+ 5, 5×	RA-2 vs DR2	4	1	3	32	10^{-2}
w6, w8 + w6, w8×	HA-1 vs DR3	7	1	0	32	10^{-6}
5, w6 + w6, w6×	HA-2 vs DR3	4	1	1	18	10^{-2}
1, w6 + w6, w6×	HA-3 vs DR3	5	2	0	20	10^{-3}
1, 1+ 1, 1×	MA-1 vs DRw6	5	2	4	32	10^{-2}

Analysis of associations between "new" PLT-defined non-D/DR, DP, DQ determinants and HLA-D/DR antigens

Histocompatibility Testing 1984
Edited by E. D. Albert et al.

LB-Q1 and LB-Q2: Population Genetics in Dutch Caucasoids and Inhibition Studies with Monoclonal Antibodies

A. Termijtelen, S. Naipal-van den Berge, F. Koning, and J.J. van Rood

Dept. of Immunohematology and Blood Bank, University Hospital, 2333 AA Leiden, The Netherlands

Introduction

Using primed lymphocytes (PLT reagents) generated between HLA-D/DR identical responder and stimulator lymphocytes, we identified two new determinants, referred to as LB-Q1 and LB-Q2. Both determinants are distinct from the established HLA antigens [1]. We have since studied the population genetics of LB-Q1 and LB-Q2 and investigated whether recognition of these structures could be inhibited by monoclonal antibodies (Moabs) directed against different HLA molecules.

Typing a Random Panel. A random panel of 84 unrelated Dutch Caucasoids was typed for LB-Q1 and LB-Q2. The gene frequency for LB-Q1 was 0.23, and that for LB-Q2 was 0.18. LB-Q1 is significantly associated with ($P < 0.001$) but distinct from DRw52, while LB-Q2 is significantly associated with ($P < 0.0001$) but distinct from HLA-B8.

Typing Families. Six families informative for LB-Q1 and/or LB-Q2 were tested. The typing results showed that both LB-Q1 and LB-Q2 segregate with HLA. One recombination between HLA-A and B and one between HLA-B and DR mapped LB-Q1 between HLA-A and HLA-DR. One recombination between HLA-A and B and two between HLA-B and DR mapped LB-Q2 between HLA-A and HLA-DR.

PLT Inhibition with Moabs. We tried to inhibit the recognition of these antigens by PLT reagents with Moabs directed against a class I backbone structure, against β_2-mircoglobulin, against HLA-DR, against HLA-DR + DQ, and against DRw52. We found that recognition of LB-Q1 was inhibited by α class I and/or by α class II Moabs. Recognition of LB-Q2 was always inhibited by α class I, and most strongly by α β_2-microglobulin, but never by the α class II Moabs.

Discussion and Summary

We were able to prepare a set of PLT reagents recognizing two new determinants, referred to as LB-Q1 and LB-Q2. These antigens are associated with but distinct from DRw52 and HLA-B8, respectively. Recognition of LB-Q1 can be inhibited by α class I and/or α class II Moabs. Recognition of LB-Q2 can only be inhibited by α class I Moabs. Our findings imply new polymorphisms in HLA, and their nature needs to be investigated further. The possible role of LB-Q1 in antigen presentation to PPD and tetanus toxoid-specific T cell lines is discussed elsewhere (T. H. M. Ottenhoff et al., Function of DRw52 and LB-Q1 in Antigen Presentation, this volume).

Reference

1. Termijtelen A, van den Berge SJ, Van Rood JJ (1983) LB-Q1 and LB-Q2: Two determinants defined in the primed phocyte test and independent of HLA-D/DR, MB/LB-E, or SB. Hum Immunol 8:1 – 15

 Histocompatibility Testing 1984
Edited by E. D. Albert et al.

Allelic Class II Determinants Defined by PLT Typing

L. Legrand, M.P. Font, J. Hors, D. Cohen, and J. Dausset

Institut de Recherches sur les maladies du sang, Hôpital Saint-Louis, 2, place du Docteur Fournier, 75475 Paris, Cedex 10, France

The HLA-D/DR region in man is complex, containing several closely linked genes which control a number of different cell surface antigens. Among these, some determinants can be detected by primed lymphocyte typing (PLT). In the present study, 50 PLTs were generated between pairs of healthy individuals sharing the same DR allele and, in 2 cases, a blank allele at the DR locus. The PLTs were obtained using classic techniques [1] and were tested against a panel of 81 normal individuals typed for HLA-DR (DR1-w10) and, in some cases, also for DP. Comparisons were also

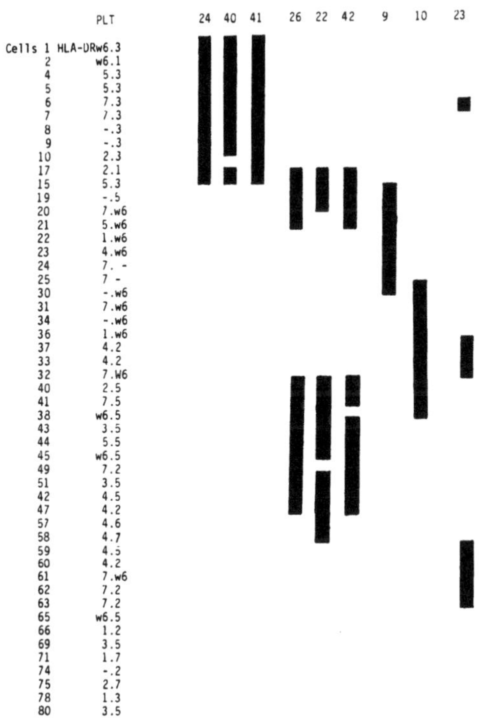
PLT
24 40 41 26 22 42 9 10 23
Cells 1 HLA-DRw6.3
2 w6.1
4 5.3
5 5.3
6 7.3
7 7.3
8 -.3
9 -.3
10 2.3
17 2.1
15 5.3
19 -.5
20 7.w6
21 5.w6
22 1.w6
23 4.w6
24 7. -
25 7 -
30 -.w6
31 7.w6
34 -.w6
36 1.w6
37 4.2
33 4.2
32 7.W6
40 2.5
41 7.5
38 w6.5
43 3.5
44 5.5
45 w6.5
49 7.2
51 3.5
42 4.5
47 4.2
57 4.6
58 4.7
59 4.5
60 4.2
61 7.w6
62 7.2
63 7.2
65 w6.5
66 1.2
69 3.5
71 1.7
74 -.2
75 2.7
78 1.3
80 3.5

Fig. 1. Pattern of reactivity of ten PLT reagents against a panel of cells from 50 unrelated individuals. *Vertical bars* indicate positive results with 50 of 81 normal individuals. PLTs 24 and 26 were obtained with two different DR5s vs the same DR5 situation; PLTs 9 and 10 in a reciprocal DRw6 vs DRw6 (haplo-identical related individuals); PLTs 40–42 with DR3 vs DR3; and PLTs 22 and 23 in an unrelated pair of DR4, 5 individuals

made with DNA restriction fragments using a β DQ probe. The PLT activity was extremely reliable, using 25×10^3 PLT cells against 1×10^5 restimulating cells. The level of MLC reactivity (10,000–25,000 cpm) appeared to be predictive of the PLTs obtained: reliable results were observed only in the case of reactive reagents giving $\geq$ 10,000 cpm. The nine PLT reagents (single or clusters), selected because they demonstrated a pattern of reactivity, recognized five allelic determinants (no triplets) and were correlated ($P < 10^{-8}$) with splits of DR specificities: short DR3 (PLTs 24, 40, 41), short DR5 (PLTs 26, 22, 42); and with two different parts of DRw6 (PLT 9 and PLT 10). (The patterns against 50 cells are shown in Fig. 1.) The determinant recognized by PLT 9 is correlated ($P = 0.003$) with a split of DQw1 determined by β DQ restriction fragments. No correlation with the pattern given using specific PLTs developed against DPw1–5.

PLTs 22 and 23 were generated by two different cells from unrelated individuals – cell 59 and cell 42, respectively, both bearing DR4 and DR5 antigens. It is postulated that cell 59 recognized in cell 42 a split of DR5 or another determinant closely linked to this part of DR5. A similar interpretation can be made concerning DR4, since both PLT 22 and 23 recognized two allelic series of four DR4 cells out of a total of nine DR4 cells.

Family studies, including two informative recombinants, clearly map the recognized target among class II products of the HLA-D/DR region.

Cloning of these PLT reagents, blocking experiments using monoclonal antibodies and further correlation studies with DNA polymorphism are in progress, with the aim of better definition of these determinants either as splits of DR5 specificities or as closely related determinants.

Reference

1. Sheehy MJ, Bach FH (1976) Tissue Antigens 8:157

Histocompatibility Testing 1984
Edited by E. D. Albert et al.

HLA-D and DR in Different Populations

D. Jaraquemada, R. Okoye, W. Ollier, J. Awad, and H. Festenstein

Dept. of Immunology, The London Hospital Medical College, Turner Street, London E1 2AD, UK

The HLA-D-segregant series of lymphocyte activating determinants (Lads) was originally described by using homozygous cells as reagents in mixed lymphocyte cultures (MLC). Later, the serological definition of the HLA-DR antigens was established by using HLA-D homozygous cells (HTCs) as reference cells. It appeared in Caucasoid panels that the two techniques were detecting the same antigenic determinants. Further serological, biochemical, and DNA studies have now revealed the complexity of the HLA-D region, but the relationship between D and DR remains unresolved.

The high correlation of D and DR in Caucasoids presents serious limitations to the further study of their relationship. An additional approach is to investigate other ethnic groups in which association patterns may be different. Figure 1 shows phenotype frequencies and a comparison of DR/D association patterns in five different populations. In British Caucasoids the correlation between DR and D for all specificities is extremely high and the D antigens are included in the corresponding DR antigen. DR1, 2, 3, 5, and 7 and DRw9 show association with their respective D specificities, i.e., Dw1, 2, 3, 5, and 7 and DB5. Dw4 is the most frequent specificity "included" within DR4, followed by Dw13 and Dw14. Dw6 and Dw9 are included in DRw6 and both Dw8 and DB7 in DRw8. No Dw antigen associated with DRw10 has been defined.

Our mixed European Caucasoid panel consists predominantly of English subjects, with some southern and central Europeans. The phenotype frequency distributions and the D/DR association patterns in this panel are very similar to those seen in the British panel. However, an additional DR4-associated antigen, Dw10, is present, and the correlation between D and DR is lower in this group than in the more homogeneous British sample.

The Saudi Arabs show an extremely high frequency of DR7 and Dw7 (46% and 42%, respectively). Their D/DR association pattern is similar to that in the previous groups, although there are some discrepancies between DR5/Dw5, DRw6/Dw6, and DR1/Dw1. DR1/Dw1 do not show any significant associations. Dw10, and not Dw4, is the most common D antigen associated with DR4.

Phenotype frequencies of DR in the Chinese are very different from those seen in Caucasoid populations. DRw9 and DR2 are the most common DR antigens; DR1 is absent; and Dw1 present at low frequency. DR2/Dw2, DR5/Dw5 and DR7/Dw7 show a clear inclusion pattern of D in DR, and their correlation is significant. An additional D antigen, Dw12, described in Japanese subjects, was found at a low frequency and included within DR2. A similar correlation is seen for DRw9 and DB5, with some discrepancies. Dw3, although included in DR3, was present at a much lower frequency. DRw8 was observed but no Dw specificity was associated with it. A further complication is seen with the DR4 related group of specificities. A "Japanese" antigen, Dw15, is the most frequent D antigen in association with DR4. Other antigens of the group, i.e., Dw4, Dw13, and DKT2, are not significantly associated with DR4, and Dw10 and Dw14 could not be detected.

DR2/Dw2; DR5/Dw5 and DR7/Dw7 are the most common antigens found in the Nigerian population, and with DRw9/DB5 are the only specificities showing high association and inclusion patterns. DR1/Dw1 and DR3/Dw3 show only partial association, and DRw8 and Dw8 are totally dissociated. An interesting observation is that 33% of the DRw8 individuals are Dw3 positive. DR4 was only found in one individual and Dw4 and Dw10 are totally absent. Dw13 was found at a low frequency and is not associated with DR4.

In conclusion, the high association and total inclusion of D and DR in Caucasoids breaks down when examined in other populations, with several instances of complete dissociation. Whereas DR antigens can be defined in a majority of individuals, the Dw series shows greater polymorphism, part of which is still to be defined in non-Caucasoid populations. This supports the hypothesis that D and DR are different entities which may reside on the same molecule. Study of these cells at the molecular and DNA levels will help to resolve the problem.

Histocompatibility Testing 1984
Edited by E. D. Albert et al.

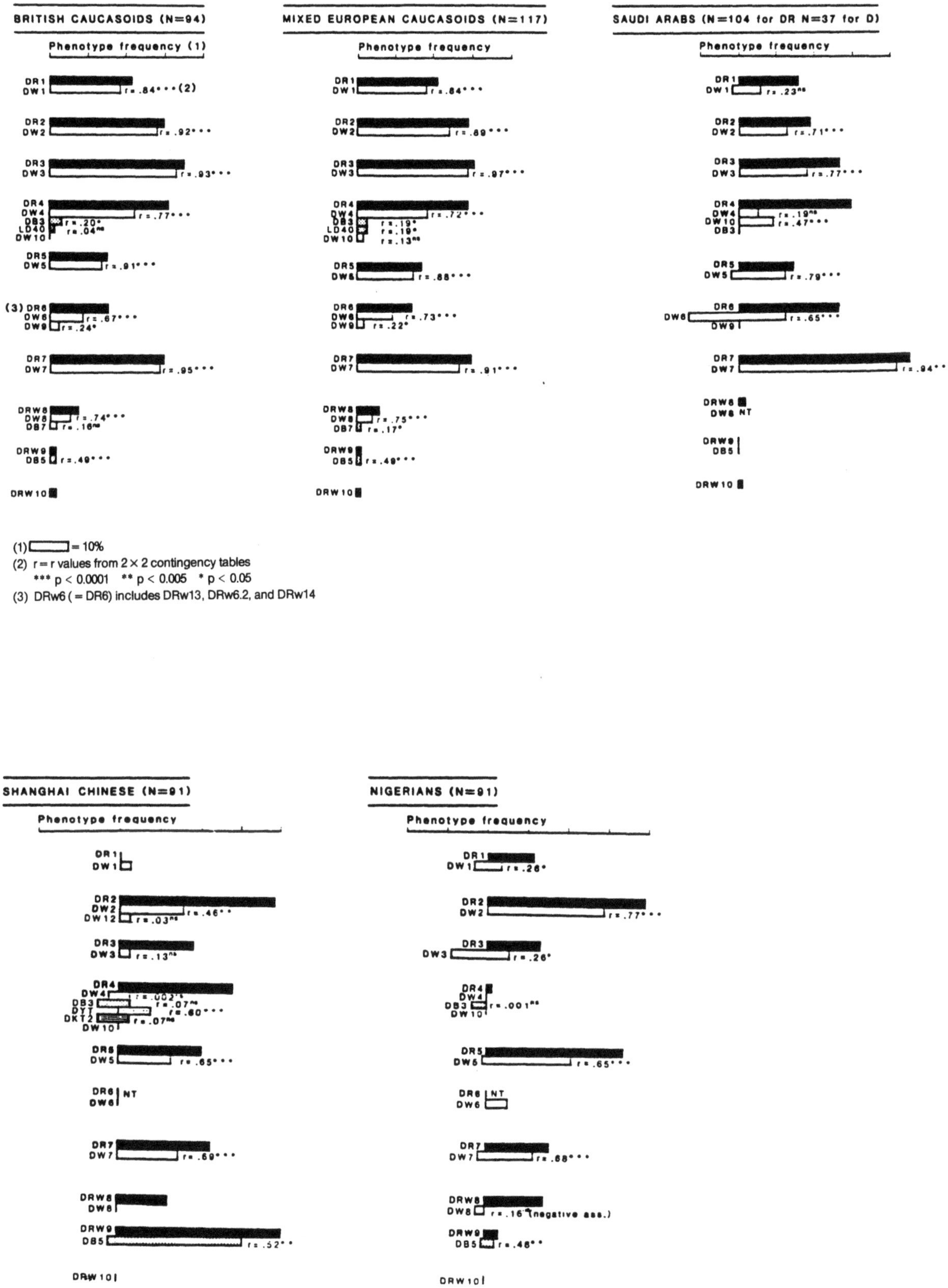

Fig. 1. The distribution of HLA-DR and D phenotype frequencies in various ethnic groups: differences in their patterns of association (DB3 = Dw13; LD40 = Dw14; DYT = Dw15; as in the text)

Private Specificities of Human IA-Like Molecules Detected by T Cell Lines

E. J. Ball, L. Myers, G. Nunez, and P. Stastny

Dept. of Internal Medicine, University of Texas Health Science Center, Southwestern Medical School Dallas, TX 75235, USA

Summary

Among a number of human T cell lines tested, two alloreactive and two GAT-specific, HLA-restricted lines were found to be inhibited by monoclonal antibodies against human IA-like (DQ) molecules. When tested in panel studies, the specificities detected were distinct from any known HLA antigens, but were associated with DR and DQ antigens. This indicates that, in addition to the "supertypic" or public specificities, the human IA-like molecules carry *private* specificities recognized by T cells.

The HLA-D region encodes class II molecules of three types; DR, DQ, and DP. By amino acid sequence, DR-like molecules are homologous to murine IE products and DQ molecules to IA products. No murine homologue of DP is known [1, 2]. In addition to the known HLA antigens (DR, DQ, BR), both the IE- and IA-like molecules have structural polymorphisms not currently recognized serologically [3, 4]. T cell sublines specific for allogeneic cells or the polypeptide antigen GAT were tested for inhibition by monoclonal antibodies against human IA-like molecules (e.g., IVD12). Table 1 shows the results of a representative experiment with the GAT-specific T cell line PT104.2 using the DQw3-specific antibody IVD12 [5] and the DRw53-specific 109d6 [6]. The strong inhibition by IVD12 (74%–93%), but not 109d6 (4%–16%), suggested that the determinant was on IA-like molecules.

Lines inhibited by anti-IA-like antibodies were tested in panel studies (Table 2). The reactivity pat-

Table 1. Monoclonal antibody inhibition of PT104.2

Monoclonal antibody		Antigen-induced response 3H-TdR uptake (cpm)			
Name	Dilution^{-1}	No Ag	+Ag	Delta	% Inh
None	–	978	15 026	14 048	–
IVD12	500	452	1 483	1 031	93
	1 000	675	1 958	1 283	91
	2 000	578	2 188	1 611	89
	4 000	834	2 392	1 558	89
	8 000	584	3 514	2 930	79
	16 000	348	4 049	3 702	74
109d6	500	954	12 690	11 736	16
	1 000	1 014	12 785	11 771	16
	2 000	1 194	13 055	11 862	16
	4 000	841	14 301	13 460	4

Ascites antibody was added to accessory cells 1 h prior to the addition of responding cells and antigen

Table 2. Panel studies

D reg	++	+–	–+	––	χ^2	r
PT126.B8			(DST1.B8)			(GAT)
DR1	6	9	0	12	4.07	.39
DR2	5	10	3	9	.00	.01
DRw6	2	13	4	8	.60	.15
DRw10	3	12	0	12	1.05	.20
DRw52	7	8	3	9	.57	.14
DRw53	5	10	7	5	.83	–.17
DQw1	15	0	6	6	6.97	.51
DQw2	6	9	5	7	.09	–.58
DQw3	6	8	8	5	.34	–.11
PT104.2			(DST4.GAT)			(GAT)
DR4	5	4	6	21	2.14	.24
DR5	5	4	5	22	2.95	.29
DRw52	6	3	11	16	.93	.16
DRw53	6	3	14	13	.15	.06
DQw1	3	6	21	6	4.17	–.34
DQw2	1	8	12	15	1.97	–.23
DQw3	9	0	10	17	8.37	.48
PT9.25.E11			(DST5.E11)			(Allo)
DR4	0	9	9	31	1.21	–.16
DR5	8	1	4	36	20.65	.65
DRw52	9	0	28	12	2.14	.21
DRw53	2	7	14	26	.12	–.05
DQw1	3	6	27	13	2.32	–.22
DQw2	3	6	12	28	.04	.03
DQw3	9	0	11	29	13.12	.52
PT31.C3			(DST6.C3)			(Allo)
DR1	3	6	6	34	.65	.12
DR2	2	7	10	30	.06	–.04
DRw6	8	1	11	29	9.22	.43
DRw10	0	9	2	38	.06	–.04
DRw52	9	0	28	12	2.14	.21
DRw53	5	4	15	25	.38	.09
DQw1	9	0	25	15	3.26	.26
DQw2	3	6	19	21	.16	–.06
DQw3	2	7	13	27	.04	–.03

++ = positive response and positive for antigen
+– = positive response and negative for antigen
–+ = negative response and positive for antigen
–– = negative response and negative for antigen

Histocompatibility Testing 1984
Edited by E. D. Albert et al.

terns were distinct from known HLA antigens, but associated with both DR and DQ. The specificities seen by the four lines were tentatively named DST1.B8, DST4.GAT, DST5.E11, and DST6.C3, referring to a T-cell-defined determinant of DS, the DR typing of the priming cell, and a T cell line identifier. Others have described human T cells with patterns similar to the "supertypic" specificities carried by IA-like molecules [7, 8]. Our results indicate that these molecules also carry *private* specificities recognized by T cells.

References

1. Tanigaki N, Tosi R (1982) The genetic control of human Ia alloantigens: a three loci model derived from the immunochemical analysis of 'supertypic' specificities. Immunol Rev 66:5–37
2. Shackelford D, Kaufman J, Korman A, Strominger J (1982) HLA-DR antigens: structure, separation of subpopulations, gene cloning and function. Immunol Rev 66:133–187
3. Groner J, Watson A, Bach F (1983) Dw/LD-related molecular polymorphism of DR4 B-chains. J Exp Med 157:1687–1691
4. Nepom G, Nepom B, Antonelli P, Mickelson E, Silver J, Goyert G, Hansen J (1984) The HLA-DR4 family of haplotypes consists of a series of distinct DR and DS molecules. J Exp Med 159:394–404
5. Giles R, Nunez G, Hurley C, Nunez-Roldan A, Winchester R, Stastny P, Capra JD (1983) Structural analysis of a human I-A homologue using a monoclonal antibody that recognizes an MB3-like specificity. J Exp Med 157: 1461–1470
6. Nunez-Roldan A, Szer I, Toguchi T, Cuttner J, Winchester R (1982) Association of certain Ia allotypes with the occurrence of chronic lymphocytic leukemia. J Exp Med 156:1872–1877
7. Zeevi A, Annen K, Bass G, Marrari M, Duquesnoy R (1982) Association of the PLT specificity of alloreactive clones with HLA-DR, MB and MT determinants. Immunogenetics 16:209–218
8. Berle E, Thorsby E (1982) Both DR and MT class II HLA molecules may restrict proliferative T-lymphocyte responses to antigen. Scand J Immunol 16:543–547

PLT Analysis of D Region Complexity by Cloned Cells: A New Non-DP Antigen *

Y. Nose, T. Sukegawa, F. Tsuchida, T. Nakatsuji, and K. Tsuji

Department of Transplantation, Tokai University School of Medicine, Bhoseidai, Isehara, Kanagawa 259-11, Japan

The HLA-D region is very complex. HLA-D specificity is not identical to DR. It is not known whether the difference in HLA-D of cells with the same DR can be supposed to be due to one antigen determinant. To resolve the problem, PLT clones were used. From the MLC of cells with the same DR, DQ, DP antigens but with different D antigens, Dw15-specific PLT clones and a Dw4-specific clone were established.

PLT clones were established as described by Inouye et al. [1]. KN (HLA-Dw1, Dw15, DR1, DR4, DRw53, DQw1, DQw3, DPw2, DPw4) and OS (HLA-Dw1, Dw4, DR1, DR4, DRw53, DQw1, DQw3, DPw2, DPw4) were used as stimulator cells or responder cells. PLT assay was done using the standardized technique of the Ninth International Histocompatibility Workshop. When the relative reference response exceeded 80%, then the reaction was counted as positive [2]. 32 panel cells of Caucasian origin and nine panel cells of Japanese origin were used to characterize cloned PLT cells. Also 14 HTCs were used; there were three types of Dw15, three types of Dw4, three types of Dw10, three types of Dw14, and two types of Dw12.

Four Dw15-specific PLT clones, C-4, C-11, C-14, and C-17, were established using KN as stimulator cells and OS as responder cells in MLC. From the reverse combination of MLC, the Dw4-specific PLT clone, 1–3, was obtained. These clones were characterized using the 41 panel cells and 14 HTCs described above. It was found that C-4, C-11, C-14, and C-17 belonged to one cluster ($r > 0.73$). C-4, C-11, C-14, and C-17 can specifically recognize Dw15 but no other HLA antigens (Table 1). Clone 1–3 has a high r value with only Dw4 (Table 1). Figs. 1 and 2 show the relationship of antigen phenotypes of stimulator cells and ^{3}H-thymidine uptake of C-11 and 1–3. These data clearly indicate that the response of the clones are very specific to Dw15 or Dw4. As shown above, Dw15 and Dw4 specific PLT cells were established. Recombination

* This work is supported in part by the Japanese Ministry of Health and Welfare and the Ministry of Education

Table 1. Correlation coefficient (r) values ($\times 100$) of PLT cells and DR, D and DP antigens

	C-11	C-14	C-17	1-3
C-4	73	73	73	13
C-11		91	83	18
C-14			83	18
C-17				18
1-3				

DR	C-4	C-11	C-14	C-17	1-3
DR1	15	6	25	6	15
2	15	21	22	21	6
3	10	13	13	13	1
4	19	26	26	26	32
5	5	7	7	7	9
w6	10	13	13	13	1
7	6	12	12	12	1
w8	5	7	7	7	9
w9	0	0	0	0	0
w10	0	0	0	0	0
6Y	3	35	0	5	6
blank	17	0	0	0	29

D	C-4	C-11	C-14	C-17	1-3
Dw1	19	10	31	10	13
2	10	14	15	14	24
3	10	14	15	14	4
4	13	18	18	18	[100]
5	5	7	7	7	9
6	9	12	12	12	1
7	8	10	11	10	4
8	5	7	7	7	9
9	5	7	7	7	9
10	10	13	13	13	15
11	0	0	0	0	0
12	6	9	9	9	11
14	11	16	0	0	6
13	6	9	9	9	11
MN2	5	7	7	7	9
NTR	3	5	5	5	6
15	[73	100	91	83]	19
KT2	6	9	9	9	11
En	3	35	0	5	6
blank	17	0	0	0	29

DP	C-4	C-11	C-14	C-17	1-3
DPw1	4	5	5	5	6
2	1	11	12	1	6
3	14	19	5	5	9
4	26	36	25	36	9
5	37	34	34	34	11
6	0	0	0	0	0
Cp63	7	9	10	9	11
blank	26	36	25	24	9

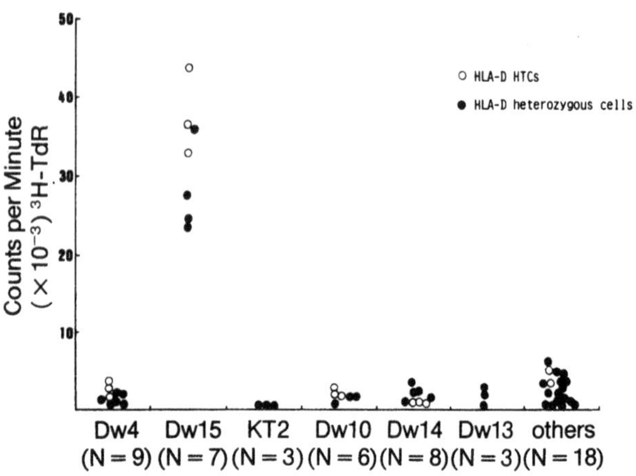

Fig. 1. ^{3}H-thymidine uptake of clone C-11 and antigen phenotypes of stimulation cells

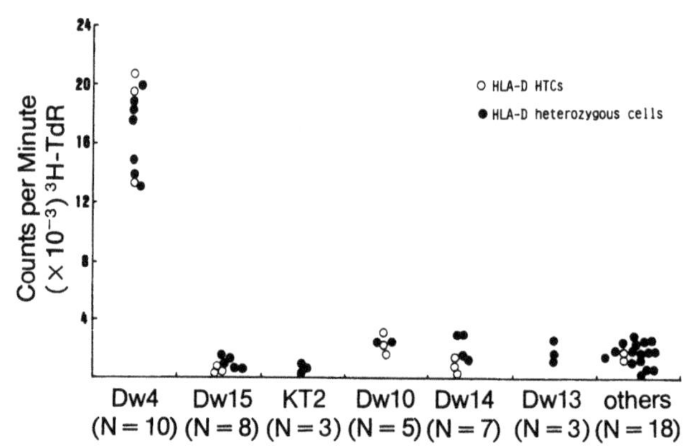

Fig. 2. ^{3}H-thymidine uptake of clone 1 – 3 and antigen phenotypes of stimulation cells

specific PLT cells were established. Recombination between D and DR has been reported [3]. There are some reports of D-specific PLT cells [4, 5] or clones [6, 7]. These results suggest the existence of D-specific antigen determinants. The data presented here confirmed that one antigen determinant defines Dw15 or Dw4 in a DR4-positive population. The antigen was tentatively named Sp. Based upon reports of DR- and DQ-specific PLT cells [8, 9], it is considered that the combination of DR, DQ and DP defines D antigenicity.

Summary

PLT clones which could specifically react with Dw15 or Dw4 were established from MLR between cells with different D and the same DR, DQ, DP. The new antigen, which is in the HLA-D region, may be involved in MLR.

Acknowledgement. The authors would like to thank Dr. Nancy L. Reinsmoen for supplying Caucasian cells.

References

1. Inouye H, Hank JA, Chardonnens X, Segall M, Alter BJ, Bach FH (1980) Cloned primed-lymphocyte-test reagent in the dissection of HLA-D. J Exp Med 152:143s–155s
2. Wank R, Schendel DJ, Hansen JA, Dupont B (1978) The lymphocyte restimulation system. Evaluation of intra-HLA-D group priming. Immunogenetics 6:107–115
3. Reinsmoen N, Noreen HJ, Friend PS, Gibiette R, Greenberg LJ, Kersey JH (1978) Positive mixed lymphocyte reactivity between HLA-DR identical siblings. Transplant Proc 10:793–795
4. Moen T, Nousiainen H, Bratlie A, Solheim G, Thorsby E (1981) Detection of HLA-D region products by primed lymphocyte typing (PLT). Hum Immunol 2:287–294
5. Suciu-Foca N, Godfey M, Khan R (1980) HLA-D-DR relationships: PLT studies of HLA-D specificities associated with DR1, DR2 and DR4. Hum Immunol 2:295–304
6. Pawelec G, Rehbein A, Kahle P, Muller C, Wernet P (1981) Restimulation properties of cloned alloactivated lymphocytes: detection of a novel type of HLA-D/DR region determinant and allelic subtypes for HLA-Dw3 using cloned reagents. Hum Immunol 2:315–324
7. Zeevi A, Annen K, Scheffel C, Duquesnoy RJ (1983) Detection of HLA-DR associated PLT determinants by alloreactive lymphocyte clones. Immunogenetics 18: 205–220
8. Bach FH, Inouye H, Hank JA, Alter BJ (1979) Human T-lymphocyte clones reactive in primed lymphocyte typing and cytotoxicity. Nature 281:307–309
9. Zeevi A, Annen A, Bass G, Marrari M, Duquesnoy RJ (1982) Association of the PLT specificity of alloreactive lymphocyte clones with HLA-DR, MB and MT determinants. Immunogenetics 16:209–218

Correlation Between PLT and CML Specificity of Alloreactive T Cell Clones*

A. Zeevi[1] and R.J. Duquesnoy[2]

1 The Histocompatibility Research Laboratory, The Blood Center of Southeastern Wisconsin Inc., Milwaukee, Wisconsin 53233, USA
2 The Department of Pathology, University of Pittsburgh School of Medicine, Room 406 Scaife Hall, Pittsburgh PA 15261, USA

Alloreactive T cell clones were grown from soft agar colonies generated from different MLR combinations according to previously described methods [1, 2]. After 6–8 weeks long-term culture, each clone was tested against the original stimulator for secondary proliferative responsiveness in a 3-day primed lymphocyte test (PLT) assay and for cytolytic activity in a cell-mediated lympholysis (CML) assay using PHA blasts and/or B-lymphoblastoid cell lines (B-LCL) as targets. Several clones displayed both PLT and CML activity towards the original stimulator and these dual reactive clones were further studied with selected cell panels to determine their alloantigenic specificity. The data summarized in Table 1 showed perfect correlations between the PLT and CML specificities of both class I and class II specific alloreactive clones. Two clones exhibited PLT and CML activity specific for class I antigens B21 and B17. Four clones had PLT and CML activity specific for various class II (I-E and I-A-like) HLA antigens, namely DR1, DR5, DRw53 and DQw3 (Table 1).

* This work was supported by AI-18923, ACS-IM 373, and AA-93

In order to further analyze the relationship between the determinants recognized in PLT and CML, we have employed a battery of class I- and class II-specific monoclonal antibodies (mAbs) in inhibition studies of the reactivity of these clones. In these studies, the PLT stimulators or the CML target cells were pretreated with mAbs prior to testing in the two different assays. Identical mAb inhibition profiles were observed for the PLT and CML activity of class I- and class II-specific T cell clones. This similarity in mAb inhibition profiles for CML and PLT provided additional evidence that the PLT and CML determinants recognized by allo-

Table 1. Perfect correlation between PLT and CML specificity of alloreactive T cell clones

Clone	Class	Specificity	PLT vs. CML			
			++	+-	-+	--
DD13	I	B17	7	0	0	13
DR3	I	B21	6	0	0	8
DL65	II	DR1	3	0	0	9
DS56	II	DR5	6	0	0	8
DD56	II	DQw3	10	0	0	9
HT72	II	DRw53	12	0	0	14

reactive T cells reside on the same HLA molecule and may even represent the same cellular epitope. In context with our findings regarding PLT and CML specificity, we have studied the alloantigenic specificity of the stimulator necessary to induce interleukin 2 (IL2) release by T cell clones. It was observed that the specificity of IL2 release was identical to the PLT specificity of both class I- and class II-specific alloreactive T cell clones. This suggests the same HLA determinant can induce a PLT response and the release of IL2 by a T cell clone. This concept was further strengthened by the results of mAb studies of PLT and IL2 release of our clones. Linear regression analysis showed a highly significant correlation ($p < 0.001$) between the mAb inhibition profiles of PLT and IL2 release of these clones.

These findings suggest that the same MHC molecule and even the same cellular epitope may trigger three properties of alloactivated T cells, namely, secondary proliferation, cytolytic activity, and IL2 release.

References

1. Zeevi A, Scheffel A, Annen K, Bass G, Marrari M, Duquesnoy RJ (1982) Association of the PLT specificity of alloreactive lymphocyte clones with HLA-DR, MB and MT determinants. Immunogenetics 16:209–218
2. Zeevi A, Scheffel C, Annen K, Duquesnoy RJ (1983) Primed lymphocyte testing specificity of alloreactive lymphocyte clones for HLA-B locus determinants. Proc Natl Acad Sci USA 80:1440–1444

Heterogeneity of DR5-Associated Alloantigens Detected by Human T Lymphocyte Clones

S. Rosen-Bronson, A.H. Johnson, R.J. Hartzman, and D.D. Eckels

Lombardi Cancer Center, 3800 Reservoir Rd., N.W., Washington DC 20007, USA

We have used monoclonal T cells (i.e., T lymphocyte clones, TLCs) to investigate the fine specificities of HLA-D region alloantigens. The results presented confirm the existence of heterogeneity within the DR5 specificity [1] and also reflect the complexity observed with other D region haplotypes [2].

The panel of TLCs was generated by stimulating PBLs from a DR2, Dw2, DQw1; DPw4 donor with irradiated PBLs from a heterozygous donor (DR3, 5; Dw3, w5; DQw2, w3; DPw2, w4) in a primary MLC for 4 days. Viable cells were subsequently cloned by limiting dilution at 0.3 cells/well in the presence of 20% TCGF and irradiated stimulator PBLs. After 7 days, wells containing clones were transferred to 96-well U-bottom trays with irradiated stimulators 1×10^5/well in 0.1 ml). Clones were maintained on a regular schedule of 20% TCGF on day 3 followed by irradiated feeder cells plus 20% TCGF on day 7. Further methodological details can be found elsewhere [3].

Resulting clones were initially screened in proliferation assays on a panel of four stimulator cells. Functional clones were expanded and again tested in a proliferation assay against a panel of 22 PBLs positive for DR3 and/or DR5. Ten clones recognizing DR5-associated alloantigens split DR5 into seven potential subtypes and were selected for further analysis on an expanded panel (Table 1).

Our results are consistent with the existence of allotypic heterogeneity within an HLA-DR5 haplotype. After ruling out association with other known loci (i.e., DQ and DP) there are three DR5-associated subtypes. Clone S3.32 reacts positively on all the DR5 stimulators tested, whereas S3.13 and S3.75 show identical patterns which are different from S3.32 and S3.113. S3.113 demonstrates a unique pattern of reactivity. More extensive panel studies should clarify and better define the subsets which exist within DR5. Similar to the results with DR5, six clones from Table 1 which appear to recognize DQw3-associated epitopes (S3.22, S3.47, S3.91, S3.78, S3.69, S3.125) suggest that there is heterogeneity associated with the DQ series also. Four different reaction patterns were observed. Additional studies are needed to clarify the nature of the heterogeneity described; however, in view of data from molecular genetic and protein chemistry experiments as well as early serological data, the technique of using TLCs to detect HLA-D region polymorphism should prove useful in attempts to define those structures important for cellular recognition, immune regulation, and tissue engraftment.

Table 1. Heterogeneity of DR5- and DQw3 associated PLT clones

			Clones (cpm)										PLT line
			DQw3-associated						DR5-associated				
	DR	DQw	S3.22	S3.47	S3.91	S3.78	S3.69	S3.125	S3.32	S3.113	S3.13	S3.75	S3
64	(5, w6)	(1, 3)	16 777[a]	18 409[a]	25 501[a]	4 977[a]	327[a]	637[a]	4 905[a]	8 237[a]	6 755[a]	699[a]	9 791
197	(5, w8)	(4, –)	12 923[a]	4 212[a]	234	1 375[a]	611[a]	2 640[a]	4 317[a]	81	8 902[a]	1 476[a]	13 687
1 003[b]	(3, 5)	(2, 3)	9 493[a]	7 938[a]	1 935	4 373[a]	2 644[a]	1 409[a]	1 861[a]	4 310[a]	14 025[a]	599[a]	11 210
1 199	(3, 5)	(3, –)	13 463[a]	11 786[a]	9 635[a]	1 747[a]	862	1 169[a]	5 395[a]	429[a]	9 579[a]	900	7 655
101	(5, w6)	(1, 3)	11 196[a]	8 899[a]	18 736[a]	5 318[a]	1 018[a]	456	3 347[a]	10 076[a]	3 259[a]	388[a]	9 273
65	(5, w6)	(NT)	4 389[a]	2 403[a]	666[a]	20[a]	24[a]	51[a]	1 284[a]	1 518	255[a]	42[a]	657
1 220	(4, 5)	(3, –)	5 705[a]	8 297[a]	23[a]	406[a]	823[a]	473	1 812[a]	4 659	61[a]	50[a]	2 523
126	(5, –)	(1, 3)	2 295[a]	1 358[a]	1 069[a]	439[a]	122[a]	169[a]	1 628[a]	169	3 571[a]	815[a]	6 703
1 059	(2, 5)	(1, 3)	5 953[a]	5 265[a]	13 864[a]	35[a]	33[a]	51[a]	2 614[a]	18[a]	35[a]	19[a]	7 894
1 193	(5, –)	(NT)	5 749[a]	5 548[a]	10[a]	17[a]	13[a]	23[a]	1 499[a]	22[a]	9[a]	21[a]	3 058
1 022	(2, 4)	(1, 3)	1 417	8 276	18	3 750	21	57	13	19	20	15	601
1 256	(4, –)	(NT)	4 239	16	22	15	11	11	37	21	19	11	116
128	(4, w6)	(1, 3)	4 632	10 347	3 359	17	1 305	2 320	15	538	28	14	2 320
2[c]	(2, 2)	(1, –)	16	7	159	103	10	16	15	357	19	14	7

[a] Results confirmed in two separate experiments
[b] Original stimulator cell
[c] Autologous responder cell
Proliferation assays were performed by incubating 5×10^4 irradiated stimulators with 1×10^4 clones in 96 well U-bottom trays for 72 hours followed by pulsing with tritiated methylthymidine for 16 hours. Results are expressed as the mean cpm of triplicate cultures. Underline indicates positive response determined by maximized T-test

References

1. Zeevi A, et al (1983) Detection of HLA-DR associated PLT determinants by alloreactive lymphocyte clones. Immunogenetics 18:205–220
2. Rosen-Bronson S, et al (1984) # 3274. Fed. Proc. 43:1981
3. Eckels DD, Hartzman RJ (1982) Characterization of human T-lymphocyte clones (TLCs) specific for HLA-region gene products. Immunogenetics 16:117

Heterogeneity of HLA-B7 as Detected by Cytotoxic T Cell Clones

G. van Seventer[1], H. Ijssel[2], M. Breuning[1], H. Spits[2], B.S. Breur[1], A. van Poelgeest[1], B. Huis[1], A. Voordouw[2], and P. Ivanyi[1]

1 Division of Hematology, Central Laboratory, Netherlands Red Cross Blood Transfusion Service, Amsterdam, The Netherlands
2 Division of Tumor Biology, The Netherlands Cancer Institute, Amsterdam, The Netherlands

Cytotoxic T cells (CTCs) activated in an allogeneic mixed lymphocyte culture generally recognize products coded for by the major histocompatibility complex. In this study we examined the serologically defined HLA-B7 with alloreactive CTC clones. Four cloned lines of CTCs were isolated by limiting dilution from T cells which were stimulated with the HLA-B7 homozygote EVC-transformed cell line JY (HLA-A2,2; B7,7; C–,–; DR4,w6). The clones HG-31 and HG-61 were isolated from the responder HG (HLA-A2,23; B40,44 Cw4,–; DRw6,7), and the clones LIV-7 and LIV-8, from the responder LIV (HLA-A2,31; B44,w60; Cw3,–; DR2,–). The specificity of the clones was determined with panel studies involving a large number of third-party lymphocytes. (PBL

Histocompatibility Testing 1984
Edited by E. D. Albert et al.

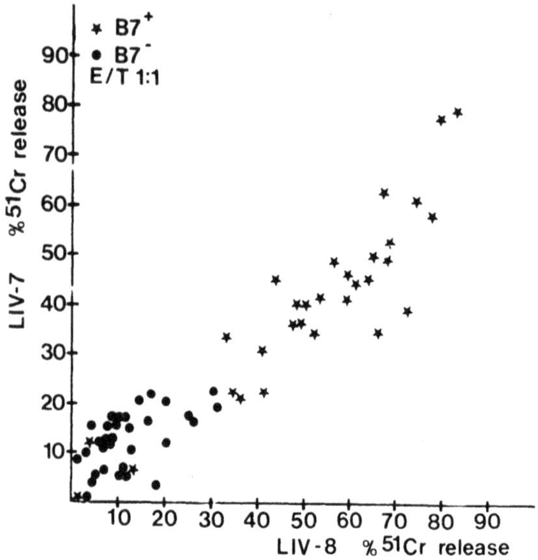

Fig. 1. Reactivity pattern of two CTC clones (LIV-7 and LIV-8) tested on B7-positive and B7-negative target cells

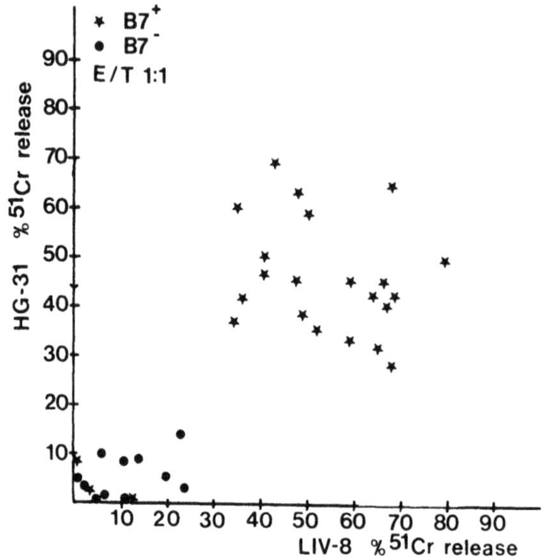

Fig. 2. Reactivity pattern of two CTC clones (HG-31 and LIV-8) tested on B7-positive and B7-negative target cells

cultured for 6 days in the absence of mitogen were used as targets.) The clones HG-31 and HG-61 have already been described [1, 2]. Briefly, HG-31 has a clear HLA-B7 specificity and was also positive on two HLA-Bw56-containing cells. HG-61 gave positive lysis on 30% of B7-positive and 50% of B40-positive lymphocytes, and on all cells carrying a previously described subtype of HLA-B27. All clones could be blocked by the MoAb W6/32, which is specific for a monomorphic determinant on class 1 HLA gene products, and MoAb SPVL8, which is specific for all HLA-B locus products (H. Spits, manuscript in preparation). The clones were phenotypically characterized as OKT3$^+$, 4$^-$, 8$^+$. In panel studies, LIV-7 and LIV-8 showed a specificity that is in good agreement with HLA-B7. Both clones gave the same reactivity on the panel cells. LIV-8 had a higher cytotoxic activity but both recognized the same panel cells as positive (Fig. 1). When the specificity of the LIV clones is compared with the specificities of HG-31 and HG-61 we can conclude that they match with the reaction pattern of HG-31 (Fig. 2). This means that we can confirm one of the subtypes of HLA-B7 earlier defined by

Table 1. Three HLA-B7 subtypes, defined by CTC clones

HG-31	LIV-7/8	HG-61	Proposed HLA-B7 subtypes	Frequency in random (Caucasian) HLA-B7 panel
+	+	+	7.2	30%
+	+	–	7.1	60%
–	–	–	7.3	10%

CTC clones. As shown in Table 1, we can split HLA-B7 into three subtypes. The position of JY is interesting, who is included in subtype 7.2, which is not the common subtype. The generally used DNA probe of HLA-B7 can therefore not be considered the best representive for HLA-B7. The subtypes 7.2 and 7.3 are biochemically confirmed (Strominger, personal communication).

References

1. Spits H, Breuning MH, Ivânyi P, Russo C, De Vries JE (1982) Immunogenetics 16:503–512
2. Breuning MH, Spits H, De Vries JE, Ivânyi P (1984) Hum Immunol 9:231–242

Analysis of Cytolytic Clones Directed at Class I and Class II Antigens Using HLA Loss Mutants of a Lymphoblastoid Cell Line*

N. Ohta, N.L. Reinsmoen, A. Anichini, and F.H. Bach

Immunobiology Research Center, Box 724 Mayo, University of Minnesota, Minneapolis, MN 55455, USA

One useful approach to analysis of the human major histocompatibility complex is to generate somatic cell variants with altered expression of HLA gene products. It is possible to generate not only a single HLA antigen loss, but also variants with simultaneous loss of two or three HLA antigens, by gamma ray irradiation. These HLA loss variants have enabled us to study the antigenic specificities detected by alloreactive responses in man.

We have utilized cloned T cell reagents and ionizing radiation-induced mutants of an HLA heterozygous lymphoblastoid cell line (LCL) to investigate the determinants detected by the cell-mediated lympholysis assay. The HLA loss mutant LCLs used were mostly generated in our laboratory by the method of Kavathas et al. [1]. Cells of an HLA haplotype loss mutant LCL, # AA2 (expressing the HLA-A2, B51, DR1, Dw1, DQw1, DPw2 haplotype), derived from LCL-721: (HLA-A2, B51, DR1, Dw1, DQw1, DPw2 A1, B8, DR3, Dw3, DQw2, DPw4), were used as the sensitizing cells for HLA-disparate responder cells in vitro. Cloned reagents were generated by single-cell deposition utilizing a fluorescence activated cell sorter, and those "clones" were tested for cytolytic activity against various HLA loss mutant targets derived from LCL-721 of four different categories; loss of HLA-A2 only, loss of A2, B51, loss of A2, B51, DR1, DQw1, and loss of the whole haplotype.

Of 36 cytolytic clones, three were anti-HLA-A2, five anti-B51, 12 anti-DR1/DQw1, 13 anti-DP/FA region associated with DPw2, and three of undetermined specificities based on cytolytic patterns against the HLA loss mutant targets. Of 25 anti-HLA class II clones, 23 (92%) were proliferative, thus having the characteristics of helper cell-independent cytolytic T cell clones (HITc), while two of eight (25%) anti-class I clones were HITc. It should be noted that 25 of 36 cytolytic clones (69.4%) were anti-class II, while only eight (22%) were anti-class I. Both the specificities studied and the type of stimulator cells used for sensitization (LCL vs PBL) may influence the predominant specificities recognized by CTL.

The anti-DP/FA clones were investigated by blocking experiments using various monoclonal antibodies (mcAb), such as w6/32, L243, anti-FA [2], and Tu39 (kindly supplied by Dr. P. Wernet) [3]. Preliminary results indicate that those clones detecting the DP/FA region associated with DPw2 could be divided into subgroups defined by blocking by anti-FA and not Tu39, Tu39 and not FA, or both sera at the serum concentrations tested to date (Table 1). Studies are in progress to investigate the relationship between the DP allospecificities and the determinants detected by anti-FA or Tu39 monoclonal antibodies using those T cell clones.

Table 1. Blocking of cytotoxicity of anti-DP/FA clones by monoclonal antibodies

Clone	w6/32	L243	Anti-FA	Tu39
# B1	21	29	<u>92</u>	NT
# B6	-12	18	<u>147</u>	<u>135</u>
# B13	-5	24	14	<u>91</u>
# B17	9	16	-9	<u>73</u>
# B26	14	24	<u>97</u> (87-97)[a]	36
# B79	8	<u>88</u>	8	<u>117</u>
# S1	20	5	10	<u>100</u>

Results expressed as % blocking of cytotoxicity calculated for the dilution of monoclonal antibodies showing the highest blocking. Underscored numbers indicate significant blocking of cytotoxicity.
NT, not tested
[a] Range of % blocking of repeated testing

References

1. Kavathas P, Bach FH, DeMars R (1980) Gamma ray-induced loss of expression of HLA and glyoxalase I alleles in lymphoblastoid cells. Proc Natl Acad Sci USA 77:4251-4255
2. Watson AJ, DeMars R, Trowbridge IS, Bach FH (1983) Detection of a novel human class II HLA antigen. Nature 304:358-360
3. Pawelec GP, Wernet P, Rosenlund R, Blaurock M, Schneider EM (1984) Strong lymphoproliferative suppressive function of PLT clones specific for SB-like antigens. Hum Immunol 9:145-157

This is paper # 389 from the Immunobiology Research Center, and was supported in part by NIH grants AI 17687, AI 18326, AM 13083, AI 19007, and the National Multiple Sclerosis Society grant # RG 1505-A-1 and the March of Dimes Birth Defects Foundation grant # 1-887

HLA Mutants of Lymphoblastoid Cell Lines: Generation of New Mutants and Analysis by Southern Blotting *

J.A. Nicklas [1], H. Noreen [1], N. Ohta [1], F.C. Grumet [2], and F.H. Bach [1]

1 Immunobiology Research Center, University of Minnesota, Minneapolis, MN 55455, USA
2 Department of Pathology, Stanford University, Stanford, CA 94305, USA

The study of the MHC of the mouse was greatly facilitated by the use of congenic and coisogenic strains; unfortunately, such tools are of course not available in man. The development of γ-ray-induced mutant cell lines deleted for HLA specificities by Kavathas et al. [1] created a human analog of coisogenic mouse strains. These mutants are extremely valuable for a number of immunologic and biochemical experiments, such as selection of specific cytotoxic T cell clones and definition of new genes in the HLA region.

This report describes additional mutants of the LCL 721 used by Kavathas et al. and mutants derived from a new cell line, LCL 526. The mutants were all derived using the method of Kavathas et

* This is paper # 390 from the Immunobiology Research Center. This work was supported in part by National Institutes of Health grants # RO1 AI 17687, AI 19007, and 2PO1 AM 13083; March of Dimes Birth Defects Foundation grant # A-188; National Multiple Sclerosis Society grant # RG 1505-A-1 to JAN, HN, NO, and FHB and grant HL 2972 to FCG

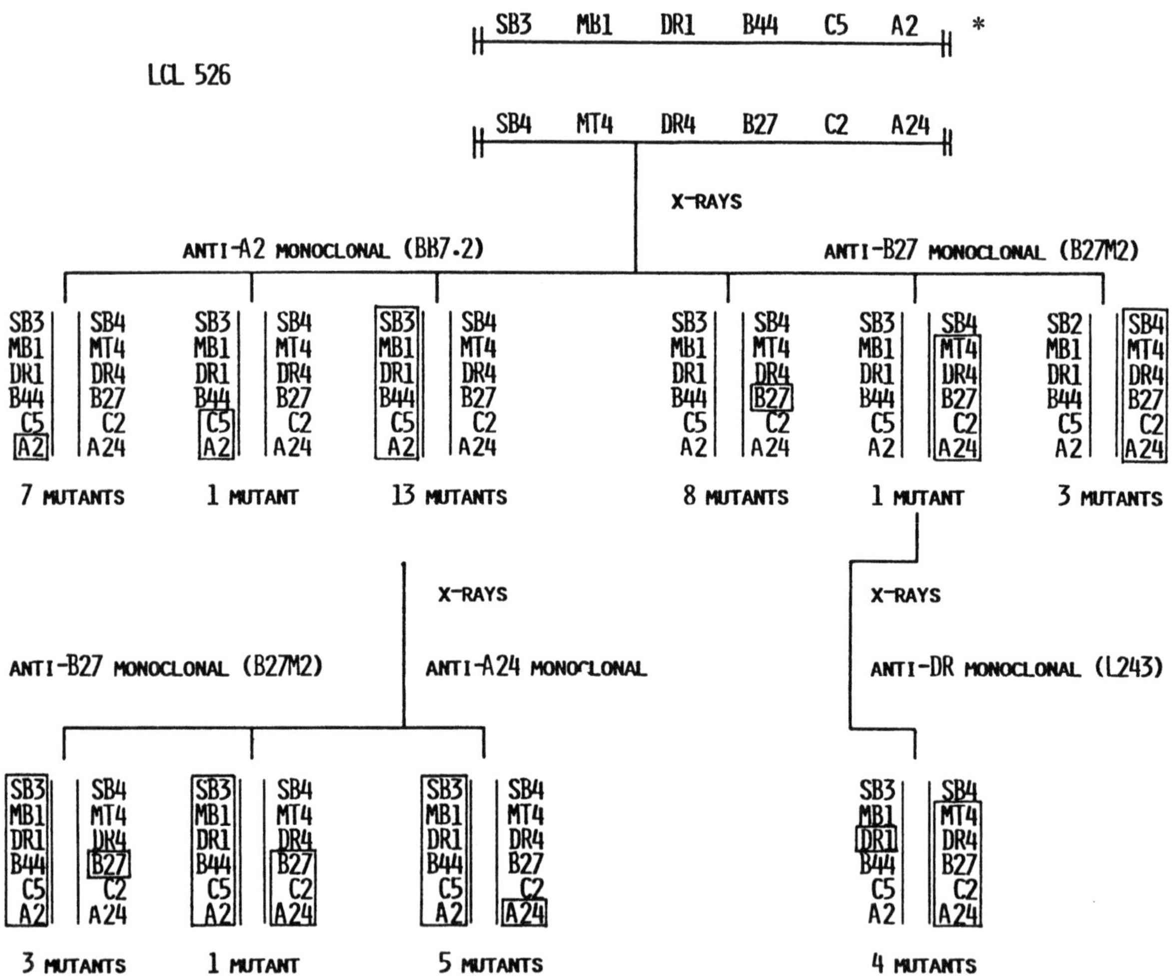

Fig. 1. The selection of HLA mutants of LCL 526 using X-irradiation to induce mutations and anti-HLA monoclonals and C′ for selection. The primary mutants were selected with either an anti-A2 monoclonal [2] or an anti-B27 monoclonal [3]. Subsequent X-ray treatment of primary mutants and selection with anti-B27, anti-A24, or anti-DR [4] monoclonals led to the induction of secondary loss mutants (A null, B null, and DR null). **Boxed specificities are lost.** *SB = DPw; MB = DQw; MT4 = DQw3; C = Cw

Histocompatibility Testing 1984
Edited by E. D. Albert et al.

al. [1], which consists of 300 rads γ-irradiation, a 5-day rest, treatment with an anti-HLA monoclonal and complement, and then plating in soft agar over irradiated fibroblasts. Growing colonies should be derived from cells which have lost the HLA specificity to which the monoclonal was directed. Expanded clones were typed using two-stage microcytotoxicity tests.

An anti-A2 monoclonal, BB7.2 [2] was used against LCL 721 (DPw4, DRw52, DR3, B8, A1/DPw2, DQw1, DR1, B5, A2). This treatment generated 13 A2 loss, 19 A2-B5 loss, 17 A2-B5-DR1-DQw1 loss, and 10 A2-B5-DR1-DQw1-DPw2 loss mutants. Figure 1 shows the mutants of LCL 526 that were obtained in several rounds of selection. These include both haplotype loss mutants, A2 loss, B27 loss, and A null, B null, A-B-C null and DR null mutants.

Preliminary Southern blots of haplotype loss variants of LCL 526, using both class I [5] and class II [6] probes, allowed the mapping of certain restriction fragments to each HLA haplotype. Additional Southern blots are planned with both the LCL 721 and the LCL 526 mutants, using DRβ, DQβ, DRα, and DPβ probes to elucidate the number and order of class II genes in man.

The induction of mutations in LCL 526 demonstrates the general applicability of the Kavathas method and allows the study of two new haplotypes. LCL 526 has the advantages of two defined C alleles and contains B27, which has relevance for disease studies. These mutants are generally available.

References

1. Kavathas P, Bach FH, DeMars R (1980) Gamma ray-induced loss of expression of HLA and glyoxalase I alleles in lymphoblastoid cells. Proc Natl Acad Sci USA 77:4251–4255
2. Parham P, Brodsky FM (1981) Partial purification and some properties of BB7.2 – A cytotoxic monoclonal antibody with specificity for HLA-A2 and a variant of HLA-A28. Hum Immunol 3:277–299
3. Grumet FC, Fendley BM, Fish L, Foung S, Engleman EG (1982) Monoclonal antibody (B27M2) subdividing HLA-B27. Hum Immunol 5:61–72
4. Lampson LA, Levy R (1980) Two populations of IA-like molecules on a human B cell lines. J Immunol 125:293–299
5. Sood AK, Pereira D, Weissman SM (1981) Isolation and partial nucleotide sequence of a cDNA clone for human histocompatibility antigen HLA-B by use of an oligodeoxy nucleotide primer. Proc Natl Acad Sci USA 78:616–620
6. Long EO, Wake CT, Strubin M, Gross N, Accolla RS, Carrel S, Mach B (1982) Isolation of distinct cDNA clones encoding HLA-DRβ chains by use of an expression assay. Proc Natl Acad Sci USA 79:7465–7469

Mutant Cell Lines as Means of Resolving HLA Gene Products

C. Müller, B. Spring, A. Ziegler, G. Pawelec, C. Fonatsch, and P. Wernet

Immunology Laboratory, Medical Clinic II, 7400 Tübingen, Federal Republic of Germany

Introduction

Mutants of lymphoblastoid cell lines have helped to identify, dissect, and locate genes of defined HLA products particularly within the HLA-D region [1]. They can be used to characterize still unknown human MHC antigens and genes.

Methods

Fifteen mutants were established from a clone of the B lymphoma cell line BJAB.B95.8.6 after mutagenization with γ-ray irradiation and subsequent immunoselection with the monoclonal antibodies TÜ101, TÜ109, and TÜ48. Ninth Workshop alloantisera and monoclonal reagents were used to define their HLA phenotype. Immunoprecipitation followed by IEF analysis was applied for further study of expressed MHC products.

Results and Discussion

The parental cell clone BJAB. B95.8.6 typed as HLA-A1, A2, B13, B35, Bw4, Bw6, Cw4, DR5, DRw52, DQw1, DQw3, DPw2, DPw4. No second HLA-DR allele could be unequivocally defined, although reactivity both with anti-DRw10 alloantisera and with the anti-DR2 monoclonal antibody NDS15.38 [2] was found. The mutants lacked reactivity with all monospecific anti-HLA-A2, B13, and Bw4 alloantisera, but retained HLA-A1, B35, Bw6, Cw4, DR5, DRw52, DQw3 and DPw4 de-

Histocompatibility Testing 1984
Edited by E. D. Albert et al.

fined by cellular studies. Loss of HLA-A2, B13 was confirmed by biochemical analysis. HLA typing thus suggested HLA-A2, B13, Bw4, DR –, DQw1, DPw2 as a mutated, and HLA-A1, B35, Bw6, Cw4, DR5, DRw52, DQw3, DPw4 as an unchanged haplotype of the parental cell line. Three different patterns of HLA-D region antigen alterations could be distinguished by serological and cellular analysis: (a) DQw1$^+$, DPw2$^+$ (6 mutants); (b) DQw1$^-$, DPw2$^+$ (3 mutants); and (c) DQw1$^-$, DPw2$^-$ (4 mutants). Loss of HLA antigens appeared to correlate with different deletions in the 6p21.3 – 6p23.0 regions on one of the no. 6 chromosomes according to karyotype analysis. Retention of an unexpected cytotoxicity of alloantisera directed against HLA-B13-related CREG specificities or of anti-DRw10 antisera indicated either contaminating antibodies specific for antigens of the unchanged haplotype or continued expression of still undefined molecules encoded by genes on the mutated chromosome 6. Thus these mutants could be of value for the serological characterization of HLA gene products that are still unknown or have so far been detected only by cellular analysis.

Summary

MHC mutants with multilocus deletions were established from a clone of the B lymphoma cell line BJAB.B95.8 by γ-ray irradiation and subsequent immunoselection with monoclonal antibodies. Fifteen loss mutants all lacking the expression of HLA-A2, B13, and Bw4 but retaining HLA-A1, B35, Bw6, Cw4, DR5, DRw52, and DQw3 of the parental cell line showed three different patterns of HLA-DQw1/DPw2 antigen alterations. These changes in the HLA phenotype appeared to correlate with gene duplications and/or deletions on one of the no. 6 chromosomes.

References

1. Pious C, Krangel M, Dixon L, Parham P, Strominger J (1982) HLA antigen structural gene mutants selected with an allospecific monoclonal antibody. Proc Natl Acad Sci USA 79:7832 – 7836
2. Suggle S, Kirkley J, Ting A, Morris P (1983) A monoclonal antibody recognizing HLA-DR2 on malignant and activated cells. Immunogenetics 18:415 – 418

Human T Cell Clone Inhibition by Distinct Monoclonal Anti-HLA-DR Antibodies

F. Triebel, D.J. Charron, and P. Debré

Laboratoire d'Immunogénétique, CHU Pitié-Salpétrière, 91 boulevard de l'Hôpital, 75013 Paris, France

Inhibition studies of the specific proliferative response of T cell clones with different anti-HLA-DR monoclonal antibodies (moAb) should help to relate the structure and the function of multiple DR epitopes. We now describe the inhibition of diphtheria toxoid- and Varidase-specific T cell clone proliferative responses in a single DRw6/7 donor by eight distinct monoclonal anti-HLA-DR moAbs. These moAbs were selected because they have already been biochemically characterized. MoAbs 141, D1.12, VI-15 C, and 157, which detected very similar epitopic specificities, immunoprecipitated only DR molecules on DR 1 – w8. MoAbs 206 and 135, which detected different epitopes, recognized DR (I-E-like) molecules in most of the alleles and also DQ (I-A-like) molecules in DR7 individuals. BM 50 recognized molecules of all alleles except DR7 and the corresponding subgroup of DRw6. MoAbs 141 and 135, 157, and BM 50 shared idiotypic specificities. BM Mag 8 had a cross-reactive idiotope in common with 141 and 135. Our results showed a distinct inhibition pattern of specific proliferative response for each clone. Furthermore, the various moAbs could be classified into three groups according to their inhibitory effect on T cell proliferation: BM Mag 8, BM 50, 141, and 135 moAbs had little or no effect on T cell proliferation. In contrast, VI-15 C, D1-12, and to a lesser extent 157 moAbs had a marked or pronounced blocking effect. The 206 moAb gave intermediate results (Table 1). In other experiments, the proliferative responses specific for diphtheria toxoid of T cell clones from another DRw6/7 individual were shown to be genetically restricted by the DR7 haplotype. Responses of these clones were inhibited by 135 and D1-12 but not by BM 50. Since 135 and D1.12 recognize two different Ia epitopes on DR7, these results indicate that at least two different epitopes on the DR7 molecule participate in the clonal proliferative response. Together these

Histocompatibility Testing 1984
Edited by E. D. Albert et al.

Table 1. Effects of anti-DR moAbs on specific T cell clones

moAb	Number of clones with relative response > 50%	Number of clones with relative response 20% – 50%	Number of clones with relative response < 20%
BM Mag 8	11	0	0
BM 50	11	0	0
141	10	1	0
135	9	2	0
206	7	2	2
157	4	4	3
VI-15 C	1	0	10
D1.12	2	4	5

data suggest (a) an epitopic restriction by class II antigens of specific human T cell clone proliferation; (b) the recognition of functional epitopes on the human Ia by some but not all moAbs studied; and (c) the participation of more than a single functional Ia determinant in class II restricted proliferative responses to soluble antigens.

Variation in the Epitopes on the HLA-A2 Molecule as Recognized by HLA-A2-Restricted and Alloimmune HLA-A2-Specific Cytotoxic T Lymphocytes*

J.J. van der Poel, E. Goulmy, M.J. Giphart, and J.J. van Rood

Department of Immunohaematology, University Medical Center, 2333 AA Leiden, The Netherlands

Introduction

Serologically defined HLA specificities can be subdivided by biochemical and immunobiological techniques. Especially the use of cytotoxic lymphocytes (CTLs) has been shown to be effective in this regard. Polymorphism within the serologically defined HLA-A2 antigen was demonstrated by means of HLA-A2-restricted influenza virus-specific CTLs [1], Epstein-Barr virus (EBV)-specific CTLs [2], HLA-A2-restricted H-Y-specific CTLs [3], and HLA-A2-specific alloimmune CTLs [4, 5]. Analysis of the heterogeneity of the HLA-A2 antigen in a combined biochemical and alloimmune CTL study revealed the existence of four distinct HLA-A2 subtypes. The major HLA-A2 subtype, designated HLA-A2.1, includes 89% of the serologically defined HLA-A2 antigen. The remaining 11% could be divided into three minor HLA-A2 subtypes, designated HLA-A2.2, HLA-A2.3, and HLA-A2.4 [6]. Previously, we have shown that HLA-A2-restricted anti-H-Y CTLs failed to recognize lymphocytes of the male HLA-A2 variant "M7" [3]. Recently, we analyzed the reaction patterns of HLA-A2-restricted minor histocompatibility (minor H) antigen-specific CTLs against lymphocytes from individuals who carried the HLA-A2.2, HLA-A2.3, or HLA-A2.4 subtypes. The results indicated that the minor HLA-A2 subtype antigens have, generally speaking, lost the relevant epitope(s) for associative recognition of minor H antigens by minor H antigen-specific CTLs [7].
Nevertheless, one exception was found. An HLA-A2.4 subtype positive individual was recognized by HLA-A2-restricted anti-H-Y CTLs [7]. Subsequently, the HLA-A2.4 subgroup was analyzed with HLA-A2-restricted minor H antigen-specific CTLs and alloimmune HLA-A2.4 subtype-specific CTLs. The results reported here show that using different types of HLA-A2-specific CTLs, ad-

* Supported in part by the Dutch Foundation for Medical Research (FUNGO), which is subsidized by the Dutch Organisation for the Advancement of Pure Research (ZWO), the J.A. Cohen Institute for Radiopathology and Radiation Protection (IRS), and the Dutch Kidney Foundation

Histocompatibility Testing 1984
Edited by E. D. Albert et al.

Table 1. HLA-A and B phenotypes of the anti-HLA-A2.4 CTL combinations

Responder cells	Stimulator cells
CTL 4: A1, A9; B8, Bw50	Individual 3 A1, A2.4; B8, Bw50
CTL 5: A1; B8, B35	Individual 4 A2.4, A24; B8, B35
CTL 6: A1, Aw19; B8, B27	Individual 1 A1, A2.4; B8, B27
CTL 7: A2.1, A24; B8, B35	Individual 4 A2.4, A24; B8, B35

ditional polymorphism can be demonstrated within the heterogeneous HLA-A2 specificity. The relationship between the recognition patterns of both types of CTLs at the level of the HLA-A2 target molecule will be discussed.

Materials and Methods

The HLA-A2-restricted minor H antigen-specific CTLs used were as follows:
CTL 1: HLA-A2-restricted anti-H-Y CTLs
CTL 2: HLA-A2- and B7-restricted anti-H-Y CTLs
CTL 3: HLA-A2-, B27-, and Bw62-restricted anti-minor HA CTLs
These CTLs have been described in detail [8 – 10].
Alloimmune CTLs directed against the HLA-A2.4 subtype were made using the cell donors listed in Table 1. CTLs were established by standard mixed lymphocyte cultures for 6 days, followed by T cell growth factor expansion [5].
Cell-mediated lympholysis (CML) was performed as described in detail [4, 5]. Experimental results for the alloimmune CTLs were normalized to a percent relative cytotoxic response (RCR), based on the specific response of a given CTL by the formula:

$$\frac{\text{percent release of experimental target}}{\text{percent release of specific target}} \times 100 = \%\text{RCR}$$

RCR values up to 25% were considered as negative cytotoxic reactions. Values greater than 60% were considered as positive, while values ranging from 25% to 40% were considered as weak cytotoxic reactions [5].

Results

Analysis of HLA-A2-Restricted Anti-Minor H Antigen-Specific CTLs Against the HLA-A2.1, A2.2, and A2.3, Subtypes

The anti-minor H CTLs themselves carried the HLA-A2.1 major subtype antigen and are therefore HLA-A2.1 restricted. As shown in Table 2, the three anti-minor H CTLs recognized, as expected, the HLA-A2.1 antigen when the appropriate minor H antigens (i.e. H-Y or minor HA) were present. The reactivity pattern of the HLA-A2-restricted minor H-specific CTLs was analyzed on lymphocytes from individuals carrying the HLA-A2.2 and A2.3 minor subtypes. No reactivity was found on the A2.2 and A2.3 subtype-positive individuals (Table 2). These data confirmed and extended the observation made with the HLA-A2-restricted anti-H-Y CTL 1 on the male HLA-A2 variant "M7" [3]. The results indicated that the absence of the target determinant, as expressed on the HLA-A2.1 molecule, led to the loss of the epitope(s) necessary for the associative recognition of the minor H antigens by minor H-specific CTLs [7].

Table 2. Reactivity pattern of HLA-A2.1-restricted anti-minor H antigen-specific CTLs against the HLA-A2.1, A2.2, and A2.3 subtypes

Target cell specificity	Sex/no of target cell tested	Reactivity pattern with		
		CTL 1	CTL 2	CTL 3
HLA-A2.1	Male/50	+	+	+
	Female/20	–	–	+
HLA-A2.2[a]	Male/3	–	–	–
	Female/4	–	–	–
HLA-A2.3[a]	Male/2	–	–	–
	Female/2	–	–	–

[a] Individuals carrying other antigens (i.e., HLA-B7, Bw62, and B27) which can function as restricting molecules for associative recognition of minor H-Y or minor HA were excluded

Table 3. Reactivity patterns of the minor H antigen-specific CTLs on the HLA-A2.4 subtype-positive individuals

Target cell individual	Presence (+) or absence (–) of restricting molecule				Reactivity pattern with		
	A2.4	B7	B27	Bw62	CTL 1	CTL 2	CTL3
2	+	–	+	+	–	–	+
3	+	–	–	–	–	–	–
4	+	–	–	–	+	+	–
5	+	+	–	–	+	+	–
6	+	–	–	–	+	+	+

All target cells were obtained from males

Reactivity of HLA-A2-Restricted Anti-Minor H Antigen-Specific CTLs on the HLA-A2.4 Subtype

The reactivity pattern obtained with the HLA-A2-restricted minor H CTLs against the HLA-A2.4 subtype-positive individuals, as shown in Table 3, is more complex. As expected, negative reactions were found on several HLA-A2.4-positive individuals. However, positive reactions were also observed against the lymphocytes from some individuals carrying the HLA-A2.4 subtype. Apparently, the restricting epitope(s) necessary for the recognition by the minor H CTLs, as present on the HLA-A2.1 molecule, were retained in those individuals.

When the reactivity pattern of the two anti-H-Y CTLs 1 and 2 was analyzed, positive reactions were observed on lymphocytes from individuals 4, 5, and 6. The lymphocytes from individuals 2 and 3 were not recognized. Thus, by using the anti-H-Y CTLs, the HLA-A2.4 subgroup can be subdivided. When the reactivity pattern of the HLA-A2-, B27-, and Bw62-restricted anti-minor HA CTL 3 was analyzed, fewer positive reactions were observed.

Only the lymphocytes from individuals 2 and 6 were recognized by CTL 3. The positive reaction of CTL 3 on individual 2 was caused by the presence of another restricting molecule, namely HLA-Bw62, in addition to the HLA-A2.4 molecule. This is supported by segregation studies (data not shown). As far as the recognition of the HLA-A2.4 subtype antigen is concerned, only one (i.e., individual 6) out of the five individuals tested, were recognized by the minor HA-specific CTL 3. Individuals 4 and 5, lysed by the anti-H-Y CTLs 1 and 2, have lost the epitope(s) necessary for the recognition by the anti-minor HA CTL 3.

Thus, the A2.4 subgroup can also be subdivided by using the anti-minor HA CTL 3. Apparently, the anti-minor H-Y CTLs and the anti-minor HA CTL do not always use the same restricting epitope(s) on the HLA-A2 molecule. The cytotoxic reactions of the HLA-A2-restricted anti-minor H antigen-specific CTLs against the A2.4 subtype can be divided into three patterns:

1. Absence of recognition by anti-H-Y- and anti-minor HA specific CTLs, thus loss of the epitope(s) for associative recognition of minor H-Y and minor HA
2. Recognition by anti-H-Y-specific CTLs only, thus retention of epitope(s) for associative recognition of minor H-Y, but loss of epitope(s) for associative recognition of minor HA.
3. Recognition by anti-H-Y- and anti-minor HA-specific CTLs, indicating, despite the presence of the A2.4 subtype molecule, the presence of epitope(s) for the associative recognition of both minor H antigens, H-Y and HA.

The latter situation is in fact identical with the reaction pattern obtained in the HLA-A2.1 subtype-positive individuals (see previous section).

Alloimmune HLA-A2.4 Subtype-Specific CTLs

We have previously shown that the HLA-A2.4 subtype was defined by a lack of recognition by HLA-A2.1 and A2.2 subtype-specific CTLs [6].

We have been able to show that also HLA-A2.3-specific CTLs failed to lyse HLA-A2.4 subtype-positive individuals (van der Poel et al., manuscript in preparation). It should be emphasized that the HLA-A2.1-, A2.2-, and A2.3-specific CTLs clearly identified individuals carrying the relevant subtype antigen. Since this approach was successful, CTLs were made against A2.4 subtype-positive individuals in order to positively select for the A2.4 antigen. Four CTLs could be made against three of the A2.4 subtype-positive individuals identified (Table 1).

The alloimmune CTLs 4 to 7 were tested against six HLA-A2.4 subtype-positive individuals. As shown in Table 4, the reactivity patterns of CTL 4 to 7 within the HLA-A2.4 subgroup were complex. CTL 4 reacted with all individuals carrying the HLA-A2.4 subtype antigen.

CTL 5 recognized individuals 4 (specific stimulator), 5, and 6. Lymphocytes from individuals 1, 2, and 3 were only weakly lysed. CTL 7, which was made against the same stimulator cell (i.e., individual 4) as CTL 5, showed the same reactivity pattern as CTL 5. Thus, using CTL 5 and CTL 7, the A2.4 subgroup could be subdivided.

CTL 6 recognized individuals 1 (specific stimulator), 2, 4, and 5. Lymphocytes from individual 3 were not recognized at all, while targets from individual 6 were weakly lysed by CTL 6. Thus, the A2.4 subgroup could also be subdivided by using

Table 4. Reactivity patterns of HLA-A2.4 subtype-specific alloimmune CTLs on HLA-A2.4 subtype-positive individuals

Target cell individual	CTL 4	CTL 5	CTL 6	CTL 7
1	87[a]	25	100	17
2	97	40	98	21
3	100	32	7	20
4	78	100	77	100
5	71	90	82	87
6	66	85	35	74

[a] Results are expressed as mean % RCR obtained with the alloimmune CTL indicated

CTL 6. CML analysis of the HLA-A2.4 subtype antigen with the alloimmune HLA-A2.4 subtype-specific CTLs demonstrated that further heterogeneity in the A2.4 subgroup existed.

Discussion

The reaction patterns of HLA-A2-restricted minor H antigen (minor H-Y and minor HA)-specific CTLs and alloimmune HLA-A2 subtype-specific CTLs against lymphocytes from individuals carrying different HLA-A2 subtypes have been analyzed. The presence of the minor H-Y antigen, a prerequisite for recognition by CTL 1 and 2, is easily controllable since it is sex-linked. The minor HA antigen, recognized by CTL 3, is present in 95% of the HLA-A2.1 subtype-positive individuals and can, furthermore, be verified by family studies in most cases [7]. The minor H-specific CTLs 1 and 2 (anti-minor H-Y) and CTL 3 (anti-minor HA), which were HLA-A2.1 restricted, recognized A2.1 subtype-positive individuals carrying the relevant minor H antigen. Absence of lysis was observed when lymphocytes from individuals carrying the HLA-A2.2 and A2.3 subtype were tested with the two types of HLA-A2-restricted anti-minor H CTLs. The A2.2 and A2.3 subtype molecules must have lost the epitope(s) necessary for associative recognition by the minor H antigen-specific CTLs. The cytotoxic reactions of the anti-minor H CTLs on the HLA-A2.4 subtype can be divided into three patterns:

1. Loss of epitope(s) necessary for recognition by both minor H antigen-specific CTLs
2. Loss of epitope(s) for minor HA recognition but retention of epitope(s) for minor H-Y recognition
3. Retention of epitope(s) for recognition by both anti-minor H CTLs despite the presence of an HLA-A2.4 subtype antigen.

For the A2.4-positive individuals 4 and 5, belonging to the second category, the absence of the minor H antigen HA could not be excluded. This might explain the lack of recognition by CTL 3. However, since the minor H antigen HA is present in 95% of the HLA-A2.1-positive individuals tested, we favor the interpretation that the epitope(s) necessary for associative recognition were absent. One explanation would be that the minor H-Y and minor HA CTLs use different epitope(s) on the HLA-A2.4 molecule for associative recognition.

An alternative explanation would be that the A2.4 subgroup can be divided into three subtypes. In order to prove the latter assumption, alloimmune HLA-A2.4 subtype-specific CTLs were generated.

It should be noted that the definition of the A2.4 subtype was essentially based on the lack of recognition by HLA-A2.1-, A2.2-, and A2.3-specific alloimmune CTLs. The finding that the A2.4 subtype is not lysed by A2.1 subtype-specific CTLs was confirmed independently by Brenner and Strominger using a cytotoxic T cell clone which was A2.1 specific (M. Brenner and J. L. Strominger, personal communication). This confirmation reinforces the notion that the A2.4 subtype is genuine.

Further heterogeneity was found within the A2.4 subtype using A2.4-specific alloimmune CTLs. Three types of reaction patterns were observed (see Table 4). In fact, it seems that the four unrelated A2.4-positive individuals 1, 3, 4, and 6 differ from each other with respect to the epitopes recognized by the anti-A2.4 subtype-specific CTLs tested. When the relationship between the alloimmune CTLs and the anti-minor H CTLs within the A2.4 subgroup is compared, it is seen that the reaction pattern of alloimmune CTLs 4 and 6 do not correlate with the reaction pattern of the anti minor H CTLs. However, the reaction pattern of alloimmune CTLs 5 and 7 are identical to that of the anti-H-Y CTLs 1 and 2, since these CTLs recognized the A2.4-positive individuals 4, 5, and 6. The epitope(s) which these CTLs recognize on the A2 molecule may be identical, but this can probably only be stated with certainty when the reactivity pattern is analyzed at the clonal level. Biochemical analyses may eventually bring answers to this problem. Amino acid differences have been shown to exist in the tryptic peptide spanning residues 147–157 in the A2 heavy polypeptide chains of the A2.1, A2.2 and A2.3 subtype [11, 12] (J. L. Strominger, personal communication). These differences have been postulated to be of functional relevance for the recognition by CTLs [12]. The results obtained with CML analysis of the HLA-A2.4 subtype predict that differences in amino acid sequence would have to be found within the A2.4 subgroup and between the A2.4 and the other A2 subtypes. Amino acid sequence data should clarify this issue.

One other point should be taken in consideration. Additional polymorphism might be generated by differences in folding of the A2 molecule, resulting in conformational changes. The conformation of molecules seems to be important for the recogniton by CTLs [13].

Therefore conformational changes in the different HLA-A2 subtype molecules may explain the reaction patterns obtained with the minor H antigen-specific CTLs and the alloimmune HLA-A2.4-specific CTLs.

References

1. Biddison WE, Ward FE, Shearer GM, Shaw S (1980) The self determinants recognized by human virus immune T cells can be distinguished from the serologically defined HLA antigens. J Immunol 124:548–552
2. Gaston JSH, Rickinson AB, Epstein MA (1983) Epstein-Barr virus specific cytotoxic T lymphocytes as probes of HLA polymorphism. J Exp Med 158:280–293
3. Goulmy E, Van Leeuwen A, Blokland E, Van Rood JJ, Biddison WE (1982) MHC restricted H-Y specific antibodies and cytotoxic T lymphocytes can recognize different self determinants. J Exp Med 155:1567–1572
4. Horai S, Van der Poel JJ, Goulmy E (1982) Differential recognition of the serologically defined HLA-A2 antigen by allogeneic cytotoxic T cells. I. Population studies. Immunogenetics 16:135–142
5. Van der Poel JJ, Pool J, Goulmy E, Van Rood JJ (1983) Differential recognition of the serologically defined HLA-A2 antigen by allogeneic cytotoxic T cells. II. Definition of three HLA-A2 subtypes by CTLs. Immunogenetics 17:599–608
6. Van der Poel JJ, Mölders H, Thompson A, Ploegh HL (1983) Definition of four HLA-A2 subtypes by CML typing and biochemical analysis. Immunogenetics 17:609–621
7. Goulmy E, Van der Poel JJ, Giphart MJ, Van Rood JJ (1984) Analysis of the functional epitopes on different HLA-A2 molecules. Immunogenetics 20:13–21
8. Goulmy E, Termijtelen A, Bradley BA, Van Rood JJ (1977) Y antigen killing by women is restricted by HLA. Nature 266:544–545
9. Goulmy E, Hamilton JD, Bradley BA (1979) Anti-self HLA may be clonally expressed. J Exp Med 149: 545–550
10. Goulmy E, Gratama JW, Blokland E, Zwaan FE, Van Rood JJ (1983) A minor transplantation antigen detected by MHC restricted cytotoxic T lymphocytes during graft versus host disease. Nature 302:159–161
11. Krangel MS, Taketani S, Biddison WE, Strong DM, Strominger JL (1982) Comparative structural analysis of HLA-A2 antigens distinguishable by cytotoxic T lymphocytes: Variants M7 and DR1. Biochemistry 21:6313–6321
12. Krangel MS, Biddison WE, Strominger JL (1983) Comparative structural analysis of HLA-A2 antigens distinguishable by cytotoxic T lymphocytes. II. Variant DK1: evidence for a discrete CTL recognition region. J Immunol 130:1856–1862
13. De Waal LP, Nathenson SG, Melief CJM (1984) Direct demonstration that cytotoxic T lymphocytes recognize conformational determinants and not primary amino acid sequences. J Exp Med 158:1720–1726

Cloned Cytotoxic T Cells Which May Define a Minor Transplantation Antigen and a Variant of the HLA-B8 Molecule

P.F. Pfeffer, E. Qvigstad, and E. Thorsby

Institute of Transplantation Immunology, The National Hospital, 0027 Oslo 1, Norway

A male patient (HLA-A3,9; B8,15; DR3,w6) first rejected a female cadaveric kidney (HLA-A1,10; B8,40; DR3,8) and then a kidney from his HLA identical sister. The recipient and his sister typed identically with Ninth Workshop antisera and pretransplant MLC tests were reciprocally negative. Six weeks after the rejection the recipient responded weakly to the sister in MLC tests and he formed cytotoxic T cells (CTLs) reactive with his sibling donor. These T cells were then cloned.

Two clones with different specificities (clones 20 and 23) were tested (Table 1). Clone 20 lysed target cells from the HLA identical donor, from some family members, and from approximately 50% of unrelated individuals carrying HLA-B15. This clone probably recognizes a minor transplantation antigen and is restricted by B15.

Table 1. Specificity of donor-specific cytotoxic T cell clones

Target cells	HLA-A,B specificities shared with the recipient	Clones tested 20	Clones tested 23
Donor	3, 9; 8, 15	81[a]	73
Mother	9; 8	0	37
Father	3, ; 15	64	5
Sibling 1	9; 8	1	32
Sibling 2	3, 9; 8, 15	0	37
Sibling 3	3, ; 15	65	0
Unrelated ($U_1 - U_{10}$)	; 8	0–10	22–44
Unrelated ($U_{11} - U_{15}$)	; 15	50–87	0–14
Unrelated ($U_{16} - U_{20}$)	; 15	0–8	0–2
Unrelated ($U_{21} - U_{29}$)	3, 9;	0–14	0–7

[a] % Cytotoxicity

Histocompatibility Testing 1984
Edited by E. D. Albert et al.

Clone 23 lysed target cells from the HLA identical donor and all family and unrelated individuals carrying HLA-B8. This clone may recognize an almost ubiquitous minor transplantation antigen (which the recipient lacks), and be restricted by B8. Alternatively, the recipient may have inherited a "variant" B8 molecule from his mother (by point mutation or gene conversion), thereby being able to recognize the nonvariant B8 antigen of the sibling donor and most others (including the first cadaveric donor) as foreign. When CTLs were generated toward ("non-variant") B8 using third-party responding and stimulating cells, they lysed target cells from all B8 family members, except those from the recipient. This suggests, but does not prove, that the recipient may have inherited a "variant" of B8, which may be recognized by CTLs but not by available antisera. Biochemical studies are under way.

Construction and Expansion of CTLs for HLA Typing: Definition of B44 Subtypes by Cellular Typing

P.W. Hansen, S.E. Christiansen, F. Kissmeyer-Nielsen, and T. Kristensen

The Tissue Typing Laboratory, University Hospital of Aarhus, 8000 Aarhus, Denmark

Introduction

The polymorphic gene products of the human HLA region can be identified both by serological and cellular typing techniques. Although the definition of the system, its loci, and their antigenic determinants is in essence based on serological studies and analyses, it is now evident that a determinant primarily described by one technique, e.g., serology, may be detected similarly by the other, viz cellular typing (MLC, PLT, or CML). Thus, serological and cellular typing studies are equally precise with regard to specificity and must supplement each other.

This paper concerns the definition of the serologically defined HLA-A, B, C antigens by cytotoxic T lymphocytes (CTLs) and focuses on the definition of antigenic subtypes not as yet defined by serology. Such observations are not new. Mawas et al. [1], Kristensen et al. [2], Schendel et al. [3], and Goulmy et al. [4] all published similar results, but tended to interpret them as evidence for new loci in the HLA region. Recent studies extending our biochemical knowledge of the HLA molecules suggest that a majority of the discrepancies observed earlier can in all probability be attributed to CTL recognition of epitopes on classical HLA molecules not as yet defined by antibodies [5–11].

Cellular typing research in this area, however, has until recently been impeded by the fact that only small numbers of CTLs could be produced at a time, resulting in considerable experimental variance due to the use of different CTL batches. Further, the relatively low numbers of active CTLs in classical CML effector combinations called for high effector-to-target (E/T) ratios or extensive E/T titrations.

Initiated by our participation in the European CML Study Group, we have developed methods for production of interleukin-2 (IL-2)-conditioned media and expansion of classical CML effector combinations into T cell lines based on the studies of Gillis et al. [12]. Consequently, large batches of CTL-enriched effector combinations may be ready at any time, enabling cellular typing of selected panels, populations, and families with identical CTLs. We used this approach to study the serological HLA-B44 determinant. (For an extensive review on the CTL approach to HLA typing, see [13].)

Material and Methods

Cells were prepared from defibrinated blood using Isopaque-Ficoll separation. Donors were selected from our files of HLA-typed healthy individuals, in some special cases including their family.

CTL Generation

Primary cultures were set up according to the protocol adopted by the European CML Study Group [14]. In brief, equal numbers of responding and 4000-rad-irradiated stimulating cells were mixed in

Histocompatibility Testing 1984
Edited by E. D. Albert et al.

culture medium [RPMI, 20% v/v human heat-inactivated serum (pool of 25 male donors regardless of AB0 Type), antibiotics, and L-glutamine]. Cultures were established in vertically placed Falcon flasks (3013) or 2 ml/well cluster plates (NUNC) (final cell concentration 10^6/ml), and incubated for 6 days at 37 °C, 5% CO_2 in a humidified atmosphere.

Short-term expansion: On day 6 the cell concentration in primary culture was determined. After transfer to larger flasks, the cultures were diluted by addition of IL-2-conditioned medium (see below) to a final concentration of 0.2×10^6 cells/ml. Every 3–4 days this procedure was repeated. After 2–3 feedings (day 14–17) the total of cells exceeded the initial number of responding cells by a factor of 10–20. Immediately prior to the assay, growing cells were washed once and resuspended to the desired effector cell concentration in culture medium.

Preparation of IL-2-Conditioned Medium by PHA Stimulation

Fifty to sixty milliliters of defibrinated blood was obtained from each of five donors. Mononuclear cells were isolated, lightly irradiated (900 rad), and resuspended at 10^6 cells/ml in RPMI supplemented with 1% human serum pool + antibiotics + L-glutamine. PHA (Wellcome) was added to each culture at a final concentration of 1% v/v. After 24 h, individual cultures were harvested, cells removed by centrifugation and the culture supernatants were pooled, sterile filtered (0.22 µm), and freeze stored (−20 °C). These culture supernatants were used at a final concentration of 40% v/v for preparation of the IL-2-conditioned medium.

PHA Targets

Three days before the CML assay the cell panel to be typed was thawed and stimulated with 1% v/v PHA.

CML Assay

A standard [14] 4-h ^{51}Cr release assay was performed in V-bottomed microplates. Tests were done in duplicate at varying effector : target ratios. Maximum release was determined with Zaponin, spontaneous release was determined by incubating cells in medium alone. The maximum and spontaneous releases were performed in quadruplicate. Plates were centrifuged at 500 *g* for 5 min and half the test volume was transferred to plastic tubes using a four-channel Titertek multipipette. Tubes were sealed and counted in a Packard Autogamma Counter.

Calculation

Percentage cytotoxicity =

$$\frac{\text{experimental (cpm)} - \text{spontaneous (cpm)}}{\text{maximum (cpm)} - \text{spontaneous (cpm)}} \times 100\%$$

Autologous and specific targets (i.e., targets autologous to the responder and the stimulator respectively) were included in the panels. The relative response was expressed as:

$$\frac{\text{Percentage cytotoxicity (experimental target)}}{\text{Percentage cytotoxicity (specific target)}} \times 100\%$$

Results and Discussion

Specificity of CTL P/Jx

In a collaborative CML study, a CTL (P/Jx) was constructed which was anticipated to contain mainly anti-HLA-B7 components (responder: HLA-A1,2; B8,44; Cw–; stimulator: HLA-A1,2; B7,44; Cw5). In each laboratory participating in the European CML Study Group this CTL was tested against selected, local panels consisting of five B7-negative and five B7-positive targets using a standardized method. The CTL was tested after primary culture as well as after short-term expansion in different local and commercial IL-2-conditioned media. The anti-B7 specificity was amply confirmed: ++ 20, +– 0, –+ 2, –– 18. The two extrareactions concerned two HLA-B44-positive targets and were reproducible. The 18 negative targets were B44 negative, indicating the extrareactivity to be B44 associated.

Testing CTL P/Jx in a Selected B7-Negative, B44-Positive Panel

CTL P/Jx was subsequently tested against a local panel of ten B7-negative, B44-positive individuals. Testing was done after primary culture of CTL P/Jx and repeated after expansion. Results are shown in Fig. 1. In primary culture discrimination is poor at E/T = 10 : 1, but a dichotomy becomes apparent at E/T = 40 : 1, dividing the panel into five positive and five negative targets. After expansion of the CTL, the same dichotomy is already apparent at E/T = 10 : 1, where the general level of cytotoxicity is clearly higher. At E/T = 40 : 1, the

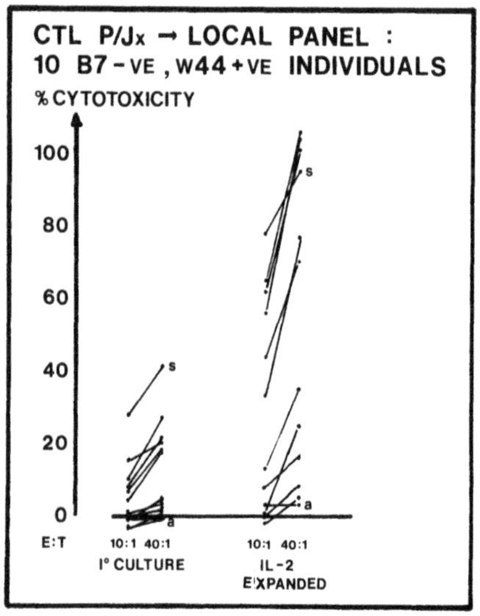

Fig. 1. CTL P/Jx tested against a selected panel of ten B7-negative, B44-positive individuals. Results are shown as percentage cytotoxicity at E/T ratios of 10 : 1 and 40 : 1, both after 1 ° culture and after IL-2 expansion *s*, specific target; *a*, autologous target

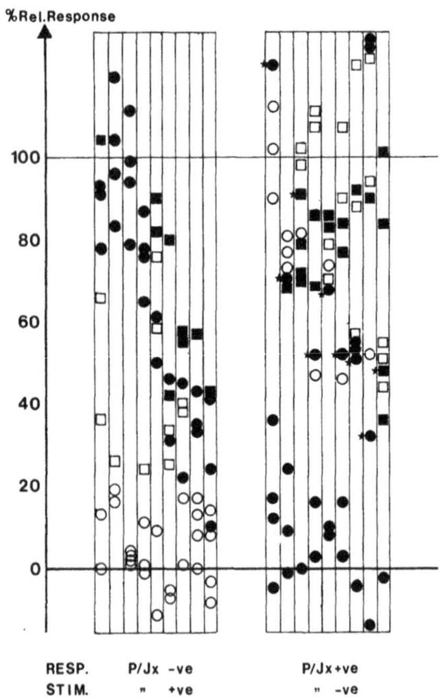

Fig. 2. Relative responses against the panel of Fig. 1 of nine CTLs generated by combinatorial mixing of three B44.1-negative cells against three B44.1-positive cells (*left column*) and nine CTLs obtained by reciprocal priming (*right column*). For further details see text. ●, B44.1-positive cell; ○, B44.1-negative cell; ■, B44.1-positive cell, additional cytotoxicity expected due to other recognized HLA antigens; □, B44.1-negative cell, additional cytotoxicity expected due to other recognized HLA antigens; *, see text, beginning of Family Study section

level of cytotoxicity against the five negative targets is comparable to the cytotoxicity obtained with unexpanded CTL against the five positive targets, but remains fully negative against the autologous target. The dichotomy is still apparent, since cytotoxicity is remarkably increased against the five targets in the "high-level" group.

Construction of CTL By Combined Mixing Within the Panel

The simplest interpretation of these data is that CTL-P/Jx defines one B44-associated epitope (B44.1) which is consequently shared by the five positive target cells but absent in the five negative targets. To test the validity of this interpretation, nine CTLs were generated by combinatorial priming of three B44.1 negative cells against three B44.1 positive cells from the panel. Further, in order to investigate potential other B44-associated epitope(s) in a positive way, nine reciprocal primings were performed. In this way 18 CTLs were generated and were subsequently tested back on the original panel. The results are given in Fig. 2, in which percentage cytotoxicity has been converted to a relative response. The impression from Fig. 2 is that the generated CTLs obtained by priming of P/Jx-negative cells against P/Jx-positive cells generally define the same epitope (B44.1) as CTL P/Jx. Further, reciprocal combinations seem to define at least one epitope (B44.2) possessed by the B44.1-negative cells. Individual CTL reagents vary in their value as typing reagents, some being highly discriminative, others much less so. This is partly ascribable to the fact that the latter, in addition to the component studied, contains reactivity against other serologically identified HLA-A or B antigens.

Family Study

One target cell – marked by a star in Fig. 2 – was peculiar in the sense that it was positive with the CTL anti-B44.1 as well as with the reciprocal combinations (anti-B44.2), suggesting that this individual might possess both the B44-associated epitopes.
To test this suggestion, we generated CTL in all possible combinations within the family of this individual, who is the father of the family depicted in Fig. 3. This figure shows the HLA-A, B, Cw, and DR types in the family, as well as the deduced haplotypes. The HLA typing of the family was performed with international reagents and was unequivocal. Child 2 has a maternal HLA-B-DR recombination. The father is either HLA-B44 homo-

zygous or carries a blank allele in the B locus of the b haplotype. All children are HLA-B44 positive. Child 3 is a paternal recombinant: if the father carries a blank allele in the B locus, the recombination must have occurred between the HLA-B and the HLA-DR loci; if he is B44 homozygous the recombination might also have taken place between HLA-A and HLA-B.

All CTLs generated within the family were tested back on the family as well as on the original panel. Figure 4 displays the results of the two most clearcut CTLs generated, viz the reciprocal combinations between child 1 and child 3, who are HLA-A, B seroidentical. Child 3 anti-child 1 produces a clear anti-B44.1 pattern in the panel, whereas the reciprocal combination produces a clear anti-B44.2 pattern. These results strongly suggest that the paternal a haplotype encodes the B44.1 epitope and that the b haplotype encodes the B44.2 epitope. Further, since child 3 inherited the B44.2 gene from the b haplotype, the recombination must have taken place between HLA-A and the gene encoding the molecule carrying the B44.2 epitope.

This conclusion was amply confirmed by the other CTLs generated: in combinations where the responder was negative for the b haplotype (or the centromeric part of it) and was stimulated with cells positive for this haplotype, the B44.2 pattern was discernible. The same was true concerning the a haplotype and the B44.1 pattern. The mother as responder was an exception. On challenge with both the a and the b haplotypes, CTLs were generated that were equally strongly positive against all B44-positive cells, which might indicate the existence of a distinct B44 common epitope recognized only and predominantly by B44-negative individuals.

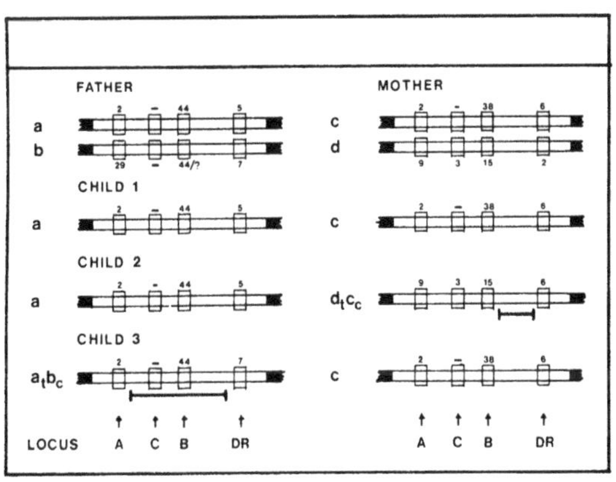

Fig. 3. HLA-A, B, Cw, and DR types and deduced haplotypes in the family of the target cell donor (the father), who, based on results from Fig. 2, is both B44.1 positive and B44.2 positive. *Horizontal bars* indicate sites of recombination

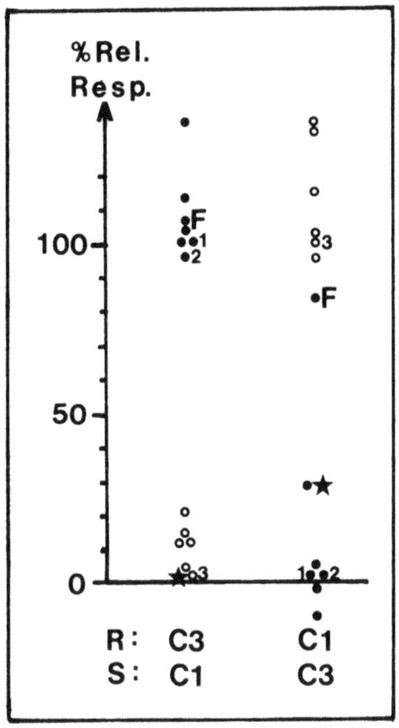

Fig. 4. Percentage relative response obtained by testing CTLs generated in reciprocal combinations between child 1 and child 3 from the family depicted in Fig. 3. Both CTLs were tested against the family members as well as the selected panel (Fig. 1). *Filled* and *open symbols* have the same meaning as in Fig. 2. The *star* represents the mother. *F, 1, 2,* and *3* identify the father, child 1, child 2, and child 3 respectively as targets. For further details see text

Summary

Initiated by our participation in the European CML Study Group, we have developed methods for production of interleukin-2 (IL-2)-conditioned media and short-term expansion of classical CML effector combinations. Consequently, large batches of CTL-enriched effector combinations may be ready at any time, enabling cellular typing of selected panels, populations, and families with identical CTLs. By the use of this approach we studied the serological HLA-B44 determinants:

1. For a collaborative CML study one anti-B7 CTL was constructed (HLA-A1,2; B8,44; Cw– anti-HLA-A1,2; B7,44; Cw5). On testing in selected panels, extrareactions were observed with B7–, 44+ target cells.
2. Testing in panels of selected B7–, 44+ unrelated cells revealed some target cells to be clearly CTL+, others CTL–.
3. Construction of CTLs by combinatorial mixing of the unrelated cells of 2. and back-testing on the panel corroborated this in as much as CTLs –anti+ combinations yield the original pattern (B44.1), while CTLs +anti– yield a complementary pattern (B44.2). CTLs +anti+ or –anti– were generally negative.

4. The CTLs constructed in 3. indicated one individual to be both B44.1 and B44.2 positive. This was amply confirmed by generating new CTLs within the family of this individual by combinatorial mixing. Among these CTLs two were highly discriminating and thus valuable typing reagents defining the B44.1 and B44.2 types.

References

1. Mawas C, Christen Y, Legrand L, Sasportes M, Dausset J (1974) Cellular and humoral response against determinants other than the classical HL-A specificities. Transplantation 18:256–266
2. Kristensen T, Grunnet N, Kissmeyer-Nielsen F (1974) Occurrence of unexpected HL-A (LA and FOUR) irrelevant lympholysis. Tissue Antigens 4:378–382
3. Schendel DJ, Wank R, Hansen JA, Dupont B (1977) Cell-mediated lympholysis in man: identification of a common target determinant associated with HLA-B12 and Bw35. Transplant Proc 9:1777–1780
4. Goulmy E, Termijtelen A, Bradley BA, van Rood J (1976) HLA restriction of non-HLA-A, -B, -C and -D cell mediated lympholysis. Tissue Antigens 8:317–326
5. Biddison WE, Krangel MS, Strominger JL, Ward FE, Shearer GM, Shaw S (1980) Virus-immune cytotoxic T cells recognize structural differences between serologically indistinguishable HLA-A2 molecules. Hum Immunol 1:225–232
6. Kato S, Iványi P, Lacko E, Breur B, du Bois R, Eijsvoogel VP (1982) HLA-B locus (B12) antigen variants defined by CTL generated between B locus-identical (B12) responder-stimulator pairs. J Immunol 128: 949–955
7. Breuning MH, Lucas CJ, Breur BS, Engelsma MY, de Lange GG, Dekker AJ, Biddison WE, Iványi P (1982) Subtypes of HLA-B27 detected by cytotoxic T lymphocytes and their role in self-recognition. Hum Immunol 5:259–268
8. van der Poel JJ, Mölders H, Thompson A, Ploegh HL (1983) Definition of four HLA-A2 subtypes by CML typing and biochemical analysis. Immunogenetics 17:609–621
9. Goulmy E, van Leeuwen A, Blokland E, van Rood JJ, Biddison WE (1982) Major histocompatibility complex – restricted H-Y-specific antibodies and cytotoxic T lymphocytes may recognize different self determinants. J exp Med 155:1567–1579
10. Tekolf AW, Biddison WE, Aster RD, Shaw S (1982) Two subgroups of HLA-Bw44 defined by cell-mediated lympholysis that differ in Bw44 expression on platelets and in patterns of genetic linkage disequilibrium. J Immunol 129:1474–1478
11. Hahn AWA, Schendel DJ, Hansen PW, Ploegh HL (1984) Biochemical and cellular identification of HLA-Bw44 subtypes. Hum Immunol 11:69–76
12. Gillis S, Baker PE, Ruscetti FW, Smith KA (1978) Long-term culture of human antigen specific cytotoxic T cell lines. J Exp Med 148:1093–1101
13. Kristensen T, Malissen B, Johnsen HE (1982) Histocompatibility typing by polyclonal and cloned human cytotoxic T lymphocytes. In: Ferrone S, Solheim BG (eds) HLA typing: methodology and clinical aspects, vol 2. CRC Press, Florida, pp 123–150
14. European CML Study Group (1980) Human histocompatibility testing by T cell-mediated lympholysis: a European standard CML technique. Tissue Antigens 16:335–367

Frequencies of Proliferative and Cytotoxic Precursor T Cells During a Course of Active Immunization as Analysed by Limiting Dilution

T. Kristensen[1], M. Madsen[1], P. Platz[2], and L.P. Ryder[2]

1 Dept of Clinical Immunology, The Tissue Typing Laboratory, University Hospital of Aarhus, 8000 Aarhus C, Denmark
2 Dept of Clinical Immunology, The Tissue Typing Laboratory, University Hospital of Copenhagen, Tagenvej 20, 2200 Copenhagen N, Denmark

In limiting dilution assays, mixed lymphocyte cultures grown with a limiting number of responding cells allow direct estimation of proliferative and cytotoxic precursor cells. The basis of the assay is the culture of many replicates of a range of responder cells in the presence of an excess of stimulating cells. The doses of responder cells are chosen so that a fraction of the cultures contains no precursor cells. The fractions of nonresponding cultures for each responding cell dose are scored. From these the frequencies of precursor cells are calculated using the zero-order term of the Poisson distribution.

The range of responding cells was estimated in preliminary experiments using cells from the recipient isolated prior to immunization. The informative range was found to be doses of 10–100 cells, i.e., cell doses at which a considerable fraction of the cultures contain no responding cells. The number of stimulator cells, i.e., cells from the immunizing donor, was constant at 5×10^4. Primary culture was performed in U-bottomed microtiter wells (72 wells

Histocompatibility Testing 1984
Edited by E. D. Albert et al.

per responder cell dose). Proliferative cultures were identified by ^{3}H-thymidine uptake from day 6 to day 7. Cytotoxic cultures were identified by direct addition of 10^4 ^{51}Cr-labeled PHA blasts (3 days) from the immunizing donor to each well at day 6. Supernatants were harvested 4 hours later. At each responder cell dose appropriate negative controls containing either autologous or no stimulator and target cells were included.

Results

With the aim of producing anti-HLA-DR antisera, eight healthy human volunteers were immunized by repeated ID injections of lymphocytes. One donor was immunized against the following incompatibilities: HLA-A2; B40 (w60); Cw3; and D/DRw6. A total of six immunizations was performed.

During and after immunization, the donor developed several high-titered anti-donor antibodies: anti-HLA-A2 strongly cross-reacting with HLA-A28; anti-HLA-B40; and unidentified components, possibly specific for B cells. No anti-HLA-C antibodies were identified. T-cell cloning performed on several occasions after immunization repeatedly revealed the presence of highly specific anti-HLA-A2, anti-HLA-Bw60, anti-HLA-Cw3, and anti-HLA-D/DRw6-like cytotoxic clones in the donor. Proliferative clones were never demonstrated after immunization.

Limiting dilution experiments were performed on lymphocytes isolated and frozen prior to, during, and after immunization. Screening and frequency analyses were performed for cellular proliferation and cytotoxicity using donor lymphocytes as stimulators and targets in PLT and CML assays. Basic frequencies of anti-donor proliferative and cytotoxic precursors prior to immunization are approx. 1%. During immunization the frequency of proliferative precursors rises quickly to a maximum of approx. 5% after the third immunization, with a subsequent decline to below preimmunization levels. By contrast, the frequency of cytotoxic precursors rises more slowly, reaching a maximum of approx. 14% after the fifth immunization, followed by a plateau of approx. 8%, which is also detectable after the period of immunization.

HLA Class II Alloantigens Defined by Cytotoxic T Cell Clones and Monoclonal Antibodies*

N. Flomenberg, K. Horibe, R.W. Knowles, D. Williams, K. Rosenkrantz, and B. Dupont

Human Immunogenetics Section, Sloan-Kettering Institute for Cancer Research, 1275 York Avenue, New York, NY 10021, USA

Introduction

Biochemical studies of HLA-DQ molecules have revealed polymorphisms which have not been previously recognized with alloantisera. HLA-DQ molecules from individuals homozygous for DR1, DR2, or DRw6 can all be distinguished from one another, despite the fact that all three bear the DQw1 determinants [1]. These findings suggest that the DQ determinants represent supertypic specificities associated with the HLA-DQ molecules, and that these molecules exhibit a finer level of polymorphism as well. Allospecificities associated with these fine HLA-DQ polymorphisms have not been detected to date. This may reflect the fact that HLA-DQ is closely linked to and in strong linkage disequilibrium with HLA-DR. It is thus possible that some "HLA-DR alloantisera" may actually recognize unique HLA-DQ determinants which cosegregate with the relevant HLA-DR specificities in the population.

In the present report, we have begun to address two related questions: (1) Do the fine biochemical polymorphisms associated with HLA-DQ evoke an alloresponse? (2) What is the relative functional contribution of HLA-DR, DQ, and DP in the subdivision of serologically DR-identical individuals into mutually MLC-reactive groups? For this purpose, we have raised a panel of T cell clones and monoclonal antibodies (MoAbs) to HLA class II molecules and have analyzed the effects of these antibodies on the cytolytic activity of the T cell clones.

* Supported by NCI Grants CA-22507, CA-08748, CA-19267, CA-23766, and CA-33050

Material and Methods

Isolation and Characterization of Monoclonal Antibodies

MoAbs PL3, PL5, PL8, PL12, and PL18 were generated from mice immunized with the PLH B-lymphoblastoid cell line (B-LCL) (HLA-A3; Cw6; Bw47; DR7 homozygous). The HLA class II molecules bound by these antibodies were characterized by immunoprecipitation, SDS gel electrophoresis, and 2-D gel analysis using previously described techniques. MoAb 4E [2] recognizing HLA-B molecules as well as HLA-A29, A30, A31, and A32, MoAb CR1 [3] recognizing an HLA class I monomorphic determinant, MoAb SG157 [1] recognizing HLA-DR molecules, and MoAb SG171 [1] recognizing HLA-DR molecules as well as the DQ molecules present on DR7-positive cell lines have all been described previously. MoAb M101 binds to all peripheral blood mononuclear leukocytes (PBL) (R. Knowles, unpublished observations).

Isolation and Characterization of Allocytoxic T Cell Clones

T cell clones were derived from a mixed lymphocyte culture performed utilizing 8000 R irradiated stimulator cells from the PLH cell line (HLA-A3; Cw6; Bw47; DR7 homozygous). Equal numbers of irradiated PLH cells and responder cells from an unrelated individual, RK (HLA-A2; Cw7; B7; DR2/Aw33; B35; DRw6) were cocultured for 10 days. Clones were then derived from limiting dilution cultures seeded at 0.3 cells per well [4]. Cell-mediated cytotoxicity studies were performed using previously described techniques [4].

Results

The patterns of cytolytic activity observed for six interesting T cell clones are summarized in Table 1. Clones K1I and K1T reacted broadly with all cells tested from the DR7 cluster. Clones K1D and K1P lysed only B-LCL expressing the sensitizing haplotype. Clone K1Q lysed B-LCL expressing either DR3 or DR7 and clone K1X lysed B-LCL expressing DR3, DR4, DR5 or DR7.

In order to characterize the specific families of HLA class II molecules recognized by these clones, a series of blocking studies were performed utilizing MoAbs to HLA class II molecules. The antibodies utilized for these studies were characterized biochemically with regard to the molecules recognized on HLA-DR7 homozygous cell lines. Based on sequential immunoprecipitation studies as well as 1- and 2-D gel electrophoresis, these antibodies were grouped into two clusters. The first cluster, including PL3 (anti-DRw53) as well as PL8, PL12, and PL18 (anti-HLA class II monomorphic) binds exclusively to the HLA-DR family of molecules. PL5 and SG171 constitute the second cluster. These two antibodies bind to DR, DQ, and DP molecules on DR7-positive cell lines (data not shown).

Clones K1I and K1T recognize a determinant closely related to the serologically-defined DR7 specificity, in that they lysed 11 of 11 DR7-positive cell lines and failed to lyse any of 18 DR7-negative cell lines. As illustrated in Fig. 1, target cells which were preincubated with the HLA-DR specific cluster of MoAbs were not lysed by these clones, while the other MoAbs studied did not produce similar blocking effects. Thus the target antigen for these clones indeed appears to be a determinant associated with HLA-DR molecules. The behavior of clones K1I and K1T was representative of six additional clones broadly reactive with DR7-positive B-LCL, all of which could be blocked by MoAb binding only to DR molecules.

Clones K1Q and K1X lysed target cells in a pattern consistent with recognition of supertypic specificities expressed by HLA class II molecules. Clone K1Q appeared to recognize an DQw2-like determinant in that it lysed six of ten lines expressing HLA-DR7 and three of four cell lines expressing HLA-DR3. It should be noted that three of the four DR7 cell lines which this clone failed to lyse were from the Bw57; DR7; Dw11 cluster, which has been shown by several groups to express DQw3 rather than DQw2 determinants [5, 6]. Unlike clones K1I and K1T, the cytolytic activity of this clone was not blocked by preincubating target cells with MoAb PL3, PL8, PL12, or PL18 or with MoAb recognizing HLA class I molecules (Fig. 1). In contrast, MoAb PL5 and SG171, which bind to HLA-DQ and DP demonstrated strong blocking effects.

Clone K1X recognizes a supertypic specificity distinct from any of the DQ or DRw52,53 specificities in that it lyses B-LCL expressing DR3, DR4, DR5, or DR7. B-LCL expressing DR1, DR2, or DRw6 are not lysed by this clone, indicating that it recognizes a determinant which is complementary to DQw1. The cytolytic activity of this clone was also inhibited by MoAb PL5 (Fig. 1), but not by the DR-specific MoAbs, nor by MoAbs recognizing HLA class I molecules. (MoAb SG171 was not tested). These data suggest that clone K1X, like clone K1Q, recognizes a target determinant present on the HLA-DQ molecule of DR7 haplotypes.

Clones K1D and K1P exhibited identical patterns of cytolytic activity in panel studies. These clones lysed three cell lines expressing the HLA-A3; Cw6; Bw47; DR7 haplotype, including the original sen-

Table 1. Target antigen specificity of cytotoxic T cell clones

Clone ID	Sensitizing haplotype									
	A3; Bw47; DR7	DR7; Dw7	DR7; Dw11	DR3	DR4	DR5	DR1	DR2	DRw6	NK
K1I	+	+	+	–	–	–	–	–	–	–
K1T	+	+	+	–	–	–	–	–	–	–
K1D	+	–	–	–	–	–	–	–	–	–
K1P	+	–	–	–	–	–	–	–	–	–
K1Q	+	+	–	+	–	–	–	–	–	–
K1X	+	+	+	+	+	+	–	–	–	–

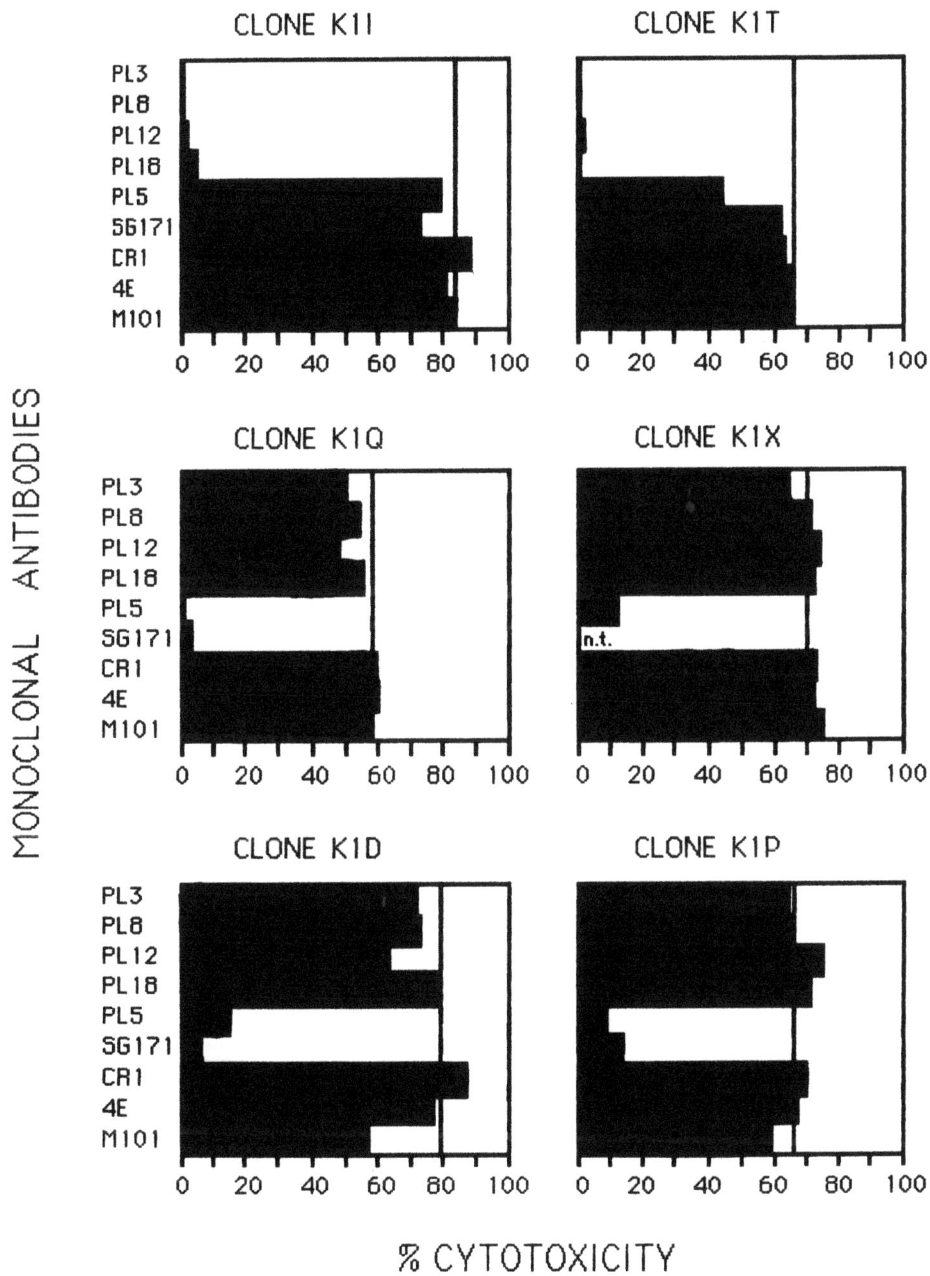

Fig. 1. Blocking of anti-HLA class II specific cytotoxicity. Cytotoxicity in the absence of antibody is indicated by the vertical line. Cytotoxicity in the presence of a 1 : 40 dilution of ascites of each MoAb is indicated by the solid horizontal bars. n.t. = not tested

sitizing cell line, PLH. They failed to lyse any of 26 additional cell lines lacking this haplotype, including other B-LCLs expressing HLA-A3, Cw6, or DR7. This finding initially suggested that HLA-Bw47 might be the target molecule. This possibility was ruled out based on two independent findings. First, these clones lysed B-LCL but not PHA-activated lymphoblasts from individuals with the A3; Cw6; Bw47; DR7 haplotype. Second, the cytolytic activity of these clones could not be blocked by any of 7 MoAb recognizing HLA class I molecules (data not shown). The cytolytic activity of clones K1D and K1P was also not inhibited by MoAbs binding to the DR family of molecules (Fig. 1). In contrast, however, PL5 and SG171 produced strong blocking effects. Taken together, these findings indicate that clones K1D and K1P recognize target determinants on HLA-DQ or DP molecules.

Discussion

Functional analyses of HLA-DR and DQ are frequently complicated by the fact that these two molecules do not segregate independently in the population. Therefore, the in vivo sensitizations which generate alloantisera and the in vitro sensitizations which generate proliferative and cytotoxic T cells are not restricted to one or the other of these HLA-class II molecules. For this reason, the immunologic dissection of human class II alloantigens is greatly facilitated through analyses of T cell clones and monoclonal antibodies.

In the present study, we have reported two clones which react broadly with DR7-associated determinants. These clones recognize B-LCL derived from the Dw7 cluster, the Dw11 cluster, or expressing the unique A3; Cw6; Bw47; DR7 haplotype. The cytolytic activity of these clones can be blocked by MoAbs recognizing only DR molecules, and the degree of blocking by these antibodies may approach 100%. Six additional clones broadly reactive with DR7-associated determinants have shown similar blocking effects. We have not identified a T cell clone which reacts broadly with DR7-associated determinants which is blocked preferentially by DQ rather than DR-specific antibodies.

Clones recognizing both broad supertypic and fine, haplotype-specific determinants on HLA-DQ molecules have been identified, however. Clone K1Q recognizes a specificity which appears related to the serologically-defined DQw2-specificity. Clone K1X recognizes an DQw2 + DQw3 specificity. The blocking studies of these clones are in agreement with biochemical studies which have suggested that the DQw1, w2, and w3 determinants are indeed carried on HLA-DQ molecules.

In addition, we have described two clones which recognize determinants associated only with the HLA-A3, Cw6, Bw47, DR7 haplotype. These clones do not lyse PHA-activated lymphoblasts, and their allocytotoxicity cannot be blocked by MoAbs to class I HLA molecules. These findings indicate that the target molecule is not an HLA class I alloantigen. In contrast, antibodies binding to DQ molecules (but not antibodies binding exclusively to DR molecules) dramatically inhibit the cytotoxicity of these clones. Thus, these clones detect a DQ or DP target determinant which appears thus far to be specific for a single haplotype.

The fact that these clones recognize a target determinant which is restricted only to this one haplotype is not altogether surprising. This haplotype is also associated with an unusual HLA-B locus antigen, with unusual C4 complotypes, as well as with 21-hydroxylase deficiency, and it exhibits an extreme degree of positive genetic linkage disequilibrium. This haplotype is thus associated with unusual alleles at several loci held together by strong linkage disequilibrium [7].

The present findings suggest a model for the subdivision of DR7 into its distinct subclusters. Our analysis of eight clones which react broadly with DR7-associated determinants has revealed that these clones can be inhibited by antibodies which react only with DR molecules (PL3, PL8). None of these broadly reactive clones would appear to recognize determinants unique to the DQ molecules associated with DR7 haplotypes. Similarly, we have not identified any clones recognizing target determinants associated with DR molecules which subdivide the DR7 cluster. In contrast, we have presented evidence for recognition of a DQ or DP associated determinant unique to one particular DR7 haplotype. This suggests that such DQ-associated determinants may be responsible for the various splits of DR7, wherein the determinants carried on the DR family of molecules are the same or quite similar throughout the entire DR7 cluster, while the DQ and DP determinants vary between the Dw11, Dw7, and other (e.g., Bw47-associated) subgroups. Testing this hypothesis will require characterization of additional clones generated by primings against other DR7-associated haplotypes and additional biochemical analysis of the DR, DQ, and DP families from each DR7 subcluster. In this way, it may ultimately be possible to distinguish the roles played by HLA-DR, DQ, and DP molecules in allorecognition and immunity.

Acknowledgments. We thank Doctors Goyert, Silver, Russo, Ferrone, Collins, Hansen, and Duffy, who provided antibodies and cell lines for these studies.

References

1. Goyert SM, Moriuchi J, Winchester R, Silver J (1983) HLA-DS molecules and their relation to supertypic specificities. Hum Immunol 8:53–63
2. Yang SY, Morishima Y, Collins NH, Alton T, Pollack MS, Yunis EJ, Dupont B (1984) Comparison of one-dimensional IEF patterns for serologically detectable HLA-A and B allotypes. Immunogenetics 19:217–231
3. Russo C, Pellegrino MA, Ng AK, Wilson BS, Ferrone S (1982) Antigenic constitution of HLA-A, B, C molecules: immunochemical analysis with monoclonal xenoantibodies. In: Ferrone S, Solheim BG (eds) HLA typing: methodology and clinical aspects, vol 1. CRC Press, Boca Raton, p 77
4. Flomenberg N, Naito K, Duffy E, Knowles RW, Evans RL, Dupont B (1983) Allocytotoxic T cell clones: both Leu 2^+3^- and Leu 2^-3^+ T cells recognize class I histocompatibility antigens. Eur J Immunol 13:905–911
5. Schreuder I, Parlevliet J (1983) HLA-DR, LB, MB, MT and 8w13 with 9th Workshop HTCs. In: Albert E (ed) Newsletter V, Ninth International Histocompatibility Workshop and Conference, p 41
6. Honeyman M, Hakos G, Hsu S, Bias W (1984) Pretesting of Dw7 HTCs: four subtypes of Dw7. In: Albert E (ed) Newsletter VIII, Ninth International Histocompatibility Workshop and Conference, p 26
7. Fleischnick E, Raum D, Alosco SM, Gerald PS, Yunis EJ, Awdeh ZL, Granados J, Crigler JF, Giles CM, Alper CA (1983) Extended MHC haplotypes in 21-hydroxylase-deficiency congenital adrenal hyperplasia: Shared genotypes in unrelated patients. Lancet 22:152–156

Biochemistry of HLA Antigens

Structural Analysis of the Polymorphism of HLA Class I Antigens*

J.A. Lopez de Castro, R. Bragado, A. Ezquerra, and M.A. Vega

Department of Immunology, Fundación Jiménez Diaz, Avda. Reyes Católicos, 2, 28040 Madrid, Spain

The exceptional polymorphism of HLA class I antigens is relevant to immunologists because (a) HLA class I molecules are able to elicit strong antibody and cytolytic T lymphocyte (CTL) responses upon allogeneic stimulation, such as in allografting; (b) T cell receptors on the surface of CTLs and their precursors are restricted in their capacity for antigen recognition of virus-infected or otherwise modified cells, by the associative recognition of self-HLA class I molecules; and (c) it appears that some HLA class I specificities are more efficient than others in restricting T cell recognition of a given foreign antigen. A definition of the structural features of HLA polymorphism seems essential for establishing the molecular basis of the function of HLA class I molecules.

Much information has been accumulated recently on the nature and location of polymorphic areas, as well as on their putative relevance as alloantigenic sites. This information has been derived mainly from three types of approaches: (1) structural analysis of cross-reactive alloantigens; (2) sequence determination of HLA class I genes; (3) biochemical analyses of HLA variants and mutants.

In this communication, some structural studies concerning HLA class I polymorphism will be reviewed to present a current evaluation of putative functional sites as well as a biochemical interpretation of various features of HLA class I serology.

Structure and Variability of Polymorphic Regions

A comparison of available protein sequences for the extracellular portions of HLA-A, B, C antigens is presented in Fig. 1. It includes three alloantigens from the HLA-A locus: A2 [1], A28 [1] and A3 [2]; two from the HLA-B locus: B7 [3] and B40 [4]; and one from the HLA-C locus: Cw3 [5]. There are 65 nonidentity positions. All but six of them are located in the N-terminal 194 residues, which encompass α1 (residues 1–90) and α2 (residues 91–182) domains as well as the most N-terminal part of the α3 domain (residues 182–271). Most variable positions (85%) are clustered in eight segments. Of these, three are located in α1 and span residues 9–12, 40–45, and 62–80. Three more lie in α2, spanning residues 94–97, 105–116, and 137–163. Another segment spans residues

* This work has been partially funded by grants from the Fondo de Investigaciones Sanitarias (F.I.S.) de la Seguridad Social of Spain (No. 10/81 and 12/81). M.A.V. is a fellow of the F.I.S.

Histocompatibility Testing 1984
Edited by E. D. Albert et al.

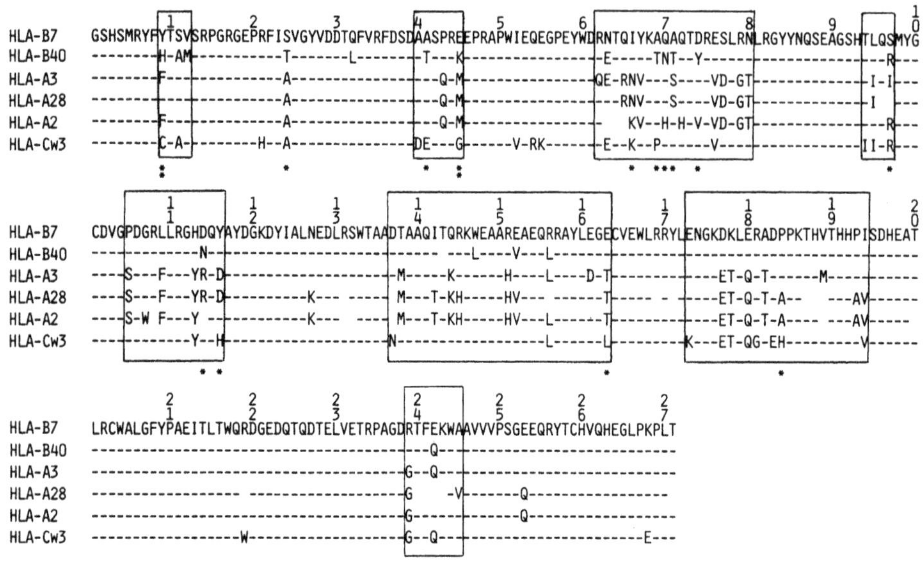

Fig. 1. Amino acid sequences of the extracellular portion of HLA class I antigens [1–5]. Regions of variability are boxed. *Asterisks* denote variable positions with three (*) or four (**) different residues among the molecules being compared. *Blanks* correspond to nonassigned residues. The following one-letter code for amino acids is used: A: Ala; B: Asx; C: Cys; D: Asp; E: Glu; F: Phe; G: Gly; H: His; I: Ile; K: Lys; L: Leu; M: Met; N: Asn; P: Pro; Q: Gln; R: Arg; S: Ser; T: Thr; V: Val; W: Trp; Y: Tyr; Z: Glx

173–194, that include the α2/α3 interdomain junction, and a final one is located in α3, at residues 239–245. Together, they encompass 101 residues, or 37% of the extracellular portion of the chain and 45% of the length of α1 and α2 domains. Clearly, such a large extent of variability areas endows these molecules with the potential for a great number of polymorphic epitopes and correlates well with the complexity of their antigenic structure as envisaged by serological studies.

A remarkable feature of the variability pattern presented in Fig. 1 is that the amount of different residues in most individual positions is very low. Thus, 50 of 65 nonidentity positions show only two different amino acid residues among the six molecules being compared. Of the remaining 15 positions, 13 have three different amino acid residues, and only two (positions 9 and 45) show four different residues. The variability clusters outlined above differ in their inclusion of positions of various degrees of variability (Fig. 1). For instance, the segment 62–80 includes five positions of higher variability, whereas in the segments 138–163 and 173–194 all but one position in each segment are of low variability.

The possibility that gene conversion may occur in HLA class I genes [1, 2] provides a genetic argument for the low variability of many positions, through segmental sequence homogenization among various members of the multigene family. In addition, there may be structural constraints imposed by the folding of the protein chain that limit the extent of variability in individual positions (see below). Whatever the mechanisms involved, the pattern of structural polymorphism that emerges from these sequence comparisons is one that involves generally low variability in many different positions. This pattern provides the basic interpretation for the complexity of serological cross-reactions commonly observed in conventional typing serology as well as with HLA monoclonal antibodies. Thus, much antigenic polymorphism can be generated by a combinatorial effect in epitopes formed by various positions, each one of them being of low variability. Furthermore, the restricted variability of most polymorphic positions implies that many epitopes will be shared by different subsets of specificities, frequently involving products of different class I loci. Conceivably, most antibodies generated in response to HLA class I antigens will be directed against antigenic structures which are not unique to a single allelic product, which explains the difficulty of finding truly monospecific antisera for most "private" specificities.

The Nature of Alloantigenic Epitopes

After the above considerations, it is easy to see that the search for structures that define single HLA allospecificities is exceedingly difficult. First, some substitutions might not be necessarily relevant in generating antigenic polymorphism. Second, it is not clear whether or not various polymorphic segments are equally important as putative alloantigenic sites for antibodies, CTLs, or both. In fact, there is increasing evidence that the antibody and the cellular immune responses for a given alloantigen may be directed, at least in some cases, against different determinants [6, 7]. Third, a given allospecificity may be the result of a unique combination of variable residues, each one of them being identical to other class I molecules, so that its structure may not become readily evident upon structural analysis. A way to approach these problems is through sequence comparison of cross-reactive alloantigens, in combination with biochemical analyses of HLA variants that have lost their capability of being recognized by either allospecific monoclonal antibodies or CTLs. The best-studied example is the HLA-A2 system [8–11]. A comparison between HLA-A2 and HLA-A28 (see Fig. 1) shows that they differ in at least ten positions. Five of them are clustered in the segment 66–74. Two more are at positions 107 and 116, within one of the variability clusters outlined above. The remaining three substitutions are very conservative and are scattered through the sequence, at positions 9, 95, and 245. This result suggests that polymorphic segments 62–80 and/or 105–116 are major contributors to the alloantigenic determinants that define the A2 and A28 specificities. The biochemical analysis of two independent HLA-A2 mutants that have a greatly decreased reactivity with the A2 allospecific antibody BB7.2 shows that both of them have one or more mutations in the segment 98–108 [8], thus confirming that at least one alloantigenic site of HLA-A2 is contributed to by residues in or close to the cluster 105–116. The epitope defined by a different A2 allospecific monoclonal antibody, MA21, is not affected in these mutants, suggesting that the A2 specificity may be composed of several different epitopes, which is compatible with the pattern of differences between A2 and A28, involving various areas in the amino acid sequence.

It is conceivable that the alloantigenic sites of different HLA-A specificities are located in different areas of the molecule. Thus, the segment 105–116 is probably not an alloantigenic site for HLA-A28 and HLA-A3 as suggested by the fact that these two antigens have an identical sequence over its entire length (Fig. 1). In addition, A3 and A28 differ in at least 11 substitutions, five of them being located at positions 127, 142, 145, 152, and 161. In all these positions A28 and A2 are identical (Fig. 1). Some or all of these residues may be spatially related by the three-dimensional folding of the $\alpha 2$ domain [12]. Hence, they may contribute to an antigenic site in which A3 differs from both A2 and A28. It is striking that the number of amino acid differences between A3 and A28 is analogous to that between A2 and A28. However, A28 is significantly more cross-reactive with A2 than with A3. This indicates that it is not only the number of substitutions which is important in determining serological cross-reactivity, but also their location and/or chemical nature. In this respect, some of the substitutions in which A3 differs from both A28 and A2 may be more significant as antigenic allodeterminants than are the differences between A2 and A28.

The relationship between serologically defined allodeterminants and the recognition sites for allospecific and virus immune, HLA-restricted CTLs is a matter of critical importance in understanding the functional basis of HLA polymorphism. The serologically immunoselected HLA-A2 mutants discussed above are killed very efficiently by HLA-A2 allospecific [6] as well as by Epstein-Barr virus immune, HLA-A2-restricted CTL lines [13]. Although the polyclonal nature of the CTL effectors may hide effects over the reactivity at a clonal level, this result suggests that mutations in the area 105–116, especially at residues 105–108 [see 8], may more efficiently affect a serologically defined allodeterminant than a CTL recognition site. In addition, the structural analysis of two different HLA-A2 variants with impaired capability for being recognized by both allospecific and influenza-virus immune, HLA-A2 restricted CTL shows that they differ from a "reference" HLA-A2 antigen at various positions in the region 147–157 [10, 11]. This area is identical between A2 and A28 (Fig. 1), and is therefore unlikely to be the site of a serological allodeterminant. Hence, conventional typing allosera would not be expected to distinguish between these variants. Taken together, these data suggest that CTL and antibody recognition of class I antigens may involve different antigenic structures. A corollary of this conclusion is that typing serology may overlook structural differences among HLA class I antigens that may still be able to elicit CTL responses upon allogeneic immunization in apparently matched donor-recipient combinations.

The structural analysis of some HLA-B specificities suggest that the main conclusions obtained from the HLA-A2 system are likely to have a more general character. Unfortunately, there are as many as 19 differences between cross-reactive HLA-B7 and HLA-B40 [4], which makes it difficult to make a reliable outline of putative alloantigenic sites. However, as with A2 and A28, the most conspicuous cluster of differences lies in the segment 63–74 (Fig. 1). B27 differs from both B7 and B40 as much as these two specificities differ among themselves. Areas of nonidentity between B27, B7, and B40 fall within the variability clusters outlined in the first paragraph (A. Ezquerra and J. A. Lopez de Castro, unpublished work). In addition, preliminary analysis of a HLA-B27 CTL variant indicates that it differs from a "reference" B27 antigen at least in one substitution in the segment 152–157 (M. Vega and J. A. Lopez de Castro, unpublished work), supporting the suggestion [11] that this area may be critical in determining CTL recognition.

Polymorphism and Conformation: Prediction Studies

In an attempt to place the polymorphic regions of HLA class I antigens in the context of their spatial structure, the chain folding was estimated by various predictive methods [14–16] and variable positions were correlated with the distribution of areas of defined secondary structure (Figs. 2, 3). A detailed report of these studies has been published [12]. Only the most relevant aspects concerning the conformation of polymorphic regions will be mentioned here. The analysis predicts a high probability for β structure in $\alpha 1$, $\alpha 2$ and $\alpha 3$ domains. As expected from sequence analyses [17], the predicted secondary structure of $\alpha 3$, with seven β strands, is strongly reminiscent of that of immunoglobulin C domains. Five β strands are predicted in $\alpha 1$, flanked by a number of β turns. The three N-terminal strands, which lie within residues 1–37, involve the most hydrophobic segments of $\alpha 1$. Hence, it is likely that a significant number of residues in these segments are buried, forming the domain core. The reduced number of variable positions in this area (Fig. 3) is compatible with this assumption. The two remaining β strands predicted in $\alpha 1$ lie within the hypervariable region at residues 62–80. They are predominantly formed by polar residues and have the features of peripheral β strands [18] that are found at the protein surface, shielding the hydrophobic core.

There are six predicted β strands in the $\alpha 2$ domain. As in the case of $\alpha 1$, the 37 N-terminal residues present a well-defined structure consisting of three β strands flanked by β turns. The analogy in their location and length (Fig. 2) suggests that these two domains might have some similarities in their tertiary folding. Strands A, C, D, and E (Fig. 2) correlate with areas of highest local hydrophobicity [12], suggesting that a number of their residues may be buried. As in $\alpha 1$, variability in these more hydrophobic strands is low (Fig. 3).

A single α helix of 11–14 residues is predicted within the segment 146–160. It is remarkable that this apparent structural singularity lies in a segment that appears to be critical for CTL recognition, as suggested by the fact that substitutions in this area drastically abrogate recognition and killing of targets by specific CTLs, both in HLA (see above) and H-2 class I antigens [19, 20]. The pattern of restricted variability in this segment adjusts to the steric restrictions of α helices. For instance, the two differences between HLA-B7 and HLA-B40 at positions 152 and 156 (Fig. 1) would be brought into proximity by the helical turn that relates residues at positions i, i + 3, and i + 4. The same is true for the three substitutions of the HLA-A2 variant DK1 at positions 149, 152, and 156 [11]. Similarly, the murine bm1 mutant differs from the parental H-2K^{b} molecule at positions 152, 155, and 156 [19]. This mutant is one of the most conspicuously different of the bm series as judged by grafting and by cellular assays.

Figure 3 shows that many variable positions lie in areas of defined secondary structure. These positions may have restricted possibilities for variation due to the constraints imposed by the conformational requirements of the α helix, β strands, and β turns. Thus, much of the limited polymorphism of individual positions (Fig. 1) could possibly be explained by selection against mutations that would introduce changes leading to disruption of defined structures. The distribution of variable residues through areas of well-ordered conformation suggests that most substitutions in HLA class I antigens are accommodated within a more or less rigid framework, so that variation at a few positions (such as that occurring in HLA mu-

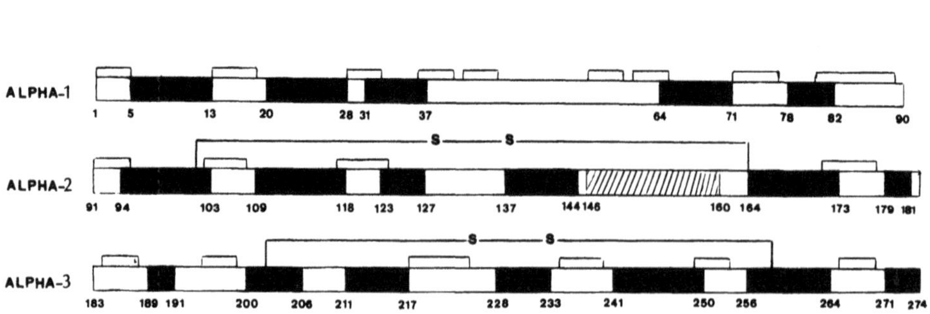

Fig. 2. Prediction of secondary structure for HLA- B7 heavy chain domains. Predicted β strands and α helix [14] are represented as *solid* and *diagonally hatched* segments respectively. β strands in each domain are denoted from the N-terminus as A, B, C, D, E, etc. β turns are marked as lines over the bar diagram. Overlapping β turns are drawn together

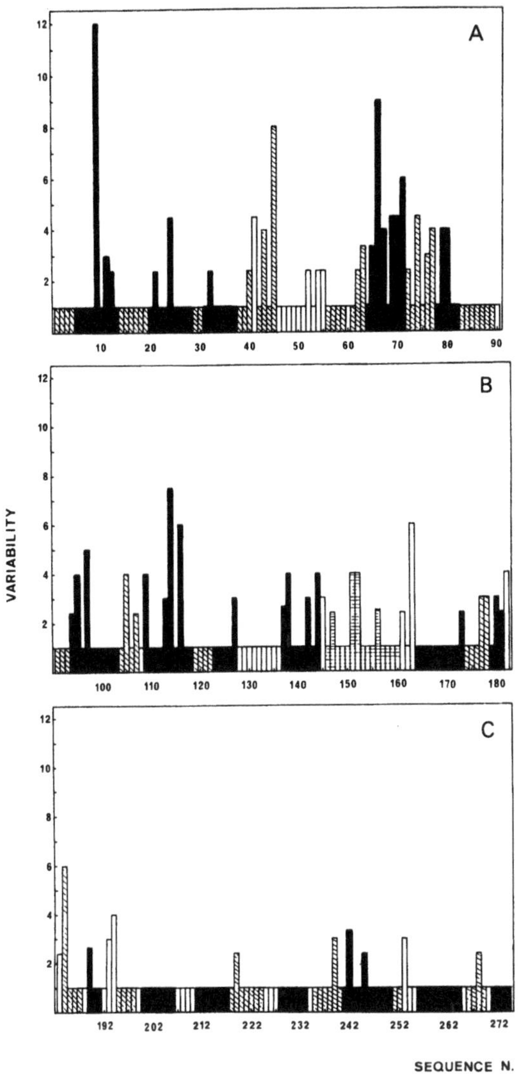

Fig. 3 A–C. Variability of amino acid residues, in **A** α1, **B** α2, and **C** α3 domains of HLA class I antigens, calculated from the data in Fig. 1. Superimposed are β strands (*solid*), β turns (*diagonally hatched*), and α helix (*horizontally hatched*) as predicted for HLA-B7 [14, 16]

tants) would probably not produce gross conformational changes in the molecule. This is supported by the fact that such variation often produces a selective alteration of antigenic sites while leaving other epitopes unchanged [6, 8, 10, 11, 21].

In conclusion, the biochemical analysis of HLA class I antigens is providing a definition of the polymorphic regions of the molecule and a progressive correlation of these areas with putative antigenic or functional sites. The nature of the structural polymorphism being unveiled by sequence comparisons and other structural studies, provides a molecular interpretation for the complexity of serological cross-reactions in the HLA system.

Acknowledgments. The authors thank Drs. R. Sodoyer, T. Strachan and B. Jordan for pre-prints, Dr. J. Strominger for critically reading the manuscript, and Ms. Alice Furumoto-Dawson for secretarial assistance.

References

1. Lopez de Castro JA, Strominger JL, Strong DM, Orr HT (1982) Structure of cross-reactive human histocompatibility antigens HLA-A28 and HLA-A2: Possible implications for the generation of the HLA polymorphism. Proc Natl Acad Sci USA 79:3813–3817
2. Strachan T, Sodoyer R, Damotte M, Jordan BR (1984) Complete nucleotide sequence of a functional class I HLA gene, HLA-A3: implications for the evolution of HLA genes. EMBO J 3:887–894
3. Orr HT, Lopez de Castro JA, Lancet D, Strominger JL (1979) Complete amino acid sequence of a papain-solubilized human histocompatibility antigen, HLA-B7. 2. Sequence determination and search for homologies. Biochemistry 18:5711–5719
4. Lopez de Castro JA, Bragado R, Strong DM, Strominger JL (1983) Primary structure of papain-solubilized human histocompatibility antigen HLA-B40 (-Bw60). An outline of alloantigenic determinants. Biochemistry 22:3961–3969
5. Sodoyer R, Damotte M, Delovitch TL, Trucy J, Jordan BR, Strachan T (1984) Complete nucleotide sequence of a gene encoding a functional class I histocompatibility antigen (HLA-Cw3). EMBO J 3:879–885
6. Ware CF, Krangel MS, Pious D, Biddison WE, Burakoff SJ, Strominger JL (1983) Recognition of HLA-A2 mutant and variant target cells by an HLA-A2 allospecific human cytotoxic T lymphocyte line. J Immunol 131: 1312–1317
7. Sherman LA, Vitiello A, Klinman NR (1983) T-cell and B-cell responses to viral antigens at the clonal level. Ann Rev Immunol 1:63–86
8. Krangel MS, Taketani S, Pious D, Strominger JL (1983) HLA-A2 mutants immunoselected in vitro: definition of residues contributing to an HLA-A2 specific serological determinant. J Exp Med 157:324–336
9. Taketani S, Krangel MS, Pious D, Strominger JL (1983) Structural analysis of HLA-A2 antigen from immunoselected mutant 8.6.1: further definition of an HLA-A2 specific serological determinant. J Immunol 131:2935–2938
10. Krangel MS, Taketani S, Biddison WE, Strong DM, Strominger JL (1982) Comparative structural analysis of HLA-A2 antigens distinguishable by cytotoxic T lymphocytes: Variants M7 and DR1. Biochemistry 21: 6313–6321
11. Krangel MS, Biddison WE, Strominger JL (1983) Comparative structural analysis of HLA-A2 antigens distinguishable by cytotoxic T lymphocytes. II. Variant DK1: evidence for a discrete CTL recognition region. J Immunol 130:1856–1862
12. Vega MA, Bragado R, Ezquerra A, Lopez de Castro JA (1984) Variability and conformation of HLA class I antigens: A predicative approach to the spatial arrangement of polymorphic regions. Biochemistry 23:823–831
13. Gaston JSH, Pious D, Rickinson AB, Epstein MA (1983) Mutant HLA-A2 antigens as restricting elements for cytotoxic T cells. Poster abstract 21st Harden Conference,

Structure and Biology of Lymphocyte Membranes, 19–23 September 1983
14. Garnier J, Osguthorpe DJ, Robson B (1978) Analysis of the accuracy and implications of simple methods for predicting the secondary structure of globular proteins. J Mol Biol 120:97–120
15. Lim VI (1974) Algorthims for prediction of α-helical and β-structural regions in globular proteins. J Mol Biol 88:873–894
16. Chou PY, Fasman GD (1979) Prediction of β turns. Biophys J 26:367–384
17. Orr HT, Lancet D, Robb RJ, Lopez de Castro JA, Strominger JL (1979) The heavy chain of a human histocompatibility antigen (HLA-B7) contains an immunoglobulin-like region. Nature 282:266–270
18. Lim VI (1974) Structural principles of the globular organization of protein chains. A stereochemical theory of globular protein secondary structure. J Mol Biol 88: 857–872
19. Schultze DH, Pease LR, Geier SS, Reyes AA, Sarmiento LA, Wallace RB, Nathenson SG (1983) Comparison of the cloned H-2K^{bm1} variant gene with the H-2K^{b} gene shows a cluster of seven nucleotide differences. Proc Natl Acad Sci USA 80:2007–2011
20. Melief C (1983) Remodelling the H-2 map. Immunol Today 4:57–61
21. Pious D, Krangel MS, Dixon LL, Parham P, Strominger JL (1982) HLA Structural gene mutants selected with an allospecific monoclonal antibody. Proc Natl Acad Sci USA 79:7832–7836

Molecular and Functional Analysis of Class II Molecules Characteristic to HLA-Dw2 and Dw12 *

Y. Nishimura [1]**, K. Tsukamoto [1], T. Sone [1], K. Hirayama [1], T. Takenouchi [2], K. Ogasawara [2], M. Kasahara [2], A. Wakisaka [2], M. Aizawa [2], and T. Sasazuki [1]**

1 Department of Human Genetics, Medical Research Institute, Tokyo Medical and Dental University, 1-5-45 Yushima, Bunkyo-Ku, Tokyo 113, Japan
2 First Department of Pathology, Hokkaido University, School of Medicine, Sapporo 060, Japan

Introduction

HLA-D specificities determined by mixed lymphocyte reaction (MLR) correlate to the serologically determined HLA-DR specificities. However, it was noticed that there are several different HLA-D specificities sharing the same HLA-DR. For example, HLA-Dw2 and Dw12 are both typed as DR2 serologically, but they mutually provoke a strong primary MLR [1]. We investigated the molecular basis of the difference between Dw2 and Dw12 and the functions of class II molecules characteristic to HLA-Dw2 and Dw12.

Materials and Methods

Monoclonal Antibodies

Anti-DR framework monoclonal antibody (MoAb) HU-4 (synonymous with 3G7 in [2]) and anti-DR2 MoAb HU-30 [3] were produced by hybridomas between murine myeloma cell line P3-X63-Ag8 and spleen cells of BALB/c mouse immunized with human B lymphoblastoid cell line.

Cells

HLA-Dw2 homozygous B lymphoblastoid cell lines EB-CMG, GAY and PGF were used in this study. EB-CMG and GAY were kindly donated by Dr. J. A. Hansen of the Fred Hutchinson Cancer Institute, Seattle, Washington, USA. PGF established by Dr. H. Festenstein of London Hospital Medical College was distributed for the Ninth International Histocompatibility Workshop (9th IHWS). HLA-Dw12 homozygous B lymphoblastoid cell lines EB-AKIBA and EB-KT were from our laboratory (SAS). HLA-D and DR phenotypes of donors of peripheral blood lymphocytes (PBLs) were as follows: TOK (9w1202): DR2-Dw12 homozygous typing cell (HTC); Len-2: DR2-Dw2 HTC; SM: DR2-Dw12/DRw6-D blank heterozygote; HU: DR1-Dw1/DR4-Dw15 heterozygote. Dw2 HTC Len-2 was kindly donated by Dr. N. Reinsmoen of Minnesota University.

Two-dimensional PAGE

B lymphoblastoid cell lines were metabolically labeled with L-[^{35}S]methionine for 4 h or for 30 min. In order to detect the unglycosylated precursor of class II molecules the B cell lines were incubated with 5 μg/ml tunicamycin for 30 min before the

* This work was supported in part by grants-in-aid from the Ministry of Education, Culture and Science, Japan, a grant for research into intractable disease from the Ministry of Health and Welfare, Japan, and the Mitsubishi Science Foundation
** Present adress: Dept. of Genetics, Medical Institute of Bioregulation. Kyusku University, 3-1-1 Maldaski, Higashi-Ku, Fukuoda 812, Japan

Histocompatibility Testing 1984
Edited by E. D. Albert et al.

labeling of lines with [^{35}S]methionine for 4 h. Immunoprecipitates from the B cell lines with MoAbs were collected by the method described by Jones et al. [4]. Two-dimensional (2D) PAGE was performed by the method of O'Farrell [5] with minor modification [6]. Nonequilibrium pH gradient electrophoresis (NEPHGE) was adopted as the first dimension using tube gels (4% polyacrylamide, 2% pH 3.5–10 and 2% pH 5–7 ampholine, 9.2 *M* urea and 2% NP-40), and the sample was electrofocused at a constant 500 V for 6 h. Sodium dodecyl sulfate slab gel (10% polyacrylamide, 0.5 mm thickness) electrophoresis was performed as the second dimension.

Mixed Lymphocyte Culture

One-way mixed lymphocyte culture (MLC) was performed by the method described elsewhere [7]. In the blocking study of MLR with MoAbs, 20 µl of the ascites form of MoAbs diluted with culture medium was added into each culture well. As a control, ascites of BALB/c mouse injected intraperitoneally with P3-X63-Ag8 myeloma cell line was used at the final dilution of 10^2.

Immune Response to Streptococcal Cell Wall Antigen

The assay system of the proliferative response of T cells to streptococcal cell wall antigen (SCW) was described elsewhere [7]. In the blocking study, MoAb was added to the culture of PBL (1×10^5) with 0.5 µg/ml SCW by the same method as in the blocking study of MLR. An IL-2-dependent T cell line which showed specific immune response to SCW was established as described elsewhere [8]. The SCW-specific IL-2-dependent T cell line (1×10^4) was cocultured with autologous or allogeneic irradiated PBL (5×10^4) as the source of antigen-presenting cells (APCs) and with 5 µg/ml SCW. Proliferative response of the T cell line was assayed after 60 h by counting the incorporated [^{3}H]thymidine into T cells. The blocking study of the immune response of the T cell line to SCW with MoAbs was performed as described above.

Results

Two-dimensional PAGE

Immunoprecipitates of 4-h-labeled Dw2 or Dw12 homozygous cell lines with MoAb HU-4 consisted of actin (a, 44K), invariant chain (Ii, 31–32K) and two distinct β chains (basic β^1, 28–30K, and acidic β^2, 27–29K) and one α chain (α^1, 32–34K) of human class II molecules (Fig. 1) The α chain and β chain showed a series of two to four distinct spots due to the difference in glycosylation of each polypeptide. The α^1 chains and β^1 chains of all five lines (Dw2 or Dw12) were identical in molecular weight and in charge. The β^2 chains (28.5–30K) from the three independent Dw2 homozygous lines EB-CMG, GAY, and PGF were electrophoretically identical and they were distinct from β^2 chains (28–30K) of two independent Dw12 homozygous lines EB-KT and EB-AKIBA. The β^2 chain of EB-KT had a charge identical to that of EB-AKIBA.

In order to avoid the complex pattern of glycosylated class II molecules, 30-min pulse labelling of the lines with [^{35}S]methionine was performed. One glycosylated precursor was observed for α^1 (32K), β^1 (28.5K) and β^2 (28–28.5K) chains. The α^1 and β^1 chains showed no difference among all five lines but the β^2 chain of Dw2 was more acidic than that of Dw12 line (Fig. 2). The β^2 chain (28K) of Dw12 is slightly smaller than the β^1 (28.5K) chains of both Dw2 and Dw12. The β^2 (28.5K) chain of Dw2 has the same molecular weight as the β^1 chain of Dw2. Difference of the β^2 chain between two HLA-D specificities was confirmed by comparing the nonglycosylated polypeptides of tunicamycin-treated lines (data not shown).

Effect of MoAbs on MLR

Effect of anti-HLA-DR framework MoAb HU-4 or anti-DR2 MoAb HU-30 on the MLR between Dw2

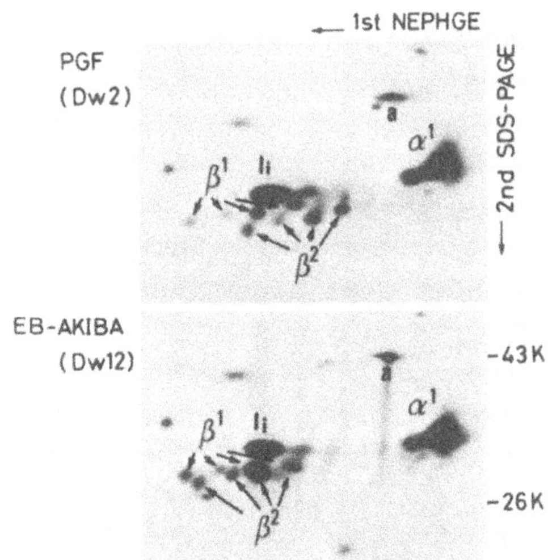

Fig. 1. 2D-PAGE profiles of immunoprecipitates from 4-h-labeled Dw2 homozygous line PGF or Dw12 homozygous line EB-AKIBA with MoAb HU-4

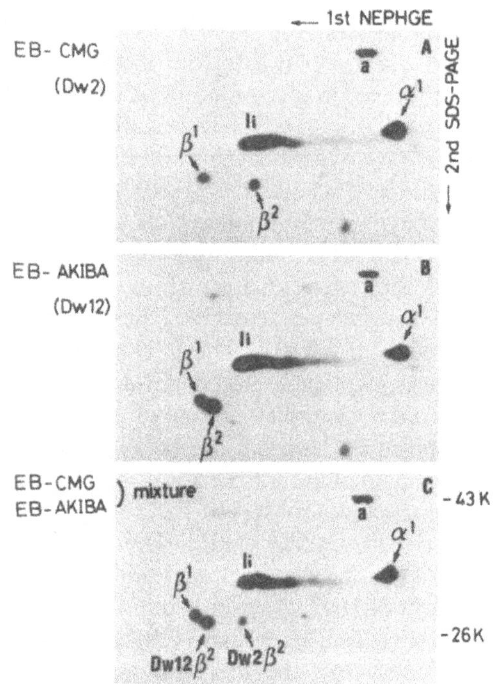

Fig. 2 A–C. 2D-PAGE profiles of immunoprecipitates from 30-min pulse-labeled cell lines with MoAb HU-4. **A**: Dw2 homozygous EB-CMG. **B**: Dw12 homozygous EB-AKIBA and **C**: mixture of A and B

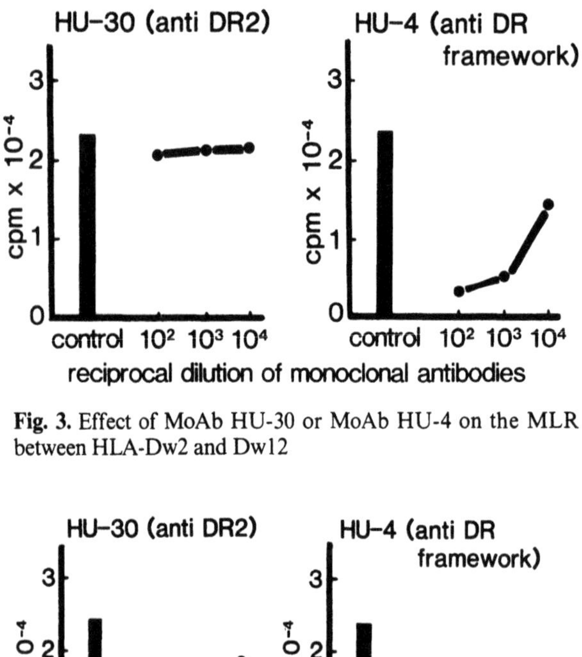

Fig. 3. Effect of MoAb HU-30 or MoAb HU-4 on the MLR between HLA-Dw2 and Dw12

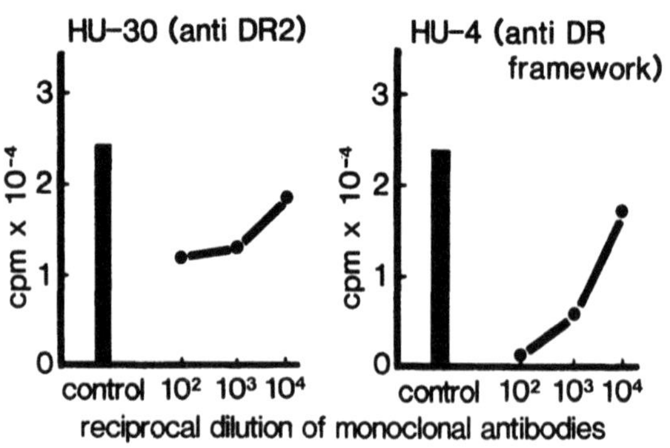

Fig. 4. Partial inhibition of the MLR between HLA-Dw12 homozygous PBL as a stimulator cell and Dw1/Dw15 heterozygous PBL as a responder cell with MoAb HU-30

and Dw12 was investigated using Dw2 homozygous Len-2 as a stimulator cell and Dw12 homozygous TOK as a responder cell (Fig. 3) and vice versa. HU-4 completely inhibited the MLR between Dw2 and Dw12, but HU-30 had no effects on this MLR. The MLR between Dw2 and Dw12 was inhibited by HU-4 by 73.5%–98.4%. This inhibition was not due to the antibody-dependent cell-mediated cytotoxicity, since no killing was observed by the chromium release assay.

Effect of MoAbs HU-4 or HU-30 on the MLR between Len-2 (Dw2) or TOK (Dw12) as stimulator cells and HU (Dw1/Dw15 heterozygote) as a responder cell were then investigated. In this case, HU-4 completely and HU-30 partially inhibited the MLR (Fig. 4). The range of the inhibition of MLR by HU-4 was 85.7%–97.2% and that of HU-30 was 33.7%–53.0% in two independent experiments.

Restriction Molecule of the Antigen Presentation of SCW to T Cells

As described before [9], proliferative response of PBL to SCW was controlled by an HLA-linked immune suppression gene and the antigen presentation of SCW to T cells by monocytes was strictly restricted by HLA-DR. MoAb HU-4 completely blocked the immune response to SCW of PBL from 30 unrelated healthy panels. The effect of HU-4 or HU-30 on the proliferative immune response to SCW of PBL from Dw2 or Dw12 homozygote is shown in Fig. 5. The immune response of PBL from TOK (Dw12) was markedly blocked by both HU-4 (82.2%–96.5% inhibition) and HU-30 (60.0%–82.2% inhibition). The immune response of Len-2 (Dw2) to SCW was also markedly inhibited by both HU-4 and HU-30 (data not shown).

The SCW-specific T cell line from a high-responder SM (DR2-Dw12/DRw6-D blank heterozygote) showed proliferative response to SCW in the presence of autologous APC. The genetic restriction between the T cell line and allogeneic APC was tested and the strength of the immune response of the T cell line with allogeneic APC was expressed by the percent autologous cooperation (%AC), which was estimated by calculating percentage of the cpm observed in a allogeneic combination to that observed in autologous combination. As shown in Fig. 6, the T cell line showed marked immune response in the presence of APCs from seven unrelated Dw12-positive panels without showing any MLR, and mean %AC was 32.6 ± 9.8. Decreased but apparently positive immune response (10.0 ± 3.7 %AC) was observed when the T cell line was cultured with APC from six unrelated

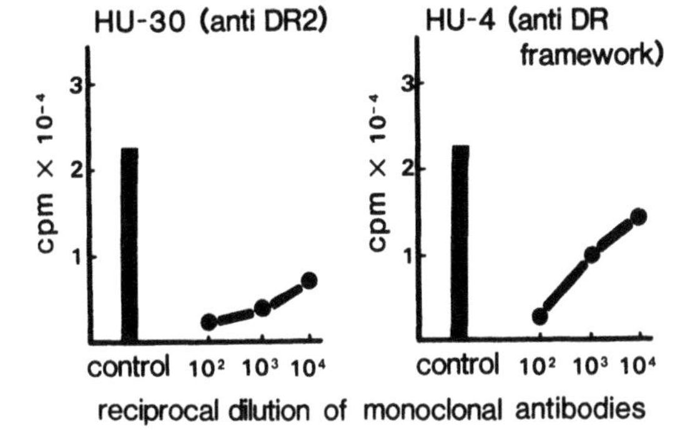

Fig. 5. Inhibition of the immune response of *Dw12* homozygous PBL to SCW by MoAb HU-30 or by MoAb HU-4

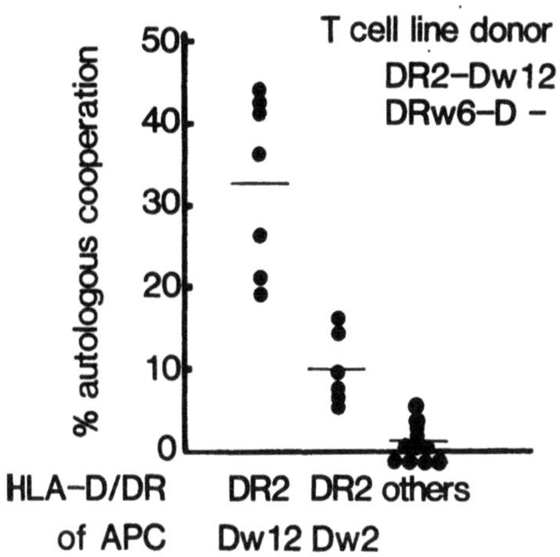

Fig. 6. Genetic restriction of the antigen presentation of SCW by allogeneic APC to the IL-2-dependent T cell line established from a *Dw12* heterozygote

Dw2-positive panels. No immune response (1.46 ± 1.79 %AC), on the other hand, was detected in the coculture of the T cell line with 11 unrelated DR-nonsharing APCs. Differences of mean %AC between DR2-Dw12-sharing combination and DR2-sharing but D-nonsharing combination, or between the latter combination and DR-nonsharing combination were both statistically significant ($p < 0.0005$ and $p < 0.002$ respectively). The immune response of the T cell line cocultured with *Dw12* heterozygous allogeneic APCs was markedly inhibited by HU-4 (60.5% – 84.0% inhibition).

Discussion

We have clearly presented the molecular difference between Dw2 and Dw12 using 2D-PAGE and functional assay. Two distinct β (β^1 and β^2) chains and one α (α^1) chain of human class II molecules were identified in both Dw2 and Dw12 by using anti-HLA-DR framework MoAb HU-4. The α^1 and β^1 chains were shared, but the β^2 chain was distinct between Dw2 and Dw12. Since only one α chain is detected, the same α chain is used to express two distinct dimers of $\alpha^1\beta^1$ and $\alpha^1\beta^2$ in Dw2- or Dw12-positive B cells.

Recently, Takenouchi et al. [10] reported that only α^1 and β^1 chains were precipitated with anti-DR2 MoAb HU-30 and that the DR2 molecule of Dw2 was identical with that of Dw12. The $\alpha^1\beta^1$ dimer should be, therefore, the DR2 molecule. Concerning the correlation between the $\alpha^1\beta^2$ dimer, DQw1, DP, and FA molecules, we identified the DQw1 and FA molecules using workshop MoAbs (anti-DQw1 MoAbs: SDR4.1 and Tü22; anti-DP MoAb: Tü39 and MHM-4; and anti-FA MoAb: FA) and proved that the $\alpha^1\beta^2$ dimer was distinct from DQw1 and FA molecules [6]. Since we cannot so far identify the DP molecules of Dw2 or Dw12 in 2D-PAGE, the possibility that $\alpha^1\beta^2$ dimer is identical to the DP molecule cannot be excluded. However, it is most likely that the $\alpha^1\beta^2$ dimer is distinct from the DP molecule for the following reasons: (1) HU-4 which precipitates the $\alpha^1\beta^2$ molecule cannot inhibit the response of DP-primed lymphocytes to five known DP antigens (data not shown). (2) There is no evidence that any DP allele is in complete linkage disequilibrium with *HLA*-Dw2 or Dw12 [11], whereas $\alpha^1\beta^2$ is always associated with Dw2 or Dw12. (3) Known DP antigens never stimulate the strong primary MLR [12], whereas the $\alpha^1\beta^2$ molecule provokes strong primary MLR between Dw2 and Dw12. The $\alpha^1\beta^2$ dimers of Dw2 and Dw12 thus seems to be novel class II molecules distinct from DR2, DQw1, FA, and probably DP molecules.

Since HU-4 completely blocked and HU-30 failed to block the MLR between Dw2 and Dw12, we concluded that the $\alpha^1\beta^2$ dimer is the stimulating molecule of the MLR between two HLA-D specificities. HU-4 completely inhibited and HU-30 partially inhibited the MLR between Dw2 or Dw12 as stimulator and Dw1/Dw15 heterozygote as responder, indicating that both $\alpha^1\beta^1$ and $\alpha^1\beta^2$ dimers have the activity of stimulating primary MLR.

The marked inhibition of the immune response of Dw2 or Dw12 homozygous PBL and of the IL-2-dependent T cell line established from the Dw12 heterozygote to SCW with HU-4 or HU-30 proved that the $\alpha^1\beta^1$ dimer is recognized by T cells as a restriction molecule at the antigen presentation by APC. Our IL-2-dependent T cell line showed proliferative immune response in the presence of DR2-shared APCs and clearly distinguished Dw12 from Dw2 expressed on APCs. This observation proved the existence of the T cell clones recognizing SCW in the context of the $\alpha^1\beta^2$ dimer.

This is the first report that a human class II molecule, which is distinct from HLA-DR, stimulates primary MLR, and is recognized by T cells as a restriction molecule at the antigen presentation of SCW by APC.

Summary

We investigated the molecular basis of the difference between HLA-Dw2 and Dw12 using two-dimensional PAGE. A novel class II molecule which is distinct from DR2, DQw1, and FA molecules and which stimulates the primary mixed lymphocyte reaction between Dw2 and Dw12 was identified. This novel class II molecule consists of a novel β chain (29K) and a DR α chain (34K), and was recognized by T cell line specific to streptococcal antigen as a restriction molecule at the antigen presentation.

References

1. Sasazuki T, Kohno Y, Iwamoto I, et al (1977) The relationship between HLA-D and WIA specificities in the Japanese population. In: Bodmer WF (ed) Histocompatibility Testing 1977. Muncksgaard, Copenhagen, pp 489–498
2. Koide Y, Awashima F, Yoshida TO, Takenouchi T, Wakisaka A, Moriuchi J, Aizawa M (1982) The role of three distinct Ia-like antigen molecules in human T cell proliferative responses. J Immunol 129:1061–1069
3. Kasahara M, Ogasawara K, Ikeda H, Okuyama T, Ishikawa N, Takenouchi T, Wakisaka A, Kikuchi Y, Aizawa M (1983) A monoclonal antibody that detects a polymorphic determinant common to HLA-DR1 and 2. Tissue Antigens 21:105–113
4. Jones PP (1980) Analysis of radiolabeled lymphocyte proteins by one- and two-dimensional gel electrophoresis. In: Mishell BB, Shiigi SM (eds) Selected methods in cellular immunology. Freeman, San Francisco, pp 398–440
5. O'Farrell PZ, Goodman HM, O'Farrell PH (1979) High resolution 2-dimensional electrophoresis of basic as well as acidic proteins. Cell 12:1133–1141
6. Sone T, Tsukamoto K, Hirayama K, Nishimura Y, Takenouchi T, Aizawa M, Sasazuki T (1984) A nobel class II molecule responsible for the primary MLR between HLA-Dw2 and Dw12. J Immunol (in press)
7. Sasazuki T, Kaneoka H, Nishimura Y, Kaneoka R, Hayama M, Ohkuni H (1980) An HLA-linked immune suppression gene in man. J Exp Med 152:297s–313s
8. Sasazuki T, Nishimura Y, Muto M, Saito Y (1984) MHC-linked immune suppression genes and their role in immunological disorders. In Sasazuki T, Tada T (eds) Immunogenetics – its applications to clinical medicine. Academic Japan, Tokyo pp 21–37
9. Nishimura Y, Sasazuki T (1983) Suppressor T cells control the HLA-linked low responsiveness to streptococcal antigen in man. Nature 302:67–69
10. Takenouchi T, Hawkin S, Kasahara M, Ishikawa N, Ogasawara K, Ikeda H, Wakisaka A, Kikuchi Y, Aizawa M (1984) Electrophoretic analysis of HLA-DR2 molecules isolated from two HLA-D clusters associated with HLA-DR2. Immunogenetics (submitted)

10a. Hawkin S, Ishikawa N, Kasahara M, Ikeda H, Ogasawara K, Wakisaka, Aizawa M (1984) Two-dimensional gel analyses of DR2 and DQwl molecules isolated from Dw2 and Dw12 homozygous cell lines. In: Albert ED et al. p 508 (this volume)

11. Shaw S, Duquesnoy RJ, Smith PL (1981) Population studies of the HLA-linked SB antigens. Immunogenetics 14:153–162
12. Shaw S, Johnson AH, Shearer GM (1980) Evidence for a new segregant series of B cell antigens that are encoded in the HLA-D region and that stimulate secondary allogeneic proliferative and cytotoxic responses. J Exp Med 152:565–580

Two-dimensional Gel Analyses of DR2 and DQw1 Molecules Isolated from Dw2 and Dw12 Homozygous Cell Lines

S. Hawkin, N. Ishikawa, M. Kasahara, H. Ikeda, K. Ogasawara, A. Wakisaka, and M. Aizawa

Department of Pathology, Hokkaido University School of Medicine, Sapporo 060, JAPAN

DR2 and DQw1 (DC1) antigens were isolated from a panel of cell lines homozygous for DR2, Dw2, DQw1, or DR2, Dw12, DQw1 and were compared by two-dimensional (2-D) gel electrophoresis.

Two homozygous typing cell lines PGF (DR2, Dw2, DQw1 homozygous) and EB-KT (DR2, Dw12, DQw1 homozygous) were used in this study. The monoclonal antibodies (MoAbs) used are as follows: HU-30, operationally monospecific for DR2 [1]; and HU-11, anti-DQw1-like [2]. 2-D gels were performed as previously described [3].

DR2 molecules isolated from PGF and EB-KT cells are electrophoretically indistinguishable (Fig. 1). HU-30 preferentially precipitated DR2 molecules that consisted of one heavy and one light chain subunits denoted α and β_1 from PGF and EB-KT cells. When the DR2 molecules (the α and β_1 subunits) of the two cell lines were compared, no electrophoretic difference was noted (Fig. 1).

DQw1 molecules isolated from PGF and EB-KT cells are structurally different in both their heavy and light chain subunits (Fig. 2): HU-11, primarily

Histocompatibility Testing 1984
Edited by E. D. Albert et al.

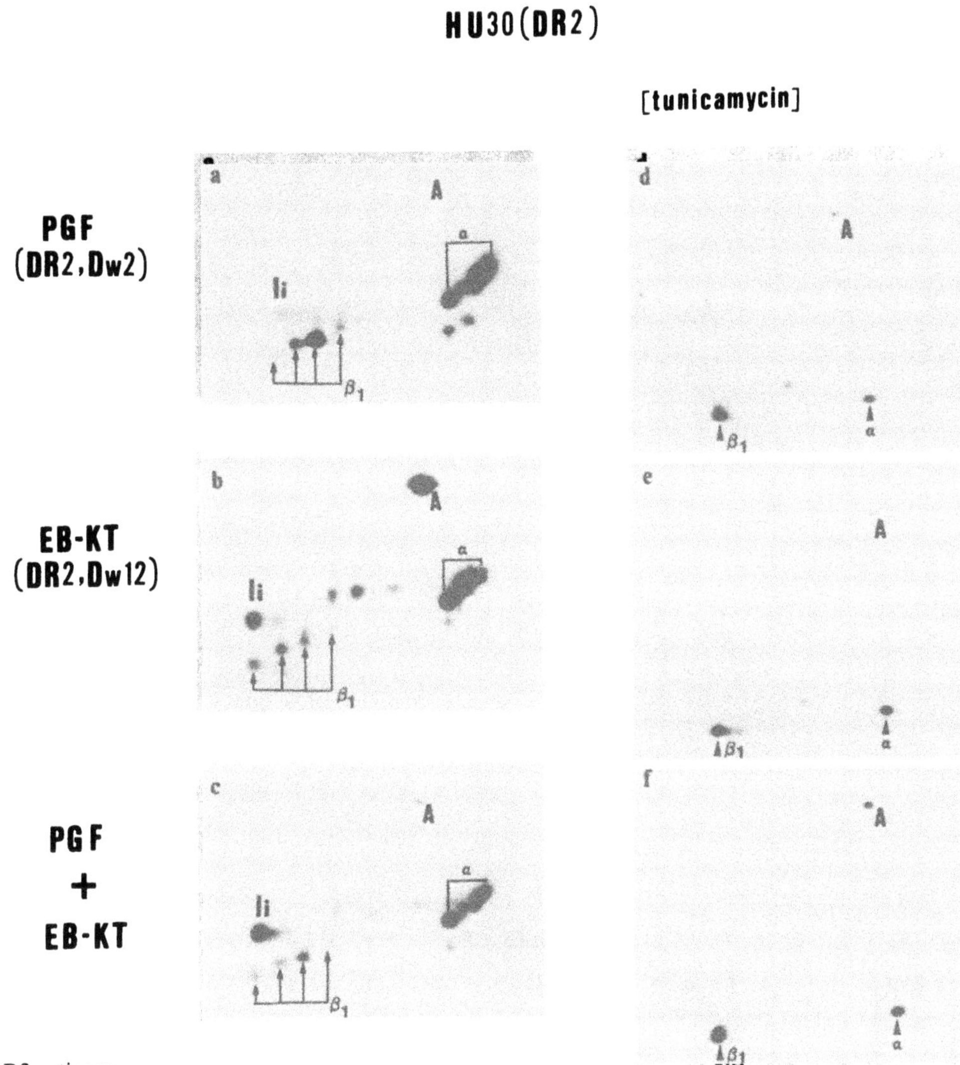

Fig. 1. Comparison of DR2 antigens

specific for DQw1, precipitated two heavy and two light chain subunits denoted α, α′, β_1, and β_2 from PGF cells (Fig. 2). Of them, the α and β_1 subunits were considered to be the heavy and light chains of the DR2 molecules because they were identical with those precipitated with HU-30 (Fig. 1). Unlike this rather simple pattern, HU-11 precipitated two heavy and at least five light chain subunits from EB-KT cells (Fig. 2). Although the β_1 subunit was clearly distinguishable, the remaining four light chain subunits were observed as closely situated spots with minor molecular weight differences but with apparently identical isoelectric points. Because it was not possible to identify the true light chain subunit of the DQw1 antigens, we called them collectively the β_2 subunits. When the α′ and β_2 subunits from PGF and EB-KT cells were compared, both were polymorphic; the α′ subunit from EB-KT cells was more basic than that of PGF cells, the β_2 subunits from EB-KT cells more acidic than that of PGF cells. These electrophoretic differences were still retained when tunicamycin-treated cell lysates were subjected to 2-D gel analyses. Taken together, our results raise the possibility that, unlike DR4-associated HLA-D clusters where the polymorphism of the DR4 light chain subunits is supposed to be responsible for mutual MLR stimulation, DQw1 rather than DR2 polymorphisms are the basis for the assignment of DR2-associated Dw specificities.

Figure 2 and References see on page 510.

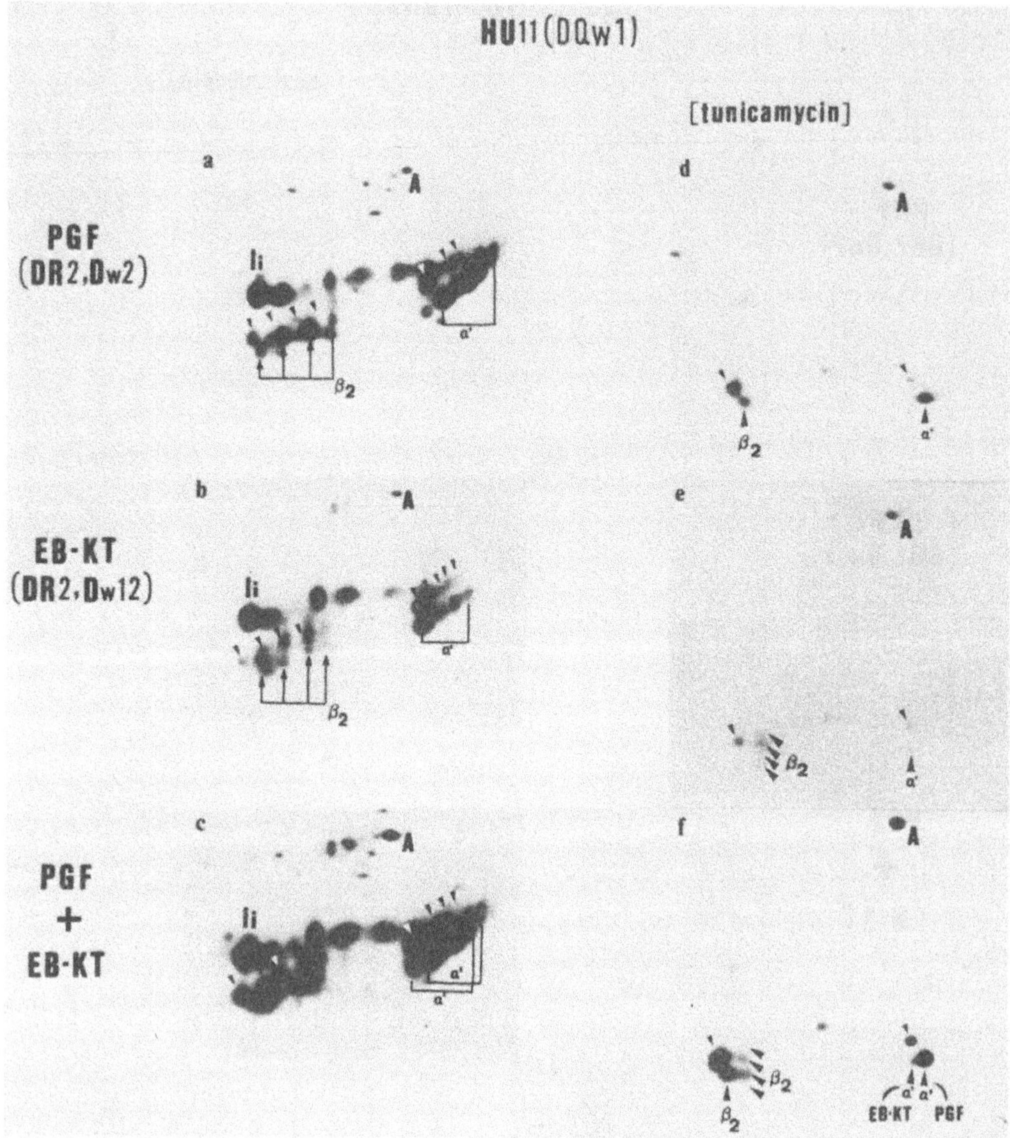

Fig. 2. Comparison of DQw1 antigens

References

1. Kasahara M, Ogasawara K, Ikeda H, Okuyama T, Ishikawa N, Takenouchi T, Wakisaka A, Kikuchi Y, Aizawa M (1983) A monoclonal antibody that detects a polymorphic determinant common to HLA-DR1 and 2. Tissue Antigens 21:105–113
2. Kasahara M, Takenouchi T, Ikeda H, Ogasawara K, Okuyama T, Ishikawa N, Wakisaka A, Kikuchi Y, Aizawa M (1983) Serologic dissection of HLA-D specificities by the use of monoclonal antibodies. II. Distinction between HLA-Dw2 and HLA-Dw12. Immunogenetics 18:525–536
3. Ikeda H, Kasahara M, Ogasawara K, Takenouchi T, Okuyama T, Ishikawa N, Wakisaka A, Kikuchi Y, Aizawa M (1984) Evidence for polymorphism of MB3 antigens among three HLA-D clusters associated with HLA-DR4. Immunogenetics 19:381–390

Separation of Three Human B-Cell Alloantigens, DR4, DRw53, and DQw3 (TB21), by Two-dimensional Gel Electrophoresis: Comparison of Alloantibodies and Monoclonal Antibodies

H. Maeda[1], R. Hirata[1], and R. Mukai[2]

1 Blood Transfusion Service, Tokyo University Hospital, Hongo 7-3-1, Bunkyo-ku, Tokyo 113
2 Department of Human Genetics, University of Tsukuba, Ibaragi, Japan

Introduction

The HLA-DR antigens are the major human class II molecules which behave as alleles encoded at a single locus [1]. To date, fourteen alleles at the DR locus have been recognized [2]. The heavy chain of the DR antigens shows no variability, whereas the light chain exhibits a marked polymorphism [3]. By the amino acid sequence analysis, the DR antigens have been shown to be homologous to the murine I-E molecules [4].

Besides the DR antigens, several "supertypic" specificities, i.e., DQ (DC) [5], MB [6], LB [8] and DRw52, w53 [7], series, are found in linkage disequilibrium with two or more DR specificities. The relationships of these class II molecules on some haplotypes have been analyzed and it was demonstrated that the DC1, MT1, and LB12 antigens (now DQw1) are identical to each other but different in both the heavy and light chains from the DR antigen [9, 10]. Thus, the existence of a second family of class II molecules, a DQ ("DC") locus, on DR2 and DRw6 haplotypes was established. Another "supertypic" specificity DQw3 (MB3 [6], MT4 [11], TB21 [12]) is primarily found on cells carrying DR4 and DR5 haplotypes, and is expressed on a subset of class II molecules [13 – 15], which belongs to the DQ ("DC") locus, since the structural characteristics of this antigen is quite similar to the DQw1 (DC1) antigen and the murine I-A molecule [16].

The MT system (now DRw52 and DRw53) included the specificity, DRw53, which was found in association with DR4, DR7, and DRw9 [7]. The same kind of specificity as DRw53, Hon7 [17], and BR4 × 7 [18] was previously shown to be carried on separate molecules from the DR antigens. More recently, we have directly demonstrated by two-dimensional (2-D) gel electrophoresis that the DRw53 molecule was distinct from the DR4 molecule in its light chain [15, 19]. However, the overall relationship of these three molecules, DR4, DRw53, and DQw3, on the DR4 haplotype was not well established.

In the present study, we have isolated DR4, DRw53, and DQw3 antigens from a DR4 homozygous cell line by using alloantisera. These molecules were also compared with those detected by various monoclonal antibodies.

Materials and Methods

Cells and Antisera

The human B lymphoid cell line BSM was established by Epstein-Barr virus from an individual of a consanguineous marriage and is homozygous for the HLA antigens (A2, B15, DR4, and Dw4) [20]. The cell line was obtained from Dr. J. J. van Rood (Leiden, the Netherlands). The human alloantisera used were obtained from the authors' laboratory and were well characterized by extensive serological and immunochemical testing [12, 15, 19]. The monoclonal antibodies NC1 and PLM12 were previously characterized [20]. The reference antibodies IVD12 [16], Tu22 [21], and FA [22] from the 9th Biochemical Workshop held in München were used for comparison. The antibody 109d6 [23] was a gift from Dr. R. Winchester (New York, NY).

Immunoprecipitation and 2-D Gel Analysis on Class II Molecules

The BSM cell line was internally radiolabeled with [^{35}S]methionine. Two different procedures of isolation of antigen molecules were used: (1) The human alloantisera were first reacted with the intact labeled cells, followed by solubilization and immunoprecipitation by protein A-Sepharose as described [15]. This procedure detected the cell surface antigen and increased the sensitivity of antigen detection by alloantisera. (2) The radiolabeled cell lysates were used for immunoprecipitation by monoclonal antibodies, in which the intracytoplasmic antigens were also detected. 2-D gel analysis was performed as described [20].

Histocompatibility Testing 1984
Edited by E. D. Albert et al.

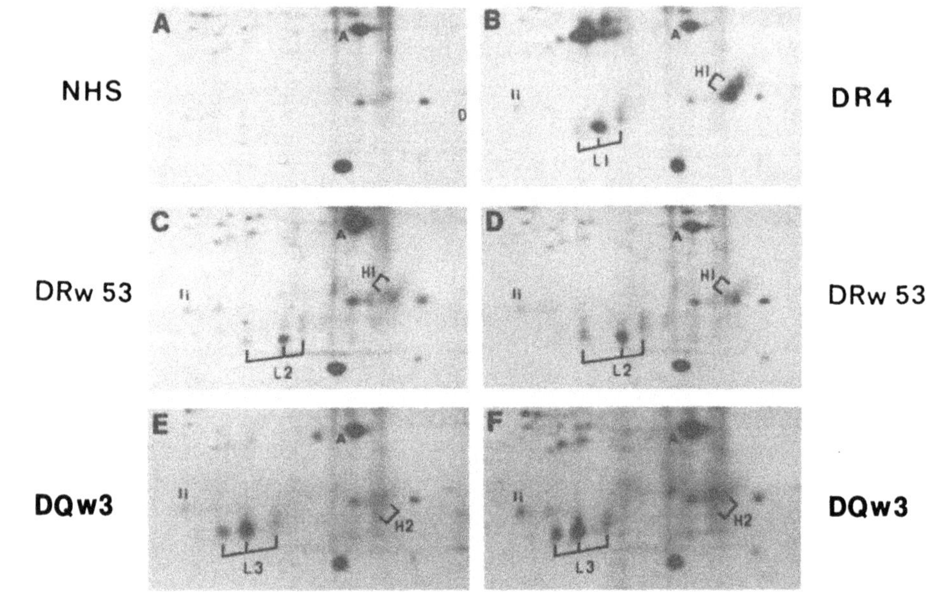

Fig. 1A–F. 2-D gel patterns of class II molecules from a DR4 cell line immunoprecipitated with alloantisera. The intact [^{35}S]methionine-labeled cells were incubated with alloantisera. After washing the unbound antibodies, the cells were solubilized and immunoprecipitated by protein A-Sepharose. The samples were analyzed by 2-D gel electrophoresis. The NEPHGE gel is oriented with the acidic end on the right and the basic end on the left. The range of m.w., 20 000–50 000 daltons, is shown from bottom to top. The antisera used are **A** NHS; **B** T2297; **C** T1065; **D** TD148; **E** T383; F T2200. *H1*, DR4 and DRw53, heavy chains; *H2*, TB21 heavy chain; *L1*, DR4 light chain; *L2*, DRw53 light chain; *L3*, TB21 light chain; *Ii*, invariant protein; *A*, actin. A dense spot of m.w. ~ 22 000 daltons is immunoglobulin light chain

Results

Identification of DR4, DRw53, and DQw3 (TB21) from a DR4 Homozygous Cell Line

To define the molecular relationship of the DR4, DRw53, and DQw3 (TB21) antigens, a radiolabeled DR4 homozygous cell line, BSM, was immunoprecipitated with alloantisera: T2297 (anti-DR4), T1065 and TD148 (anti-DRw53), T383 and T2200 (anti-DQw3). The immunoprecipitates were analyzed by 2-D NEPHGE/SDS-PAGE gel electrophoresis (Fig. 1). All the immunoprecipitates obtained by alloantisera were composed of one heavy chain of m.w. ~ 33 000–34 000 daltons at the isoelectric point (pI) of ~ 5.0, a set of three light chains of m.w. 27 000–29 000 daltons with variable pI, and an invariant polypeptide (Ii) of m.w. 31 000 daltons at the pI of ~ 7.0. However, the structural differences of the light chains among DR4, DRw53, and DQw3 antigens were clearly demonstrated. The DQw3 light chain (L3) was most basic, whereas that of DR4 (L1) was slightly different in charge. The DRw53 light chain (L2) was very acidic in charge and therefore different from the former two. In addition, the m.w. of the DR4 light chain was relatively larger, by approximately 2000 daltons, than those of DRw53 and DQw3. The heavy chain (H1) of the DR4 molecule was not resolved from the DRw53 heavy chain, but appeared to be greater in m.w. and more acidic in charge than that of DQw3 (H3). Thus, the results indicated the existence of three loci that encode three distinct alloantigens, DR4, DRw53, and DQw3.

Comparison of DR4, DRw53, and DQw3 Molecules Precipitated by Alloantisera and Mouse Monoclonal Antibodies

The 2-D gel patterns of the antigen molecules precipitated by various monoclonal antibodies are shown in Fig. 2. The antibody NC1 reacted with B cells of all DR haplotypes and immunoprecipitated two forms of DR-like molecules with varying intensity of the minor light chain on different haplotypes. The major antigens of NC1-reactive molecules were essentially identical to the DR4 molecule (H1L1) detected by alloantiserum on the BSM cell line. The weak cross-reactive light chain corresponded to that of the DRw53 molecule (L2). The antibody 109d6 showing the DRw53 specificity mainly precipitated the DRw53 heavy and light chains (H1L2). In contrast, two antibodies reactive with DRw53-like antigens, PLM12 and IVD12, and one other antibody Tu22 precipitated molecules essentially identical to each other and to the DQw3 molecules (H2L3) detected by alloantisera. The

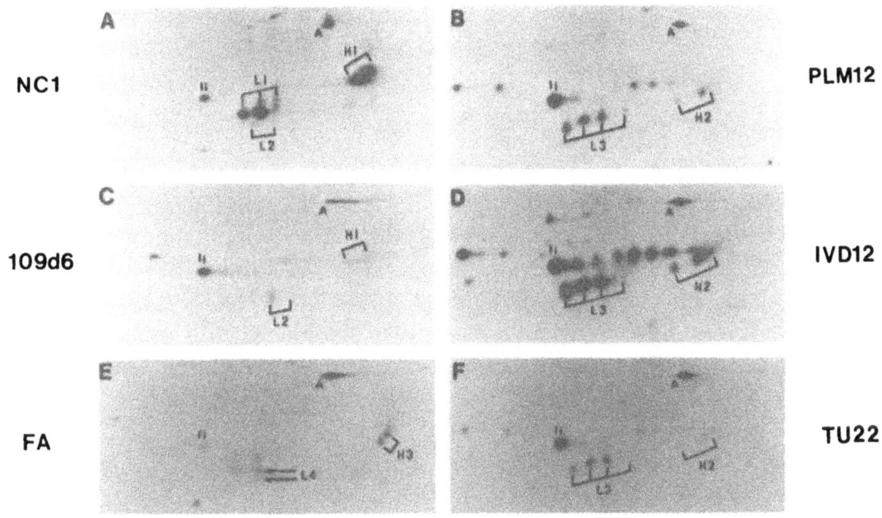

Fig. 2A–F. 2-D gel patterns of class II molecules detected with monoclonal antibodies. The [^{35}S]methionine-labeled cell lysates were immunoprecipitated with various antibodies: **A** NC1; **B** PLM12; **C** 109d6; **D** IVD12; **E** FA; **F** Tu22. Each immunoprecipitate was compared with those of the alloantisera presented in Fig. 1 and was given the label of H1, H2, L1, L2, or L3 when they were identical. H3 and L4 were given to the heavy and light chains precipitated with FA (**E**). The gel orientation is identical to that in Fig. 1. *A*, actin; *Ii*, invariant protein

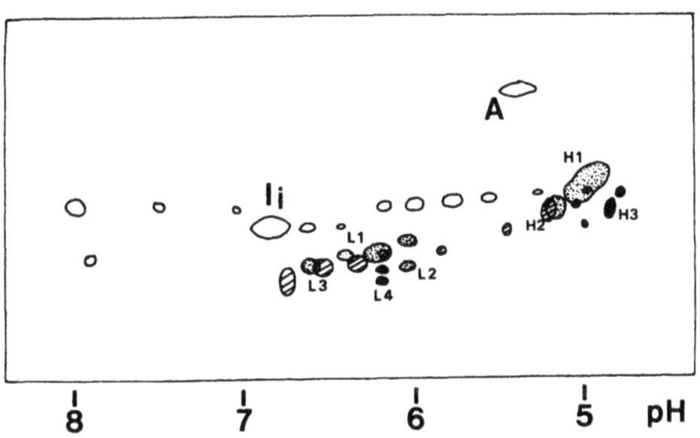

Fig. 3. Scheme of 2-D gel patterns of four class II molecules from a DR4 cell line. The heavy and light chains of DR4 are designated H1 and L1, those of DRw53 H1 and L2 (*stippled spots*). The heavy and light chains of TB21 are designated H2 and L3 (*oblique lines*), those of FA H3 and L4 (*closed spots*). *Open spots* are invariant, including an invariant protein (*Ii*) and actin (*A*)

most basic extra spot seen in the precipitate by the monoclonal antibodies was the biosynthetic intermediate form of the DQw3 light chain, which, along with other invariant spots of m.w. of around 35 000 daltons, was not detected on the cell surface. At least the three most acidic spots of the light chains were identical between the monoclonal antibodies and alloantisera. A fourth class II molecule, FA, was immunoprecipitated by the anti-FA antibody. The heavy chain (H3) of FA was more acidic in charge and lower in m.w. than the DR heavy chain (H1). The light chain (L4) was also distinguished from the former three light chains. The relationships of these four molecules are schematically illustrated in Fig. 3. Thus, we have isolated three heavy chains and four light chains, which possibly form four class II molecules, DR4, DRw53, DQw3, and FA, coded in the HLA-D/DR region.

Discussion

Three HLA-linked class II antigens, DR4, DRw53, and DQw3, from a DR4/Dw4 homozygous cell line were isolated by alloantisera. Two heavy chains and three light chains were identified. The DR4 antigenic determinant resided on a bimolecular complex of H1L1. Since the heavy chain of the DR antigens (H1) does not exhibit any polymorphism [3], the light chain (L1) would be possibly encoded by the DR locus. The DRw53 molecule was composed of a distinct light chain (L2) from that of DR4 but the heavy chain was indistinguishable from the DR4 heavy chain, suggesting that the DRw53 determinant is also expressed on the light chain.

Thus far, it has been believed that the DR antigens detected by alloantisera are controlled by a single locus. However, carefully selected alloantisera specific for some DR alleles, i.e., DR2 and DRw6, immunoprecipitated two light chains and one heavy chain [24] (unpublished work). On other DR alleles, DR4, DR7, and DRw9, anti-DR alloantibodies only precipitated one heavy and one light chain. Instead, some antisera containing DRw53 activity detected the DRw53 molecule from DR4, DR7, and DRw9 cell lines which is essentially identical to that described in this report (manuscript submitted). Thus, the biochemical definition of DR molecules is rather more complex than has been thought.

Interestingly, the monoclonal antibody NC1 immunoprecipitated two forms of DR-like molecules from all DR alleles tested. The major antigen of NC1-reactive molecules from DR4, DR7, and DRw9 cell lines corresponded to the DR antigen and the minor one to the DRw53 antigen. In addition, two forms of NC1-reactive molecules from DR2 and DRw6 cell lines are identical to those detected by anti-DR2 and anti-DRw6Y alloantisera, respectively (unpublished work). From these observations, we emphasize that both DR4 and DRw53 belong to a "DR" family of class II molecules.

The DQw3 molecule was also composed of a bimolecular complex. Both chains (H2L3) were distinct from and slightly smaller than those of the DR4 antigen (H1L1). Two monoclonal antibodies, PLM12 and IVD12, reactive with DQw3-like antigens immunoprecipitated identical molecules to the DQw3 antigen. Since the antigen molecule detected by IVD12 showed more similarity to the DQw1 antigen than DR and was the murine I-A like molecule [16], the TB21 antigen might well belong to the DQ ("DC") family. The structural polymorphism of the DQw3 light chains was previously demonstrated by using the PLM12 antibody [20]. The heavy chain also appeared to be polymorphic. Therefore, which of the two chains carry the DQw3 determinant is not yet determined.

A fourth class II molecule, FA, was identified by the novel monoclonal antibody [22]. Both chains were distinct from the former three antigens on the BSM cell line. Although the FA heavy chains were indistinguishable among those from DR2, DR4, and DRw6 cell lines, the light chains were apparently distinct from each other and therefore polymorphic (unpublished work). No available alloantisera have detected this molecule. Further, structural analysis on FA and its association with the DP polymorphism would greatly assist our understanding of the functions of a wide array of human class II molecules.

Summary

Three HLA-linked class II molecules, DR4, DRw53, and DQw3, from a DR4/Dw4 homozygous cell line were isolated by alloantibodies and mouse monoclonal antibodies. A fourth class II molecule, FA, was also isolated by the novel monoclonal antibody. Three heavy chains and four light chains were identified. The DR4 and DRw53 antigens appeared to share the same heavy chain but carried distinct light chains. Both antigens were detected by the monoclonal antibody NC1 and formed a "DR" family of class II molecules. The DQw3 antigen was distinct in both the heavy and light chains from those of DR4 and DRw53 and was identical to those detected by the monoclonal antibodies PLM12 and IVD12. Thus, the DQw3-like TB21 antigen would possibly belong to a "DQ" ("DC") family. The FA antigen was a "new" class II molecule that has not been detected by alloantisera and was polymorphic in its light chain.

References

1. Bodmer JG, Pickbourne P, Richards S (1978) Ia serology. In: Bodmer WF, Batchelor JR, Bodmer JG, Festenstein H, Morris PJ (eds) Histocompatibility Testing 1977. Munksgaard, Copenhagen, pp 35–84
2. Terasaki PI, Park MS, Bernoco D, Opelz G, Mickey MR (1980) Overview of the 1980 International Histocompatibility Workshop. In: Terasaki PI (ed) Histocompatibility Testing 1980. UCLA Press, Los Angeles, pp 1–17
3. Shackelford DA, Strominger JL (1980) Demonstration of structural polymorphism among HLA-DR light chains by two-dimensional gel electrophoresis. J Exp Med 151:144–165
4. Silver J, Walker LE, Reisfeld RA, Pellegrino MA, Ferrone S (1979) Structural studies of murine I-E and human DR antigens. Mol Immunol 16:37–42
5. Tosi R, Tanigaki N, Centis D, Ferrara GB, Pressman D (1978) Immunological dissection of human Ia molecules. J Exp Med 148:1592–1611
6. Duquesnoy RJ, Marrari M, Annen K (1979) Identification of an HLA-DR-associated system of B-cell alloantigens. Transplant Proc 11:1757–1760
7. Park MS, Terasaki PI, Nakata T, Aoki O (1980) Supertypic DR groups: MT1, MT2, and MT3. In: Terasaki PI (ed) Histocompatibility Testing 1980. UCLA Press, Los Angeles, pp 854–857
8. Termijtelen A, Boettcher B, Bradley BA, D'Amaro J, van Leeuwen A, van Rood JJ (1980) DR typing in Australian Aborigines. An indication for a second locus in the HLA-D region defined by serology. Tissue Antigens 16:140–146
9. Corte G, Garabi F, Damiani G, Bargellesi A, Tosi R, Sorrentino R (1981) Human Ia molecules carrying DC1 determinants in both α- and β-subunits from Ia molecules carrying DR determinants. Nature 292:357–360
10. Shackelford DA, Mann DL, van Rood JJ, Ferrara GB, Strominger JL (1981) Human B-cell alloantigens DC1, MT1, and LB12 are identical to each other but distinct from the HLA-DR antigen. Proc Natl Acad Sci USA 78:4566–4570
11. Park MS, Terasaki PI, Bernoco D (1980) Relationship between MT and DR antigens. In: Terasaki PI (ed) Histocompatibility Testing 1980. UCLA Press, Los Angeles, pp 572–573
12. Maeda H, Juji T (1982) A new B-cell alloantigen, TB21, coded for in the HLA-D/DR region. Tissue Antigens 20:327–334
13. Karr RW, Kannapell CC, Stein JA, Gebel HM, Mann DL, Duquesnoy RJ, Fuller TC, Rodey GE, Schwartz BD (1982) Molecular relationships of the human B cell alloantigens MT2, MB3, MT4, and DR5. J Immunol 128: 1809–1818

14. Tanigaki N, Tosi R, Sagawa K, Minowada J, Ferrara GB (1983) The distribution of DR5, MT2, and MB3 specificities on human Ia subsets. Immunogenetics 17: 371–386
15. Maeda H, Hirata R (1984) Molecular identifications of HLA-DR4, MT3, and TB21 antigens on HLA-DR4 homozygous cell lines. J Immunol 132:574–577
16. Giles RC, Nunez G, Hurley CK, Nunez-Roldan A, Winchester R, Stastny P, Capra JD (1983) Structural analysis of a human I-A homologue using a monoclonal antibody that recognizes an MB3-like specificity. J Exp Med 157:1461–1470
17. Katagiri M, Ikeda H, Maruyama N, Moriuchi J, Wakisaka A, Kimura S, Aizawa M, Itakura K (1979) Evidence for two B-cell alloantigen loci in the HLA-D region. Immunogenetics 9:335–351
18. Tanigaki N, Tosi R, Pressman D, Ferrara GB (1980) Molecular identification of human Ia antigens coded for by a gene locus closely linked to HLA-DR locus. Immunogenetics 10:151–167
19. Suzuki M, Maeda H, Mukai R, Yabe T, Hamaguchi H (1983) Identification of the MT3 molecule using two-dimensional gel electrophoresis and alloantisera. Immunogenetics 18:575–583
20. Maeda H, Hirata R, Okuyama M, Thompson A, Tohyama H (1984) Two-dimensional gel analysis of a second family of class II molecules by polymorphic HLA-DR4, 5, and w9 monoclonal antibodies, J Immunol 132: 2478–2484
21. Pawlec GP, Shaw S, Ziegler A, Muller C, Wernet P (1982) Differential inhibition of HLA-D- or SB-directed secondary lymphoproliferative responses with monoclonal antibodies detecting human Ia-like determinants. J Immunol 129:1070–1075
22. Watson AJ, DeMars R, Trowbridge IS, Back FH (1983) Detection of a novel human class II HLA antigen. Nature 304:358–361
23. Nunez-Roldan A, Szer I, Toguchi T, Cuttner J, Winchester R (1982) Association of certain Ia allotypes with the occurrence of chronic lymphocytic leukemia. J Exp Med 156:1872–1877
24. Shackelford DA, Lampson LA, Strominger JL (1983) Separation of three class II antigens from a homozygous human B cell line. J Immunol 130:289–296

Serological and Structural Heterogeneity of HLA-DR4 Alloantigens

M. Igarashi[1], M. Yoshii[2], N. Kashiwagi[2], T. Crepaldi[1], and S. Ferrone[1]

1 Dept. of Microbiology and Immunology New York Medical College, Valhalla, NY 10595, USA
2 Dept. of Transplantation Immunology, Kitasato University, School of Medicine, Sagamihara, Kanagawa, 228, Japan

Testing of a large panel of anti-class II monoclonal antibodies (MoAb) with the lymphoid cell lines FS, L-KT9, L-KT13, THO, and WALK carrying serologically indistinguishable DR4 allospecificities but different cellularly defined HLA-D allospecificities showed that the anti-HLA-DR MoAb Q2/80 displayed differential reactivity with the cell lines (Table 1).

2D-PAGE analysis of antigens immunoprecipitated with the anti-HLA-DR MoAb I2 showed marked and reproducible differences in the profile of the β chains isolated from the cell lines FS, L-KT9, L-KT13, and WALK, but did not detect any difference between the β chains isolated from the cell lines THO and WALK. No significant difference was detected in the profile of the α and γ chains isolated from the panel of cell lines. The differences in the profile of β chains were not due to glycosylation, since they were detected also in β chains synthesized by B lymphoid cells in the presence of tunicamycin. Furthermore, 2D-PAGE analysis of antigens immunoprecipitated with the anti-DQ MoAb B2 from the panel of lymphoid cell lines showed that the profiles of the β chains isolated from the cell lines L-KT9 and WALK are different from each other and from those of the β chains isolated from the cell lines L-KT13 and THO. The profile of the β chains from the last two cell lines were not significantly different from each other. These results indicate that the high discriminatory power of MoAb can detect serological differences among DR4 cell lines which are indistiguishable with conventional antisera. Serologically and cellularly defined differences are associated with marked differences in the structural profile of β chains of class II antigens immunoprecipitated with anti-HLA-DQ and anti-DQ MoAb. HLA-DR4 cell lines which carry different cellularly defined HLA-D allospecificities may carry structurally indistinguishable HLA-DR alloantigens. The latter conclusion is in agreement with the data of Groner et al. [1], but in conflict with those of Nepom et al. [2].

Table 1. Reactivity of monoclonal antibodies with homozygous HLA-DR4 cell lines

MoAb	L-KT9 Dw15[a]	L-KT13 KT2	FS Dw10	WALK Dw4	THO Dw14
Q2/80	8[b]	1024	256	256	16
Q5/6	256	256	256	256	128
CR12-356	32	64	32	64	32

[a] HLA-D specificity
[b] Reciprocal of titer

Histocompatibility Testing 1984
Edited by E. D. Albert et al.

References

1. Groner JP, Watson AJ, Bach FH (1983) Dw/LD-related molecular polymorphism of DR4 β-chains. J Exp Med 157:1687–1691
2. Nepom BS, Nepom GT, Mickelson E, Antonelli P, Hansen JA (1983) Electrophoretic analysis of human HLA-DR antigens from HLA-DR4 homozygous cell lines: Correlation between β-chain diversity and HLA-D. Proc Natl Acad Sci USA 80:6962–6966

Molecular Polymorphism of DR and DQ Products*

F.H. Bach, K.M. Linner, S.A. Choong, and J.P. Groner

Immunobiology Research Center, Box 724, University of Minnesota, Minneapolis, MN 55455, USA

In an attempt to obtain a molecular localization of determinants on HLA class II products recognized by T lymphocytes (the LD determinants), as distinct from the serologically defined DR/DQ determinants, we have studied DR and DQ β-chains using two-dimensional gel analysis (SDS-PAGE: IEF). Cells used for study of the DR product were homozygous for DR. Our primary focus has been on the DR4 product, of which there are at least five LD/Dw subtypes (Dw4, Dw10, Dw13, Dw14, and Dw15) [1]. Our findings [2, 3], illustrated in Fig. 1, are the following: The IEF position of DR4 β-chains from cells expressing different LD/Dw subtypes varies, showing a correlation between the IEF pattern and the LD/Dw phenotype. Shown in the top of Fig. 1 are IEF patterns for DR4 cells expressing Dw10, Dw4, Dw14, and Dw15, respectively. (DR4-Dw13 β-chains migrate between Dw4 and Dw10, data not shown). No difference was seen in the IEF patterns of Dw4 and Dw14 β-chains, whereas the other DR4-associated LD/Dw subtypes could be distinguished. Differences in IEF patterns were maintained following treatment with neuraminidase [3].

Treatment of the DR product with α-chymotrypsin allows individual evaluation of N-terminal and C-terminal fragments [4]. Shown in the bottom two parts of Fig. 1 is evidence that the protein difference leading to IEF positional variation which correlates with the Dw/LD phenotype resides in the N terminal portion of the DR β-chain. Analysis of N-terminal β-chain fragments from three DR4 subtypes (Dw4, Dw14, and Dw10) was also done, utilizing high-performance liquid chromatography (HPLC). Preliminary results indicate that there are differences in peptide patterns in all three cell lines, as shown in Fig. 2.

We have obtained some data suggesting a similar picture for DR2 β-chains from cells carrying different DR2-associated subtypes (Dw2, Dw12, and LD-MN2). Certain of the results discussed above have been confirmed by Nepom et al. [5].

We have extended our studies to the DQw1 molecule associated with different DR (DR1, DR2, or DRw6) specificities or with the different subtypes of DR2. Consistent with the findings of others [6], we found that the DQw1 β-chain associated with

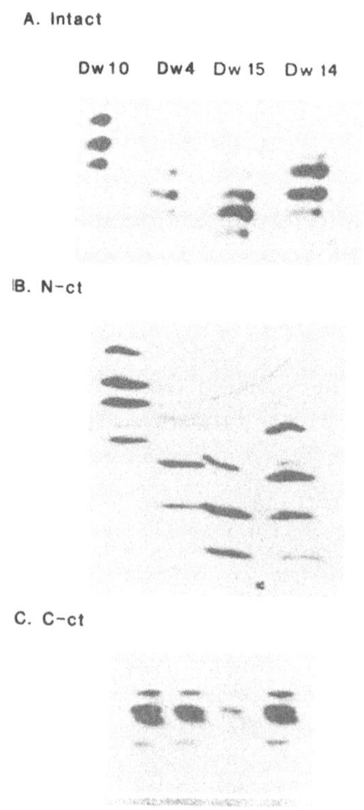

Fig. 1. Dw/LD-associated polymorphisms reside in N-ct fragments. Dw15 = DYT and Dw14 = LD40

* This is paper # 387 from the Immunobiology Research Center. This work was supported in part by NIH grants # RO1 AI 17687, AI 18326, AI 19007, and 2PO1 AM 13083, the March of Dimes Birth Defects Foundation grants # 6-255 and # 1-887, and the National Multiple Sclerosis Society grant # RG 1505-A-1

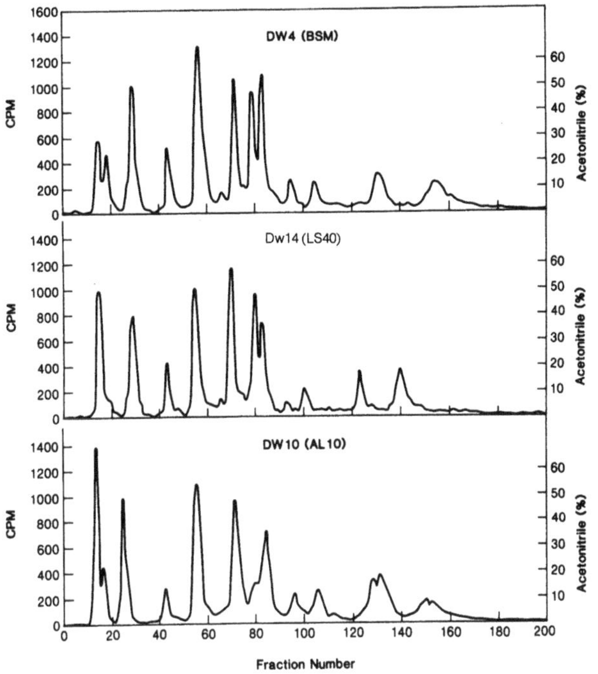

Fig. 2. HPLC: tryptic digestion of ^{3}H-arginine labeled N-terminal β-chain fragments

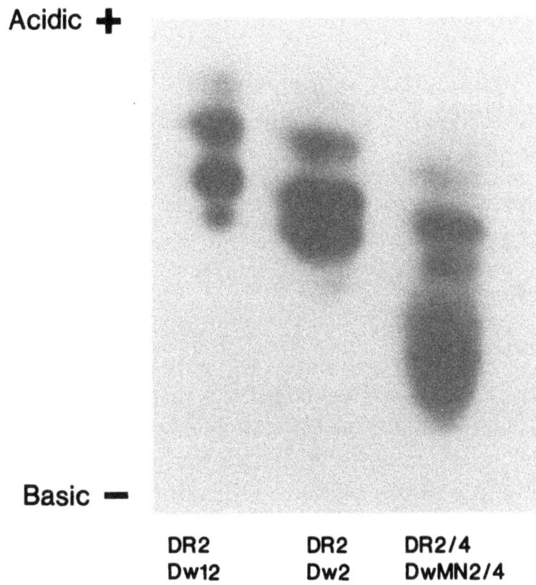

Fig. 3. DQw1 β-chain IEF polymorphism

different DR specificities migrates differently in IEF [7]. Shown in Fig. 3 are the IEF patterns of DQw1 β-chains obtained when the DQw1 molecule is associated with different LD/Dw subtypes of DR2.

The findings described above, which add a dimension to the study of HLA class II polymorphism, are primarily of import in terms of the correlation between molecular polymorphism and the polymorphism recognized by T lymphocytes, i.e., the LD polymorphism. A further understanding of which products, and which portions of which products, stimulate which functional subpopulations of T lymphocytes will greatly advance our overview of the very intimate relationship between the MHC-encoded molecules and T lymphocyte response.

References

1. Reinsmoen NL, Bach FH (1982) Five HLA-D clusters associated with HLA-DR4. Human Immunol 4:249–258
2. Groner J, Watson A, Bach FH (1983) Dw/LD related molecular polymorphism of DR4 beta chains. J Exp Med 157:1687–1691
3. Bach FH, Watson AJ (1983) Dw/LD associated molecular polymorphism of DR-4 β-chains: intramolecular localization of polymorphic sites. J Immunol 131:1622–1625
4. Kaufman JF, Strominger JL (1982) HLA-DR light chain has a polymorphic N-terminal region and a conserved immunoglobulin-like C-terminal region. Nature 297:694–697
5. Nepom BS, Nepom GT, Mickelson E, Antonelli P, Hansen JA (1983) Electrophoretic analysis of human HLA-DR antigens from HLA-DR4 homozygous cell lines: correlation between β-chain diversity and HLA-D. Proc Natl Acad Sci USA 80:6962
6. Nepom GT, Nepom BS, Antonelli P, Mickelson E, Silver J, Goyert SM, Hansen JA (1983) The HLA-DR4 family of haplotypes consists of a series of distinct DR and DS molecules. J Exp Med 159:394–404
7. Bach FH, Groner J, Watson AJ, Reinsmoen N, Segall M (1984) HLA class II molecules: T cell response and molecular characterization. In: Sasazuki T, Tada T (eds) Immunogenetics: its application to clinical medicine. Academic Press, New York (in press)

Structural Polymorphism in DQw3 Light Chains

N. Ishikawa, M. Kasahara, H. Ikeda, K. Ogasawara, S. Hawkin, T. Takenouchi, A. Wakisaka, I. Kikuchi, and M. Aizawa

Address correspondence to: Dr. Naoshi Ishikawa, Department of Pathology, Hokkaido University School of Medicine, Sapporo 060, Japan

Introduction

The DQ alloantigen system, originally described by Duquesnoy et al. [1], encodes three distinctive allelic antigens that are closely associated with particular HLA-DR antigens. Although the molecular relationship between DQ and DR antigens has long been a matter of controversy because of extremely strong linkage disequilibria between DQ and DR loci, recent biochemical evidence unequivocally shows that DQ antigens are molecularly separate from DR [2] and that they represent the human homologues of murine I-A antigens [3], whereas DR antigens are the human counterparts of murine I-E antigens [4].

However, the apparent paucity of serologically detectable polymorphism in the DQ system stands in sharp contrast with a high degree of allelic polymorphism known in genes in the murine *I-A* subregion. If DQ antigens really correspond to murine I-A antigens, they too should be polymorphic. Recently, a solution to this apparent discrepancy was provided by several investigators [5, 6]; they found the DQw1 light chain subunits derived from DR1-, DR2-, and DRw6-positive cells to be structurally different, indicating that DQw1 is a public serologic specificity shared by at least three distinct DQ (human I-A-like) molecules and that the DQ system is much more polymorphic than serologically defined. Thus, the remaining two allelic specificities, DQw2 and DQw3, may also represent public serologic specificities similar to DQw1.

In the present study, in order to assess the extent of structural polymorphism among DQw3 antigens and to compare it with that among DR antigens, DQw3 and DR antigens were isolated from a panel of homozygous typing cell (HTC) lines with DR4, DR5, DRw6.2, and DRw9 specificities and their electrophoretic mobilities were compared by two-dimensional (2-D) gel electrophoresis.

Materials and Methods

Human Cell Lines. Table 1 summarizes the HLA phenotypes of the DQw3-homozygous human B cell lines used in this study. All cell lines except Ky are homozygous for the whole HLA complex, whereas Ky (now designated EBV-Ky in order to distinguish it from the original HTC) is heterozygous for HLA-A and -B but homozygous for HLA-DR, -DQ, and -D.

Monoclonal Antibodies (MoAbs). The MoAbs used in this study are shown in Table 2. HU-18 reacts

Table 1. Lymphoblastoid cell lines used in this study

Cell lines	HLA phenotype						Reactivity of	
	A	B	DR	DRw	DQ	D	HU-18	HU-20
EBV-Wa	24	w54	4	53	w3	Dw15	–	+
KT2	2	51	4	53	w3	DKT2	+	+
ER	2	44	4	53	w3	Dw4	+	+
JMe	2	39	5	52	w3	Dw5	+	+
EBV-Sh	2	15	w6.2	52	w3	DSh	+	+
Ky	26, 11	w61, w48	w9	53	w3	DKy	+	+

Table 2. Monoclonal antibodies used in this study

Monoclonal antibodies	Workshop number	Ig class, subclass	Specificity	References
HU-18	9w915	IgG2b	DQw3	[7, 8]
HU-20	–	IgG2	all DR except DR7	[9]

 Histocompatibility Testing 1984
Edited by E. D. Albert et al.

with B cells typed as DR4, DR5, DRw6.2, or DRw9, and its serologic specificity is identical with the supertypic specificity DQw3 defined with alloantisera [7]. This MoAb recognizes human Ia-like molecules carrying the conventional DQw3 determinant on the basis of sequential coprecipitation test using an DQw3-specific alloantiserum KY-10 [8]. HU-20, initially reported as monomorphic anti-DR [9], was found in further population studies not to react with B cells typed as DR7, a DR specificity virtually absent in the Japanese. Thus, this MoAb recognizes a broadly polymorphic DR determinant shared by all B cells negative for DR7.

Isolation and 2-D Gel Analysis of Human Ia-Like Molecules. Full details of the procedure have been described previously [9]. 2-D nonequilibrium pH-gradient gel electrophoresis (NEPHGE)/sodium dodecyl sulfate-polyacrylamide gel electrophoresis (SDS-PAGE) was performed according to the method of O'Farrell et al. [10].

Results

Structural Polymorphism of DQw3 Antigens

Figure 1 shows 2-D NEPHGE/SDS-PAGE profiles of Ia-like molecules immunoprecipitated with HU-18 that has been characterized to recognize an antigenic determinant on DQw3 molecules. With the exception of EBV-Wa cells that do not react with HU-18 (panel *a*), the following specific immunoprecipitates were obtained from each of the [^{35}S]methionine-labeled cell lines shown in panels *b* to *f*: two heavy chain subunits of 32 000 – 34 000 daltons (α) and 31 000 – 33 000 daltons (α'); and one light chain subunit of 27 000 – 30 000 daltons (β') with variable isoelectric points. In all cell lines examined, the mobility of the α subunits was exactly identical with that of the heavy chain subunits immunoprecipitated with the DR-specific MoAb HU- 20 (Fig. 2). Thus, the α subunits in Fig. 1 most likely represent cross-reactively precipitated heavy chains of DR antigens, leading to the conclusion that the α' and β' subunits correspond to the heavy and light chains of the DQw3 antigens. We next compared the electrophoretic mobility of the α' and β' subunits from KT2, ER, JMe, EBV-Sh, and Ky cells (Fig. 1 panels b – f). No difference in charge or molecular weight was noted in the α' subunits. In contrast, the β' subunits from the cell lines KT2 (panel *b*), ER (panel *c*), and Ky (panel *f*) were clearly different in terms of their isoelectric points; the KT2 β' subunit was most basic, the ER β' subunit most acidic, and the Ky β' subunit had an in-

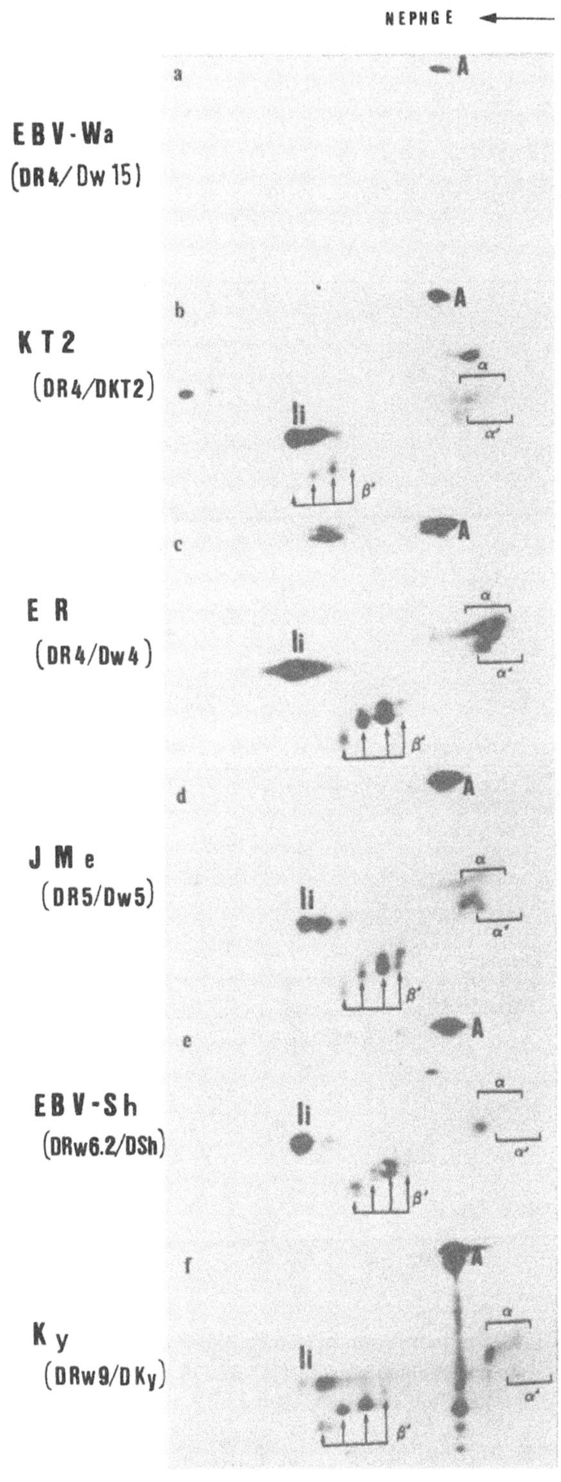

Fig. 1a – f. 2-D NEPHGE/SDS-PAGE profiles of DQw3 molecules immunoprecipitated with HU-18. DQw3 molecules were isolated from [^{35}S]methionine-labeled KT2 (**b**), ER (**c**), JMe (**d**), EBV-Sh (**e**), and Ky (**f**) cells. Because HU-18 did not react with EBV-Wa cells, no specific immunoprecipitates were obtained in panel **a**. The direction of SDS-PAGE is from top to bottom and the acidic end of the NEPHGE gel is on the right. *A*, actin; *Ii*, invariant polypeptide

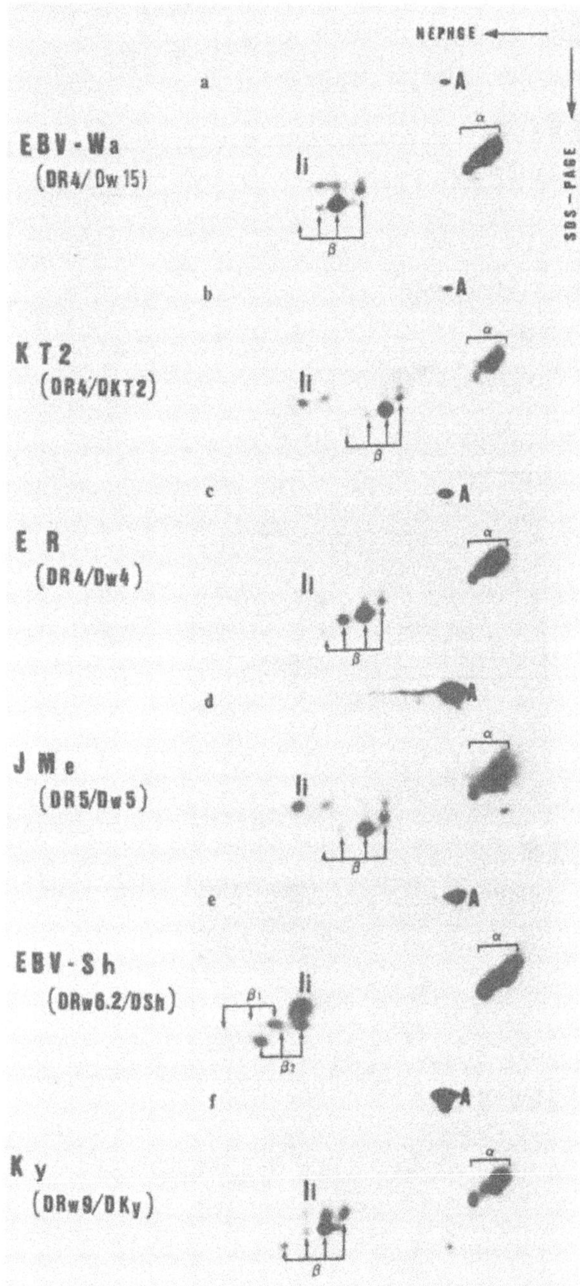

Fig. 2a–f. 2-D NEPHGE/SDS-PAGE profiles of DR molecules immunoprecipitated with HU-20. DR molecules were isolated from [^{35}S]methionine-labeled EBV-Wa (**a**), KT2 (**b**), ER (**c**), JMe (**d**), EBV-Sh (**e**), and Ky (**f**) cells. Gels are orientated as described in Fig. 1 legend. For abbreviations, see Fig. 1 legend

termediate isoelectric point. However, the β' subunits from ER, JMe, and EBV-Sh cells were electrophoretically indistinguishable. The polymorphism of the β' subunits was not due to glycosylation processes, because it was still retained when tunicamycin-treated cell lysates were subjected to 2-D gel analyses (data not shown). Because HU-18 does not react with EBV-Wa cells, the DQw3 molecules of EBV-Wa cells are considered to be structurally different from those of the other HU-18-positive HTCs. Thus, the results presented here indicate the existence of at least four structurally distinct DQw3 molecules.

It should be noted that the β' subunits of ER, JMe, and EBV-Sh cells consistently focused as two series of closely situated spots with minor molecular weight differences but with apparently identical isoelectric points. Because it was not possible to determine which one of these two adjoining spots really corresponded to the light chain of the DQw3 molecules, we did not provide them with separate designations and simply called them the β' subunits.

Structural Polymorphism of DR Antigens

The D/DR-related structural polymorphism of the DR light chain subunits is well established [11]. To compare the extent of structural polymorphism among DR antigens with that among DQw3 antigens, DR antigens were immunoprecipitated with HU-20 from the six HTC lines shown in Fig. 2. In all cell lines except EBV-Sh (panel *e*), HU-20 precipitated one heavy chain subunit of 32 000 – 34 000 daltons (α) and one light chain subunit of 28 000 – 31 000 daltons (β). The molecular weights and isoelectric points of these α and β subunits were clearly different from those of the α' and β' subunits precipitated with HU-18 (Fig. 1), providing the basis for our interpretation that the α subunit in Fig. 1 represents the heavy chain of the DR antigens that were cross-reactively precipitated with HU-18. In EBV-Sh cells (panel *e*), consistent with our earlier observation [8], two light chain subunits denoted β_1 and β_2 were precipitated with HU-20. Although this suggests the existence of two DR-like molecules in this cell line, it remains to be answered which light chain subunit carries the serologically defined DR alloantigenic determinant.

Comparisons of the DR heavy and light chain subunits (α and β subunits) from the six cell lines revealed that the α subunits were virtually invariant, whereas the β subunits were different in their isoelectric points from cells to cells (Fig. 2). Although we could not determine the true light chain subunit of the EBV-Sh DR antigens, both of the β_1 and β_2 subunits differed from the β subunits of the remaining five cell lines. Similar to the DQw3 antigens, the DR light chain polymorphism was not affected after tunicamycin treatment, indicating that the DR light chain polypeptides were structurally polymorphic (data not shown).

Thus, the results presented here show that all of the six cell lines express structurally different DR light chain subunits. Because the four out of the six cell lines examined were found to express structurally distinct DQw3 molecules (Fig. 1), the DR light chain subunits are apparently more polymorphic than the DQw3 light chain subunits.

Of interest is the finding that the DR4 light chains isolated from EBV-Wa, KT2, and ER cells are structurally different (Fig. 2). This is consistent with the results of Groner et al. [12] and Nepom et al. [13] and indicates that DR4 is a public serologic specificity shared by at least three structurally distinct DR molecules. This structural polymorphism of the DR light chains was further confirmed by using HU-48, a MoAb specific for DR4 and DR5 (data not shown). Taken together, our results in Figs. 1 and 2 demonstrate that HTCs defining Dw15, DKT2, and Dw4, though equally typed as DR4 and DQw3, differ from one another in both their DQ and DR molecules.

Conclusions

Four out of the six cell lines were found to express structurally distinct DQw3 (human I-A-like) molecules. These results, in combination with the observations of other investigators that DQw1 light chain subunits derived from DR1-, DR2-, and DRw6-positive cells are structurally different, demonstrate that the serologically detectable DQ specificities DQw1 and DQw3 are supertypic to several DQ molecules and that the *DQ* system, which has been believed to be composed of only three alleles, DQw1, DQw2, and DQw3, is in reality much more polymorphic.

The DR light chain subunits were apparently more polymorphic than the DQw3 light chain subunits. However, because the electrophoretic identity does not immediately mean structural identity of the molecules compared, further work is needed to assess the exact extent of structural polymorphism among the DQw3 and DR antigens.

References

1. Duquesnoy RJ, Marrari M, Annen K (1979) Identification of an HLA-DR-associated system of B-cell alloantigens. Transplant Proc 11:1757–1760
2. Tosi R, Tanigaki N, Centis D, Ferrara GB, Pressman D (1978) Immunological dissection of human Ia molecules. J Exp Med 148:1592–1611
3. Bono MR, Strominger JL (1982) Direct evidence of homology between human DC-1 antigen and murin I-A molecules. Nature 299:836–838
4. Allison JP, Walker LE, Russell WA, Pelligrio MA, Ferrone S, Reisfeld RA, Frelinger JA, Silver J (1978) Murine Ia and human DR antigens: homology of anti-terminal sequence. Proc Natl Acad Sci USA 75:3953–3958
5. Shackelford DA, Mann DL, van Rood JJ, Ferrara GB, Strominger JL (1981) Human B-cell alloantigens DC1, MT1, and LB12 are identical to each other but distinct from the HLA-DR antigen. Proc Natl Acad Sci USA 78: 4566–4570
6. de Kretser TA, Crumpton MJ, Bodmer JG, Bodmer WF (1982) Two-dimensional gel analysis of the polypeptides precipitated by a polymorphic HLA-DR1, 2, w6 monoclonal antibody: Evidence for a third locus. Eur J Immunol 12:214–221
7. Kasahara M, Takenouchi T, Ogasawara K, Ikeda H, Okuyama T, Ishikawa N, Moriuchi J, Wakisaka A, Kikuchi I, Aizawa M, Kaneko T, Kashiwagi N, Nishimura Y, Sasazuki T (1983) Sereologic dissection of HLA-D specificities by the use of monoclonal antibodies. Immunogenetics 17:485–495
8. Ikeda H, Kasahara M, Ogasawara K, Takenouchi T, Okuyama T, Ishikawa N, Wakisaka A, Kikuchi I, Aizawa M (1984) Evidence for polymorphism of MB3 antigens among three HLA-D clusters associated with HLA-DR4. Immunogenetics (in press)
9. Kasahara M, Ogasawara K, Ikeda H, Okuyama T, Ishikawa N, Takenouchi T, Wakisaka A, Kikuchi I, Aizawa M (1983) A monoclonal antibody that detects polymorphic determinant common to HLA-DR1 and DR2. Tissue Antigens 21:105–113
10. O'Farrell PZ, Goodman HM, O'Farrell (1977) High resolution two-dimensional electrophoresis of basic as well as acidic proteins. Cell 12:1133–1141
11. Charron DJ, McDevitt HO (1980) Characterization of HLA-D-region antigens by two-dimensional gel electrophoresis. Molecular genotyping. J Exp Med 152:18s–36s
12. Groner JP, Watoson AJ, Bach FH (1983) Dw/LD-related molecular polymorphism of DR4 β-chains. J Exp Med 157:1687–1691
13. Nepom BS, Nepom GT, Mickelson E, Antonelli P, Hansen JA (1983) Electrophoretic analysis of human HLA-DR4 homozygous cell lines: correlation between β-chain diversity and HLA-D. Proc Natl Acad Sci USA 80:6962–6967

Molecular Dissection of DRw6

A. Haziot[1,2], V. Lepage[2], L. Degos[2], and D.J. Charron[1]

1 Laboratoire d'Immunogénétique, Département d'Hématologie CHU Pitié Salpétrière, 91 boulevard de l'Hôpital, 75013 Paris, France
2 INSERM U.93, Hôpital Saint-Louis, 2, Place du Dr. Fournier, 75475 Paris Cedex 10, France

The complex HLA-DRw6 specificity was first described at the Seventh Histocompatibility Workshop according to the reactivity of a set of polyspecific sera (DR2 + w6; DR3 + w6). While the DR specificities 1 to 5 and 7 were clearly defined during the following workshop, no monospecific anti-DRw6 sera were found. HLA-DRw6 was therefore only defined by a serie of supertypic sera. These include anti-DQw1, which react with DR1, DR2, and DRw6; anti-DRw52 which react with DR3, DR5, DRw6, and DRw8; and sera with shorter reactivity: anti-DR2 + w6, anti-DR3 + w6, anti-DR5 + w6, anti-DR3 + 5 + w6. DRw6 specificity was thus assigned to cells reacting with the above supertypic sera but negative with monospecific sera anti-DR1, 2, 3, 5, and w8. Subdivisions of DRw6 were proposed following combinations of reactivities with clusters of supertypic sera as reviewed in a recent report [7]. Because of the absence of monospecific DRw6 sera the existence of the DRw6 molecule itself has been a matter of controversy. We investigated the molecular nature of the DRw6 antigens in 15 individuals and four families using a monomorphic monoclonal anti-HLA-DR antibody and two-dimensional gel electrophoresis (2D-PAGE).

Materials and Methods

Sera. Cells were typed by lymphomicrocytotoxicity with alloantisera of the Ninth Histocompatibility Workshop. The following supertypic sera were used to assign the DRw6 specificity: DR2 + w6: sera 652, 653, 654, 655, 656; DR1 + 2 + w6: sera 657, 661, 662, 663, 664, 667, 668; DR1 + 2 + w6 + w10: sera 669, 670, 671, 672, 674; DR3 + w6: sera 677, 678, 679, 680, 712, 713, 714, 715; DR5 + w6: sera 681, 682, 683, 684; DR3 + 5 + w6: sera 685, 687, 688, 689; DR3 + 5 + w6 + w8: sera 692, 693, 694, 696, 697, 698, 699. The monoclonal antibodies (moAbs) D1.12 and SG 157 were used for immunoprecipitation. Both moAbs react with a monomorphic epitope of the DR antigens [2, 6, 8].

Cells. B-lymphoblastoid cell lines (B-LCL) or PHA-stimulated peripheral blood lymphocytes (PBL) of 15 different unrelated individuals and members of four informative families were used in this study.

Radiolabelling, Extraction, and Immunoprecipitation of DR Antigens. Cells were internally labeled with [^{35}S]methionine for 4–5 h. The cell proteins were solubilized with 0.5% NP 40 and the membrane extracts collected. Five microliters of monoclonal anti-HLA-DR ascites was used for immunoprecipitation. *Staphylococcus aureus*-precipitated antigen-antibody complexes were eluted in reducing and denaturing conditions for gel migration [4].

2D-PAGE. This was performed as previously described [4, 15]. Briefly, non-equilibrium pH-gradient electrophoresis (NEPHGE) was used in the first dimension to obtain a good resolution of the β chain area. The second dimension was a 10% SDS-PAGE. The autoradiographs presented are the result of exposure for 7–36 days.

Results and Discussion

Previous studies showed that HLA-DR antigens are composed of a complex of two chains, the α-chain (33K) and the β-chain (29K). Analysis of DR antigens by 2D-PAGE has precised the heterogeneity of this complex with an acidic α chain and a basic β chain. In addition, while the α chain pattern is constant from one cell to the other, typical β chain profiles were described for each well-defined DR allele [4]. An invariant third chain (Ii) of 31K is coprecipitated with the DR complex and focusses in the basic area of the gel [5], and can serve as internal marker for β chain comparisons. In our study, cells from 15 individuals and four informative families were operationally defined as DRw6 for at least one haplotype. Because the 2D-PAGE β chain patterns of DR1 to 5, DR7, and DRw8 are known and because the moAbs used in this study would only react with the HLA-DR molecules, it has been possible to assign a DR β chain to the HLA-DRw6 haplotype. In cells typed DRw6/DR blank, when one of the β chains was identical to one of the previously defined DRw6 β chains, the second β chain was considered to represent the serological DR blank. In family studies, each β chain pattern segregates according to the serological markers defining the haplotypes. It was thus possible to associate one of the DR β chains the

Histocompatibility Testing 1984
Edited by E. D. Albert et al.

DRw6 haplotype. In this study, four different DRw6 antigens were identified by the electrophoretic mobility of their DR β chain. The first DRw6 β chain pattern consists of a set of four spots. Two spots are more basic than the invariant chain, the two other more acidic (Fig. 1A). In this molecular group, DQw1-positive reaction is associated with three DRw6 haplotypes, two of which are positive for the serum 9W781. However, one cell is DQw1 negative. These four cells have positive and informative serological reactions with anti-DRw52 sera and with DR3 + 5 + w6 sera. Preliminary results indicate that this β chain is present in a Dw9 HTC (A. Haziot, H. Betuel, D. Charron, unpublished observation). The second β chain pattern observed on DRw6 cells is more acidic and of lower molecular weight (Fig. 1B). Biochemical and serological family studies associate this β chain with positive reactions with DRw52 sera and anti-DR5 + w6 sera and with negative reactions with DQw1 sera. The third β chain profile immunoprecipitated from DRw6 cells is defined by three spots in the basic end of the gel (Fig. 1C). All cells in this group are DQw1 negative. In one family and in several cases where DRw52 typing is informative, positive reactions are found with DRw52 sera and weaker reactions with anti-DR3 + 5 + w6 sera. Informative reactions with short DRw52 sera are variable from one cell to another in this molecular group. A fourth β chain pattern was identified in

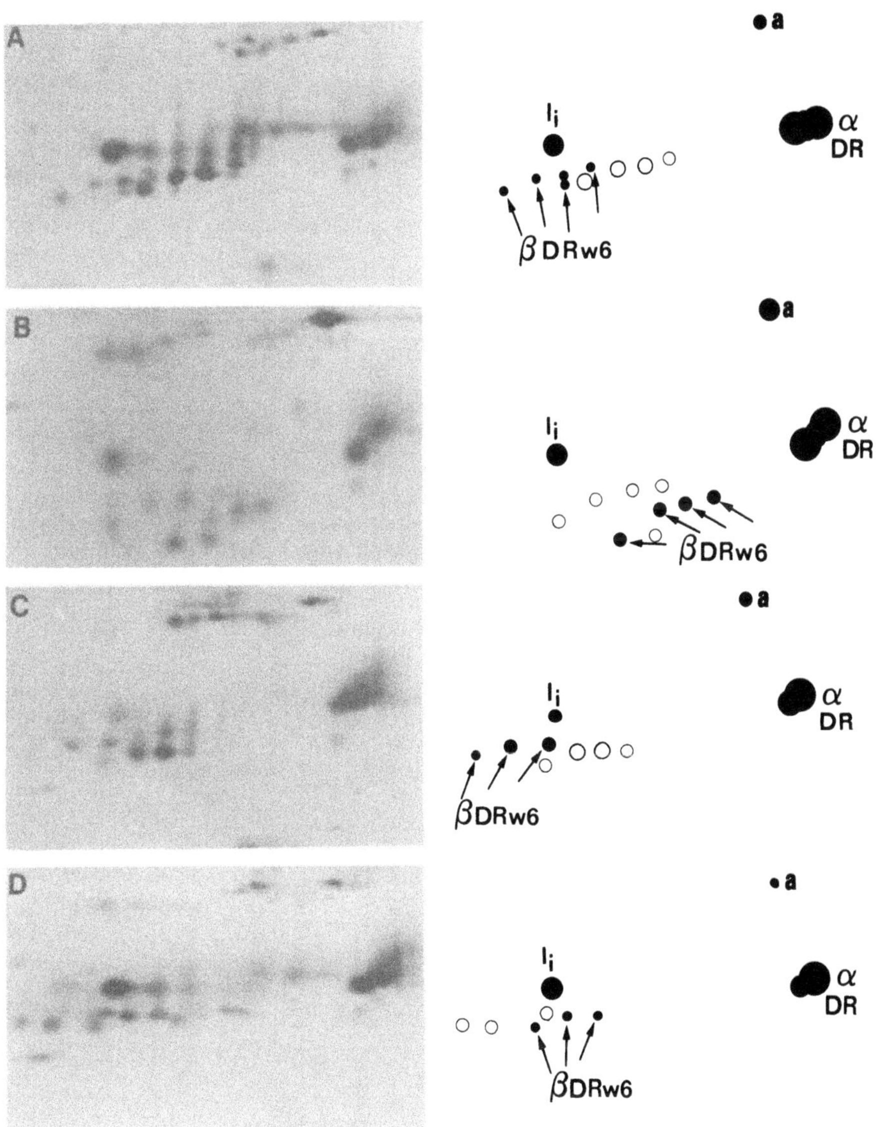

Fig. 1A–D. 2D-PAGE profiles of the different HLA-DRw6 molecules immunoprecipitated with moAbs D1.12 (**A, C, D**) and SG 157 (**B**) from [^{35}S]methionine-labeled cells. **A** B-LCL family PER patient J. F. (DRw6/DR7); **B** PHA-activated PBL from family PRE father (DRw6/DR2); **C** B-LCL 545 (DRw6/DR5); **D** B-LCL 560 (DRw6/DR3). The basic end of the NEPHGE gel is on the left and the direction of SDS electrophoresis is from top to bottom. *a*, actin

five DRw6 cells and is composed of three spots. The two most basic spots are located below, one each side of, the Ii chain (Fig. 1D). The cells expressing this HLA-DR β chain have only in common positive reactions with DRw52 sera. Reactivities with short DRw52 sera are variable among these cells, and one cell is weakly positive with DR2 + w6 sera.

Of particular interest are two cells which were previously typed DR7/w6 and DR5/w6 with the Eighth Histocompatibility Workshop sera and are presently typed DR7/5 and DR5/blank with the Ninth Workshop sera. In 2D-PAGE, the DR5/blank cell possess one typical DR5 β chain. The second set of β chain spots (Fig. 2), corresponding to the DR blank, is identical to the DR5 β chain pattern of the cell typed DR7/5. The DR5/blank cell is thus serologically DR5 homozygous with sera of the Ninth Workshop, but expresses two different molecular forms of the DR5 β chain. Moreover, this cell was weakly positive with DQw1 local sera, suggesting a possible association of this specificity with a particular DR5 haplotype.

In one cell typed DR4/DRw6, no DR β chain is detected corresponding to the DRw6 haplotype (Fig. 3A). Heterozygosity was proven in this individual by segregation of the serological markers in the family. Similarly, no detectable DRw6 haplotype associated β chain was found in two additional cells (data not shown). However, for one cell, long exposition of the gel (Fig. 3B) allowed detection of two very faint spots which migrate in the position of the two most basic spots of the fourth DRw6 β chain pattern described above. Because of the serological complexity, extensive biochemical analysis of DRw6 was clearly needed to answer some puzzling questions about the existence and the polymorphism of the DRw6 products. The absence of monospecific anti-DRw6 sera led to consideration of DRw6 as a null allele. Heterogeneity of DR anti-

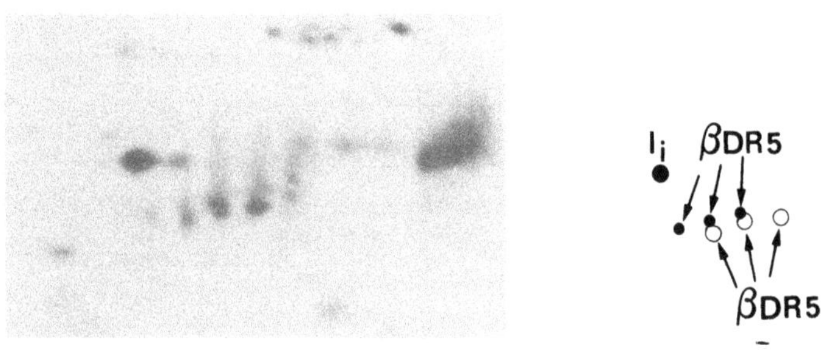

Fig. 2. 2D-PAGE of [^{35}S]methionine-labeled B-LCL 346 immunoprecipitated with D1.12. This cell was previously typed DRw6/DR5 with 8W sera and is typed DR blank/DR5 with 9W sera. *Open spots* represent a previously described DR5 β chain; *full spots* represent a new DR5 β chain pattern identified in a DR5/DR7 cell

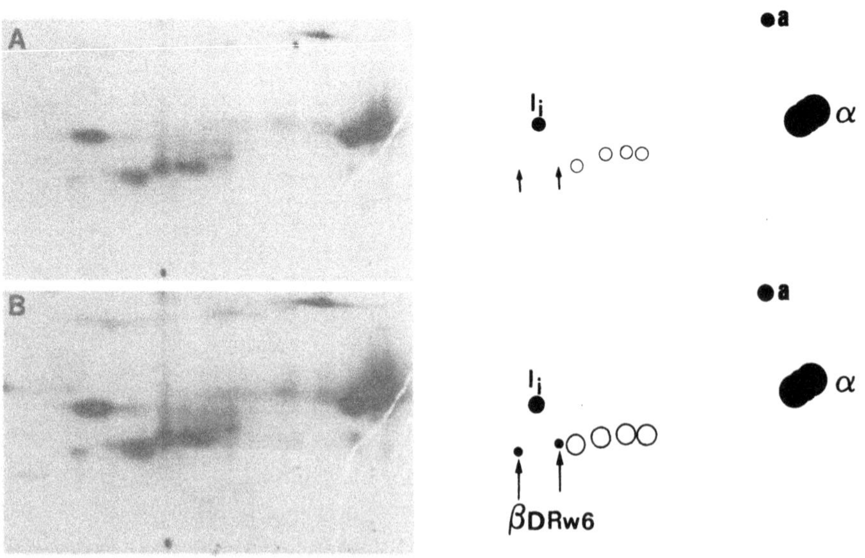

Fig. 3A, B. 2D-PAGE of [^{35}S]methionine-labeled B-LCL 432 (DRw6/DR4) immunoprecipitated with D1.12. Gels were exposed for 13 days (**A**) and 36 days (**B**). *Arrows* localize in **A** the faint additional spots detected after long exposure in **B**

gens in several DRw6 positive cells has recently been reported [16]. The results presented here show that in most but not all cases, one DR β chain is associated with DRw6 haplotypes. We were able to characterize biochemically four different HLA-DR subtypes within DRw6 cells. Structural polymorphism has been previously localized to the β chain of the HLA-DR molecule [4, 11]. No structural difference was found for the DR α chain from different alleles [3, 11]. According to these results, the molecular heterogeneity of the DRw6 antigens was assessed on the electrophoretic polymorphism of the β chain.

The DRw6 β chains described here have clearly distinct 2D-PAGE patterns. Moreover, no spot in common was found in different subtypes. Therefore it is unlikely that the observed polymorphism is due to maturation processes. No DRw6 molecular group defined here could be predicted by DRw6 serology. In the first group, the same DR antigen is associated with DQw1 positive and negative haplotypes. Similar dissociation is observed with serum 9W781. This molecularly defined DRw6 subtype does not coincide with the recently described DRw14 specificity [17, 1]. In each of the other subtypes, common serological reactivities of the cells do not fit with any DRw6 serological subdivision previously proposed: that is, cells with distinct DRw6 specificities possess clearly identical DR antigens. Conversely, and as has been reported for other DR specificities [14], different DR β chains correspond to one particular serological DRw6 specificity. However, DNA analysis has shown the complexity of the HLA-DR region genes, with at least three different loci for DR β chains [12]. Therefore, the DR β chain associated here with each DRw6 haplotype might by only one of the DR β chains which contribute to the DRw6 serological specificity. Further investigations are needed to prove the expression of each DRw6 β chain on the cell surface. These biochemical results provide a rationale for searching for and identifying allosera specific for each DRw6 molecular subtype.

Evidence for DRw6 haplotype without detectable DR β chain is given here. Biochemical family studies and immunoprecipitations with moAbs that react either with the α chain or with the β chain are in progress to confirm the nonexpression or weaker expression of the DRw6 β chain in those cells. Null I-E alleles were described in four murine haplotypes [10]. Depending on the haplotype, defect at the gene level and in mRNA processing were proposed to explain the nonexpression of I-E α chain [13]. In human heterozygous cells, absence of one DR nonpolymorphic α chain is expected to be silent, as transcomplementation might occur. Therefore, lack of detectable β chain would only be explained by defects or regulation events at the β DR gene or transcript level. An alternative possibility is the existence of some α chain polymorphism restricted to these DRw6 haplotypes.

Lack of monospecific antisera has made serological subdivisions of DRw6 arduous to outline. 2D-PAGE analysis of DR antigens from DRw6 cells provides an accurate and reproducible classification inside a complex specificity. Characterization of I-A-like (DQ) antigens in those cells is in progress to aid our understanding of the particular nature of DRw6 haplotypes. Molecular analysis in DRw6 cells may explain the high immune response of HLA-DRw6 positive recipients of kidney graft [9]. In such a complex specificity, molecular typing should be preferred to serological typing.

Summary

Due to an absence of monospecific alloantisera, the definition of DRw6 specificities remains unclear. We have analyzed the molecular heterogeneity of HLA-DRw6 antigens by two-dimensional gel electrophoresis (2D-PAGE) in 15 unrelated individuals and in four informative families, all typed with the sera of the Ninth Workshop. In most cells, a DR β chain corresponding to the DRw6 haplotype was present. Four different molecular species were identified according to the 2D-PAGE profile of the β chain. The molecular subgroups defined correlate only partially with DRw52 sera and not with DQw1 sera. In several cells, the DR β chain associated to the DRw6 haplotype was absent or weakly detected, suggesting a quantitative polymorphism. 2D-PAGE genotyping provides an appropriate approach to further definition and classification of DR specificities.

References

1. Betuel H, Gebuhrer L, Lambert J, Freidel AC, Farre A (1983) A possible new HLA-DR allele. Hum Immunol 8:227–237
2. Carrel RS, Tosi R, Gross N, Tanigaki N, Carmagnola AL, Accola RS (1981) Subsets of human Ia-like molecules defined by monoclonal antibodies. Mol Immunol 18:403–411
3. Charron DJ, McDevitt HO (1979) Analysis of HLA-D region associated molecules with monoclonal antibody. Proc Natl Acad Sci USA 76:6567–6571
4. Charron DJ, McDevitt HO (1980) Characterization of HLA-D region antigens by two dimensional gel electrophoresis. J Exp Med 152:18s–36s
5. Charron DJ, Aellen-Schulz MF, St Geme III J, Erlich HA, McDevitt HO (1983) Biochemical characterization of an invariant polypeptide associated with Ia antigens in human and mouse. Mol Immunol 20:21–32

6. Corte G, Accolla RS, Charron DJ, Köning F, Steel MC (1984) Workshop report. Monoclonal antibodies to human MHC class II antigens. Exp Clin Immunogenetics (in press)
7. Degos L, Lepage V, Raffoux C (1983) DRw6 nomenclature. 9th International Histocompatibility Workshop, Newsletter I
8. Goyert SM, Shively JE, Silver J (1982) Biochemical characterization of a second family of human Ia molecules, HLA-DS, equivalent to murine I-A sub-region molecules. J Exp Med 156:550–566
9. Hendriks GFJ, Schreuder GMT, Claas FHJ, D'amaro J, Persijn GG, Cohen B, Van Rood JJ (1983). HLA-DRw6 and renal allograft rejection. Br Med J 286:85–87
10. Jones PP, Murphy DB, McDevitt HO (1981) Variable synthesis and expression of Eα and Ae (Eβ) Ia polypeptide chains in mice of different H-2 haplotypes. Immunogenetics 12:321–337
11. Kaufman JF, Andersen RL, Strominger JL (1980). HLA-DR antigens have polymorphic light chains and invariant heavy chains as assessed by lysine containing tryptic peptide analysis. J Exp Med 152:37s–53s
12. Long EO, Gorski J, Rollini P, Wake CT, Strubin M, Rabourdin-Combe C, Mach B (1983) Molecular analysis of the genes for human class II antigens of the major histocompatibility complex. Hum Immunol 8:113
13. Mathis DJ, Benoist C, Williams II VE, Kanter M, McDevitt HO (1983) Several mechanisms can account for defective Eα gene expression in different mouse haplotypes. Proc Natl Acad Sci USA 80:273–277
14. Nepom BS, Nepom GT, Mickelson E, Antonelli P, Hansen JA (1983) Electrophoretic analysis of human HLA-DR antigens from HLA-DR4 homozygous cell lines: correlation between β chain diversity and HLA-D. Proc Natl Acad Sci USA 80:6962–6966
15. O'Farrel PZ, Goodman HH, O'Farrel PH (1977). High resolution two dimensional electrophoresis of basic as well as acidic proteins. Cell 12:1133–1142
16. Schackelford DA, Eibl B, Strominger JL (1983) Structural polymorphism of the DC1 light chains from DR1-, DR2-, and DRw6-positive cell lines. Immunogenetics 18:625–637
17. Schreuder GMT, Parlevliet J, Termijtelen A, Van Rood JJ (1983) Reanalysis of the HLA-DRw6 complex. Tissue Antigens 21:62–74

Heterogeneity of HLA Class II Gene Products as Studied in a Family by Sequential Immunoprecipitation*

R.E. Bontrop, F. Koning, R. v. Miltenburg, R. Gerrets, A. Thompson, R. Schuurman, and M.J. Giphart

Department Immunohematology and Bloodbank, University Medical Centre, Rijnsburgerweg 10, 2333 AA Leiden, The Netherlands

Abbreviations

IEF	isoelectric focusing
Ip	isoelectric point
kd	kilodalton
mCI	millicurie
MoAb	monoclonal antibody
NaNase	neuraminidase
PAGE	polyacrylamide gel electrophoresis
SDS	sodium dodecyl sulfate
V	volt

* In part supported by the Dutch Foundation for Medical Research (FUNGO), which is subsidized by the Dutch Organization for the Advancement of Pure Research (Z.W.O.) and the J. A. Cohen Institute for Radiopathology and Radiation Protection (IRS)

Introduction

The HLA class II region contains three different serologically defined loci: DR, DQ, and DP [1]. There is evidence suggesting that there are more loci than serologically detected products [2]. Despite intensive international collaboration, there are difficulties in assigning the class II loci and determinants. This might be explained by the limited knowledge of class II antigens on the product level. Amino acid sequences derived from the class II molecules of a DR2-positive cell line suggest that at least seven β chains are expressed [3]. The total number of β chains expressed on the membrane is still an enigma. We therefore undertook an investigation into the class II gene products. A panel of three MoAbs used in a sequential immunoprecipitation assay allowed us to analyze all expressed class II antigens.

Histocompatibility Testing 1984
Edited by E. D. Albert et al.

Materials and Methods

Sera. Hybridoma cells which produced the MoAb B.8.11.2 were a generous gift from Dr. B. Malissen, Marseille [4]. The MoAbs 7.3.19.1 and 7.5.10.1 were generated by F. Koning [5].

Preparation of Radiolabeled Cell Extracts. B-lymphoblastoid cells (5×10^6) were labeled for 16 h at 37 °C with 0.2 mCi [^{35}S]methionine [6]. After washing, the cells were treated with 270 µl of lysis buffer which contained: 0.01 *M* Tris-HCl pH 7.6, 1 m*M* $MgCl_2$ and 20 m*M* NaCl. After 30 min incubation on ice, 30 µl of a 10% Triton X-114 solution in H_2O was added. Membrane proteins could be selectively isolated after phase separation [7].

Sequential Immunoprecipitation. The procedure for sequential immunoprecipitation has been described [5]. The NaNase digestions were carried out with the immunoprecipitated molecules still adsorbed to the bacteria [8].

Electrophoresis. One-dimensional IEF was performed as has been described [6]. Electrophoresis was carried out for 15 h at 300 V and 1 h at 800 V at 12 °C. Gels were processed for fluorography using Kodak XS film [9].

Results

By means of sequential immunoprecipitation with three different MoAbs we have previously shown the existence of three groups of class II antigens [5] MoAb 7.3.19.1 recognizes a DRw52-like determinant on antigens that are composed of 29.5-kd light chains and 34.5-kd heavy chains. MoAb B.8.11.2 reacts with class II antigens bearing DR determinants built up of 29-kd light chains and 34-kd heavy chains. The third MoAb, 7.5.10.1, reacts in a sequential immunoprecipitation assay still with a third group of class II antigens. This group is clearly heterogeneous and is composed of 32- to 34-kd heavy chains and 27- to 29-kd light chains. After the final immunoprecipitation step, no class II antigens were left in the membrane extract. Our interest was drawn towards the question of whether each group of class II antigens is homogeneous, thus composed of only one α chain and one β chain, or whether each group of antigens represents a mixture of different α and β chains, thus being heterogeneous. Therefore, each antigen group showing characteristic molecular weights was analyzed for charge heterogeneity. IEF analysis was combined with segregation studies in families.

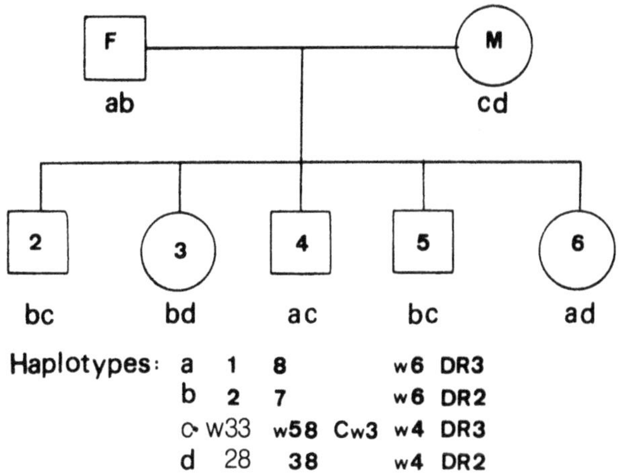

Fig. 1. Pattern of segregation of HLA antigens. Both father and mother are heterozygous for DR. Serological typing data showed that both parents are DR2,3-positive individuals. Sibling 3 (DR2,2) and sibling 4 (DR3,3) were typed as DR-homozygous individuals

The family studied (Fig. 1) had DR2,3-positive parents. There are two phenotypically DR homozygous siblings: sibling 3 (DR2,2) and sibling 4 (DR3,3). These two individuals were informative for our segregation studies. From the DR heterozygous family members, sibling 2 was chosen for further study. On 1D-IEF gels we could not detect differences between the class II antigens expressed by sibling 2 and those of the other HLA identical siblings (data not shown). Thus, the class II molecules of the father are equal to those of the mother as far as Ips are concerned. The 1D-IEF gel is shown in Fig. 2.

This type of analysis always contains radiolabeled background molecules that are not HLA class II-like. This can be shown by a so-called blank precipitation. The membrane extract derived from sibling 3 was treated with 7.3.19.1 ascites. Serologically typed DR2,2-positive individuals do not express antigens that bear the DRw52 specificity as shown by microcytotoxicity testing and FACS analysis [5]. Two background bands could be detected (Fig. 2, DR2,2 lane A). Two-dimensional gel electrophoresis showed that these molecules have molecular weights of 44-kd (data not shown). They might be actin. In this way we are able to correct for background material. Figure 3 is a schematic representation of the IEF gel shown in Fig. 2, now corrected for the radiolabeled background molecules.

The β Chains

The light chains all focused in the neutral and more alkaline region of the IEF gels. The DRw52-like determinant seems to be associated with three or four different β chains, which all have identical molecular weights but can be distinguished by their Ips. (Fig. 3; DR3,3, DR2,3 lanes A). The DR determinant seems to be associated with seven different β chains in the case of the heterozygous sibling (Fig. 3; DR2,3 lane B). Five of these β chains are also expressed by sibling 3 and should be considered as the DR2 β chains (Fig. 3; DR2,2 lane B). The remaining two or three β chains are expressed by sibling 4 and should be considered as DR3 β chains (Fig. 3; DR3,3 lane B). A β chain with the same Ip is shared among DR2 and DR3 individuals (Fig. 3; lanes B chain β 3). Most of the β chains isolated with MoAb 7.3.19.1 have Ips that are similar to β chains isolated by MoAb B.8.11.2. Although these two sets of β chains share similar Ips, they are different in molecular weight and also differ in the determinants they are asociated with.

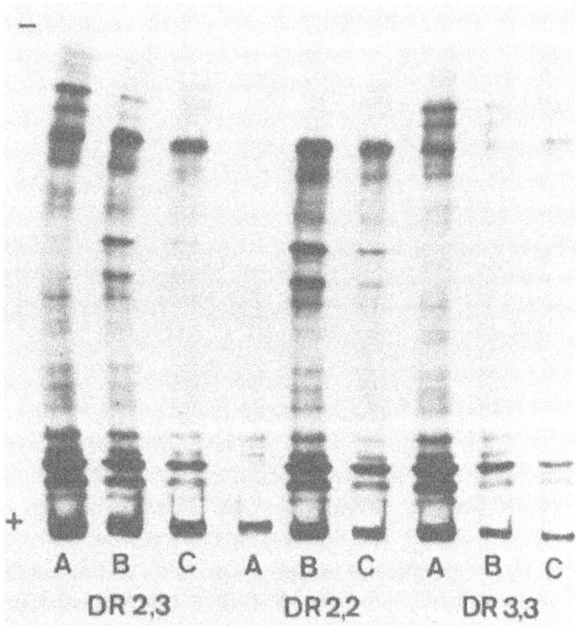

Fig. 2. 1D-IEF of NaNase-treated class II antigens. The data show the separate α and β chains that are expressed on B cells of sibling 2 (DR2,3), sibling 3 (DR2,2), and sibling 4 (DR3,3). Class II antigens were isolated by sequential immunoprecipitation. The *top* of the gel represents the alkaline part, the *bottom* the acidic part. *A*, antigens isolated with the anti-DRw52-like MoAb; *B*, antigens isolated with MoAb B.8.11.2; *C*, antigens recognized MoAb 7.5.10.1

The α Chains

The α chains focus in the acidic regions of the IEF gels. The DRw52 group of class II antigens expressed by DR3 individuals contained two or three α chains differing in Ip (Fig. 3; DR2,3, DR3,3 lanes A). With the second precipitation step with MoAb B.8.11.2 two additional α chains could be isolated, both for DR2- and DR3-positive individuals. This situation applies also to the third immunoprecipitation step with MoAb 7.5.10.1. Thus each group of class II molecules is represented by two or three α chains that are distinct in Ip but identical in molecular weight. Each α chain of each group of class II antigens has at least one other α chain partner, present in at least one other group, that shares the same Ip. Thus, the molecular weights of α chains may be variable, whereas the Ips are highly conserved.

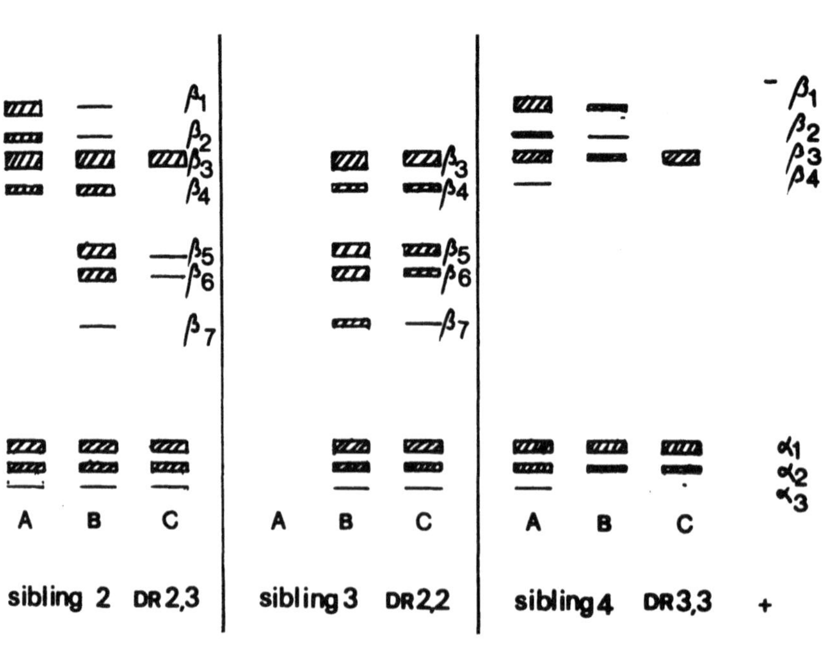

Fig. 3. Schematic representation of NaNase-digested class II antigens that are expressed on B cells of members of family A. The scheme has been corrected for background products that are not class II-like in their molecular weight or specificity. The data shown state that a DR homozygous individual expresses at least three to five different β chains. The heterozygous individual might express over seven different β chains. The minimum number of α chains that could be detected by charge heterogeneity is at least two or three. This number is expressed by both heterozygous and homozygous B cells

Discussion

Characteristics of class II antigens isolated from a membrane extract by only one selected MoAb are difficult to interpret because one β chain might be involved in the expression of other determinants, for example caused by the interaction of one β chain with different α chains. By means of sequential immunoprecipitation, the relationships of class II determinants can be analyzed. IEF studies were performed to detect charge variability. The data obtained suggest that the MHC class II region in man is far more complex than thought. Each group of class II antigens, as defined by a panel of three MoAbs, can be split into at least two distinct α chains and even more β chains. Each group represents therefore a heterogeneous set of α and β chains, with distinct but variable Ips. Thus, each α and β chain represents a different gene product.

The observed variability is not due to sialic carbohydrate variation. Removal of sialic acids was conducted by NaNase digestion and did not lead to more simplified IEF patterns.

The DR homozygous individuals express at least three to five different β chains. The two DR specificities present in this study, DR2 and DR3, can be discriminated by their β chain pattern. We have analyzed more families, and by now we are able to distinguish all DR serotypes by their β chain pattern on ID-IEF gels (Bontrop et al., manuscript in preparation). Some β chains have Ips that are typical for a certain DR specificity. The chains β_1 and β_2 have Ips that are characteristic for the serotype DR3. The chains β_5, β_6, and β_7 have Ips that are characteristic for the serotype DR2.

A large proportion of the chains recognized by MoAb 7.5.10.1 have Ips similar to those of the chains recognized by MoAb B.8.11.2. These chains are distinct in molecular weights and in determinants they are associated with. Fingerprint studies are necessary to demonstrate whether these chains carry distinct amino acid sequences. If this is so, then it implies that DR homozygous individuals might express far more than three to five different β chains. For example, sibling 3: chain β_5 lane B could be distinct from chain β_5 lane C.

The β chain pattern of DR heterozygous individuals is difficult to interpret. Some β chains that are expressed by the DR2,2 individual and the DR3,3 individual have identical Ips. The heterozygous DR2,3 individual expresses both β chains. Since they are not distinguishable on IEF gels, this heterozygous individual seems to express only one β chain (DR2,3 β_3, DR2,2 β_3, and DR3,3 β_3). If one takes these considerations into account, the heterozygous individual might express more than seven class II molecules. Heavy chains focus in the acidic regions of the IEF gels, whereas light chains focus in the alkaline zones. Heavy and light chains form noncovalently associated dimers. The IEF data suggest that this interaction might occur by charge interactions. Based upon Ips, at least two or three distinct α chains are present on the membrane. If one takes into account that there is also molecular weight variation, then a higher number of α chains is still possible. The α chains are very conservative in their Ips. Thus fingerprint studies may demonstrate heterogeneity within or between the three different groups of class II α chains.

Provisional gene counting for β chains predicts the presence of six β genes [10]. Recent DNA studies state the existence of at least four α chain genes [11]. The number of genes present at the DNA level fits well with the number of class II gene products isolated.

Two different α chains might fold one given β chain into two different tertiary structures. This might be the reason why two different epitopes can arise on class II molecules containing the same β chain. This may also be the case for the reversed situation, in which two different β chains and one α chain are involved in the formation of determinants. This would of course imply that cis complementation for the class II antigens occurs.

Summary

Isolation of class II antigens was conducted by sequential immunoprecipitation with the following MoAbs: 7.3.19.1 (anti-DRw52-like), B.8.11.2 (anti-DR backbone) and 7.5.10.1 (anti-HLA class II backbone). In the case of those individuals expressing the DRw52 determinants, i.e., those individuals of the HLA-DR3, 5, and w6 type, we were able to isolate three groups of class II antigens. SDS-PAGE showed that the α and β chains of each of the three groups were distinct in molecular weight [5]. Here we report on the molecular heterogeneity of each separate group of class II antigens and their segregation in a family. Analysis of each group was done with 1D-IEF gels. The segregation pattern of the serologically defined HLA antigens within a family enabled the characterization of the different α and β chains. Charge heterogeneity revealed that a DR homozygous individual expresses at least three to five distinct β chains. A DR heterozygous individual might express more than seven different β chains.

The two or three α chains present within each group showed different Ips, although they are identical in molecular weight. However, charge heterogeneity was not found for the α chains between the three different groups of antigens, although they differ in molecular weight. Thus the molecular weight variations do not contribute to the charge heterogeneity of the α chains.

References

1. Van Rood JJ, de Jongh B, Claas FHJ, Goulmy E, Gratama JW, Giphart MJ (1984) New facts on HLA genetics: are they relevant in bone marrow grafting? Semin Hematol 21:65–80
2. Dick H (1982) HLA-DR: more than three loci. Immunol Today 3:199–203
3. Kratzin H, Yang C, Götz H, Pauly E, Kölbel S, Egbert G, Thinnes PT, Wernet P, Altevogt P, Hilschman N (1981) Primärstruktur menschlicher Histokompatibilitätsantigene der Klasse II. Hoppe-Seylers Z Physiol Chem 362:1665–1669
4. Rebai N, Malissen B, Pierres M, Accolla RS, Corte G, Mawas C (1983) Distinct HLA-DR epitopes and distinct families of HLA-DR molecules defined by 15 monoclonal antibodies either anti-DR or allo-anti-Ia cross-reacting with human DR molecule. Eur J Immunol 13:106–111
5. Koning F, Schreuder GMT, Giphart MJ, Bruning JW (1984) A monoclonal antibody with MT2-specificity: serology and biochemistry. Hum Immunol 9:221–230
6. Shackelford DA, Strominger JL (1980) Demonstration of structural polymorphism among HLA-DR light chains by two dimensional gel electrophoresis. J Exp Med 151:144–165
7. Bordier C (1981) Phase separation of integral membrane proteins in Triton X-114 solution. J Biol Chem 256:1604–1607
8. Mölders HH, Breuning MH, Ivanyi P, Ploegh HL (1983) Biochemical analysis of variant HLA B27 antigens. Hum Immunol 6:11–117
9. Pulleyblank DE, Booth GM (1981) Improved methods for the fluorographic detection of weak β-emitting radioisotopes in agarose and acrylamide gel electrophoresis media. J Biomed Biophys Meth 4:339–346
10. Rabourdin-Combe R, Mach B (1983) Expression of HLA-DR antigens at the surface of mouse L cells cotransfected with cloned human genes. Nature 303:670–674
11. Auffray C, Koo J, De Mars R, Strominger JL (1983) A minimum of four human class II α chain genes are encoded in the HLA region of chromosome 6. Nature 304:174–177

A Supertypic DRw53 Determinant is Carried on the HLA-DR Subset of Class II Molecules on HLA-DR7 Cell Lines

R.W. Knowles[1], K. Horibe[1], T.E. Adams[2], and B. Dupont[1]

1 Memorial Sloan-Kettering Cancer Center, Box 41, 1275 New York Ave., New York, NY 10021, USA
2 Cold Spring Harbor Laboratories, Cold Spring Harbor, NY 11724, USA

The HLA class II molecules carrying a supertypic DRw53 determinant have been characterized in biochemical studies through the use of the monoclonal antibody (mAb) PL3. This mAb binds specifically to all DR4, DR7, and DRw9 cells tested. A panel of mAbs which recognize various nonpolymorphic determinants on subsets of HLA class II molecules has been used in parallel with PL3 to immunoprecipitate these ^{125}I-labeled cell surface molecules from detergent lysates of HLA-DR homozygous cell lines. Examination of HLA-DR7 cell lines showed that the two-dimensional patterns of alpha and beta chains immunoprecipitated by PL3 were identical to those immunoprecipitated by the group of mAbs specific for the HLA-DR subset of class II molecules. Furthermore, sequential immunoprecipitation studies showed that the DRw53-specific mAb completely removed the HLA-DR subset of molecules from lysates of HLA-DR7 cell lines without removing the other subsets of class II molecules. In reciprocal experiments, removal of the HLA-DR subset of molecules completely removes the PL3-reactive subset. Identical results were obtained for HLA-DR7 cells which type in mixed lymphocyte culture as Dw7 and those which type as Dw11. These results demonstrate that the supertypic DRw53 determinant defined by this mAb is carried on the DR molecule on HLA-DR7-positive haplotypes. This is in striking contrast to its expression on HLA-DR4-positive haplotypes where the DRw53 supertypic determinant is not carried on the DR molecule. This suggests that the DRw53 determinant has evolved independently from the monomorphic determinants that are specific for the DR molecule.

Histocompatibility Testing 1984
Edited by E. D. Albert et al.

The Molecular Complexity of DR7-Associated Ia Molecules

R.W. Karr[1], T.C. Fuller[2], S.H. Hsu[3], and W.B. Bias[3]

1 Veterans Administration Medical Center and the Department of Internal Medicine, University of Iowa College of Medicine, Iowa City, IA 52240, USA
2 Histocompatibility Testing Laboratory, Massachusetts General Hospital, Boston, MA, USA
3 Immunogenetics Laboratory, Johns Hopkins University School of Medicine, Baltimore, MD, USA

Recent serologic and cellular studies have demonstrated considerable heterogeneity of DR7-associated Ia antigens. Two serologically defined DR7 haplotypes have been identified: the standard DR7, DQw2, DRw53 haplotype and the alternative DR7, DQw3, DRw53 haplotype. DQw3 (equivalent to Te22 and DC4) is classically associated only with DR4 and DR5, while all DR7-positive cells were formerly said to be DQw2-positive. DQw2 and Te24 appear to be equivalent to DC3 [1], while DRw53 is equivalent to BR4 [1]. Four DR7-associated HLA-D specificities have recently been identified using HTCs: Dw7 "short" (Dw7S), Dw7 "long" (Dw7L), Dw11 "short" (Dw11S), and Dw11 "long" (Dw11L) [2]. Interestingly, the Dw7S, Dw7L, and Dw11S haplotypes bear DQw2, while the Dw11L haplotype includes DQw3, but not DQw2. These relationships are summarized in Table 1. In the studies described here, the Ia molecular basis for serologically and cellularly defined differences among DR7 cells has been investigated using two-dimensional (2-D) gel electrophoresis.

First, the Ia molecules expressed by a DR7, DQw2, DRw53, Dw7S homozygous cell line were analyzed. The β chains of Ia molecules isolated by an anti-DQw2 alloserum (9w792, 7w127, [3]) were identical to DQ β chains isolated by the Rb03 heteroserum [4] which is specific for biochemically defined DQ (I-A-like) molecules. Therefore, the DQw2 allodeterminant appears to reside on molecules encoded by the HLA-DQ (DC) loci. An anti-DRw53 alloserum isolated Ia molecules containing a non-DQ, DR-like β chain which is distinct from the major DR (I-E-like) β chain. Therefore, the DRw53 allodeterminant appears to reside on a DR-like molecule, in agreement with previous reports [5, 6].

Table 1. Subgroups of Dw7

Cellularly defined D specificities	Serologic specificities		
	DR	DRw	DQw
Dw7S	7	53	2
Dw11L	7	53	3
Dw11S	7	53	2
Dw7L	7	53	2

Comparisons by 2-D gels of Ia molecules isolated by the DR-specific monoclonal antibody (MAB) SG157 [4] from a DR7, DQw2, DRw53, Dw7S (8W156) homozygous cell line and a DR7, DQw3, DRw53, Dw11L (8W163) homozygous cell line revealed that their DR β chains are identical. These studies also indicate that both the Dw7S and Dw11L cells express two DQ β chains. The 2-D gel spots of one Dw7S DQ β chain (DQβ_1) have very basic isoelectric points, while the other Dw7S DQ β chain (DQβ_2) is more acidic. In contrast, the Dw11L cell lacks a DQ β chain that corresponds to DQβ_1 from the Dw7S cell. The Dw11L cell expresses two acidic DQ β chains: DQβ_3, which appears to be distinct from DQβ_1 and DQβ_2 from the Dw7S cell, and DQβ_2, which appears to be identical to DQβ_2 from the Dw7S cell. Importantly, the anti-DQw3-like MAB IVD12 [7] isolated only DQβ_3-containing molecules from the Dw11L cell. These data indicate that the DQw3-like determinant resides on DQ molecules from a Dw11L cell, as it does on DR4 and DR5 cells. Therefore, the Ia structural differences between Dw7S cells and Dw11L cells appear to be limited to differences in one DQ β chain expressed by each cell.

Interestingly, two MABs which are specific for DQ molecules, Leu-10 [8], and 33.1 [9], distinguish between the DQ molecules from Dw7S and Dw11L homozygous cells. These MABs reportedly recognize DQ molecules on cells of all DR types except DR3 and DR7. However, when analyzed by indirect immunofluorescence, Leu-10 and 33.1 are reactive with Dw11L cells, but not Dw7S cells. This indicates that DQ molecules from Dw7S cells lack the Leu-10 and 33.1 DQ epitopes expressed by most other DQ molecules. In contrast, three other MABs, TÜ22 [10], SG520 [11], and SG465 [11], that are specific for DQ molecules on DR7 cells are reactive with both Dw7S and Dw11L cells.

These data provide insight into the Ia structural basis for the serologic and cellular differences noted among DR7 haplotypes in two previously reported families [2, 3]. Biochemical studies of the two DR7 haplotypes in the family reported by Ful-

Histocompatibility Testing 1984
Edited by E. D. Albert et al.

ler et al. [3] have now defined the relevant haplotypes as Dw7S and Dw11L respectively. In summary, these data indicate that cellularly defined HLA-D differences (Dw7S and Dw11L) may be due entirely to structural differences in DQ molecules which bear serologically defined allodeterminants.

References

1. Tosi R, Tanigaki N, Sorrentino R, Centis D, Ferrera GB (1984) Serologically detectable polymorphism of the HLA-DC α-subunit. J Immunol 132:277–282
2. Hsu SH, Lambert P, Scribner PP, Hartzman RJ, Robbins F, Bias WB (1983) Primary and secondary MLR characterization of three allelic variants of HLA-Dw7 segregating in a single family. Hum Immunol 6:167–176
3. Fuller TC, Einarson M, Pinto C, Ahern A, Yunis EJ (1978) Genetic evidence that HLA-DR (Ia) specificities include multiple HLA-D determinants on a single haplotype. Transplant Proc 10:781–784
4. Goyert SM, Shively JE, Silver J (1982) Biochemical characterization of a second family of human Ia molecules, HLA-DS, equivalent to murine I-A subregion molecules. J Exp Med 156:550–566
5. Tanigaki N, Tosi R, Duquesnoy RJ, Ferrara GB (1983) Three Ia species with different structures and alloantigenic determinants in an HLA-homozygous cell line. J Exp Med 157:231–247
6. Goyert SM, Moriuchi J, Winchester R, Silver J (1983) HLA-DS molecules and their relation to supertypic specificities. Hum Immunol 8:53–63
7. Giles RC, Nunez G, Hurley CK, Nunez-Roldan A, Winchester R, Stastny P, Capra JD (1983) Structural analysis of human I-A homologue using a monoclonal antibody that recognizes an MB3-like specificity. J Exp Med 157:1461–1470
8. Brodsky FM (1984) A matrix approach to human class II histocompatibility antigens: reactions of four monoclonal antibodies with the products of nine haplotypes. Immunogenetics 19:179–194
9. Marti GE, Kuo MC, Shaw S, Chang CC, DeMars R, Sogn JA, Coligan JE, Kindt TJ (1983) A novel HLA-D/DR-like antigen specific for human B lymphoid cells: biochemical evidence for similarity to but nonidentity with known HLA-D/DR antigens. J Exp Med 158:1924–1937
10. Ziegler A, Uchanska-Ziegler B, Zeuthen J, Wernet P (1982) HLA antigen expression at the single cell level on a K562 × B cell hybrid: an analysis with monoclonal antibodies using bacterial binding assays. Somatic Cell Genet 8:775–789
11. Govert SM, Silver J (1983) Further characterization of HLA-DS molecules: implications for studies assessing the role of human Ia molecules in cell interactions and disease susceptibility. Proc Natl Acad Sci USA 80:5719–5723

Alloantisera and Monoclonal Antibodies Which Appear to Define the Same Ia Allospecificity in Population Studies Do Not Detect the Same Ia Molecules in Biochemical Studies

R.W. Karr

Veterans Administration Medical Center and the Department of Internal Medicine, University of Iowa College of Medicine, Iowa City, IA 52240, USA

Some anti-Ia monoclonal antibodies (mabs) define specificities similar to Ia allospecificities based on their reactions in population studies. Two anti-Ia mabs, Genox 3.53 [1] and BT3.4 [2], bind to DR1, 2, and w6 cells, and therefore define specificities (referred to as DQw1-like) similar to the DQw1 allospecificity. In addition, the anti-Ia mab IVD12 [3] binds to DR4 and DR5 cells, and therefore defines a specificity (DQw3-like) similar to the DQw3 allospecificity. The human Ia alloantigens, which were defined and categorized based on serologic testing with alloantibodies, are now being redefined in immunochemical studies with mabs. However, the possibility exists that anti-Ia allosera and mabs which have similar reactivity patterns in population studies may not recognize the same Ia molecules.

The Ia molecules isolated from a DRw6 homozygous cell line by anti-DQw1 allosera and the DQw1-like mabs were analyzed. Comparative 2-D gel studies of Ia molecules isolated with a DS-specific reagent, as well as the anti-DQw1 reagents, indicate that this homozygous cell expresses two DQ molecules. Two anti-DQw1 allosera immunoprecipitated only one of the two DQ molecules, while the DQw1-like mabs isolated both DQ molecules [4]. Therefore, the Ia molecular specificities of these DQw1 alloantisera and

Histocompatibility Testing 1984
Edited by E. D. Albert et al.

DQw1-like mabs are clearly different. The Ia molecules isolated from a DR5 homozygous cell line by anti-DQw3 allosera and the DQw3-like mab IVD12 were also compared. The DQw3 allodeterminant resides on only one of the two DQ molecules expressed by this cell [5]. However, the DQw3-like mab isolated both DQ molecules from the DR5 cell. Therefore, the Ia molecular specificities of three DQw3 allosera and an DQw3-like mab differ.

These findings underscore the importance of designating in the nomenclature of the serologically defined Ia alloantigens the potential differences between the Ia molecular specificities of alloantisera and mabs which have the same reactivity patterns in population studies. The designation of such mabs as DQw1-like or DQw3-like, for example, would seem to accomplish this goal without unduly complicating the nomenclature.

References

1. Brodsky FM, Parham P, Bodmer WF (1980) Monoclonal antibodies to HLA-DRw determinants. Tissue Antigens 16:30–37
2. Corte G, Calabi F, Domiani G, Bargellesi A, Tosi R, Sorrentino R (1981) Human Ia molecules carrying DC1 differ in both alpha and beta subunits from Ia molecules carrying DR determinants. Nature 292:357–360
3. Giles RC, Nunez G, Hurley CK, Nunez-Roldan A, Winchester R, Stastny P, Capra JD (1983) Structural analysis of human I-A homologue using a monoclonal antibody that recognizes an MB3-like specificity. J Exp Med 157: 1461–1470
4. Karr RW, Alber C, Goyert SM, Silver J, Duquesnoy RJ (1984) The complexity of HLA-DS molecules: a homozygous cell line expresses multiple HLA-DS alpha chains. J Exp Med (in press)
5. Karr RW, Kannapell CC, Zangara RJ, Goyert SM, Silver J, Schwartz BD (1983) An HLA-DR5 homozygous cell line expresses two DS (I-A-like) molecules. J Exp Med 158:1374–1379

The Polymorphism of DQ (DC) Molecules *

N. Tanigaki [1], R. Tosi [2], G.B. Ferrara [3]

1 Department of Molecular Immunology, Roswell Park Memorial Institute, 666 Elm Street, Buffalo, NY 14263 USA
2 Laboratorio di Biologia Cellulare CNR, 00196 Roma, Italy
3 Istituto Tumori, Università di Genova, 16132 Genova, and AVIS, Bergamo, Italy

Introduction

Based on the finding that previously defined DQ specificities, DQw1 (DC1, MB1, MT1, LB12), DQw2 (DC3, MB2), and DQw3 (DC4, MB3, MT4), all are "supertypic specificities", multiple linkage disequilibrium relationships can be assumed between DQ and DR alleles; the same DQ allele is linked to more than one DR allele [1]. However, structural study by 2-dimensional gel electrophoresis has indicated that this may not be the case; the DQ molecules associated with DR1, 2, and w6, though carrying DQw1 specificity, possess different isoelectric focusing patterns, particularly noticeable in the β chains [2]. Yet no serological variations which can discriminate those DQ molecules have been found.

As to the molecules sharing DQw3 specificity associated with DR4, 5, 7, and 8w13 [3], not only structural but also serological differences have been recently unveiled. The structural variations are found in both α and β chains; at least two different α chains and three different β chains can be distinguished. The serological variations are shown by three new specificities which have different distribution patterns in population. One is associated with all DR5-positive and/or 8w13-positive individuals and with some DR3-positive individuals, but not with DRw6-positive cases, differing from DRw52 [4]. This specificity is designated DCα3, because it has been shown to be an α chain specificity. One is detected in all DR5-positive and/or 8w13-positive cases and in a small fraction of DR4-positive cases [5]. This specificity is called DC5. Another is found in all DR4-positive and/or DRw9-positive individuals and is termed provisionally DC4HON, because it was defined by the use of alloantiserum HON [6]. Including the DQw1, 2 and 3 specificities, now six different specificities have been located on DQ molecules.

Thus the serological as well as structural polymorphism of DQ molecules appear to be more

* This work was supported in part by USPHS Grants AI20251 and CA17276 awarded by the National Institute of Allergy and Infectious Diseases and the National Cancer Institute, Department of Health and Human Services, and by the grant of Progetto Finalizzato CNR Ingegneria Genetica Sottoprogetto "Basi moleculari delle malattie ereditarie", the CNR Grants 820 130 504 and 820 133 696, and a grant awarded by the North Atlantic Treaty Organization

complex than once thought. It could be comparable to or higher than that of DR molecules, especially considering the presence of allotypic variations in the DQ α chains which DR molecules lack.

Material, Methods, and Results

The new DQ specificities were identified through detailed analysis of DQ-enriched Ia preparations carrying DQw3 specificity obtained from LG38 (DR5,5) and RPMI8057 (DR1,4) cells. The Ia molecules were purified and labeled with radioactive iodine ^{125}I by our standard procedures [7]. The labeled Ia preparations were then absorbed with rabbit antiserum U115-coupled Sepharose. This antiserum raised against an α chain preparation isolated from a pooled Ia preparation had been found to bind only DR molecules and DR-like molecules we call BR, and not to bind DQ molecules, and had been successfully used to delete DR and BR molecules from given labeled Ia preparations and to enrich them in the DQ molecules [1, 3]. The DQ-enriched Ia preparations, hereafter simply called LG 38-DQ and 8057-DQ preparations, were then tested for their reactivity with a panel of Eighth Workshop and local anti-Ia alloantisera by the direct binding assay [7]. This assay first allows reacting of a labeled Ia preparation with a test antiserum, and then measures the extent of binding by the double antibody technique. Results are usually expressed as percent Ia binding, i.e., the proportion of the maximum binding obtained with an excess of rabbit anti-human Ia antiserum. A positive binding with those DQ-enriched Ia preparations could be taken as indicative of anti-DQ activity present in test antiserum.

Three antisera, 8W670, 8W1062 (Balkin), and 8W614 (Andro), were found to bind about 40% of Ia molecules in the LG38-DQ preparation. The first two had been classified as anti-DR5 and the last as anti-DR3 in the Workshop analysis. The observed binding proportion was similar to that obtained with antisera 8W769 (CCB48) and Fe117/30, which had been shown to contain anti-DQw3 activity and been used for determination of DQw3 distribution in population and also for immunospecific isolation of DQw3-positive Ia molecules [3]. With the 8057-DQ preparation, two antisera, Ducouret and HON, gave a near 30% binding. The former classified as anti-DR5 had been found to contain anti-DQw3 activity [3] and the latter had been used to define a non-DR specificity HON7 which is probably identical to BR4 (DRw53) specificity [8, 9].

To define the specificities involved in these bindings, the binding inhibition assay [7] was set up using a panel of cultured human lymphoid cells and/or primary chronic lymphocytic leukemia cells which had been typed for DR specificities. The assay measures the inhibitory activity of those cell samples on the binding of a labeled Ia preparation to an antiserum. When cell samples carry a specificity of the labeled Ia preparation recognized with the antiserum, an inhibition of the radiobinding is expected. Results are given as the percent reduction of the binding which can be obtained in the absence of inhibitor.

A sharply bimodal inhibition pattern was observed for each specificity, allowing an unequivocal grouping of positive and negative cases. It was evident in the LG38-DQ preparation that 8W1062 and 8W614 defined the same specificity, whereas 8W670 detected different specificity and that their distributions only partially overlapped with that of the DQw3 specificity determined with 8W769 or Fe117/30 [4, 5]. All three specificities were present on DR5-positive and/or 8w13-positive cells. However, other associations differed; DQw3 included all DR4-positive and some DR7-positive cells, whereas DCα3, the specificity recognized with 8W1062 and 8W614, included most DR3-positive cells, and DC5, the specificity detected with 8W670, was found only in two additional cells (RPMI8057 and MT1), both DR4-positive. Five other DR4-positive cells were clearly negative. These findings were confirmed by testing a panel of 91 unrelated individuals by the same binding inhibition assays. The specificity involved in the binding with Ducouret with 8057-DQ preparation was definitely DQw3; its distribution exactly followed the DQw3 pattern obtained by the use of LG38-DQ preparation and antiserum 8W769 or Fe117/30. In the case of HON, the inhibition was obtained with DR4-positive and/or DRw9-positive cells.

It is certain that the new specificities were identified in DQ-enriched Ia preparations carrying DQw3 specificity, but this does not necessarily allow their immediate assignment to the DQw3-bearing Ia molecules. More specific data for the molecular distribution were given by the following sequential binding experiments [7]. When the LG38-DQ preparation was first treated with 8W1062 and the antigen molecules remaining were allowed to react with 8W769 or Fe117/30 (both anti-DQw3), about 90% of the reactivity was found to have been eliminated [4]. Similar results were obtained in the reciprocal setting-up; the treatment with 8W769 or Fe117/30 abolished about 90% of the reactivity with 8W1062. Since the specificity recognized by 8W769 was previously shown by peptide mapping to be carried by molecules which have all the features of DQ molecules [3], the 8W1062-defined specificity must also be located on

DQ molecules, along with the 8W769-defined DQw3 specificity. Likewise, the specificity detected with 8W670 was assigned to DQw3-bearing molecules [5]. In this case, the LG38-DQ preparation was first treated with 8W670, and then the reactivity with 8W769 and 8W1062 was determined. The pretreatment with 8W670 abolished over 90% of the reactivity with the latter two antisera. Reciprocal experiments confirmed the localization of all three specificities on the same molecules. The determinant reacting with HON antiserum in 8057-DQ preparation also was located on DQw3-positive molecules [6]; the prior treatment of the 8057-DQ preparation with HON reduced the reactivity with Ducouret (anti-DQw3) by about 90%, and reciprocally the treatment with Ducouret diminished the HON reactivity by about 80%.

Peptide mapping study provided more direct evidence for the presence of HON-defined specificity on DQ molecules. HON antiserum was allowed to react with the labeled 8057-Ia preparation, and the molecules bound by HON were recovered by protein A-coupled Sepharose. The component chains were isolated by sodium dodecyl sulfate polyacrylamide gel electrophoresis and were subjected to elastase digestion followed by microfingerprinting analysis [10]. The α chain map displayed all characteristics of DQ α chains; it possessed the marker spot found in all DQ α chains so far analyzed [1], and moreover, it showed a group of chromatographically fast-migrating peptides which had been found in the α chains of DQ molecules isolated with 8W769 from LG38-Ia preparation [3]. However, their patterns were not identical; subtle but significant differences were seen mostly restricted to a few minor spots located near the origin. The β chain map showed a resemblance to that of the DQ molecules from LG38-Ia, but there existed clear differences in some major spots. The same DQ molecules as bound by HON antiserum could be isolated by the use of Fe117/30 known to have anti-DQw3 activity, supporting the presence of DQw3 specificity on the HON-reactive DQ molecules. Thus the DQw3-bearing molecules found in 8057-Ia preparation differ in both α and β chains from those detected in LG38-Ia preparation. It should be noted here that HON antiserum reacts with Ia preparations obtained from U698M (DR2,4), BT1 (DR4, w9), and Chevalier (DR3,7) according to the known HON7 (BR4, DRw53) specificity and the reactive molecules are indeed BR molecules which have a high structural similarity to DR molecules [6].

The structural variations of DQw3-bearing Ia molecules have been confirmed and also expanded by the use of the anti-Ia monoclonal antibody IVD12. This antibody, introduced by Giles et al. [11], has been reported to have a specificity similar to DQw3 and to bind DQ molecules. As a part of the 9W Biochemistry Study, the IVD12 was tested by the direct binding assay for its reactivity with a panel of ^{125}I-labeled preparations of Ia molecules purified from cells of the Workshop core cell lines; PGF (DR2, 2), WT49 (DR3, 3), LEIF-T (DR4, 4), KT2 (DR4, 4), WT46 (DRw6, w6), and MANN (DR7, 7). In addition, two Ia preparations from local cell lines, LG2 (DR1, 1) and LG38 (DR5, 5), were included in the antigen panel. In accord with the reported specificity, IVD12 bound only to Ia preparations derived from DR4-positive cells and DR5-positive cells. The extent of Ia binding with LEIF-T-Ia and KT2-Ia was 5.4% and 5.1% respectively, and that with LG38-Ia was 9.5%. No other Ia preparations gave any significant reaction. The IVD12-reactive molecules were immunospecifically purified from those three Ia preparations and analyzed by microfingerprinting. The results can be summarized as follows: (1) The molecules isolated from LG38-Ia were identical in both α and β chains to those previously obtained with 8W769 from the same Ia preparation. (2) The molecules obtained from LEIF-T-Ia and KT2-Ia were the same in both α and β chains. (3) These two sets of DQ molecules, one from LG38-Ia and another from LEIF-T-Ia and KT2-Ia, showed differences in both α and β chains. The α chain differences reproduced those previously found between the 8W769-reactive molecules from LG38-Ia and the HON-reactive molecules from 8057-Ia. (4) Most importantly, the DQ molecules isolated from LEIF-T-Ia and KT2-Ia and from 8057-Ia shared an identical α chain but possessed different β chains. Thus a third structural variant of DQw3-bearing Ia molecules was found on LEIF-T and KT-2 cells.

The data presented here demonstrate that the DQ molecules associated with DR4, 5, 7, and 8w13, though sharing DQw3 specificity, are not a single moiety, but can be divided into at least three subsets which differ in both serological specificity and primary structure.

The serological differences are manifested by the three newly identified allospecificities. These new specificities must be located on one or more of the component subunits composing the structural variants. This subunit assignment can be made most directly by measuring the binding of antiserum or monoclonal antibody with isolated Ia chains. When a strong binding is observed, the interpretation is unequivocal. This has been the case for the 8W1062 and 8W617 antisera which defined DCα3 specificity; those antisera did bind with the α chains of DQw3-bearing molecules isolated from LG38-Ia preparation [4]. When such direct data are not available, the subunit attribution has to be made on the less direct criterion of structural comparison of molecules carrying different specificities. For example, the microfingerprinting analysis of DQ molecules from CLL46 (DR3, 5) cells showed that the molecules differing in DQw3 and DQw2 specificities but sharing the DCα3 specificity possess clearly different β chains but a very similar or identical α chain. Therefore, it was assumed that the DQw3 and DQw2 determinants are carried by the DQ β subunit [4]. Similarly, the DC5 specificity was deductively attributed to the DQ β subunit [5]. Peptide mapping also revealed that DQ molecules from DR4-positive cells, LEIF-T, KT2 and 8057, possess an identical α chain. This finding can be utilized to assign DC4HON specificity to the DQ α subunit, because this specificity is consistently associated with DR4. However, the subunit attribution based on structural comparison is not decisive; serological differences are not necessarily reflected in structural variations and vice versa.

Apart from the correlation of the observed serological and structural differences at the subunit level, the three new specificities have clearly defined four DQw3 haplotypes; DQw3$^+$/DC4HON$^+$/DC5$^-$/DCα3$^-$, DQw3/DC54HON$^+$/DC5$^+$/DCα3$^-$, DQw3$^+$/DC4HON$^-$/DC5$^+$/DCα3$^+$, and DQw3$^+$/DC4HON$^-$/DC5$^-$/DCα3$^-$. The first haplotype is detected in over 70% of DR4-positive cases (13 of 17) and the second is found in the remaining DR4-positive cases. The third is associated with DR5-positive cases (53 of 53) and with 8w13-positive cases (2 of 2). The last appears to be carried by some DR7-positive cases. These haplotypes, except for the last, have apparently one to one relationship with the three structural variants; the first haplotype corresponds to the DQw3-positive molecules found in LEIF-T and KT2 cells, the second haplotype to those identified in 8057 cells, and the third haplotype to those isolated from LG38 cells. The LEIF-T and KT2 cells have not been typed yet for the new DQ specificities, but they must have the first haplotype, because their DQw3-bearing molecules are different structurally from those of 8057 cells and among the two haplotypes linked to DR4 the second haplotype is carried by 8057 cells. The question as to whether or not this correlation can be generalized to other DR4-, DR5- or 8w13-positive cells remains to be investigated.

The characterization of DCα3 specificity has revealed the presence of structural variations in Ia molecules sharing DQw2 specificity. This specificity is known to be associated with DR3 and DR7. As described above, the DCα3 specificity is also associated with DR3, but not with DR7. This difference indicates that the DQw2-bearing molecules do not have the same α chains, clearly predicting the presence of structural differences in their α chains. More extensive analysis of various DQ-enriched Ia preparations would disclose still other serological and/or structural variations which allow further dissection of DQw3- or DQw3-bearing Ia molecules. It would be also possible to find allospecificities which can differentiate DQw1-bearing Ia molecules according to their structural differences.

The definition of those different DQw3 haplotypes linked to DR4 and DQw2 haplotypes linked to DR3 may have an implication in the study of HLA disease association. It necessitates reevaluation of various DR3- and/or DR4-associated diseases, particularly insulin-dependent diabetes. A significant shift of patients with those diseases towards any of those haplotypes may provide useful information on the primary HLA association of the diseases.

References

1. Tanigaki N, Tosi R (1982) The genetic control of human Ia alloantigens: a three loci model derived from the immunochemical analysis of 'supertypic' specificities. Immunol Rev 66:5–37
2. Shackelford DA, Mann DL, van Rood JJ, Ferrara GB, Strominger JL (1981) Human B-cell alloantigen DC1, MT1, and LB12 are identical to each other but distinct from the HLA-DR antigen. Proc Natl Acad Sci USA 78:4566–4570
3. Tanigaki N, Tosi R, Sagawa K, Minowada J, Ferrara GB (1983) The distribution of DR5, MT2, and MB3 specificities on human Ia subsets. Immunogenetics 17: 371–386
4. Tosi R, Tanigaki N, Sorrentino R, Centis D, Ferrara GB (1984) Serologically detectable polymorphism of the HLA-DC α subunit. J Immunol 132:277–282
5. Tanigaki N, Tosi R, Centis D, Ferrara GB (1984) DR5-associated DC molecules carry three different allospecificities. Hum Immunol (in press)
6. Tanigaki N, Tosi R, Katagiri M, Ferrara GB (1984) A new allodeterminant on HLA-D molecules carrying the DQw3 specificity. Hum Immunol (submitted)
7. Tanigaki N, Tosi R (1982) Assessment of the specificity of human Ia alloantisera and alloantigens by the use of radioiodinated human Ia antigens. Tissue Antigens 20:1–21
8. Katagiri M, Ikeda H, Maruyama N, Moriuchi J, Wakisaka A, Kimura S, Aizawa M, Itakura K (1979) Evidence for two B-cell alloantigen loci in the HLA-D region. Immunogenetics 9:335–351
9. Tanigaki N, Tosi R, Pressman D, Ferrara GB (1980) Molecular identification of human Ia antigens coded for by a gene locus closely linked to HLA-DR locus. Immunogenetics 10:151–167
10. Tanigaki N, Tosi R, Duquesnoy RJ, Ferrara GB (1983) Three Ia species with different structures and alloantigenic determinants in an HLA-homozygous cell line. J Exp Med 157:231–247
11. Giles RC, Nunez G, Hurley CK, Nunez-Roldan A, Winchester R, Stastney P, Capra JD (1983) Structural analysis of a human I-A homologue using a monoclonal antibody that recognizes an MB3-like specificity. J Exp Med 157:1461–1470

Comparison of Supertypic Specificities by Cytotoxicity and by Radioimmunoassay in Segregating Families

G.B. Ferrara[1], D. Centis[2], I. Cascino[3], P. Lulli[3], M. Mennucci[4], M. Morellini[3], M.P. Pistillo[1], S. Roncella[1], S. Trabace[3], C. Viviani[5], and A. Longo[1]

1 Istituto Nazionale per la Ricerca sul Cancro, viale Benedetto XV 10, 16100 Genova, Italy
2 Laboratorio di Biologia Cellulare, C.N.R., Roma, Italy
3 Cattedra di Genetica Medica, Università di Roma, Italy
4 Istituto Elaborazione dell'Informazione, C.N.R., Pisa, Italy
5 Centro Ricerche Immunoematologiche A.V.I.S. Bergamo, Italy

We have experienced serious problems in typing some of the supertypic specificities, viz. DQw2, DQw3, and DRw53, by cytotoxicity. In an attempt to analyze the reasons for these difficulties, we studied 23 families within the framework of the Ninth Workshop. Their members have been typed by RIA using purified, ^{125}I-labeled class II molecules, for DC beta 3 (~ DRw52), DC beta 4 (~ DQw3), and BR4 (~ DRw53).

DQw1 *(DC1, MT1)* and DRw52 were omitted: the former because it does not give any problem in its definition by cytotoxicity, the latter because it is a complex, bi-locus, specificity for which more precise characterization is still required. The outcome of the RIA has been arbitrarily taken to express the "real" phenotype. Based on this, the cytotoxicity reactions have been classified as positive, negative, false positive, and false negative. The advantage of studying offspring of segregating families is that a confirmation of phenotype is derived from the haplotype distribution.

Table 1. DQw2

	Cytotoxicity	9w723	727	720	726	722
RIA$^+$	+	24	30	23	12	23
(DCbeta3)	–	6	0	7	18	7
RIA$^-$	+	1	0	2	3	4
	–	19	20	18	17	16

Table 2. DQw3

	Cytotoxicity	9w746	584	745	747	748
RIA$^+$	+	11	14	11	10	9
(DCbeta4)	–	11	8	11	8	13
RIA$^-$	+	0	0	0	0	0
	–	7	7	7	7	7

Table 3. DRw53

	Cytotoxicity	9w734	743	735	753	736
RIA$^+$	+	28	26	30	29	14
(BR4)	–	2	4	0	1	16
RIA$^-$	+	1	0	0	8	0
	–	15	15	15	7	15

For each of the supertypic specificities the five best 9W antisera have been selected on the basis of their Q scores. The cytotoxicity data have been compared with the RIA typing. Positivity by cytotoxicity includes scores 8, 6, and 4. Tables 1–3 summarize these comparisons.

On the assumption, which is by no means granted, that the RIA data express the true typing, the following conclusions can be drawn:

DQw2. Only for 9W727 is there a perfect fit with DCβ3. The other antisera lack some DR3$^+$, while essentially all DR7$^+$ match. An additional presence of DR7 antibodies in most 9W DQw2 antisera is a plausible possibility.

DQw3. About half the positives are missed by cytotoxicity. When the antigen is present in a double dose (e.g., in DR4$^+$/5$^+$ individuals) it is detected (4 of 4 cases) by all antisera.

The associations of DQw3 with DR7, 8w13, and "DRw6$^+$ DQw1$^-$", which are clearly found by RIA, are not easily detected by cytotoxicity.

The most plausible explanation is that the DQw3 anti-DQw3 reaction is particularly weak in cytotoxicity, either for the low antibody concentration or, more probably, for a relative scarcity of the antigen on the cell surface.

DRw53. One antiserum (9w735) gives a perfect match. The others seem to miss the antigen either in some DR4$^+$ individuals (9w734 and 9w743) or in some DR7$^+$ individuals (9w736).

The possible presence of antibodies against one or the other subtypic component may explain the different strengths of the reactions.

In conclusion, the problems encountered in typing these specificities by cytotoxicity seem to be due to:
Generally weak reactions of the antisera.
Presence of antibodies against the associated subtypic specificities.

The first problem may be partially overcome by the use of stronger complement batches. The interferences of subtypic antibodies may be avoided by taking into consideration, for each antiserum, only the reactions with individuals negative for the corresponding subtypic specificity.

Histocompatibility Testing 1984
Edited by E. D. Albert et al.

HLA-FA: A Non-DR, Non-DQ HLA Class II Product*

K.M. Linner and F.H. Bach

Dept. of Lab. Medicine and Pathology, Box 724, Minneapolis, MN 55455, USA

We have used a monoclonal antibody (mcAb) supplied by Dr. Ian Trowbridge to define a non-DR, non-DQ HLA class II molecule which we have provisionally termed HLA-FA; certain features of this molecule are unusual as compared with HLA-DR and HLA-DQ [1]. First, there is a molecular weight polymorphism of the FA β chain, ranging from 25K to 27K; second, the FA α chain is virtually inaccessible to lactoperoxidase-catalyzed iodination (^{125}I), though it can be readily visualized with metabolic labeling.

Although FA is different from DR and DQ, FA does appear to be related to DP [2], although the exact relationship between FA and DP [3] is not known. We have previously discussed (a) that "DP" is complex as detected with "cloned" primed lymphocyte typing (PLT) reagents and thus there may be more than a single molecular product in the "DP region" [4], and (b) that the αFA mcAB may at times be reacting with a different product than that against which a given αDP PLT clone(s) is responding [3]. (N. Ohta et al., Analysis of Cytolytic Clones Directed at Class I and Class II Antigens Using HLA Loss Mutants of a Lymphoblastoid Cell Line, this volume.)

As shown in Figs. 1 and 2 both the α and β chains of FA are polymorphic in isoelectric focusing (IEF), as noted elsewhere [5]. We have attempted to evaluate further the association between DP and FA by studying the IEF patterns of the FA β chain(s) obtained from cells with different DP phenotypes. Since the intact FA β chain is difficult to focus in IEF, we have used α-chymotrypsin to cleave the β chain into two fragments, one of which (presumably the N-terminal fragment in analogy with DR) does focus [5, 6]. Our findings (Fig. 2) demonstrate that there is a strong correlation between the DP phenotype, as defined by PLT reagents, and the focusing pattern of the FA β chain fragment. We have, however, found exceptions to this correlation [5] (data not shown).

The positive correlations of DP and FAβ suggest that the FA product(s) and the DP product(s) are one and the same. The exceptions, on the other hand, could indicate either that the αDP "clone" used to define DP for a given haplotype and the anti-FA mcAb are reacting with different products of that haplotype, or that the polymorphism leading to the differential migration in IEF (for the exceptions) does not encode a portion of the molecule important for T cell recognition and thus that DP and FA determinants are expressed on the same molecule(s) despite the exceptions.

In collaboration with Dr. Peter Wernet, using his Tu39 mcAb, we have found that in one cell line, the metabolically labeled extract of which had been precleared of DR and DQ products, αFA and Tu39 appear to react with products migrating differentially in IEF (data not shown). This finding is consistent with the existence of two products.

We would propose that if there are two DP/FA products (a) they both stimulate T cells and thus contribute to the "DP phenotype" (although in any one haplotype one product may be immunodominant over the other), and (b) that αFA recognizes a determinant that is frequently shared by the two products; this determinant is, however, presumably polymorphic, so that in some haplotypes FA may react with only one of the products.

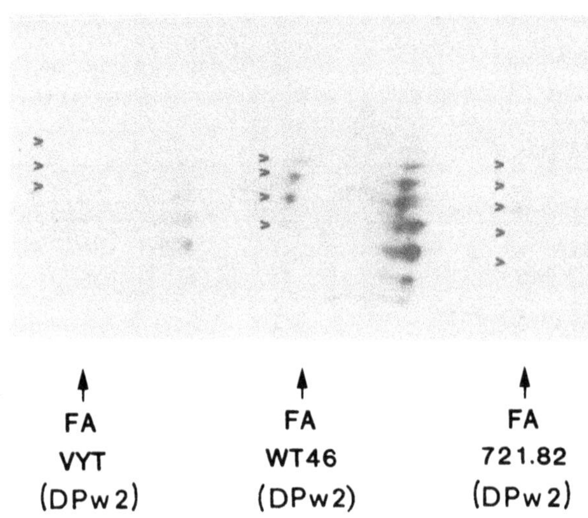

Fig. 1. The FA α chains from three different LCLs are polymorphic (*arrows*). The unidentified focusing patterns are not FA

* This is paper # 388 from the Immunobiology Research Center. This work was supported in part by NIH grants AI 17687, AI 18326, AI 19007, and AM 13083, the March of Dimes Birth Defects Foundation grants # 6-255 and # 1-887, and the National Multiple Sclerosis Society grant # RG 1505-A-1

Histocompatibility Testing 1984
Edited by E. D. Albert et al.

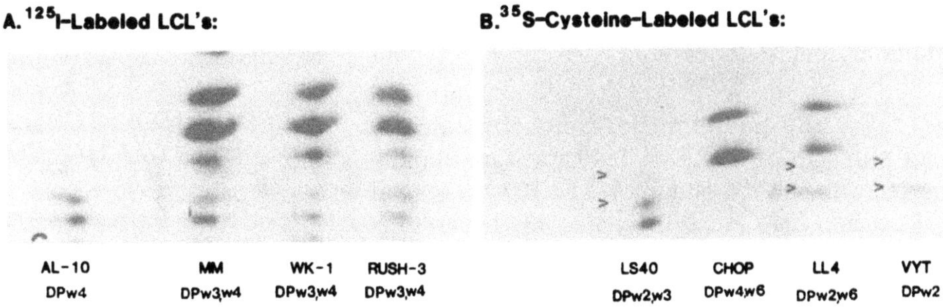

Fig. 2. IEF pattern of band α-chymotryptic fragments precipitated by FA. LCLs in *panel A* were not treated with neuraminidase. *Arrows* denote presumed DPw2 bands. DPw6 in lanes 2 and 3 are similar

References

1. Watson A, DeMars R, Trowbridge IS, Bach FH (1983) Detection of a novel human class II HLA antigen. Nature 304:358–361
2. Shaw S, Pollack MS, Payne SM, Johnson AH (1980) HLA-linked B cell alloantigens of a new segregant series: population and family studies of the SB antigens. Hum Immunol 1:177–185
3. Bach FH, Groner J, Watson AJ, Reinsmoen N, Segall M (1984) HLA class II molecules: T cell response and molecular characterization. In: Sasazuki T, Tada T (eds) Immunogenetics: its application to clinical medicine. Academic, Tokyo (in press)
4. Reinsmoen NL, Bach FH (1983) HLA-D region complexity associated with HLA-DR, Dw, and SB phenotypes. Trans Proc XV, 1:76–78
5. Watson AJ, Bach FH (1984) Structural polymorphism of FA: an HLA class II antigen with unusual molecular properties (submitted)
6. Kaufman JF, Strominger JL (1982) HLA-DR light chain has a polymorphic N-terminal region and a conserved immunoglobulin-like C-terminal region. Nature 297: 694–697

Hybrid HLA-DQ Antigens: Molecular Expression

D.J. Charron, V. Lotteau, P. Turmel

Laboratoire d'Immunogénétique. CHU Pitie Salpetrière 91, boulevard de l'Hôpital, CNRS 500, 75013 Paris, France

Introduction

Ia antigens are gene products of the I region of the H-2 complex in mouse and of the HLA-D region of the HLA complex in man. They play a crucial role in the initiation of the immune response and in the interaction of immunocompetent cells [1, 2]. Three distinct subsets of Ia molecules (HLA-DR, HLA-DQ, and HLA-DP) have been defined in man using monoclonal antibodies (mAbs) and alloantisera [3–5]. The HLA-DR and HLA-DQ antigens are biochemically analogous to the murine I-E and I-A antigens respectively [4, 6]. No DP product has been found in the mouse. The structure of Ia antigens consists of two noncovalently linked polypeptide chains: a 32- to 34-kd α chain and a 27- to 29-kd β chain. Ii, a third 31-kd basic polypeptide, is constantly associated with the α-β dimer [7]. Structural polymorphism is an essential feature of Ia antigens and provides a molecular basis for the Ir gene phenomenon. In both mouse and man, the primary source of Ia diversity resides in the structure of the genes coding for the individual chains [8]. However, genetic studies in the mouse have indicated that several loci can interact to control a given trait [9]. Hybrid I region determinants have been shown to contribute to the polymorphism of the MHC class II antigens and thus provide a molecular basis for Ir gene complementation [10, 11]. Furthermore, such determinants can stimulate in the mixed lymphocyte reaction (MLR) and can function as a restriction element for T cell recognition of antigen-specific clones [12, 13]. Although functional *trans*-complementation within the HLA-D region was recently reported [14], no biochemical evidence of HLA-D region hybrid determinants has been provided. We describe in this report the existence of hybrid HLA-DQ molecules resulting from the association of an α chain and a β chain encoded by genes located on the two haplotypes in an heterozygous cell line.

Histocompatibility Testing 1984
Edited by E. D. Albert et al.

Materials and Methods

Cell Lines. EBV-transformed B-lymphoblastoid cell lines were grown in RPMI 1640 medium supplemented with 4 m*M* L-glutamine and 10% (v/v) fetal calf serum. Cells were incubated at 37 °C in a humidified atmosphere of 5% CO_2 in air. Three different cell lines were used in this study: two homozygous lines, SC-CA (DR1/1) and GM 3163 (DR7/7), and one heterozygous line, LES (DR1/7).

Monoclonal Antibodies. The monoclonal antibodies (mAbs) used in this study were selected on the basis of their molecular reactivity with homozygous cell lines of different HLA-DR types. CA 1.41 and D1.12 are monomorphic anti-HLA-DR antibodies. CA 2.06 and SG 171 were used in several experiments. They both react with HLA-DR antigens 1–8 and additionally with HLA-DQw2 molecules when used in DR7 cells [15, 16]. Moreover, CA 2.06 and SG 171 have been shown in western blot experiments to react only with the β chains of the antigens they immunoprecipitate (V. Lotteau et al., Nonassociated HLA-DR α and β chains: Molecular Detection and Differential Cellular Expression, this volume). G25a, an γ2a spontaneous variant of Genox 3.53, is an anti-DQw1 reagent which reacts with and immunoprecipitates HLA-DQw1 molecules from DR1, 2, and w6 cells [17]. SG 465 and SG 520 have a more complex reactivity pattern. They both identify DQw2 molecules when used in DR7 cells [18].

Radiolabeling of Cells and Immunoprecipitations. 0.5×10^7 viable cells were labeled for 5 h with 500 µCi [^{35}S]methionine (Amersham) and the membranes extracted with 0.5% NP40 as previously described [3]. ^{125}I was used for surface labeling. Radiolabeled cell proteins were immunoprecipitated by addition of 3–5 µl mAb (ascites fluid or purified Ig) to 100 µl NP40 extract with 60 min incubation time. One hundred microliters of a 10% wt : vol staphylococcus cowan I strain (SaC) solution was added for 15 min. The bound antigen complexes were eluted in 40 µl isoelectrofocusing (IEF) sample buffer.

Two-dimensional Gel Electrophoresis (2D-PAGE). 2D-PAGE was performed as previously described [3]. In the first dimension IEF was used instead of nonequilibrium pH-gradient gel electrophoresis (NEPHGE) in order to maximize the resolution in the acidic α chain area. The second dimension was a 10% polyacrylamide SDS slab gel. The autoradiographs presented are the result of 10–20 days exposure.

Results

HLA-DQ α 2D-PAGE Patterns of SC-CA (DR1/1) and GM 3163 (DR7/7)

Monoclonal antibody G25a immunoprecipitates HLA-DQw1 molecules from the DR1 homozygous cell line SC-CA. Examination of the 32- to 34-kd area of the gel reveals a series of four distinct spots, the most basic being slightly lower and the most acidic slightly higher (Fig. 1). This IEF profile defines the electrophoretic patterns of the DQw1 α chain present in a DR1/1 cell line. Actin, a 44-kd protein, is a constant contaminant of HLA-DR and HLA-DQ immunoprecipitates. It can serve as a migration marker within the gel to localize other molecular species. In several experiments with the same cell line the DQw1 α chain pattern was reproducible and constant relative to the position of actin. The β chain of the DQw1 molecule was not adequately resolved because of the use of IEF instead of NEPHGE. Similarly, the Ii chain was present only as a smear at the basic end of the gel. The α chain 2D-PAGE pattern obtained from GM 3163 (DR7/7) immunoprecipitated with SG 520 is reproducibly different from the DQw1 α chain species. As shown in Fig. 1, it consists of four to five spots which are slightly more acidic and slightly higher compared to the DQw1 α chain. An identical gel pattern was obtained with SG 520 when a second DR7/7 cell line (Mann) was used. Because SG 520 had previously been reported to immunoprecipitate only DQ molecules from DR7/7 cell lines, including GM 3163, the IEF pattern obtained can be identified as the α chain of the DQw2 molecule. Difference in electrophoretic mobility of DQw1 α and DQw2 α is confirmed when DQw1 antigens immunoprecipitated from SC-CA and DQw2 antigens immunoprecipitated from GM 3163 are mixed together and analyzed on the same gel. The IEF pattern obtained is a composite of the DQw1 and of the DQw2 α chains. Both the HLA-DQw1 α chain and the DQw2 α chain IEF profiles were distinct from the HLA-DR α pattern obtained by immunoprecipitation of either CA-SC or GM 3163 cells with CA 141 or D1.12, two monomorphic anti-HLA-DR mAbs. The HLA-DR α chain has a higher molecular weight and is slightly more acidic than the DQ α chain species. Furthermore, the HLA-DR α chains are more intensely labeled with [^{35}S]methionine than the HLA-DQ α chains.

HLA-DQ α 2D-PAGE Patterns of LES (DR1/7)

Cell lysate from LES (DR1/7) cells was depleted of HLA-DR antigens by eight cycles of sequential im-

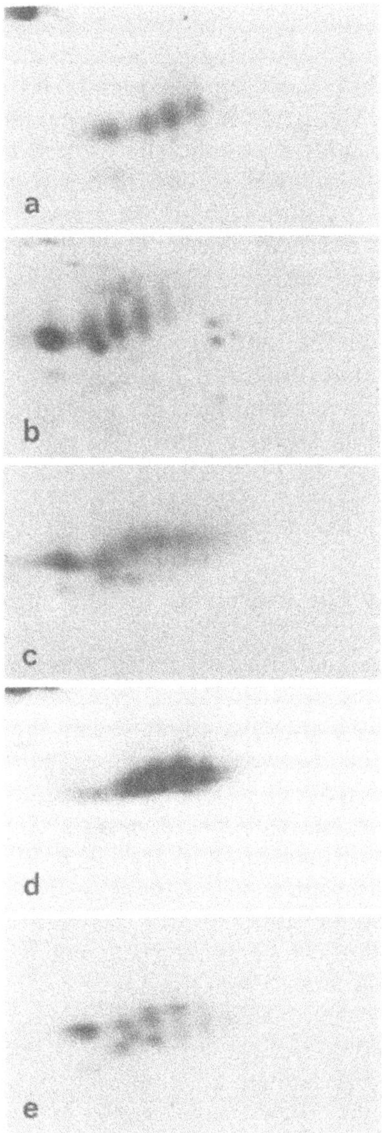

Fig. 1 a – e. IEF 2D-PAGE profiles of the DR and DQ α chains from SC-CA (DR1/1), GM3163 (DR7/7), and LES (DR1/7) cell lines. Panel *a* represents the DQw1 α chain isolated from SC-CA using the mAb G25a (anti-DQw1), panel *b* the DQw2 α chain from GM3163 immunoprecipitated with the mAb SG 520. In panel *c* DQw1 α and DQw2 α chains were coelectrophoresed on the same gel, while panel *d* shows an HLA-DR α chain pattern. In panel *e* LES DR$^-$ (DQw1, DQw2) cell lysate was immunoprecipitated by SG 171. Both the DQw1 α chain and the DQw2 α chain are present, in contrast to panel *b*. The position of actin is indicated by the letter *A* in panel *e*

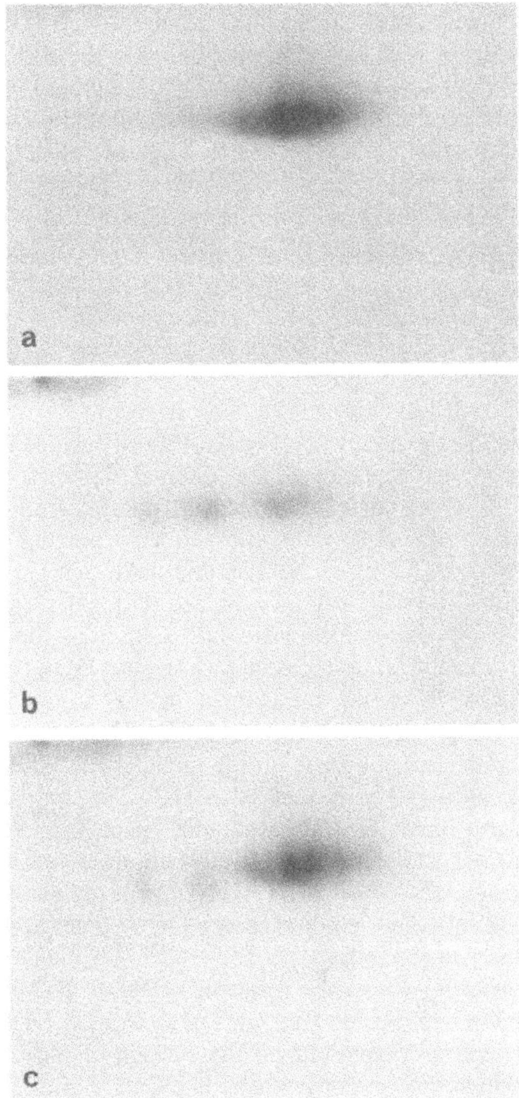

Fig. 2 a – c. IEF 2D-PAGE profiles of DR and DQ α chains from ^{125}I-surface labeled LES cells (DR1/7). Panel *a* shows the DR α chain precipitated with the mAb D1.12. Both DQw1 and DQw2 α chains immunoprecipitated with SG 465 are shown in panel *b*. As shown in panel *c* SG 171 precipitates a DQw1 α chain in addition to the DR and DQw2 α chains

munoprecipitation with D1.12, a monomorphic anti-HLA-DR antibody (Fig. 1). After such treatment the LES lysate could be operationally considered as DR1$^-$, DR7$^-$, DQw1$^+$, and DQw2$^+$. This was confirmed in the final round of immunoprecipitation with mAb D1.12. Based on data obtained in DR1/1 and DR7/7 homozygous cell lines, CA 2.06 and SG 171 are expected to immunoprecipitate only DQw2 antigens from a DR1 – 7 cell lysate previously depleted of HLA-DR antigens. Indeed, a DQw2 α chain is present, as revealed by IEF 2D-PAGE when LES DR$^-$ lysate is reacted with CA 2.06 or SG 171. However, an additonal α chain species is clearly detected in these immunoprecipitates. This second chain is slightly more acidic and slightly lower than the DQw2 α chain and has an electrophoretic mobility similar to the previously identified DQw1 α chain. Because CA 2.06 and SG 171 have been shown in western blot to react only with the β chain species (V. Lotteau et al., Nonassociated HLA-DR α and β Chains: Molecular Detection and Differential Cellular Expression, this volume) of the human Ia molecules, and because they would react only with the DQw2 β chain in the LES DR^- cell lysate, the two α chains (DQw1 α and DQw2 α) are precipitated through their molecular association with the DQw2 β chains. Thus an anti-DQw2 β chain precipitates both (DQw2 α – DQw2 β) and (DQw1 α – DQw2 β) complexes in a DR1 – 7 heterozygous cell line.

HLA-DQ Hybrid Molecules Are Present on the Cell Surface

In these experiments (Fig. 2), ^{125}I cell surface labeling was substituted for internal labeling with [^{35}S]methionine, ^{125}I-labeled cell lysates from LES (DR1 – 7) cells were subsequently reacted with mAb D1.12, mAb SG 465, and mAb SG 171. The IEF 2D-PAGE pattern obtained with D1.12 allows identification of the HLA-DR α chain as the most acidic and larger molecule, while both DQw1 α and DQw2 α chains are present in the SG 465 immunoprecipitate. When mAb SG 171 is used, the α chain electrophoretic profile includes the HLA-DR α, HLA-DQw1 α, and HLA-DQw2 α chains. Because mAb SG 171 does not react with HLA-DQw1 antigens in DR1/1 cells but does react with both HLA-DR7 and HLA-DQw2 molecules in DR7/7 cells, the presence of a DQw1 α chain in the immunoprecipitate of LES (DR1/7) cells with mAb SG 171 is the result of a DQw1 α-DQw2 β hybrid molecule. Thus, in DR1 – 7 cells, DQw2 β chains are expressed on the surface of individual cells in association with both DQw2 α chains and DQw1 α chains. These results provide the possibility for the HLA-DQ hybrid determinants to be exposed and recognized on the cell surface.

Discussion

Multiple differences present at the nucleotide and amino acid levels provide a molecular basis for the structural polymorphism observed within different alleles of the MHC class II antigens. These structural variations may affect only one of the two chains, as is the case for HLA-DR: a nonpolymorphic DR α chain is associated with a highly polymorphic DR β chain [3]. In contrast, both the α and β subunits of DQ are variable when different alleles are compared [18]. Substantial differences in the structure of either subunit result in electrophoretic variants and thus allow the identification of the haplotype of origin of each subunit by 2D-PAGE. Previous studies have focused on the analysis of the β chains. Molecular polymorphism of the DQ α chain is thus not extensively documented. However, amino acid sequences, DNA restriction fragment analysis, and peptide mapping have revealed some structural differences among several DQ α alleles [4, 19, 20]. These results constituted our rationale for searching for electrophoretic variants of the DQ α chains. While NEPHGE provides good separation of the β chains of both the HLA-DR and the HLA-DQ molecules, the α chains are not well resolved by this procedure [3, 4, 18]. IEF was substituted for NEPHGE in order to maximize resolution of the acidic area of the gel. The DQw2 α chain is slightly more basic and higher than the DQw1 α chain. This was confirmed in comigration experiments in which DQw1 α and DQw2 α were analyzed on the same gel. Furthermore, the α chain species could be precisely located according to their position relative to that of actin. DQw1 α and DQw2 α chains also differ from the DR α chain in several ways. The DR α chain is higher, more acidic, and more strongly labeled with [^{35}S]methionine than the DQ α chains, confirming previous data [17]. Since the IEF 2D-PAGE patterns of DQw1 α and DQw2 α are obviously different, they are used in this study as molecular fingerprints to identify the haplotype of origin of the spots. Although the range of electrophoretic variability appears less for DQ α than for DQ β and DR β, IEF 2D-PAGE analysis represents a simple and reproducible method of distinguishing between α chain alleles and thus can be applied to genotypes for the DQ α chain locus. From the above results we could conclude that mAbs with a biochemical specificity restricted to the light chain of the DQw2 antigen are able to precipitate a DQw1 α chain in association with the DQw2 α-β complex when used in a DR1 – 7 heterozygous cell line. The possibility that mAb CA 2.06 or SG 171 recognizes a DQw1 determinant directly can be ruled out, since the mAbs would be expected to immunoprecipitate the DQw1 molecule from a DR1/1 cell. The DQw1 α chain can only be precipitated through a molecular association with the DQw2 β chains. Taken together, our results indicates that in a heterozygous cell line, gene trans-complementation occurs and results in the expression of HLA-DQ hybrid molecules containing one subunit of maternal origin and one of paternal origin. Random association of the DQ α and β chains creates a potential for four different molecular combinations. The existence of hybrid Ia determinants was first postulated in the mouse to explain serological and functional traits expressed in F1 animals but absent from both parental strains [12]. Some MLR-stimulating determinants and restriction of T cell recognition were shown to require the presence (in cis or trans position) of at least two loci within the MHC [12,

13]. Furthermore, Jones et al. [10] and Silver [11] demonstrated that one gene product of the I-A region (A β) and a gene product of the I-E region (E α) could interact (in cis or trans position) to generate new molecules in F1 animals. Trans-complementation was also demonstrated between A α and A β polypeptides in the appropriate F1 [11]. In man, no convincing serological nor biochemical data of HLA-D region hybrid antigen is available. In a recent report, antigen-specific T cell clones obtained from an HLA-D region heterozygous individual were shown to function only when the antigen was processed by accessory cells carrying both HLA-D region antigens possessed by the donor [14]. Such T cell clones could represent the functional counterpart of the hybrid DQ antigens described here. We demonstrate in this report that additional polymorphism arises from combinatorial association of Ia chains. Such mixed haplotype hybrid molecules contribute to the qualitative diversity of human HLA-D region antigens. Increasing the number of possible functional Ia restriction sites may have important implications for the immune response potential.

Summary

At least two major subsets of human Ia molecules have been identified, DR and DQ, which correspond to the murine I-E and I-A antigens respectively. In contrast to HLA-DR molecules composed of an invariant α chain and a polymorphic β chain, both subunits of the HLA-DQ antigens are structurally variable. We used two-dimensional gel electrophoresis to further analyze DQ molecules. Isoelectrofocusing was used in the first dimension to maximize the separation of the α subunits, which were not previously well resolved when nonequilibrium pH-gradient electrophoresis was applied. Using selected monoclonal antibodies (mAbs) and homozygous typing cells, we were able to identify different DQ α chain 2D gel patterns. The DQw1 α chain immunoprecipitated by G25a is clearly distinct from the DQw2 α chain immunoprecipitated by SG 520 or SG 171. We analyzed the DQ antigens from several heterozygous cell lines typed as DR1−7. The DR antigens were previously removed from the cell lysate by sequential immunodepletion. In the DR1−7 heterozygous cell, an anti-DQw1 mAb (G25a) precipitates only the DQw1 molecule, as expected. In contrast, mAb SG 171, which recognizes DQw2 antigens but not DQw1 antigen, was able to precipitate both the DQw1 and the DQw2 α chains in association with the DQw2 β chain. Moreover, SG 171 was shown by western blot to react only with the β chain, not with the α chain. A monoclonal antibody reacting only with the DQ β chain of one haplotype is thus capable of immunoprecipitating the DQ α chains of both haplotypes. This indicates that the DQw2 β chain can freely associate with the DQ α chains of both the DQw1 and DQw2 haplotypes and therefore demonstrates that a molecular association occurs in heterozygous cells between products of the two parental haplotypes. The DQ hybrid molecules generated by unique combinations of DQ α and DQ β chains may be responsible for new antigenic specificity present in the heterozygous cells but not in their homozygous counterparts. Our results provide a structural basis for gene trans-complementation of human DQ antigens and have important implications for future serological and functional studies.

Acknowledgments. We thank J. Silver and S. Goyert for the gift of SG 171, SG 520, and SG 465, and F. Brodsky and P. Parham for the gift of G25a. We thank V. Perseil for typing the manuscript.

References

1. McDevitt HO (1976) In: Katz DH, Benacerraf B (eds) The role of the products of the histocompatibility gene complex in immune responses. Academic, New York, pp 257
2. Bach FH, Van Rood JJ (1976) N Engl J Med 295:806
3. Charron DJ, McDevitt HO (1980) J Exp Med 152:185
4. Goyert SM, Shively JE, Silver J (1982) J Exp Med 156:550
5. Nadler LM, Stashenko P, Hardy R, Pesando SM, Yunis EJ, Schlossman SF (1981) Hum Immunol 2:77
6. Allison JP, Walker LE, Russell WA, Pellegrino MA, Ferrone S, Reisfeld RA, Frelinger JA, Silver J (1978) Proc Natl Acad Sci USA 75:3953
7. Charron DJ, Schulz MF, St Geme J, Erlich H, McDevitt HO (1983) Mol Immunol 20:21
8. Lee J, Trowsdale J (1983) Nature 304:214
9. Murphy DB (1981) In: Dorf M (ed) The role of the major histocompatibility complex in immunobiology. Garland, New York, p 1
10. Jones PP, Murphy DB, McDevitt HO (1978) J Exp Med 148:925
11. Silver J, Swain SL, Hubert JJ (1980) Nature 286:272
12. Fathman G (1980) Transplantation 30:1
13. Schwartz RH, Chen C, Paul W (1980) Eur J Immunol 10:708
14. Hansen GS, Svejgaard A, Claesson MH (1982) J Immunol 128:2497
15. Corte G, Accolla R, Charron DJ, Köning F, Steel M (1984) Exp Clin Immunogenet (in press)
16. Piatier-Tonneau D, Boyer B, Debre P, Charron DJ (1983) J Immunol 131:1339
17. Bono R, Strominger JL (1984) Immunogenetics 18:453
18. Goyert SM, Silver J (1983) Proc Natl Acad Sci USA 80:5719
19. Chang HS, Moriuchi T, Silver J (1983) Nature 305:813
20. Auffray C, et al (1983) EMBO J 121

Nonassociated HLA-DR α and β Chains: Molecular Detection and Differential Cellular Expression

V. Lotteau, B. Boyer, P. Debré, and D.J. Charron

Laboratoire d'Immunogénétique, CHU Pitié Salpetrière CNRS 500-91, boulevard de l'Hôpital, 75013 Paris, France

The major histocompatibility complex plays a critical role in the control of immune phenomena. Biochemical studies of the molecular structure of Ia antigens led to the characterization of a 55-kd complex composed of two noncovalently associated polypeptides of 32–34 kd (α chain) and 27–29 kd (β chain). The subunits have been considered to be associated very early during the maturation process. Western blot experiments showed that one monoclonal antibody (moAb DA6–147) was directed against DR α chain and two others were directed against DR β chain (moAb SG 171, moAb SG 520). These anti-DR moAb, recognizing unbound α and β chains, were used to demonstrate the presence of free α and free β chains in the cell lysates of lymphoblastoid cell lines (B-LCL).

Under nondissociating conditions (no boiling and 0.6% SDS), these moAbs were able to detect a significant amount of nonassociated α and β chains, in addition to the 55-kd complex (Fig. 1). This was confirmed after complete removal of the DR complex by immunoprecipitation with an moAb, VI-15 C, which only reacts with the DR complex. After this depletion, SG 171 and DA6–147 were still able to precipitate β and α chains. The relative amounts of free α and β chains varied from experiment to experiment and could be due to cell cycle influence. In other experiments free chains were detected in PHA-induced T cell lines. During polyclonal activation of T cells by Varidase, PPD, or PHA, the nonassociated forms seemed to occur around day 10, whereas the DR complex is detected from day 3 on. In contrast, under the same conditions, these chains were absent from cell lysates of several HLA-DR⁺ antigen-specific T cell clones, unstimulated peripheral blood B and T cells, and a DR⁺ leukemia (Fig. 1).

Taken together, these results provide evidence for a new source of structural diversity. The role of these free chains in the differentiation and functions of lymphoid cells is under investigation.

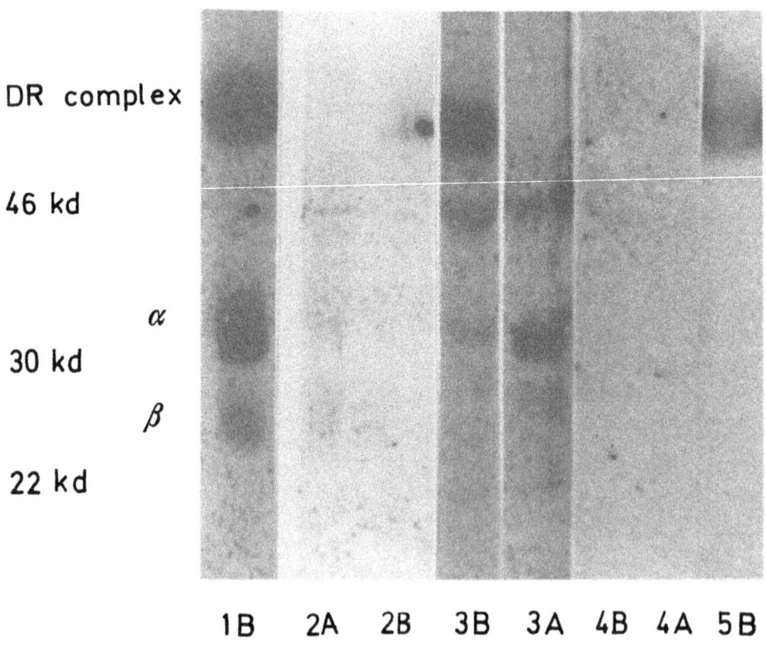

Fig. 1. Presence and absence of free chains in various cell types. *A*, dissociating conditions; *B*, nondissociating conditions. After electrophoretic transfer of total cell lysates separated by 1D gel electrophoresis no free chains were detected in unstimulated peripheral blood B (*2*) and T cells (*4*), or DR⁺ leukemia (*5*). Free chains were detected in B-LCL (*1*), PHA-induced T cell line (*3*)

Histocompatibility Testing 1984
Edited by E. D. Albert et al.

The Expression of HLA-DR, DQ and DP Antigens on the Surface of Lymphocytes as Assessed by 2-D Polyacrylamide Gel Analysis of Immunoprecipitates

C.E. Rudd, J.G. Bodmer, W.F. Bodmer, and M.J. Crumpton

Imperial Cancer Research Fund, P.O. Box 123, Lincoln's Inn Fields, London WC2A 3PX, UK

Introduction

The HLA-D region of the human major histocompatibility complex (MHC) encodes for several sets of class II antigens involved in regulating immune responses. At least three distinct subregions have been distinguished (namely HLA-DR, DQ, DP) by a combination of serology, immunoprecipitation and cellular responses [1–3].
Recent DNA cloning techniques have shown the presence of genes for at least two DR, two DQ and two DP antigens [4–6]. However, the number of distinct HLA-D region antigens that are expressed on the surface of B cells and their relative amounts have not been designated, although precipitation of class II antigens with monoclonal antibodies has allowed the identification of a minimum of two α chains and three β chains [7–9]. Both DR and DQ antigens comprise a heavy (α) chain of MW 32 000–34 000 and a light (β) chain of about 27 000 [10, 11].
In this study, monoclonal antibodies (TAL-1B5, SDR4.1, Tü22, Tü39 and B7/21) from the Ninth International Histocompatibility Workshop were used in conjunction with cell surface labelling and two-dimensional non-equilibrium pH-gradient gel electrophoresis/sodium dodecyl sulphate – polyacrylamide gel electrophoresis (2-D NEPHGE/SDS-PAGE) to identify subsets of the class II antigens expressed by B-lymphoblastoid cell lines. The use of the TAL-1B5 (monomorphic anti-DR) and SDR4.1 (anti-DQw1) antibodies allowed the α subunits of HLA-DR and DQ antigens, as well as their β subunits, to be distinguished. A minimum of two HLA-DR and DQ β chains were evident even after the removal of sialic acid by neuraminidase. Monoclonal antibody Tü39 precipitated two additional β chains (presumably β-DP) as well as two β-DR subunits and one β-DQ subunit from the surface of cells. The anti-FA monoclonal antibody (B7/21) precipitated the two β-DP subunits only, suggesting that the DP and FA antigens are equivalent. In total, one α chain and two β chains derived from each of the HLA-DR, DQ and DP subregions were detected on the surface of B cells.

Materials and Methods

Cells and Monoclonal Antibodies. The human B-lymphoblastoid cell line WT46 (HLA-DRw6, w6) was cultured in RPMI 1640 medium supplemented with penicillin (100 units/ml), streptomycin (50 µg/ ml) and 5% (v/v) foetal calf serum (Flow Laboratories, Irvine, Ayrshire, U.K.). The monoclonal antibodies TAL-1B5 (Bodmer, ICRF), SDR4.1 (Bodmer, ICRF), Tü22 and Tü39 (Wernet/Ziegler, Tübingen) and B7/21 (Bach/Trowbridge, Minnesota/California) have been described or referred to previously [12–15].

Radiolabelling and Immunoprecipitation. Biosynthetic labelling of cells with [^{35}S]methionine and neuraminidase treatment of immunoprecipitates has been described [13]. Immunoprecipitates were carried out by incubating 500 µl of cell lysates [10^7 cells lysed in 1 ml of 1% (w/v) Nonidet P40 in 10 m*M* Tris-HCl buffer, pH 8.2, containing 150 m*M* NaCl and 1 m*M* phenylmethanesulphonyl fluoride] at 4 °C for 2 h with the monoclonal antibody (5 µl of ascitic fluid or 10 µg of purified IgG) and then precipitating with 20 µl of 10% suspension of fixed *Staphylococcus aureus* (Cowan I strain) organisms. Lactoperoxidase-catalysed iodination of cells was performed under conditions of vectoral labelling [16].

2-D Electrophoresis. The procedure, which has been described previously [13], was essentially that of O'Farrell et al. [17] using ampholines of a 3.5–10 pH range (LKB Instruments, Croydon, U.K.). NEPHGE was run as the first dimension overnight for a total of 2550 V/h; the second dimension was SDS-PAGE using 10% acrylamide.

Results

2-D Gel Analysis of HLA-D Region Antigens

Figure 1A, B shows the pattern of spots revealed by 2-D NEPHGE/SDS-PAGE analyses of immunoprecipitates using the monomorphic HLA-DR monoclonal antibody TAL-1B5 and the polymorphic DQw1 monoclonal antibody SDR 4.1 re-

Histocompatibility Testing 1984
Edited by E. D. Albert et al.

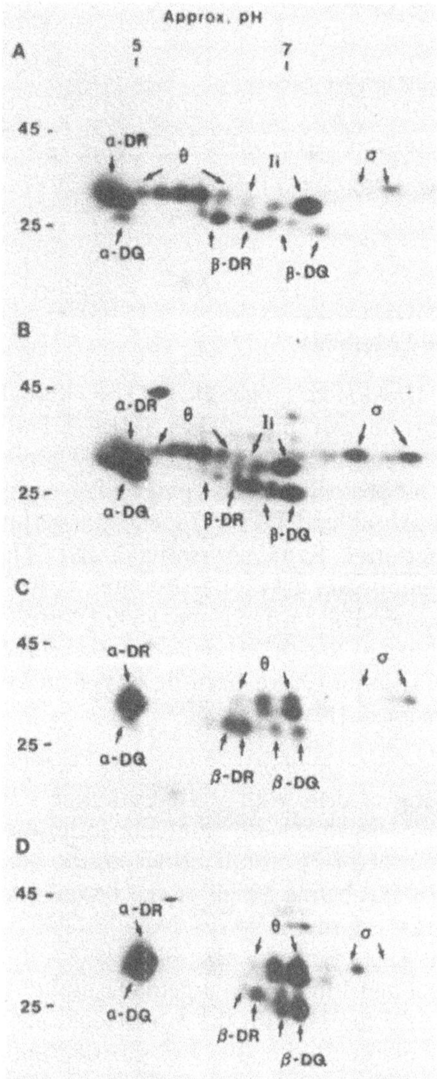

Fig. 1A–D. 2-D gel analyses of HLA-D region antigens. Immunoprecipitates were separated from detergent lysates of WT46 cells which had been labelled for 4 h with [^{35}S]methionine. Neuraminidase digestion (100 mU in 100 m*M* sodium acetate buffer, pH 5.5, containing 0.2 *M* NaCl and 0.2% $CaCl_2$) of the immunoprecipitate was carried out overnight. Digested samples were precipitated with 15% (w/v) trichloroacetic acid for 30 min at 4 °C, and washed in acetone at −20 °C. Immunoprecipitates were prepared by using the following monoclonal antibodies. **A** TAL-1B5; **B** SDR4.1; **C** TAL-1B5 + neuraminidase; **D** SDR4.1 + neuraminidase

spectively. The B-lymphoblastoid cell line WT46 (HLA-DRw6, w6) which had been labelled for 4 h with [^{35}S]methionine was used as a source of antigen. As seen in Fig. 1A, a series of polypeptides including at least two α chains of *Mr* 34 000 and 32 000 and a number of β subunits in the *Mr* range of 25 000–29 000 were precipitated by TAL-1B5. In addition, a regularly spaced series of spots extending across the pH range of 5.0–8.5 and comprising at least three Ii spots of *Mr* 31 000, five θ spots of *Mr* 34 000 and two σ spots of *Mr* 35 000 was also observed. The θ spots have been shown previously to be biosynthetically processed forms of the Ii polypeptide arising through the addition of sialylated *O*-linked oligosaccharides and the maturation of *N*-linked glycans [13, 18, 19]. The σ (35) spots comprise a subset of the invariant chain that is structurally related to Ii but processed to a series of spots of *Mr* 38 000 (C. E. Rudd and M. J. Crumpton, manuscript in preparation).

The monoclonal antibody SDR4.1 was used to identify the DQ antigens which are expressed by WT46 cells. As shown in Fig. 1B, SDR4.1 precipitated a pattern comparable with that precipitated by TAL-1B5, although the relative intensities of the individual spots differed significantly. In particular, the SDR4.1 antibody precipitated preferentially the α chain of lower molecular weight (MW 32 000; α-DQ) and the most basic β spot (β-DQ). These results are similar to those reported previously where the α and β subunits of the DQw1 antigen were shown to have a lower MW than those of the HLA-DR antigen [2]. In contrast, the position and relative intensities of the invariant chains (Ii, θ and σ) were comparable between the immunoprecipitates of the HLA-DR and DQ antigens.

In order to determine the degree to which the charge heterogeneity was due to the presence of sialic acid, the immunoprecipitates were digested with neuraminidase prior to their analysis. Figure 1C, D shows that neuraminidase digestion reduced significantly the complexity of the pattern of spots. Under these circumstances, the pattern of β polypeptides precipitated by TAL-1B5 was resolved into at least four distinct spots (or two pairs of doublets), of which the two most acidic β chains were preferentially precipitated by TAL-1B5 (Fig. 1C). The more acidic of the latter β-DR spots was previously identified as that which carries the HLA-DR serological specificity [7]. In contrast, the monoclonal antibody SDR4.1 preferentially precipitated the two most basic β subunits (Fig. 1D). These data are consistent with the presence in WT46 cells of two distinct HLA-DR antigens and two distinct DQ antigens.

In order to determine whether all these antigens are expressed on the surface of the B-lymphoblastoid cells, the monoclonal antibodies TAL-1B5 and Tü22 were used to precipitate the antigens from ^{125}I-lactoperoxidase-labelled cells. As seen in Fig. 2A, the monoclonal antibody TAL-1B5 precipitated a poorly resolved area of radioactivity in the α chain position and at least four β chains from the WT46 cells. The two most acidic β subunits were precipitated most strongly, which is similar to what was observed for [^{35}S]methionine-labelled immunoprecipitates that had been digested with neuraminidase (Fig. 1C). The monoclonal antibody Tü22 preferentially precipitated two to three of the most basic β spots as well as an α chain of lower molecular weight (Fig. 2B). These results are also comparable to the pattern revealed for neuraminidase treated immunoprecipitates isolated from [^{35}S]methionine-labelled cells by using the monoclonal antibody SDR4.1 (Fig. 1B). These data thus argue strongly that at least two HLA-DR antigens and two distinct DQ antigens are expressed on the surface of WT46 cells.

The Identity of the DP Antigen

In an attempt to study the expression of the DP antigen on the cell surface, immunoprecipitates separated from ^{125}I-lactoperoxidase-labelled cells by using the monoclonal antibody Tü39 were subjected to 2-D gel analysis. The monoclonal antibody Tü39 has been suggested to recognise products of the HLA-DP subregion [14]. As seen in Fig. 2C, this monoclonal antibody precipitated an α chain of about MW 34 000 (α-DR), as well as two of the HLA-DR β subunits (β-DR) and at least one DQ β chain (β-DQ) that were recognised previously (Fig. 2A). However, in addition two chains of MW 26 000 which were slightly more acidic than the β-DR and β-DQ polypeptides were also precipitated. The latter spots, which are provisionally designated as β-DP, were absent in immunoprecipitates obtained using the monoclonal antibodies TAL-1B5 and Tü22 (Fig. 2A, B).

The monoclonal antibody B7/21 (anti-FA) has been reported to react with a previously undefined subset of HLA-D region antigens [15]. Figure 2D shows a 2-D gel of an immunoprecipitate derived by using the anti-FA monoclonal antibody against WT46 cells which had been labelled by lactoperoxidase-catalysed iodination. In this case, only two β subunits were observed, occupying positions identical with those of the two β-DP subunits recognised by Tü39. In contrast to the other monoclonal antibodies, FA did not precipitate the α and β polypeptides previously identified as comprising the HLA-DR and DQ antigens. In addition, no α chain was detected, as previously reported [14]. The latter result suggests that the α chain of the immunoprecipitate obtained using Tü39 was associated with the β subunits of HLA-DR and DQ antigens (Fig. 2C). These data indicate that the FA antigen is a product of the DP subregion and that, as in the case of HLA-DR and DQ antigens, two DP antigens are expressed on the surface of at least some B-lymphoblastoid cell lines.

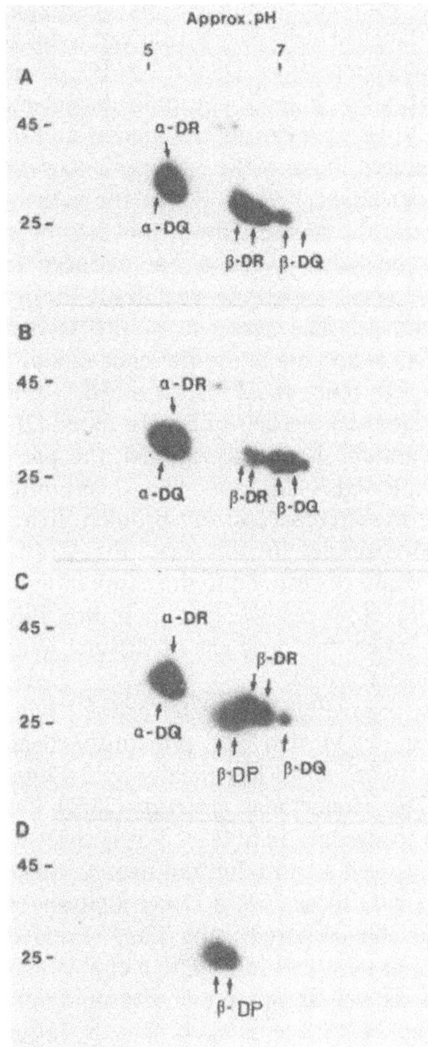

Fig. 2A–D. 2-D gel analyses of HLA-D region antigens. Immunoprecipitates were prepared from WT46 cells (96% viable) which had been labelled with ^{125}I by lactoperoxidase-catalysed iodination. The monoclonal antibodies used for precipitation were **A** TAL-1B5; **B** Tü22; **C** Tü39; **D** B7/21

Discussion

DNA cloning techniques have shown the presence of genes with the potential to encode for at least three HLA-DR, two DQ and two DP antigens [4–6]. However, evidence at the protein level regarding the expression of multiple class II antigens is limited. Previous studies using monoclonal antibodies have allowed the identification of two α chains and three β chains [7–9]. These studies have, however, been hampered by a limited range of monoclonal reagents and a failure to distinguish glycosylation differences from differences in the primary structure of HLA-D region antigens. In this study, the HLA-DR and DQ β chains that had been digested with neuraminidase and prepared from surface labelled cells, were resolved into at least two distinct spots (Figs. 1C, D; 2A, B). In the case of the HLA-DR β spots, the more basic one corresponded to that previously designated as β-1, which was deduced to carry the epitopes encoding the DR serological specificities [7]. In the case of the DQ antigens, the more acidic β spot has been previously designated as β-3 and was deduced to carry the serological supertype specificity designated as DQw1 [2]. The presence of the second β-DR and β-DQ is not due to the presence of sialic acid (Fig. 2C, D). Since the β chains of HLA-DR associated antigens are neither phosphorylated [20] nor acylated (unpublished observations), the presence of multiple HLA-DR and DQ β subunits probably reflects differences in the primary structure of the polypeptides. In this case, the second DQ β subunit could correspond to the expression of the DX gene [6]. However, whether these multiple spots actually reflect the products of distinct gene loci is at present uncertain.

The DP locus, originally defined by primed lymphocyte typing (PLT) had not previously been unequivocally identified biochemically by 2-D gel analysis [3]. The monoclonal antibody Tü39 has been reported to strongly inhibit PLT responses to the DP locus, as well as, to a limited degree, those against the HLA-D locus [14]. 2-D gel analysis of immunoprecipitates prepared using Tü39 revealed the presence of at least two HLA-DR β chains and a DQ β chain, as well as two previously unidentified chains (Fig. 2C). It seems likely that the latter are β subunits derived from the DP subregion. The monoclonal antibody B7/21 (anti-FA) precipitated only the above DP-related β subunits. This argues that the FA antigen is coded by the DP subregion. As previously noted, the α chain of the FA antigen was not detected after ^{125}I-lactoperoxidase labelling, although an α chain was recognised in immunoprecipitates prepared from [^{35}S]methionine-labelled cells [15].

The above data collectively argue for the presence of at least three distinct genes coding for the α chains of the DR, DQ and DP antigens in B cells. The fact that the monoclonal antibody B7/21 precipitated two β-DP chains without the presence of β-DR or β-DQ chains argues against the presence of DR/DQ/DP oligomers or hybrid complexes between the α and β subunits of DR/DQ/DP on the surface of cells. It is interesting that, as in the case of the HLA-DR and DQ β subunits, the DP β chains from the surface of cells focused as two distinct spots. These data are consistent with the presence of multiple HLA-DR, DQ and DP loci [4–6].

References

1. Tosi R, Tanigaki N, Centis D, Ferrara GB, Pressman D (1970) Immunological dissection of human Ia molecules. J Exp Med 148:1592–1611
2. de Kretser TA, Crumpton MJ, Bodmer JG, Bodmer WF (1982) Two-dimensional gel analysis of the polypeptides precipitated by a polymorphic HLA-DR1, 2, w6 monoclonal antibody: evidence for a third locus. Eur J Immunol 12:600–606
3. Shaw W, Kavathas P, Pollack S, Charmot D, Mawas C (1981) Family studies define a new histocompatibility locus, SB, between HLA-DR and GLO. Nature 293: 745–747
4. Trowsdale J, Lee J, Carey J, Grosveld F, Bodmer JG, Bodmer WF (1983) Sequences related to HLA-DRα chain on human chromosome 6: restriction enzyme polymorphism detected with DCα chain probes. Proc Natl Acad Sci USA 80:1972–1976
5. Auffray C, Lillie JW, Arnot D, Grossberger D, Kappes D, Strominger JL (1984) Isotopic and allotypic variation of human class II histocompatibility antigen α chain genes. Nature 308:327–333
6. Spielman RS, Lee J, Bodmer WF, Bodmer JG, Trowsdale J (1984) Six HLA-Dα chain genes on human chromosome 6: Polymorphisms and associations of DCα-related sequences with DR types. Proc Natl Acad Sci USA (in press)
7. de Kretser TA, Crumpton MJ, Bodmer JG, Bodmer WF (1983) Biochemical analysis of the polymorphism of three HLA-D region antigens. Mol Biol Med 1:59–76
8. Hurley CK, Nunez G, Winchester R, Finn OI, Levy R, Capra JD (1982) The human HLA-DR antigens are encoded by multiple β-chain loci. J Immunol 129:2103–2108
9. Shackelford DA, Lampson LA, Strominger JL (1983) Separation of three class II antigens from a homozygous human B cell line. J Immunol 130:289–296
10. Snary D, Barnstable C, Bodmer WF, Goodfellow P, Crumpton MJ (1976) Human Ia antigens – purification and molecular structure. Cold Spring Harb Sym Quant Biol XLI:379–386
11. Shackelford DA, Mann D, Van Rood JJ, Ferrara GB, Strominger JL (1981) Human B-cell alloantigens DC1, MT1 and LB12 are identical to each other but distinct from the HLA-DR antigen. Proc Natl Acad Sci USA 78:4566–4590
12. Adams TE, Bodmer JG, Bodmer WF (1983) Production and characterisation of monoclonal antibodies recognising the α-chain subunits of human Ia alloantigens. Immunology 50:613–624
13. Rudd CE, Bodmer JG, Bodmer WF, Crumpton MJ (1984) HLA-D region antigen associated invariant polypeptides as revealed by 2-D gel analysis: glycosylation and structural inter-relationships. J Biol Chem (submitted)
14. Pawelec GP, Shaw S, Zeigler A, Muller C, Wernet P (1982) Differential inhibition of HLA-D or SB-directed secondary lymphoproliferative responses with monoclonal antibodies detecting human Ia-like determinants. J Immunol 129:1070–1075
15. Watson AJ, DeMars R, Trowbridge IS, Bach FS (1983) Detection of a novel human class II HLA antigen. Nature 304:358–361
16. Walsh FS, Crumpton MJ (1977) Orientation of cell-surface antigens in the lipid bilayer of the lymphocyte plasma membrane. Nature 269:307–311

17. O'Farrell PL, Goodman HM, O'Farrell PH (1977) High resolution two-dimensional electrophoresis of basic as well as acidic proteins. Cell 12:1133–1142
18. Machamer CE, Cresswell P (1982) Biosynthesis and glycosylation of the invariant chain associated with HLA-DR antigens. J Immunol 129:2564–2569
19. Claesson L, Peterson PA (1983) Association of human γ chain with class II transplantation antigens during intracellular transport. Biochem 22:3206–3213
20. Kaufmann JF, Strominger JL (1979) Both chains of HLA-DR bind to the membrane with a penultimate hydrophobic region and the heavy chain is phosphorylated at its hydrophilic carboxyl terminus. Proc Natl Acad Sci USA 76:6304

Preferential Increase of Expression and Release of DQ Molecules in Human Cells Treated with Interferons*

F. Ameglio[1], A. Dolei[2], M.R. Capobianchi[2], and R. Tosi[1]

1 Laboratory of Cell Biology, CNR, Via Romagnosi 18A, 00100 Rome, Italy
2 Institute of Virology, University of Rome, Viale Porta Tiburtina 28, 00185 Rome, Italy

It has been suggested that among Class II HLA antigens, DQ molecules, which are the equivalent of I-A in the murine system, are involved in the generation of effector T cells mediating specific cytolytic activity and in some autoimmune disorders. It is likely that the modulation of expression of these molecules plays a role in their function(s).
Interferons (IFNs) α, β and γ exert a number of important effects in the host, among which antiviral, cell-modulating, and immunoregulatory activities are the most documented.
We have previously shown that IFNs β and γ enhance the expression of Ia molecules [1, 2]. We now present data on the expression and release of DQ molecules in human cells treated with IFN, as detected by specific radioimmunoassay [3].
On the basis of the antiviral units used, IFN γ is the most effective of the three in this respect. In the heterozygous melanoma M14 cell line, the increase due to treatment with IFN γ (Table 1) is greater for the DQ than for the DR molecules (11-fold vs 3-fold). The two allelic forms at each locus behave similarly (not shown). The shedding of these molecules from the cell membrane is also increased by IFN γ (Table 1).
These findings may be connected with the immunoregulating activities of IFN γ.

Table 1. Increase of cell-associated (A) and released (R) Ia molecules in IFN γ-treated M14 cells over control values

DRw6		DQw1	
A	R	A	R
2.8	2.6	11.2	8.0

Cells were treated with 500 U/ml IFNγ. Control values ($IU_{50}/10^6$ cells) were: DRw6: A, R6; DQw1: A15, R5. Results are expressed taking respective control values as 1

* Work supported in part by grants from CNR, Progetto Finalizzato Oncologia, Contratto 84., and Ingegneria Genetica e Basi Molecolari delle Malattie Ereditarie, Contratto 84

References

1. Dolei A, Ameglio F, Capobianchi MR, Tosi R (1981) Human β-type interferon enhances the expression and shedding of Ia-like antigens. Comparison to HLA-A, B, C and β_2-microglobulin. Antiviral Res 1:367–381
2. Dolei A, Capobianchi MR, Ameglio F (1983) Human interferon γ enhances the expression of Class I and Class II MHC products more effectively than interferons α and β. Infect Immun 40:172–176
3. Ameglio F, Capobianchi MR, Dolei A, Tosi R (1983) Differential effects of γ interferon on expression of HLA Class II molecules controlled by the DR and DC loci. Infect Immun 42:122–125

Histocompatibility Testing 1984
Edited by E. D. Albert et al.

Differential Molecular Expression of HLA-DR and HLA-DQ Antigens in Leukemic Cells

A.A. Faille[1], L. Degos[2], P. Turmel[3], J.L. Binet[3], and D.J. Charron[3]

1 Service du Pr. Y Najean (médecine nucléaire), Hôpital Saint Louis, 2, Place du Docteur Fournier, 75010 Paris, France
2 Unité de Recherche sur l'Immunogénétique de la Transplantation Humaine, Hôpital Saint-Louis, 2, Place du Docteur Fournier, 75010 Paris, France
3 CHU, Pitié-Salpétrière, 91, Boulevard de l'Hôpital, 75013 Paris, France

MHC class II antigens are mainly expressed on B cells, monocytes, and activated T cells [1, 2]. They also represent differentiation markers in hematopoiesis.

Molecular structure and expression of MHC class II antigens were analyzed by two-dimensional gel electrophoresis (2D-PAGE) in two cases of chronic lymphocytic leukemia (CLL), one of hairy cell leukemia (HCL) before and after therapy, one case of prolymphocytic leukemia (PLL), and one of erythroleukemia (EL). Internal labeling, immunoprecipitation and 2D-PAGE were performed as previously described [3]. Monoclonal antibody (Mab) VII5C is a monomorphic anti-HLA-DR. CA-206 reacts with HLA-DR and in addition with HLA-DQ molecules in the DR7 haplotype. G25A is a monoclonal anti-DQw1 and Rb03 a rabbit anti-HLA-DQ reagent. Leukemic cells were subsequently incubated with phorbol-ester (TPA: 1.6×10^{-7} *M*), 5-azacytidine (5-aza: 5 u*M*), and sodium butyrate (NA-BU: 5×10^{-4} *M*) and the HLA-DR pattern shown in Fig. 1 was revealed.

Table 1. Effects of TPA, NA-BU, and 5-AZA on DR and DQ synthesis in leukemic cells

Cells				TPA	Na-BU	5-AZA
HCL(1)[a]	DR2/DR7	DR	++	↑↑	↑↑↑	↑↑
		DQ	0	↑↑	↑↑↑	↑↑
HCL(2)	DR2/DR7	DR	++	ND	ND	ND
		DQ	++			
CLL	DR1/DR7	DR	++	++	↑↑↑	↑↑
		DQ	0	↑↑	↑↑↑	0
CLL	DR2/DR3	DR	+	++	↑↑↑	↑↑
		DQ	0	0	0	0
PLL	DR1/DR2	DR	+	+	↑↑↑	↑↑↑
		DQ	0	↑↑	↑↑	↑
EL	DR3/DR7	DR	++	ND	ND	ND
		DQ	0			

[a] Same patient before (1), and after (2) splenectomy and leukopheresis

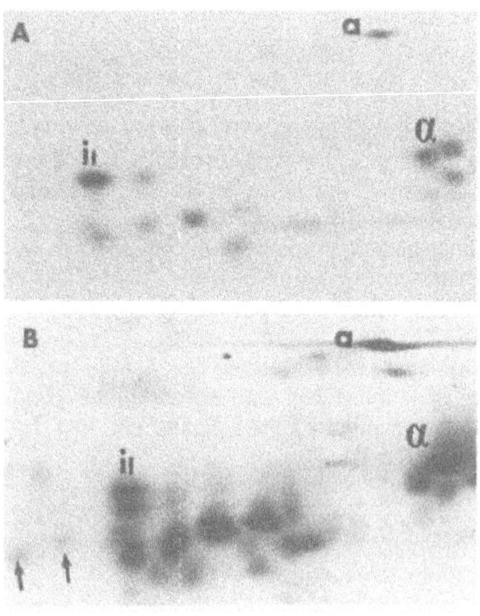

Fig. 1A, B. Differential molecular expression of HLA-DQ antigens in leukemic cells. HLA-DQ is absent (**A**) in the resting cells and is only detected (*arrows*) after induction with TPA (**B**)

Table 1 displays the effects of TPA, NA-BU, and 5-AZA on DR and DQ synthesis in leukemic cells. Our data demonstrate the absence of biosynthesis of HLA-DQ molecules in leukemic cells of various origins, while HLA-DR molecules are readily detectable and qualitatively normal compared with B lymphoblastoid cell lines and normal B cells [4]. TPA, 5-AZA, and NA-BU restored the biosynthesis of DQ molecules in some but not all cases. It is also of interest that after therapy the HCL patient had normal B cells expressing both DR and DQ molecules. The results confirm the lack of DQ expression at the molecular level in some hematopoietic malignancies. Leukemic samples provide unique material for study of the molecular processing of MHC class II antigens. MHC class II antigens may define discrete stages of differentiation in hematopoietic malignancies.

Histocompatibility Testing 1984
Edited by E. D. Albert et al.

References

1. Winchester RJ, Kunkel HG (1980) The human Ia system. Adv Immunol 28:221–228
2. Charron DJ (1981) Ia antigens on human lymphocytes: An overview. Immunol Commun 10:293–315
3. Charron DJ, McDevitt HO (1980) Characterization of HLA-D region antigens by 2-D gel electrophoresis: Molecular genotyping. J Exp Med 152:18–36
4. Faille A, Turmel P, Charron DJ (1984) Differential expression of HLA DC/DS and HLA-DR molecules in a patient with hairy cell leukemia: Restoration of HLA DC/DS expression by TPA; 5-AZA; and NA-BU. Blood. Vol. 64, No 1 (July), pp 33–37

Analysis of HLA Genes at the DNA Level

HLA Class I Gene Typing with an HLA-B-Specific DNA Probe

F.C. Grumet [1], L. Fish [1], J. Moossazedeh [1], D. Ness [1], and B. Duceman [2]

1 Department of Pathology, Stanford University School of Medicine, Stanford, CA 94305, USA
2 Yale University, New Haven, CT, USA

Introduction

HLA class I antigens and genes are of interest as markers of disease susceptibility and targets of cytolytic T lymphocytes [1, 2]. In addition to the HLA-A, B, and C loci, human analogs of the murine class I Qa and Tl loci also probably exist [3, 4]. The well-known serological polymorphism of the class I antigens forms the basis of a substantial part of this workshop; however, early studies using recombinant DNA techniques such as Southern blotting to detect restriction fragment length polymorphisms (RFLPs) suggest that even greater complexity may be found at the level of the genes themselves, with estimates of more than 20 class I loci [3]. Identification of differences at the gene level has been difficult because their great homology results in strong cross-reactivity of cloned class I gene probes with all members of this multigene family. A strategy was therefore devised to prepare a DNA probe that would be HLA-B locus specific and thus permit clear-cut characterization for RFLP of that locus. We report here the preparation and use of such a probe with preliminary results demonstrating the first intragenic DNA restriction endonuclease site specific for an HLA allele.

Materials and Methods

Homology of genomic DNA sequences was determined by a Stanford Blood Center computer program that compares, between two different genes, every set of a preselected, specified number of consecutive bases. Each time a prespecified percentage of the bases within a set match, a dot is printed on a graph in which each axis represents the sequence of one of the two genes. A perfect match (100% homology) between two genes would thus result in a line of dots running at 45°; non-homologous stretches would show up as gaps in that line.

To prepare gene fragments, the cloned B7 gene, pHLA-B7 [5, 6], was sequentially digested with restriction enzymes. The resulting fragments were electrophoretically separated and purified from 0.75% low gelling temperature agarose (FMC Corp., Rockland, Me.). For use as probes, the fragments or intact cloned genes were labeled with [^{32}P]dATP and dCTP by nick translation [7].

In addition to the B7 gene, 17 additional cloned class I genes, including HLA-A2, were available (generously provided by S. Weissman, Yale University) from the genomic library of the HLA-A2, B7 homozygous cell line JY [6]. Each is unique, based on restriction enzyme digestion patterns and/or sequencing, and therefore each represents a non-HLA-B gene.

To perform Southern blotting, DNA was extracted from either peripheral blood lymphocytes or lymphoblastoid cell lines [8]. After digestion with restriction enzymes, 10–15 µg of DNA were loaded onto each lane of 0.5% or 0.6% agarose gels and then electrophoresed. Gels were then blotted onto Genatran paper (Plasco, Woburn, Ma.), prehybridized with herring sperm DNA and then hybridized with appropriate ^{32}P-labeled probes [7]. Blots were washed under stringent conditions

Histocompatibility Testing 1984
Edited by E. D. Albert et al.

(2 × SSC at 20 °C × 10 min × 2, then 0.1 × SSC at 65 ° – 68 °C × 60 min × 2, all in 0.1% SDS) and autoradiograms were then prepared. In some experiments dot blots were prepared by directly dotting heat-denatured, cloned genomic DNA onto the Genatran paper and then probing with nick-translated probe as described above.

Results

Initial experiments utilizing pHLA-B7 as a hybridizing probe showed that, even under the most stringent washing conditions, complex banding patterns resulted, consistent with large numbers of homologous class I genes. Even when only 10 – 15 bands appeared, it was likely that some represented superimposition of different class I genes whose fragments were of similar size. In order to obtain a more selective probe, the sequences of the B7 genes and the pHLA 12.4 pseudogene [9] were compared. As seen in Fig. 1, a region of relative nonhomology was identified in and around exon 7 and intron 7 (hence the designation EI7 for the derived fragment). Sequential digestion with *Pvu*III and *Tth*111I followed by electrophoresis isolated EI7 for subsequent labelling with ^{32}P and use as a hybridization probe. An initial test of restricted specificity, obtained by dotting onto Genatran paper each of the 17 non-HLA-B genes from the JY genomic library along with the B7 gene itself as a positive control, showed the EI7 probe hybridized only to the B7 gene.

As seen in the examples shown in Fig. 2, when the EI7 fragment was used to probe Southern blots of different individuals, either one or two (but never more) bands were observed, consistent with B-locus-specific hybridization for this probe. Approximately one-fourth of the restriction enzymes tested yielded polymorphic patterns for the B locus bands (i.e., different size bands in different individuals). Analysis of families, including four with intra-HLA recombinants, showed that in all instances inheritance of polymorphic EI7-detected bands was consistent with cosegregation of the appropriate HLA- B locus marker. Examples of such patterns are shown for an HLA-A/C recombinant family (Fig. 2a) and an HLA-B/Bf recombinant family (Fig. 2b). In the A/C recombinant, the 2.0-kb band cosegregates with the maternal B44 antigen. In the B/Bf recombinant family, the paternal 17.5-kb band cosegregates with the paternal Bw41 of his e haplotype, while the maternal 21-kb band segregates with her B8 (g haplotype). The 27-kb bands found in each of the parents cosegregate appropriately with the other parental haplotypes. In each of these families the recombinant child shows

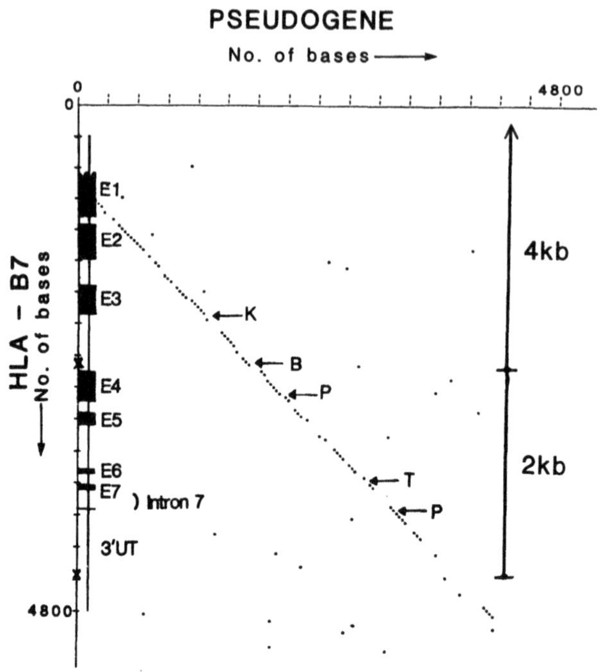

Fig. 1. Computer analysis of homologies between DNA sequences of HLA-B7 (*vertical axis*) and pHLA 12.4 (*horizontal axis*). *Black bars* on the vertical axis represent exons (E1 through E7) and *3′UT* is the 3′ untranslated region. Each *dot* represents a match of ten sequential bases, and the *capital letters* along the line of homology represent restriction enzyme cut sites (*K*, *Kpn*I; *B*, *Bst*NI; *P*, *Pvu*II; *T*, *Tth*111I)

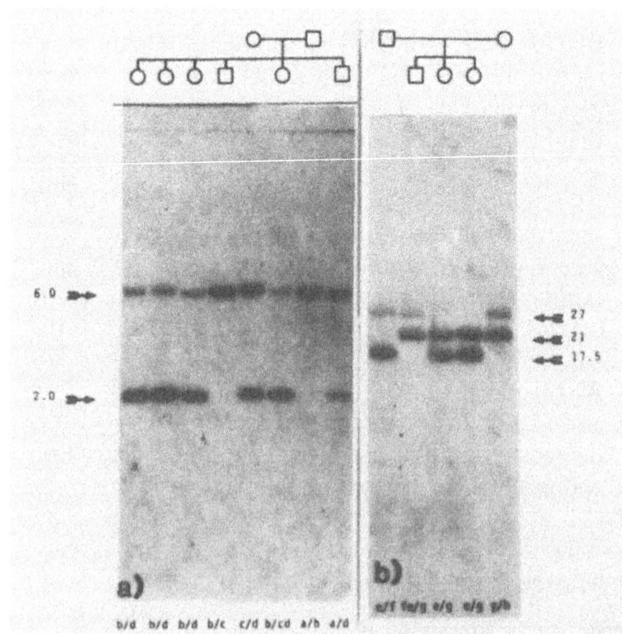

Fig. 2. **a** *Bst*EII RFLPs of HLA-A/C recombinant family DeL. B locus antigens for each haplotype are: *a*, B8; *b*, B18; *c*, B27; *d*, B44; *cd*, B44. **b** *Hin*dIII RFLPs of HLA-B/Bf recombinant family Vas. B locus antigens for the haplotypes are: *e*, B41; *f*, B39; *g*, B8; *h*, B13; *fe*, B39

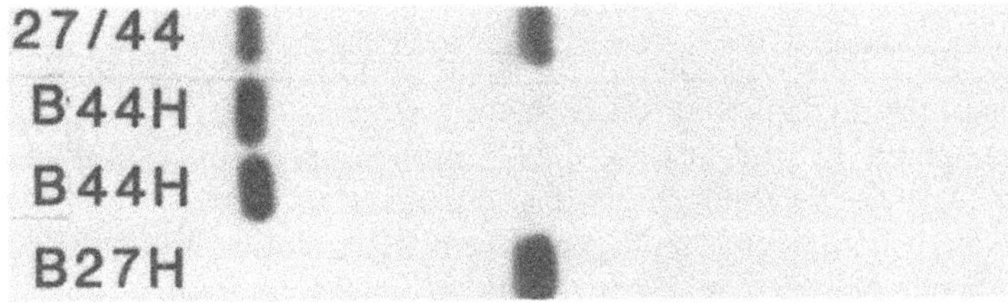

Fig. 3. *Bst*EII RFLPs of B27 and B44 homozygous (*H*) or heterozygous cells. The lower bands (nearest the labels) are 2.0-kb and the upper bands are 6.0-kb

the RFLP pattern expected for cosegregation of the polymorphic band with the appropriate parental B locus gene. From these family data, therefore, the band (i.e., gene) identified by EI7 is localized between HLA-A and Bf as would be expected for a B-locus-specific probe.

Of particular interest were the patterns observed using *Bst*EII. DNA from a total of 30 unrelated individuals, representing 21 different HLA-B antigens including B45, were digested with that enzyme, and Southern blots were probed with the EI7 fragment. Because earlier experiments indicated a correlation between B44 and a 2.0-kb band, the total population of individuals was selected to include 13 different B44 haplotypes (Caucasian and Mexican/American). Complete correlation was observed between the 2.0-kb fragment and B44 ($r = 0.95$). All other B locus genes showed only a 6.0 kb fragment; HLA-B44 homozygous individuals had only the 2.0-kb band and lacked the 6.0-kb band (Fig. 3). Further, using the intact B7 gene as a probe revealed a 4.0-kb fragment found only in B44 individuals. Reprobing with a DNA fragment derived from the fourth intron of the B7 gene (the segment between "K" and "B" along the line of homology depicted in Fig. 1) isolated by sequential digestion with *Kpn*I and *Bst*NI, hybridization was observed with the 6.0-kb band of non-B44 individuals and with the 4.0-kb but not with the 2.0-kb band of B44 individuals. Combined, these data suggest that all B locus genes are flanked by invariant *Bst*EII cut sites 6.0-kb apart, and that the B44 allele contains a unique, intervening, intragenic *Bst*EII site positioned to yield a 2.0-kb plus a 4.0-kb fragment. Although sequence data are not available for any B44 genes, the well-studied B7 gene has a *Bst*EII site in the 3′ untranslated region at position 4475 (the extreme 5′ end of that gene is not yet available for localization of the proposed upstream invariant site). Again in the B7 gene, moving 2-kb upstream a single base change at position 2485 in intron 3 would yield the proper sequence of GGTNACC to permit a *Bst*EII restriction cut site, consistent with the suggestion that the intragenic *Bst*EII site should be located in a highly homologous intron region of the Bw44 gene.

Additional studies have been initiated using the EI7 fragment to seek disease-associated RFLPs. An initial panel of DNA from two ankylosing spondylitis patients, two Reiter's syndrome patients, and two completely normal individuals, all B27+, was digested with different enzymes, run in Southern blots, and probed with EI7 to seek B locus bands that might be uniquely related to disease. Among the enzymes tested thus far, 15 (*Hgi*AI, *Acc*I, *Bcl*I, *Mst*II, *Fok*I, *Tth*111I, *Eco*RI, *Rsa*I, *Pvu*II, *Bss*HII, *Mlu*I, *Nar*I, *Sal*I, *Cla*I, *Bgl*I) revealed no polymorphisms and five (*Bst*EII, HindIII, *Bgl*III, *Eco*RV, *Taq*I) gave polymorphic bands; none showed any bands uniquely disease related.

Discussion

An HLA-B-locus-specific probe, designated EI7, has been produced by identification and isolation of a nonhomologous fragment of the HLA-B7 gene. Greatest nonhomology resides in that part of the probe derived from intron 7, consistent with the phenomenon seen in other multigene families in which intron or flanking sequences can have sufficient divergence to show locus specificity [10, 11]. In this regard the intragenic *Bst*EII site specific for B44 is also of interest. If that site does indeed reside in intron 3, then its correlation with the serologically detectable polymorphic marker of the B44 gene product would be the strongest reported to date between intron and exon allele-specific markers for any single gene [12]. The presence in introns of both locus-specific and allele-specific markers must be taken into account in any consideration of gene evolution or possible intron functions [13].

Finally, the associations of HLA antigens and diseases suggest that HLA RFLPs should be investigated to determine their value as disease markers. Several examples already exist of associations between diseases and RFLPs for genes other than those of the HLA class I family [e.g., 14, 15]. Preliminary evaluation of B locus RFLPs failed to yield any unique markers for spondyloarthropathy; however, more extensive testing will be required before any definitive conclusion can be drawn.

Summary

Study of DNA restriction fragment length polymorphisms (RFLPs) of HLA class I genes has been hampered by the lack of DNA probes specific enough to discriminate among members of this strongly homologous multigene family. By isolating a nonhomologous fragment of the HLA-B7 gene, an HLA-B-locus-specific probe has been derived, and is designated EI7. Use of this probe simplifies class I HLA RFLP patterns and has already revealed a polymorphic, intragenic *Bst*EII site specific for B44. Preliminary studies of spondyloarthropathy patients have not yet shown any correlation between disease and HLA class I RFLP.

References

1. Parham P, Strominger J (1982) Histocompatibility antigens. Structure and function. Receptors and recognition. Series B, vol 14. Chapman and Hall, London
2. Grumet FC (1983) HLA disease associations. Clin Immunol Rev 2:123–155
3. Steinmetz M, Winoto A, Minard K, Hood L (1982) Clusters of genes encoding mouse transplantation antigens. Cell 28:489–498
4. Mahoney RJ, Gazit E, McCarthy-Shanley K, Martin Alosco S, Palomaki GE, Smith ED, Yunis EJ (1982) Alloantisera detect HLA-A-B-C and non-HLA differentiation antigens on human thymocytes. J Immunol 129:2630–2635
5. Barbosa JA, Kamarch ME, Biro A, Weissman SM, Ruddle FH (1982) Identification of human genomic clones encoding the major histocompatibility antigens HLA-A2 and HLA-B7 by DNA-mediated gene transfer. Proc Natl Acad Sci USA 79:6327–6331
6. Biro PA, Reddy VB, Sood A, Periera D, Weissman SM (1981) Isolation and analysis of human major histocompatibility complex genes in recombinant DNA. Proceedings of Third Cleveland Symposium on Macromolecules. Elsevier, Amsterdam, pp 41–49
7. Erlich HA, Stetler D, Sheng-Dong R, Ness D, Grumet FC (1983b) Segregation and mapping analysis of polymorphic HLA class I restriction fragments: detection of a novel fragment. Science 222:72–74
8. Erlich HA, Stetler D, Sakai R, Gladstone P, Pious D (1983a) Mapping of the genes encoding the HLA-DR alpha chain and the HLA-related antigens to a chromosome 6 deletion by using genomic blotting. Proc Natl Acad Sci USA 80:2300–2364
9. Malissen M, Malissen B, Jordan BR (1982) Exon/intron organization and complete nucleotide sequence of an HLA gene. Proc Natl Acad Sci USA 79:893–897
10. Hayashida H, Miyata T (1983) Unusual evolutionary conservation and frequent DNA segment exchange in class I genes of the major histocompatibility complex. Proc Natl Acad Sci USA 80:2671–2675
11. Efstradiatis A, Posakony JW, Maniatis T, Lawn RM, O'Connell C, Spritz RA, DeRiel JK, Forget BG, Weissmann SM, Slighton JL, Blechl AE, Smithies O, Baralle FE, Shoulders CC, Proudfoot NJ (1980) The structure and evolution of the human beta-globin-gene family. Cell 21:653–668
12. Cann HM, Ascanio L, Paul P, Marcaded A, Dausset J, Cohen D (1983) Polymorphic restriction endonuclease fragment segregates and correlates with the gene for HLA-B8. Proc Natl Acad Sci USA 80:1665–1668
13. Cech TR (1983) RNA Splicing: Three themes with variations. Cell 34:713–716
14. Owerbach D, Lernmark A, Platz P, Ryder LP, Rask L, Peterson PA, Ludvigsson J (1983) HLA-D region beta-chain DNA endonuclease fragments differ between HLA-DR identical healthy and insulin-dependent diabetic individuals. Nature 303:815
15. Rotwein PS, Chirgwin J, Province M, Knowler WC, Pettit DJ, Cordell B, Goodman HM, Permutt MA (1983) Polymorphism in the 5′ flanking region of the human insulin gene: A genetic marker for non-insulin-dependent diabetes. N Engl J Med 308:65–71

A Study of HLA-B-Locus Polymorphism with a Specific Hybridization Probe

H.L. Coppin, S.M. Weissman, and H.O. McDevitt

Medical Microbiology Department, Fairchild Building, Stanford University, Stanford, CA 94305, USA

Introduction

The extensive polymorphism among the gene products of the major histocompatibility complex (MHC) is one of the mysteries of mammalian genetics. Serological analysis of human class I gene products has revealed a high degree of genetic polymorphism for the HLA-A, B, and C loci with 10–40 alleles for each locus. However, all these allelic products have considerable overall amino acid sequence homology [1]. At the DNA level, 20 class I genes per haploid genome, including HLA-A, B, C, Tla, and Qa, have been enumerated with a full-length cDNA class I probe [2]. The extensive sequence homology between these different genes has made it difficult to find regions of "A-ness, B-ness, or C-ness" or to correlate alleles with bands on genomic Southern blots. The obtainment of locus and

Histocompatibility Testing 1984
Edited by E. D. Albert et al.

allele specific probes is clearly desirable in order to study polymorphism of the class I genes at the DNA level.

Characterization of a Putative HLA-B-Locus-Specific Probe

To obtain a DNA fragment hybridizing to a subset of class I genes related only to the B locus, a computer dot plot analysis was used to compare the genomic nucleic acid sequences of two different class I genes: JY150, coding for HLA-B7, and a class I pseudogene, pHLA12.4 [3, 4]. A region of weak homology within the 3′ untranslated region of these genes was selected. From this region a *Pvu*II-*Pvu*II fragment of 544 base pairs, JY150/C5, was isolated and its specificity was characterized by Southern blotting.

The specificity of the JY150/C5 fragment was tested by hybridization to three genomic clones containing complete HLA class I genes. Two of these clones coded for HLA-A2 (B3.2) and HLA-B7 (JY150), and the other is of unknown specificity (LN11A). The JY150/C5 probe specifically hybridized to the HLA-B7 genomic clone, but not to the two other clones, under stringent conditions (65 °C, 0.1 × SSC). Southern blots, using the genomic DNA from one heterozygous cell line (MWF : A2, B8,35) and from one homozygous cell line (LBF : A30, B13), allowed a comparison of the hybridization pattern of the JY150/C5 probe with the hybridization pattern of a full-length class I cDNA clone (cDNA-B7). After digestion with *Bam*HI or *Hin*dIII, transfer, and hybridization, the cDNA-B7 probe detected eight to ten bands in each cell line, whereas only one band (*Bam*HI digest) or two bands (*Hin*dIII digest) were detected with JY150/C5 probe. These results showed that the JY150/C5 probe recognizes only a fraction of the class I genes that hybridize with the cDNA-B7 probe. The combination of these two experiments indicates that under stringent conditions the JY150/C5 probe recognizes a small subset of class I genes related to the B locus.

Study of the HLA-B-locus Polymorphism with a Specific Hybridization Probe

To further characterize the specificity of the JY150/C5 probe, its pattern of hybridization was examined on restriction enzyme digested DNA from human B-cell lines. The 10 cell lines used were derived from individuals typed as homozygous-consanguineous for the HLA region. DNA preparations from 8–10 cell lines were digested with four restriction endonucleases: *Eco*RI, *Bgl*II, *Hin*dIII, and *Bst*EII.

After *Eco*RI digestion, two fragments of 8 and 6.5 kb that hybridize with JY150/C5 were observed for ten cell lines tested. In contrast, polymorphism was detected in some cell lines after digestion with the other endonucleases. After *Hin*dIII digestion, two bands of 21 and 27 kb were detected for B7, B14, B17, B27, and B35 alleles. Different patterns were seen for cell lines expressing B16 (24- and 28-kb bands) and B40 (27- and 10-kb bands). After *Bst*EII digestion, a single band of 5.5 kb was observed for all the cell lines tested except those expressing the B7 and B27 alleles which gave an additional band of 1.3 kb. After *Bgl*II digestion, two patterns of hybridization were observed. One showed a single band of 7 kb and was obtained from cell lines expressing the B14, B8, B17, B35, and B40 alleles. The other pattern consisted of two bands of 7 kb and 5.3 kb and was found with cell lines expressing the B7, B13, B16, B18, Bw22, and B27 alleles. No correlation with the two serologically defined antigen families Bw4 and Bw6 could be made with these two subgroups defined by Southern blotting.

There are several points of interest in these results. Firstly, no obvious differences were found in the restriction enzyme fragment patterns of homozygous consanguineous and heterozygous cell lines. Indeed, some cell lines were indistinguishable in their patterns of hybridization after digestion with all four of the restriction enzymes employed. This shows that the flanking region around the B locus has been highly conserved, at least for these sites.

Secondly, the JY150/C5 probe hybridizes with two different DNA fragments obtained from homozygous consanguineous cell lines. Thus, in addition to the B-locus gene, a second gene or pseudogene sharing a homologous sequence with the JY150/C5 probe is present in the genome. It has been hypothesized that the class I multigene family could have arisen from the duplication of one ancestor gene and that the allelic polymorphism could have been generated later by mutation or gene conversion mechanisms. One explanation for the presence of these two homologous sequences is that a duplication at the B locus has occurred, generating a new B-locus-like gene or pseudogene. Similar phenomena have already been observed for the mouse class I gene family [5].

Our results indicate that probes of restricted specificity may be derived from the 3′-untranslated region of class I genes, where homology between members of this multigene family is low. Single or low copy probes will be useful to study the class I gene polymorphism and the association between HLA and diseases.

References

1. Kimball ES, Coligan JE (1983) Structure of class I major histocompatibility antigens. Top Mol Immunol 9:1–62
2. Orr HT, Buck FH, Ploegh HL, Strominger JL, Kavathas P, De Mars R (1982) Use of HLA loss mutants to analyse the structure of the MHC. Nature 296:454–459
3. Barbarosa JA, Kamark ME, Biro PA, Weissman SM, Ruddle FH (1982) Identification of human genomic clones coding for the major histocompatibility antigens HLA-A2 and HLA-B7 by DNA mediated gene transfer. Proc Natl Acad Sci USA 79:6237–6331
4. Malissen M, Malissen B, Jordan BR (1982) Exon-intron organisation and complete nucleotide sequence of an HLA gene. Proc Natl Acad Sci USA 79:893–897
5. Steinmetz M, Winoto A, Minard K, Hood L (1982) Cluster of genes encoding mouse transplantation antigens. Cell 28:489–498

HLA Gene Polymorphism: Class I

D. Cohen, I. Legall, M.P. Font, A. Marcadet, C. Massart, J. M. Lalouel, and J. Dausset

INSERM U93, Hôpital Saint Louis, 75010 Paris, France

Restriction fragment length polymorphism was analyzed in 92 independent chromosomes. For this purpose, DNA samples from 23 families were digested with five restriction enzymes: *Eco*RI, *Eco*RV, *Bam*HI, *Hin*dIII, and *Pvu*II. More than 60 restriction fragments, variable in the population, were detected. Each fragment was assigned to the corresponding parental haplotype in almost all cases (99%). Each fragment segregates with HLA, and band intensity suggests homozygosity (strong) or heterozygosity (weak).

The data were analyzed by computer. The results can be summarized as follows:

1. More than 50% of the variable fragments correlate (positively or negatively) with HLA-A alleles. Twenty percent of the variable fragments correlate with HLA-B alleles, but less strongly than for the A series, and approximately 10% correlate with HLA-C. About 30% of variable bands do not correlate with serologically defined HLA alleles; some of these occur at low frequencies.
2. Specific clusters of variable restriction fragments correlate positively with alleles HLA-A1, A3, A11, A9 (A23 and A24), and some of the Aw19 subseries (A30, A31, Aw33). Four other clusters found in most haplotypes are defined by negative correlations with HLA-A1, A11, and A9; A3 and A11; A3, A9, and A11; and A9 respectively, but not with the Aw19 subseries. Two HLA-Aw19-negative haplotypes (one with A2 and one with A28) carry these four clusters *and* the Aw19-specific cluster. These observations suggest that Aw19 haplotypes carry more class I gene copies than the other haplotypes. The data for the single HLA-A2 and A28 haplotypes also carrying the Aw19-specific cluster may indicate that these are recombinant haplotypes. This cluster may not originate from the HLA-A region.
3. We note that HLA-A9 (A23 and A24) haplotypes are positively associated with relatively few restriction fragments. This suggests that these haplotypes carry fewer gene copies than the others.

We have used these new MHC markers for:

1. Analysing associations with HLA-associated diseases (see below)
2. HLA genotyping of patients where classical tissue typing was impossible, such as in the bare lymphocyte syndrome
3. Identification of genes isolated from cosmid libraries (see below)

Histocompatibility Testing 1984
Edited by E. D. Albert et al.

HLA Gene Polymorphism: Class II

D. Cohen, M.P. Font, I. Legall, A. Marcadet, C. Massart, J.M. Lalouel, and J. Dausset

INSERM U93, Hôpital Saint Louis, 75010 Paris, France

Restriction fragment length polymorphism was analyzed in 92 independent chromosomes. DNA samples from 23 families were digested with restriction enzymes, as specified below. Various restriction fragments showed variation in these families. Each fragment was assigned to the corresponding parental haplotype according to its segregation. Assignment of restriction fragments to haplotypes was almost complete (99% of haplotypes). Each fragment segregated with HLA, and band intensity suggests homozygosity (strong) or heterozygosity (weak) of haplotypes.

Blots of genomic DNA were hybridized with β-DQ and β-DR (Peterson) cDNA probes and an α-DQ probe (Strominger).

With the β-DQ probe and the four restriction enzymes, 52 variable restriction fragments were detected. We considered β-DQ fragments to be (1) those which were seen with the β-DQ probe but not with the β-DR probe, and (2) those which showed a more intense signal with the former probe. Analysis of β-DQ variable restriction fragments revealed ten groups of these markers, each group clustering with a subset from all the haplotypes studied. Of four restriction fragment clusters, one correlates with HLA-DR3, one with DR4, one with DR5, and one with DR7. Another cluster is associated with the HLA-DQw1 related DR specificities DR1, DR2, DRw6 and DR– (blank). Two other restriction fragment clusters split the DQw1-related cluster. Another cluster is correlated with the DQw3-associated DR specificities DR4 and DR5. In addition, a single restriction fragment correlates with DR3- and DR7, DQw2-associated specificities. Finally, two β-DR clusters correlate with DRw53, one cluster positively associated and one negatively associated with this specificity. It is of interest that another β-DR restriction fragment also correlated positively with DRw52.

With the α-DQ probe, four variable *Hin*dIII restriction fragments were noted. These four fragments behave as alleles in the population. They may define a locus (DR?). One fragment correlates with DR4 and DR7 (DRw53), another with DR3 and DR5 (DRw52), the other two with DR1, DR2, DRw6 and DR–, representing a split of DQw1. This split differs from that found with the β-DQ probe in three ways: (1) by haplotype comparisons, and by different restriction fragment patterns for (2) *Hin*dIII and (3) *Eco*RV. β-DQ, *Hin*dIII fragments do not split DQw1, *Eco*RV fragments do. α-DQ, *Hin*dIII fragments split M1, *Eco*RV fragments are not polymorphic.

Association of Class I and Class II MHC Restriction Fragment Polymorphism with HLA-Related Diseases

D. Cohen, O. Cohen, A. Marcadet, M.P. Font, C. Massart, J. Hors, I. Deschamps, and J. Dausset

INSERM U93, Hôpital Saint Louis, 75010 Paris, France

Three diseases were studied – ankylosing spondylitis (AS), multiple sclerosis (MS), and insulin-dependent diabetes mellitus (IDDM).

1. *AS.* Sixteen HLA-B27+ patients, 16 HLA-B27+ control individuals, and 16 other control individuals who were HLA-B27– were the subjects of this study. The HLA-B7 cDNA clone (Sood et al.) was used to probe cellular DNA from these subjects. A 9.6-kb *Pvu*II fragment occurred more frequently in the patients than in the latter control group but not in the former control group. This fragment occurs in 4% of normal individuals.
2. *MS.* Cellular DNA from 32 patients and 52 control individuals was digested with the restriction enzyme *Eco*RV. A 12.8-kb β-DQ fragment was

Histocompatibility Testing 1984
Edited by E. D. Albert et al.

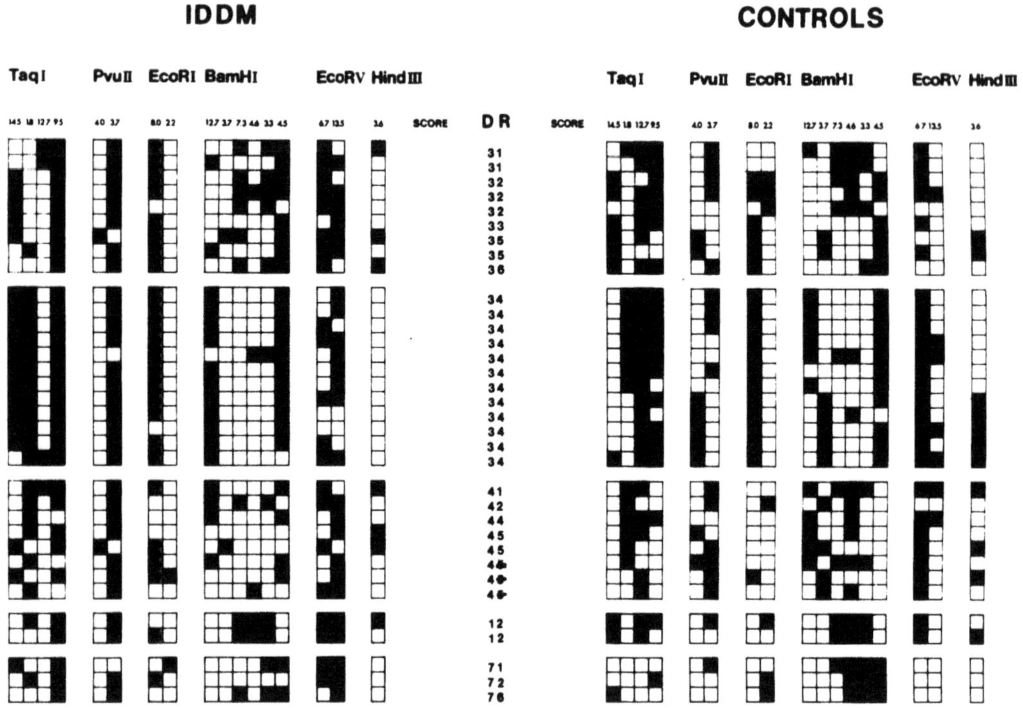

Fig. 1. β-DQ or β-DR restriction enzyme fragment patterns in DR3, 4

found in 22 patients and 26 controls. Among the HLA-DRw6 or DR− (blank) individuals, 12 of 16 controls and none of seven patients carried this fragment, a significant difference.

3. *IDDM.* Thirty-five patients with IDDM were matched for HLA-DR with an equal number of control individuals. Comparison of HLA-DR2 individuals for β-DQ restriction fragments revealed a 2.2-kb *Eco*RV fragment in 14 of 15 controls and in none of seven patients.

Comparison of 12 IDDM and 12 control HLA-DR3, 4 individuals for β-DQ restriction enzyme fragments showed only three patterns of fragments among the patients and seven patterns among controls. The most frequent pattern seen in DNA from 10 of 12 patients consisted of the following fragments: *Taq*I 14.5, 1.8, 6.4 kb; *Pvu*II 3.7 kb; and *Bam*HI 12.0 kb (Fig. 1). This pattern was not generated from cellular DNA of any control individual. The relative risk for IDDM among HLA-DR3, 4 individuals carrying this pattern is over 400, about 10 times higher than the risk using serologically defined DR3, 4 as a marker.

Cloning and Expression of the Gene Encoding HLA-A11

P. Paul[1], B. Sayagh[1], D. Beaud'hui[1], J.J. Metzger[2], M. Pla[1], V. Lepage[1], J.P. Levy[1], L. Degos[1], J. Dausset[1], and D. Cohen[1]

1 INSERM U93, Hôpital Saint Louis, 75010 Paris, France
2 Hôpital Cochin, 75674 Paris, Cedex 14, France

A cosmid library was constructed with DNA from a healthy heterozygous individual (A11, A26, Cw7, Cw−, B38, B51). This library was screened with an HLA class I probe (Weisman et al.). The positive cosmids were digested by *Hin*dIII and probed with the same probe. One of them contained a *Hin*dIII 4.8-kb fragment, previously correlated in a population study with HLA-A11 and A1 ($r = 1$). This gene was transfected in mouse L cells which had been transformed with human β2-microglobulin (P. Kavathas). The transformed cells reacted with monoclonal anti-A11.
Interestingly, this A11 gene is totally included in the 4.8-kb fragment. On the other hand, Jordan et al. have shown that the gene expressing HLA-A3 is also totally included in a *Hin*dIII 5.2-kb fragment. This shows that the polymorphism detected by restriction fragment length polymorphism in these two cases is located outside the genes, since it correlates perfectly ($r = 1$) with the specificities encoded by the gene. This suggests that these two related polymorphisms (extragenic detected by restriction fragment length polymorphisms and intragenic detected serologically) could be derived from the same mutational event, for example gene conversion.

Isolation and Characterization of the cDNA Clones and the Genomic Clones of the HLA Class II Antigen Heavy Chains

H. Inoko[1], A. Ando[1], M. Kimura[1], S. Ogata[2], and K. Tsuji[2]

1 Department of Molecular Biology, School of Medicine, Keio University, 35 Shinamimachi, Shinjukuku, Japan
2 Department of Transplantation, School of Medicine, Tokai University, Kanagawa, Japan

Introduction

The class II HLA antigens, Ia antigens, are essential for cellular recognition and cooperation in immune response [1, 2]. A cluster of genes encoding these class II antigens has been mapped in the HLA-D region of human chromosome 6. Serological as well as cellular reagents allowed the identification of two sets of molecular entities that display a similar function and tissue distribution to HLA-D products. These antigens, named DR and DQ, are composed of two noncovalently associated glycosylated 33 000 dalton α (heavy) and 28 000 dalton β (light) chains. The latter carries the main polymorphic determinants. Recently, another human class II antigen, named DP, has been defined by cellular assay which is encoded in subregions distinct from DR and DQ [3, 4]. DP antigens control a secondary lymphocyte reaction and are encoded in a region centromic to the DR loci. Further, biochemical data and genetic approach with cloned DNA probes provide evidence for several other distinct α and β chains of human Ia molecules [5–9]. However, information on the number of genes encoding α and β chains of DR, DQ, DP, and other Ia antigen(s), regulation of their expression and α-β subunit association, and the extent of allelic polymorphism in each gene is virtually lacking. To clarify these problems we have recently isolated and characterized a number of cDNA and genomic DNA clones for α and β chains of human class II antigens. In this study, we report the isolation and characterization of cDNA clones for the DAα1 chain which presumably corresponds to the DPα chain and for a new class II antigen heavy chain (designated DTα*) and their genomic clones.

Histocompatibility Testing 1984
Edited by E. D. Albert et al.

Results

Several phage clones containing sequences related to the DRα chain were isolated from a human genomic library [10] by plaque hybridization under low-stringent conditions with a cDNA clone for the DRα chain, pDRH2 [11], as a probe. One clone, called λHMC3, was chosen for further analysis. It contained a 2.3 kilobase-pair (kb) *Bgl*II fragment which hybridized to the DRα cDNA at low stringency, but not at high stringency. This DRα-related gene was found to correspond neither to the DRα chain gene nor to the DQα chain gene by Southern blot hybridization and nucleotide sequence analysis (manuscript in preparation) and so was named DAα1 (see Fig. 2). In order to characterize this DAα1 gene, the 2.3-kb *Bgl*II fragment was used as a probe in an attempt to isolate a cDNA clone corresponding to a transcript from the DAα1 gene if present.

A poly $(A)^+$ fraction enriched for the α and β mRNAs through sucrose density centrifugation was used to construct a cDNA library from the consanguineous HLA-homozygous lymphoblastoid cell line AKIBA (HLA-A24, Bw52, DR2, Dw12, DQw1) using the dG · dC homopolymer tailing method. This cDNA library was screened by colony hybridization with a nick-translated 2.3-kb *Bgl*II fragment from the DAα1 genomic clone, λHMC3, under low-stringent conditions, and more than 500 positive clones were obtained from about 3×10^5 clones thus screened. Among them, more than 80 clones gave strong hybridization signals even under high-stringent conditions, and were expected to encode the DAα1 chain. Two clones, pDAα1 − 4 and pDAα1 − 5, among those thus obtained were further analyzed in detail because these overlapping clones together cover an almost full-length cDNA copy of a transcript coding for the DAα1 chain. The size of the cDNA insert was 286 base pairs (bp) for pDAα1 − 5 and 1100 bp for pDAα1 − 4. The restriction mapping and sequence analysis strategy are shown in Fig. 1A, and the complete nucleotide sequence of pDAα1 − 5 and partial nucleotide sequence of pDAα1 − 4 are presented in Fig. 1B. The two clones were identical over the 110 overlapping bases. The pDAα1 − 4 insert encodes the amino acids starting with residue +35, and presumably terminating with the termination codon around nucleotide position 610, if the DAα1 chain is composed of 229 ∼ 232 amino acids as in the case of DRα and DQα [12, 13], followed by a 3′ untranslated region of about 410 nucleotides and a poly-(A) tail of 80 nucleotides. The pDAα1 − 5 insert encodes the amino acids from residue −24 of the signal peptide to +71 of the α1 domain, but lacks the initiation codon.

The amino acid sequence deduced from part of the nucleotide sequence is shown and compared to the DRα and DQα chain sequence in Fig. 2 [12 − 14]. Three sequences can be aligned by matching the first codon of the pDAα1 − 5 insert with amino acid residue −24 of the signal peptide of the DAα1 chain which have the strongest homology, but are clearly distinct from each other. In contrast, the sequence of five amino acids at the N-terminal region is in complete agreement with the limited N-terminal amino acid sequence of the DPα chain determined by Hurley et al. [4] (tyr-9, phe-12, phe-22, phe-24, and phe-26). It can be concluded that the cDNA clone pDAα1 corresponds to the DPα or DP-like α chain.

We have isolated seven overlapping phage clones that can be arranged into a 41-kb length of continuous genomic DNA around the DAα1 gene by successive screening of the human genomic DNA library [10] (Fig. 3). Southern blot hybridization with several Ia molecule cDNA clones such as DRα, DRβ, DQα, DQβ, and DAα1 as probes revealed that a β chain gene, named DAβ, is located 9 kb upstream from the DAα1 gene and a second α chain gene, named DAα2, the DAα1-related gene, is situated a further 7 kb from the DAβ gene. The DAα2 gene hybridized more efficiently to the N-terminal portion of DAα1 cDNA probe than to the C-terminal portion under low-stringent conditions. However, it did not hybridize with either of them at high stringency, suggesting that the DAα1 and DAα2 genes are related, but different from each other at the nucleotide level.

During the course of isolation of the DAα1 cDNA clones, we have isolated cDNA clones specifying a novel class II antigen α chain. This cDNA clone, named pDTα20 *, gave a very weak hybridization signal to DRα, DQα, and DAα1 cDNA probes even under relaxed conditions, implying that pDTα20 represents a new Ia antigen α chain (Fig. 4A). To examine this possibility directly, pDTα20 was subjected to nucleotide sequence analysis (Fig. 4B). The cDNA insert of pDTα20 consists of 490 bp, and the first 150 bp encode the portion of a class II antigen α chain from residue +172 of the α2 domain through the C-terminus (see below), terminating with the TAA and TGA codon. This is followed by a 3′ untranslated region of about 280 nucleotides and a poly(A) tail of 18 nucleotides. Twenty-five bases upstream of the poly(A) tail is the canonical polyadenylation signal ATTAAA. The amino acid sequence predicted from part of the nucleotide sequence is shown and compared to the DRα, DQα, and DAα1 chain sequence in Fig. 4B. Four sequences can be most convincingly aligned by matching the first codon of the pDTα20 insert with amino acid residue +172 of the α2 do-

A

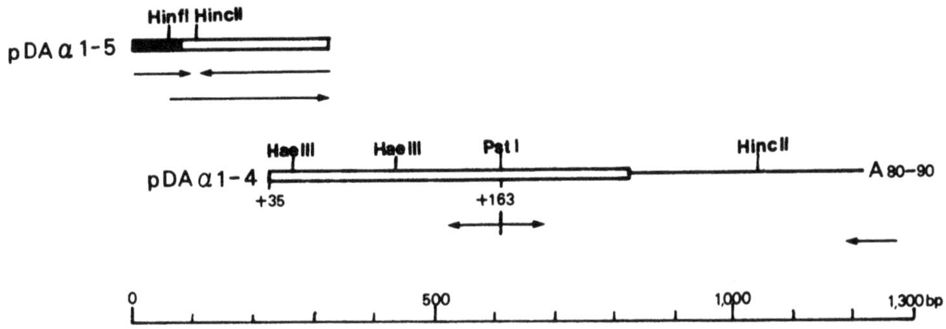

B

```
-24          -20                                -10                               -1  +1
 F   H   I   R   A   V   I   L   R   A   L   S   L   A   F   L   L   S   L   R   G   A   R   A   I
TTC CAT ATC AGA GCT GTG ATC TTG AGA GCC CTC TCC TTG GCT TTC CTG CTG AGT CTC CGA GGA GCT AGA GCC ATC

                             +10                                         +20
 K   A   D   H   V   S   T   Y   A   A   F   V   Q   T   H   R   P   T   G   E   F   M   F   E   F
AAG GCG GAC CAT GTG TCA ACT TAT GCC GCG TTT GTA CAG ACC CAT AGA CCA ACA GGG GAG TTT ATG TTT GAA TTT

             +30                                     +40                                     +50
 D   E   D   E   Q   F   Y   V   D   L   D   K   K   E   T   V   W   H   L   E   E   F   G   R   A
GAT GAA GAT GAG CAG TTC TAT GTG GAT CTG GAT AAA AAG GAG ACC GTC TGG CAT CTG GAG GAG TTT GGC CGA GCC

                             +60                                         +70
 F   S   F   E   A   Q   G   G   L   A   N   I   A   I   L   N   N   N   L   N
TTT TCC TTT GAG GCT CAG GGC GGG CTG GCT AAC ATT GCT ATA TTG AAC AAC AAC TTG AAT A - - - - - - - - -

                             +170                                        +180
 D   C   R   V   E   H   W   G   L   D   Q   P   L   L   K   H   W   E   A   Q   E   P
GAC TGC AGG GTG GAG CAC TGG GGC TTG GAC CAG CCG CTC CTC AAA CAC TGG GAG GCC CAA GAG CCG - - - - - -
```

Fig. 1. A Restriction map and strategy of nucleotide sequence analysis of the pDAα1−4 and pDAα1−5 inserts. *Solid bar* and *open bar* indicate the signal sequence and the coding region, respectively. The *number* below the bar refers to the amino acid number of the mature DR heavy chain [12, 14]. Nucleotide sequence was determined by the chemical degradation procedure of Maxam and Gilbert [18]. **B** The complete nucleotide sequence of the pDAα1−5 insert and partial nucleotide sequence of pDAα1−4 and the predicted amino acid sequence of the DAα1 chain. The 110 bases of the overlapping region between pDAα1−4 and pDAα1−5 are identical

```
        -24     -20                 -10                1                 10                  20
DAα1    F H I R A V I L R A L S L A F L L S L R G A R A|I K A D H V S T Y A A F V Q T H R P T G
DRα     A I S G V P V - G F F I I - V - M - A Q E S W -|- - E E - - I I Q - E - Y L N P D Q S -
DQα                                                    |- V A - S - A QLG V N L Y - S Y G - S -
                          SP

                       30                  40                  50                  60
DAα1    E F M F E F D E D E Q F Y V D L D K K E T V W H L E E F G R A F S F E A Q G G L A N I A
DRα     - - - - D - - G - - I - H - - M A - - - - - - R - - - - - - F A - - - - - - A - - - - -
DQα     Q Y S H - - - G - - E - - - - - - E R - - - - - Q - P L - R - F R R - D P - F A - T - - -
                                            α1

                    70                                     170                   180
DAα1    I L N N N L N - -|- - - - - - - -  D[C]R[V]E[H]W G[L]D Q[P]L L K H[W]|E A Q E P - - - -
DRα     V D K A - - E    |                 -[-]-[-]-[-]- -[-]- E[-]- - - - -[-]|- F D A -
DQα     V - K H - - -    |                 -[-]K[-]-[-]- -[-]- E[-]- - - - -[-]|- P E I -
                                                α2                              CP
```

Fig. 2. Comparison of DA, DR, and DQ heavy chain amino acid sequences. The amino acid sequences of DR and DQ are derived from references 14 and 13 respectively. *SP,* signal peptide; *α1* and *α2,* regions coding for the first and second extracellular domains respectively; *CP,* connecting peptide. The *dash* indicates an identical residue with that of the DAα1 chain. Highly conserved residues in the immunoglobulin-like regions are *boxed* [12, 15]

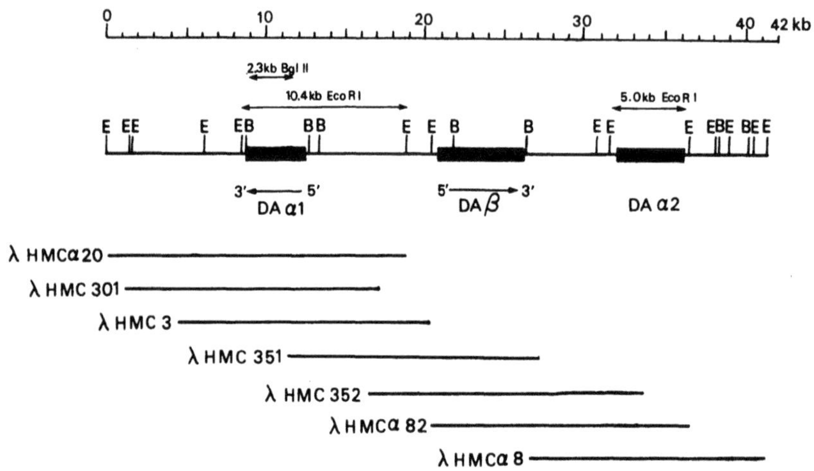

Fig. 3. Molecular map of 41 kb of the DA region defined by seven overlapping phage clones and containing two class II antigen α chains and one β chain. These phage clones were isolated from the human gene library constructed by Lawn et al. [12]. The location and orientation of the class II genes, shown as *blank boxes*, was determined by Southern blot analyses of restriction fragments from the phage clones with the separated 5′- and 3′-end fragments from respective cDNA clones as hybridization probes and also nucleotide sequence analysis. *E, Eco*RI, *B, Bam*HI

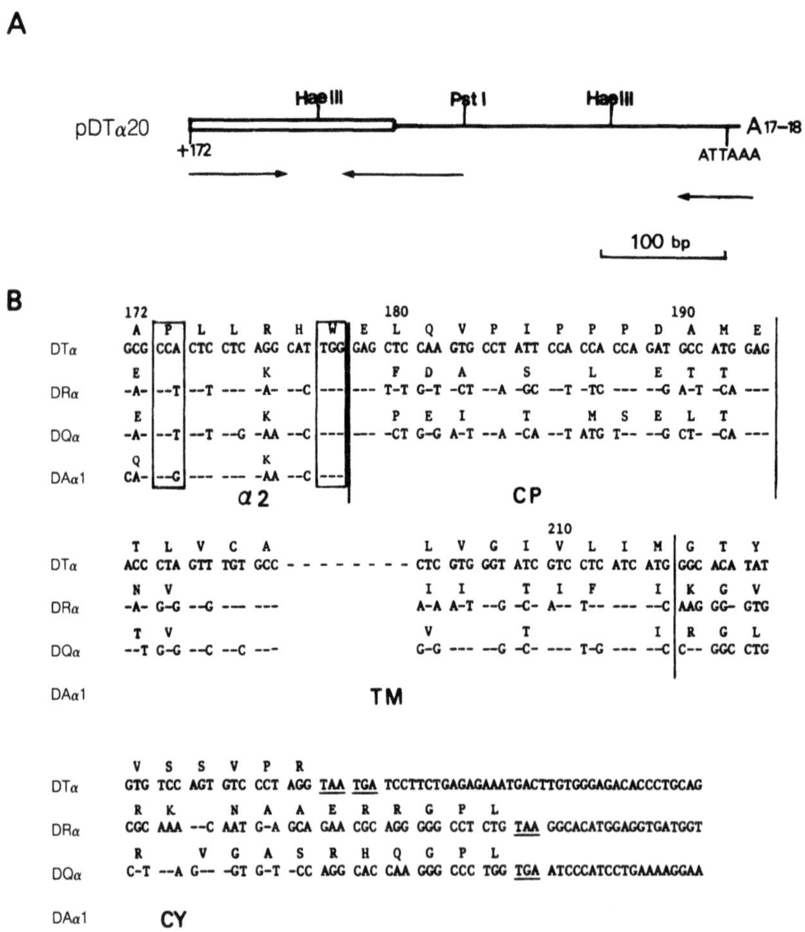

Fig. 4. A Restriction map and strategy of nucleotide sequence analysis of the pDTα20 insert. The *open bar* indicates the coding region. The amino acid number shown by the number below the bar refers to that of the mature DR heavy chain [12, 14]. The nucleotide sequence was determined by the method of Maxam and Gilbert [18]. **B** Part of the nucleotide sequence of the pDTα20 insert and the homologous sequences from the cDNA clones for DRα [14], DQα [13], and DAα1 (this chapter). *α2*, region coding for the second extracellular domain; *CP*, connecting peptide; *TM*, transmembrane region; *CY*, intracytoplasmic region. The dash in the nucleotide sequence indicates no change from the DTα chain sequence. Highly conserved residues in the immunoglobulin-like regions are boxed [12, 15]

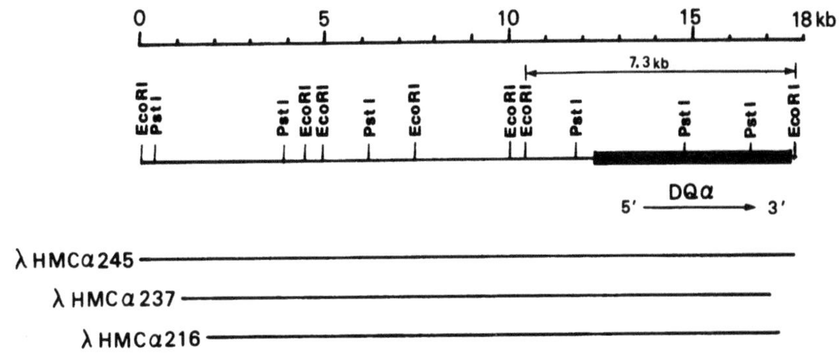

Fig. 5. Molecular map of 18 kb of the DQ region defined by three overlapping clones; for details see legend to Fig. 3

main. From this comparison, it can be concluded that the DTα chain encoded by pDTα20 is completely different from the DRα, DQα, and DAα1 chains and represents a new class II antigen heavy chain. However, the DTα chain bears some characteristic features of the class II antigen α chains. Two amino acid residues (proline-173 and tryptophan-178) which are highly conserved in the α2 domain of DRα, DQα, and DAα [12, 13, 14] and are needed for adoption of an immunoglobulin-like structure [15] are found in the C-terminal region of the α2 domain of DTα. The DTα chain bears a hydrophilic connecting peptide rich in proline, followed by a transmembrane hydrophobic region as in the case of other class II heavy chains. Thus the DTα chain displays remarkable homology with DRα, DQα, and DAα1 in the α2 domain and the transmembrane region, but there is no detectable homology among them in the cytoplasmic region.

Three overlapping phage clones containing a DTα gene were isolated using the pDTα20 insert, and 17.6 kb continuous genomic DNA around the DTα gene was cloned (Fig. 5). The DTα gene was found to be located in a 7.3-kb *Eco*RI fragment by DNA blot analysis. The pDTα20 insert was hybridized to the Southern blot of digested cellular DNAs from a number of homozygous human B-cell lines with different HLA-DR serotypes. When digestion was performed with *Eco*RI, only a single band (about 7.3 kb) to homologous DTα cDNA was detected at high stringency with respect to all of the cell lines (data not shown). This result, together with the simple pattern of bands seen with other restriction endonucleases, is compatible with the existence of a single DTα chain gene and also suggests that the sites around the DTα chain gene are nonpolymorphic as DRα [11], but not as DQα [8].

Discussion

Two kinds of the cDNA clones and genomic clones encoding heavy chains of MHC class II molecules, designated DA and DT, were isolated and characterized. The nucleotide sequence of the C-terminal region of the α2 domain and the connecting peptide region encoded by the pDAα1−4 insert was in complete agreement with that of the corresponding region of the DAα1 gene around the internal *Pst*I site carried by the genomic clone λHMC3, except for one nucleotide (data not shown), suggesting that pDAα1−4 corresponds to a transcript from the DAα1 gene. A comparison of the limited N-terminal amino acid sequence which is encoded by the DAα1 cDNA with that of the DPα chain [4] implied that DAα1 is identical to DPα, but it is possible that the DAα2 gene, a DAα1-like gene, located 20 kb upstream from the DAα1 gene may specify the DPα chain. Further, it appears that the DAβ gene situated between the DAα1 and DAα2 gene represents DPβ. These possibilities are now being tested by characterization of the recently isolated cDNA clones falling in the category of sequences strongly hybridizing with the DAα2 and DAβ genes even at high stringency.

The DTα chain has been demonstrated to be derived from a novel and new HLA class II antigen. Nucleotide sequence analysis shows that the DTα chain is clearly distinguished from DRα, DQα, and DAα1 and represents a fourth isotypic form of a class II antigen heavy chain. We have recently isolated long cDNA clones covering an almost full-length transcript, and determination of their nucleotide sequence is now in progress. It must be noted that genomic blot analyses demonstrate the existence of a single DTα chain gene which has revealed no restriction enzyme polymorphism so far. The genetic and biochemical traits and the function of the DT antigen, together with the problem of what sort of β chain is associated with DTα, remain to be clarified. The number of expressed α chain genes is at least five, i.e., DRα, DQα, DQα-related (unpublished data), DAα1, and DTα. In addition, we have isolated some other possible new α chain cDNA clones. This is in marked contrast with the situation in the mouse, where only two α chain genes have been found in the I region [16, 17].

Summary

A human cDNA library was constructed from partially purified poly(A)$^+$RNA from a consanguineous HLA-homozygous cell line AKIBA (HLA-A24, Bw52, DR2, Dw12, DQw1) using the dG · dC tailing technique. From this cDNA library, cDNA clones encoding the DP- or DP-like α chain and a new HLA class II antigen, named DTα, have been isolated and analyzed by restriction enzyme mapping, Southern blot hybridization, and nucleotide sequence determination. We have also isolated and characterized seven overlapping genomic phage clones spanning 41 kilobase pairs of the DP region which were found to contain one DPα gene, one DP-like α gene, and one β chain gene (presumably DPβ), and three overlapping genomic phage clones encoding the DTα chain gene. Genomic blot analyses with different HLA-DR serotype cell lines indicate the existence of a single DTα chain gene which reveals no restriction enzyme polymorphism.

Acknowledgments. We thank M. Katsuki, K. Tsukamoto, and T. Sasazuki for their valuable discussions and W. Bodmer for generously providing the cDNA clone pDRH2.

References

1. Benacerraf B (1981) Role of MHC gene products in immune regulation. Science 212:1229–1238
2. Schackelfold DA, Kaufman JF, Korman AJ, Strominger J (1982) HLA-DR antigens: structure, separation of subpopulations, gene cloning and function. Immunol Rev 66:133–187
3. Shaw S, DeMars R, Schlossman SF, Smith PL, Lampson LA, Nadler LM (1982) Serological identification of the human secondary B cell antigens: correlations between function, genetics and structure. J Exp Med 156:731–743
4. Hurley CK, Shaw S, Nadler L, Schlossman S, Capro JD (1982) Alpha and beta chains of SB and DR antigens are structurally distinct. J Exp Med 156:1557–1562

* The designations DTα and pDTα20 were substituted by the editors for DQα and pDQα20 chosen by the authors because this would have created confusion with the official WHO nomenclature of DQ for the genes formerly called DC, DS

5. Accolla RS, Gross N, Carrel S, Corte G (1981) Distinct forms of both α and β subunits are present in the human Ia molecular pool. Proc Natl Acad Sci 78:4549–4551
6. Karazin H, Yang C, Gotz H, Pauley E, Korbel S, Egert G, Thinnes FP, Wernet P, Altevogt P, Hilshmann N (1981) Primärstruktur menschlicher Histokompatibilitätsantigen der Klasse II. Hoppe Seylers. Z Physiol Chem 362:1665–1669
7. Goyert SM, Shively JE, Silver J (1982) Biochemical characterization of a second family of human Ia molecules, HLA-DS, equivalent to murine I-A subregion molecules. J Exp Med 156:550–566
8. Trowsdale J, Lee J, Carey J, Grosveld F, Bodmer J, Bodmer W (1983) Sequence related to the HLA-DRα chain on chromosome 6: restriction enzyme polymorphism detected with DCα chain probes. Proc Natl Acad Sci 80:1972–1976
9. Auffray C, Kuo J, DeMars R, Strominger JL (1983) A minimum of four human class II α-chain genes are encoded in the HLA region of chromosome 6. Nature 304: 174–177
10. Lawn RM, Fritsch EF, Parker RC, Blake G, Maniatis T (1978) The isolation and characterization of linked δ- and β-globin genes from a cloned library of human DNA. Cell 15:1157–1174
11. Lee JS, Trowsdale J, Bodmer W (1982) cDNA clones coding for the heavy chain of human HLA-DR antigen. Proc Natl Acad Sci 79:545–549
12. Korman AJ, Auffray C, Schamboeck A, Strominger JL (1982) The amino acid sequence and gene organization of the heavy chain of the HLA-DR antigen: homology to immunoglobulins. Proc Natl Acad Sci 79:6013–6017
13. Auffray C, Korman AJ, Rowx-Dosseto M, Bono R, Strominger JL (1982) cDNA clone for the heavy chain of the human B cell alloantigen DC1: strong sequence homology to the HLA-DR heavy chain. Proc Natl Acad Sci 79:6337–6341
14. Lee JS, Trowsdale J, Travers PJ, Carey J, Grosveld F, Jenkins J, Bodmer WF (1982) Sequence of an HLA-DRα chain cDNA clone and intron-exon organization of the corresponding gene. Nature 299:750–752
15. Orr HT, Lancet D, Robb RJ, Lopez JA, Castro L, Strominger JL (1979) The heavy chain of human histocompatibility antigen HLA-B7 contains an immunoglobulin-like region. Nature 282:266–270
16. Steinmetz M, Minard K, Horvath S, McNicholas J, Srelinger J, Wake C, Long E, Mach B, Hood L (1982) A molecular map of the immune response region from the major histocompatibility complex of the mouse. Nature 300:35–42
17. Steinmetz M, Hood L (1983) Genes of the major histocompatibility complex in mouse and man. Science 222:727–733
18. Maxam ML, Gilbert W (1980) Sequencing end-labelled DNA with base-specific chemical cleavages. Meth Enzymol 65:499–560

DNA Polymorphism of HLA-DRβ and HLA-DPβ Genes

A.K.L. So, J. Trowsdale, J.G. Bodmer, and W.F. Bodmer

Imperial Cancer Research Fund Laboratories, Lincoln's Inn Fields, London WC2A 3PX, UK

Introduction

The existence of at least three sets of cell surface products encoded by the HLA-D region – DR, DQ and DP – has been established by serological, cellular biochemical and molecular studies [for reviews see 1, 2]. The initial definition of DR was based on alloantisera reactive against B cell determinants, which showed extensive polymorphism. Serological and biochemical studies of the cross-reactive determinants detected within the DR series indicated the existence of a second allelic series of cell surface products, DQ (DC or MB), which are in strong linkage disequilibrium with DR alleles. Subsequently, a third series, DP (SB), was defined by primed lymphocyte typing [3], and available biochemical studies show that it is distinct from DR and DQ [4]. A fourth set of products, closely related to DR, has been described [5]. They are probably the antigens recognised by the MT or BR group of apparently cross-reactive sera [6], and are also coded for in the DR subregion.

Molecular cloning of D region genes has resulted in the isolation of both cDNA and genomic clones for α and β chain genes of DR, DQ and DP. Analysis of these clones has revealed an even greater complexity of the region. Thus it is now clear that there are at least six α chain genes [9, 10], and probably seven or more β chain genes [14, 15]. We have used both cDNA and genomic clones as probes to study the restriction fragment length DNA polymorphism of DR β, DP β and other genes in a panel of predominantly homozygous typing cells covering the DR, DQ and DP specificities.

Materials and Methods

The homozygous cell lines studied are mainly derived from EBV transformation of homozygous typing cells [9–11]. Extraction of genomic DNA, restriction enzyme digestion and Southern blotting were as previously described [8, 10].

The probes used were (a) a 530-bp *Pst* fragment of a DR-β cDNA clone pDRβ2 [12] encoding the β2 (membrane proximal), transmembrane and cytoplasmic domains and a part of the 3′ untranslated region of the DR β chain gene, and (b) a 900-bp *Pst*I fragment of a genomic clone covering the first intron and part of the β1 (membrane distal, terminal) exon of the DP β chain [13]. Probes were nick-translated to a specific activity of $> 10^8$ cpm/μg and used for hybridisation at 5×10^5 cpm/ml in standard hybridisation buffer. Filters were then washed at 6 × SSC for 15 min; 2 × SSC for 20 min; and 0.2 × SSC for 45 min, all at 65 °C; and exposed to Kodak XAR-5 film for 3–7 days [9, 10].

Results

The DNA polymorphism associated with the DR β gene was studied using the enzyme *Eco*RI. The resulting restriction band sizes observed with different cell lines are listed in Table 1 according to DR type, and representative band patterns for each type are shown in Fig. 1. A striking observation from this analysis was that cell lines with the same DR type had identical restriction band patterns. Furthermore, the patterns for DR4 and DR7 associated with DRw53 (MT3) were the same, as were those for DR3, DR5 and DRw6 associated with DRw52 (MT2). The two DRw8 cell lines shared a 10.0-kb band which was also seen in the

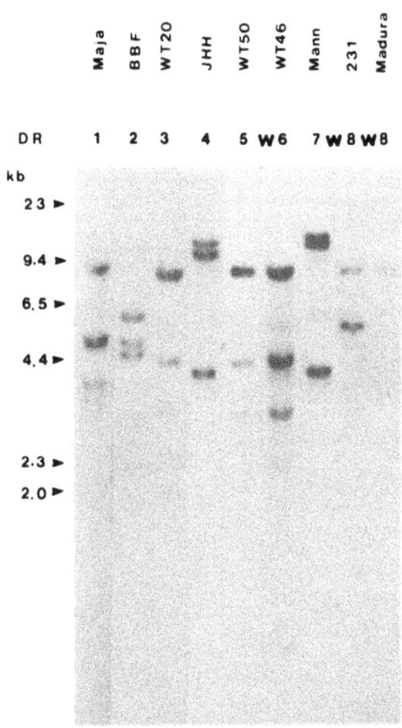

Fig. 1. Southern blot of *Eco*RI digests of cell lines of DR specificities 1–w8, probed with the DR-β probe

Histocompatibility Testing 1984
Edited by E. D. Albert et al.

Table 1. Restriction band sizes (kb) of *Eco*RI digests probed with DR-β

Cell line	DR	15.0	13.0	11.0	10.0	6.5	5.5	5.4	5.0	4.4	4.2	3.2
Maja	1			+			+					
Mette	1			+			+					
IBW4	1			+			+					
MST	2					+		+	+			
WT18	2					+		+	+			
BBF	2					+		+	+			
JHH	4	+	+								+	
1296S	4	+	+								+	
MTF	4	+	+								+	
SJAH	4	+	+								+	
KT2	4	+	+								+	
KT9	4	+	+								+	
KT3	4	+	+								+	
Mann	7	+	+								+	
IBW9	7	+	+								+	
WT20	3				+					+		+
SCTA	3				+					+		+
WT49	3				+					+		+
IDF	5				+					+		+
Baan	5				+					+		+
WT50	5				+					+		+
WVB	w6				+					+		+
Daudi	w6				+					+		+
WT46	w6				+					+		+
WT52	w6				+					+		+
231[a]	w8				+							
Madura	w8				+							
Herluf	w12				+					+		

Filters were washed to high stringency. Some weakly hybridising bands were also seen, but are not listed. The DR-β probe used was a 530-bp *Pst* fragment from the pDRβ2 cDNA clone [12]. + indicates presence, a space absence of the respective band. Note that DR4 and DR7 are included in DRw53 (MT3), while DR3, DR5, and DRw6 are included in DRw52 (MT2).

[a] 231 has in addition a band of 6 kb

Table 2. Restriction band sizes of HindIII digests probed with DR-β

Cell line	DR	8	7	6.5	3.2	3	2.8	2.5	2.3
Mette	1			+		+			
IBW4	1			+		+			
BBF	2				+			+	+
PGF	2				+			+	+
MST	2				+			+	+
WT18	2				+			+	+
JHH	4	+	+			+		+	
1296S	4	+	+			+		+	
Mann	7	+	+			+		+	
IBW9	7	+	+			+		+	
WT49	3						+	+	
WT20	3						+	+	
IDF[a]	5						+	+	
Daudi	w6						+	+	
WT46	w6						+	+	
WT52	w6						+	+	
Madura	w8						+		
231[b]	w8						+		
Koz	w9		+			+		+	

Only strongly hybridising bands are listed

[a] IDF has in addition a 2.6-kb band

[b] 231 has in addition a 1.9-kb band

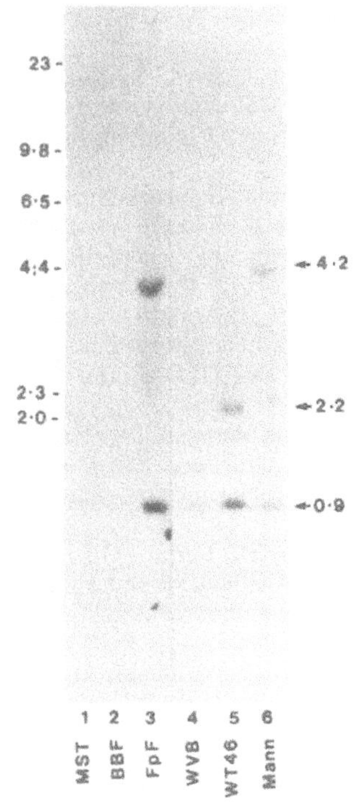

Fig. 2. Southern blot of *Pst* I digests of DNA from cell lines probed with DP-β, showing the 4.2-kb polymorphic band which correlates with the DPw2 phenotype. Blots were washed to stringent conditions (0.2 × SSC, 65 °C). FpF, WVB, WT46 and MANN are DPw2; MST and BBF are DPw4. The very faint bands in the WVB track are due to low DNA concentration

Table 3. Correlation between presence of 4.2-kb band and DPw2

4.2-kb band		+	–
DPw2	+	8	1
	–	0	10

DP typing of homozygous and heterozygous cell lines correlated with presence of a 4.2-kb band on *Pst* digest, probed with DP genomic fragment

other DRw52 (DR3, 5, w6) cell lines. However, LCL 231 had in addition a 6.0-kb band which was not seen in Madura.

The restriction bands seen with *Hin* dIII-digested DNA probed with DR-β are listed in Table 2. Once again, cell lines with the same DR type had the same restriction pattern, and the patterns for DRw53 (DR4, 7) and DRw52 (DR3, 5, w6) were also the same. However Koz (DRw9) lacked the 8.0-kb band present in the other DRw53 cell lines. Similarly, the two DRw8 lines lacked the 2.5-kb band seen with the other DRw52 lines. LCL 231 also differed from Madura in having an additional 1.9-kb band.

The restriction patterns obtained with the DP-β probe were studied using the enzymes *Eco* RI, *Hin* dIII, *Taq* I, *Bam* HI and *Pst* I. Only digestion with *Pst* I showed a polymorphic band, of 4.2 kb, which correlated with the DPw2 type in the cell lines (Fig. 2). A panel of 13 additional DP-typed cell lines (a gift from S. Shaw) was also studied. This confirmed the correlation of the 4.2-kb band with the DP phenotype, with the exception of WT46, which, though typed as DPw2, lacked the 4.2-kb band (Table 3).

Discussion

Studies of DNA polymorphism using cloned probes have already indicated that there is extensive polymorphism of the β chain genes [7, 14, 15]. Using the DR-β probe under stringent conditions, we have shown considerable polymorphism in the restriction fragment sizes, which correlates with the DR serological specificity. Southern blots carried out under varying stringencies and with various probes indicate that, under the conditions used here, the bands seen with the DR-β probe most probably represent DR-β-related sequences, and not cross-hybridising β genes from other loci. The variation in band sizes and numbers is readily accounted for, firstly by polymorphism of restriction enzymes sites in the coding and non-coding regions of the various DR β genes, and secondly by possible variation in the number of DR β genes between different DR types. The results of our experiments are probably mainly explained by the former, although there are some hints from our data (see Tables 1 and 2) of variation in the number of genes in different cell lines. This can only be conclusively demonstrated by comparison of the genomic maps between different haplotypes.

The correlation of the band patterns obtained using the DR-β probe with the DR serological types is consistent with the evidence that the main DR specificities are determined by one of the two or three DR subregion β genes. The fact that the patterns are generally the same within the DRw52 and DRw53 supertypic specificities is also consistent with the evidence that these are determined by one of the DR β genes (see the report on the Ninth Workshop biochemistry exchange by Crumpton et al. in this volume). Though further work is needed to locate the restriction enzyme polymorphic sites precisely, the pattern of band size variation makes it very unlikely that these in general fall within the coding regions determining serological specificity. Thus the patterns of association between DNA polymorphisms and serological specificities are best explained by extreme disequilibrium between variations within and outside the coding regions, as expected for such exceedingly closely linked differences. Similar strong linkage disequilibrium has been previously described between most of the DNA polymorphisms detected using DQα probes and both DR and DQ serological specificities [9]. The detailed patterns of combinations of DNA bands and serological specificities define complex haplotypes which, at least in some cases, subdivide genetically the known serological types. The difference in band pattern, for example, between Herluf (DRw12) and the other DRw52 (DR3, 5 or w6) lines may reflect the fact that monoclonal antibodies to DRw52 do not necessarily react with Herluf. There is, similarly, variation in the association of DRw8 with DRw52.

The DPβ gene showed little DNA polymorphism with the enzymes studied. Only one polymorphism using *Pst*I was detected which correlated with DPw2. This lack of extreme polymorphism, in comparison with that detected using DQ-α, DQ-β and DR-β probes may reflect the fact that the DP genes are less likely to give rise to selectively advantageous variation. Preliminary results suggest similarly that one of the DQ-β genes (DX-β) is less polymorphic than the other (DQ-β).

DNA probes can now be used to identify extensive HLA-D region polymorphism that associates with serological specificities. Inevitably, the data will have to be interpreted in the light of the very high linkage disequilibrium expected between the genes of the various loci in the DR and DQ subregions. It should, however, soon become possible to identify the specific DNA sequences that determine the serological specificities.

These molecular tools greatly extend the potential for studying genetic variation in the HLA region and provide the basis for identifying the DNA sequences that determine disease susceptibility and immune response differences.

Acknowledgments. We should like to thank E. Long for the gift of pDRβ2, S. Shaw for DP (SB) typing of cell lines, and C. Figg and J. Heyes for technical help.

References

1. Bodmer WF, Bodmer JG, Lee J, So A, Spielman R, Travers P, Trowsdale J (1984) Molecular genetics of the HLA-D region. Gorer Symposium. J Immunogenet (in press)
2. Kaufman JF, Auffray C, Kouman AJ, Shackelford DA, Strominger JL (1984) The class II molecules of the human and murine major histocompatibility complex. Cell 36:1–13
3. Shaw J, Kavathas P, Pollack MA, Charmot D, Mawas C (1981) Family studies define a new histocompatibility locus SB, between HLA-DR and GLO. Nature 293: 745–747
4. Shackelford DA, Kaufman JF, Kouman AJ, Strominger JL (1982) HLA-DR antigens: structure, separation of subpopulations. Gene cloning and function. Immunol Rev 66:133–187
5. Tanigaki N, Tosi R, Duquesnoy RJ, Ferrara GB (1983) Three Ia species with different structures and alloantigenic determinants in an HLA-homozygous cell line. J Exp Med 157:231–247
6. Shackelford DA, Strominger JL (1984) Identification of three class II antigens, DR7, MB2, and MT3 from a homozygous human cell line. Hum Immunol 9:159–174
7. Wake CT, Long EO, Mach B (1982) Allelic polymorphism and complexity of the genes for HLA-DRβ chains. Nature 300:372–374
8. Southern EM (1975) Detection of specific sequences among DNA fragments separated by gel electrophoresis. J Mol Biol 98:503–517
9. Spielman R, Lee J, Bodmer WF, Bodmer J, Trowsdale J (1984) Six HLA-D region α chain genes on human chromosome 6. Proc Natl Acad Sci USA 81:3461–3465
10. Trowsdale J, Lee J, Carey J, Grosveld F, Bodmer J, Bodmer WF (1983) Sequences related to HLA-DRα chains on human chromosome 6. Proc Natl Acad Sci USA 80: 1972–1976
11. de Kretser TA, Crumpton MJ, Bodmer JG, Bodmer WF (1982) Two-dimensional gel analysis of the polypeptides precipitated by a polymorphic HLA-DR1, 2 and w6 monoclonal antibody. Eur J Immunol 12:600–606
12. Long EO, Wake CT, Strubin M, Gross N, Aciolla R, Carrel S, Mach B (1982) Isolation of distinct cDNA clones encoding HLA-DRβ chains by use of an expression assay. Proc Natl Acad Sci USA 79:7465–7469
13. Trowsdale J, Kelly A, Lee J, Carson S, Austin P, Travers P (1984) A linkage map of two SBα and β related genes. Cell 38:241–249
14. Owerbach D, Lernmark A, Rask L, Peterson PA, Platz P, Svejgaard A (1983) Detection of HLA-D/DR-related DNA polymorphism in HLA-D homozygous typing cells. Proc Natl Acad Sci USA 80:3758–3761
15. Bodmer WF, Bodmer J, Lee J, Spielman R, Travers P, Trowsdale J (1984) Structure, evolution and polymorphism of the HLA-D region. Immunogenetics – its application to clinical medicine. Academic, London (in press)

Molecular Complexity of the HLA-DR, DQ, and DP Genes and Genotypic Split of HLA-DR Serological Specificities by "DNA Typing"*

C. de Préval, J. Gorski, and B. Mach

Department of Microbiology, University of Geneva School of Medicine, 64, Avenue de la Roseraie, 1205 Geneva, Switzerland

Introduction

Class II or Ia antigens encoded within the D region of the major histocompatibility complex are composed of two transmembrane glycoproteins, the α chain (35 kd) and the β chain (29 kd). They are expressed on macrophages, certain lymphocytes, and some epithelial cells. The Ia molecules are characterized by extensive allelic polymorphism, which is responsible for the self-restriction of cell–cell interactions within the immune system. In the human MHC, several biochemically distinct groups of polymorphic class II antigens have been described: HLA-DR [1], DQ (DC) [2], and DP (SB) [3]. The functional properties of HLA class II molecules map in the D region of this complex. Several lines of evidence suggest that the biochemically defined surface antigens HLA-DR, DQ, and DP might be responsible for the functional properties of the D region [4, 5]. Our laboratory has exploited the methodology of gene cloning to isolate, identify, and study the genes coding for human class II antigens. We have concentrated on the study of β chain genes, which, in the case of HLA-DR, form the polymorphic component of greatest importance. The initial steps of that study have led to the cloning of HLA-DR and DQ β chain cDNA [6] and to the determination of the DNA sequence of a DR β chain cDNA [7]. These cDNA clones have then been used to identify the genomic genes for the HLA-DR, DQ, and DP β chains.

Multiplicity of the Class II Genes in Man and Structural Comparisons

In the haplotype DRw6, evidence for three nonallelic DR β chain genes or three DR β chain loci was obtained on the basis of extensive structural homology [8, 9] (Gorski et al., in preparation). In the case of HLA-DQ, the same structural analysis allowed us to conclude the presence of two DQ β chain loci [9]. Finally, we have identified two nonallelic β chain genes corresponding to HLA-DP [10]. In certain cases, the molecular linkage map has been established, giving us the distance and the orientation of the genes. Evidence was obtained for the existence of one DRα chain gene [11, 12], two DP-like [10], and two DQ-like α chain genes plus another unmapped α chain gene [13]. The combination of these results allows us to tentatively propose the map shown in Fig. 1 for the human D region. The most striking finding was the extent of genetic complexity: Seven β chain genes and six α chain genes. This gene multiplicity may not be fixed and identical in every haplotype, and it is possible that variations in gene number might be found as part of the D region polymorphism.

The identification of probes for class II β chain genes has allowed us to isolate and sequence HLA-DR, DQ, and DP β chain genes from both cDNA and genomic clones. A comparison of DR β chain sequences reveals more than 90% sequence homology over the entire coding and noncoding (3′ UT) regions. The pattern of sequence conservation extends within introns and flanking region, suggesting a fairly recent gene duplication. The sequence diversity among different DR β chain genes is primarily in the exon coding for the first extracellular domain, and clusters of hypervariable amino acid positions can be identified. These hypervariable segments are good candidates for recognition sites by T cell receptors. The 3 DR β chain loci differ in a similar way from alleles of a given DR β locus.

The β chain genes of DR, DQ, and DP differ from one another by about 72%–76% throughout the coding region, are equally related, but are clearly different in the 3′ UT region. The two DQ and the two DP β chain genes differ much more in sequence than the three DR β chain genes. This data allows us to present in Fig. 2 a tentative model for the evolution of β chain gene evolution. Three short DNA segments in the first domain are totally conserved in DR, DQ, and DP β chain genes. Both DP β chain genes have a deletion of six base pairs in the 5′ portion of the first domain. The homology of DR and IE and of DQ and IA β chain genes respectively is maximal in the second domain and is greater than the homology among the genes of different subregions in a given species. This suggests that the genes for IE-DR and IA-DQ result from a duplication that preceded the events which led to human and mouse speciation.

* This work was supported by the Swiss National Foundation. CP was supported by the EMBO

Histocompatibility Testing 1984
Edited by E. D. Albert et al.

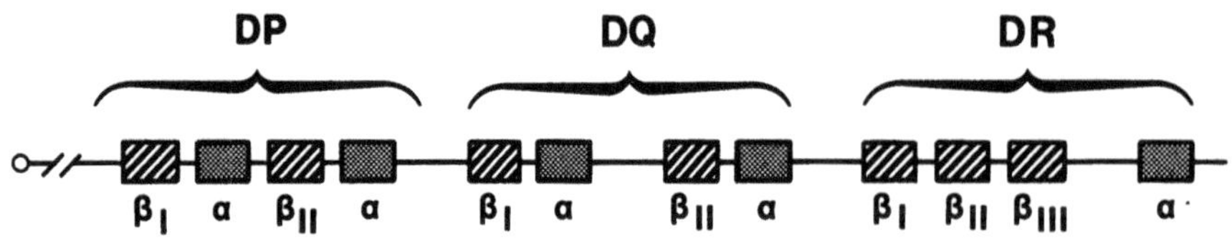

Fig. 1. Schematic representation of the human HLA-D region. A sixth α chain gene cannot be located yet [13]. The relative order of DR and DQ subregions is still tentative

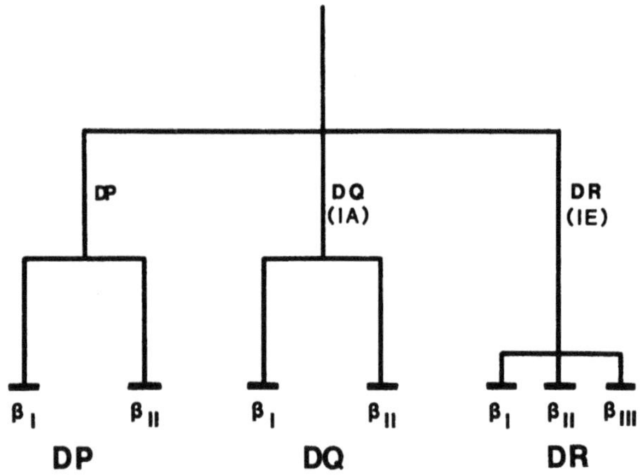

Fig. 2. Schematic representation of the evolution of class II genes

Allelic Polymorphism and DNA Typing

We have previously shown that the structural polymorphism of the HLA DR and DQ β chain genes can be analyzed directly at the DNA level by Southern blot hybridization of restriction enzyme fragments, a procedure we termed DR DNA typing [14]. We have now extended this observation, and at the gross level of restriction site polymorphism have observed a hierarchy of DR β gene polymorphism, the most polymorphic being the DR β chain genes, followed by DQ β [14] and finally DP β [10]. Another report in this workshop presents a detailed analysis of the DR β chain gene allelism and the segregation of DR β chain genes in family studies (G. Angelini et al., Analysis and Segregation of HLA-DR by DNA Typing: Correlation with Supertypic Specificities, this volume; de Préval et al. submitted). We report here evidence for the split of serological specificities at the DNA level. We first studied the DNA of DR2/3 unrelated heterozygous donors. One series of lymphocyte samples collected in Reggio Calabria, Italy, was provided by G. B. Ferrara, and a series of EBV-transformed lines was established in the USA from local donors by S. Shaw [15]. When digested with *Bgl*I, the DNA from the Italian donors presented an extra 4.7-kb band. This result indicates that different human subpopulations possess genomic differences within the D region which are not detected at the serological level. Further family studies are necessary to find out if the extra *Bgl*I band comes from the DR2 or the DR3 haplotype. Furthermore, it was observed that some DR2-specific bands or DR3-specific bands were absent from certain DNA samples after digestion with *Bgl*I and *Eco*RI. This indicates that the genomic polymorphism is larger than the serological polymorphism. This last observation was confirmed when DNA of genetically homozygous DR3/DR3 donors, provided by M. Giphart, was analyzed. With *Bgl*I and *Bam*HI, it was possible to split the DR3 pattern, whereas with *Eco*RI and *Pvu*II, unique DR3 patterns were observed.

Serological and Functional Analysis of a Single DR Molecule

Mouse L cells transformed with HLA-DR genes can express HLA-DR antigen on their membrane [16, 17]. These cells gave us the opportunity to analyze the product of a single gene of the three DR β chain genes, an analysis which by definition cannot be performed with normal DR-positive cells. Such transfected clones will be very useful to study the recognition of Ia antigens by T cells in various contexts. However, mouse L cells do not seem to be the appropriate cells for such studies, as reported by Moen et al. (Mouse L Cells Expressing Human DR Antigens After Transfection with Class II Genes Do Not Stimulate Human Lymphocytes, this volume). Transfection of human cells is in progress to offer an alternative model for functional analysis.

The DR^+-L cells transfected with a DRw6 β chain gene were extensively analyzed with antisera and monoclonal antibodies [16, 17] (Gorski et al., in preparation), including MCS 7 [18]. This latter reagent recognizes a public specificity, Pub-3, on $DRw52^+$ cell lines. It was used by Tanigaki and Tosi to split $DRw52^+$ Ia molecules isolated from DR3 and DR5 cell lines into two groups: DR^+-$DRw52^+$-$Pub3^+$ molecules, and DR^-DRw52^+-$Pub3^-$ molecules, called BR3 [18]. We extended this observation to the DRw6 haplotype. The DR^+-transfected mouse L cells were found to be DRw52 positive and Pub-3 negative; this phenotype indicates that the cloned DRw6 β gene used for transformation codes for a BR3 molecule.

Coordinate Regulation of Human Class II Gene Expression

Class II genes in man constitute a multigene family which are only expressed in certain cell types. Because of these two features, genetic complexity and regulated expression, the mechanisms involved in the control of the expression of this entire region are of special interest. We have described two instances where a coordinate regulation of the entire HLA-D region was documented: induction by interferon, and repression as the result of a trans-acting mutation. (a) Exposure of human monocyte macrophages to interferon results in the induction of the expression of mRNA for HLA-DR, DQ, and DP genes. Furthermore, the gene for the DR-associated invariant chain (which is on another chromosome) is also induced (de Préval et al. submitted). The same observation was made with melanoma and glioma cell lines. (b) Patients with severe combined immune deficiency, a congenital and usually lethal disease, have a defect in the expression of HLA-DR antigen. In collaboration with B. Grospierre and C. Griscelli, we have shown that the defect results from a lack of expression of the HLA-DR genes, accompanied by a similar block of DQ and DP gene expression (B. Grospierre et al., Defect of Gene Expression Responsible for Negative HLA-DR Phenotype of Lymphocytes from Combined Immunodeficiency Patients, this volume). The fact that the mutation maps outside the MHC and that the class II genes are structurally intact (reversions in established lines) suggests a model of regulation of class II genes based on the existence of a class II regulator gene. The nonresponsiveness of the patients' lymphocytes to interferon (M. R. Hadam et al., Defective Expression of HLA-D Region Determinants in Children with Congenital Agammaglobulinaemia and Malabsorption: A New Syndrome, this volume) suggests that the class II regulator gene or its product could be the target for this lymphokine.

Conclusion: Toward a Correlation Between Individual Class II Genes and Antigenic Class II Specificities

In a multigene family, it is not simple to trace the molecular basis of allelism. The available DR β sequences do not yet allow us to recognize the structure of allelic DR β genes from the structure of adjacent genes on a single haplotype. However, it will become easier to understand the class II polymorphism when results of serological typing, Southern blotting, and gene transfection experiments are correlated. As a preliminary contribution to this understanding, the genetic meaning of supertypic specificities can be discussed. Supertypic specificities are defined as antigenic determinants common to several haplotypes. Two interpretations could be given to explain this finding: (1) Supertypic specificities could be attributed to framework determinants common to the products of the three DR β genes (Fig. 1); indeed, nucleotide sequences show that the DR β genes are very closely related and could have appeared upon recent gene duplications (Fig. 2). (2) Supertypic specificities could also be the product of a single locus which exhibits only a limited polymorphism. If so, the few allelic forms of that locus will be found associated with several alleles of the more polymorphic DR β locus. (These two interpretations are not mutually exclusive.) Two of our findings could support the second hypothesis: First, when mouse L cells were transfected with DR genes [16] cloned from a DRw6 haplotype, the Ia antigen expressed was recognized as BR ($DRw52^{+}$, $Pub\text{-}3^{-}$) [17] (Gorski et al., in preparation). This result agrees with the proposal that one of the three DR β gene codes for the BR allelic series, which, so far, is less allelic than the DR series [18]. Second, when DR polymorphism was analyzed at the DNA level by Southern blotting experiments (G. Angelini et al., Analysis and Segregation of HLA-DR by DNA Typing: Correlation with Supertypic Specificities, this volume; de Préval et al., submitted), it became clear that some haplotypes, while differing in certain restriction fragments, do share several other bands. These shared fragments allow the grouping of haplotypes according to the supertypic series DRw52/DRw53 (DR3, 5, w6, 8w13 vs DR4, 7). The conserved patterns of restriction fragments may reflect the existence of one or two DR β loci with limited polymorphism; the more variable DNA bands would then represent restriction fragments from one or two more polymorphic DR β chain loci.

References

1. Springer TA, Kaufman JF, Terhorst C, Strominger JL (1977) Purification and structural characterization of human HLA linked B cell antigens. Nature 268:213–218
2. Shackelford DA, Mann DL, van Rood JJ, Ferrara GB, Strominger JL (1981) Human B-cell alloantigens DC 1, MT 1, and LB 12 are identical to each other but distinct from the HLA-DR antigen. Proc Natl Acad Sci USA 78: 4566–4570

3. Shaw S, Kavathas P, Pollack MS, Charmot D, Mawas C (1981) Family studies define a new histocompatibility locus, SB, between HLA-DR and *glo*. Nature 239:745–747
4. Thorsby E, Berle B, Nouisainen H (1982) HLA-D region molecules restrict proliferative T-cell responses to antigens. Immunol Rev 66:39–56
5. Shaw S, DeMars R, Schlossman SF, Smith PL, Lampson LA, Nadler LM (1982) Serological identification of the human secondary B cell antigens. Correlation between function, genetics and structure. J Exp Med 156:731–741
6. Long EO, Wake CT, Strubin M, Gross N, Accolla RS, Carrel S, Mach B (1982) Isolation of distinct cDNA clones encoding HLA-DR β chains by use of an expression assay. Proc Natl Acad Sci USA 79:7465–7469
7. Long EO, Wake CT, Gorski J, Mach B (1983) Complete sequence of an HLA-DR β chain deduced from a cDNA clone and identification of multiple non-allelic DR β chain genes. EMBO J 2:389–394
8. Long EO, Gorski J, Rollini P, Wake CT, Strubin M, Rabourdin-Combe C, Mach B (1983) Molecular analysis of the genes for human class II antigens of the major histocompatibility complex. Hum Immunol 8:113–121
9. Gorski J, Rollini P, Kawashima E, Long EO, Mach B (1984) Regulation of the Immune System. In: Sercaz E, Cantor H, Chess L (eds) UCLA symposia on molecular and cellular biology, new series, vol 18. Liss, New York (in press)
10. Gorski J, Rollini P, Long EO, Mach B (1984) Molecular organization of the HLA-SB region of the human major histocompatibility complex and evidence for two SB β chain genes. Proc Natl Acad Sci USA 81:3934–3938
11. Lee JS, Trowsdale J, Bodmer WF (1982) cDNA clones coding for the heavy chain of human HLA-DR antigen. Proc Natl Acad Sci USA 79:545–549
12. Wake CT, Long EO, Strubin M, Gross N, Accolla RS, Carrel S, Mach B (1982) Isolation of cDNA clones encoding HLA-DR α chains. Proc Natl Acad Sci USA 79:6979–6983
13. Auffray C, Lillie JW, Arnot D, Grossberger D, Kappes D, Strominger JL (1984) Isotypic and allotypic variation of human class II histocompatibility antigen α-chain genes. Nature 308:327–333
14. Wake CT, Long EO, Mach B (1982) Allelic polymorphism and complexity of the genes for HLA-DR β-chains-direct analysis by DNA-DNA hybridization. Nature 300:372–374
15. Shaw S, Johnson AH, Shearer GM (1980) Evidence for a new segregant series of B cell antigens that are encoded in the HLA-D region and that stimulate secondary allogeneic proliferative and cytotoxic responses. J Exp Med 152:565–580
16. Rabourdin-Combe C, Mach B (1983) Expression of HLA-DR antigens at the surface of mouse L cells cotransfected with cloned human genes. Nature 303: 670–674
17. de Préval C, Rabourdin-Combe C, Gorski J, Mach B (1984) Expression of a single HLA-DR antigen on DNA transfected mouse cells: analysis by a panel of monoclonal antibodies. In: Disease markers, vol 2, special issue: Human MHC class II antigens; genetics, structure, and function. Wiley, New York 207–221
18. Tanigaki N, Tosi R (1982) The genetic control of human Ia alloantigens: a three-loci model derived from the immunochemical analysis of "supertypic" specificities. Immunol Rev 66:5–37

HLA Class II Polymorphism: Restriction Fragment Patterns Correlated to Ninth Workshop Serology and Function

J. Wallin[1], J. Böhme[2], B. Carlsson[1], E. Möller[1], P.A. Peterson[2], and L. Rask[3]

1 Department of Clinical Immunology, Huddinge University Hospital, Karolinska Institute, Stockholm, Sweden
2 Department of Cell Research, Wallenberg Laboratory, Uppsala University, Uppsala, Sweden
3 Swedish University for Agricultural Sciences

Introduction

Recent studies have vastly expanded our knowledge of MHC gene organization and structure [for review see 6, 7, 13]. The HLA class II gene map is presently thought to contain at least three DRβ, one DRα, two DQβ, two DQα, two DPβ, and two DPα genes. Serological studies indicate at least four distinct class II antigens: DR, supertypic DR (DRw52, w53), DQ and DP [12; for review see 10]. It is now possible to isolate HLA class II cDNA and genomic clones with recombinant DNA techniques. With the use of cDNA specific for DRβ, DQβ, and DQα and a genomic clone corresponding to an DPβ chain first domain as probes in genomic hybridizations, we have investigated the class II gene polymorphism. The cDNA and genomic clones used as probes are described elsewhere for DRβ [1], DQβ [8], DQα [3], and DPβ (K. Gustafsson, unpublished results). As the HLA glycoproteins retain their antigenic specificities even in the absence of carbohydrate moieties [11], it can be expected that all biologically relevant polymorphism can be detected at the DNA level.

Histocompatibility Testing 1984
Edited by E. D. Albert et al.

DRβ and DQβ Polymorphism

Southern blotting analyses with DRβ and DQβ probes have previously been shown to discriminate between homozygous typing cells (HTCs) with specificities Dw1–8 [1]. Hybridization with DRβ and DQβ probes to genomic DNA digested with *Bam*HI or *Pvu*II gives rise to 15–30 bands in the population. A marked extent of cross-hybridizations can be found between the probes under the stringency conditions adopted. Allele-specific bands can only be assigned to DR1, 2, and 4, while the other specificities can be determined by a certain combination of bands where each band can be common to several alleles. These complex sets of bands make the interpretation of restriction fragment length polymorphisms (RFLPs) from heterozygous cells difficult, but it remains feasible. When comparing the number of bands detected with a DRβ probe in different alleles, clear discrepancies are found which may indicate different numbers of genes corresponding to specific DR alleles. Whether these disparities are also expressed at the cell surface level is not known.

We have employed this method to analyze genomic DNA in lymphocytes from a panel of 43 healthy donors. These cells were also typed with Ninth Workshop antisera. When grouping the cells for DR identity, the RFLP diversity within the groups is very limited with both DRβ and DQβ probes (Fig. 1), indicating that genetic polymorphism detected in this assay is closely correlated to serology and that the DRβ and DQβ loci are situated close to each other. The linkage disequilibrium is in fact so strong that it is possible to "type" for DR with a DQβ probe, this phenomenon also being due in part to cross-hybridizations.

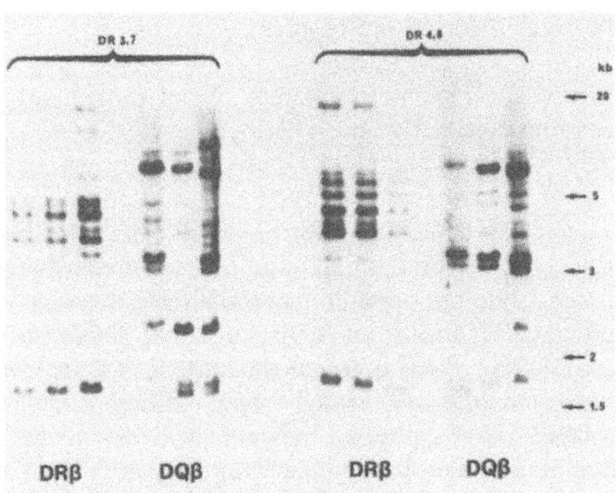

Fig. 1. Linkage between DRβ and DQβ probe hybridization patterns shown in three unrelated DR3, 7-typed individuals and three unrelated DR4, w8-typed individuals

When considering the potential of this type of study for revealing relevant polymorphism, one must bear in mind that the restriction enzymes used are estimated to recognize sequences approximately every 4 kb. Considering that a class II gene including introns is roughly 7 kb long (the figure varies owing to variable intron sizes) and that the expressed parts of it account for around 10%, it is obvious that a few restriction enzymes cannot detect all the expressed polymorphic sites. The strong correlation between RFLP and serology in spite of these conditions establishes that intron and flanking sequences are well conserved with the alleles. Although we register only a few disparities between serologically identical individuals, it can be expected that additional relevant information can be disclosed if restriction enzymes and new probes are used optimally. It is plausible that application of intron-specific probes, which are apparently locus specific, e.g., distinguish between two different DRβ genes, may be informative.

Thus, it can be concluded that Southern blotting analyses can be used in tissue typing. However, at present the methods are too time-consuming to equal serological test systems as a method of choice. Nevertheless, these tests will be useful in cases when conventional typing is hard to perform, e.g., in testing cells with a low molecular density of cell surface Ia molecules.

With regard to RFLP, some DR alleles resemble each other more than DR alleles do in general. This is true for DR4 and 7 and for DR3, 5, and w6, and may reflect the mechanism of generation of diversity in the MHC proposed to be events of gene duplication and gene conversion. A conceivable interpretation of these findings is that all alleles have emerged from one primordial gene sequence, and that the similarity with regard to RFLP detected between these specificities is a result of more recent diversifications.

DQα Polymorphism

Hybridizations with a DQα probe to *Bam*HI- and *Pvu*II-digested genomic DNA reveal a limited picture of polymorphism. Only four distinct bands are detected in the population with *Pvu*II. Also with this probe, we find a correlation to DR serology, which could be expected considering the strong linkage between DR and DQ specificities.

Restriction Fragment Patterns Related to DRw52, w53 and DQ Specificities

An examination of the material to find associations between RFLP and the "supertypic" specificities

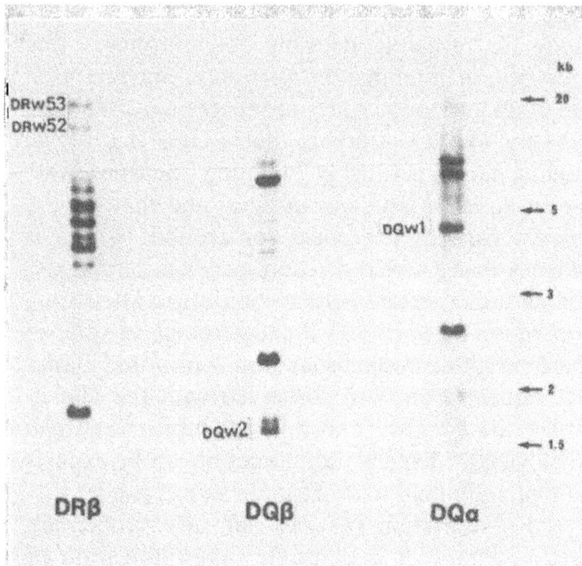

Fig. 2. DRw52, w53 and DQ specificities detected with DRβ, DQβ, and DQα probes separately hybridized to *Pvu*II-digested genomic DNA

Table 1. Chi-square analysis of association between serological specificities and certain *Pvu*II restriction fragments

Serological type	cDNA probe used	Fragment length (kb)	Significance level
DQw1	DQα	4.5	$p<0.001$
DRw52	DRβ	11	$p<0.01$
DRw53	DRβ	14	$p<0.001$
DQw2	DQβ	1.6	$p<0.001$

DRw52, w53 and DQ revealed specific bands which were significantly correlated to DQw1, DRw52 and DRw53 and DQw2 (Table 1). In *Pvu*II digestions the DRβ probe detects two bands, 11 and 14 kb in size, which parallel the serological presence of DRw52 and DRw53 respectively. With the DQβ probe a 1.6-kb *Pvu*II band correlating to DQw2 is found, and the DQw1 specificity is detected with the DQα probe as a 4.5-kb *Pvu*II band (Fig. 2).

A correlation between band patterns obtained with *Hin*dIII and a DQα probe and DQw1, DRw52 and DRw53 has been published [2]. Two antisera with specificity for DQα chains were recently described to be inhibited by cells from DR3-positive, DR5-positive, and 8w13-positive individuals, thus defining a specificity included in the DRw52 reactivity pattern. Interestingly, specific reactivity to these two antisera correlated to the presence of a 7-kb *Hin*dIII band [16]. Moreover, a comparison of nucleotide sequences of cDNA clones obtained from Dw4 and Dw7 HTCs shows a striking sequence homology to each other compared to the extent they resemble DQα sequences in general (the DQα cDNA clone derived from the Dw7 HTC has been described by Chang et al. [4]). These data agree in part with our results, e.g., regarding the DQw1 band, but contrast with our findings that the DRw52- and DRw53-associated bands are specifically detected with the DRβ probe, displaying no cross-hybridization. The reason for association of DQw1, DRw52 and DRw53 types to both DQα- and DRβ-specific bands remains to be elucidated. Interpretation of these results may be highly facilitated by the identification of genomic cosmid clones with overlapping sequences, thus achieving mapping of the entire distance between DR and DQ.

DPβ Polymorphism

RFLPs obtained with the DPβ probe show less polymorphism than the other β chain probes. The limited variability detected may be due to the facts that the DP genes are located close to each other, hence accompanied by limited flanking sequence polymorphism, and that thorough use of different restriction enzymes can better distinguish between allelic forms. Analysis of clusters of Dw3- and Dw4-positive HTCs showed that the DRβ and DQβ patterns were very similar, but the DPβ-derived pattern showed dissimilarities that were as extensive within the clusters as between them. This argues in favor of the finding that DP alleles occur only in limited linkage disequilibrium with DR and DQ alleles [14], and indicates that the DP genes are located at some distance from DR and DQ.

DR "x,x" Restriction Fragment Patterns

In order to elucidate the extent of polymorphism yet to be detected in the DR locus, we have also analyzed approximately 20 individuals to whom none of the antigens DR1 – w8 and w10 could be assigned consequently referred to as DR "x,x". Both DNA hybridization studies and extensive serology were performed on material from these individuals. Hybridization with DRβ and DQβ on *Bam*HI- and *Pvu*II-digested genomic DNA from these individuals revealed some entirely new RFLPs. These patterns indicate at least three "new" DR alleles. Some "new" patterns were, however, present several times when all samples were analyzed, and formed groups with similar RFLPs (Fig. 3). This probably reflects a limited number of new alleles among these cells and a maximum

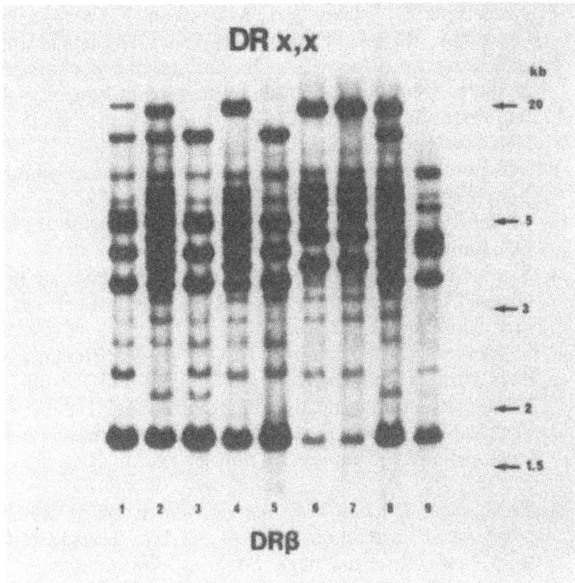

Fig. 3. Hybridization patterns in individuals serologically typed as DR "x,x" detected with a DRβ probe

Table 2. One-way MLC between unrelated individuals typed as DR2, 5

	AF*	SN*	HN*	LR*
AF		107	129	46
SN	63		55	49
HN	45	28		60
LR	61	300	178	

Results expressed as percent relative response against fully incompatible cells
* Stimulator

number of DR alleles of about 15. Among these individuals, several had a distinct 5.4-kb *Bam*HI band with both DRβ and DQβ probes significantly associated with DR4. When reanalyzed serologically with Ninth Workshop antisera, all these cells displayed a weak reactivity with DR4 antisera, but serological patterns were not sufficient for a definite assignment.

Mapping of Loci

In our analyses of families with diabetic members and the studies of HLA-identical sibs (donor-recipient pairs) in clinical transplantations we have searched for evidence of DR/DQ recombinations. The 14 diabetic families studied showed none, but the transplantation pairs revealed one possible recombination between DRβ and DQβ in a HLA-A, B, C, DR-identical pair of sibs. This would locate the DQ locus centromeric to the DR locus, in agreement with the findings of De Mars et al. in chromosomal loss mutant cells [5], but in contradiction to an earlier family published by van Leeuwen et al. [9].

Functional Aspects

In order to elucidate the predictive value of RFLP studies in functional terms we have performed MLC and PLT tests between individuals with identical RFLPs obtained with DRβ and DQβ probes. These combinations were also serologically HLA-DR identical. As stated, the genetic polymorphism detected in this assay is well correlated to serology. As expected, we found that this method cannot predict MLC non-reactivity between unrelated individuals (Table 2). Whether these results can be explained by HLA class II molecules other than DRβ and DQβ acting as MLC-stimulating determinants or by relevant polymorphism that has not yet been detected residing in these loci is not understood. Our material has not yet been evaluated with a DPβ probe, but cellular typing for DP has only yielded marginal additional information [15]. In this context, we conclude that genomic hybridization with present assay conditions do not add information to serologic analyses when selecting recipients for necro-kidney transplantations. On the other hand, RFLP analysis can give additional information in investigations of intrafamilial transplantations. As demonstrated by Carlsson et al. (HLA-DR and DQ Studied with Genomic Blotting in Diabetic Families and Transplant Donor-Recipient Pairs; this volume), it has been informative in bone marrow transplantation.

Conclusions

Southern blotting used for the detection of HLA class II polymorphism has already proven very useful. We want to stress that so far the theoretical possibilities of these experiments have been exploited to only a limited extent. The main possible applications are:
- As an alternative to tissue typing
- In definition of new alleles
- As a tool to explore the functional properties of different HLA class II molecules
- In determination of the origin of cells not expressing class II antigens
- In studies of association between HLA and disease
- In obtaining further information on the organization and number of class II genes

References

1. Andersson M, Böhme J, Andersson G, Möller E, Thorsby E, Rask L, Peterson PA (in press) Genomic hybridization with class II transplantation antigen cDNA probes as a complementary technique in tissue typing. Hum Immunol
2. Auffray C, Ben-Nun A, Roux-Dosseto M, Germain RN, Seidman JG, Strominger JL (1983) Polymorphism and complexity of the human DC and murine I-A α chain genes. EMBO J 2:121–124
3. Auffray C, Korman AJ, Roux-Dosseto M, Germain RN, Seidman JG, Strominger JL (1982) cDNA clone for the heavy chain of the human B-cell alloantigen DC1: strong sequence homology to the HLA-DR heavy chain. Proc Natl Acad Sci USA 79:6337–6341
4. Chang H-C, Moriuchi T, Silver J (1983) The heavy chain of human B-cell alloantigen HLA-DS has a variable N-terminal region and a constant immunoglobulin-like region. Nature 305:813–815
5. DeMars R, Chang CC, Rudersdorf RA (1983) Dissection of the D-region of the human major histocompatibility complex by means of induced mutations in a lymphoblastoid cell line. Hum Immunol 8:123–140
6. Kaufman JF, Auffray C, Korman AJ, Shackelford DA, Strominger JL (1984) The class II molecules of the human and murine major histocompatibility complex. Cell 36:1–13
7. Larhammar D, Andersson G, Andersson M, Bill P, Böhme J, Claesson L, Denaro M, Emmoth E, Gustafsson K, Hammerling U, Heldin E, Hyldig-Nielsen JJ, Lind P, Schenning L, Servenius B, Widmark E, Rask L, Peterson PA (1983) Molecular analysis of human class II transplantation antigens and their genes. Hum Immunol 8:95–103
8. Larhammar D, Schenning L, Gustafsson K, Wiman K, Claesson L, Rask L, Peterson PA (1982) Complete amino acid sequence of an HLA-DR antigen-like β chain as predicted from the nucleotide sequence similarities with immunoglobulins and HLA-A-B and -C antigens. Proc Natl Acad Sci USA 79:3687–3691
9. Van Leeuwen (1980) In: Terasaki PI (ed) Histocompatibility Testing 1980. UCLA, Los Angeles, pp 853
10. Möller G (ed.) (1982) Structure and function of HLA-DR. Immunol Rev 66
11. Shackelford DA, Strominger JL (1983) Analysis of the oligosaccharides on the HLA-DR and DC1 B-cell antigens. J Immunol 130:274–282
12. Shackelford DA, Strominger JL (1984) Identification of three class II antigens, DR7, MB2, and MT3, from a homozygous human cell line. Hum Immunol 9:159–174
13. Steinmetz M, Hood L (1983) Genes of the major histocompatibility complex in mouse and man. Science 222:727–733
14. Termijtelen A, Khan PM, Shaw S, van Rood JJ (1983) Mapping SB in relation to HLA and GLO1 using cells from first-cousin marriage offspring. Immunogenetics 18:503–512
15. Termijtelen A, Naipal van den Berge S, Suwandi-Thung L, van Rood JJ (1984) The influence of matching for SB on MLC typing is significant but marginal. Scand J Immunol 19:265–268
16. Tosi R, Tanigaki N, Sorrentino R, Centis D, Ferrara GB (1984) Serologically detectable polymorphism of the HLA-DCαsubunit. J Immunol 132:277–282

HLA-DRw6: A Molecular Approach *

M.L. Bosch, M.G.J. Tilanus, and M.J. Giphart

Dept of Immunohematology and Blood Bank, University Medical Center, Rijnsburgerweg 10, 2333 AA Leiden, The Netherlands

An analysis of the genes that make up the DRβ region will extend our information about the complexity of the HLA class II system, since the serologically detectable polymorphism is located mainly on the DRβ chain. Probably this analysis will be most informative if we look at the 5′ ends of the genes coding for the variable stretches of a DRβ chain [1].

One of the serologically detectable HLA-DR specificities is DRw6. There are no monospecific alloantisera for DRw6, and DRw6 is defined by the reactivities of various antisera that have a wide range of reactions and recognize determinants not necessarily located on DR antigens. In this respect, DRw6 is markedly different from the other DR specificities. This difference is underlined by observations on renal transplantation [2, 3]. It has been postulated that DRw6 either induces immunosuppression, both in the mother of a DRw6 positive child and in the recipient of a kidney transplant, or does not express the determinants to which a normal immunoresponse can be mounted.

* This work was supported in part by the Dutch Foundation for Medical Research (FUNGO), which is subsidized by the Dutch Organization for the Advancement of Pure Research (ZWO), and the J. A. Cohen Institute for Radiation Protection (IRS)

Table 1. Southern blot patterns of the various DR specificities

RE	*Kpn* I	*Pst* I	*Pvu* II	*Bgl* II	*Eco* RI	*Bam* HI
Non-DRw6	qi	rstuvwyz	x	bcd	efhlmo	a
DRw6	q	r	x	b	N	aa'

If this last assumption is true we would expect to find a molecular basis for it at the DNA level. We studied the DNA of 19 B lymphoblastoid cell lines homozygous for DRw6 by direct DNA–DNA hybridization. The DNA was digested with several restriction enzymes and, after Southern blotting, hybridized with the LIM4 cDNA probe specific for the 5' end of a DRβ gene (manuscript submitted). Each specific restriction fragment length pattern can be denominated by a character, and these are shown in Table 1, together with those obtained for DR specificities 1, 2, 3, 4, 5, 7, and w8. Several restriction enzymes (REs) yielded restriction fragment length patterns with a comparable number of bands for all DR specificities ("x", "a"), while other REs, e.g., EcoRI, produced different patterns that discriminated partly between the DR serotypes [5]. Pattern "N" comprises hybridizing bands at 4.2, 4.0, 1.2 and 0.5 kb (kilobases), of which the 4.0-kb band and the 0.5-kb band occurred in all DRw6 individuals tested and in none of the samples expressing other DR specificities, thus being apparently unique for DRw6.

We concluded from these data that the coding potential for DRβ chains is identical in DRw6 and non-DRw6 individuals, and it may be possible to type for DRw6 at the DNA level. In these respects DRw6 appears to be a regular DR specificity. In addition to this, subdivisions could be made within the DRw6 serotype, as has been accomplished for the other DR specificities (see M. G. J. Tilanus et al., Molecular Analysis of HLA: Haplotype-Specific DNA Hybridization Patterns Using Class II cDNA Probes, this volume)

References

1. Gustafsson K, Wiman K, Larhammar D, Rask L, Peterson P (1984) Scand J Immunol 19:91
2. Hendriks GFJ, Schreuder GMT, Claas FHJ, D'Amaro J, Persijn GG, Cohen B, Van Rood JJ (1983) Br Med J 8:83
3. Hendriks GFJ, Persijn GG, Lansbergen Q, D'Amaro J, Schreuder GMT, Cohen B (1983) Lancet 23:187

Molecular Analysis of HLA: Haplotype-Specific DNA Hybridization Patterns Using Class II cDNA Probes*

M.G.J. Tilanus, M.L. Bosch, R. Gerrets, and M.J. Giphart

Department of Immunohematology and Blood Bank, University Hospital, 2333 AA Leiden, The Netherlands

Introduction

Originally, the HLA-D/DR region was described by cellular and serological techniques [1], but since the introduction of the Southern blot technique [2] this region can be analyzed directly at the level of the genes themselves.

The complexity of the HLA-D/DR region is based upon the polymorphism of the β chain and on the existence of at least three loci: DR, DQ, and DP [1, 3]. It is generally accepted that the class II region encompasses more genes in each of these loci, particularly genes coding for the β chains. In order to study the genes of the class II loci, cDNA and genomic probes have been constructed [4–9]. In contrast to the full-length cDNA probes for DRβ, the LIM4 cDNA probe [9] contains the leader and signal sequence and only the first 29 bases of the N-terminal protein coding sequence. This LIM4 cDNA probe has been derived from mRNA isolated from a B-lymphoblastoid cell line of an individ-

* In part supported by the Dutch Foundation for Medical Research (FUNGO), which is subsidized by the Dutch Organization for the Advancement of Pure Research (ZWO), and the J. A. Cohen Institute for Radiation Protection (IRS)

Histocompatibility Testing 1984
Edited by E. D. Albert et al.

ual homozygous for HLA-DR4, which was of consanguineous origin. This leaves no doubt about the haplotype-specific identification of this probe.

To analyze the class II gene system, homozygous typing cells were used in Southern blot analysis. These cells were selected from cousin marriage offspring for true homozygosity of the HLA complex [10]. After digestion of the DNA from these cell lines with various restriction enzymes their HLA-DR haplotypes were analyzed using the LIM4 cDNA probe in Southern blot hybridizations. Special attention was given to HLA-DR4 and -w6 (M. L. Bosch et al., HLA-DRw6: A Molecular Approach, this volume) [11]. In this way a haplotype-specific pattern for each of the HLA-DR serotypes 1 – w8 could be recognized.

Materials and Methods

Cell Lines

B-lymphoblastoid cell lines from individuals homozygous for a given HLA-DR type were established by EBV transformation. Table 1 shows the cell lines for each of the HLA-DR serotypes used in this study. All of them are of consanguineous origin except those of the DR4 serotype. These cells were selected for their HLA-DR homozygosity (BSM, however, is of consanguineous origin).

The characteristics of the homozygous cells have been described by Termijtelen [12].

Southern Blot Analysis

DNA was isolated according to the method of Gross-Bellard [13] with minor modifications. The DNA (10 – 15 μg) was digested with the restriction enzymes *Bam*HI, *Bgl*II, *Eco*RI, *Hin*dIII, *Kpn*I, *Pst*I, and *Pvu*II. The fragments obtained in this way were separated on submarine agarose gels (0.7%) and subsequently transferred to nitrocellulose filters (Schleicher and Schüll PH 79) as described by Southern [2]. Conditions for prehybridization, hybridization, and washes were as published previously [14], using a cDNA probe which was ^{32}P-labelled by nick translation [15].

Table 1. Cell lines homozygous for HLA-DR

DR1	DR2	DR3	DR4	DR5	DRw6	DR7	DRw8
CJO	NOL	QBL	BSM	THR	APD	EKR	LUY
BVR	PHS	CAA	JB[a]	ATH	HHK		
EDR	IWB	HAR	JSM[a]				
OOS	WIB	AVL	LRM[a]				
MVL	VYF		MWM[a]				
			SG1[a]				
			VABR[a]				
			WEN[a]				

[a] Not of consanguineous origin

Results

One of the Southern blots obtained after digestion of the DNA with *Hin*dIII is shown in Fig. 1. The hybridizing bands are identical in size in individuals of the DR1, 2, 3, and 4 serotypes, but different in a DRw8 individual.

In order to describe and compare all hybridization patterns obtained with seven restriction enzymes, each pattern was given a symbol. Thus, in Fig. 1 the pattern for DR1, 2, 3, and 4 with *Hin*dIII was designated "p" and the DRw8 pattern "k". A combined picture of the analysis is shown in Fig. 2. Each symbol represents a specific hybridization pattern characterized by a number of hybridizing bands with specific molecular weights. In the case of *Hin*dIII (Fig. 1), the number of hybridizing bands of pattern "p" is three, of pattern "k" only two. The molecular weights of the hybridizing bands by which pattern "p" is characterized are 4.1, 2.8, and 1.8 kb, whereas pattern "k" is characterized by bands with molecular weights of 5.3 and 4.4 kb. The hybridizing patterns after digestion of DNA with restriction enzymes *Bam*HI and *Pvu*II are similar in all DR serotypes tested (patterns "a" and "x" respectively). The patterns obtained with restriction enzymes *Eco*RI, *Pst*I, *Kpn*I, and *Bgl*II, however, showed extensive variability.

Next we analyzed the relation of the serologically defined DR types with the hybridization patterns. This is shown in Fig. 3. The molecular weights of the hybridizing bands and their respective pattern symbols after digestion with *Eco*RI, *Pst*I and *Kpn*I of the DR1 to DRw8 haplotypes are indicated. Unique patterns are obtained for HLA-DRw6 (pattern "n") and DRw8 (pattern "o") with *Eco*RI, for DR3 (pattern "y" and "t"), DR4 (pattern "u"), DR5 (pattern "v" and "z"), and DRw8 (pattern "w") with *Pst*I, and for DR2 (pattern "r") with *Kpn*I. Some patterns are shared among different haplotypes, e.g. pattern "h" among DR1, 2, and 3, pattern "q" among DR1 and DR3 – w8. In order to find a haplotype-specific pattern for DR1 and DR7, combinations of hybridization patterns should be used.

Apart from this "typing at the DNA level" a striking phenomenon is observed, namely the occurrence of additional restriction fragment length variation (RFLV). Thus, with the five DR1 indi-

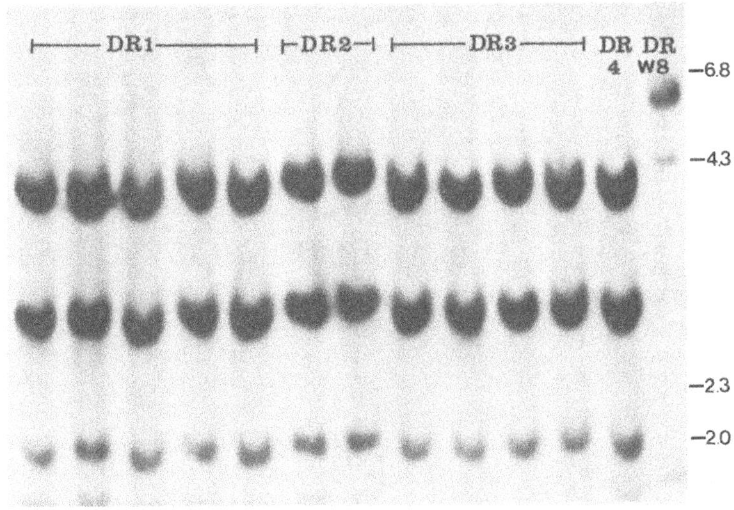

Fig. 1. Autoradiography of DNA from homozygous cell lines of consanguineous origin hybridized with the LIM4 cDNA probe after digestion with *Hind* III. Molecular weight markers are as indicated (in kb). From left to right: BVR, EDR, MVL, OOS, CJO (all DR1); NOL IWB (both DR2); AVL, CAA, HAR, QBL (all DR3), BSM (DR4) and LUY (DRw8)

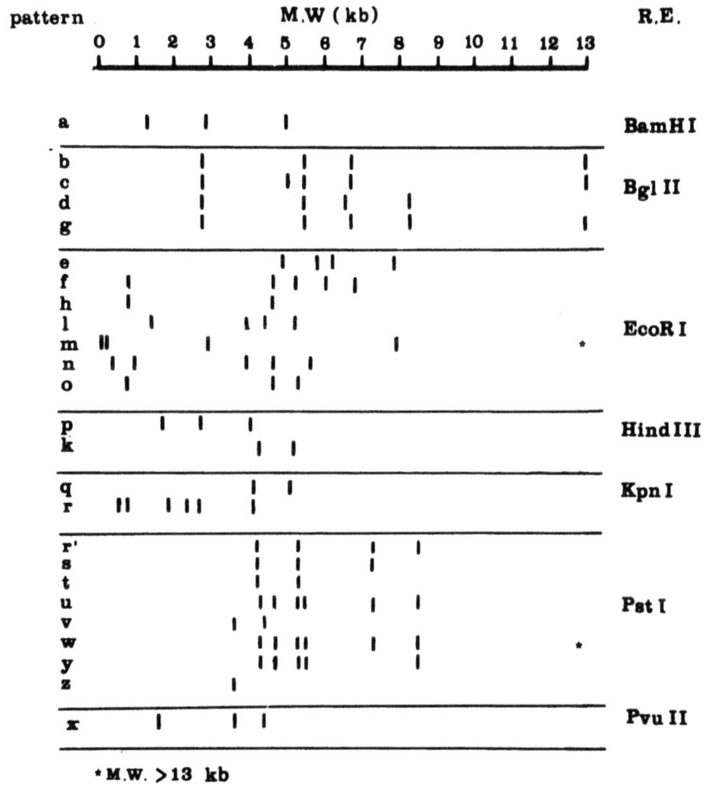

Fig. 2. Characteristic molecular weights of restriction fragments hybridizing with the LIM4 cDNA probe

viduals tested, two patterns were obtained using *Eco*RI, namely patterns "h" and "e". Similar and sometimes more RFLVs are observed: within DR3 (*Eco*RI), DR1 (*Pst*I), DR3 (*Pst*I) and DR5 (*Pst*I). The results obtained with the DRβ_2 cDNA probe are comparable (data not shown). It should be stressed that the number of individuals of a given haplotype tested is still very limited (yet there is extensive RFLV). More studies have to be carried out to confirm or extend the haplotype-specific hybridization and its relationship to RFLV.

We therefore tested two additional panels of individuals. One consisted of eight individuals homozygous for DR4 by serotyping, the other of 19 DRw6 homozygous individuals. Within the DR4 individuals, the cellularly determined HLA-Dw4

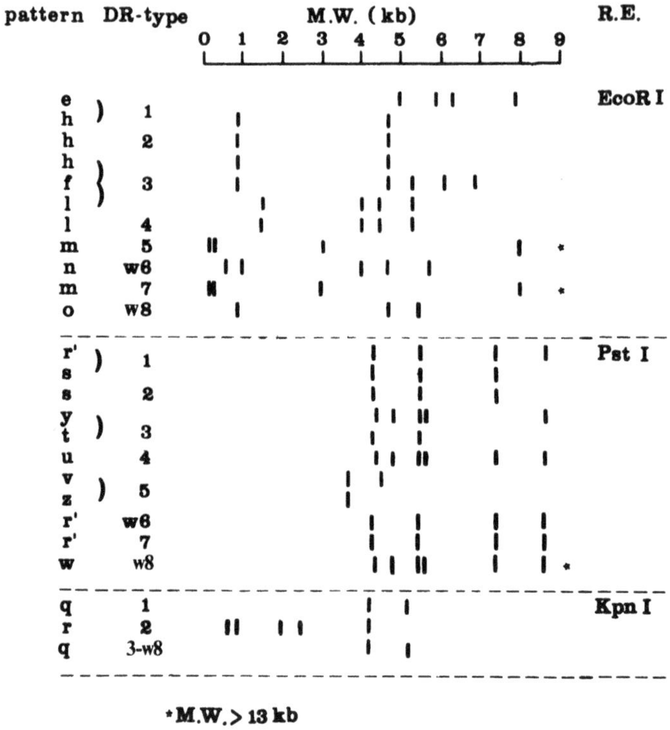

Fig. 3. Correlation of RFLV patterns with the DR1–w8 serotypes after digestion of DNA with *Eco*RI, *Pst*I, and *Kpn*I

and Dw10 specificities could be recognized by a specific hybridization pattern. Within the Dw4 individuals, separate and unique RFLVs were found with the LIM4 cDNA probe. This subdivision was not seen when using the DRβ_2 probe [9, 11]. The analysis of the 19 DRw6 individuals confirms the haplotype-specific hybridization pattern as indicated in Fig. 3 (M. L. Bosch et al., HLA-DRw6: A Molecular Approach, this volume). The hybridizing bands which are unique for DRw6 haplotypes within the pattern "n" are characterized by concomitant occurrence of bands at 4.0 kb and 0.5 kb (M. L. Bosch et al., HLA-DRw6: A Molecular Approach, this volume).

Discussion

The HLA-D/DR region can be described and possibly dissected by hybridization patterns obtained from Southern blot analysis using the LIM4 cDNA probe. However, from the homozygous typing cells tested, some haplotypes were only represented by a very limited number of individuals. The results as obtained so far have indicated the possibility of characterizing a given serologically defined HLA-DR haplotype by RFLV. Moreover, additional RFLVs were detected, illustrating a greater resolving power of DNA analysis. Enlargement of the homozygous typing cell panel with DR4 homozygous individuals led to a subdivision of RFLVs relating to the cellularly defined Dw4 and Dw10 alleles. The Dw4 group could be subdivided into two or three RFLVs depending on the restriction enzyme used. This frequent occurrence of RFLV was not found with DRβ_2 cDNA probe [9, 11]. This raises the question of how far we should proceed in determining and producing RFLVs, in other words how far to go in complicating the already extreme polymorphism. In our view, it now seems logical to proceed to analyze DNA RFLVs in relation to function, e.g., gene products.

The analysis of the 19 individuals homozygous for DRw6 confirms the typing pattern "n" (Fig. 3), thus allowing the conclusion that haplotype-specific hybridization patterns for the class II system can be found. Our results have shown that the DNA analysis may be powerful as a supplementary assay to serotyping.

However, the individuals tested are at the moment limited in number and are all homozygous. It remains to be ascertained how easily the haplotype-specific hybridization patterns can be found in a random population sample or how easily hybridization patterns can be "translated" into serotypes.

RFLVs have been found in most DR haplotypes. Whether this variation has any significance remains unknown. Our first aim is to answer the question of whether these variations can be used as better markers for HLA and disease predisposition. It would then tell us whether these RFLV's bear any relation with function.

We are now studying patients suffering from diseases which are associated with HLA-DR3 and 4, the haplotypes having the greatest variation in terms of RFLV. It has already been shown that some variation in hybridizing patterns may have a higher frequency in a diabetic patient group than in a control group [16].

Summary

The HLA class II cDNA probes LIM4 and DRβ_2 were used to study the genes of HLA by Southern blotting. The serologically defined alleles HLA-DR1 to HLA-DRw8 seem to have a haplotype-specific hybridization pattern. It is therefore possible to determine the HLA-D/DR region at the DNA level. Moreover, additional variation of restriction fragment length was detected within serologically identical individuals, suggesting the presence of subtypes (at the gene level). These subtypes occurred in the HLA-DR haplotypes DR1, 3, 4, 5, and w6, some of them correlating with other immunogenetic parameters.

Acknowledgements. The technical assistance of A. Thompson and M. van Eggermond is gratefully acknowledged. The HLA-DRβ_2 cDNA probe was a generous gift from E. Long and B. Mach.

References

1. Van Rood JJ, De Jongh B, Claas FHJ, Goulmy E, Gratema JW, Giphart MJ (1984) New facts on HLA genetics: are they relevant in bone marrow transplantation. Sem Hematol 21:65–80
2. Southern EM (1975) Detection of specific sequences among DNA fragments separated by gel electrophoresis. Mol Biol 98:503–519
3. Hurley CK, Giles RC, Capra JD (1983) The human MHC: evidence for multiple HLA-D region genes. Imm Today 4:219–226
4. Long EO, Wake CT, Strubin M, Gross N, Acolla RS, Carrel S, Mach B (1982) Isolation of distinct cDNA clones encoding HLA-DRβ chains by use of an expression assay. Proc Natl Acad Sci USA 79:7465–7469
5. Wake CT, Long EO, Strubin M, Gross N, Acolla R, Carel S, Mach B (1982) Isolation of cDNA clones encoding HLA-DR chains. Proc Natl Acad Sci USA 79:6979–6983
6. Lee JS, Throwsdale J, Bodmer WF (1982) cDNA probes coding for the heavy chain of HLA-DR antigens. Proc Natl Acad Sci USA 79:545–549
7. Auffrey C, Kuo J, De Mars R, Strominger JL (1983) A minimum of four human class II α chain genes are encoded in the HLA region of chromosome 6. Nature 304: 174–177
8. Wiman K, Larhammer D, Claesson L, Gustafsson K, Schenning L, Bill P, Böhme J, Denaro M, Dobberstein B, Hammerling U, Kvist S, Servenius B, Sundelin J, Peterson PA, Rask L (1982) Isolation and identification of a cDNA clone corresponding to an HLA-DR antigen β chain. Proc Natl Acad Sci USA 79:1703–1707
9. Tilanus MGJ, Vijg J, Van Boom JH, Thompson A, Giphart MJ (1984) The production and identification of HLA DR specific cDNA probes by selective primer extension and its relevance for the analysis of the HLA-D region genes (submitted)
10. Keuning JJ, Termijtelen A, Blusse van Oud-Alblas A, Gabb BW, D'Amaro J, Van Rood JJ (1975) LD (MLC) population and family studies in a Dutch population. In: Kissmeyer-Nielsen F (ed) Histocompatibility Testing 1975. Munksgaard, Copenhagen
11. Tilanus MGJ, Bosch ML, De Vries RRP, Giphart MJ (1984) Analysis of the HLA-DR region by DNA–DNA hybridization with special reference to the HLA-Dw4/DR4 region (submitted)
12. Termijtelen A, Van Leeuwen A, Van Rood JJ (1982) HLA linked lymphocyte activating determinants. Imm Rev 66:79–101
13. Gross-Bellard M, Oudet P, Chambon P (1973) Isolation of high molecular weight DNA from mammalian cells. Eur J Biochem 36:32–38
14. Böhme J, Owerbach D, Denaro M, Lernmark A, Peterson PA, Rask L (1983) Human class II major histocompatibility antigen β chains are derived from at least three loci. Nature 301:82–84
15. Rigby PWJ, Dieckmann M, Rhodes C, Berg P (1977) Labeling deoxyribonucleic acid to high specific activity in vitro by nick translation with DNA polymerase I. J Mol Biol 113:237–251
16. Owerbach D, Lernmark A, Platz P, Ryder LP, Rask L, Peterson P, Ludvigsson J (1983) HLA-D region β chain DNA endonuclease fragments differ between HLA-DR identical healthy and insulin dependent diabetic individuals. Nature 303:815–817

Analysis and Segregation of HLA-DR by DNA Typing: Correlation with Supertypic Specificities

G. Angelini [1, 2], C. de Préval [2], G.B. Ferrara [1], and B. Mach [2]

1 Istituto Nazionale per la ricerca sul cancro, Viale Benedetto XV, 10 Genova, Italy, and
Centro Ricerche Immunoematologiche, A.V.I.S., Bergamo
2 School of Medicine, University of Geneva, Switzerland

We have analyzed the structural polymorphism of the HLA-DR beta chain genes at the DNA level by Southern blot hybridization of restriction enzyme fragments with a DNA probe specific for DR beta chain genes. The probe, called Φ 14 *Bam* G, derives from the DNA of a heterozygous cell line typed DR4, DRw6, partially digested with *Sau* 3AI and cloned in the *Bam* HI site of the vector Charon 30 (J. Gorski, in preparation). The probe contains the exons coding the first domain, the second domain, the transmembrane region, and the cytoplasmic portion of the protein and the intercalated introns. The "Southern blot hybridization" procedure is referred to as "DNA typing" [1]. The conditions used are specific for DR loci and exclude cross-hybridization with the other class II beta chain genes of the D region (DQ and DP).

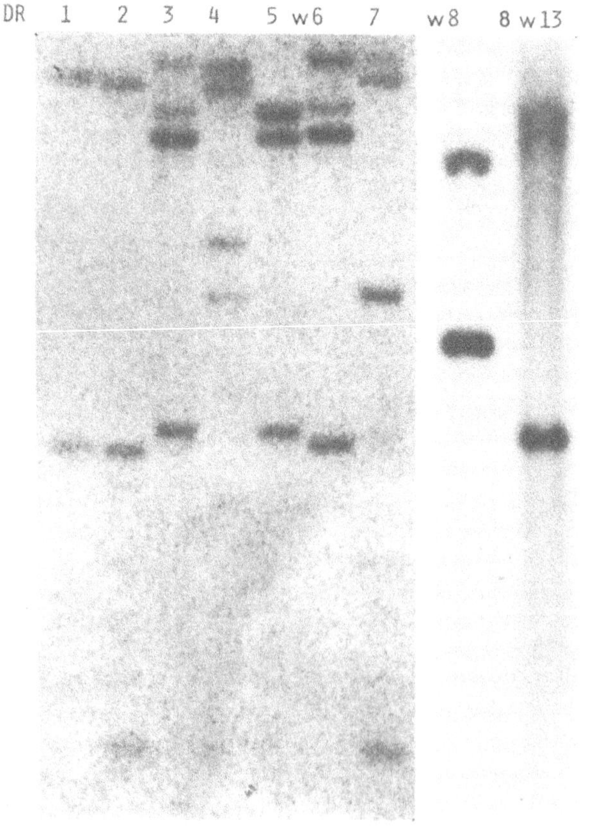

Fig. 1 Restriction patterns of different homozygous cell lines digested with *Bgl*I

We have experience so far of four restriction enzymes: *Eco* RI, *Bgl* I, *Pvu* II and *Pst* I. The clearest differentiation between the DR genotypes was obtained by *Bgl* I. Fig. 1 shows the restriction pattern obtained by digesting with *Bgl* I a series of DNA samples obtained from HLA homozygous offspring of first-cousin marriages. In addition to the commonly recognized DR specificities, a cell homozygous for 8w13 was available. The typing of this specificity was performed by radioimmunoassay, a method by which 8w13 can be confidently assessed [2]. As apparent from Fig. 1, though some bands are shared, each DR phenotype can be distinguished by at least one restriction fragment.

Next, the segregation of each restriction fragment was followed in the offspring of selected families. Six families have been studied so far, including two first-cousin marriages. In Fig. 2, family PA is shown as an example. The distribution pattern of the bands is unequivocal and perfectly fits the segregation of HLA antigens, so that each fragment can be labelled "a", "b", "c", or "d" according to the segregating haplotype. As expected, the fragment expressed by the HLA-A/B recombinant haplotype c−d is that corresponding to the d end. To be noted is the clear differentiation of 8w13 from DR5 for the 2.45-kb fragment. Family segregation could also be followed after cleavage by *Pvu* II, *Eco* RI, and *Pst* I. This study of families and of homozygous cells has permitted establishment, for each enzyme and each DR haplotype, of a defined restriction pattern.

Because we have been studying mainly families, the number of independent samples analyzed is not large. However, we have so far a solid indication of a good correspondence between DR haplotypes as defined by serology and restriction patterns, which are constant and reproducible. Some exceptions, which can be attributed to "DR splits" have been found, which will be reported elsewhere (B. Mach, in preparation).

Some restriction fragments were found in more than one DR haplotype. The analysis of the shared patterns has been as interesting as the analysis of

Histocompatibility Testing 1984
Edited by E. D. Albert et al.

bands specific for a single DR haplotype. The most remarkable observation was that two "groups" of genotypes could be clearly distinguished: DR4 and DR7 on one side, and DR3, 5, w6, w8, 8w13 on the other side. Figure 3 shows schematically the fragments in common between DR4 and DR7 as detected by three different enzymes. Here and in Figs. 4 and 5 fragments are referred to in terms of their kb's. Fragments shared by two or more DR phenotypes are boxed. The similarity is especially evident in the pattern produced by *Pvu*II where six of seven fragments are in common. Very similar patterns are also produced by the two other enzymes (three shared fragments out of five). In the DR3, 5, w6, w8, 8w13 group almost all fragments are shared by two or more haplotypes after *Pvu*II and *Eco*RI digestion. With *Bgl*I digestion, the DRw8 genotype becomes independent. The complex patterns in this group are summarized in Fig. 4. It must be stressed that none of the fragments generated by any of these enzymes is the same in the two groups.

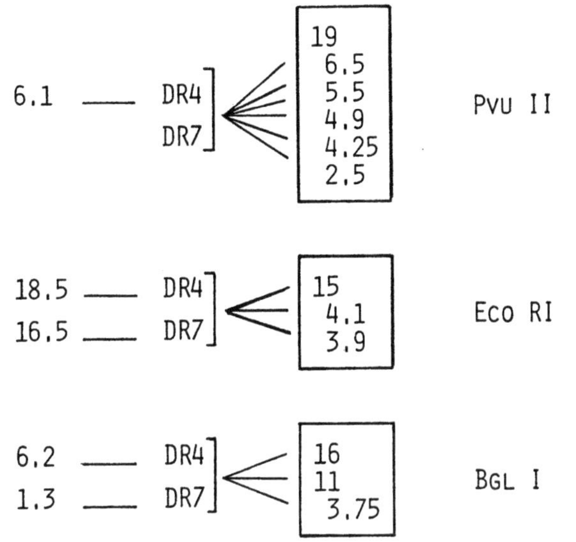

Fig. 3. Restriction pattern homology between haplotypes sharing the BR4 (~ DRw53) supertypic specificity

These two groups find their obvious correspondence in the DRw52 and DRw53 supertypic specificities. Both these specificities have been previously shown to be localized on BR molecules and have been given the names BR3 and BR4 respectively [3]. BR molecules do not possess the classical DR determinants; they are composed of an alpha subunit which is probably identical to that of DR molecules and a beta subunit which is structurally some what different [4]. BR molecules probably represent the product of one of the several beta chain genes localized in the "DR region". It is not surprising that restriction pattern similarities corresponding to DRw52 and DRw53 supertypic specificities are found by hybridization with a DR-beta probe. A consistent picture is appearing which fits with serology, immunochemistry, and molecular biology.

The remaining DR haplotypes, DR1 and DR2, also possess some resemblance. As shown in Fig. 5, while *Bgl*I digestion produces an entirely different pattern for DR1 and DR2, with *Pvu*II and *Eco*RI digestion about half of the restriction bands are shared. A serological correlate of this homology is more difficult to assess. DR1 and DR2 are both included in the DQw1 supertypic specificity. The latter was shown to be localized on DQ molecules and should not have anything to do with the present restriction pattern similarity, since DR-DQ cross-hybridization does not take place with the adopted experimental conditions. A DR1 + DR2 supertypic specificity has been described by Park and Terasaki [5] and named Te21. Its molecular localiza-

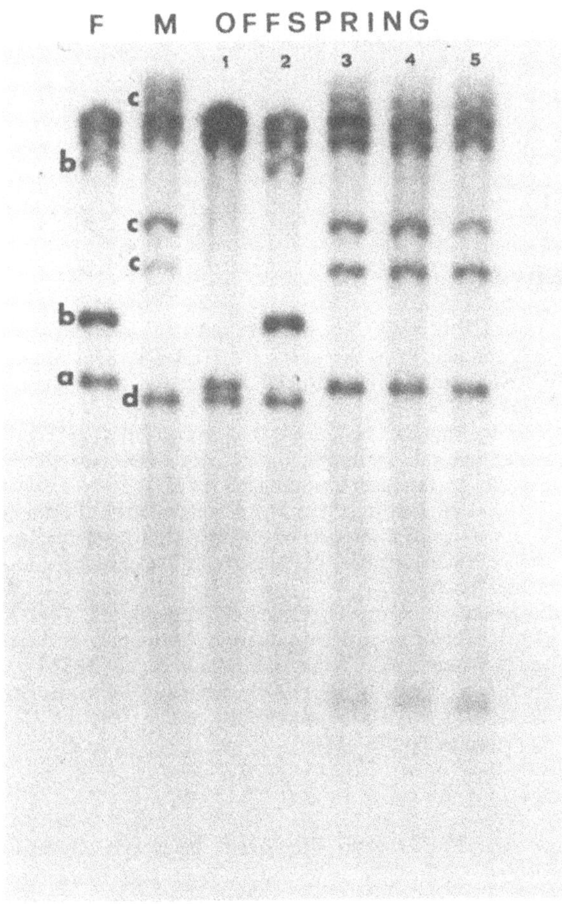

Haplotypes:
a = A2, B35, Cw4, DR5, BR3, DQβ4, DQβ5, DQα3;
b = A2, B51, –, DRw8, –, –, –, –;
c = A24, Bw61, Cw2, DR4, BR4, DQβ4, –, –;
d = A11, B51, –, 8w13, BR3, DQβ4, DQβ5, DCα3;
c–d = A24, β51, –, 8w13, BR3, DQβ4, DQβ5, DCα3
Offspring:
1 = a/d; *2* = b/c–d; *3* = a/c; *4* = a/c; *5* = a/c

Fig. 2. Segregation of restriction fragments in family PA

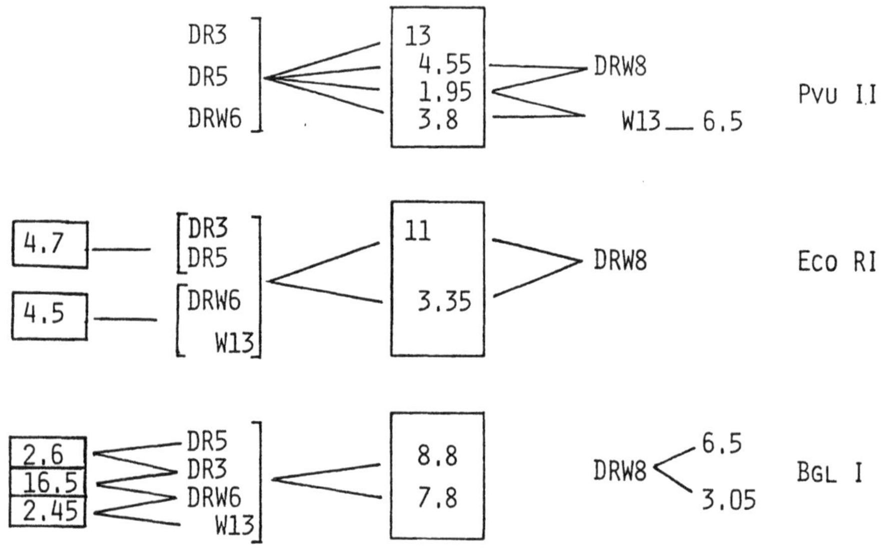

Fig. 4. Restriction pattern homology between haplotypes sharing the DRw52 supertypic specificity (W13 = 8w13)

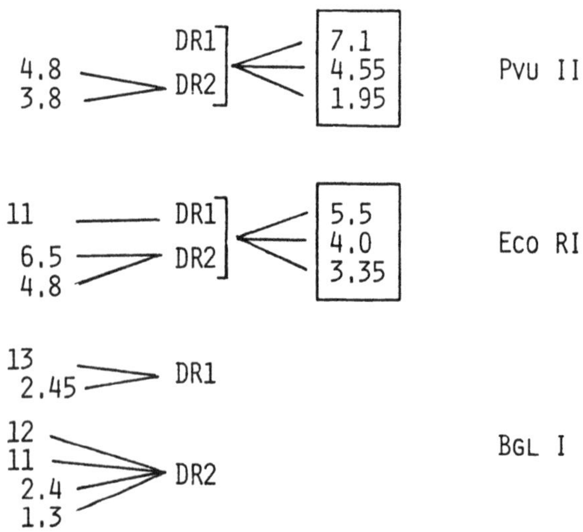

Fig. 5. Restriction pattern homology between DR1 and DR2 haplotypes

tion is not defined. Moreover, it is difficult to exclude that Te21 antisera are simply weak DQw1 antisera, since they seem to react also against some DRw6 individuals. Another candidate is the DRPub1 specificity described by Tanigaki and Tosi [3] as associated with DR1, DR2, and DRw9 and shown to be localized on DR molecules. The DRw9 haplotype has not been analyzed yet. If it turns out to share restriction fragments with DR1 and DR2, the possibility of a correspondence with DRPub1 will be strengthened.

In general, the establishment of a correlation with serological and with protein structure data is a necessary requirement for a correct interpretation of the DNA patterns.

References

1. Wake CT, Long EO, Mach B (1982) Allelic polymorphism and complexity of the genes for HLA-DR beta-chains. Direct analysis by DNA–DNA hybridization. Nature 300:372–374
2. Tosi R, Tanigaki N, Centis D, Ferrara GB (1981) Immunochemical definition of a new DR specificity 8WDRw13. Immunol Commun 20(3):275
3. Tanigaki N, Tosi R (1982) The genetic control of human Ia alloantigens: a three-loci model derived from the immunochemical analysis of "supertypic" specificities. Immunol Rev 66:5–37
4. Sorrentino R, Corte G, Calabi F, Tanigaki N, Tosi R (1983) Microfingerprinting analysis of human Ia molecules favours a three loci model. Mol Immunol 20:333
5. Park MS, Terasaki PI (1980) Second DR locus. In: Terasaki PI (ed) Histocompatibility testing 1980. UCLA, Los Angeles, pp 578–582

Supported by "Progetto Finalizzato Ingegneria Genetica CNR"

Recombinant DNA Technology: Its Use in the Study of HLA

D. Cohen, E. Robbins, and J. Dausset

Institut de Recherches sur les Maladies du Sang, Hôpital Saint Louis, 2, Place du Docteur Fournier, 75475 Paris Cedex 10, France

Introduction

Since the 1970s tremendous progress has been made in the development of techniques which allow the study of the HLA system to be undertaken directly at the level of the gene. This new recombinant DNA technology makes possible the production of virtually unlimited quantities of any desired DNA segment for analysis. These techniques provide a powerful approach to the study of gene expression, and have greatly advanced our knowledge of the structure and function of the HLA system. Among the most useful techniques are:

1. The cutting of DNA into multiple fragments by restriction enzymes
2. The transfer of size-separated fragments onto nitrocellulose filters
3. The hybridization of fragments with specific, complementary radiolabeled probes
4. The isolation and cloning of specific fragments of interest
5. The localization of a given fragment to a particular position on the chromosome
6. The determination of the DNA sequence of a fragment

Restriction Enzymes and Restriction Maps

The first step in the analysis of a segment of DNA is the cutting of extracted genomic DNA into multiple fragments of various sizes by restriction enzymes. Restriction endonucleases are enzymes made in bacteria which serve to protect bacteria from invasion by foreign DNA. Restriction enzymes cut DNA at specific recognition sites of four to six nucleotides in length; bacterial DNA recognition sequences are protected from autodigestion by methylation of adenine or cytosine bases. The distribution of the sizes and number of restriction fragments produced by a given enzyme will be identical for two identical DNA strands, while nonidentical strands may differ in their pattern of restriction fragments.

The analysis of these genomic segments includes the establishment of a restriction map, a schema showing the location on the gene of the cutting sites of several enzymes with respect to each other. This is obtained by studying the numbers and sizes of restriction fragments using several different restriction enzymes singly and in combination. Chromosomal regions with similar DNA sequences will have similar restriction maps. The restriction map permits the localization of the genes of the HLA on the segment of DNA isolated; this is done by identifying the size, and therefore position, of the restriction fragments of the segment that are capable of hybridizing to a specific complementary DNA (cDNA) probe.

Nucleic Acid Hybridization with cDNA Probes

Nucleic acid hybridization is the process which permits the precise identification and isolation of specific gene sequences. One strand of a single-stranded DNA or RNA molecule will pair, base by base, with a second strand provided that its sequence is complementary to that of the first strand. This pairing can occur even if the strands are not entirely homologous, as long as at least 70% of the base pairs are complementary; these hybrids are somewhat less stable, however, and can only be maintained in so-called relaxed physicochemical conditions of low temperature and high salt concentration. Hybridization can be carried out on cellular DNA, isolated and digested by restriction enzymes, and transferred to nitrocellulose filters (Southern blot), or in situ, which permits the localization of a particular sequence to a specific chromosome. The most commonly used procedure is the Southern blot [1]. Double-stranded restriction fragments are arranged by size on an agarose gel by electrophoresis. Following denaturation, the single-stranded fragments are transferred by diffusion to a nitrocellulose filter, which is then exposed to a single-stranded ^{32}P-labeled cDNA probe. The locations of the fragments capable of hybridizing with the probe are revealed by autoradiography.

The careful construction of the radiolabeled probe is important for successful hybridization; it is the sequence of the probe which determines which segments of the genome will be identified and isolated. A probe is any isolated, cloned, single-stranded DNA fragment containing all or part of a gene; it can be radioactively labeled with ^{32}P. One method

Histocompatibility Testing 1984
Edited by E. D. Albert et al.

of obtaining a probe involves the synthesis and cloning of a cDNA molecule using messenger RNA (mRNA) from HLA genes as a template. mRNA can be extracted from cells, and a complementary, single-stranded DNA copy can be made using the enzyme reverse transcriptase. The RNA matrix is eliminated by alkaline hydrolysis; the single-stranded DNA is then made into a double-stranded molecule using the enzyme DNA polymerase. The resulting double-stranded DNA molecule can be inserted into a plasmid or cosmid and cloned in an appropriate bacterial host. Selection of cDNA clones that are potentially useful for probes for the HLA region is performed using synthetic oligonucleotides. The oligonucleotide sequence is obtained from the previously determined protein sequence of HLA molecules. Short, radiolabeled synthetic oligonucleotide sequences are then used for in situ hybridization in bacterial colonies carrying cDNA clones, and positive clones are selected for use as probes.

Construction of Genomic Libraries

Cloning of DNA molecules in bacteriophage, plasmid, or cosmid vectors is necessary for the production of specific probes; it is also an essential procedure for the isolation and study of any specific gene segment, as it allows the production of unlimited quantities of the segment. DNA cloning consists of the amplification in a bacterial or yeast host of a segment of DNA inserted into an appropriate vector. A plasmid is a circular, double-stranded DNA molecule that is capable of independent replication inside a bacterial or yeast host. Plasmids frequently carry genes for antibiotic resistance, a property which is exploited in the selection of transformed bacterial colonies. A cosmid is a hybrid vector between the bacteriophage and plasmid, carrying the "cos" sequence specific for phage and the origin of replication and the genes coding for antibiotic resistance of the plasmid. It is 5–10 kilobases in length and can combine with a genomic fragment of 35–45 kilobases. Like the bacteriophage, it can be encapsulated. Plasmids and cosmids are more useful in eucaryotic gene cloning than bacteriophages because they permit the cloning of larger fragments of DNA.

The construction of a cosmid genomic library for the study of the HLA region passes through many stages. Genomic DNA is first extracted from cells and then digested with a restriction enzyme, chosen such that fragments will be between 35 and 45 kilobases long. The cosmid vector is also cut with the same restriction enzyme; cohesive ends that can either self-anneal or combine with a genomic DNA fragment are created. DNA ligase seals the ends by creating covalent phosphodiester bonds between the opposing ends of each strand of DNA, thereby completing the graft of eukaryotic DNA onto the vector. These hybrid or recombinant molecules are then reintroduced into an appropriate bacterial host by making the bacterial cells temporarily permeable to large molecules. Successfully transformed bacteria can be selected by the antibiotic resistance conferred by the cosmid. The cosmid is capable of independent replication within the bacterial host, and large numbers of the DNA fragments are produced.

A mammalian genome cloned in this manner will produce between 10^5 and 10^7 different fragments. The selection of the bacterial colonies of interest requires in situ hybridization with a ^{32}P-labeled probe specific for the region of interest. Bacteria colonies that hybridize with specific probes are lysed, and cosmid DNA is separated from host DNA. The DNA fragments cloned in each colony are recovered by treatment with the same restriction enzyme originally used for the construction of the hybrid molecule.

"Walking Along the Chromosome"

A technique of considerable utility in the study of HLA genes is that of "walking along the chromosome". After a given gene segment has been identified as a particular HLA gene, the gene segments immediately adjacent to either end can be identified, isolated, and studied. This is done by excising the end of the initial segment for use as a probe of the genomic library to identify the next adjacent segment. The new segments obtained with this probe are located on a restriction map in order to establish their degree of overlapping with the initial segment. The new segment which overlaps the least with the original segment is retained. The most distal end of this fragment then serves as the probe for the next step along the chromosome; the process can be repeated indefinitely.

Approaches to Gene Structure and Function

The availability of unlimited quantities of cloned DNA fragments has greatly facilitated the study of the HLA region. Gene fragments can be localized to a particular chromosomal segment. Sufficient DNA fragments can be produced to determine the nucleotide sequence using the technique of Sanger [2] or Maxam and Gilbert [3]. The sequence of the protein coded for by the gene fragment can then be deduced.

In addition to position and structure, the function of a given gene fragment can be studied by transfection experiments in which the gene is introduced into an eukaryotic cell of murine or human origin. The foreign DNA is introduced into the host cell cytoplasm by calcium phosphate precipitation. It then enters the host nucleus and inserts itself into the host genome where it is transcribed. The corresponding mRNA is translated into a protein product which undergoes post-translational modification within the cytoplasm. The final product may then be expressed on the surface of the cell, where it can be detected and identified by immunological methods. Both class I and class II HLA genes have been successfully transfected into mammalian cells [4, 5].

Applications to the Study of HLA

Number and Position of Class I and Class II Genes

Southern blot analyses and cloning studies have been useful in the determination of the precise number of class I and class II genes, as well as their chromosomal position. In man, between 20 and 40 genes exist for class I. For class II, between five and six alpha chain genes and seven beta chain genes have been found [6, 7]. Restriction maps demonstrate the chromosomal location of each gene (Fig. 1); structural studies demonstrate similarities and differences between the human HLA complex and that of the mouse.

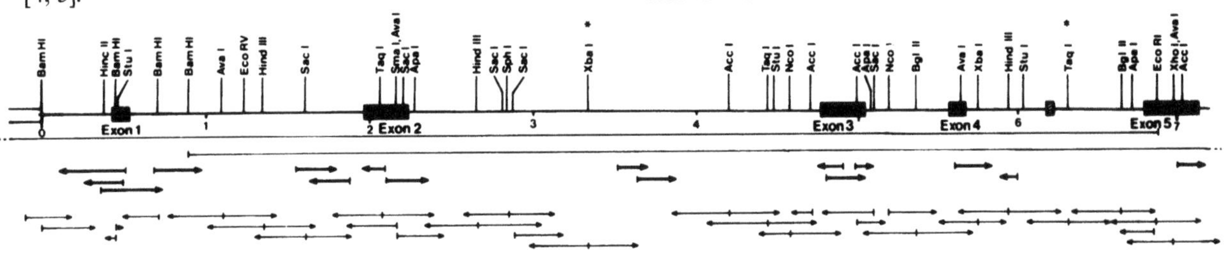

Fig. 1. Restriction map of a β-DQ gene. Entire length is 7 kilobases. Exon organisation provides evidence for a relationship between class II β chains and members of the immunoglobulin family. *Arrows* indicate sequences determined after labeling at 5′ or 3′ ends (provided by P. A. Peterson)

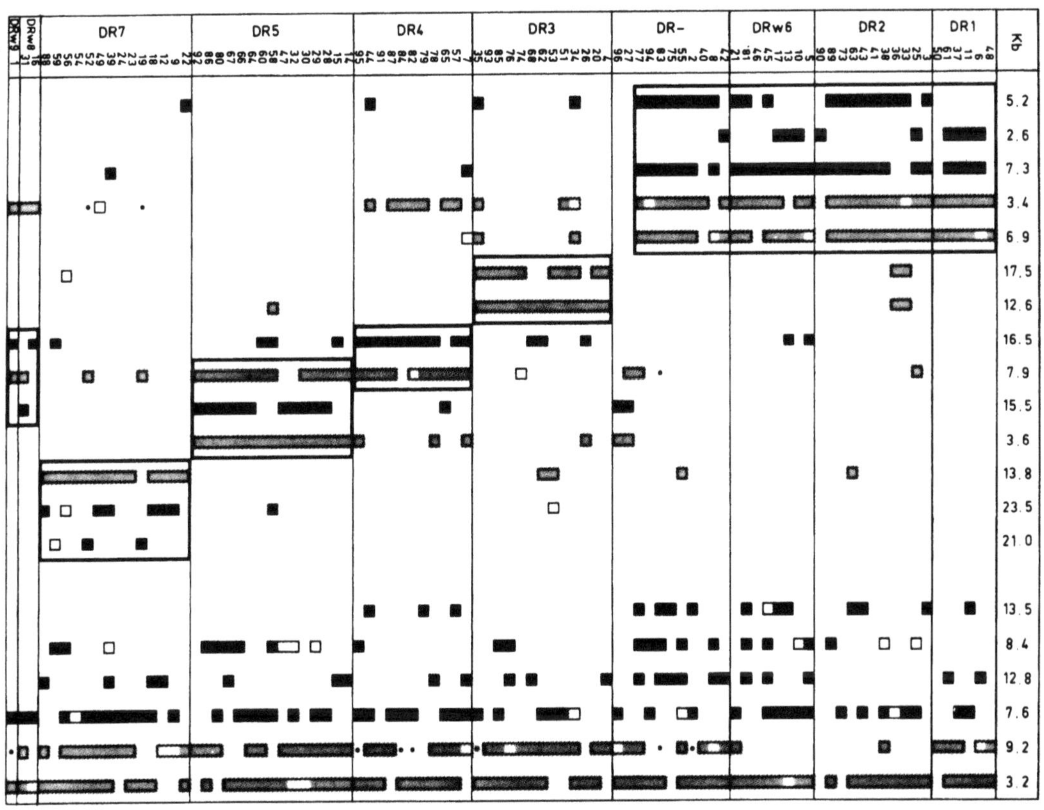

Fig. 2. Correlation of restriction fragments with HLA-DR types. DNA was digested with *Hin*dIII (*black boxes*) or *Eco*RV (*grey boxes*) and hybridized with a β-DQ probe. DR haplotypes are identified at *left.* Clusters of bands that correlate with particular DR specificities are shown in *boxes*

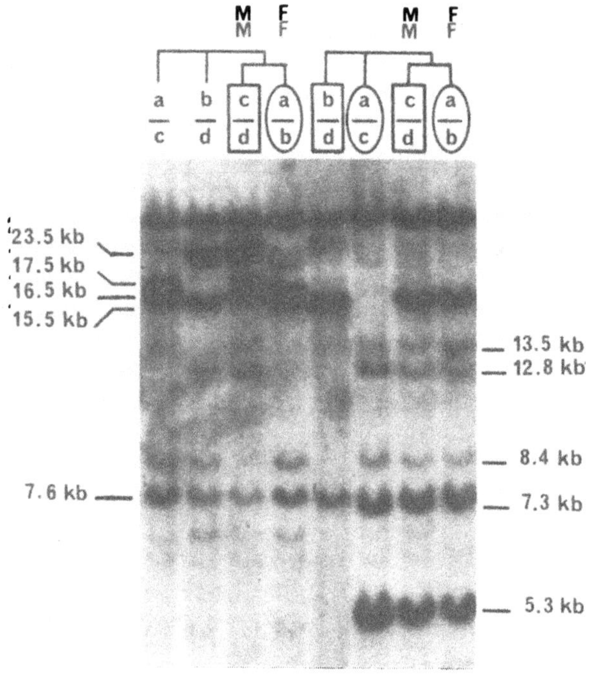

Fig. 3. HLA polymorphism at the gene level. Each lane consists of genomic DNA digested with *Eco* RV from individuals of two unrelated families. Hybridization with a β-DQ probe illustrates the previously known HLA polymorphism at the gene level. The segregation of a group of fragments as a haplotype can be observed in these family studies

Polymorphism at the Gene Level: Allogenotopes

Molecular genetic analyses have contributed to a new appreciation of the complexity of the HLA region. An even greater polymorphism can be detected at the gene level than was previously seen at the cell surface. Restriction fragments can be shown to correlate with serological defined HLA alleles; these are called allogenotopes [8]. Other polymorphic bands do not correlate with any known specificity, and may represent new specificities or noncoding elements of the genome. Single bands or clusters of bands can sometimes be shown to correlate closely with a known HLA specificity (Fig. 2).

Restriction fragments can be observed to segregate with haplotypes in family studies (Fig. 3). Recombination can also be observed. Such family studies can be useful in determining the HLA type of an individual.

The recombinant DNA techniques developed over the past decade have greatly facilitated the study of the polymorphism of HLA molecules. The correlation of some restriction fragments with serologically-defined alleles is the first stage in the synthesis of the two approaches. The extensive polymorphism of the HLA system will ultimately be more completely and precisely defined. Finally, the ability to work directly at the gene level may mean that certain diseases that are linked to HLA will also be better understood.

References

1. Southern EM (1975) Detection of specific sequences among DNA fragments separated by gel electrophoresis. J Mol Biol 98:503–517
2. Sanger F (1981) Determination of nucleotide sequences in DNA. Science 214:1205–1210
3. Gilbert W (1981) DNA sequencing and gene structure. Science 214:1305–1312
4. Lemonnier FA, Malissen M, Goldstein P, et al (1982) Expression of human class I histocompatibility antigens on the surface of DNA-transformed mouse cells. Immunogenetics 16:355–361
5. Rabourdin-Combe C, Mach B (1983) Expression of HLA-DR antigens at the surface of mouse L cells co-transfected with cloned human genes. Nature 303:670–674
6. Steinmetz A, Hood L (1983) Genes of the major histocompatibility complex in mouse and man. Science 222:727–733
7. Auffray C, Kuo J, DeMars R, Strominger JL (1983) A minimum of four human Class II α-chain genes are encoded in the HLA region of chromosome 6. Nature 304:174–177
8. Cohen D, Paul P, Font M-P (1983) Analysis of HLA Class I genes with restriction endonuclease fragments: implications for polymorphism of the human major histocompatibility complex. Proc Natl Acad Sci USA 80: 6289–6292

HLA-DR and DQ, Studied with Genomic Blotting, in Diabetic Families and Transplant Donor-Recipient Pairs

B. Carlsson[1], J. Böhme[2], B. Kalm[2], G. Lundgren[3], E. Möller[1], B. Persson[4], P.A. Peterson[2], L. Rask[5], and J. Wallin[1]

1 Department of Clinical Immunology, Huddinge University Hospital, 14186 Huddinge, Sweden
2 Department of Cell Research, Wallenberg Laboratory, Uppsala University, Uppsala, Sweden
3 Department of Transplantation, Surgery, Huddinge University Hospital, Huddinge, Sweden
4 Department of Pediatrics, St. Göran University Hospital, Stockholm, Sweden
5 Swedish University for Agricultural Sciences, Uppsala, Sweden

The DNA–DNA hybridization technique was employed to investigate the possible role of HLA class II genes other than DR in clinical kidney and bone marrow transplantation. Using cDNA probes corresponding to the polymorphic DRβ, DQβ, and DQα chains (Wallin et al., this volume), we examined the restriction fragment length polymorphism (RFLP) in *Pvu*II- or *Bam*HI-digested genomic DNA in bone marrow and kidney transplant donor-recipient pairs, and in 14 diabetic families. The RFLP detected is adequate to type for DR and DQ specificities [1; Wallin et al., this issue]. The bone marrow transplant donor-recipient pairs examined are all serologically HLA-A, B, C, DR identical sibs. Among those patients with good clinical outcome it was not possible to detect any difference in RFLP between the donor and the recipient with either DRβ or DQβ probes. However, in one donor-recipient pair a 1.6-kb *Pvu*II fragment visualized with the DQβ probe was present in the recipient and absent in the donor. In our material this band is strongly correlated with DQw2 ($P < 0.001$). Hybridization patterns with the DRβ probe were identical. These two sibs also differed in hybridization pattern when *Pvu*II-digested genomic DNA was hybridized with the DQα probe. The outcome of this transplantation was fatal due to a severe graft-versus-host (GvH) reaction. These data indicate that the difference at the genomic level is also reflected phenotypically and that this difference caused the GvH reaction and the strongly positive MLC that was observed prior to transplantation. According to the HLA genotypes of the parents, the observed difference might be the result of a recombination between the DR and DQ loci. In one case of intrafamilial living-donor kidney transplantation between a donor (mother) and a recipient (daughter) identical for DR and DQ, we detected additional polymorphism with genomic hybridization that might explain the graft rejection observed. Thus, relevant and new biological information pertinent to transplantation has been obtained with this technique. Hybridization with DRβ, DQβ, and DQα probes was also performed to *Pvu*II or *Bam*HI restriction enzyme-digested genomic DNA from individuals in 14 families, serologically studied in the present workshop, who had one or more diabetic children. In all families it was obvious that a certain band pattern always segregated with one of the parental haplotypes, regardless of the probe and endonuclease used. No crossing over was detected with either serological or hybridization techniques. It could also be ascertained that no difference was detectable at the genomic level between healthy and diabetic HLA identical sibs. A significantly reduced frequency of a 3.7-kb *Bam*HI fragment detected with the DQβ probe was observed in the DR4-positive diabetic families compared with healthy DR4-positive controls, as described earlier [2].

References

1. Andersson M, Böhme J, Andersson G, Möller E, Thorsby E, Rask L, Peterson PA (1984) Genomic hybridization with class II transplantation antigen cDNA probes as a complementary technique in tissue typing. Hum Immunol 11, 2:57–68
2. Owerbach D, Lernmark Å, Platz P, Ryder LP, Rask L, Peterson PA, Ludvigsson S (1983) HLA-D region chain DNA endonuclease fragments differ between HLA-DR identical healthy and insulin-dependent diabetic individuals. Nature 303:815–817

Histocompatibility Testing 1984
Edited by E. D. Albert et al.

DNA Restriction Fragment Length Polymorphism of the Human Class II Genes as Analyzed by Southern Blotting Technique*

K.M. Hui [1], A.V. Groves [1], D. Jaraquemada [1], F. Grosveld [2], J. Awad [1], C. Navarrete [1], J. Trowsdale [3], E. Murray [2], and H. Festenstein [1]

1 Department of Immunology, The London Hospital Medical College, Turner Street, London E1 2AD, U.K.
2 Laboratory of Gene Structure and Expression, National Institute for Medical Research, The Ridgeway, Mill Hill, London, U.K.
3 Imperial Cancer Research Fund, 44 Lincoln's Inn Fields, London, U.K.

Introduction

The human HLA-D region class II antigens each consist of two non-covalently linked trans-membrane glycoprotein subunits: an α heavy chain of 32−35 kd and a β light chain of 28−30 kd [1]. They are encoded by a complex multigene family consisting of several loci within the major histocompatibility complex on chromosome 6 [1]. Their products, which are primarily represented on B cells, monocytes and activated T cells, participate in several cellular immune functions. These include antigen presentation and cell−cell recognition. They are also associated with susceptibility/resistance to some diseases [1]. There are at least three distinct class II allelic series − HLA-DR, BR and DQ − all detectable by molecular and serological assays [2]. A fourth serologically defined class II system has been called "SB" (now DP) because it is thought by some to correspond to the antigens defined by primed lymphocyte typing [5]. In addition, there are the HLA-D specificities which are defined by mixed lymphocyte culture testing. Most of these specificities correlate closely with HLA-DR in Caucasoids but not in Negroids and Mongoloids [3]. The precise relationship between these "MLC determinants" and the molecules described above has not yet been established.

Ten WHO-designated HLA-DR specificities have so far been characterized using alloantisera obtained from multiparous women [4]. The remaining class II allelic series have also been defined serologically [2]. The DQw1 (MB1, MT1, DC1) specificity is found in strong linkage disequilibrium with DR1, DR2 and DRw6 in Caucasoids; DRw52 (which includes BR3 and DR Pub3) is associated with DR3, DR5, DRw6 and DRw8; DRw53 is associated with DR4, DR7 and DRw9. DQw2 (DC3) is associated with DR3 and 7; and DQw3 (DC4) is associated with DR4, DR5 and a split of DR7. There is no clear linkage disequilibrium between the DP and the DR, DQ specificities.

The structural genes for several human class II products have recently been isolated and sequenced [6−9]. Thus far, at least six class II α chain genes (two DP-α, one each of DR-α, DQα, DX-α and DZ-α) and at least seven non-allelic β chain genes (three DR-like, two DQ-like and two DP-like) have been identified. Using these cloned class II genes, we have studied the structural polymorphism of a panel of selected homozygous typing cells at the DNA level by Southern blot analyses of gene fragments produced following digestion with restriction enzymes and hybridizing with DNA probes specific for the genes encoding the following class II α and β chains: DR-α, DR-β, DQ-α, DQ-β, DP-α and DP-β.

Materials and Methods

Homozygous Typing Cells

The HLA-D region phenotypes of the homozygous typing cells (HTCs) used in this study are listed in Table 1.

Southern Blot Analysis

Ten micrograms of genomic DNA was completely digested with the different restriction enzymes as indicated. The resulting DNA fragments were separated by electrophoresis on 0.5% agarose gels and transferred to nitrocellulose filters [10]. The different probes used for hybridization and their sources are described in Table 2.

The DNA fragments isolated from the different probes were labelled with [α ^{32}P]dATP and [α ^{32}P]dTTP by nick translation [11]. Before hybridization, the nitrocellulose filters were pre-hybridized for 2 h at 65 °C in 0.45 *M* NaCl, 45 m*M* trisodium citrate (pH 7.0) and 10× concentrated Denhardt's reagent. The filters were then hybri-

* These studies were supported by the Cancer Research Campaign (KH), the Medical Research Council (FG, JA), the Nuffield Foundation (HF), the Leukaemia Research Fund (CN) and the Multiple Sclerosis Society (AVG)

Histocompatibility Testing 1984
Edited by E. D. Albert et al.

dized with the ^{32}P-labelled heat-denatured probe in 0.45 *M* NaCl/45 m*M* trisodium citrate (pH 7.0)/ 10× concentrated Denhardt's reagent/10% sodium dextran sulfate (SDS) and 500 μg denatured salmon sperm DNA per ml hybridization mix.

After 16–24 h at 65 °C, the filters were washed three times at 65 °C for 15 min each with 0.45 *M* NaCl/45 m*M* trisodium citrate (pH 7.0)/0.1% SDS, three times at 65 °C for 15 min each with 0.15 *M* NaCl/15 m*M* trisodium citrate (pH 7.0)/0.1% SDS, and three times at 65 °C for 15 min each with 50 m*M* NaCl/5 m*M* trisodium citrate (pH 7.0)/ 0.1% SDS. Labelled fragments were detected by exposing X-ray films to the radioactive filters at −70 °C with intensifying screens.

Table 1. HLA-D region phenotypes of the cells used for southern blot hybridization

Cells	DR	Dw	DQw	DRw	DPw
AHA	2, 7	2, 11	1, 3	53	2, 4
APD*	w6	6.1	1	52	"blank"
AS(ASJ)	3	NT	2	52	NT
CHA	2, 7	2, 11	1, 3	53	2, 4
DAUDI	w"6"	NT	1	52	NT
DHI*	5	5	3	52	4
FJO*	2	DB9	1		4
FPA*	"5"	"FS"	1	52	2
GEV	w6.9	9	1	52	NT
GHA	1, 7	1, 11	1, 3	53	4
HOM II*	1	1	1		4
I10W10	4	10	3	53	4
JLO	4	4	3	53	4
JMF*	7	7	2	53	4
KCAR	2	2	1		NT
KRO	5	5	3	52	2, 4
LBU*	7	DB1	2	53	NT
MADURA	w8	8	blank	52	NT
PGF*	2	2	1		4
SHA*	7, 7	11, "1"	3	53	4

*, consanguineous HTCs; NT, not tested

Results

The DR-α probe detected no DNA structural polymorphism with the selected HTCs of phenotypes DR1 through DRw8 after digestion with the restriction enzymes *Eco*RI and *Msp*I. In all cases, a single *Eco*RI fragment of 6.7 kb or a single *Msp*I fragment of 6.5 kb was observed (data not shown).

With the DR-β probe, the restriction fragment length polymorphism (RFLP) patterns obtained with *Eco*RI digest showed a distinctive pattern which is identical for HTCs with the same phenotype. Different patterns were observed for HTCs of phenotypes DR1, DR2, DR3, DR4, DR7 and DRw8 (Fig. 1a). In contrast, the *Eco*RI RFLP patterns are similar between the limited number of selected HTCs of the phenotypes DR3, DR5 and DRw6 (Fig. 1a). It is also interesting to note that the same RFLP pattern was obtained for the three DR2-positive HTCs, despite one of them (FJO) having a different HLA-D phenotype. These similarities may be attributed to common *Eco*RI sites in the different genes encoding these specificities. While the RFLP patterns of the DR3 (AS) and DR5 (DHI) DNAs are also the same following *Msp*I digestion (data not shown), the RFLP patterns of the DNAs of the DR3 (AS) and DRw6 (APD) cells and those of the DR4 (I10W10) and DR7 (JMF, LBU) cells are different (Fig. 1b). Furthermore, the RFLP patterns for the DNAs of the DR3 (AS) and DR5 (DHI) cells are also different when *Pst*I is used (Fig. 1c). It is therefore possible to establish unique RFLP patterns for DNA isolated from cells of different DR phenotypes using a combination of several restriction enzymes.

The DQ-α related products and genes have both been reported to be polymorphic. With a DQ-α probe, a constant *Pst*I-produced fragment of about 9.6 kb was observed in all the DNA digests of the HTCs except that of FPA. This gene fragment of restricted polymorphism is referred to as DX-α [7].

Table 2. DNA probes used for Southern blot hybridization

Probes	Description	Source (designation)
DR-α	cDNA, two *Pst*I fragments of about 500 bp each	P. Peterson (pDR-α-1)
DR-β	cDNA, *Pst*I fragment of about 650 bp	J. Silver, S. Goyert
DQ-α	Genomic, *Pst*I fragment of about 2 kb	J. Trowsdale, W. Bodmer (10.8)
DQ-β	cDNA, *Ava*I fragment of about 850 bp	P. Peterson (pDR-β-1)
DP-α	Genomic, *Pst*I fragment of about 2 kb	J. Trowsdale, W. Bodmer (11-α-1, SB-α-1)
DP-β	Genomic, *Pst*I fragment of about 1 kb	J. Trowsdale, W. Bodmer (11.13)

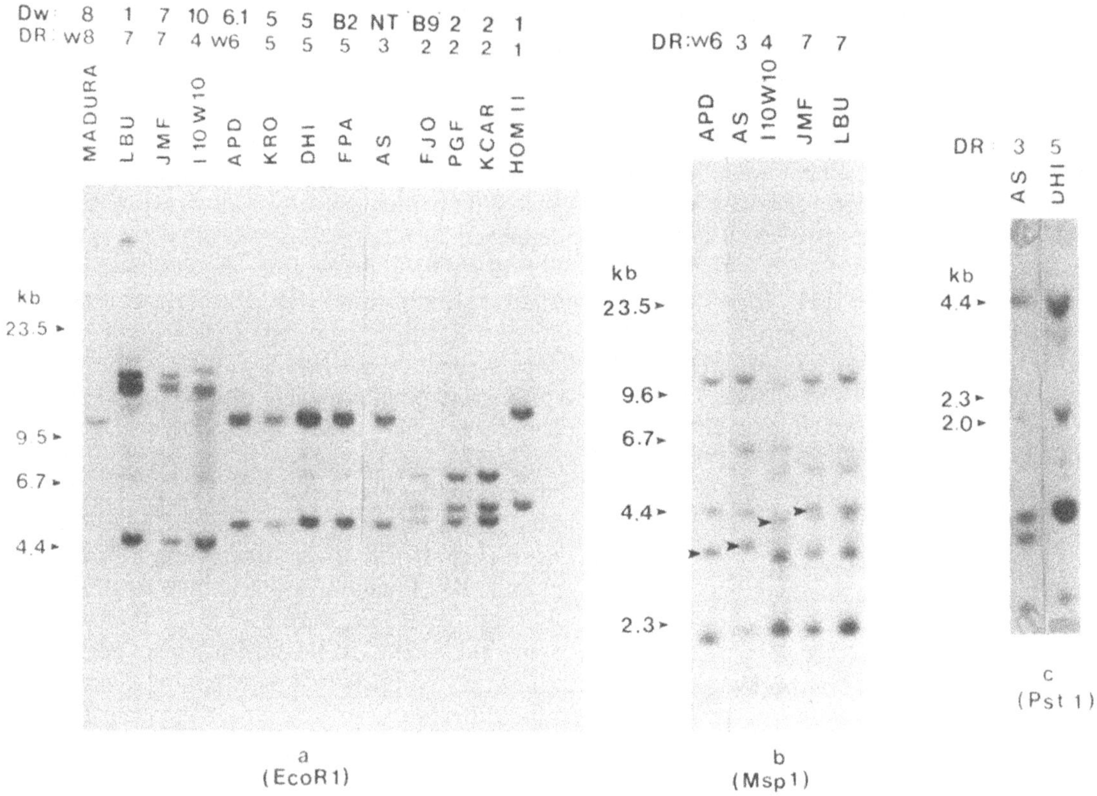

Fig. 1a–c. Southern blot obtained after hybridization of the DR-β cDNA probe to genomic DNA isolated from various human HTCs after digestion with, **a** *Eco*RI; **b** *Msp*I; **c** *Pst*I

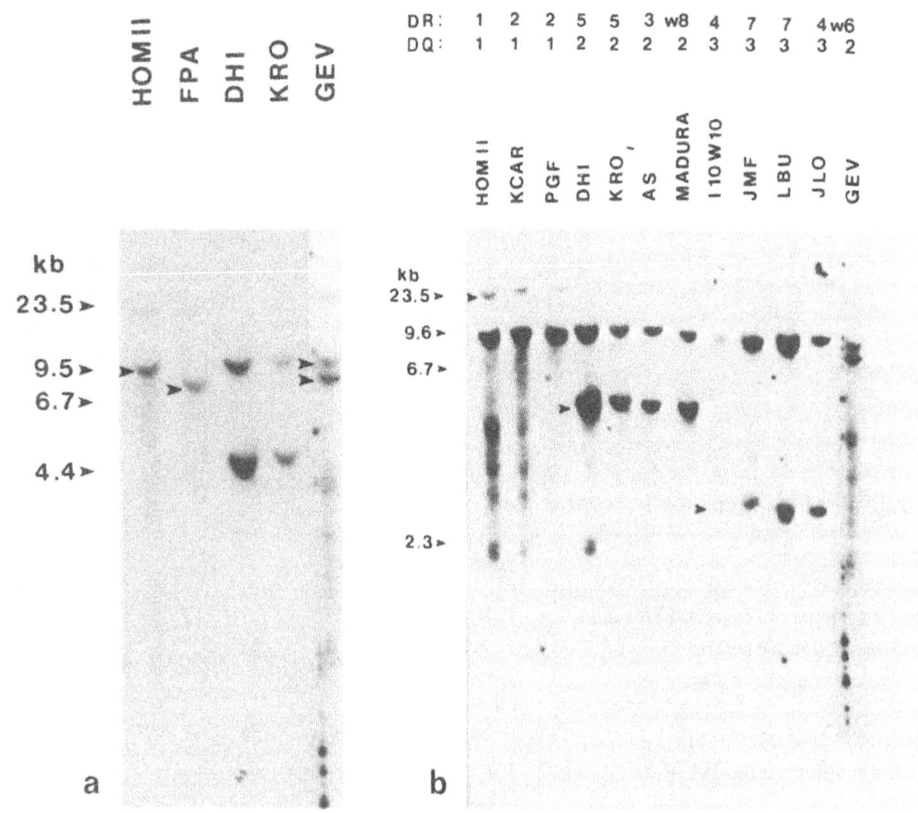

Fig. 2a, b. Southern blot obtained after hybridization of the DQ-α genomic DNA probe to genomic DNA isolated from various human HTCs after digestion with *Pst*I

The DNA produced from FPA has a smaller *Pst*I DX-α fragment than the DNA from all the other cells tested (Fig. 2a). This polymorphism could be due to mutation of the *Pst*I sites or it could be that these two different *Pst*I fragments are alleles. The latter explanation is preferred, as the *Pst*I digest of the DNA of cell line GEV has both these DX-α fragments (Fig. 2a). The cell line GEV could be heterozygous for the DX-α locus. More extensive polymorphism was observed with a second *Pst*I fragment using the DQ-α probe (Fig. 2b). The polymorphism appears to correlate best, but only partially, with the DR, DQ specificities obtained by serotyping. The DQw1 specificity (of the DR1 and DR2 cells) is associated with a *Pst*I-produced DNA fragment (*Pst*I fragment) of about 24 kb, the DRw52 specificity (of DR3, DR5 and DRw8 cells) with a *Pst*I fragment of about 5 kb and the DRw53 specificity (of DR4 and DR7 cells) with a *Pst*I fragment of about 3 kb (Fig. 2b). However, there are some important exceptions to this rule. The cell lines FPA and GEV, which typed as DQw1, DRw52, have different RFLP patterns from those of the other DRw52 cells tested. Both cell lines have the 24-kb *Pst*I fragment that is associated with the DQw1 specificity (Fig. 2a). However, the 5-kb *Pst*I fragment (which associates with the other DRw52-positive cells tested) is absent in both FPA and GEV (Fig. 2a). It is therefore likely that the DNA fragment that associates with the DRw52 specificity for GEV and FPA has "*Pst*I sites" which differ from those of the other DRw52-positive cells. Alternatively, the anti-DRw52 reagents used in phenotyping these cells cross-react with non-DRw52 determinants.

Some of these gene fragments which seem to be associated with certain DR, DQ specificities segregate independently within families. Figure 3 shows the DR, DQ typings of the cells and the RFLP of their DNA from a selected family as analyzed by Southern blotting. Family members who are DQw1, DRw53 have the *Pst*I fragments of 24-kb and 5-kb respectively, but one of the offspring, SHA, who is DRw53 homozygous, has only the *Pst*I fragment of 5-kb (Fig. 3), as expected. This confirms that the *Pst*I fragment which appears to be associated with DR, DQ specificities is an independent gene fragment.

Three different *Pst*I RFLP patterns were obtained with the different HTCs studied using the DQ-β DNA probe (Fig. 4). A split of the DQw1 specificity with different DR-phenotyped HTCs can be distinguished: the DQw1 RFLP pattern of DR1 cells (Hom II) is the same as the DQw1 RFLP patterns of DRw6 cells (GEV and Daudi), whereas a different DQw1 pattern is obtained for DR2 cells (KCAR) and the unusual DR5/DQw1-positive

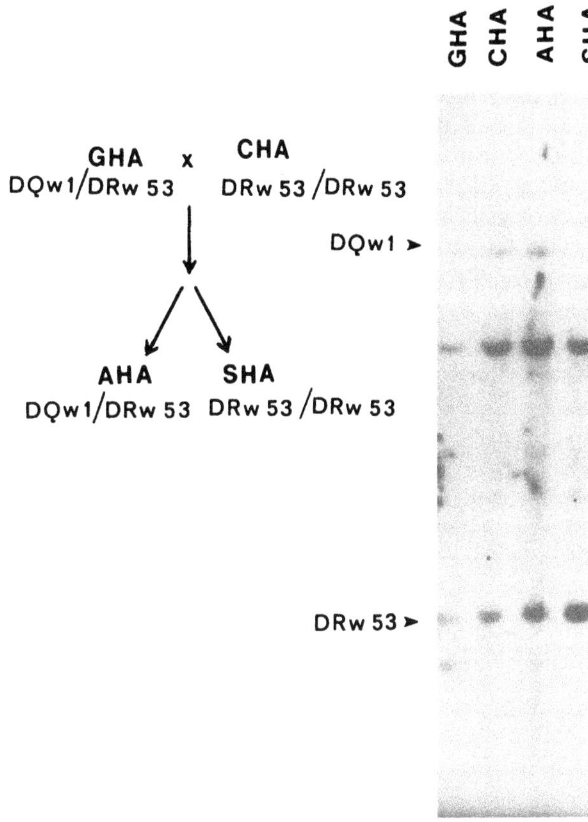

Fig. 3. Southern blot obtained after hybridization of the DQ-α genomic DNA probe to genomic DNA isolated from members of a selected family after digestion with *Pst*I

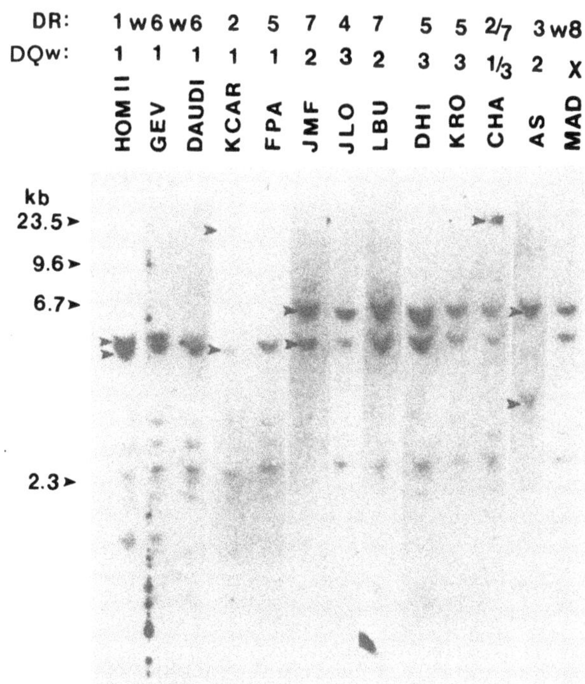

Fig. 4. Southern blot obtained after hybridization of the DQ-β cDNA probe to genomic DNA isolated from various human HTCs after digestion with *Pst*I

cells (FPA) (Fig. 4). The RFLP patterns for most DQw2- and DQw3-positive cells are similar (Fig. 4). The cell line AS, which is DQw2, has a unique RFLP pattern different from the other DQw2 cells (Fig. 4). It would be interesting to see if this difference is reflected in the antigenic profile of this particular cell line. In addition, the cell line Madura, which typed DQ-"X" has the same RFLP pattern as most DQw2- and DQw3-positive cells. This similarity can be attributed to common *Pst*I sites shared by these cells.

The DP-α DNA probe does not detect any polymorphism with a selected panel of HTCs employed in this study: fragments of about 23 kb, 4.3 kb and 2.5 kb were seen when using *Eco*RI, *Msp*I and *Pst*I respectively.

The DP-β probe detected two DP-β-like genes for each of the HTCs studied. One of these two fragments is constant (about 1 kb) whereas the other is polymorphic (either 2 or 4 kb; Fig. 5). The 4-kb fragment appears to be present in DPw2-positive HTCs as defined by primed lymphocyte typing, but the 2-kb fragment does not correlate with any DP phenotype.

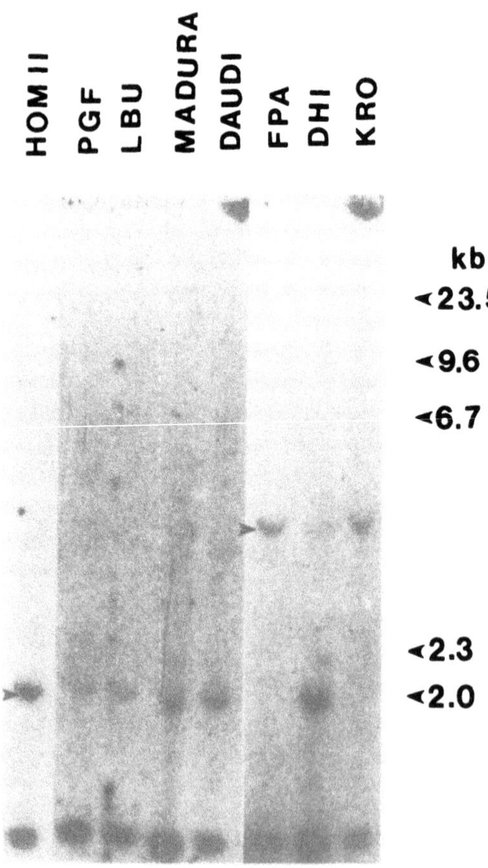

Fig. 5. Southern blot obtained after hybridization of the DP-β genomic DNA probe to various HTCs after digestion with *Pst*I

Discussion

In this study, we have compared the RFLP patterns for a selected panel of HTCs after Southern blot hybridization with different class II DNA probes. We have not been able to detect any structural polymorphism at the DNA level for the DR-α and DP-α genes. On the other hand, the DR-β, DQ-α, DQ-β and DP-β genes show various degrees of polymorphism. We have tried to correlate the polymorphism with specificities detected by conventional serotyping methods. Although correlations can be seen in some cases, we have always been able to find some exceptions. It is possible that serological determinants are encoded by different genes which will consequently give different RFLP patterns with some of the DNA probes used in this study. It may be helpful to use a combination of approaches in order to associate serological specificities and RFLP patterns. For example, Southern blot analysis of deletion mutants and family members are most valuable in this context. Moreover, serologically defined specificities are possibly determined by both the class II α and β chains. It may be difficult, therefore, to compare serological determinants and RFLP patterns which only consider one individual chain of a particular gene at a time. The solution to this problem may be obtained through molecular cloning studies of these genes.

Acknowledgments. We wish to thank P. Peterson, J. Silver, S. Goyert and W. Bodmer for providing the DNA probes used in this study.

References

1. Kaufman JF, Auffray C, Korman AJ, Shackelford DA, Strominger J (1984) Cell 36:1
2. Tanigaki N, Tosi R (1982) Immunol Rev 66:5
3. Jaraquemada D, Okoye R, Ollier W, Awad J, Festenstein H (1984) This volume, p 472
4. Terasaki PI, Park MS, Bernoco D, Opelz G, Mickey MR (1980) In: Terasaki PI (ed) Histocompatibility testing 1980. UCLA, Los Angeles, p 1
5. Shaw S, Kavathas P, Pollack MS, Charmot D, Mawas C (1981) Nature 293:745
6. Auffray C, Lillie JW, Annot D, Grossberger D, Kappes D, Strominger J (1984) Nature 308:327
7. Trowsdale J, Lee J, Carey J, Grosveld F, Bodmer J, Bodmer W (1983) Proc Natl Acad Sci USA 80:1972
8. Larhammer D, Schenning L, Gustafsson K, Wiman K, Claesson L, Rask L, Peterson PA (1982) Proc Natl Acad Sci USA 79:3687
9. Wiman K, Larhammer D, Claesson L, et al (1982) Proc Natl Acad Sci USA 79:1703
10. Southern EM (1975) J Mol Biol 98:503
11. Rigby PWJ, Diekmann M, Rhodes C, Berg P (1977) J Mol Biol 113:237

Mouse L Cells Expressing Human HLA-DR Antigens After Transfection with Class II Genes Do Not Stimulate Human T Lymphocytes

T. Moen[1], C. de Préval[2], C. Rabourdin-Combe[2], B. Mach[2], G. Gaudernack[1], E. Bondevik[1], and E. Thorsby[1]

1 Institute of Transplantation Immunology, The National Hospital, Oslo 1, Norway
2 Department of Microbiology, University of Geneva Medical School, 1205 Geneva, Switzerland

Introduction

The HLA class II determinants are involved in activation of T4 lymphocytes. These dimeric cell membrane molecules are glycoproteins comprised of one α and one β chain subunit and are expressed mainly on B cells and accessory lymphoid cells [7]. Recent data has revealed that the class II region most probably encompasses a complexity of loci: DR coding for three β and one α chain, DQ and DP each coding for two β and two α chains [2, 11].
Recently it was possible to co-transfect the mouse L cell line LMTK− with cloned human genes for DRβ, DRα, and the DR associated invariant chain. The resulting cell line 22.9.1 expresses human DR molecules at a high concentration and as a stable trait [15, 1]. The transfected DR β chain gene originated from a DR4, w6 gene donor and has been identified as the DRw52 (BR3)-positive β chain coded for on the DRw6-carrying haplotype [2, 4].
The present functional studies were performed to test if the DR-expressing 22.9.1 cell line was capable of activating human T cells in analogy with human DR-expressing cells.

Material and Methods

Cells: The thymidine kinase-deficient murine L cell line LMTK−, its DR-transfected derivate 22.9.1, and a lymphoid cell line (LCL) from the gene donor (DR4, w6) were prepared as described [15]. A homozygous LCL, HHK, shown to carry the same β chain as the 22.9.1 cell line [3], was provided by M. Giphardt, Leiden, and LCLs expressing the DRw6 subspecificities were made locally by EBV transformation of homozygous typing cells (HTCs). The cell lines were cultured in RPMI 1640 supplied with glutamine and 10% FBS, penicillin, and streptomycin. Purified T cells and non-T cells were made from peripheral blood mononuclear cells (PBMs) by rosetting with AET-treated sheep red blood cells. The T cells were subsequently incubated for 1 h for removal of remaining adherent cells.
IL-1 was made by stimulating adherent cells (2×10^6/ml) with lipopolysaccharide (LPS) 10 µg/ml [8] for 48 h in the presence of indomethacine 5 µg/ml. The crude supernatant was subsequently added to the cell cultures by substituting one-third of the culture medium.
Proliferative assays were mainly performed as described elsewhere [14]. PBMs (5×10^4) or T cells (4×10^4) were used as responding cells. Stimulating cells were treated with mitomycin (Medac) for 20 min at 37 °C, 100 µg/ml, and mainly used at concentrations of 2.5×10^4 (L cells and non-T cells) and 6×10^3 (LCLs).
Assays for measuring induction of IL-2 receptor were performed using the monoclonal antibody (Moab) anti-Tac kindly provided by Thomas A. Waldman [10, 18]. 5×10^5 T cells in tissue culture flasks (25 cm^2 growth area) were incubated with 25 µl Moab on ice for 60 min. The second step was performed with 50 µg radioiodinated $F(ab)_2$ rabbit antimouse IgG [17].
Detection of DR on the transfected L cells: Binding of Moabs specific for different epitopes on DR molecules was quantitated by an indirect radioimmunoassay (see above). The results (not shown) were consistent with earlier reports [15].

Results

Activation of Nonprimed Allogeneic T cells

Figure 1 depicts data from one of three experiments giving similar results. It can be seen that within the stimulating cell concentrations tested, allogeneic PBMs stimulate strongest at a high concentration (1×10^5) and LCLs at a lower concentration (6×10^3). In contrast, neither the DR-transfected L cell line 22.9.1 nor the untransfected cell line LMTK− demonstrate any stimulation above the autologous control.
The lack of stimulating capacity could possibly be explained by lack of IL-1 induction or by an inhibitory effect of the L cells. To study these possibilities, purified T cells were stimulated in parallel with a Dw6 homozygous LCL and the L cell lines 22.9.1 and LMTK−. For each combination, tests were also carried out in the presence of added IL-1 con-

Histocompatibility Testing 1984
Edited by E. D. Albert et al.

taining supernatants, and both induction of IL-2 receptor and incorporation of ^{3}H-thymidine were measured on days 3–5 of culture. Figure 2 depicts the results on day 5 (similar findings were made on days 3 and 4). The LCLs activate T cells strongly, and this effect can be somewhat augmented by adding exogenous IL-1. No activation was exerted by the DR-transfected L cell line or by the untransfected control, even in the presence of IL-1-containing medium. The kinetics of IL-2 receptor induction and ^{3}H-thymidine incorporation were found to be very similar.

Next we studied whether the 22.9.1 cell line had an inhibitory effect on T cell activation. The results are shown in Fig. 3. Neither the induction of IL-2 receptors nor the incorporation of ^{3}H-thymidine when confronted with allogeneic LCLs were significantly reduced in the presence of the 22.9.1. cells.

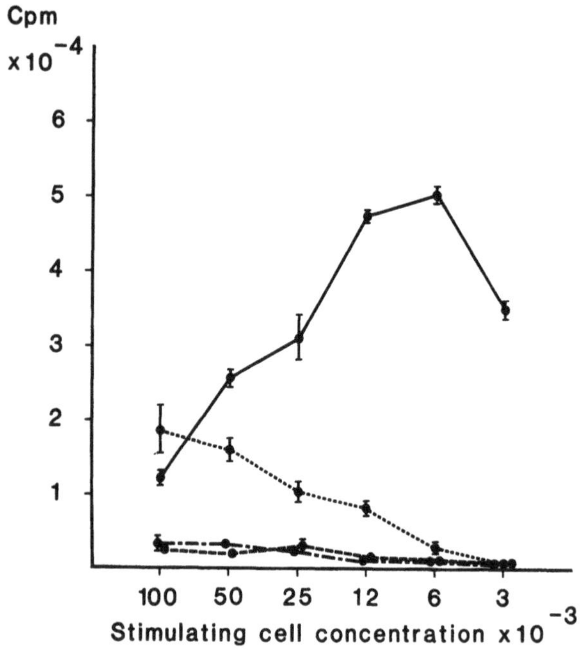

Fig. 1. Lymphocyte-stimulating capacity of different cells: ——•—— LCLs (Dw6 homozygous), ----•---- PBMs (Dw4, 6), -—-•—- L cells (22.9.1), — —•— — L cells (LMTK–). Responding cells were 5×10^4 PBMs. Proliferation given as mean ± s.e. of triplicates harvested on day 5 of culture after 16 h incorporation of ^{3}H- thymidine

Activation of Primed T Cells

We first attempted to prime T cells to the 22.9.1 cell line. However, upon restimulation, no response was seen. We then primed PBMs to the different Dw6 subtypes, using as stimulating cells LCLs made from HTC. The primed cells were restimulated by the same cell lines and by the L cells 22.9.1 and LMTK–. The LCLs restimulated the primed PBMs strongly and showed extensive cross-reactivity. However, no proliferative response to the DR-transfected 22.9.1 cells could be seen (not shown). Experiments with priming specifically to DRw52 are continuing. Adding the 22.9.1 cell line to the culture did not inhibit the proliferative response to LCLs.

Use of 22.9.1 Cells as Antigen-Presenting Cells to Sensitized T Cells

We then tested in repeated experiments the responses of purified T cells to antigens such as herpes simplex virus (HSV) and PPD. The response of an individual (Dw3, w6) to the HSV antigen is shown in Fig. 4. It can be seen that the Dw6 homo-

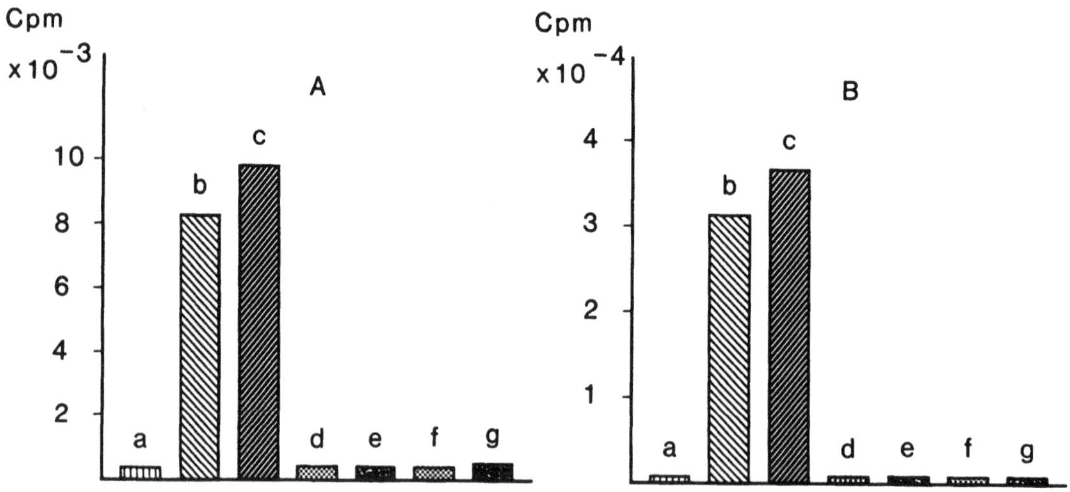

Fig. 2 A, B. T cell activation measured by induction of IL-2 receptor (**A**) and proliferation (**B**) on day 5 of culture. Columns depict T cells plus *a*, IL-1; *b*, LCL; *c*, LCL + IL-1; *d*, LMTK–; *e*, LMTK– + IL-1; *f*, 22.9.1; *g*, 22.9.1 + IL-1

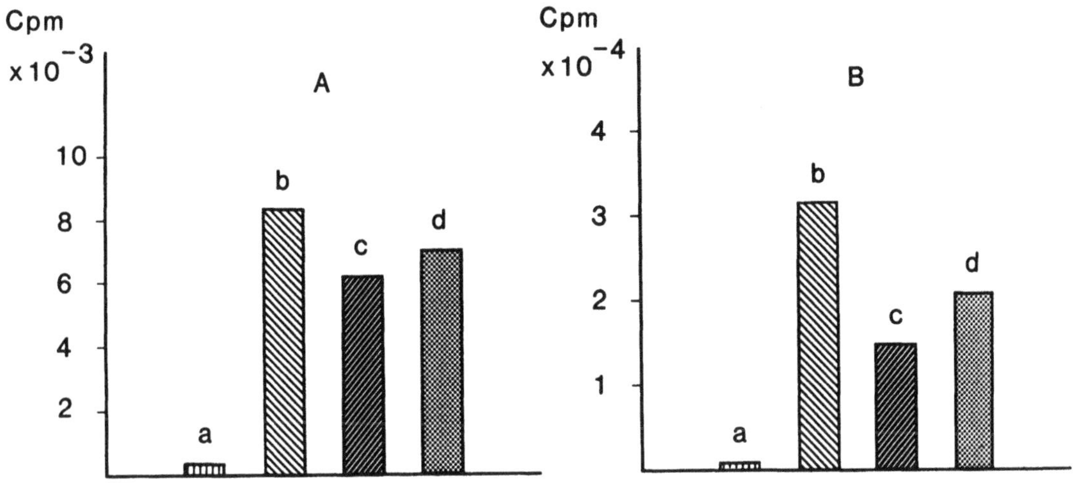

Fig. 3A, B. Attempted inhibition of IL-2 receptor LMTK-induction (**A**) and proliferation (**B**). Columns depict T cells plus: *a*, IL-1; *b*, LCL; *c*, LCL +; *d*, LCL + 22.9.1

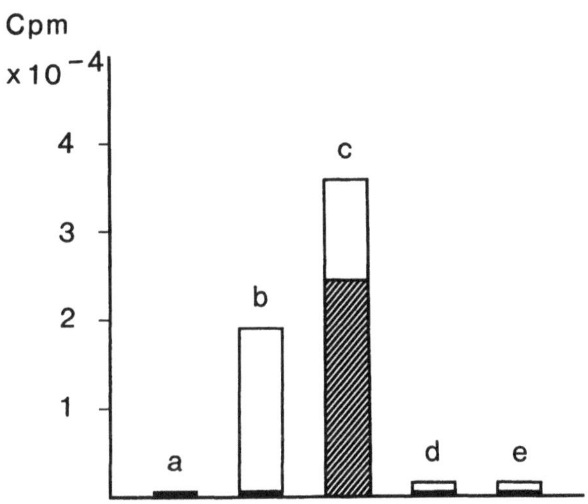

Fig. 4. Presentation of HSV antigen to T cells measured by proliferation. Columns depict T cells plus: *a*, HSV; *b*, autologous non-T cells + HSV; *c*, B-LCL HHK + HSV; *d*, LMTK− + HSV; *e*, 22.9.1 + HSV

zygous cell line HHK, in addition to inducing allogeneic stimulation, was also able to induce a superimposed HSV-specific response of a magnitude similar to that of autologous non-T cells. The 22.9.1 and LMTK− cell lines were not able to induce any significant HSV-specific responses.

Discussion

The 22.9.1 cell line has been found to express human DR molecules as a stable trait through months of culture [15]. Using serological techniques, as well as by analysis of the cloned genes, indications have been found that the DR β chain expressed on the transfected cell line is BR3, which is one of three DR β chains of the DRw6 haplotype [4, 6, 11, 16]. However, as reported here, we are unable to demonstrate any alloactivating ability of the 22.9.1 cell line, nor it was able to present antigens in a DR-restricted way to sensitized T cells.

The explanation for this lack of function is not evident. The expression of a human DR molecule in a xenogeneic cell may possibly modify the structure so much that function is disturbed even if the serotype (i.e., DRw52) is conserved. The seemingly inadequate functional expression of the DR molecule on the 22.9.1 cell line might be due to disturbances in transcription or splicing of the DNA or to other metabolic failures or interactions with murine genes. Alternatively the L cell could be inadequate for some auxiliary function in T cell activation. Both murine [12] and human [5] class I α chain genes have been introduced into the LMTK− cell with subsequent clear expression of class I antigens that could be recognized both in serological tests and by CTLs. Lemonnier et al. [9], however, found that after corresponding transfection of the LMTK− cell line with cloned human class I α chain genes, the structure of the associated murine β_2-microglobulin expressed on these cells was changed so that it reacted with murine anti human β_2-microglobulin. In contrast, when introducing a murine IA β chain gene into a murine B cell tumor line, Germain et al. [3] could demonstrate alloactivation by this gene, and Norcross et al. [13] have shown that L cells transformed with murine IA α and β genes can present antigen to cloned T cells and T cell hybridomas.

Further experiments with gene cloning and transfection of cells will probably solve these problems.

Summary

A mouse L cell line, 22.9.1, which permanently expresses human DR molecules at high concentration after transfection, was studied to see if it could stimulate human T cells. We found that the DR-expressing cell line did not induce proliferation or expression of IL-2 receptors of human T cells, nor was it able to present antigen (HSV or PPD) to T cells from sensitized DRw6-positive donors. The reason why the 22.9.1 mouse cell line cannot replace human DR-expressing cells in these functional tests is not clear, but may be explained by modification of the DR molecule when expressed in the foreign cell membranes or by insufficient function of a particular kind of DR molecules in the cells.

References

1. dePreval C, Rabourdin-Combe C, Gorski J, Mach B (1984) Expression of a single HLA-DR antigen on DNA transfected mouse cells: analysis by a panel of monoclonal antibodies. In: Disease markers, vol. 2, special issue: human MHC class II antigens; genetics structure and function. Wiley, New York (in press)
2. dePreval C, Gorski J, Mack B (1984) Molecular complexity of the HLA-DR, DC, and SB genes and genotypic split of HLA-DR serological specificities by "DNA typing" (this volume)
3. Germain RN, Norcross MA, Margulies DH (1983) Functional expression of a transfected murine class II MHC gene. Nature 306:190–194
4. Gorski J, et al. Manuscript in preparation
5. Herman A, Parham P, Weissman SM, Engelhard VH (1983) Recognition by xenogeneic cytotoxic T lymphocytes of cells expressing HLA-A2 or HLA-B7 after DNA-mediated gene transfer. Proc Natl Acad Sci USA 80:5056–5060
6. Hurley KC, Giles RC, Capra JD (1983) The human MHC: evidence for multiple HLA-D region genes. Immunol Today 4:219–226
7. Kaufman JF, Auffrey C, Korman AJ, Shackelford DA, Strominger J (1984) The class II molecules of the human and murine major histocompatibility complex. Cell 36:2–13
8. Pollach S, Micali A, Kinne DW, Enker WE, Geller N, Oettgen HF, Hoffman MK (1983) Endotoxin-induced in vitro release of interleukin-1 by cancer patients' monocytes: relation to stage of disease. Int J Cancer 32:733–736
9. Lemonnier FA, le Bouteiller PP, Malissen B, Golstein P, Malissen M, Mishal Z, Caillol DH, Jordan BR, Kourilsky FM (1983) Transformation of murine LMTK-cells with purified HLA class I genes. I. Modification of confirmation of murine β_2-microglobulin upon its association with HLA heavy chains. J Immunol 130:1432–1437
10. Leonard WJ, Depper JM, Uchiyama T, Smith KA, Waldmann TA, Greene WC (1982) A monoclonal antibody that appears to recognize the receptor for human T cell growth factor: partial characterization of the receptor. Nature 300:267–269
11. Long EO, Gorski J, Mach B (1984) Structural relationship of the SB β-chain gene to HLA-D-region genes and murine I-region genes. Nature 310:233–235
12. Malissen B, Steinmetz M, McMillan M, Pierres M, Hood L (1983) Expression of I-A^k class II genes in mouse L cells after DNA-mediated gene transfer. Nature 305:440–443
13. Norcross MA, Bentley DM, Margulies DH, Germain RN (1984) Membrane Ia expression and antigen-presenting accessory cell function of L cells transfected with class II major histocompatibility complex genes. J Exp Med 160:1316–1337
14. Moen T (1982) Primed lymphocyte typing (PLT): application in typing for HLA-D locus determinants. In: Ferrone S, Solheim BG (eds) HLA typing: methodology and clinical aspects. II. CRC Press, Boca Raton pp 71–81
15. Rabourdin-Combe C, Mach B (1983) Expression of HLA-DR antigens at the surface of mouse L cells cotransfected with cloned human genes. Nature 303:670–674
16. Tanigaki N, Tosi R (1982) The genetic control of human Ia alloantigens: a three-loci model derived from immunological analysis of supertypic specificities. Immunol Rev 66:5–37
17. Qvigstad E, Gaudernack G, Thorsby E (1984) Antigen-specific T cell clones restricted by DR, MT or SB class II HLA molecules. Inhibition studies with monoclonal HLA-specific antibodies. Hum Immunol (in press)
18. Uchiyama T, Broder S, Waldmann TA (1981) A monoclonal antibody (anti-Tac) reactive with activated and functionally nature human T cells. J Immunol 126:1393–1397

Modification of Immunogenicity of Leukaemic Cells by DNA Mediated Gene Transfer *

K.M. Hui [1], F. Grosveld [2], and H. Festenstein [1]

1 Dept. of Immunology, London Hospital Medical College, Turner Street, London E1 2AD, UK
2 Dept. of Gene Structure and Expression, National Institute for Medical Research, Mill Hill, London, UK

The spontaneous AKR leukaemia K36 has been extensively studied in our laboratories. This tumour does not express the H-$2K^k$ gene product and is resistant to T cell cytolysis. The H-$2K^k$ antigen is the restriction element for T cell killing of Gross virus-infected AKR cells [1]. We have now introduced a normal H-$2K^k$ cloned gene c27.2 (M.

* These studies were supported by the Cancer Research Campaign and the Medical Research Council of Great Britain

Steinmetz), together with the G418-resistant plasmid pTCF into this tumour by calcium phosphate-mediated gene transfer. Between 8 and 20 transformants per 10^6 cells were selected in medium containing 800 μg/ml G418. From over 300 transformants we selected a series of clones that expressed different amounts of H-$2K^k$ molecule on the cell surface for study. DNA was isolated from each of the selected transformants and analysed by Southern blot. Hybridisation of the plasmid pTCF (vector), or an H-$2K^k$ DNA probe to the blots, showed that each of the transformants contained one to three copies of the exogenous H-$2K^k$ gene. Moreover, the presence of H-$2K^k$-specific mRNA was demonstrated by SI núclease protection mapping using an H-$2K^k$-specific DNA probe (S. Kvist, personal communication) from the third exon-intron boundary of the H-$2K^k$ gene and mRNA isolated from these transformed clones. Subsequently, we showed the presence of the H-$2K^k$ gene products in the transformed cells by radiobinding and immunoprecipitation studies with monoclonal antibodies. Large variations in the amount of the gene products were detected in different transformed clones when they were analysed by radiobinding assays. Those clones, which express a relatively high level of the H-$2K^k$ gene products, were rejected by syngeneic AKR mice (Table 1). The ease of rejection corresponded to the amount of detectable H-$2K^k$ antigen in the various clones studied (Table 1). The ability of these transformed cells to grow was regained when the H-$2K^k$ gene product was "blocked" with anti-H-$2K^k$ monoclonal antibodies before injection into the recipient mice. Mice that had rejected these transformed clones were also immune against the original, unmodified, K36.16 tumour cells. These experiments show the importance of the expression of MHC Class I products (both quantitative and qualitative) in host-tumour interactions.

Table 1. Correlation of H-$2K^K$ expression and clone rejection

Clones	^{125}I-Sheep anti-mouse Ig $F(ab')_2$ fragments (net cpm) using 11.41 (anti-H-$2K^k$)	Tumour incidence in AKR mice
K36.16	0	10/10
pTCF.K36.16	92	10/10
c27-2-11	364	0/10
c27.2-14	376	1/5
c27.2-34	1 334	0/5
c27.2-58	257	4/5
c27.2-72	320	0/5
369	19 416	NT

Acknowledgments. We would like to thank M. Steinmetz for the cosmid c27.2 and S. Kvist for information on the preparation of the H-$2K^k$ sequence DNA probe for the SI nuclease protection analysis.

Reference

1. Festenstein H, Schmidt W (1981) Immunol Rev 60: 85–127

Genetics of HLA

Precise Location of HLA Genes on Chromosome 6

V. Lepage[1], N. Leporrier[2], M. Sasportes[1], G. Hauptmann[3], A. Marcelli-Barge[1], and L. Degos[1]

1 INSERM U93, Hôpital Saint-Louis, 2, Place du Docteur Fournier, 75010 Paris, France
2 CHU de Caen, Laboratoire de Cytogénétique, 14000 Caen, France
3 C.T.S. de Strasbourg, 68000 Strasbourg, France

The location of HLA on the short arm of chromosome 6 was ascertained by several studies on cases of 6 trisomy. Two recent reports have pin-pointed the position of HLA: Berger et al. [1] observed a 6p 2105 GpTer trisomy with an HLA-A, B, C, and DR trisomy, but they found a positive MLR between the trisomic patient and her mother, who transmitted both HLA haplotypes.
Conversely, Ferrando et al. [2] studied a 6pTer trisomy with no HLA-A, B trisomy.

Table 1. Genetic profile of Family B

	A	C	B	Bf	C2	C4	DR	DQw	GLO
Grand-	1	w4	12	F	1	A3B1	7, w53		1
father	32	w6	37	F	1	A3B1	2	1	2
Grand-	24	w6	21	S	1	AQ0B1	2	1	2
mother	30	w5	18	F1	1	A6BQ0	3, w52		2
Father	1	w4	12	F	1	A3B1	7, w53		1
	24	w6	21	S	1	AQ0B1	2	1	2
Mother	2	w7	7	S	1	AQ0B1	7, w53		1
	w33	–	14	S	1	A3B1	1	1	2
Trisomic	1	w4	12	F	1	A3B1	7, w53		1
patient	24	w6	21	S	1	AQ0B1	2	1	2
	w33	–	14	S	1	A3B1	1	1	2

We present a case with the 6p trisomy restricted to the 6p12–6p221 region. HLA-A, B, C, and DR polymorphisms were informative. The propositus also received a rare C4 allele from the first haplotype of the father and a Bf polymorphic allele from the second haplotype of the father. Intrafamilial MLR confirmed the presence of both paternal haplotypes. Table 1 gives the family details. This case confirms the presence of HLA-A, B, C, DR, C4, and Bf on the short arm of chromosome 6. The position of the breakpoint means that the structural and regulatory genes are located between 6p12 and 6p22. The presence of a trisomy for MRL reaction, compared with the case reported by Berger et al., locates a gene involved in the MLR distinct from HLA-DR between 6p12 and 6p2105.

References

1. Berger R, Bernheim A, Sasportes M, Hauptmann G, Hors J, Legrand L, Fellons M (1979) Regional mapping of the HLA on the short arm of chromosome 6. Clinical Genetics 15:245–251
2. Ferrando P, San Koman C, Rodriguez de Cordoba S, Arnaiz-Villena A (1981) Partial trisomy 6p: 46, XX, –10, der (10), t (6; 10) (p22; q26) pat and HLA localisation

A Structural Locus for Coagulation Factor XIIIA (*F13A*) Is Located Distal to HLA on the Short Arm of Chromosome 6 in Man

B. Olaisen[1], T. Gedde-Dahl Jr.[2], E. Thorsby[3], and P. Teisberg[4]

1 Institute of Forensic Medicine, University of Oslo, 0027 Oslo, Norway
2 Dept. of Genetics, NHIK, Radiumhospitalet, 0027 Oslo, Norway
3 Tissue Typing Laboratory, Rikshospitalet, 0027 Oslo, Norway
4 Medical Dept. Rikshospitalet, 0027 Oslo 1, Norway

In 1979, Board [1] described a genetic polymorphism of coagulation factor FXIIIA of plasma and platelets (the a2 subunit, FXIIIA). We report linkage and association studies with this new polymorphic gene marker. The family material studied (Oslo-NHIK material) comprises a total of 375 matings with 1295 offspring. This material has been typed in some 40 polymorphic gene marker systems, including chromosome 6 markers PGM3; GLO; HLA-A, B, C, DR; C4A, C4B; C2; and Bf. *FXIIIA* typing was performed by high-voltage agarose gel electrophoresis followed by passive transfer of protein bands to nitrocellulose sheets. FXIIIA bands were visualized through the use of specific anti-FXIIIA antibody and peroxidase-conjugated anti-IgG antibody. *F13A* linkage information was obtained in altogether 111 matings. There is linkage between *F13A* and HLA region genes with maximum lod score 7.60 at a recombination fraction $\theta = 0.18$ in males. Given linkage, the 95% confidence limits are $\theta = 0.12$ and $\theta = 0.26$. Lod scores rule out linkage between *F13A* and *PGM3* at all θ's below 0.12. Taken together this means that *F13A* is located distal to the HLA region on chromosome 6p. In females, the maximum lod score between *F13A* and HLA region genes is 0.19, $\theta = 0.42$,

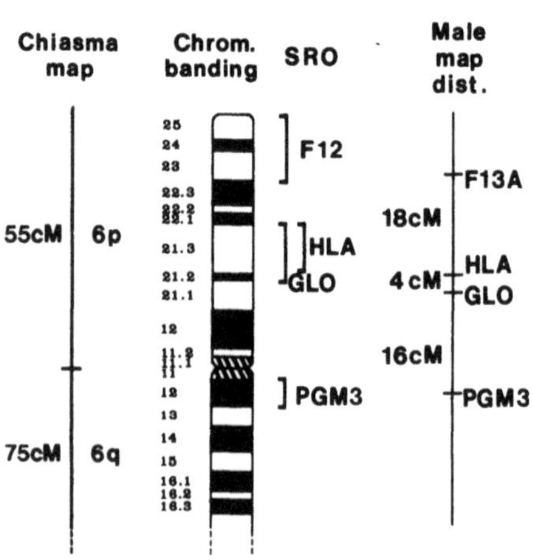

Fig. 1. Genetic map of some parts of chromosome 6

Histocompatibility Testing 1984
Edited by E. D. Albert et al.

thus indicating a considerable sex difference in recombination in this chromosome region. Haplotype association studies have been performed in 336 haplotypes with deducable *F13A* alleles. No indication of association between *F13A* alleles and any of the alleles within 6p complement genes, HLA genes, or *GLO* was found. Gene distances between *F13A* and these genes are far too large for linkage disequilibrium to occur. Figure 1 shows a genetic map of parts of chromosome 6; for all genes except *F13A* the data have been taken from published reviews [2, 3]. The existence of a polymorphic marker gene towards 6pter will be of considerable value in future gene mapping work. Furthermore, the known existence of another coagulation factor gene, *F12*, in the same region may indicate a cluster of related genes within mappable distance of the HLA region.

References

1. Board PG (1979) Polymorphism of the A subunit of coagulation factor XIII. Am J Hum Genet 31:116–124
2. Weitkamp LR, Lamm LU (1982) Report of the Committee on the Genetic Constitution of Chromosome 6. Cytogenet Cell Genet 32:130–143
3. Robson EB, Lamm LU (1984) Report of the Committee on the Genetic Constitution of Chromosome 6. Cytogenet Cell Genet 37:47–70

The Selective Origin of Linkage Disequilibrium in the HLA Region

W. Klitz and G. Thomson

Genetics Department, University of California, Berkeley, CA 94720, USA

The linkage disequilibrium patterns observed between tightly linked loci, such as the HLA loci, can indicate the nature of evolutionary events, particularly selection events, acting on the region. We have developed a method, disequilibrium pattern analysis, for examining the disequilibrium distribution of a population of two-locus haplotypes. Specific quantifiable patterns are predicted as a result of selective events.

Results have been obtained for deterministic models in which the haplotype A_1B_1 increases in frequency due to selection. All linkage disequilibrium values between the alleles at the two loci of interest are initially assumed to be zero:

1. The positive disequilibria of the favored haplotype A_1B_1, and the unrelated haplotypes A_iB_j ($i = 2, \ldots, r$, $j = 2, \ldots, s$) will be balanced by the negative disequilibria of the related A_iB_1 and A_1B_j haplotypes.
2. The negative disequilibria of the A_iB_1 haplotypes will be proportional to the A_i allele frequency. The normalized disequilibria values will be equal. Equivalent results hold for the A_1B_j haplotypes.
3. If selection is operating on k haplotypes concurrently, we except $k(r+s) - 2\,(1+2+\ldots k)$ haplotypes in the negative space and the remainder in the positive space.

A published report of HLA-A and B locus haplotypes from a large ($n = 5202$) Danish study [1] has been analyzed. Subdivision of the linkage disequilibria revealed cases where patterns indicative of a strong selection event were apparent, as well as cases which did not exhibit such patterns.

Haplotype A1, B8, which has the highest positive disequilibrium ($D = 0.0766$, $D' = 0.728$) reveals a pattern indicative of selection. For the B8 graph, A1, B8 is the only haplotype in the positive space, while all related haplotypes with B8 but not A1 fall in the negative space with disequilibria values approximately proportional to the frequency of the unshared A allele. The presence or absence of patterning is not a function of high or low frequencies of the constituent alleles. We have identified six haplotypes which show in varying extents the patterning of a selected event. These haplotypes are A1, B8 and A3, B7 (selection pattern observed for both the A and B alleles), A25, B18 and A29, B44 (patterning only for the A alleles) and A2, B15 and A1, B17 (patterning only for the B alleles).

Reference

1. Hansen HE, Larsen SO, Ryder LP, Nielsen LS (1979) HLA-A, B haplotype frequencies in 5202 unrelated Danes by a maximum likelihood method of gene counting. Tissue Antigens 13:143–153

Histocompatibility Testing 1984
Edited by E. D. Albert et al.

HLA-A, B Genes in the World and the Effect of Climate

A. Piazza [1], and P. Menozzi [2]

1 Istituto di Genetica Medica, Università di Torino, 10100 Torino, Italy
2 Istituto di Ecologia, Università di Parma, 43100 Parma, Italy

Material and Methods

The information contained in the HLA-A (A1, A2, A3, A9, A10, A11, A28) and HLA-B (B5, B7, B8, B12, B13, B14, B15, B16, B17, B18, B21, Bw22, B27, B35, B40) gene frequencies from 213 world aboriginal populations has been condensed in trichromic maps using techniques described elsewhere [1]. Global trends in variation are substantially similar to those already published on the basis of half of the populations [2], and they are being combined in map form and will be published elsewhere.

Table 1. Corrected correlations between HLA allele frequencies and climatic factors

Allele	Temperature [a]		Humidity [b]		Precip. [c]	Rainy days [d]
	Min.	Max.	Min.	Max.		
HLA-A1	−0.30				−0.40	
HLA-A3	−0.36	−0.30			−0.50	−0.30
HLA-A9					0.50	0.30
HLA-A10			−0.30	−0.40		
HLA-A11	0.30		0.40		0.40	
HLA-B7				−0.30	−0.40	
HLA-B8					−0.40	
HLA-B15			0.30			
HLA-B21						−0.30
HLA-Bw22	0.40		0.30		0.40	
HLA-B27			0.35			
HLA-B35				0.30		0.30

[a] Average min./max. value in the coldest/hottest month
[b] Min./max. relative humidity in the driest/most humid month
[c] Maximum fall in 24 hours in a year
[d] Average number of days with more than 0.01 in. of rain

Temperature and humidity indicators [3] measured at 1584 meteorological stations are correlated with the values of each allele frequency map at the same locations. Conventional correlation coefficients have to be "corrected" by ad hoc statistical techniques to take account of the effect of the non-random spatial distribution of sampling points on correlation estimates [4]. The HLA genes whose world frequency variation is associated with climatic factors are likely to be affected by natural selection.

Results

Table 1 shows a summary of the results. Only the corrected correlations greater than 0.30 are reported. Some of the alleles in Table 1 are known to be associated with susceptibility to various diseases, but with the exception of B27, which is associated with joint diseases, it is rather implausible to interpret their etiology in terms of climatic factors.

References

1. Piazza A, Menozzi P, Cavalli-Sforza LL (1981) The making and testing of geographic gene frequency maps. Biometrics 37:635–659
2. Piazza A, Menozzi P, Cavalli-Sforza LL (1980) The HLA-A, B gene frequencies in the world: migration or selection? Hum Immunol 4:297–304
3. Tables of temperature, relative humidity and precipitation for the world. Great Britain: Meteorological Office (1958) Air Ministry M.O. 617a, London
4. Menozzi P, Piazza A, Cavalli-Sforza LL (to be published) Correlation between biological characteristics of population and environmental variables: importance of their distribution in space. Ecology

Histocompatibility Testing 1984
Edited by E. D. Albert et al.

Glyoxalase I (GLO I) Phenotyping by Isoelectric Focusing

P.T. Klouda and J.L. Bidwell

U.K. Transplant Service, S.W. Regional Transfusion Service, Southmead, Bristol BS10 5ND, U.K.

The polymorphism of the red cell enzyme glyoxalase I (GLO-I), first described by Kömpf et al. [1] using starch gel electrophoresis, was investigated by isoelectric focusing (IEF) on polyacrylamide plates at pH 4–5 (LKB, PAG plates). Briefly, 20 µl red cell lysate was applied near the cathode. Following the focusing, the gels were incubated for 20 minutes at 37 °C in a 0.2 *M* phosphate buffer containing 257 m*M* methylglyoxal and 16.3 m*M* reduced glutathione. The detection gel consisted of 1% agarose in 0.1 *M* Tris buffer with 0.06 m*M* DCIP and 2.4 m*M* MTT poured on a GelBond film.

In general, the phenotypes detected by IEF showed the same patterns as those detected by gel electrophoresis with two main bands of approximately pI = 4.3 and 4.4 corresponding to the GLO phenotypes GLO-1 and GLO-2, respectively.

In a family studied by the two methods, regular GLO phenotypes were observed by agarose electrophoresis. With IEF, weak GLO activity was observed in the parents and no activity in one child. The other sib showed normal activity. After fixing and staining of the PAG plates, two intensely staining protein bands were detected in the GLO region in the child with no GLO activity and light bands in the parents. No bands were detected in the child with normal activity. The HLA typing showed that the sibs inherited different haplotypes.

These results revealed the existence of a GLO phenotype, which was active in gel electrophoresis but inactive after IEF. In the family described both parents were heterozygous for this GLO phenotype. One child inherited the IEF-inactive alleles from both parents, while the other inherited the two active allelomorphs.

GLO typing of a panel of blood donors by the two techniques revealed further examples of such IEF-inactive, but gel electrophoresis-active GLO phenotypes.

Recently, GLO "null" alleles were described [2–4] in families with abnormal segregation following gel electrophoresis. IEF of GLO on PAG plates in addition to gel electrophoresis can identify phenotypes that are inactive after IEF but have normal activity on gel electrophoresis. Thus the combination of the two techniques reveals further GLO polymorphism.

Table 1. GLO phenotypes and HLA segregation in BOR family

	GLO agarose	GLO IEF	IEF bands	HLA haplotypes
Father	2-1	2-1	Weak	ab
Mother	2-1	2-1	Weak	cd
Sib 1	1	Null	Strong	ac
Sib 2	2	2	Absent	bd

References

1. Kömpf J, Bissbort S, Gussman S, Ritter H (1975) Polymorphism of a new genetic marker in man. Hum Genet 27:141–143
2. Rittner C, Weber W (1978) Evidence for a "silent allele" Glo^0 at the glyoxalase I locus. Hum Genet 42:315–318
3. Rubinstein P, Suciu-Foca N (1979) Glyoxalase I: a possible "null" allele. Hum Hered 29:217–220
4. Sparkes RS, Sparkes MC, Crist M, Anderson CE (1983) Glyoxalase I "null" allele in a new family. Hum Genet 64:146–147

Histocompatibility Testing 1984
Edited by E. D. Albert et al.

C4 Haplotypes with Duplicated C4A or C4B: Frequency and Associations with Bf, C2, and HLA-A, B, C, DR Alleles with Special Reference to the Duplication C4B1, 2 *

B. Uring-Lambert [1], C.M. Giles [2], J. Goetz [1], M.M. Tongio [1], S. Mayer [1], and G. Hauptmann [1]

1 Institut d'Hématologie, C.H.U. Strasbourg and Centre de Transfusion Sanguine, Strasbourg, France
2 Royal Postgraduate Medical School, Hammersmith Hospital, London, England

Introduction

The fourth component of human complement (C4) is encoded by two separate genes, C4A and C4B, located between the HLA-B and HLA-DR loci [4]. The recent technology of C4 typing has allowed the identification of 12 alleles at the C4A locus and 18 alleles at the C4B locus [12]. In addition, "null alleles", AQ0 and BQ0, are relatively common at both loci. Duplications at C4A or C4B have also been described [2, 3, 7, 11, 13, 16, 18], and it has been proposed that they have arisen by unequal crossing-over between chromosomes with two expressed genes [1].

The gene products of C4A and C4B carry the Rodgers (Rg) and Chido (Ch) antigens respectively, but qualitative and quantitative differences exist in the expression of these antigens [17].

We have found a number of duplicated C4A or C4B in the course of the study of normal French families and of families with cases of insulin-dependent diabetes (IDDM), psoriasis, or leukemia. We report below the frequency of these duplications and their associations with C2, Bf, and HLA-A, C, B, DR alleles.

Four families were studied for plasma or serum Rg/Ch determinants and immunochemical and functional serum C4 levels. Individuals bearing the duplication at C4B were investigated together with the other family members.

Material and Methods

The family material consisted of:
- Two hundred normal French families studied within the INSERM project "HLA-Provinces Françaises"
- Twenty-five families of patients with IDDM
- Thirteen families with one or several cases of psoriasis

A duplication at C4B was also found in the family of a patient with leukemia.

HLA-A, B, C, DR typing was done in several laboratories using standard methods. Some HLA-B14-positive individuals could be subtyped using Ninth Workshop split antisera.

Bf, C2, and C4 allotyping was performed with methods previously described [10].

Rg/Ch typing was performed with serum or EDTA plasma samples using the inhibition method [9].

C4 titration: C4 protein levels were measured on commercial immunoplates (ICL Scientific, Fountain Valley, California). C4-deficient guinea pig serum was used for the functional titration according to the method of Gaither et al. [8].

Results and Discussion

We have observed six duplications at C4A and eight duplications at C4B on a total of 800 haplotypes in the normal family material, which represents a frequency of 0.0075 for C4A and a frequency of 0.010 for C4B.

The duplications at C4A were of different types (four C4A3, 2; three C4A3,3; one C4A3,13) associated with either C4B1 or C4BQ0, C2C, BfF or BfS, and various HLA haplotypes. One example of the "extended" HLA-B35, BfF, C4A3,2 BQ0, DR1 haplotype reported by Awdeh et al. [2], Bruun-Petersen et al. [3], Fielder et al. [7], Raum et al. [16], and Rittner et al. [18] was observed in a normal family.

In contrast, the duplications at C4B were with one exception all of the same type, C4B1,2, and always associated with C2C, BfS, and C4A2 (Table 1). The complotype C2C, BfS, C4A2, C4B1,2 was always found in association with HLA-B14. The B14 subtype could be defined in five cases and in each of them it was Bw65. However, considering the linkage disequilibrium between Bw65 and the HLA-A alleles [5], we would expect the existence of Bw65 in five other cases. HLA-DR1 was only observed in

* This work was supported in part by INSERM grants CRL 818003 and 821015

 Histocompatibility Testing 1984
Edited by E. D. Albert et al.

four haplotypes. However, we noticed the absence of DR7 usually in significant association with Bw64 [6, 14]. Our results are in agreement with the recent findings of O'Neill et al. [15] who found a strong association between Bw65 and BfS, C2C, C4A2B2, but the duplication at the C4B locus was not evidenced in O'Neill's study.

Figures 1–4 show the inheritance of the duplication C4B1,2 in four families. An additional duplication, C4A3,2, was observed in family MI (Fig. 4). Some duplications at C4B were evidenced by the quantitative increases of the C4B2 or C4B1 bands on immunofixation patterns in individuals expressing respectively two C4B2 or two C4B1 alleles. This was the case in families BRA (Fig. 2), CA (Fig. 3), and MI (Fig. 4). In family BER (Fig. 1) the duplication at C4B was evidenced by the observation of a quantitative increase of the

Table 1. HLA-A, C, B, C2, BF, C4A, C4B, HLA-DR haplotypes with duplications at C4B

HLA-A	HLA-C	HLA-B	C2	Bf	C4A	C4B	HLA-DR	Family material
28	w8	w65	C	S	2	1, 2	ND	Normal
28	w8	w65	C	S	2	1, 2	w6	Leukemia
w33	ND	14	C	S	2	1, 2	3	IDDM
28	ND	14	C	S	2	1, 2	5	Normal
–[a]	ND	14	C	S	2	1, 2	5	Normal
31	ND	14	C	S	2	1, 2	3	Normal
28	w8	w65	C	S	2	1, 2	w6	Normal
w33	ND	14	ND	S	2	1, 2	1	Normal
w33	ND	14	ND	S	2	1, 2	1	Psoriasis
w33	ND	14	C	S	2	1, 2	1	Normal
1	ND	8	ND	S	3	1, 6	3	Normal
w33	w8	w65	C	S	2	1, 2	1	Psoriasis
28	w8	w65	C	S	2	1, 2	ND	Psoriasis

The order of the C2, Bf and C4 genes is that reported by Carrol et al. [4], but the order with respect to HLA-B and HLA-DR is unknown.
ND, not done
[a] Possibly blank

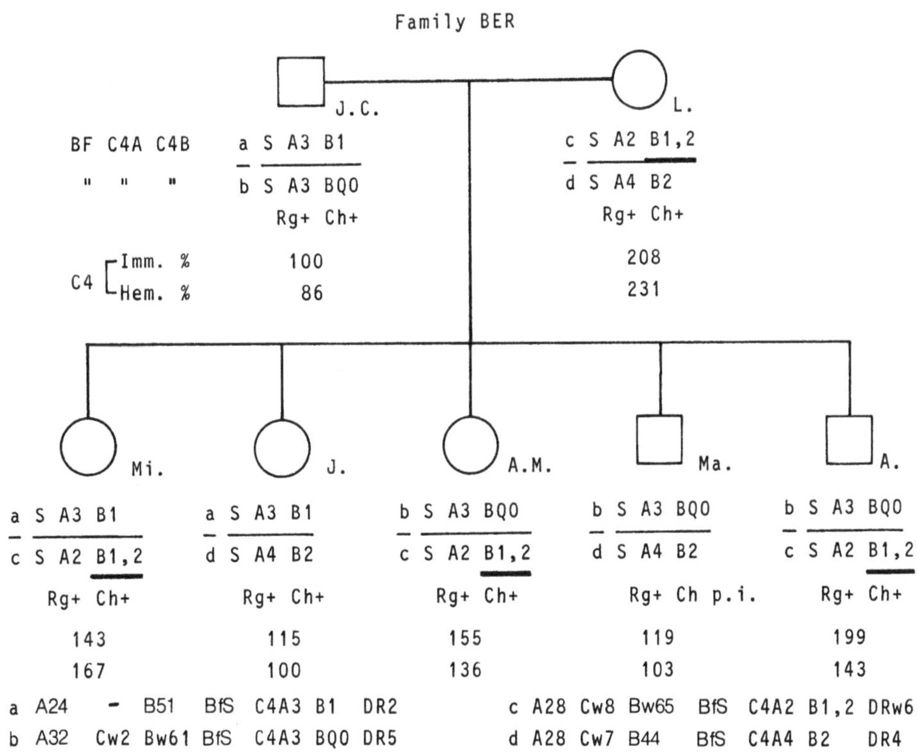

Fig. 1. Pedigree of family BER showing the segregation of the Bf, C4A, C4B haplotypes. The HLA-A, C, B, Bf, C4A, C4B, HLA-DR haplotypes are given below the pedigree. The duplicated gene C4B1,2 is underlined. C4 immunochemical and hemolytical levels are given as percent of the mean normal level (pool of 30 normal serum specimens stored at −70 °C). *Rg+*, *Ch+*, Rg or Ch complete inhibitors; *Ch p.i.*, Ch partial inhibitor

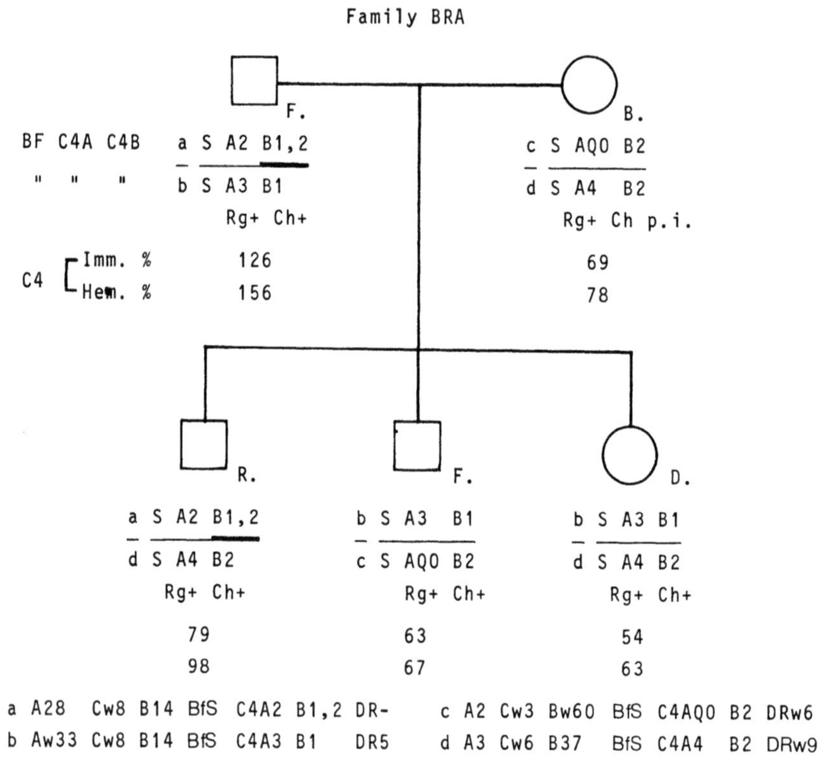

Fig. 2. Pedigree of family BRA

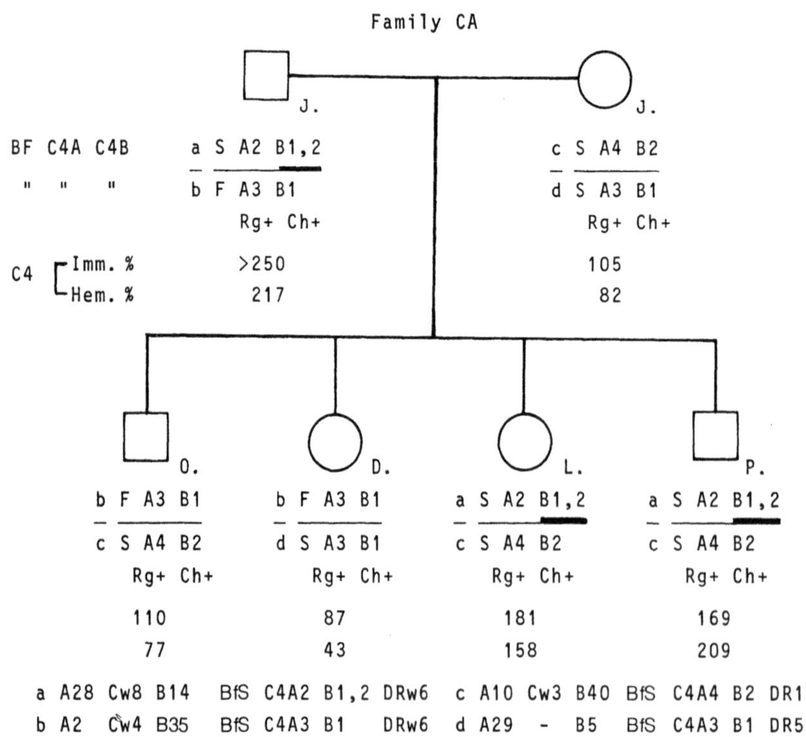

Fig. 3. Pedigree of family CA

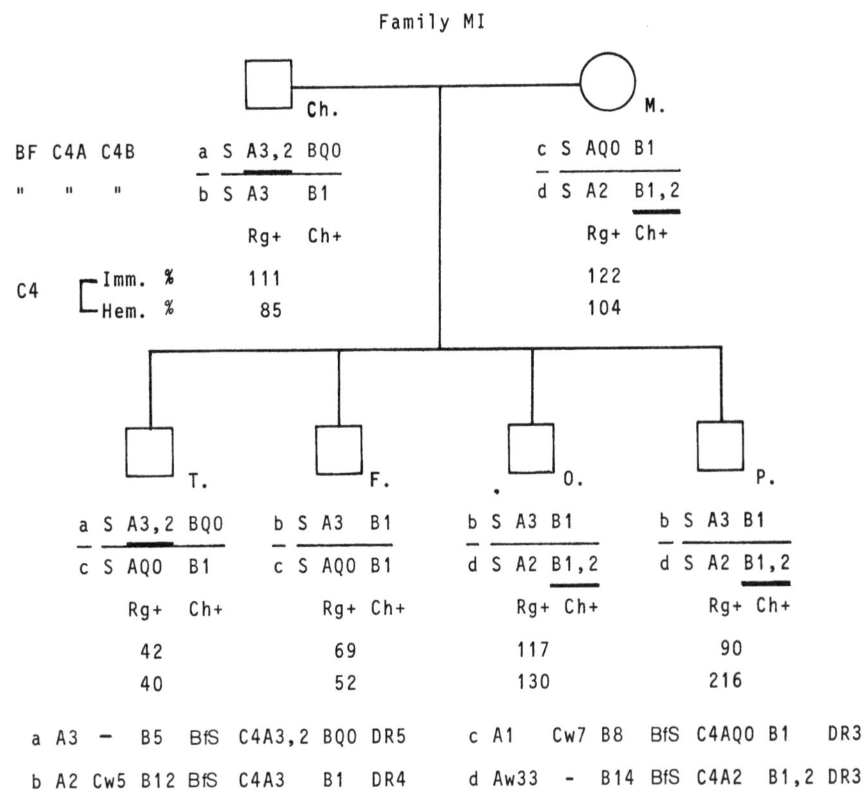

Fig. 4. Pedigree of family MI

C4B1 (child Mi.) or C4B2 (mother L.) bands. Such patterns were not observed in children A. M. and A., who express two C4B alleles, B1 and B2, but they received a C4BQ0 allele with the paternal sixth chromosome. The C4 patterns observed in the families were always in accordance with a genetic transmission linked to HLA.

Several individuals expressing three C4B alleles (two C4B1 plus one C4B2 or one C4B1 plus two C4B2) were found to have high immunochemical and functional C4 levels. The results given in Fig. 5 show that individuals expressing five C4 alleles (two at C4A and three at C4B) have significantly higher immunochemical and functional C4 levels than individuals expressing four C4 genes. However, as was found by others [13, 18], the serum C4 levels are not strictly correlated to the number of C4 genes expressed.

Rg/Ch typing by the inhibition technique showed that partial inhibition of anti-Ch was only observed in individuals homozygous C4B2/B2 (B. in family BRA, Fig. 2) or heterozygous C4B2/Q0 (Ma. in family BER, Fig. 1). Individuals having the duplication C4B1,2 in association with C4BQ0 on the other chromosome were found to be complete Ch inhibitors. This is in contrast to the products of the C4A3,2 duplication, which are responsible for par-

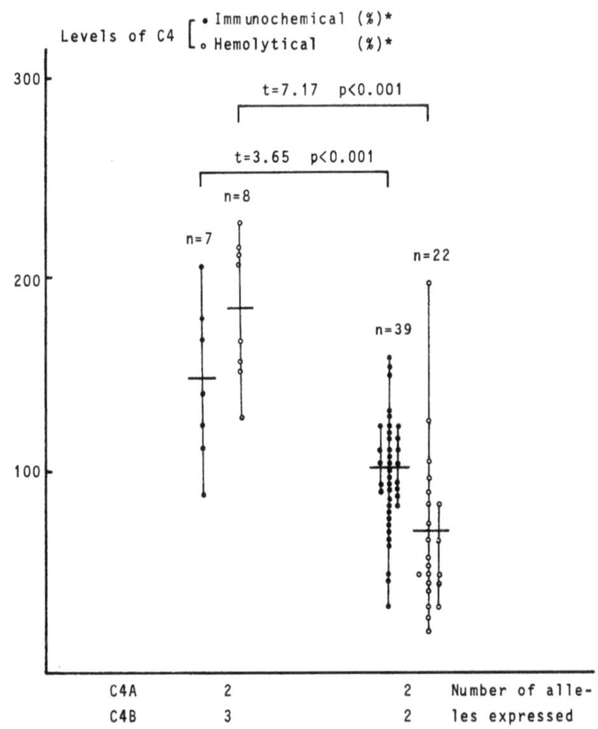

Fig. 5. Immunochemical and hemolytical levels of serum C4 in individuals expressing four or five C4 genes. The levels are given as percent of the mean normal level (pool of 30 normal specimens stored at –70 °C). Comparison of the levels is by Student's t test

tial inhibition of anti-Rg [17]. However, the child T. in family MI (Fig. 4), who inherited the duplication C4A3,2 together with a C4AQ0 allele, was not found to be a partial inhibitor of anti-Rg.

In this study, the duplicated C4B1,2 gene was observed within two kinds of "extended" HLA haplotypes: A28, Cw8, Bw65, C2C, BfS, C4A2, C4B1,2 and Aw33 (C– not done in this part of the material), B14 (subtype not defined in this part of the material), C2C, BfS, C4A2, C4B1,2, DR1.

The products of the duplicated C4B1,2 gene were found to be hemolytically active and to express a normal Ch antigenicity.

Summary

Several examples of duplications at C4A or C4B were encountered in the course of the study of families for the sixth chromosome markers HLA-A, C, B, Bf, C2, C4A, C4B, HLA-DR. In the normal family material the frequency of the duplications at C4A or C4B was respectively 0.0075 and 0.010. The duplications at C4A associated various alleles occurring with different C2, Bf, C4B, and HLA haplotypes. The duplications at C4B were with one exception all of the same type, C4B1,2, and were always associated with C2C, BfS, C4A2, and HLA-B14. The HLA-B14 subtype was defined as Bw65. The products of the duplicated C4B1,2 gene are hemolytically active and express a normal Chido antigenicity.

Acknowledgments. We are indebted to A. Y. Mercier and J. P. Saleun (Brest), F. Guignier (Dijon), J. Arvieux (Grenoble), H. Betuel und L. Gebuhrer (Lyon), and D. Alcalay (Poitiers) for providing blood samples of normal families.

References

1. Awdeh ZL, Alper CA (1980) Inherited structural polymorphism of the fourth component of complement (C4). Proc Natl Acad Sci USA 77:3576–3580
2. Awdeh ZL, Raum D, Yunis EJ, Alper CA (1983) An extended major histocompatibility haplotype with duplicated C4A. Immunobiol 164:317
3. Bruun-Petersen G, Lamm LU, Jacobsen BK, Kristensen T (1982) Two homoduplication haplotypes C4SC4S and C4FC4F in a family. Hum Genet 61:36–38
4. Carroll MC, Campbell RD, Bentley DR, Porter RR (1984) A molecular map of the major histocompatibility complex class III region linking complement genes C4, C2 and factor B. Nature 307:237–241
5. Darke C (1980) Further evidence for the partition of HLA-B14. Tissue Antigens 15:25–30
6. Dewar J (1983) HLA-B14.1 in linkage disequilibrium with HLA-DR7. Tissue Antigens 22:310–311
7. Fielder AHL, Walport MJ, Batchelor JR, Rynes RI, Black CM, Dodi IA, Hughes GRV (1983) Family study of the major histocompatibility complex in patients with systemic lupus erythematosus: importance of null alleles of C4A and C4B in determining disease susceptibility. Br Med J 286:425–428
8. Gaither TA, Alling DW, Frank MM (1974) A new one-step method for the functional assay of the fourth component (C4) of human and guinea pig complement. J Immunol 113:574–583
9. Giles CM (1980) Antigens in plasma. A seminar on antigens on blood cells and body fluids. Am Ass of Blood Banks, pp 33–49
10. Hauptmann G, Tongio MM, Goetz J, Mayer S, Fauchet R, Sobel A, Griscelli C, Berthoux F, Rivat C, Rother U (1982) Association of the C2-deficiency gene (C2*Q0) with the C4A*4, C4B*2 genes. J Immunogenet 9:127–132
11. Hauptmann G, Mauff G, Tongio MM, Goetz J, Seger J (1982) Evidence for the presence of two structurally different C4A genes on one chromosome in a caucasoid family. Fourth International Workshop for the Genetics of Complement, Boston (abstract)
12. Mauff G, Alper CA, Awdeh ZL, Batchelor JR, Bertrams J, Bruun-Petersen G, Dawkins RL, Demant P, Edwards J, Grosse-Wilde H, Hauptmann G, Klouda P, Lamm L, Mollenhauer E, Nerl E, Olaisen B, O'Neill GJ, Rittner C, Roos M, Skanes V, Teisberg P, Wells L (1983) Statement on the nomenclature of human C4. Immunobiology 164:184–191
13. Mauff G, Bender K, Giles CM, Goldmann S, Opferkuch W, Wachauf B (1984) Human C4 polymorphism: pedigree analysis of qualitative, quantitative, and functional parameters as a basis for phenotype interpretations. Hum Genet 65:362–372
14. Mueller-Eckhardt G, Mayr WR, Prel L, Mueller-Eckhardt C (1983) New evidence for the existence of HLA-B14 subtypes. Tissue Antigens 21:58–61
15. O'Neill GJ, Mueller-Eckhardt G, Prel L, Schendel DJ (1984) C4 allotyping distinguishes HLA-B14.1 and B14.2 subgroups. Immunogenet 19:335–341
16. Raum D, Awdeh Z, Anderson J, Strong L, Granados J, Teran L, Giblett E, Yunis EJ, Alper CA (1984) Human C4 allotypes with duplicated C4A or C4B. Am J Hum Genet 36:72–79
17. Rittner C, Tippett P, Giles CM, Mollenhauer E, Berger R, Nordhagen R, Buskjoer L, Bruun-Petersen G, Lamm L, Roos MH (1984) An international reference typing for Ch and Rg determinants on rare human C4 allotypes. Vox Sang 46:224–234
18. Rittner C, Giles CM, Roos MH, Demant P, Mollenhauer E (1984) Genetics of human C4 polymorphism: detection and segregation of rare and duplicated haplotypes. Immunogenet 19:321–333

Gene Duplication of C4A in the Lancaster County, Pennsylvania, Old Order Amish: C4A*2A*3 is in Coupling with HLA A3, Cw4, B35, BfF, DR1, GLO2

R.H. McLean, P.F. Howard, and W.B. Bias

Dept. of Pediatrics, Johns Hopkins University School of Medicine, Baltimore, MD 21205, USA

Eight families (76 individuals) of the Old Order Amish religious isolate of Lancester County, Pennsylvania, were selected for complement phenotype analysis. Gene duplication at the C4A locus was detected in three families. The duplication (*C4A*2A*3*) was present on the same HLA haplotype in all cases and could be traced to one founder. The phenotype for the two loci of the fourth component of complement (C4A and C4B) were determined by electrophoresis in agarose, immunofixation with anti-C4 antiserum, crossed-gel immunoelectrophoresis, and hemolytic overlay. Factor B (Bf) phenotype was determined by immunofixation. The order of genes in haplotypes is written HLA-A, Cw, B, C4A, C4B, Bf, DR, DQ, GLO.

Families 259, 4154, and 4507 had normal individuals who carried the duplicated C4A gene (*C4A*2A*3*). The duplication was found on the HLA-A3, Cw4, B35, C4A2, A3, C4BQ0, BfF, DR1, DQw1, GLO2, haplotype in all pedigrees. *C4B*Q0* on this haplotype was confirmed to be a null allele by the finding of homozygosity for *C4B*Q0* in one individual in family 259. Both parents in family 4154 carry the C4A duplication. One of their children is homozygous for the haplotype that carries the duplication. The fathers in families 259 and 4507 are first cousins. Pedigree analysis revealed multiple lines of descent from a common ancestor for the four carrier parents (Fig. 1).

A similar C4A duplication and complotype (*C4A*2,A*3,B*Q0,Bf*F*) has been reported in other studies [1, 2] where the C4A duplication was also in coupling with B35, BfF, DR1 (or DR4). We conclude that duplicated C4 loci are not rare [3], and that the B35, C4A2, A3, BQ0, BfF, DR1 haplotype may be particularly common.

* This work was supported by a National Institutes of Health Grant AM31920 and 5RO1AI17431

References

1. Arnason A, Fossdal R, Thorsteinsson J, Teitsson I, Skaftadottir I, Palsdottir A, Jensson O (1983) HLA-haplotypes and complotypes in a large inbred Icelandic family with a variety of rheumatological disorders demonstrating duplication of C4A locus, acquired deficiency of C4 proteins, high frequency of C4BQ0 and HLA B27. Immunobiology 164:206
2. Braun-Petersen G, Lamm LU, Jacobsen BK, Kristensen T (1982) Genetics of complement C4. Two homoduplication haplotypes C4S C4S and C4F C4F in a family. Hum Genet 61:36–38
3. Raum D, Awdeh Z, Anderson J, Strong L, Granados J, Teran L, Giblett E, Yunis EJ, Alper CA (1984) Human C4 haplotypes with duplicated C4A or C4B. Am J Hum Genet 36:72–79

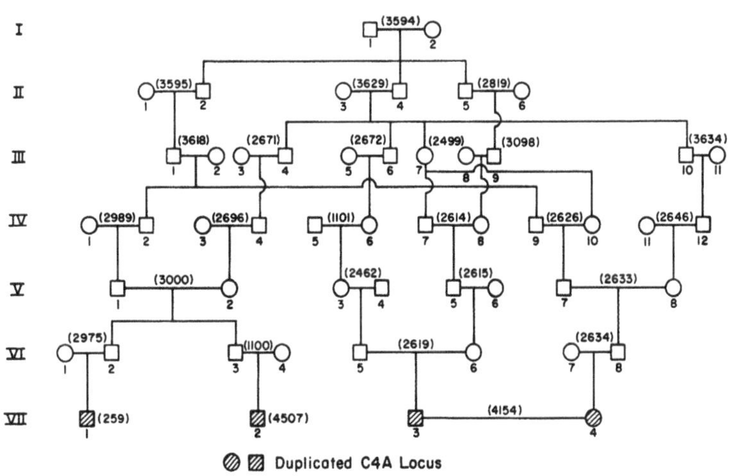

Fig. 1. Pedigree analysis

Distinct Complotypes Are Associated with HLA-B14 Subgroups

G. Mueller-Eckhardt[1], D.J. Schendel[2], L. Prel[3], C. Darke[4], and G.J. O'Neill[2]

1 Institute of Clinical Immunology and Blood Transfusion, Justus Liebig University, Langhansstraße 7, 6300 Giessen, Federal Republic of Germany
2 Institute for Immunology, University of Munich, 8000 Munich 2, Federal Republic of Germany
3 German Red Cross Blood Transfusion Centre, 2130 Rotenburg/Wümme, Federal Republic of Germany
4 Tissue Typing Laboratory, Welsh Regional Blood Transfusion Centre, Cardiff, U.K.

Up to the Ninth IHW, the subdivision of HLA-B14 [3] has not been widely accepted, due to the lack of appropriate antisera. However, the observation of linkage disequilibrium between the postulated B14 splits and determinants of the HLA-A, DR, and Bf loci [1–4] has contributed additional evidence for the partition of B14. In this study the value of the HLA-linked complement components C4 for the discrimination of B14 splits was investigated.

Materials and Methods

Sixty unrelated B14-positive individuals, fifteen normal families, and two families of patients with congenital adrenal hyperplasia (CAH) were investigated. Both unrelated individuals and normal families were included in the *Special B14 Study* of the Ninth IHW (Mueller-Eckhardt et al., this volume). The class III gene markers C4A, C4B, C2, and Bf were determined as recently described elsewhere [5].

Results and Discussion

According to the serological definition of the B14 subtypes Bw64 (14.1) and Bw65 (14.2) by 9WS sera (Mueller-Eckhardt et al., this volume), 15 (25%) of the unrelated panel typed as Bw64 and 45 (75%) as Bw65. No statistically significant difference between Bw64 and Bw65 individuals was detected for the frequencies of Bf and C2 alleles. However, comparison for C4 determinants revealed the strongest association with B14 subgroups observed so far, i.e., of C4A2 and of C4B2 with Bw65 (Fisher's test: $P = 2.9 \times 10^{-8}$ and 6.3×10^{-6}) and C4A3 with Bw64 ($P = 0.0003$). From the family study it appeared that the SC31 complotype is almost exclusively associated with Bw64 (5/6 families), whereas in the Bw65 subgroup two distinct complotypes can be demonstrated, i.e., the more frequent SC22 (5/7 families) and a less common FC31 type (2/7 families).

The two CAH families, both belonging to the Bw65 subgroup, were of particular interest, as the C4B locus appeared to be duplicated on the B14-positive haplotypes (SC22/1). It is not known whether this is restricted to HLA-Bw65 haplotypes that carry a defective 21-OH gene or whether other, "normal" Bw65-positive haplotypes also carry a duplicated C4B locus.

References

1. Darke C (1980) Further evidence for the partition of B14. Tissue Antigens 15:25–30
2. Darke C (1984) Linkage disequilibrium between HLA-B14 subdivisions and HLA-A, DR and properdin factor B alleles. Tissue Antigens 23:68–71
3. Dewar PJ, Coates E, Murray S (1977) Subdivision of the antigen HLA-B14. Tissue Antigens 10:345–347
4. Mueller-Eckhardt G, Mayr WR, Prel L, Mueller-Eckhardt C (1983) New evidence for the existence of HLA B14 subtypes. Tissue Antigens 21:58–61
5. O'Neill GJ, Mueller-Eckhardt G, Prel L, Schendel DJ (1984) C4 allotyping distinguishes HLA-B14.1 and B14.2 subgroups. Immunogenetics 19:335–341

 Histocompatibility Testing 1984
Edited by E. D. Albert et al.

Bf Polymorphism Studied by Isoelectrofocusing

V. David[1], M. Leroux[1], R. Fauchet[2], H. Phensavath[2], M. Gueguen[2], and J.-Y. Le Gall[1]

1 Laboratoire de Biochimie Médicale B, CHU Pontchaillou, 35043 Rennes Cedex, France
2 Laboratoire d'Histocompatibilité, Centre Régional de Transfusion Sanguine, Rue Pierre Jean Gineste, 35000 Rennes, France

The genetic polymorphism of the factor B (Bf) [1–3] of the alternative complement pathway has been studied hitherto by means of a technique of immunofixation electrophoresis on agarose gels. We studied this polymorphism using the isoelectrofocusing technique: this technique is more sensitive and therefore could be considered preferable for demonstration of a new polymorphism.

Sera were first selected by agarose gel electrophoresis according to the technique of Alper et al. [1]. After 1 : 3 dilution, the sera were submitted to isoelectrofocusing on thin-layer polyacrylamide gels in the pH range 3.5–9.5 (Power 30 W, time 2 h 45 min). After incubation with an anti-Bf immune serum in a moist atmosphere for 2 h, the polyacrylamide plates were washed for 48 h in 0.15 *M* NaCl, and stained with a Coomassie brilliant blue solution.

In all, 121 sera of unrelated individuals presenting the SS phenotype were studied; all these sera seemed similar when studied by electrophoresis on agarose gel; but when studied by isoelectrofocusing they appeared to vary in both the number and the relative intensity of the major bands.

Three phenotypes (S_A–S_A, S_B–S_B, S_A–S_B) were identified, corresponding to the homozygous or heterozygous expression of the two alleles S_A and S_B. The genetic frequencies of S_A and S_B in the tested population were 0.57 and 0.43, respectively.

This technique was also used in the study of 60 SF and 5 FF sera; no additional polymorphism of the F allele has yet been demonstrated further to those already described [4, 5]. However, in the SF phenotypes, expression of the S_A or S_B alleles could be shown. Thus, two new phenotypes (S_AF and S_BF) were recognized (Fig. 1).

Family studies showed segregation, with the markers of the HLA complex in six families. One of these families had a known locus B–locus C4 recombination; isoelectrofocusing allowed location of the crossing-over between the Bf locus and the C4 locus. Transmission abnormalities were observed in three families; in each of these three families one of the parents was phenotyped S_A–S_B. The genetic transmission of the Bf factor should perhaps be studied in these cases, keeping in mind the possibility of a locus duplication.

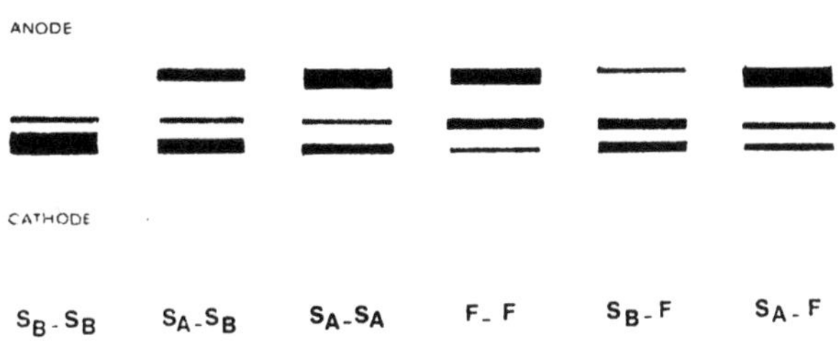

Fig. 1. Properdin factor B (Bf) polymorphism

References

1. Alper CA, Boenisch T, Watson L (1972) Genetic polymorphism in human glycine-rich beta-glycoprotein. J Exp Med 135:68–80
2. Hauptmann G, Sasportes M, Tongio M, Mayer S, Dausset J (1976) The localization of the Bf locus within the MHS region on chromosome no. 6. Tissue Antigens 7:52–54
3. Hauptmann G, Tongio M, Mayer S (1976) Bf polymorphism: study of a new variant (F.0.55). Hum Genet 33:275–278
4. Teng YS, Tan SG (1982) Subtyping of Properdin factor B (Bf) by isoelectrofocusing. Hum Hered 32:362–366
5. Geserick G, Patzelt D, Schröder A, Nagaï T (1983) Isoelectrofocusing in the study of the Bf system: Existence of two common subtypes of the Bf F allele. Vox Sang 44:178–182

Histocompatibility Testing 1984
Edited by E. D. Albert et al.

Genetic Control of HLA-Linked Immune Responsiveness to Synthethic Polypeptides in Healthy Individuals and Patients with Autoimmune Diseases

C. Brautbar [1], D. Katz [2], Z. Bentwich [3], and E. Mozes [2]

1 Laboratory of Immunohematology and the Lautenberg Center for General and Tumor Immunology, Hadassah Hebrew University Medical Center, Jerusalem, Israel
2 Department of Chemical Immunology, The Weizmann Institute of Science, Rehovot 76100, Israel
3 R. Ben Ari Institute of Clinical Immunology, Kaplan Hospital, Rehovot 76100, Israel

Introduction

The association between the HLA system and susceptibility to various diseases and in particular diseases with immunological disorders is well known [13]. However, the identification of the mechanisms by which various HLA factors cause susceptibility to a variety of diseases is yet to be clarified. The existence of immune response genes and their linkage to the major histocompatibility complex has been established in many species [2, 9, 12]. For a better understanding of HLA and disease associations it is of importance to elucidate the function of immune response (Ir) genes in man. However, in the human, studies on Ir genes have been limited due to genetic heterogeneity of the random population, complexity of the antigens relevant to diseases, constraints of immunization with foreign antigens, and lack of adequate in vitro systems for these studies.
To this end we have established an in vitro system for the activation of human peripheral blood T cells, choosing as model antigens synthetic polypeptides that are well characterized and the response to which has been demonstrated to be genetically regulated in all species studied [10, 11]. Human peripheral blood T cells of normal donors were activated in vitro with autologous adherent cells pulsed with either poly(LTyr, LGlu)-poly(DLAla) – poly(LLys), [(T,G)-A–L], or poly(LHis, LGlu)-poly(DLAla)-poly(LLys), [(H,G)-A–L]. The activated T cells were tested for their ability to produce an antigen-specific T-cell-replacing factor in cooperation with B cells for in vitro antibody responses [7]. Results of screening of over 100 healthy unrelated donors demonstrated that 50% of the tested individuals responded to (T,G)-A–L by the production of an antigen-specific T-cell-helper factor suggesting differences between donors in their capability to respond to (T,G)-A–L. The (T,G)-A–L-specific helper factor has been shown to be antigen specific in its helper activity and also by the fact that it could be absorbed by a column of Sepharose coupled to the specific antigen, namely (T-G)-A–L [7].
Since antigen-specific T-cell-replacing factors of murine origin were shown to possess Ia determinants, the (T,G)-A–L-specific helper T cell factors of human origin were passed on immunoadsorbents built of anti-DR antisera. The activity of the antigen-specific factors could be removed and eluted from columns of anti-DR antibodies relevant to the donors' DR phenotype.
Furthermore, the same factors were also removed by a monoclonal antibody (anti-Ia) which recognizes a monomorphic determinant on HLA-DR, but not by monoclonal anti-β_2-microglobulin [8].
In the present study we report the use of the antigen-specific helper T cell factor production system for the study of the genetic regulation of the immune response potential to (T,G)-A–L and (H,G)-A–L in family members, and for the investigation of the ability of patients with autoimmune diseases to respond to a genetically controlled immunogen.

Genetic Control of HLA-Linked Immune Responsiveness to (T,G)-A–L and (H,G)-A–L

The screening of a random population of healthy donors for their ability to respond to (T,G)-A–L by the production of an antigen-specific T cell helper factor has demonstrated that humans differ in their immune response potential to this antigen [7], as do all other species studied [2, 10]. However, for formal demonstration of an HLA-linked genetic regulation, family studies were required.
Peripheral blood lymphocytes obtained from 174 donors belonging to 24 different branched families with two to three generations were activated to (T,G)-A–L on autologous antigen pulsed adherent cells. The supernatants obtained from these activated PBL were tested for their antigen specific helper activity in a hapten-carrier in vitro antibody pro-

Histocompatibility Testing 1984
Edited by E. D. Albert et al.

duction system. Thus, NIP-ovalbumin-primed B cells (of murine H-2^b high responder origin) were cultured in vitro together with the supernatants of the (T,G)-A–L-activated T cells in the presence of NIP-(T,G)-A–L. As specificity controls either NIP-human-γ-globulin (HGG) or NIP-fowl-γ-globulin (FGG) were used. The number of plaque-forming cells (PFC) was determined after 5 days of culture using NIP-derivatized sheep erythrocytes as target cells [7]. All family members investigated were studied for class I (HLA-A, B, C) and class II (HLA-DR) antigens, enabling the assignment of HLA haplotypes to each individual. The results obtained in this study indicated that the ability to respond to (T,G)-A–L by the production of an antigen-specific T cell helper factor is inherited as a dominant trait linked to the responder HLA haplotype.

Fifty-three donors belonging to seven families of those tested for their immune response potential to (T,G)-A–L were also tested for their ability to respond to the synthetic antigen (H,G)-A–L. We chose to study the immune response to the latter antigen as well because in the mouse, different pattern of immune responses were shown to (T,G)-A–L and (H,G)-A–L. A comparison of the pattern of the murine immune responses to the two polypeptides resulted in the precise mapping of the genes controlling the responses to these antigens. In all the families tested in the present study, it has been clearly shown that the ability to respond to (H,G)-A–L is inherited as a dominant trait linked to the responder HLA haplotype, as shown for the (T,G)-A–L system.

The pattern of immune responses of part of the family members to (T,G)-A–L and (H,G)-A–L was found to differ, indicating that the immune responses to these antigens are controlled by independent alleles. These results are similar to those previously shown for other rodents [10, 12].

Some of the family members studied were found to produce helper factors to both (T,G)-A–L and (H,G)-A–L. These results can be explained, since in an outbred population like that studied here, it is expected to find heterozygous individuals that carry haplotypes with distinct alleles for the responsiveness to (T,G)-A–L and (H,G)-A–L.

The survey of family members led to the demonstration of HLA-linked genetic regulation of the ability to respond to (T,G)-A–L and (H,G)-A–L; however, it did not enable the mapping of the relevant genes. So far, we have studied two families with recombinant individuals. The results with the two recombinants suggest that at least one of the genes controlling the immune responses to (T,G)-A–L and (H,G)-A–L is mapped between HLA-A and HLA-B. The possibility that gene complementation is required for the immune response to (T,G)-A–L and that the second gene is located close to the HLA-DR region was also raised while investigating one of the recombinants. Hsu et al. [6] also provided evidence, with intra-HLA recombinants, that localizes the immune response genes controlling lymphocyte proliferation to (T,G)-A–L and (H,G)-A–L between HLA-A and HLA-B. They also suggested gene complementation for the proliferative responses to these antigens.

The Ability of Patients with Autoimmune Diseases to Respond to (T,G)-A–L

Autoimmunity is characterized by immunoregulatory disorders [14]. It is most likely that T cells play a major role in autoimmune diseases. Thus, the deranged immune reaction against self components might be triggered by an aberrant set of regulatory T-cell signals, and these signals are probably mediated through factors. Therefore, our above described system for activation of peripheral blood T cells to (T,G)-A–L and the production of antigen-specific T-cell-replacing factors, appeared to be adequate for investigating the immune response potential of patients with autoimmune diseases.

Systemic lupus erythematosus (SLE) is considered to be a systemic autoimmune disease, in distinction from other autoimmune diseases, such as the thyroid autoimmune diseases (TADs), which involve one organ and are therefore defined as organ-specific autoimmune diseases. We have applied our system to patients with both types of autoimmune diseases.

So far we have tested the immune response potential to (T,G)-A–L of 40 patients with SLE. All patients fulfilled four or more of the criteria of the American Rheumatism Association (ARA) for the classification of SLE [3]. The patients were divided into two groups according to the severity of their disease. Thus, patients in the first group had an active disease at the time of the study. This group was on regular treatment with steroids and/or cytotoxic drugs. Patients in the second group had been in remission for at least a year up to the time of the study.

All SLE patients responded to (T,G)-A–L by the production of an antigen-specific helper T cell factor. This observation is in contrast to a 50% response in a random population of healthy donors [7]. Neither the severity of the disease, nor the drug treatment, had any observed effect either on the ability of the patients to respond or on the efficiency of the help provided by the T cell factors produced by the activated T cells. Twenty-seven of the SLE patients were tested for their class I (HLA-A, B, C) and class II (HLA-DR) antigens. On the whole, none of the antigens tested showed a significant association with the disease. However, our results suggested a possible association between an HLA-DR antigen and the course of the disease. Thus, a high frequency (75%; 9/12) of DR5 was present in SLE patients with the mild disease in comparison to 26.6% (4/15) in patients with a severe disease. The frequency of HLA-DR5 in the Israeli healthy population is 46%. Of the patients with an active course of disease, 53.3% (8/15) carried DR7, while only 16.6% (2/12) of the patients in remission were positive for DR7. In the Israeli population the frequency of HLA-DR7 was found to be 21.8%. Although our group consisted of only 27 HLA-typed patients, the results suggest that in Israeli Jewish SLE patients, HLA-DR5 may be associated with a milder course of the disease and HLA-DR7 with a more severe disease.

Peripheral blood T cells of 27 patients with TADs were activated to (T,G)-A–L and tested for the production of antigen-specific T cell helper factor by the stimulated cells. Fifty-five percent (15/27) of the patients responded to (T,G)-A–L, similarly to the results observed (50%) in the control population. The distribution of HLA class I (A, B, C) and class II (DR) antigens in these patients did not differ from that shown in healthy Israeli donors. The results presented above clearly indicate a difference between the immune response potential to (T,G)-A–L of patients with the systemic autoimmune disease, SLE, and patients with organ-specific TADs. It is possible that in the case of the TADs a lack of T-cell regulation is expressed only towards the antigen(s) relevant to the disease, whereas in SLE patients a more general alteration of immune regulation is present and therefore the patients are expected to respond to a broad range of antigens, such as (T,G)-A–L in the present investigation. Further studies with patients affected with systemic autoimmune diseases and with organ-specific autoimmune disorders should clarify whether the differences observed between the immune response potential of patients with SLE and TADs is a general phenomenon.

Concluding Remarks

In the present report we have demonstrated the existence of immune response genes in man, using an in vitro system for T-cell activation to the synthetic polypeptide antigens (T,G)-A–L and (H,G)-A–L, the responses to which have been shown to be genetically regulated in all experimental animal species studied [2, 9, 12]. Family studies indicated that the ability to respond to these antigens is inherited as an autosomal, dominant trait. HLA genotyping showed that the immune response potential to (T,G)-A–L and (H,G)-A–L segregates in linkage to the responder HLA haplotype. Our results suggested that at least one of the genes controlling the immune responsiveness to these antigens is mapped between HLA-A and HLA-B. The active (T,G)-A–L-specific helper factors were shown to possess HLA-DR determinantes of the responder type. However, no linkage could be detected between the ability to respond to (T,G)-A–L by the production of an helper factor and a distinct DR specificity. It is possible that a gene(s) regulating the ability to respond to (T,G)-A–L is linked to a D-region determinant other than DR (e.g., DQ, DP) and only by utilizing monoclonal antibodies [1] combined with gel analysis [5] will more precise mapping be possible.

The study of patients with SLE indicated lack of immune regulation of the response to (T,G)-A–L, in contrast to patients with TADs, who responded to this antigen similarly to healthy donors. It will be of interest to follow the immune response potential to (T,G)-A–L of family members of the SLE patients, in order to find out whether the defect in immune regulation correlates with the clinical manifestations [4].

Bearing in mind the results of the present study, it would be of importance to study similarly the generation of T-cell factors specific to antigens relevant to both types of autoimmune diseases, namely systemic and organ specific. It would be of interest to study suppressor factors in addition to helper factors specific to such antigens, since it is possible that the absence of regulatory suppressor T cells, and therefore lack of such factors, is on the one hand responsible for the onset or activity of the diseases, and may on the other hand offer a potent and specific therapeutic tool in the future.

References

1. Beckmann I (1984) Monoclonal antibodies to HLA-DR antigens. Immunology 5:29–32
2. Benacerraf B, Katz DH (1975) The histocompatibility linked immune response genes. Adv Cancer Res 21:121–173
3. Cohen AS, Reynolds EW, Franklin EC, Kulka JP, Ropes NW, Shulman LE, Wallace SL (1971) Preliminary criteria for the classification of systemic lupus erythematosus. Bull Rheum Dis 21:643–645
4. Fielder AHL, Walport NJ, Batchelor JR, Rynes RI, Black CM, Dodi IA (1983) Family study of the major histocompatibility complex in patients with systemic lupus erythematosus: importance of null alleles of C4A and C4B in determining disease susceptibility. Brid Med J 286:425–428

5. Goyert S, Silver J (1983) Further characterization of HLA-DS molecules implication for studies assessing the role of human Ia molecules in cell interactions and disease susceptibility. Proc Natl Acad Sci USA 80:5719–5723
6. Hsu SH, Chan MM, Bias WB (1981) Genetic control of major histocompatibility complex linked immune responses to synthetic polypeptides in man. Proc Natl Acad Sci USA 125:352–358
7. Katz D, Bentwich Z, Eshhar N, Lowy I, Mozes E (1981) Immune response potential to poly(TyrGlu)-poly-(DLAla)–poly(Lys) of human T cells of different donors. Proc Natl Acad Sci USA 78:4505–4509
8. Katz D, Brautbar C, Bentwich Z, Mozes E (1983) Genetically regulated human (T,G)-A–L specific helper T cell replacing factors possess HLA-DR and V_H determinants. Human Immunol 7:217–227
9. McDevitt HO, Benacerraf B (1969) Genetic control of specific immune responses. Adv Immunol 11:31–74
10. McDevitt HO, Chinitz A (1969) Genetic control of the antibody response: relationship between immune response and histocompatibility (H-2) type. Science 163:1207–1537
11. McDevitt HO, Sela M (1965) Genetic control of the antibody response. I. Demonstration of determinant-specific differences in response to synthetic polypeptide antigens in two strains of inbred mice. J Exp Med 122:517–531
12. Mozes E (1975) Expression of immune response (Ir) genes in T and B cells. Immunogenetics 2:397–410
13. Svejgaard A, Platz P, Ryder LD (1983) HLA and disease 1982 – a survey. Immunol Rev 70:193–218
14. Talal N (1977) Autoimmunity: genetic, immunologic, virologic, and clinical aspects. Academic, New York

HLA-Linked Immune Suppression Genes: A Mechanism for the Statistical Association Between HLA and Disease

T. Sasazuki*, Y. Nishimura*, M. Muto, and N. Ohta

Department of Human Genetics, Medical Research Institute, Tokyo Medical and Dental University, Tokyo 113, Japan

Genetic control of immune response to cedar pollen (CP) antigen (M.W. 45 K) was analyzed using 165 families with allergy to CP antigen (cedar pollinosis). IgE response to CP antigen both in vivo and in vitro was shown to be an autosomal recessive trait, and nonresponsiveness is dominant. The gene controlling the nonresponsiveness to CP antigen was closely linked to HLA (maximum lod score was 3.20 at $\theta = 0.05$). Leu $2^{+}3^{-}$ T cell from healthy individuals (nonresponders to CP antigen) completely suppressed the IgE response of allergic patients (responders) in vitro. This suppressor T cell is both antigen and isotype (IgE) specific. Thus the HLA-linked gene controlling nonresponsiveness to CP antigen was designated as an HLA-linked immune suppression gene (Is-gene) [1]. It was clearly demonstrated that the HLA-linked Is-gene for CP antigen controlled the resistance to cedar pollinosis, and the lack of this gene in the homozygous state might predispose to cedar pollinosis. The patients with cedar pollinosis showed statistical association with HLA-DQw3. This association was unambiguously explained by the presence of an HLA-linked Is-gene in negative linkage disequilibrium with HLA-DQw3. The statistical association between HLA-DRw6 and postschistosomal liver cirrhosis [2] was also clearly explained by the existence of an HLA-linked Is-gene for schistosomal worm antigen in negative linkage disequilibrium with HLA-DRw6. Along this line, the HLA-linked gene which has a major effect on the pathogenesis of Graves' disease [3] might be an HLA-linked Is-gene for an unknown environmental agent, and the statistical association of Graves' disease with HLA-DR5 might be due to the negative linkage disequilibrium of the HLA-linked Is-gene with HLA-DR5. HLA-linked Is-genes thus explain at least a part of the associations between HLA and disease.

* Present address: Dept of Genetics, Medical Institute of Bioregulation, Kyushu University, 3-1-1 Maidashi, Higashi-Ku, Fukuoka 812, Japan

References

1. Sasazuki T, Nishimura Y, Muto M, Saito Y (1984) MHC-linked immune suppression genes and their role in immunological disorders. In: Sasazuki T, Tada T (eds) Immunogenetics: its applications to clinical medicine. Academic, Tokyo (in press)
2. Ohta N, Nishimura YK, Iuchi M, Sasazuki T (1982) Immunogenetic analysis of patients with post-schistosomal liver cirrhosis in man. Clin Exp Immunol 49:493–499
3. Uno H, Sasazuki T, Tamai H, Matsumoto H (1981) Two genes, linked to HLA and Gm, control the susceptibility to Graves' disease. Nature 292:768–770

Histocompatibility Testing 1984
Edited by E. D. Albert et al.

Effects of Anti-DQ (MB) and Anti-DR Monoclonal Antibodies on In Vitro Immune Responses

M. Kasahara, Y. Fukasawa, K. Ogasawara, H. Kojima, H. Ikeda, N. Ishikawa, T. Okuyama, H. Kunikane, S. Hawkin, A. Wakisaka, I. Kikuchi, and M. Aizawa

Department of Pathology, Hokkaido University School of Medicine, Sapporo 060, Japan

Recent studies at both the protein and DNA levels suggest that human DQ antigens are homologues of murine I-A antigens. In mice, the functional significance of I-A antigens in immune responsiveness is well established. There are, however, only a few studies on the functional role of DQ antigens in the human immune response. In the present study, we investigated the effects of an anti-DQw3 monoclonal antibody (MoAb) on various in vitro immune responses and its effects were compared with those of an anti-DR MoAb.

The following MoAbs were used in this study: HU-2, anti-HLA-A, B, C framework [1]; HU-4 (3G7), anti-DR framework [1, 2]; and HU-18, anti-DQw3 monomorphic [3, 4]. All cultures were set up as described in the figure legends.

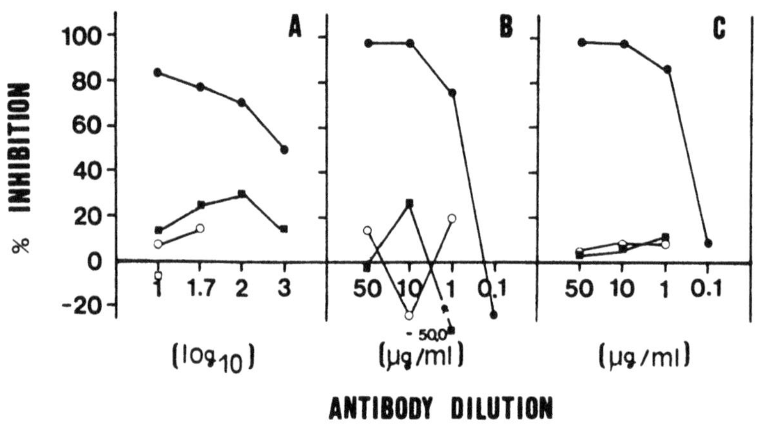

Fig. 1A–C. Effects of MoAbs on T cell proliferative responses to PPD (**A**), autologous non-T cells (**B**), and autologous EBV-transformed B cells (**C**). Mononuclear cells (*MNCs*) supposed to be homozygous for the HU-18 determinant were used in all three cases. Progressive dilutions of MoAbs (HU-2, ○–○; HU-4, ●–●; HU-18, ■–■) or control ascites (□–□) were added (50 μl/well) at the initiation of the culture and left throughout the incubation period. The mean cpm in the presence of control medium (RPMI 1640) were 60 799 ± 4907 (**A**), 67 231 ± 18 349 (**B**), and 167 653 ± 2931 (**C**). % inhibition was calculated according to the following formula: % inhibition = (1 − mean cpm in the presence of MoAbs/mean cpm in the presence of control medium) × 100

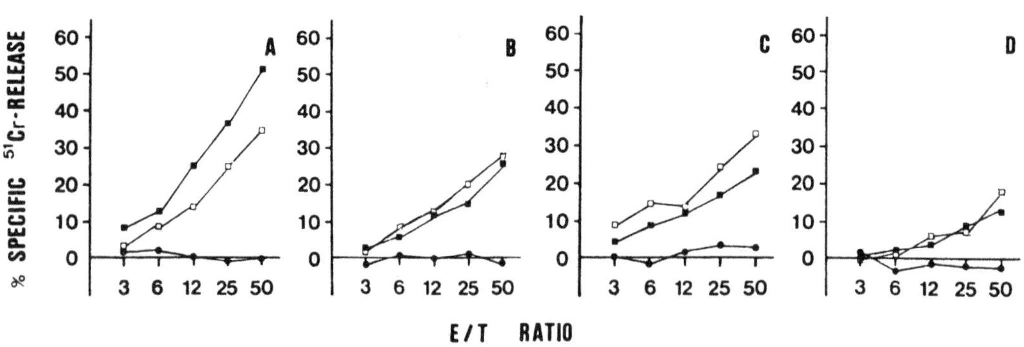

Fig. 2. A–D. Effects of MoAbs on the generation of killer T cells in MLR. MNCs (1.5×10^6/well) were cultured with 3000 rad-irradiated stimulator MNCs (1.5×10^6/well) in Linbro multiwell plates in a total volume of 2 ml RPMI 1640 supplemented with 20% FCS. Cultures were incubated at 37 °C for 7 days in the presence of 0.5 ml 1 : 10 diluted control ascites (□–□), HU-4 (●–●), and HU-18 (■–■). The resultant cytolytic activity was tested against PHA-activated blasts derived from the stimulator cells in MLR. **A** An MLR combination where both stimulators and responders are positive (homozygous) for HU-18; **B** only stimulators positive for HU-18; **C** only responders positive for HU-18; **D** both negative for HU-18

Histocompatibility Testing 1984
Edited by E. D. Albert et al.

As shown in Fig. 1, HU-4 strongly inhibited T cell proliferative responses to PPD (A), autologous non-T cells (B), and autologous EBV-transformed B cells (C). This MoAb also suppressed T cell proliferative responses to alloantigens (data not shown) and generation of killer T cells specific for alloantigens (Fig. 2). In contrast, none of these immune responses were significantly affected by HU-2 or HU-18 (Figs. 1, 2).

The inability of HU-18 to inhibit T cell proliferative responses is consistent with the results of Corte et al. [5] who used an anti-DQw1 MoAb, BT3/4. However, unlike BT3/4, HU-18 had no effect on the generation of killer T cells in MLR.

Our results presented above indicate that DR (murine I-E-like) rather than DQ (murine I-A-like) antigens play a major role in the in vitro systems studied here. These results differ from those obtained in mice, because murine I-A antigens act as potent stimulators in MLR and autologous MLR and play a critical role in the induction of killer T cells. It remains to be discovered why there are such striking differences in the functional properties of "I-A" antigens between man and the mouse.

References

1. Kasahara M, Ikeda H, Ogasawara K, Ishikawa N, Okuyama T, Fukasawa Y, Kojima H, Kunikane H, Hawkin S, Ohhashi T, Natori T, Wakisaka A, Kikuchi Y, Aizawa M (1984) Inhibition of autologous mixed lymphocyte reaction by monoclonal antibodies specific for the β chain of HLA-DR antigens. Immunology 53:79–86
2. Koide Y, Awashima F, Yoshida TO, Takenouchi T, Wakisaka A, Moriuchi J, Aizawa M (1982) The role of three distinct Ia-like antigen molecules in human T cell proliferative responses: effect of monoclonal anti-Ia-like antibodies. J Immunol 129:1061–1069
3. Kasahara M, Takenouchi T, Ogasawara K, Ikeda H, Okuyama T, Ishikawa N, Moriuchi J, Wakisaka A, Kikuchi Y, Aizawa M, Kaneko T, Kashiwagi N, Nishimura Y, Sasazuki T (1983) Serologic dissection of HLA-D specificities by the use of monoclonal antibodies. Immunogenetics 17:485–495
4. Ikeda H, Kasahara M, Ogasawara K, Takenouchi T, Okuyama T, Ishikawa N, Wakisaka A, Kikuchi Y, Aizawa M (1984) Evidence for polymorphism of MB3 antigens among three HLA-D clusters associated with HLA-DR4. Immunogenetics 19:381–390
5. Corte G, Moretta A, Cosulich ME, Ramarli D, Bargellesi A (1982) A monoclonal anti-DC1 antibody selectively inhibits the generation of effector T cells mediating specific cytolytic activity. J Exp Med 156:1539–1544

Individual Differences in the In Vitro (CTC) Immune Response to HLA Antigens

P. Ivanyi and B.S. Breur

Division of Immunohematology, Central Laboratory Netherlands Red Cross Blood Transfusion Service Laboratory for Experimental and Clinical Immunology of the University of Amsterdam, Amsterdam, The Netherlands

We refer to experiments which allow classification of individuals as narrow and broad responders to HLA antigens. The immune response of 12 healthy individuals was examined by their CTC response to four to six different HLA antigens. CTCs were generated in MLR-positive responder–stimulator combinations, always differing only in one HLA-A or HLA-B antigen. Each responder was stimulated independently by four to six different stimulator cells. From each combination the CTCs were tested against a panel of third-party cells, which expressed the same specific antigen as the stimulator, or cross-reacting antigen(s), or neither (specific, CREG, and non-CREG third-party cells, respectively). Different types of responders could be identified:

1. Those who generated CTCs only against the specific HLA antigen in all combinations (narrow or specific responders)
2. Those who generated CTCs only to the specific HLA antigen in some combinations, but showed a broader reaction pattern in other combinations
3. Those who generated broadly reacting CTCs in all combinations (broad responders)

The differences found in the in vitro immune response to HLA-A and B antigens among individuals were not dependent on the HLA-A or B phenotype of the responder, because HLA-A, B identical individuals responded differently to the same stimulator cell (Fig. 1). However, the identical response of monozygotic twins (Fig. 2) indicates that the type of response is influenced by some other, still unknown genetic factors.

Figure 1 and 2 see p. 618

Histocompatibility Testing 1984
Edited by E. D. Albert et al.

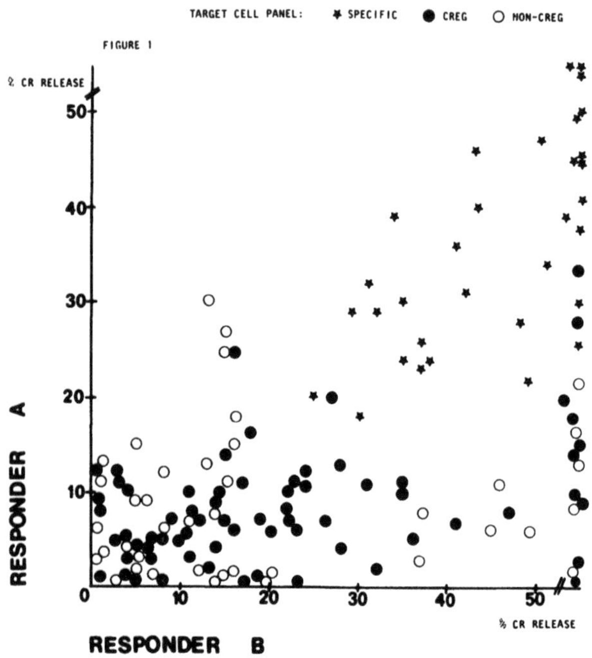

Fig. 1. Two unrelated HLA-A, B identical responders. Responder A reacted specifically (narrow responder) and responder B reacted broadly (broad responder) to all antigens

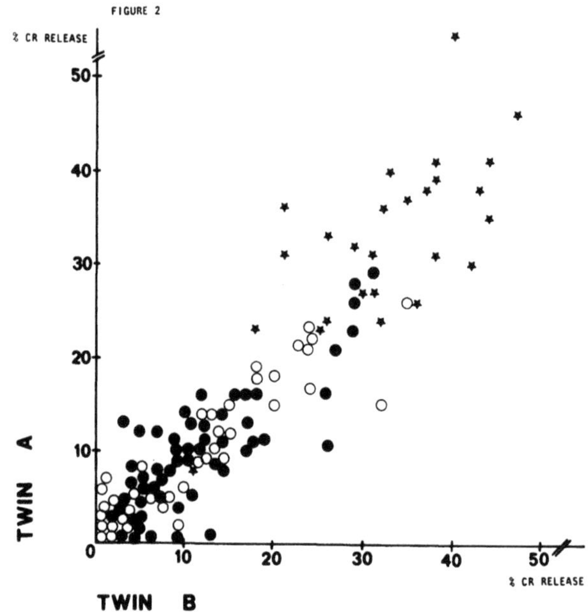

Fig. 2. Monozygotic twins. This response of both (twins A and B) is almost specific and identical

HLA-Linked Gene Regulation of the Immune Response to Nitrofurantoin-Albumin

J. Valtonen and S. Koskimies

FRC Blood Transfusion Service, Kivihaantie, 7, 00310 Helsinki 31, Finland

We have earlier found high responders to nitrofurantoin-albumin (NF-alb) antigen among healthy blood donors and observed an increased frequency of HLA-DR3 antigen among those with no sufficient T suppressor cell activity. In this study DR3+ and DR3– individuals were compared in their alloreactivity and immune response to NF-alb or NF in vitro in order to analyze the function of separate cell populations. Peripheral blood mononuclear cells from ten healthy blood donors were fractionated by Percoll gradient centrifugation into monocytes (Mo), T helper (T_h) and T suppressor (T_s) cells. Comparisons were made in pairs of DR3+ and DR3–, both sharing one DR antigen to fulfill requirements for cell collaboration. Cells were cultured separately or mixed in various combinations. Proliferative response with and without antigen was measured.

Generally the alloreaction prevailed; antigen-specific response was weakly detectable under it. A marked analogy in the function of DR3+ cells in various combinations was observed, as shown in Table 1.

It seems that monocytes do not play a decisive role, but that T_h cells may be regulated by HLA-linked genes. The possibility that both T_h and T_s cells are regulated by HLA is not totally ruled out.

Table 1. Responses in different combinations

T_hDR3	T_sDR3	Mo DR3	Response
+	+	+	strong
–	–	–	weak
+	–		strong
–	+		weak
+	–	–	strong
–	+	+	weak
+	–	+	strong
–	+	–	weak
+		+	strong
–		–	weak

Histocompatibility Testing 1984
Edited by E. D. Albert et al.

Phenotype and Specificity of MLR-Generated Suppressor Cells

H. Choremi, E.L. Milford, and C.B. Carpenter

Brigham & Women's Hospital, Harvard Medical School, Boston, MA, USA

The allogeneic MLR is being used as a model for generation of suppressor T cells which induce feedback inhibition of naive responder cells. We have been employing monoclonal antibodies to lymphocyte subsets and HLA-typed panels of stimulator cells in order to discern the phenotype and antigen specificity of such suppressor cells. One-way (A + Bx) MLR bulk cultures at 10^6 cells/ml in 50-ml flasks were incubated for 8–10 days, 2 days after the peak of ^{3}H-TdR incorporation had been reached. These primed cells were washed and added in various amounts to test micro-MLRs (A + Bx, A + Cx, A + Dx, etc.) and ^{3}H-TdR uptake was measured at 6 days. Primed cells were affinity-fractionated, employing monoclonal antibodies, anti- T4, T8, and MO1. Negatively selected T4$^+$ or T8$^+$ cell populations contained 2%–5% cross-contamination. In most combinations in which two D/DR incompatibilities were present in the generating culture, 50% suppression of the test MLR was produced at dilutions of 1 : 8–1 : 16 with respect to the total cells present, and all suppression was contained in the T8$^+$ population, while the T4$^+$ fraction caused augmentation. On some occasions when overall suppression was stronger, T4$^+$ fractions suppressed. The latter could not be eliminated by removal of MO1$^+$ contaminating cells (macrophages and/or null cells), and was accounted for by contaminating T8$^+$ cells. Kinetic analysis showed that while primed T8$^+$ cells showed minimal proliferation when re-exposed to stimulator cells, T4$^+$ cells first responded as in PLT, and then prevented proliferation on day 6. This apparent T4$^+$ suppressor effect might be due to early recruitment of unprimed cells; alternatively, there could be induction of T8$^+$ suppressor cells by primed T4$^+$ inducers.

Although it has been reported that allosuppression is directed to HLA-DR, we find several examples of patterns which do not fit this hypothesis. When the A + Bx generating cells shared one D/DR antigen, a reproducible polymorphic pattern of suppression against a selected nine-member panel was obtained, but as shown in Table 1, was not related to sharing of D/DR (or DQ, DRw53, DRw52) antigens with the original stimulator.

Hence, allosuppressive T cells in this MLR system are T8$^+$ and their specificity is not related to HLA-DR antigens.

Table 1. Suppression by T8$^+$ primed cells (A + Bx)

	HLA-Dw	HLA-DR	Suppression
A	3/x	3/6	
B	3/4	3/4	++
C	2/4	2/4	++
D	x/x	2/4	–
E	x/x	4/5	+
F	x/x	4/6	–
G	–	3/7	++
H	1/7	1/7	++
I	–	2/6	–
J	–	1/6	++
K	3/5	3/5	+

Alloproliferative T4+ T8– Human T Cell Clones with Suppressive, Not Helper, Function *

G. Pawelec, E.M. Schneider, and P. Wernet

Immunology Laboratory, Medizinische Universitätsklinik, 7400 Tübingen, Federal Republic of Germany

The existence of at least three distinct subsets of human MHC class II molecules encoded by discrete genetic loci has been clearly established, namely HLA-DR, DQ, and DP. Products of each of these loci have been shown to function as alloantigens and as restriction elements in lymphoproliferative (LP) responses of T cells to al-

* This work was supported by the Deutsche Forschungsgemeinschaft through SFB 120 (A1)

logeneic cells and to nominal antigens. However, it remains to be determined whether T cells reactive to the different subsets of class II molecules are endowed with different functional activities, since it cannot be assumed that proliferating lymphocytes are necessarily "helper" cells. Thus, the immunoregulatory activities of alloproliferative (primed lymphocyte typing, PLT) clones on lymphoproliferative (LP) responses were studied. The clones were derived as described [1] by limitation of dilution and expansion of clonal progeny in interleukin 2 (IL 2) from lymphocyte populations sensitized in (1) primary mixed lymphocyte cultures (MLCs) between HLA-D-mismatched donors: the majority of PLT clones (> 60% in several priming combinations) recognized lymphocyte-activating determinants (LADs) closely associated with HLA-D region products [1]; (2) tertiary MLCs between HLA-D-matched, DP-mismatched donors: the majority (> 90%) recognised LADs closely associated with DP products [2]; and (3) primary MLCs between HLA-D-matched, DP-mismatched donors: the majority (> 70%), on the basis of population studies and stimulation inhibition with monoclonal antibodies against different class II molecules [3], recognised LADs similar to, but different from, alleles of the DP series, which have therefore been termed "DP-like" [4] and may represent the products of a second DP-related locus (1). The PLT clones had a "helper" OKT4+, OKT8–, Leu8– cell surface phenotype, proliferated strongly, and secreted IL 2 after specific restimulation, but had markedly different effects when titrated into MLC or PLT assays. Thus, clones specific for DP-like LADs strongly suppressed primary (1′) and secondary (2′) LP responses, whereas most HLA-D-, one available DQ-, and all DP-specific clones either enhanced or had no effect on LP responses. Table 1 summarizes these results. There was no obvious difference in the recognitive specificity for HLA-D-associated determinants between the single suppressive and the nonsuppressive PLT clones, whereas the DP-like determinants were novel. The inhibitory activity of these suppressive PLT clones was radioresistant (20 Gy), and not restricted by the MHC type of either responding or stimulating cells in the test assay. Suppression was not caused by absorption of IL 2, since the clones themselves could secrete this growth factor, and, moreover, addition of exogenous IL 2 failed to abrogate suppression. Lysis of responding or stimulating cells in the test MLC was excluded as a mechanism of suppression, since no cytotoxicity against normal or activated T and B cells or against natural killer-susceptible leukemic target cells by these suppressive PLT clones could be demonstrated, and since suppressed cultures retained viability but failed to undergo blast transformation.

Table 1. Functional characteristics of allospecific PLT clones

Specificity	n	Effect on			
		PLT activity[a]	1′ LP	2′ LP[b]	IL 2 production[c]
HLA-D/DR	30	56	+35	+27	11.3
DP	18	63	+39	+45	12.4
DQ	1	25	+28	nt	7.2
DP-like	8	31	−85	−83	10.5

nt, not tested

[a] Mean stimulation in PLT, calculated as the ratio of specific stimulated/unstimulated responses

[b] Mean relative response of 1′ LP (measured in MLC) and 2′ LP (measured in PLT), calculated as a percentage change on addition of one irradiated cloned cell per ten responders compared to the value in the absence of added cells. Positive values represent enhancement, negative values represent suppression

[c] Mean IL 2 production 24 h after specific stimulation of PLT clones, measured by the ability of culture supernatants to support growth of IL 2-addicted indicator cells, calculated as the ratio of specifically stimulated responses to unstimulated responses

Suppression was mediated by at least two different mechanisms: (1) MHC-unrestricted induction of similarly unrestricted suppressor effector cells in naive lymphocyte populations, and (2) a direct inhibitory effect of the suppressive clones on LP responses of PLT clones stimulated by B lymphoblastoid cell lines. The induced suppressor effectors were also radioresistant (20 Gy) and capable of inhibiting both 1′ and 2′ LP responses even in the presence of IL 2. By propagating the induced cells with IL 2 it was excluded that the inducing clones surviving the first culture period were carried over into the assay and were responsible for its suppression, confirming that the induced cells themselves exerted the observed effects. Direct suppression was demonstrated by using PLT clones, presumed to be free of inducible suppressor precursors as the responders and a B lymphoid cell line as stimulator in the test assays. Furthermore, culture supernatants of suppressive, but not nonsuppressive, PLT clones also strongly inhibited 1′ and 2′ LP responses, although they were unable to induce suppressor effectors in normal lymphocyte populations. The inhibitory factor(s) was not destroyed at pH 2, was not heat labile (56 °C, 30 min), and was not lymphocytotoxic.

It is therefore concluded that suppressive function may be performed by cells possessing a number of "helper/inducer" phenotype-related characteristics, namely alloproliferative capacity, the ability to secrete IL 2, and the presence of OKT4– but not OKT8– or Leu8– defined cell surface antigens. Moreover, while the majority of HLA-D/DR-specific, all DP-specific, and the one DQ-specific clone failed to suppress LP responses, all PLT clones responding to "DP-like" determinants exerted strong direct and indirect suppressive influences, indicating that T cells stimulated by different subsets of class II molecules may mediate different functions. The role of the DP-like, in contrast to DP, determinants therefore seems to be predominantly in the control of nonspecific suppression. Hence, the type of MHC antigen responsible for stimulation of alloproliferative T cells correlates better with their functional status than does the presence of "helper" (T4), "suppressor" (T8), or "suppressor-inducer" (Leu8) surface structures.

Acknowledgment. The assistance of Mss A. Rehbein, I. Balko, and C. Miller is greatly appreciated.

References

1. Pawelec G (1983) Allogeneically primed T lymphocyte clones in the analysis of lymphocyte stimulatory determinants. Human Immunol 8:239–247
2. Pawelec G, Shaw S, Schneider EM, Rehbein A, Wernet P (1983) Homogeneity of the HLA-linked SB2 and SB3 specificities demonstrated by cloned alloreactive T cells. Immunogenetics 17:179–188
3. Pawelec G, Shaw S, Ziegler A, Müller C, Wernet P (1982) Differential inhibition of HLA-D or SB directed secondary lymphoproliferative responses with monoclonal antibodies detecting human Ia-like determinants. J Immunol 129:1070–1075
4. Pawelec G, Wernet P, Rosenlund R, Blaurock M, Schneider EM (1984) Strong lymphoproliferative suppressive function of PLT clones specific for SB-like antigens. Human Immunol 9:145–157

Relationship Between the OKT Phenotype of Alloreactive Human T Cell Clones and Their Specificity for HLA Class II Antigens

X. Chardonnens, G. Morgan, and M. Jeannet

Transplantation Immunology Unit, Division of Immunology and Allergology, Hôpital Cantonal Universitaire, 1211 Geneva, Switzerland

Introduction

It has recently been suggested that the phenotype of T cells is not associated with their function but with the class of MHC antigens they recognize, and that OKT4 and OKT8 molecules function as receptors for distinct classes of HLA alloantigens. The recent development of techniques allowing the cloning and proliferation of functional T cells, coupled with the use of monoclonal antibodies, allows us to examine whether a relationship exists between surface markers of the clones, their functional activity, and their specificity for class I or II HLA antigens.

Materials and Methods

Three pairs of MLC-activated lymphocytes from HLA-A, B, and/or DR-identical, unrelated individuals were cloned by limiting dilution in round-bottom microtiter plates as described previously [1]. After 1–2 months of culture with IL-2- and X-irradiated feeder cells, individual clones were tested for proliferation in response to a small panel of X-irradiated allogeneic stimulator cells using the primed lymphocyte test (PLT), and for cytotoxicity against a few selected PHA-stimulated lymphoblasts using the CML assay. Thirteen clones were selected for a more extensive study of their PLT and/or CML specificity and of their surface markers, using a standard complement-dependent microcytotoxicity test.

Results and Discussion

Five of six clones with the OKT8 phenotype demonstrated both proliferative and cytotoxic reactivity. They were all significantly stimulated to proliferate by the relevant class II specificity (DR5, DPw2, or DRw6). In panel studies, they also demonstrated class II-directed cytotoxicity, and their reactivity was often, but not always, restricted to the relevant DR or DP antigen. One additional OKT8 clone demonstrated an anti-DPw2 cytotoxicity, but no significant proliferative reactivity. Three of seven clones with the OKT4 phenotype also demonstrated both proliferative and cytotoxic reac-

Histocompatibility Testing 1984
Edited by E. D. Albert et al.

tivity, with a clear specificity towards the relevant class II determinant. Three additional OKT4 clones were significantly stimulated to proliferate by most cells bearing the relevant antigen DRw6; however, their cytotoxic reactivity was not tested. Finally, one OKT4 clone was not proliferative but demonstrated a clear DRw6 reactivity in cytotoxicity. A majority of clones thus had both proliferative and cytotoxic activities, like the recently described helper-cell-independent cytotoxic clones [2]. Although they all had a clear class II specificity, nearly half of them had the OKT8 marker, which is often considered as a recognition structure for class I antigens. Taken together, our results suggest that the expression of OKT markers is not necessarily associated with the recognition of class I or class II HLA antigens.

References

1. Chardonnens X, Froment Y, Morgan G, Jeannet M (1983) Human T cell clones allospecific for HLA-DR5 antigen with the OKT8 phenotype. Tissue Antigens 22:76–81
2. Wee SL, Chen LK, Strassmann G, Bach FH (1982) Helper-cell-independent cytotoxic clones in man. J Exp Med 156:1854–1859

Functional Heterogeneity of Human T Cell Responses to Class I and Class II MHC Antigens

N.E. Goeken, M.K. Eckerle, P.J. Lioubin, and T.S. Staggs

Departments of Medicine, Veterans Administration and University of Iowa Medical Centers Iowa City, IA 52240, USA

Class II MHC antigens have been previously demonstrated to play a crucial role in T cell activation by alloantigen and in T-B collaboration in response to soluble antigen. To investigate the role of these antigens in greater detail, we have employed four in vitro models that allow differential presentation of class I and class II antigen [1–3]. These are heat-treated lymphocytes, highly purified T cells, purified platelets, and D/DR-compatible lymphocytes. As we have reported previously, lymphocytes heated to 45 °C for 60 min completely lose their ability to stimulate an allogeneic MLR response. They do, however, retain all their serologically identified HLA-DR and DQ antigens and are equivalent to untreated cells in their ability to absorb such anti-class II activity from alloantisera. We refer to this as a model for class I plus nonimmunogenic class II antigen. D/DR (MLC-compatible) cells also fall into this category. T cells extensively purified in the absence of foreign protein (fetal calf serum) are $\gg$95% DR negative, and thus we use these cells as a model for class I antigen alone. Platelets also possess class I antigen only.

These four models were employed as stimulators in vitro in the MLR. All failed to stimulate proliferation in either the primary or the secondary MLR. Four-day culture supernatants from all of these experimental MLRs also had significantly reduced ability to support continued Con A blast proliferation when compared to conventional MLR supernatants. This indicates a reduction of IL2 synthesis or release. They also had diminished capacity to support proliferation of murine thymocytes to a submitogenic dose of PHA (costimulator assay), i.e., IL1 was also reduced. Thus, it appears that lymphokine production and consequently, cell proliferation, requires intact and unmodified class II antigen. Further, heat-treated non-T cells (B cells + monocytes) cannot present soluble antigen to purified T cells. This function also requires intact class II antigen.

Other features of activation are not affected in this way. Both heat-treated cells and D/DR-compatible (HLA A, B incompatible) cells will cause the responding cells to proliferate in the presence of exogenous IL2. IL2 receptors are generated. Platelets will not stimulate such receptors. This implies that some form of Ia antigen, even though it may be modified or even syngeneic, must be recognized together with the class I antigen to stimulate expression of these receptors.

Finally, there are at least two important functions that are triggered by all of these models, including platelets. These are suppressor cell activation and memory cell priming. Cells isolated on day 10 from any of these experimental MLRs will produce 80%–95% reduction in proliferation when added to a fresh conventional MLR employing the original responder and stimulator. In addition, even though no proliferation occurs in the primary experimental

Histocompatibility Testing 1984
Edited by E. D. Albert et al.

Table 1. Human T cell activation

	Requirement for class II antigen		
	Intact	Modified (nonimmunogenic)	Class I only
Primary MLR	Yes		
Secondary MLR	Yes		
IL2 synthesis	Yes		
IL2 receptors	Yes	Yes	
IL1 synthesis	Yes		
Antigen presentation	Yes		
Suppressor cell activation	Yes	Yes	Yes
Priming of memory cells	Yes	Yes	Yes
Model	Allogeneic Cells	1. Heat Treated 2. D/DR Compatible	1. T Cells 2. Platelets

MLRs, when these cells are subsequently *re*-stimulated with conventional irradiated lymphocytes from the original donor, they show a vigorous, accelerated (day 3) anamnestic response. Suppressor activation and memory cell priming thus require only class I MHC antigen differences.

These data, summarized in Table 1, illustrate the functional heterogeneity of T cell responses to Ia-like antigens. Some responses (suppression induction and memory cell priming), can occur independently of class II antigen, others require a non-allogeneic but heat-stable component of the class II molecule (induction of IL2 receptors), and finally, some appear to require intact and unmodified Ia molecules. (IL1 synthesis, IL2 synthesis, antigen presentation, and cell proliferation.) Further investigations on the contribution of various T cell subsets to this functional heterogeneity are currently underway.

References

1. Goeken NE (1983) Preferential activation of human suppressor cells in vitro by heat modified stimulators. Trans Proc 15:780–783
2. Goeken NE (1984) Human suppressor cell induction in vitro: preferential activation by class I MHC antigen. J Immunol 132:2291–2299
3. Goeken NE (1984) Differential stimulatory requirements and regulation of naive and primed human lymphocytes. Human Immunol 10:251–263

Restriction of Human Influenza A Virus-Specific T Cell Clones by HTC-Defined Subtypes of HLA-Dw6

B. Fleischer[1], M. Blaurock[2], P. Wernet[2], and G. Pawelec[2]

1 Department of Immunology, Universität Ulm, 7900 Ulm, Federal Republic of Germany
2 Immunology Laboratory, Medizinische Klinik, 7400 Tübingen, Federal Republic of Germany

Introduction

Human antigen-specific proliferative T lymphocyte clones (TLCs) generally recognize nominal antigen in association with self class II MHC molecules on the antigen-presenting cell (APC). Alloantisera against HLA-DR antigens could inhibit antigen recognition, and studies using panels of APCs have shown that the restriction elements (REs) for the recognition of antigen were strongly correlated with HLA-DR/D antigens [1]. The use of cloned lines of antigen-specific TLCs has suggested that several class II HLA-antigens can act as REs for antigen recognition by T cells [2, 3]. However, the question is still open of whether the HLA determinants activating alloreactive T cell responses are recognized as REs by self-restricted antigen-specific TLCs. In this report we demonstrate a close relationship between the REs for influenza virus-specific TLCs and the allodeterminants defined by HTCs.

Histocompatibility Testing 1984
Edited by E. D. Albert et al.

Materials and Methods

Cells. All experiments were done with cryopreserved PBMCs. T cell-depleted PBMCs (E^-) were prepared and infected as described [4] and used as APCs.

TLCs. The four TLCs used in this study were obtained by limiting dilution from PBMCs stimulated three times with influenza A/USSR virus-infected autologous PBMCs [4]. The clones showed distinct specificities for influenza A viruses of different subtypes. They were propagated by weekly restimulation with irradiated, infected, HLA-matched PBMCs. The clones have the $T4^+8^-$ phenotype and are capable of producing interleukin-2 after stimulation.

HLA Typing. Serological typing was performed on nylon wool-isolated B cells in a standard NIH microlymphocytotoxicity test, using Eighth and Ninth Workshop as well as local alloantisera. Cellular typing for products of the HLA-D region was performed in standard MLC checkerboard experiments, using local, exchanged, and Ninth Workshop HTCs to stimulate panels of responding lymphocytes. Data reduction of raw cpm was performed following the protocol of previous workshops by generating double normalized values (DNV) at the 75th percentile. DNV $\leq$ 40 was taken as an unequivocal typing response and formed the basis for assignation of HLA-Dw specificities. In typing for the Dw6 cluster, a larger range of HTCs was employed, including those provided by the Ninth Workshop, and specificity assignment was made when possible on the basis of the pre-workshop-defined "splits" Dw6.1, 6.2 and 6.3. In cases where such an assignment was not possible, Dw6 "broad" was assigned.
Cellular typing for DP antigens was performed as described [5].

Assay for Specific Proliferative Activity. This was performed as described [4]. Briefly, 10^4 E^- infected with A/USSR virus or the unrelated influenza B/Lee virus as a control were incubated with 10^4 TLCs for 3 days. A ^{3}H-thymidine pulse was given 18 h before the cells were harvested. Each experiment included the autologous APCs. For blocking with the monoclonal antibodies (moAbs) MHM5 [6] and DA6.231 [7], a dialyzed hybridoma supernatant was added to a final concentration of 25%. Data are given as cpm incorporated by the TLC or as percent relative response (%RR), taking the response to autologous infected APCs as 100% and the cpm of the medium control as 0%.

Statistical Analysis. Proliferative responses of the TLCs on different infected APCs were analyzed by clustering responses into positive and negative groups on the basis of minimizing variance between the two groups. A comparison of the results obtained with log-transformed and arithmetic data points was used to indicate which responses should be considered equivocal. In panel studies, the significance of association of a stimulatory RE with the APCs' HLA antigens was evaluated by Fisher's exact test.

Results

Class II HLA Molecules Carry the RE for the TLCs

Monoclonal antibodies specific for nonpolymorphic determinants of class I or class II molecules were used to block the antigen-specific proliferation of the TLC. As shown in Table 1, the anti-class II moAb DA6.231 [7] blocked antigen recognition by all TLCs. The moAb MHM5, specific for a monomorphic determinant on HLA-A, B, C molecules that blocks class I-restricted cytotoxic T

Table 1. Blocking of specific proliferation by moAbs

Antibody	Clone response (cpm)			
	GR1	GR24	GR28	GR41
Medium	3 065	2 709	2 386	1 946
MHM5	4 062	3 385	2 228	3 070
DA6.231	119	229	114	138

TLCs were incubated with hybridoma supernatants at a concentration of 25% and the autologous E^- were infected with A/USSR virus. The response to uninfected E^- was less than 200 cpm

Table 2. Segregation of REs in family R

APC	Antigen	%RR by clone			
		GR1	GR24	GR28	GR41
G.R.[a] (c/b)	A/USSR	100	100	100	100
	B/Lee	4	8	7	5
Father (a/b)	A/USSR	2	105	2	150
	B/Lee	2	4	2	4
Mother (c/d)	A/USSR	129	3	280	1
	B/Lee	4	1	0	2
Brother (a/d)	A/USSR	3	1	1	1
	B/Lee	0	0	0	0

Haplotypes: a Dw4, DP–; b Dw6, DPw3; c Dw1, DP–; d Dw3 DPw4
[a] Autologous APCs

Table 3. Association of REs with HLA specificities

Clone	Association with	Allele/response				n	Fisher's exact p
		+/+	+/−	−/+	−/−		
GR1, GR28	DR1	8	2	2	20	32	0.329×10^{-3}
GR1, GR28	Dw1	10	0	0	22	32	0.310×10^{-7}
GR24	DRw6	14	12	6	16	48	0.116
GR24	Dw6 broad	19	9	1	19	48	0.169×10^{-4}
GR24	Dw6.1	20	0	1	28	49	0.149×10^{-11}
GR41	DRw6	21	7	4	12	44	0.003
GR41	Dw6 broad	25	2	1	17	45	0.520×10^{-8}

Table 4. Association of REs for GR24 and GR41 with Dw6 subtypes in HTCs

APCs[a]	Tentative subtype	%RR by clone	
		GR24	GR41
Autologous APCs		100	100
HBS (9W0601)	Dw6.1	51	49
HHK (9W0602)	Dw6.1	41	32
J. Ted (9W0603)	Dw6.1	89	109
SCL (9W0604)	Dw6.1	123	119
WDV (9W0605)	Dw6.1	56	68
EMJ (9W0606)	Dw6.2	24	112
KRA (9W0607)	Dw6.2	14	119
SLE (9W0608)	Dw6.2	5	148
KT11 (9W0610)	Dw6.3	30	139
Steph (9W0611)	Dw6.3	40	101

[a] Local identification (Ninth Workshop number)

cells [6], did not inhibit. The specificity of blocking by moAb DA6.231 was confirmed by the finding that the moAb did not affect the mitogen-induced proliferation of the TLCs (not shown).

HLA Specificity of the TLCs

In the donor's family the TLCs GR1 and GR28 were found to proliferate against infected APCs carrying a DR1, Dw1 haplotype and TLC GR24 and GR41 against DRw6, Dw6-carrying APCs (Table 2). Panels of HLA-typed APC were employed to investigate further the genetic control of the structures functioning as REs. There was no significant association between the REs and DP, DRw52, DRw53 and DQ specificities (not shown). In the population, REs for the two DR1, Dw1-restricted TLCs showed perfect correlation with Dw1 rather than DR1 (Table 3). The situation with the DRw6, Dw6-restriced TLCs was interesting with respect to current difficulties in defining these specificity clusters. The response of both clones, GR24 and GR41, failed to correlate significantly with the presence of HLA-DRw6. However, REs for these TLCs did correlate significantly with HLA-Dw6 as defined by HTCs. Moreover, using APCs carrying the provisionally defined Dw6 subtypes, it was found that GR24 was stimulated only by cells carrying the Dw6.1 subtype, whereas GR41 recognized the viral antigens on all Dw6 APCs. This was confirmed using Ninth Workshop HTCs as APCs. As shown in Table 4, only HTCs expressing the Dw6.1 subspecificity could stimulate GR24 and GR41 to the same degree; APCs of other Dw6 subtypes could stimulate GR41 only. There was no correlation of the reactivity of clone GR24 with putative serological splits of HLA-DRw6 (data not shown).

Discussion

A number of reports have assigned the REs for antigen-specific TLCs to the HLA-DR specificities [8–10]. However, it is evident from the present study that a large panel of APCs is required to discriminate between restriction by serologically defined DR specificities and HTC-defined Dw specificities. The clones described here are clearly restricted by determinants on class II HLA molecules defined by cellular typing. The specificity of TLC GR24 for a HTC-defined subspecificity indicates that antigen-specific T cells can indeed recognize the same determinants as alloreactive T cells. Antigen-specific TLCs such as those reported here will be helpful in defining new specificities on HLA molecules and in correlating structural and functional aspects of T cell recognition.

Summary

Influenza A virus-specific T lymphocyte clones (TLCs) with proliferative activity were derived from peripheral blood mononuclear cells (PBMCs) of a normal donor (HLA-DR1, Dw1, DP−/DRw6, Dw6, DPw3) by limiting dilution in the presence of irradiated feeder cells and interleukin-2. Four clones with the OKT4+8− phenotype that showed high antigen-specific proliferation were selected for further investigation. These TLCs did not show alloreactivity and were specific for influenza A but not influenza B virus antigens presented by monocytes carrying one or other haplotype of the donor. The proliferative response of all TLCs could be specifically inhibited by monoclonal antibodies against nonpolymorphic determinants on class II HLA molecules. In the population, the restriction elements (REs) of two clones correlated better with HLA-Dw1 than DR1, the REs of the two other TLCs better with Dw6 than DRw6. These latter TLC showed differential recognition of HLA-Dw6 subtypes as defined tentatively by homozygous typing cells (HTCs) without relationship to putative serological splits of DRw6. One of the TLCs was stimulated by cells carrying the Dw6.1 but not 6.2 or 6.3 subtypes of Dw6, the other reacted with antigen on all Dw6 cells. These results indicate a remarkable concordance between the structures recognized by alloreactive T cells as HTC-defined Dw specificities and the structures acting as REs for antigen recognition by virus-immune T cells.

References

1. Thorsby E, Berle E, Nousiainen H (1982) HLA-D region molecules restrict proliferative T cell responses to antigen. Immunol Rev 66:39–56
2. Eckels DD, Lake P, Lamb JR, Johnson AH, Shaw S, Hartzman RJ, Woody JN (1983) SB-restricted presentation of influenza and herpes virus antigens to human T lymphocyte clones. Nature 301:716–718
3. Ball EJ, Stasny P (1984) Antigen-specific HLA-restricted human T cell lines. 1. An MT3-like restriction determinant distinct from HLA-DR. Immunogenetics 19:13–26
4. Fleischer B (1983) Human influenza virus-specific T helper cell clones can be restricted by MHC products different from serologically defined HLA-DR antigens. Tissue Antigens 21:238–245
5. Pawelec G, Shaw S, Wernet P (1982) Analysis of the HLA-linked SB-gene system with cloned and uncloned alloreactive T cell lines. Immunogenetics 15:187–198
6. Hildreth JHK, Gotch FM, Hildreth PDK, McMichael AJ (1983) A human lymphocyte-associated antigen involved in cell-mediated lympholysis. Eur J Immunol 13:202–208
7. Van Heyningen V, Guy K, Newman R, Steel CM (1982) Human MHC class II molecules as differentiation markers. Immunogenetics 16:459–469
8. Sredni B, Volkman D, Schwartz RH, Fauci AS (1981) Antigen-specific human T cell clones: development of clones requiring HLA-DR compatible presenting cells for stimulation in presence of antigen. Proc Natl Acad Sci USA 78:1858–1862
9. Schmitt C, Ballet JJ, Agraport M, Bizzini B (1982) Human T cell clones specific for tetanus toxoid: characterization of antigen specificity and HLA-restriction. Eur J Immunol 12:849–854
10. Sterkers G, Henin Y, Lepage D, Fradelizzi C, Levy JP (1984) Influenza A hemagglutinin specific T cell clones strictly restricted by HLA-DR. Eur J Immunol 14:125–131

Antigen-Specific T Cell Clones Restricted by DR, DQ, or DP Class II HLA Molecules*

E. Qvigstad, G. Gaudernack, T. Moen, and E. Thorsby

Institute of Transplantation Immunology, The National Hospital (Rikshospitalet), Oslo 1, Norway

Introduction

Human T4 cells corecognize antigenic epitopes together with restriction elements on class II HLA molecules in membranes of antigen-presenting cells (APCs). In man, at least three different class II HLA molecules have been detected: DR, DQ, and DP. Antigen-specific (i.e., *Chlamydia trachomatis*-specific) proliferative T4 clones (TLCs) may be restricted by elements on DR, DQ, or DP molecules [9, 12]. The inhibitory effect of a panel of murine monoclonal antibodies (Mabs) directed against HLA molecules of the APCs was studied to further dissect the restriction specificities of the TLCs.

Materials and Methods

Monoclonal Antibodies. The murine monoclonal antibodies were kindly provided by Drs. Soldano Ferrone (Valhalla, USA), Steinar Funderud (Oslo, Norway), John Hansen (Seattle, USA), Andrew McMichael (Oxford, UK), Robert Winchester (New York, USA), and Andreas Ziegler (Tübingen, FRG).

* This work was supported by grants from the Norwegian Cancer Society

Antigen Preparation. A suspension of partially purified *C. trachomatis* subtype LGV-2 was used [11].

HLA Typing. All cell donors had previously been HLA-ABC, DR, and DQ typed by highly selected alloantisera. The broad specificities (DRw52, w53, DQw1 – 3) were also based on the close association to short DR determinants (i.e., DRw53 is closely associated with DR4 and DR7). The DP antigens (DPw1 – 4) were detected by cloned primed lymphocyte typing [6].

Preparation of APCs. Details appear elsewhere [9 – 12]. Peripheral blood mononuclear cells (PBMs) from Lymphoprep flotation were rosetted with AET-treated sheep erythrocytes, and the non-T cells were harvested from the interphase. In some experiments the non-T cells were antigen pulsed before use and the nonadherent cells then removed by washing. The APC were irradiated (20 Gy) before use.

Generation of Chlamydia-*Specific Clones.* Details are given elsewhere [9 – 12]. Briefly, PBMs were obtained from a donor, BS (HLA-A3; B7, 15; DR1, 4; DQw1, DRw53; DPw4), who had previously been sensitized to *C. trachomatis* in vivo. Following in vitro stimulation with chlamydial antigen, T cell blasts were separated from small T cells on Percoll density gradients (Pharmacia, Uppsala, Sweden). The blast-enriched suspension was then cloned by a limiting dilution technique, using antigen, irradiated autologous PBMs as feeder cells, and 20% TCGF in serum-supplemented medium [10]. TLCs were later transferred and expanded. To prepare antigen-specific DP-restricted TLCs, a slightly modified technique was employed [12]. Briefly, the T cell blasts (obtained as above) were restimulated twice with antigen and a pool of allogeneic PBMs as feeders before cloning. The pooled PBMs were DR disparate but DP identical with the T cell donor BS.

Proliferative Assays. Ten thousand non-T cells together with 20 µl chlamydial antigen were added directly to U-bottomed wells (Costar), or antigen-pulsed monocytes were used as APCs [11]. In some experiments 20 µl of Mabs in different dilutions was then added and was present throughout the assay. Control wells received no Mabs. Finally, 1×10^4 TLCs were added to each well. Incorporation of ^{3}H-thymidine was assessed by liquid scintillation counting, and the results were expressed as mean cpm ± SEM for triplicates. In inhibition studies the percent relative response (RR) was expressed according to the following formula:

$$RR = \frac{\text{Mean cpm with Mab}}{\text{Mean cpm without Mab}} \times 100\%$$

Results and Discussion

All tested clones were antigen specific and did not respond to allogeneic APC without antigen, as reported previously [10]. Table 1 gives some limited

Table 1. Class II HLA restriction of TLCs from a single donor

APC[a]				Ag[b]	TLC's[c, d]			
	DR	DQ	DP		BS24	BS5	BS37	BS110
Autologous	1, 4, w53	w1	w4, 0	–	354[e]	246	141	394
				+	7 587	3 895	4 341	9 913
Allogeneic	1	w1		+	8 405	322	204	316
Allogeneic	1	w1		+	11 472	176	263	295
Allogeneic	4, w53			+	595	3 379	4 604	246
Allogeneic	4, w53			+	198	6 642	8 337	344
Allogeneic	w53			+	178	230	2 173	304
Allogeneic	w53			+	250	187	5 977	377
Allogeneic	w53			+	182	240	304	266
Allogeneic			w4	+	342	190	263	7 146
Allogeneic			w4	+	402	222	301	11 426
Allogeneic	1	w1		+	NT	237	306	6 821
Restriction molecule					DR1	DR4	DRw53	SB4

Different APC donors were used to screen the different TLCs

[a] Ten thousand non-T cells as APCs (irradiated 20 Gy); only the class II determinants shared with autologous APCs are indicated for allogeneic APCs

[b] Chlamydial antigen concentration in wells 2×10^6 IFU/ml

[c] Ten thousand cloned T cells

[d] Results expressed as mean cpm: SEM usually < 20% of mean

data on the restriction specificites of representative TLCs from donor BS [details in 9, 12]. Of the 17 TLCs from BS examined extensively for HLA restriction, ten appeared to be restricted by elements on molecules expressing DR1 (illustrated by clone 24 in Table 1), while four were restricted by DR4 (clone 5). In addition, two TLCs were probably restricted by elements on the DRw53 molecule (clone 37) and one by elements on molecules expressing DPw4 (clone 110). Thus, DR (including broad specificities such as DRw53) and DP class II molecules appeared able to express restricting elements for the chlamydia-specific T cells, of which a given clone was only able to "use" one. TLCs specific for virus antigens may also be restricted by APCs expressing DRw53 or DP molecules, as shown by others [1, 2]. As illustrated by clones BS37 and BS110 and reported in detail elsewhere [9, 12], our data also provide evidence that class II molecules may express several and different restriction elements, which often may be different from determinants recognized by alloantibodies (i.e., DR4 and DRw53) or T cells primed to alloantigens (i.e., DPw4). Possibly, different epitopes on *C. trachomatis* are selectively recognized together with the different restriction elements, as has been shown using antigens expressing a more limited number of epitopes [7]. This is an object of further studies.

We then studied the inhibitory effect of Mabs on these clones. The Mabs used are shown in Table 2. Figure 1 illustrates the effects of the Mabs on the proliferative responses of representative TLCs showing a DR4 (BS5 clone) or DRw53 (BS37 clone) restriction pattern. It can be seen that the Mabs reactive with monomorphic DR determinants inhibited both TLCs, while Mab 109d6, which is putatively DRw53 specific [14], only inhibited the DRw53-restricted TLC. Mabs reactive with DP molecules (Tü39 and MHM4) and Mabs reactive with class I molecules (Q6/64 and E2.14) demonstrated no inhibitory activity on any of the tested TLCs.

Table 2. The murine HLA-specific Mabs used in inhibition experiments

Mab	"Reactivity"	Specificity	Source
7.2	Monomorphic	DR	J. Hansen [3]
17.15	Polymorphic	DR supertypic	J. Hansen [4, 13]
109d6	Polymorphic	DRw53	R. Winchester [14]
Tü22	Monomorphic	DQ	A. Ziegler [15]
Tü39	Monomorphic	DR+DP	A. Ziegler [15]
MHM4	Monomorphic	DP	A. McMichael [5]
Q6/64	Monomorphic	AB	S. Ferrone [8]
E2.14	Monomorphic	β_2 microglobulin	S. Funderud
D-54	Monomorphic	DR	S. Funderud

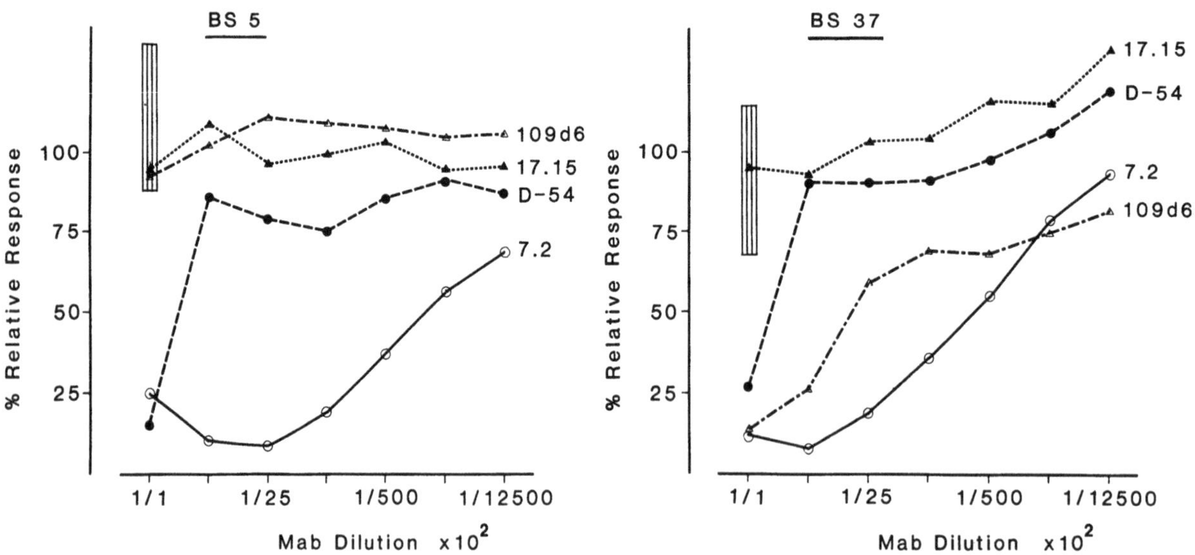

Fig. 1. Effect of different diluations of a panel of Mabs on the proliferative responses of TLCs with DR4 (BS5; *left*) or DRw53 (BS37; *right*) restriction patterns, using antigen-pulsed monocytes as antigen-presenting cells. Final dilution of Mabs in the wells is shown on the *abscissa*. Mabs (specificity in parenthesis): ○——○ 7.2 (DR); ▲·····▲ 17.15 ("DR"); ●---● D-54 (DR); △-·-·-·-△ 109d6 (DRw53); ◫ Q6/64 (AB), E2.14 (β-2-m), Tü22 (DQ), Tü39 (DR + DP), MHM4 (DP)

Antibodies directed to cell-membrane components may cause inhibition of APC–T cell interactions via several different mechanisms. Firstly, an inhibitory effect of Mabs may result from binding or interference with HLA molecules expressed in the membrane of the T cells. Activated *Chlamydia*-specific TLCs express both HLA class I and II antigens (DR, DQ, and DP; unpublished data). Since the HLA class I-specific Mabs (Q6/64 and E2.14) did not inhibit the response, binding to HLA-ABC molecules in T cells apparently does not disturb antigen activation in our studies. Mab 17.15 has been reported to bind to DR determinants expressed on B cells and activated T cells but not on monocytes [13]. Since this antibody also did not inhibit the responses, it provides additional evidence that binding to DR molecules in the T cell membrane does not in itself cause inhibition. In addition, DP-reactive Mabs did not inhibit.

Secondly inhibition could be caused by an unspecific effect of binding of antibodies to different molecules in the APC membrane. This is unlikely, since class I-specific Mabs did not inhibit and only some class II-specific Mabs were effective.

The most likely explanation of the inhibitory effects is a specific effect on the class II molecules in the APC membrane expressing the relevant restricting elements. Mabs directed to DR molecules (7.2 and D-54) inhibited DR- and DRw53-restricted clones, but not DP-restricted clones. Recent data indicate that Mab 7.2 reacts with DR framework determinants (Nepom, personal communication). Since Mab 109d6 only inhibited the DRw53-restricted clones, without any effect on DR-restricted TLCs, the epitope recognized by this Mab may be unique for the DRw53 specificity [14]. None of the other Mabs tested inhibited the TLCs significantly. The DPw4-restricted TLC was not inhibited by any Mabs, including the DP-reactive Mabs MHM 4 (DP) and Tü39 (DR + DP) (data not shown). This lack of inhibition may be caused by the Mabs binding to different "DP-like" molecules or to parts of the DP molecule other than those responsible for the restriction specificity.

In conclusion, our studies demonstrate that T cell clones from a single donor with specificity for antigens on *C. trachomatis* may be restricted by broad or narrow DR-determinants or by HLA-DP class II molecules. The results of the inhibition experiments using Mabs against different HLA molecules correlated with the restriction specificities of the clones. Our data strongly suggest that the inhibition is caused by interference with expression of the correct restriction element in the APC. More studies, using several well-defined Mabs and cloned T cells of other antigen and restriction specificities, will be necessary to further clarify these aspects.

Summary

T lymphocyte clones (TLCs) specific for *Chlamydia trachomatis* were obtained by limiting dilution of in vitro activated T cells from a single donor, BS (DR1, 4; DQw1, DRw53; DPw4). Most of the TLCs obtained were only able to recognize antigen together with restriction elements on DR1 or DR4 molecules, expressed in the antigen-presenting cells (APCs). The restriction pattern of two TLCs closely followed the expression of DRw53 in the APCs, while one TLC seemed to be restricted by elements on DPw4 molecules. A panel of murine HLA-specific monoclonal antibodies (Mabs) was employed to further dissect the restriction specificities. Two Mabs, 7.2 and D-54, which were reactive with monomorphic DR determinants inhibited DR1, 4 as well as DRw53-restricted TLCs. One Mab, 109d6, which reacts with a DRw53 determinant, selectively inhibited the DRw53-restricted TLCs. The DP-restricted TLC was not inhibited significantly by any tested Mabs.

Acknowledgment. The generous gifts of monoclonal antibodies (Table 2) are greatly appreciated.

References

1. Ball EJ, Stastny P (1984) Antigen-specific HLA-restricted human T-cell lines. I. An MT3-like restriction determinant distinct from HLA-DR. Immunogenetics 19:13–26
2. Eckels DE, Lake P, Lamb JR, Johnson AH, Shaw S, Woody JN, Hartzmann RJ (1983) SB-restricted presentation of influenza and herpes simplex virus antigens to human T-lymphocyte clones. Nature 301:716–718
3. Hansen JA, Martin PJ, Nowinski RC (1980) Monoclonal antibodies identifying a novel T-cell antigen and Ia antigens of human lymphocytes. Immunogenetics 10:247–260
4. Hansen JA, Martin PJ, Kamoun M, Nisperos B, Thomas ED (1981) A supertypic HLA-DR specificity (DR4 + 5) defined by a murine monoclonal antibody. Hum Immunol 2:103–111
5. Makgoba MW, Hildreth JEK, McMichael AJ (1983) Identification of a human Ia antigen that is different from HLA-DR and DC antigens. Immunogenetics 17:623–635
6. Moen T, Bratlie A, Kiss E, Bruserud Ø, Thorsby E (1983) Identification of four SB antigens by cloned cells. Tissue Antigens 22:298–309
7. Nagy ZA, Baxevanis CN, Ishii N, Klein J (1981) Ia antigens as restriction molecules in Ir-gene controlled T-cell proliferation. Immunol Rev 60:59–83
8. Quaranta V, Pellegrino MA, Ferrone S (1981) The monoclonal xenoantibody Q6/64 recognizes a determinant expressed by certain gene products of the A and B loci of the HLA region. Immunogenetics 14:403–413
9. Qvigstad E, Thorsby E (1983) Class-II HLA restriction of antigen-specific human T-lymphocyte clones. Evidence of restriction elements of both DR and MT molecules. Scand J Immunol 18:299–306

10. Qvigstad E, Digranes S, Thorsby E (1983) Antigen-specific proliferative human T-lymphocyte clones with specificitiy for *Clamydia trachomatis*. Scand J Immunol 18:291–297
11. Qvigstad E, Skaug K, Thorsby E (1983) Proliferative human T cell responses to *Chlamydia trachomatis* in vitro. Acta Pathol Microbiol Immunol Scand Sect C 91:203–209
12. Qvigstad E, Moen T, Thorsby E (1984) T-cell clones with similar antigen specificity may be restricted by DR, MT (DC), or SB class II HLA molecules. Immunogenetics (in press)
13. Torok-Storb B, Nepom GT, Nepom BS, Hansen JA (1983) HLA-DR antigens on lymphoid cells differ from those on myeloid cells. Nature 305:541–543
14. Winchester R, Toguchi T, Szer I, Burmester G, Galbo PL, Cuttner J, Capra JD, Nunez-Roldan A (1983) Association of susceptibility to certain hematopoietic malignancies with the presence of Ia allodeterminants distinct from the DR series: utility of monoclonal antibody reagens. Immunol Rev 70:155–166
15. Ziegler A (1984) Analysis of the specificities of monoclonal antibodies directed against human HLA class II antigens by sequential immunoprecipitations. Hum Immunol (submitted)

HLA-DR Typing by Restriction Specificity. A Functional Approach Using PPD-Specific CTLs and Antigen Presenting Monocytes

P.W. Hansen, S.E. Christiansen, L.U. Lamm, F. Kissmeyer-Nielsen, and T. Kristensen

The Tissue Typing Laboratory, University Hospital of Aarhus, 8000 Aarhus C, Denmark

Initial studies in our laboratory [1] have shown that PPD-specific CTLs from presensitized individuals can be generated in vitro, as demonstrated by the ability of such cells to lyse antigen-pulsed autologous monocyte targets but not unpulsed targets. These studies have further indicated that such CTLs are restricted by HLA-D/DR-associated determinants.

With the purpose of determining the restriction pattern more precisely, we generated large amounts of PPD-specific CTLs from each of 20 fully HLA-typed healthy individuals. These 20 CTLs were tested against PPD-pulsed vs unpulsed monocyte targets from a panel of 50 unrelated donors including the 20 CTL donors. Thus, each CTL was tested against autologous as well as 49 allogeneic targets.

Generation of CTLs in sufficient amounts was accomplished by stimulating in vitro PBM with an antigenic dose of PPD (2.5 μg/ml). After 6 days IL-2-conditioned medium was added for two or three cycles (each of 3–4 days' duration). The expanded CTLs were subsequently distributed to 15–25 aliquots and cryopreserved. One thawed aliquot contained enough cells to test six target cell donors in a standard ^{51}Cr-release assay. In individual experiments all 20 CTLs were used simultaneously. The 50 target donors were all tested twice in independent experiments. Based on a histogram of the percent PPD-specific cytotoxicity obtained in the 1000 combinations, assignments were made: –, cytotoxicity < 20%; (+), cytotoxicity (20%–30%; +, cytotoxicity > 30%. The level of cytotoxicity was

Table 1. PPD-specific cytotoxicity of CTLs generated from healthy individuals

No. and specificity of HLA-DR antigens shared											
No.:	2	1								0	
Specificity	–	1	2	3	4	5	w6	7	w8	–	Total
+	53	21	61	85	48	7	29	27	5	37	373
(+)	1	5	11	3	11	0	9	2	8	63	112
–	1	5	13	2	3	7	21	0	8	454	515
Total	55	31	85	90	62	14	58	29	21	554	1000

PPD-specific cytoxicity

Histocompatibility Testing 1984
Edited by E. D. Albert et al.

subsequently related to the number and specificity of HLA-DR antigens shared between CTL and target cell donor.

As seen from the results shown below (Table 1), the general correlation between the restriction specificity and the serologically defined HLA-DR specificity is of a magnitude that justifies consideration of PPD-specific CTLs as HLA-DR-typing reagents. The agreement is particularly convincing concerning HLA-DR1, 2, 3, 4, and 7, whereas the correlation is much less pronounced for HLA-DR5 and w8 and also for the serologically ill-defined DRw6 specificity.

Reference

1. Hansen PW, Madsen M, Christensen SE, Johnsen HE, Kissmeyer-Nielsen F (1984) Cell-mediated PPD specific cytotoxicity against human monocyte targets: Evidence for restriction by class II HLA antigens. Tissue Antigens 23:171–180

Cytotoxic T Cells Generated During GvHD Can Detect Minor Histocompatibility Antigens in an HLA-Restricted Fashion*

E. Goulmy, E. Blokland, J.W. Gratama, F.E. Zwaan, and J.J. van Rood

Department of Immunohematology and Blood Bank, Isolation Pavilion, University Hospital, 2333 AA Leiden, The Netherlands

Abbreviations

GvHD: Graft-versus-Host-Disease; minor H antigen: minor Histocompatibility antigen; CTLs: cytotoxic T lymphocytes.

In an earlier report [1] we demonstrated the identification of a minor histocompatibility (minor H) antigen with the use of posttransplant cells derived from a bone marrow-grafted patient suffering from severe chronic graft-versus-host-disease (GvHD). After the transplant the patient's lymphocytes showed in vitro cytotoxicity against a non-HLA target determinant (designated HA-1) in an HLA-restricted fashion. The latter observation prompted us to continue our search for minor H antigens and their role in bone marrow transplantation. To that purpose, we studied the posttransplant lymphocytes of 13 HLA-matched bone marrow recipients: two with no GvHD, seven with acute GvHD, and four with chronic GvHD. The effector cells harvested at day 6 were tested in the CML assay for specific cytotoxic activity. They were also expanded to obtain cytotoxic T cell lines. Posttransplant lymphocytes from five patients (four of whom suffered from chronic GvHD) showed marked cytotoxicity, which was directed against the pretransplant lymphocytes of these patients. We used those in vitro-generated CTLs for the identification of other minor H antigens. Analysis of the cytotoxic activity using a limited panel of target cells from healthy unrelated individuals identified five different CTL populations directed against different minor H antigens. The recognized structures (designated minor HA-1, minor HA-2, minor HA-3, minor HA-4, and minor HA-5) and the restricting MHC molecules necessary for their associative recognition are shown in Table 1. The large-scale expansion of these minor H-specific CTLs enabled us to store enough minor H reagents to serve as typing reagents. Retrospective typing of HLA-identical bone marrow donor/recipient pairs (recipients without GvHD, with acute GvHD, or with chronic GvHD) is now in progress with the object of more precise

Table 1. MHC restricted anti-minor H antigen CTLs generated during GvHD

		MHC-resticting molecules	Non-HLA antigens
CTLs	1	A2, B27, Bw62	Minor HA-1
	2	Not yet known	Minor HA-2
	3	A2	Minor HA-3 and allo-HLA-B8
	4	A2	Minor HA-4
	5	A2, B44	Minor HA-5

* This work was supported in part by the Dutch Foundation for Medical Research (FUNGO), which is subsidized by the Dutch Organization for the Advancement of Pure Research (Z.W.O.), and the J.A. Cohen Institute for Radiation Protection (IRS)

definition of the effect of minor transplantation antigens on the occurrence of acute or chronic GvHD. Hopefully, minor H antigen typing with CTLs may mitigate at least one of the obstacles to successful bone marrow transplantation.

References

1. Goulmy E, Gratama JW, Blokland E, Zwaan FE, van Rood JJ (1983) A minor transplantation antigen detected by MHC restricted cytotoxic T lymphocytes during graft-versus-host disease. Nature 302:159–161

Clonal Distribution of Human T Cells Recognizing PPD in the Context of Each of Two Distinct Ia Molecules

Y. Koide and T.O. Yoshida

Dept. of Microbiology and Immunology, Hamamatsu University School of Medicine, Hamamatsu, Japan

Participation of two of three distinct human Ia molecules, HLA-DR and the Ia molecule detected by monoclonal antibody (MoAb) 1B4 (1B4 molecules), in antigen presentation for T cell responses to purified protein derivative (PPD) and herpes simplex virus (HSV) was first suggested from studies on the inhibition of proliferative responses of whole T cell populations with MoAb against human Ia molecules [1].

To determine whether a single T cell recognizes the antigen in the context of both Ia molecules or in the context of each one of two Ia molecules, we isolated and propagated PPD-reactive T cell clones from an HLA-DR heterozygous individual. The clones fell into four different restriction patterns (Table 1): Type I clones (2B3 and 1E1) recognized PPD presented by a part of a panel of APC-sharing DR4. Type II clone (3E6) appeared to restrict to DRw9. The response of both type I and II clones was blocked by MoAbs to DR molecules (Table 2). Type III clone (1D5) appeared to give anomalous patterns of response and seemed to recognize PPD in the context of non-DR antigens. Correspondingly, the response of type III clone was blocked by MoAb 1B4. Type IV clone (2A3) responded to PPD only when presented by APCs carrying both of the HLA-DR antigens and the response was blocked by MoAbs to DR molecules. Type IV T clone may, therefore, be restricted to hybrid interaction molecules of DR as observed in the mouse and in man [2, 3]. Thus, restriction molecules involved in T cell clones that belong to types I, II, and IV appeared to be DR molecules and those involved in T cell clones of type III were 1B4 molecules.

Taken together, these data suggest that DR-restricted and 1B4-restricted T cells, both specific to PPD, are clonally distinct. Similar observations were made by Eckels et al. [4], employing influenza virus

Table 1. The proliferative response of T cell clones to PPD-pulsed allogeneic APC

Type	T cell clone	PPD-pulse	APC: Auto DR4/w9	TF DR4/w9	TM DR4/w8	FA DR4/w8	HM DR2/w9	YK DR2/w6
I	2B3	–	89 (11)	76 (3)	46 (8)	169 (15)	151 (11)	223 (25)
		+	2858 (52)	2746 (221)	2622 (161)	242 (17)	207 (92)	120 (9)
	1E1	–	78 (3)	45 (31)	24 (7)	33 (4)	184 (38)	171 (56)
		+	2239 (665)	2800 (904)	1759 (77)	71 (18)	114 (12)	149 (28)
II	3E6	–	34 (9)	42 (6)	16 (2)	40 (9)	20 (5)	37 (6)
		+	1594 (211)	1861 (270)	19 (6)	38 (3)	2331 (43)	40 (3)
III	1D5	–	46 (7)	31 (10)	87 (16)	77 (36)	86 (18)	56 (13)
		+	1836 (347)	103 (21)	1011 (135)	51 (14)	153 (40)	1604 (443)
IV	2A3	–	107 (11)	93 (6)	84 (26)	141 (61)	188 (74)	107 (37)
		+	1316 (519)	1523 (436)	121 (54)	73 (21)	114 (59)	64 (2)

Results are expressed as the mean cpm (SEM) of triplicate cultures

Table 2. Effect of monoclonal anti-Ia antibodies on the proliferative response of T cell clones to PPD-pulsed APC

Clone	Response	MoAb added[b]				
		αDR			αMB	α?
		4F6	7B2	2E11	5F6	1B4
2B3	2237	115	372	281	2339	1974
3E6	2702	740	136	472	2942	2160
1D5	2348	1625	1874	1744	2004	375
2A3	2012	374	406	822	2413	2116

Results are expressed as Δcpm

[a] Cloned T cells (5×10^3) were cultured with autologous PPD-pulsed APC (5×10^3) for 3 days

[b] MoAb were added to the culture giving a final dilution of 1/500

and HSV in which the majority of T cell clones recognized influenza virus and HSV in the context of DR molecules, whereas a few clones recognized them in the context of DP molecules distinct from DR or DQw1 molecules. DP molecules have recently been described as a second homologue of the murine I-E molecules [5]. Therefore, it would be of obvious interest to study whether DP is the same molecule that was detected by MoAb 1B4.

References

1. Koide Y, Awashima F, Yoshida TO, Takenouchi T, Wakisaka A, Moriuchi J, Aizawa M (1982) The role of three distinct Ia-like molecules in human T cell proliferative responses: Effect of monoclonal anti-Ia-like antibodies. J Immunol 129:1061
2. Kimoto M, Fathman CG (1980) Antigen-reactive T cell clones. I. Transcomplementing hybrid I-A-region gene products function effectively in antigen presentations. J Exp Med 152:759
3. Hansen GS, Svejgaard A, Claesson MH (1982) T cell clones restricted to "hybrid" HLA-D antigens? J Immunol 128:2497
4. Eckels DD, Lake P, Lamb JR, Johnson AH, Shaw S, Woody JN, Hartzman RJ (1983) SB-restricted presentation of influenza and herpes simplex virus antigens to human T-lymphocyte clones. Nature 301:716
5. Shaw S, Kavathas P, Pollack MS, Charmot D, Mawas C (1981) Family studies define a new histocompatibility locus, SB, between HLA-DR and GLO. Nature 293:745

Function of DRw52 and LB-Q1 in Antigen Presentation*

T.H.M. Ottenhoff, B.G. Elferink, A. Termijtelen, F. Koning, and R.R.P. de Vries

Dept. of Immunohematology and Blood Bank, University Hospital of Leiden, Rijnsburgerweg 10, 2333 AA Leiden, The Netherlands

We have investigated the possible role of DRw52 and LB-Q1, a new PLT-defined lymphocyte-activating determinant [1] in strong linkage disequilibrium with DRw52, in antigen (Ag) presentation to T cells. Two PPD- or tetanus toxoid-specific IL-2-propagated T cell cultures (T) were generated from different donors. Because Ag presentation to these T cells was mainly HLA-DR restricted, 42 DR fully mismatched T-APC combinations were tested. All cells had been typed for DR, DQ, DP, and LB-Q1. Triplicate cultures with 5×10^3 T, 5×10^4 PBL as APC (40 Gy), and Ag were set up for 72 hours, after which ^{3}H-thymidine was added. Mean cpm in the absence of Ag was 309 ± 332. When both cpm > 1000 (range: 1055 – 17 206) and stimulation index > 4.0 (range: 4.1 – 67.3) tests were regarded as positive. Positive responses were seen in 7/15 T-APC combinations in which Ag was presented by DRw52+/LB-Q1– APC to DRw52+/LB-Q1+ T whereas no responses were observed in 9 DRw52 and LB-Q1 mismatched combinations (Table 1).

* This work was supported in part by the Dutch Foundation for Medical Research (FUNGO), which is subsidized by the Dutch Organization for the Advancement of Pure Research (ZWO) and the J.A. Cohen Institute for Radiopathology and Radiation Protection (IRS)

Table 1. T-responses upon Ag presentation by APC in relation to DRw52 and LB-Q1

DRw52 sharing		+	–	–	–	+	–
LB-Q1 sharing		–	–	+	–	+	–
T response	+	7	0	2	0	15	0
	–	8	9	0	9	1	9
		$P < 0.02$		$P < 0.02$		$P < 10^{-6}$	

Proliferation could be inhibited by an anti-DRw52 moab [2] and a monomorphic anti-class II moab, but not by an anti-class I moab (B 9.12.1, Malissen) (data not shown). Both LB-Q1 sharing and DRw52 mismatched T-APC combinations the 9 showed proliferation, in contrast to LB-Q1 and DRw52 mismatched combinations (Table 1). The responses could be blocked by the anti-class II moab, but not by the anti-DRw52-like or the anti-class I moab. Because no anti-LB Q1 moab is available, specific blocking studies could not be performed. No significant influence was observed for sharing of DQ or DP between T-APC. These data indicate that DRw52 and LB-Q1 are markers for one – and possibly two – and hitherto unknown restriction determinant in Ag presentation to T cells.

References

1. Termijtelen A, et al (1983) LB-Q1 and LB-Q2: two determinants defined in the PLT and independent of HLA-D/DR MB/LB-E or SB. Hum Immunol 8:11 – 15
2. Koning F, et al (1984) A mouse monoclonal antibody detecting a DR-related MT2-like specificity: Serology and biochemistry. Hum Immunol 9:221 – 230

Subdivision of DRw6 by Influenza-Specific Proliferative Cloned Cell Lines

G. Sterkers[1], J.M. Michon[1], V. Lepage[2], Y. Henin[1], J.Y. Muller[3], L. Degos[2], and J.P. Levy[1]

1 Laboratoire Immunologie et Virologie des Tumeurs, INSERM U.152, Hôpital Cochin, 27 rue du fg st Jacques, 75014 Paris, France
2 Unité de Recherche sur l'Immunogénétique de la Transplantation Humaine, INSERM U.93, Hôpital Saint Louis, 2 place du Docteur Fournier, 75010 Paris Cedex 10, France
3 Centre National de Transfusion Sanguine, 6 rue Alexandre Cabanel, 75015 Paris, France

We regularly produce anti-influenza A/Texas cloned cell lines selected for clear-cut HLA restriction. By this method we have recently shown a strict correlation between serological and functional definition of DR1 and DR7 molecules. Taking these results into account, HLA restriction analysis of clones issued from an HLA-DRw6 donor was studied, since the HLA-DRw6 molecule remains one of the most poorly defined. Restriction analysis of one of these clones, CotC2, showed a clear correlation with HLA DRw6 serological definition, since, as shown in Fig. 1A, among 22 DRw6 (+) APCs, 18 (82%) presented the A/Texas virus to CotC2, resulting in a strong proliferation, while 4 (18%) could not induce any proliferative response in the same culture conditions. When the same allogeneic cells were used to present the viral antigen to another clone, CotC6, none of them could induce any proliferative response. Interestingly, as shown in Fig. 1B, when we used allogeneic cells which were possibly DRw6 (+) [since they were DQw1 (+) but also DR1 (+) or DR2 (+), or DRw52 (+) but also DR3 (+), DR5 (+) or DRw8 (+)] as APCs, 4/12 (33%) presented the specific antigen. As shown in Fig. 1C, when allogeneic DRw6 (–) cells bearing all known DR specificities were used as APCs none of 18 could present the specific antigen, indicating that no extra-reaction was observed with this cell line. Blocking experiments were performed with monoclonal antibodies. Only DR-specific MoAb blocked the specific response, while class I- or DQ- specific MoAb did not. In conclusion, this monospecific reagent allows (a) the definition of a predominant subgroup of HLA-DRw6 molecule [82% of DRw6 (+) cells tested] and (b) the phenotyping of DRw6 (+) cells that could not be defined by serology.

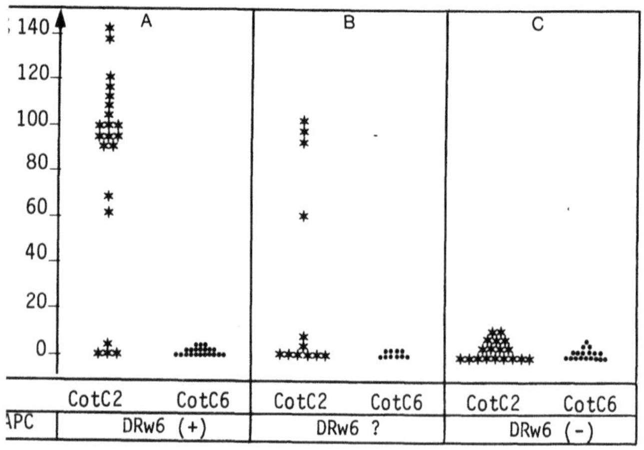

Fig. 1. Induction of proliferative responses. Results are expressed for each allogeneic APC as follows:

$$\% \text{ response} = \frac{\text{cpm observed with allogeneic APC}}{\text{cpm observed with autologous APC}} \times 100$$

Histocompatibility Testing 1984
Edited by E. D. Albert et al.

Human T Cell-MΦ Collaboration Across Allogeneic Barrier

S.H. Hsu, M.M. Chan, and W.B. Bias

Department of Medicine, Johns Hopkins University School of Medicine, 720 Rutland Ave., Baltimore, MD 21205, USA

We have documented the existence of HLA-linked Ir genes to (H,G)-A–L, (T,G)-A–L [1], (Phe,G)-A–L, GAT [2] and GLO MΦ (antigen-presenting cells, APC) are required for specific lymphoproliferative responses to these antigens, as illustrated in Table 1. We have observed that GAT and (T,G)-A–L induced lymphoproliferation was achieved by the addition of either nonirradiated or irradiated autologous MΦ, or by coculturing with 24-h antigen-pulsed autologous MΦ. Antigen-pulsed MΦ elicited lymphoproliferation comparable to that of unseparated PBLs cultured continuously with free antigen. Heat-killed MΦ (63 °C for 1 h) were incapable of restoring the proliferative response.

In contrast to other reports that DR identity is required for T-MΦ collaboration [3], we showed that responding T cells can collaborate with allogeneic responding MΦ irrespective of HLA, if one abrogates alloreactivity with BUdR and light treatment. These studies were carried out to investigate the underlying mechanism(s) for genetic nonresponsiveness. Our protocol is as follows: PBLs from responder were cocultured with PBLs from either responding or nonresponding individuals. The MLR cultures were then treated with BUdR and light to abrogate alloreactivity. The treated cultures were then passed over a Percoll gradient to eliminate MΦ, B cells, and dead T cells. Viable T cells were recovered and cultured with/without APC in the presence of serial dilution of antigens. Table 2 gives an example of one such experiment.

Table 1. Antigen-induced lymphoproliferation in various cell preparations

(T, G) AL (μg/well)	Unseparated PBLs	MΦ-dep. PBLs	MΦ-dep. PBLs + auto. MΦ	MΦ-dep. PBLs + irr. auto. MΦ	MΦ-dep. PBLs + heat-killed MΦ	(T, G) AL-pulsed MΦ
0	2 542	902	3 000	2 600	907	12 710 (5.0)
6	2 908 (1.1)	323 (0.4)	8 645 (2.8)	–	–	–
24	12 227 (4.8)	103 (0.1)	12 782 (4.2)	9 988 (3.0)	1 293 (1.0)	–
48	8 643 (3.4)	310 (0.3)	12 786 (4.9)	17 009 (6.6)	1 040 (1.0)	–
96	7 471 (2.9)	1 759 (1.9)	10 004 (3.3)	–	–	–

Values are given as CPM with S.I. in parentheses

Table 2. Human T cell-macrophage collaboration across allogeneic barrier

Treatment	(H, G) AL conc. μg/well	AxBx				AxDx			DxEx	
		no MΦ	AMΦx	BMΦx	no MΦ	AMΦx	DMΦx	no MΦ	DMΦx	EMΦx
10 μg BUdR 0 min light exposure	0	4 674*	12 189	9 893	8 272	9 746	21 123	9 009	9 576	12 724
	20	4 206	9 751	14 839	5 790	9 750	19 018	7 207	5 745	7 634
	40	4 200	12 190	14 344	4 100	8 771	14 786	7 207	8 618	8 907
	80	6 545	8 532	12 850	7 279	9 755	12 674	4 505	8 618	8 907
10 μg BUdR, 37 min light exposure	0	3 187	921	1 315	4 787	1 283	2 331	537	1 164	3 736
	20	3 824	4 236[a]	7 496	4 596	12 573	9 580	161	815	3 362
	40	2 231	3 868	12 493	957	7 570	12 122	430	1 164	4 110
	80	2 868	1 657	5 655	1 723	4 233	6 993	161	1 513	5 604

A: A2, A10, B7, B27, Cw–, Cw–, DR2, DR1 (Responder); B: A3, A11, B35, B38, Cw4, Cw–, DR7, DR– (Responder); D: A26, A2, B17, B27, Cw2, Cw–, DR4, DR5 (Nonresponder); E: A26, A30, B44, B17, Cw6, Cw–, DRw6, DR7 (Nonresponder).

* counts per minute

[a] maximum positive responses

Histocompatibility Testing 1984
Edited by E. D. Albert et al.

From these data we concluded that (a) responder T cells can collaborate with allogeneic APC provided that alloreactivity has been blocked; (b) genetic defects of nonresponsiveness do not reside on MΦ, since nonresponder MΦ can present antigen to responder T cells; (c) nonresponder T cells do not respond with either syngeneic nor allogeneic nonresponder MΦ. Thus, antigen-specific human immune responses are not HLA restricted, and genetic control appears to be exerted on the T cell rather than the APC.

References

1. Hsu SH, Chan MM, Bias WB (1981) Genetic control of major histocompatibility complex-linked immune responses to synthetic polypeptides in man. Proc Natl Acad Sci 78:440
2. Chan MM, Bias WB, Hsu SH, Meyers DA (1984) Genetic control of major histocompatibility complex-linked immune responses to synthetic polypeptides in man: (Phe,G)-A–L and GAT. Proc Natl Acad Sci (in press)
3. Thorsby E, Berle E, Nousiainen H (1982) HLA-D region molecules restrict proliferative T cell responses to antigen. Immunol Rev 66:39

Expression of HLA-DQ Molecules on Human Monocytes: Identification of Two Phenotypically Different Monocyte Populations with Distinct Accessory Cell Function

G. Nunez, E.J. Ball, L.K. Myers, and P. Stastny

Department of Internal Medicine, The University of Texas Health Science Center at Dallas, Southwestern Medical School, 5323 Harry Hines Boulevard, Dallas, TX 75235, USA

Introduction

Class II major histocompatibility antigens (MHC) play a fundamental role for both antigen presentation to T cells and stimulation in mixed lymphocyte reactions. Recent progress in the understanding of human class II MHC antigens has provided evidence for at least three types of Ia molecules: HLA-DR, DQ, and DP.

These class II MHC antigens have a restricted tissue distribution. They are primarily expressed on B lymphocytes, monocytes, macrophages, and dendritic cells [1]. In mice, only a fraction of the macrophages express Ia antigens. In the Ia-positive macrophage population, two subsets have been observed in mice: one expresses both I-A and I-E products, the other only I-A antigens [2]. Functionally active accessory cells appear to express both I-A and I-E molecules [3].

A similar heterogeneity exists in human monocytes [4, 5]. Thus, two main types of human monocytes have been identified: One subset expresses HLA-DR and DP antigens and a smaller subset additionally expresses HLA-DQ molecules [5].

In this report, we provide evidence that these phenotypically distinct human monocyte populations are also functionally different. The monocyte population that expresses DQ molecules is more active in accessory cell functions than the population that does not express DQ molecules.

Materials and Methods

Isolation of Cells. Peripheral blood mononuclear cells (PBMC) were obtained by centrifugation on Ficoll-Hypaque. Monocyte-enriched populations were purified from PBMCs by adherence to plastic as previously described [6].

Monoclonal Antibodies. L203 recognizes human HLA-DR molecules, and was a gift of Dr. R. Levy. TU22 identifies a monomorphic determinant on HLA-DQ molecules, and was a gift of Dr. A. Ziegler. Leu 10 also recognizes DQ molecules on all cells except DR3 and DR7, and was purchased from Becton-Dickinson (Mountain View, CA). 63D3 is a monocyte-specific antibody that has been previously described.

Immunofluorescence Studies. Determination of binding of monoclonal antibody to the cell surface was performed in an indirect immunofluorescence assay by flow cytometry (FACS III) as previously reported [6]. Background fluorescence was determined with a control antibody using the same settings as those used for relevant antibodies.

Isolation of Cells by Sorting in the FACS. Highly purified DQ+ and DQ– monocyte populations were prepared by labeling the monocyte-enriched cells with monoclonal antibody TU22, followed by

Histocompatibility Testing 1984
Edited by E. D. Albert et al.

incubation with $F(ab')_2$ FITC goat anti-mouse IgG. Sorting of TU22+ and TU22− cell populations was performed in the FACS III. Postsorting analysis of such populations showed that DQ+ cells were > 95% TU22+ and DQ− cells were < 2% TU22+.

T Cell Lines and Clones. Several alloreactive T cell lines were derived by primary allogeneic stimulation, followed by blast isolation and expansion in T cell growth factor as previously described [7]. Some of these T cell lines were cloned by limiting dilution as described [7]. Data on their panel specificity and class II molecules recognized have been published [7].

Proliferative Assay. Primary MLR proliferation was determined after 7-day incubation in round-bottom microtiter plates (Falcon, Oxnard, CA). Cultures contained responding cells which were PBMC (50×10^3/well) and stimulating cells at different concentrations. For secondary allogeneic responses obtained with T cell lines, a 3-day incubation with 20×10^3 responding cells/well was used. Proliferation was determined by adding ^{3}H-TdR during the final 18–24 h of culture.

Results

Differential Expression of Class II Molecules in Monocytes

We have previously shown that practically all monocytes express DR and DP antigens and only a subset (10%–40%) expresses DQ molecules detectable with monoclonal antibodies specific for DQw1 and DQw3. In Fig. 1, we show staining of a cell of a population that consisted of B cells and monocytes with monoclonal antibody TU22, known to react with a monomorphic determinant on DQ molecules. It can be seen that most smaller cells, which are predominantly B cells, were brightly stained, while only a subset of the larger cells, which are mostly monocytes, were stained with TU22. Similar results have been obtained with monoclonal antibodies, Leu 10, BT3/4, Genox 3.53, and IVD12, which react with polymorphic determinants on DQ molecules.

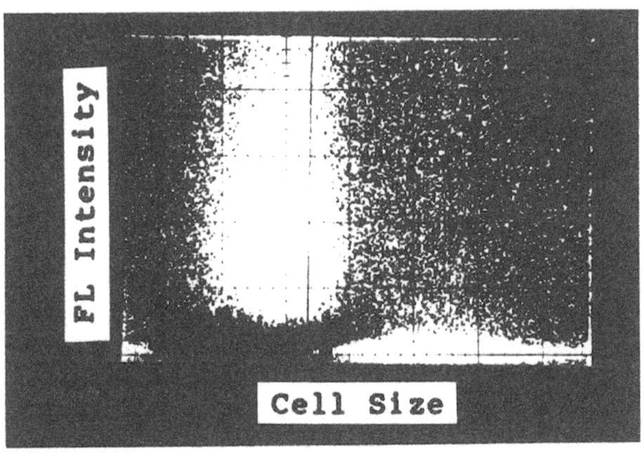

Fig. 1. Dot plot of cell population consisting of freshly isolated B cells and monocytes stained with TU22, a monoclonal antibody that reacts with DQ molecules. Smaller cells that are highly stained represent mostly B cells, the larger cells are primarily monocytes. Both DQ+ and DQ− monocyte subsets can be identified

Induction of DQ Molecules on DQ-Negative Monocytes

We and others [6, 8] have shown an increase in staining for DR molecules on monocytes by both mitogen-induced T cell supernatants and gamma-interferon. We have recently reported that supernatants from mitogen and allogeneic MLR-stimulated T cells were able to induce DQ molecules on a small subset of DR+, DQ− monocytes [5]. However, most DQ− monocytes remained DQ− after incubation with such supernatants. We have now studied the effect of purified gamma-interferon on the expression of DQ molecules on monocytes. As with crude T cell supernatants, we detected an increase in the percentage of DQ-positive monocytes after incubation with gamma-interferon (49 ± 12% vs 22% ± 7%, mean ± SD of five experiments; data not shown). Thus, even after treatment with interferon a sizable monocyte population remained DR+, DQ−.

Allogeneic Stimulation by Phenotypically Distinct Monocyte Populations

Highly purified DQ+ and DQ− monocyte populations were prepared by cell sorting. A typical postsorting analysis of these cell populations is shown in Fig. 2. Preparations of DQ-negative sorted cells were found to be > 90% DR-positive and 63D3-positive. Using these cells as stimulators, we studied primary MLR and allogeneic T cell line responses. We found that the DR+, DQ+ monocyte population was very effective in the primary MLR (Table 1). The DR+, DQ− cell population, was considerably (5–20 times) less effective. Control populations included untreated cells and cells treated with monoclonal antibody and run through the FACS without sorting (Table 1).

Other experiments with alloreactive T cell lines specific for distinct class II molecules were also conducted. In Table 2 are shown results with T cell line PT31.5C3, which has been shown to react with

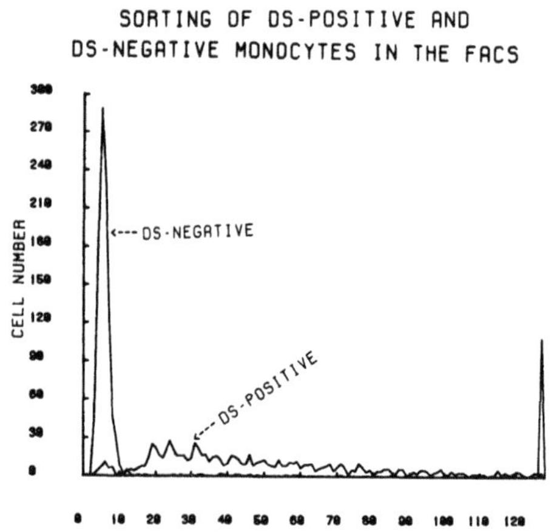

Fig. 2. Post-sorting FACS analysis of DQ+ and DQ− monocyte populations based on staining with antibody TU22. 1×10^3 cells of each sorted population were analyzed in the FACS

Table 1. Primary allogeneic stimulation by different monocyte populations

Exp	Stimulating cell population	Number of accesory cells ($\times 10^{-3}$)		
		10	5	2.5
1	Untreated	58 103	16 410	10 683
	Unsorted	15 481	5 730	1 852
	DQ−	1 388	1 073	390
	DQ+	53 274	37 576	14 519
2	Untreated	46 026	42 026	29 436
	Unsorted	NT	NT	NT
	DQ−	13 312	6 238	2 631
	DQ+	39 643	25 963	25 963

Results expressed as means of triplicate counts; proliferation was obtained at day 7 of culture
Untreated, monocyte-enriched population not treated with monoclonal antibody; unsorted, monocyte-enriched population treated with monoclonal antibody TU22 and then run through the FACS without sorting; DQ−, FACS-sorted TU22-negative monocytes; DQ+, FACS-sorted TU22-positive monocytes; NT, not tested

DQ molecules of DRw6 haplotypes [7]. Also shown is the "bulk" T cell line PT916, which recognized a DR7-associated determinant. DR+, DQ− monocytes induced a significant proliferative response with PT916 but failed to induce proliferation of the DQ-restricted T cell clone PT31.5.C3 (Table 2).
These results indicate that expression of DQ molecules identifies a monocyte subset associated with more active accessory cell function in both the primary and secondary MLR. Alternatively, the DQ+ subset may include cells other than monocytes which are very active in allogeneic stimulation. In addition, our results show that DQ+ accessory cells are absolutely required for the activation of DQ-restricted allogeneic T cells.

Discussion

Previous studies have concluded that virtually all human monocytes and tissue macrophages express surface HLA-DR antigens [4, 5] and human monocytes also express determinants associated with DP and DR molecules (including DRw52, w53) [5]. In addition, recent work has indicated that DQ molecules are expressed only on a subset of the monocyte population [4, 5]. This differential expression of DQ molecules has also been recently reported in other tissues [9].
In the present report we have studied primary and secondary allogeneic T cell responses using accessory cells separated according to their expression of DQ in the FACS. Our results have shown that: (1) DQ+ monocytes are functionally more active stimulating cells (5−20 times) compared to the DQ− monocyte subset in the primary MLR, (2) DQ+ monocytes but not DQ− monocytes elicited DQ-specific allogeneic T cell proliferation, and (3) although DR+, DQ− monocytes were able to trigger DR-specific T cell proliferation, DR+, DQ+ monocytes were more powerful in eliciting such responses.
In preliminary experiments we have also found that DQ+ monocytes are more active in presenting antigen to T cells (G. Nuñez et al., in preparation). These results are similar to those of Gonwa et al. [4]; however, in contrast to these authors we have found that the DR+, DQ+ monocyte subset also contains the main stimulatory cells in the primary allogeneic MLR.
In our experiments the DR+, DQ− monocyte population failed to induce DQ-restricted allogeneic proliferation and stimulated primary MLR and DR-restricted proliferation only weakly. Whether the active cell in the DR+, DQ+ accessory cell population was a monocyte or a cell that belongs to a different lineage needs further investigation.

Summary

Two types of circulating human monocytes have been defined based on their expression of class II molecules. Most (60%−90%) of the monocytes (type I) express DR and DP, while a smaller subset (type II) additionally expresses DQ molecules. Type II monocytes were more effective than type I monocytes in inducing primary MLC and bulk allogeneic T cell line responses. Type II monocytes were absolutely required for DQ-restricted al-

Table 2. Proliferation of alloreactive T cell lines induced by different monocyte populations

Responding T cell line[a]	Molecules recognized	Stimulating cell population[b]	Number of accessory cells (× 10^{-3})		
			10	5	2.5
PT916	Multiple	Untreated	34 172	23 251	18 752
		Unsorted	23 636	16 396	NT
		DQ−	4 931	3 008	1 528
		DQ+	44 351	34 691	12 924
PT31.5.C3	DQ	Untreated	7 133	2 507	949
		Unsorted	2 844	1 802	0
		DQ−	127	0	195
		DQ+	8 203	3 728	1 425

Results expressed as means of triplicate counts

[a] Line PT916 was an uncloned T cell line that recognized a DR7-associated determinant. Line PT31.5.C3 was a cloned line reacting with DQ molecules associated with DRw6 [7]. Proliferation was determined at day 3 of culture

[b] Stimulating cell populations as in Table 1. Proliferation was determined at day 3 of culture

Table 3. Expression of MHC antigens and allogeneic stimulating capacity of human monocytes

Monocyte type	Expression of MHC antigens				Allogeneic stimulting capacity		
	A, B, C	DR	DP	DQ	Primary MLR	DR restricted	DQ restricted
I	+	+	+	−	+	+/++	−
II	+	+	+	+	+++	+++	+++

logeneic T cell line responses. These results indicate that phenotypically distinct human monocytes are also functionally different.

References

1. Frelinger JA (1982) Tissue distribution and cellular expression of Ia antigens. In: Ferrone S, David CS (eds) Antigens, vol 1. CRC Press, Boca Raton, pp 37–54
2. Cowing C, Schwartz BD, Dickler HB (1978) Macrophage Ia antigens. I. Macrophage populations differ in their expression of Ia antigens. J Immunol 120:378–384
3. Pettinelli CB, Ahmann GB, Shearer G (1980) Expression of both I-A and I-E/C subregion antigens on accessory cells required for in vitro generation of cytotoxic T lymphocytes against alloantigens or TNBS-modified syngeneic cells. J Immunol 124:1911–1916
4. Gonwa T, Picker L, Raff H, Goyert S, Silver J, Stobo J (1983) Antigen-presenting capabilities of human monocytes correlates with their expression of HLA-DS, an Ia determinant distinct from HLA-DR. J Immunol 130:706–711
5. Nuñez G, Giles RC, Ball EJ, Hurley CK, Capra JD, Stastny P (1984) Expression of HLA-DR, MB, MT, and SB antigens on human mononuclear cells: identification of two phenotypically distinct monocyte populations. J Immunol 133:1300–1306
6. Nuñez G, Stastny P (1983) Cytofluorometric analysis of major histocompatibility antigens on human monocytes using monoclonal antibodies. Hum Immunol 6:1–11
7. Myers LK, Ball EJ, Stastny P (1984) Different specificities of an HLA-DRw6 haplotype detected by alloreactive T lymphocytes. Hum Immunol (in press)
8. Basham TY, Merigan TC (1983) Recombinant interferon-gamma increases HLA-DR synthesis and expression. J Immunol 130:1492–1494
9. Natali PG, Segatto O, Ferrone S, Tosi R, Corte G (1984) Differential tissue distribution and ontogeny of DC-1 and HLA-DR antigens. Immunogenetics 19:109–116

Differential Expression of the HLA-DQ Antigens on Acute Leukaemic Blasts

C. Navarrete, N. Fernandez, A.V. Groves, and H. Festenstein

Department of Immunology, London Hospital Medical College, Turner Street, London E1 2AD, UK

The class II HLA-DQ alloantigenic system encoded by genes within the HLA-D region is separate from but in strong linkage disequilibrium with antigens of the HLA-DR series.

We first demonstrated by using alloantisera in a complement-dependent cytotoxic test that the HLA-DR, but not the HLA-DQ antigens, were expressed on the blast cells from patients with acute myeloid leukaemia [1, 2]. We have now compared the expression of these antigens on acute myeloid and lymphoid blasts (ALLs and AMLs), chronic lymphocytic leukaemias (CLLs) and Epstein-Barr virus (EBV)-transformed cell lines with HLA-DR and HLA-DQ monoclonal antibodies (MoAbs).

By indirect immunofluorescence binding, the monomorphic HLA class I MoAb W6/32 reacted strongly with all cells tested (Table 1). EBV-transformed cell lines reacted strongly with all HLA class II MoAbs used in the assay (monomorphic DR and DQ, allospecific DQw1, and DQw3). CLLs reacted strongly with the monomorphic DR MoAb but there was a reproducible heterogeneity in the intensity of the staining with both the monomorphic and the allospecific DQ MoAbs. In addition, the number of cells that were stained varied from 12% to 28% in sample from different individuals. The acute myeloid or lymphoid blasts stained strongly with the monomorphic DR MoAbs, but, in contrast failed to react with the monomorphic and allospecific DQ MoAbs.

SDS-PAGE of biosynthetically labelled and affinity-purified glycoproteins from EBV and AML blasts, precipitated with HLA-DQ MoAbs, confirmed the absence of the DQ antigens from the blast cells. Southern blot comparisons of the DNA extracted from acute leukaemic blast cells and the autologous EBV cell lines showed no differences in the DNA restriction fragment banding patterns when hybridised with an HLA-DQ β probe. Thus in AML cells the HLA-DQ genes are present although the products are not expressed. These results indicate that the HLA-DQ antigens are differentiation markers which become expressed later in cell maturation. The absence of the HLA-DQ antigens from acute leukaemic blast cells suggests that these cells are an immature population frozen in

Table 1. Immunofluorescence binding results with monoclonal antibodies

Cell type	Phenotype		Class I	Class II				
	DR	DQ	ABC W6/32	DR DA6-231	DQ TU22	DQw1 Genox 3.53	SDR1.2	DQw3 IVD12
EBV								
HOM 2	1, 1	w1	95	92	96	93	97	–
HOM 1	2, 2	w1	100	96	100	94	86	–
DHI	5, 5	w3	95	86	96	–	–	86
CLL								
S.J.	2, 4	w1, w3	96	80	18	14	18	13
C.K.	7, w6	w1	98	65	28	8	10	–
COOK	3	–	100	96	27	–	–	–
AML								
S.C. M1*	4, X	–	96	91	–	–	–	–
J.J. M1*	2, X	–	100	45	–	–	–	–
H.F. M1*	3, X	–	92	80	–	–	–	–
ALL								
F.M. L2*	2, 4	–	100	60	–	–	–	–
S.T. cALL	2, 3		96	73	–	–	–	–

Results are expressed as percentage of cells stained with $F(ab')_2$ FITC antimouse immunoglobulin. *, FAB classification; W6/32 (monomorphic HLA-ABC), P. Parham; DA6-231 (monomorphic HLA-DR), K. Guy; TU22 (monomorphic HLA-DQ), A. Ziegler; SDR1.2, T. DeKretser; IVD12, D. Capra; Genox 3.53, F. Brodsky

Histocompatibility Testing 1984
Edited by E. D. Albert et al.

early stages of differentiation. The mechanism by which the class II antigens are expressed selectively on some mature cells, i.e., B cells and monocytes and not granulocytes, is still not clear. The biological implications of these findings are now under investigation.

Acknowledgments. We would like to thank Dr. P. Peterson for the HLA-DQ β probe used in this study.

References

1. Navarrete C, Fainboim L, Festenstein H, Lister A, Amess J, Greaves M (1981) Selective expression of HLA-DR and HLA-MB antigens on acute leukaemic cells. In: Knapp W (ed) Leukaemia markers. Academic Press, London pp 65–68
2. Newman RA, Delia D, Greaves MF, Navarrete C, Fainboim L, Festenstein H (1983) Differential expression of HLA-DR and DR-linked determinants on human leukaemias and lymphoid cells. Eur J Immunol 13:172–176

Expression of HLA Class II Molecules on Human Monocytes and Dendritic Cells

S. Bjercke, E. Thorsby, and G. Gaudernack

Institute of Transplantation Immunology, The National Hospital, 0027 Oslo 1, Norway

By using a procedure for obtaining highly enriched dendritic cells (DRCs) and purified monocytes (MOs) from human peripheral blood, we have observed that the antigen-presenting cell (APC) function of human blood resides in the fibronectin receptor-positive, FcR-negative DRC population that lacks several monocyte/macrophage-specific differentiation antigens. On the other hand, purified MOs were not capable of presenting the soluble antigen PPD to T cells. To evaluate the expression of class II molecules from different loci (DR, DQ, and DP) on MOs and DRCs, binding of defined monoclonal antibodies (Mabs), specific for products of different HLA class II loci were quantitated by the use of ^{125}I-F(ab′)$_2$ anti-mouse Ig. On a per cell basis, MOs and DRCs expressed similar amounts of DR, DQ, and DP antigens (Table 1). The finding that DRCs and MOs both seem to express similar amounts of class II molecules is in contrast to our observation that enriched epidermal Langerhans cells contain 10–50 times more class II antigen than purified MOs from the same donors. The finding that MOs and DRCs express similar levels of class II molecules indicates that expression of such products is not sufficient for APC function, and that class II molecules must be present in the DRC membrane to function as a restriction element in T cell activation. The functional significance of class II molecules in the MOs is not clear. In mixing experiments, when graded numbers of purified MOs were added to DRCs we observed complete inhibition of the APC function with MO-to-DRC ratios of 15 : 1 to 5 : 1.

Table 1. Relative expression of HLA-class II determinants on dendritic cells and monocytes

Mab	Specificity	No. of expt.	DRC:MO-ratio
OKTa1	DR	4	1.16±0.30
D54	DR	8	1.00±0.10
B66	DR	1	1.04
Leu 10	DC	5	1.19±0.15
Tü 39	DR+DP	10	1.50±0.25

[a] Relative binding of Mabs was calculated from data obtained by radioimmunoassay with ^{125}I-F(ab′)$_2$ anti-mouse IgG by the following formula: $\frac{\text{CPM of } 0.5\times10^6 \text{ dendritic cells}}{\text{CPM of } 0.5\times10^6 \text{ monocytes}}$

Absence of DQw1 on Monocytes Depending on the DR Antigens Expressed

L. Gebuhrer, H. Bétuel, J. Lambert, and A.C. Freidel

Histocompatibility Laboratory, Blood Transfusion Center, 1–3, rue du Vercors, 69007 Lyon, France

DQw1 was originally defined serologically as a supertypic specificity comprising DR1, 2, w6, w10. DRw52 correlates with DR3, 5, w6, w8. Structural studies indicate that DQw1 represents a locus distinct from DR, controlling DQ products [2]; it seems that DRw52 products are governed by DR and by DQ [3]. HLA DRw6 is heterogeneous; at the Eighth Histocompatibility Workshop (H.W.) three subsets were proposed but not unanimously agreed on. At the Ninth H.W., serological distinction is still arduous, while two distinct DW subsets appear to exist. Monocytes and B cells from the same individuals were separated and tested by complement-dependent cytotoxicity tests with anti-class II reagents of the Ninth H.W. We examined 25 unrelated cells from our panel and four D-homozygous typing cells (HTCs): two defined the Dw6.1 subset, one recognized Dw6.2, and one typed for Dw9. We have provisionally kept the Eighth H.W. nomenclature for the HTCs defining DRw6. At the Ninth H.W. there is no serological difference between Dw6.1 and 6.2, while Dw9 is different and corresponds to DRw14 (901). DQw1, which is present on B cells, was not detected on monocytes by the Ninth H.W. alloantisera: in the two HTCs DR6.1, in some heterozygous DRw6, in HTC DR901 (Dw9), in heterozygous DRw14 and DRw10. The expression of DQw1 was normal in HTC DR6.3, and in some heterozygous DRw6. The concomitant presence of DR1 or DR2 resulted in normal reactions with anti-DQw1 sera. DQw1 of course remained negative for unassociated specificities such as DR4 and DR7.

For the expression of other DQw1 or DR specificities no discrepancy was observed between B lymphocytes and monocytes. These observations are in the line of the reported absence of class II molecules not controlled by DR on monocytes [1]. These results (Table 1) should be considered as a preliminary approach. Serological distinction between DRw6 on the basis of DQw1 expression on monocytes needs more family and population studies.

References

1. Gonwa TA, Picker LJ, Raff HV, Goyert SM, Silver J, Stobo JD (1983) J Immunol 130:706–711
2. Goyert SM, Shively JE, Silver J (1982) J Exp Med 156:550–560
3. Karr RW, Kannapell CC, Stein JA, Gebel HM, Mann DL, Duquesnoy RJ, Fuller TC, Rodey GE, Schwartz BD (1981) J Immunol 128:1809–1818

Table 1. Results

HLA DR Ag.	Number	Monocytes		B cells	
	29	DQw1	DRw52	DQw1	DRw52
w6/4, or 5, or 7, or 3	4	–	+	+	+
w6.1/w6.1 (HTC) (Dw6.1/6.1)	2	–	+	+	+
w6.3/w6.3 (HTC) (Dw6.2/6.2)	1	+	+	+	+
w6.1/w6.3 (Dw6.1/6.2)	2	+	+	+	+
w6/4 or 7	2	+	+	+	+
6/1 or 2	5	+	+	+	+
901/901 (HTC) (Dw9/Dw9)	1	–	+	+	+
w14/5 or 7	2	–	+	+	+
w14/1	1	+	+	+	+
w10/3 or w10	2	–	+	+	+
2/2 or 4 or 8	6	+	+	+	+
4/	1	–	–	–	–

Histocompatibility Testing 1984
Edited by E. D. Albert et al.

Interaction Between HLA Class I Antigens and γ-Endorphin

F.H.J. Claas[1], R. Castelli-Visser[1], B.M. de Jongh[1], J.J. van Rood[1], W.M.A. Verhoeven[2], J.M. van Ree[3], and D. de Wied[3]

1 Dept. of Immunohematology, University Hospital, Rijnsburgerweg 10, 2333 AA Leiden, The Netherlands
2 Dept. of Psychiatry, State University of Utrecht, The Netherlands
3 Rudolph Magnus Institute for Pharmacology, State University of Utrecht, The Netherlands

Treatment with γ-type endorphin has a beneficial effect in only a minority of schizophrenic patients. Genetic factors coded for within the HLA region may be associated with the response of the patients to treatment with γ-endorphin, because mainly HLA-B15 and Bw22 were increased in those patients who responded to treatment and remained free of psychosis for at least 6 months after treatment [1]. To test for a physical interaction between HLA class I antigens and γ-type endorphin, lymphocytes from healthy donors were preincubated with des-Tyr^1-γ-endorphin (DTγE), and after washing the reactivity of anti-HLA-A, B and C alloantisera with their specific antigens was tested in the standard complement-dependent cytotoxicity assay. The percentage lysis of the HLA typing sera was determined against both untreated and γ-endorphin-treated lymphocytes from the same donors. It was found that the reactivity of antibodies against some HLA antigens was partially inhibited by γ-endorphin, whereas no influence was seen on the reactivity of antibodies against other antigens. The degree of inhibition was dependent on the concentration of γ-endorphin used, maximum inhibition being seen with 3×10^{-4} *M* of the peptide.

On the basis of the reactivity of 120 HLA alloantisera with the cells of 30 healthy donors, a preferential inhibition of the sera against HLA-B15, Bw22, B13, Cw6, A11, and Cw3 was found, although some other antigens were partially masked. The in vitro inhibition capacity of γ-endorphin was then compared with the in vivo clinical response to γ-endorphin therapy in 52 schizophrenic patients. Patients were divided in high and low responders upon therapy using the Brief Psychiatric Response Score. When the HLA antigens of the high and low responders were compared it was found that a relative risk of becoming a high or a low responder could be calculated for each individual HLA antigen. A significant correlation ($r = 0.71$) was found between the level of inhibition of the cytotoxicity assay in vitro and the in vivo clinical response to γ-endorphin therapy.

These results suggest that the HLA class I antigens may function as or interfere with receptors for such endogenous substances as γ-type endorphins.

Reference

De Jongh BM, Verhoeven WMA, Van Ree JM, De Wied D, Van Rood JJ (1983) HLA and the response to treatment with γ-type endorphins in schizophrenia. J Immunogenet 9:381–388

Histocompatibility Testing 1984
Edited by E. D. Albert et al.

The Major Histocompatibility Complex as an Antibiosenescent System*

R.L. Walford[1] and T. Imamura[2]

1 Department of Pathology, UCLA Medical School Los Angeles, CA 90024, USA
2 Department of Entomology, Division of Toxicology and Physiology, University of California Riverside, CA 92521, USA

Whereas knowledge about the MHC has been accumulated chiefly by investigators oriented toward immunology, evidence exists that gene systems other than those concerned exclusively with immune function but lying in the same chromosomal region influence a number of processes involved in the biology of aging [4]. These include genes regulating the levels of free radical scavengers such as SOD and catalase. We have shown that levels of repair capacity of UV-induced DNA damage segregate with alleles of the MHC [1]. Repair of this form of damage is directly related to maximum life spans of species. Levels of mixed function oxidase (MFO) are also related to species life spans. MFOs "detoxify" the wide variety of simple organic chemicals in the environment. By contrast, the immune system must "detoxify" complex organic chemicals (proteins, etc.). The MFO system must, therefore, like the immune system, be highly polymorphic and multiple allelic. Evidence from our group now indicates that the MHC may influence basal and inducible levels of MFO, and that MFO inducers are immuno-suppressive, suggesting a complex interaction between two polymorphic systems (Table 1) [2]. We have shown, furthermore, that maximum life spans differ widely among H-2 congenic mice [3]. Thus the immunologic theory of aging, the DNA repair theory, the free radical theory, and other approaches may be grouped under the genetic umbrella of the MHC, which emerges as a general self-protective chromosomal region of which immune function is only one aspect. The MHC may have arisen from primitive self-protective systems evolved during the change from anaerobic to aerobic life forms.

* The authors were supported in this work by USPHS Research Grant AG-004419

References

1. Hall KY, Bergmann K, Walford RL (1981) DNA-repair, H-2, and aging in NZB and CBA mice. Tissue Antigens 17:104–110
2. Imamura T, Devons B, Weindruch R, Walford RL (1984) Correlation of drug metabolizing capability, immune function, and murine H-2 genetic complex. Age 7:42–47
3. Smith GS, Walford RL (1977) Influence of the main histocompatibility complex on ageing in mice. Nature 270:727–729
4. Walford RL (1983) Supergenes: histocompatibility; immunologic and other parameters in aging. In: Regelson W, Sinex FM (eds) Intervention in the aging process. Part B: Basic research and pre-clinical screening. Liss, pp 53–68

Table 1. Effect of β-naphthoflavone on monooxygenase activities of B10.F and B10.RIII H-2 congenic mice (from [2])

Strain	Pretreatment	Aryl hydrocarbon hydroxylase	Ratio	7-Ethoxy coumarin *O*-deethylase	Ratio	*P*-Nitroanisole *O*-demethylase	Ratio
B10.F	Corn oil	168 ± 13	3.0	658 ± 57	2.6	1.80 ± 0.09	1.9
	β-NF	497 ± 63		1 729 ± 319		3.43 ± 0.48	
B10.RIII	Corn oil	108 ± 7	6.0	383 ± 73	3.5	1.51 ± 0.09	1.8
	β-NF	651 ± 87		1 325 ± 123		2.80 ± 0.25	

Histocompatibility Testing 1984
Edited by E. D. Albert et al.

Defective Expression of HLA-D-Region Determinants in Children with Congenital Agammaglobulinemia and Malabsorption: A New Syndrome*

M.R. Hadam[1], R. Dopfer[2], G. Dammer[3], H.-H. Peter[4], M. Schlesier[4], C. Müller[5], and D. Niethammer[2]

1 Kinderklinik, Abteilung Kinderchirurgie, Med. Hochschule Hannover, Konstanty-Gutschow-Straße, 3000 Hannover 61, Federal Republic of Germany
2 Kinderklinik, Abteilung für Hämatologie, Universität Tübingen, 7400 Tübingen, Federal Republic of Germany
3 Rudolf-Virchow-Krankenhaus, 1000 Berlin 65, Federal Republic of Germany
4 Abteilung Immunologie und Transfusionsmedizin, Med. Hochschule Hannover, 3000 Hannover 61, Federal Republic of Germany
5 Medizinische Klinik, Abteilung II, Universität Tübingen, 7400 Tübingen, Federal Republic of Germany

Abbreviations

AG agammaglobulinemia, ID immunodeficiency, BLS bare lymphocyte syndrome, IF immunofluorescence, FCM flow cytometry, MAb monoclonal antibody, IH immunohistology, Ig immunoglobulin, IFN interferon, FITC fluorescein, TR Texas red, PWM pokeweed mitogen, CBL cord blood lymphocytes, LC Langerhans' cell, BC endothelial cell, BLCL B-lymphoblastoid cell line, PBMC peripheral blood mononuclear cells.

Introduction

Recently we have described four children with congenital AG associated with persistent diarrhea, malabsorption, and failure to thrive [5, 6]. All patients displayed a lack of expression of HLA-DR and DQ antigens, whereas HLA-ABC antigens were consistently found. In contrast to our patients, Touraine et al. [17] have described a combined ID termed "bare lymphocyte syndrome" (BLS), characterized by a lack of class I antigens and a continued expression of class II antigens. Subsequently, cases of BLS were described with defects in both class I and class II antigens [4, 7, 12, 14, 16]. In this study, cell surface antigens were quantitated on single cells by indirect IF and FCM, using well-defined MAbs. In addition, skin biopsy specimens were examined for cells bearing HLA antigens by IH. As a functional parameter, Ig production was assessed in vitro. Finally, attempts are reported to modulate class II determinants by IFN treatment in vitro.

Patients

Our patients (RS♂, SM♀, AH♂, FH♀) are now aged between 3¼ and 1 year. AH and FH were born from a consanguineous marriage. RS and SM have healthy elder brothers. Family histories and pregnancies were otherwise uninformative. In all patients AG was diagnosed before the age of 6 months after bacterial infections. In addition severe and persistent diarrhea of unknown cause developed resulting in malabsorption and failure to thrive. Whereas most infections were controlled by antibiotic and Ig replacement therapy, diarrhea remained intractable up to date. Viral infections cleared normally. Lymphocyte counts were elevated and two patients had eosinophilia. Thymic shadow and lymphnodes were present. Serum Ig levels of all classes were very low or absent and specific antibodies were not detected. Complement levels, granulocyte function, growth hormone and purine metabolism enzymes revealed no gross abnormalities. Karyotyping and cytogenetic studies, kindly performed by Dr. J. Kömpf, Tübingen, FRG, showed no defects on chromosome 6. A detailed case report will be presented elsewhere [6].

Materials and Methods

Antibodies. MAbs were from commercial sources (Leu4, Leu10, Mac-120, L243: Becton-Dickinson; 7.2: New England Nuclear; OKT6: Ortho). M522 was donated by Dr. J. Lohmeyer, Giessen, FRG [9]. W6/32 HL and HK against HLA-ABC and its negative variant [1] and TÜ-35 resp. TÜ-22 against HLA-DR resp -DQ [11] were generously provided by Dr. A. Ziegler, Tübingen, FRG. $F(ab')_2$-fragments of goat antibodies against human Ig-isotypes were purchased from Cappel Laboratories.

* Supported by the Deutsche Forschungsgemeinschaft (SFB 120: A3, B3, F1; SFB54: G13) and the Robert Bosch Foundation

Histocompatibility Testing 1984
Edited by E. D. Albert et al.

Immunofluorescence and Flow Cytometry. IF on cell suspensions of peripheral blood mononuclear cells (PBMC) was performed as described [5]. Cord blood samples were kindly provided by Dr. A. Fridrich, Stuttgart, FRG. FCM was performed on a FACS IV cell sorter and evaluation of log-amplified signals was done on at least 10 000 cells after gating on 0 °/90 ° light scatter. For two-colour IF excitation was at 488 nm and 568 nm using fluorescein (FITC) and texas red (TR) as fluorochromes. Contour plots were generated on a VAX-11 computer with the invaluable help and computer programs generously provided by Dr. L. Voet, Martinsried, FRG. IF intensity measurements were done on homogeneous peaks by visual approximation of mean fluorescence intensities and reported in channel numbers (1 – 225).

Immunoglobulin Synthesis in Vitro. The technique has previously been detailed [13]. Values are reported for fresh cell cultures and after incubation for 9 days with and without pokeweed mitogen (PWM).

Immunohistology. IH was performed on cryostat sections (4 μm) of patients' skin biopsies. MAbs were visualized with developing antibodies conjugated to peroxidase as described earlier [10].

HLA-DR Modulation by IFN-γ. PBMC of patients SM and RS were incubated in Costar plates (# 3524) for 48 hrs at 2×10^6 cells/ml in 10% FCS/RPMI 1640 (Gibco) at 37 °C/5% CO_2 with various additions. Purified human IFN-γ was kindly provided by Dr. Mohr, DRK-Blutbank, Springe, FRG. Indomethacin was used at 5 μg/ml final concentration.

Results and Discussion

In this study cord blood lymphocytes (CBL) were used as control to demonstrate differential expression of HLA-ABC on T-vs. B-lymphocytes in two-colour IF. The contour plot in Fig. 1 a shows a distinctly higher mean intensity staining for class-I-antigens on neonatal B-cells than on T-lymphocytes; this contrasts to the distribution in adults [5]. PBMC from patient SM are shown on the dot-plot in Fig. 2a: again B-lymphocytes carry more HLA-ABC-determinants than T-cells, almost identical to the distribution seen in CBL. On monocytes HLA-ABC-antigens were present in normal quantities (Table 1). Whenever platelets were detected in the samples used for FCM, they were positive for HLA-ABC-antigens (data not shown). Thus in contrast to most published cases of BLS, the four patients described here demonstrate a consistent class-I-antigen expression on all cell types investigated. The levels of antigen expression particularly on T-cells may be lower compared to healthy children or adults, but closely resemble the situation in the healthy newborn.

As opposed to class-I-antigens, HLA-D-region determinants are completely lacking from lymphocytes (Table 2) despite the presence of a sizable proportion of surface-Ig-positive B-cells. Two-colour IF was applied to unequivocally establish this finding: Fig. 1 b demonstrates a contour plot of normal CBL stained with anti-S and monoclonal anti-DR. The DR-positive B-cell cluster is clearly discernible; in addition small numbers of activated T-cells can be distinguished. PBMC of patient SM showed a complete lack of HLA-DR-antigens on all surface-IgD-defined B-cells (Fig. 2b). There was also no staining of T-cells. Though monocytes of our patients reacted strongly with HLA-ABC and monocyte-specific MAbs (Table 1), 7.2 anti-

Table 1. HLA-antigens on monocytes

Antibody	Designation	Patients[a]		
		RS	AH	FH
W6/32 HL	HLA-ABC	80[b]	90	171
M522	Monocytes	133	101	170
Mac-120	Monocytes	nd[c]	125	190
7.2	HLA-DR	8	0	6
L243	HLA-DR	nd	0	3
TÜ-35	HLA-DR	4	0	6
Leu 10	HLA-DQ	0	5	5
TÜ-22	HLA-DQ	5	0	5

[a] Patient SM was evaluated on photographs from dot-plots with similar results
[b] Results are given as mean fluorescence intensities (in channel numbers) of light scatter gated monocytes. Negative control values (W6/32 HK) have been subtracted
[c] not done

Table 2. HLA-antigens on lymphocytes

Antibody	Designation	Patients			
		RS	SM	AH	FH
w6/32 HK	neg. control	1.4[a]	2.8	0.7	0.5
w6/32 HL	HLA-ABC	94.6	94.8	83.8[b]	96.9
7.2	HLA-DR	1.4	2.4	0.6	0.5
Leu 10	HLA-DQ	1.1	2.5[c]	0.6	0.5
anti-δ	B-cells	53.1	20.0	21.6	9.0

[a] Percent lymphocytes stained; negative control not subtracted
[b] Lower value due to subpopulation weakly staining for HLA-ABC
[c] In this assay, Leu 10 was replaced by TÜ-22. In other tests from the same patient, both antibodies reacted similarly

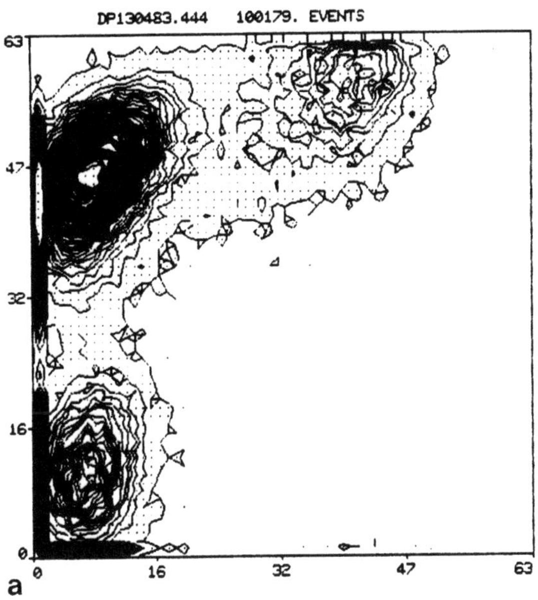

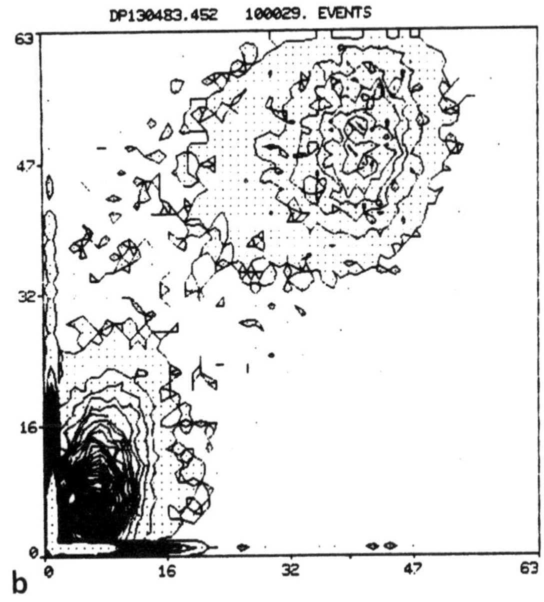

Fig. 1a, b. Two-colour IF of CBL gated on lymphocytes by forward scatter only. Contour plot with contours ranging from 1 – 500 cells/channel in steps of 10. Both axes are log scale (2.5 decades) with the cluster in the lower left corner defined as negative (channels 1 – 16 ea). With CBL, non-lymphoid cells are not completely separable from lymphocytes by light scatter only. **a** *Horizontal* axis: FITC-anti-δ. *Vertical* axis: W6/32 (HLA-ABC) followed by TR-anti-mouse-IgG. **b** *Horizontal* axis: FITC-anti-δ. *Vertical* axis: Ia-011 (HLA-DR) followed by TR-anti-mouse- IgG

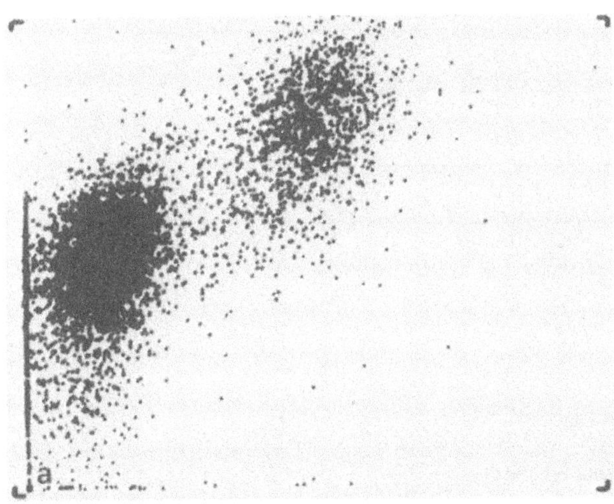

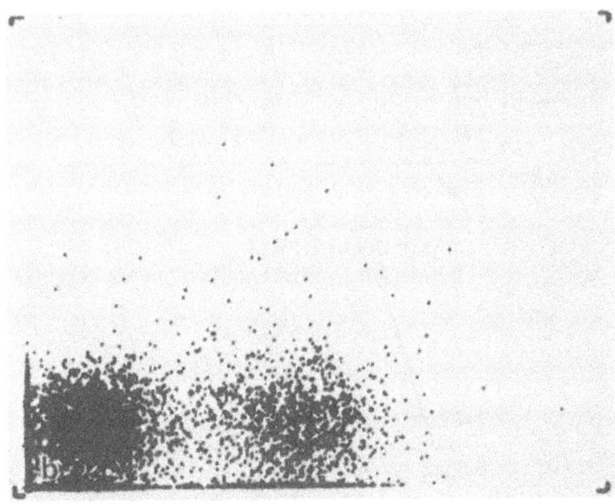

Fig. 2a, b. Two-colour IF of PBMC from patient SM gated on lymphocytes by 0 °/90 ° light scatter. Dot plot representing 4032 events; the whole experiment encompasses 50 000 lymphocytes. Both axes are log scale (2.5 decades) with the lower left corner defined as negative (channels 1 – 16 ea). **a** *Horizontal* axis: FITC-anti-δ. *Vertical* axis: W6/32 HL (HLA- ABC) followed by TR-anti-mouse-IgG. **b** *Horizontal* axis: FITC-anti-δ. *Vertical* axis: biotinylated L243 (HLA-DR) followed by TR-avidin

DR- and anti-DQ-MAbs did not result in a significant fluorescence signal. This complete lack of class-II-antigen expression is similar to what has been observed by Kuis et al. [7] and to some of the patients of Griscelli et al. [4]. However, their cases were also lacking HLA-ABC.

HLA-antigen expression in the skin was tested by IH. Representative results from patient SM are shown in Fig. 3: A typical dendritic staining pattern is obtained using the MAb OKT6 (Fig. 3a) which reacts with Langerhans' cells (LC) in the skin. Staining of a parallel section with MAb TÜ-35 against DR is quite contrasting (Fig. 3b): despite the presence of large numbers of LC only a very small proportion of LC in the skin demonstrate positive staining with anti-DR. Endothelial cells

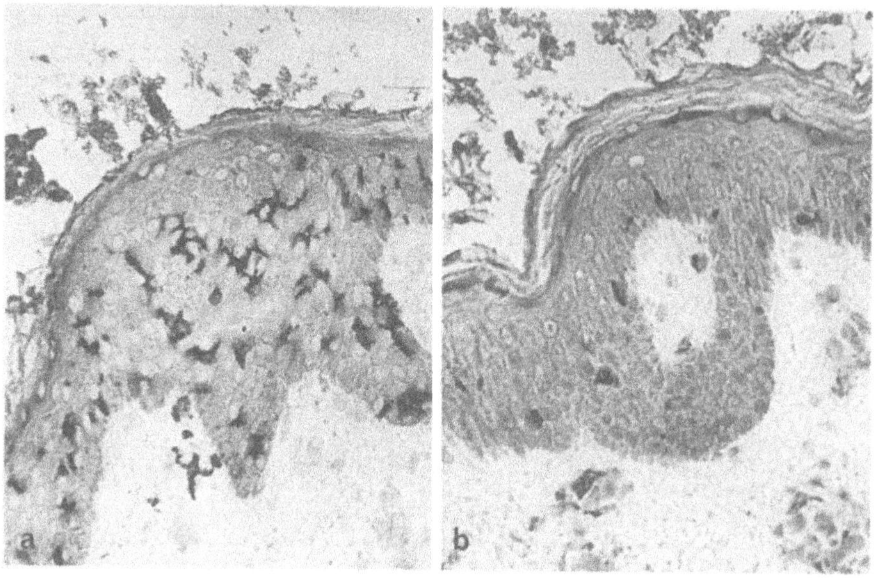

Fig. 3. Skin biopsy of patient SM stained with **a** OKT6 and **b** TÜ-35

Table 3. Immunoglobulin synthesis in vitro

Patient	IgG			IgA			IgM		
	0[a]	9	9+PWM	0	9	9+PWM	0	9	9+PWM
RS	10[b]	0	175	0	0	9	0	0	92
SM	0	72	0	0	14	14	0	135	90
AH	0	0	0	6	0	2	2	0	55
FH	0	0	0	41	8	23	66	49	88
Control	0	240	9 965	52	45	2 147	53	1 177	25 353

[a] days of culture ± PWM
[b] Results are given as ng/ml culture supernatant

Table 4. Interferon-γ and class-II-antigens on monocytes[a]

Patient	Antibody	Additions during incubation				
		ø	500 U[b]	1000 U	1000 U + Indo.	Indo.[c]
Control	Leu 10	0[d]	2	6	4	3
	7.2	97	115	128	123	100
SM	Leu 10	0	0	0	0	0
	7.2	0	0	0	0	0
RS	Leu 10	0	0	0	0	0
	7.2	0	0	0	0	0

[a] PBMC were incubated as indicated, stained and evaluated by FCM. Gating was performed on lymphocytes and monocytes. Data are shown for monocytes only
[b] Units IFN per ml culture medium
[c] Indomethacin added at 5 μg/ml final concentration
[d] Results are given as mean fluorescence intensities (in channel numbers) of light scatter gated monocytes. Negative control values (here Leu 4) have been subtracted. Difference values ≦0 were designated 0

(EC) were also negative in these sections whereas HLA-ABC-antigens were clearly present in all four patients' biopsies. Thus on LC and EC class-II-antigen expression is virtually completely lacking whereas class-I-antigens remain unaffected.

When tested for functional activities, the patients PBMC proliferated low-normally to mitogens and alloantigens and were able to generate cytotoxic T-cells. However Ig-synthesis was defective as shown in Table 3. There was no synthesis of IgG, IgA and IgM in all four patients with or without PWM. This lack of Ig-secretion is paralleled by the complete lack of terminal plasma cell maturation when examined for cytoplasmic Ig. Thus the lack of class-II-antigen expression affects primarily the capacity to produce antibodies both in vivo and in vitro. This is in accordance with the findings of Zegers et al. [18] who demonstrated defective production of helper factors in a similar patient.

The influence of exogeneous IFN-γ on class-II-antigen expression was investigated as shown in Table 4. Monocytes of adult controls increased HLA-DR-expression but not HLA-DQ in response to IFN-γ. However, patients SM and RS did not react to IFN-γ, even in the presence of indomethacin [15]. It appears from these data, that IFN-γ-treatment cannot easily reverse the defective expression of class-II-antigens, whereas class-I-antigens were shown to be readily increased by IFN-α and -β in some BLS-patients [2].

From patients RS and SM we have obtained several B-lymphoblastoid cell lines (BLCL) which are now in continuous culture for more than 140 days and are still negative for HLA-DR- and -DQ-antigens. A DR-negative T-cell line has also been established and propagated in interleukin-2. Moreover MAb CR3.43, a reagent detecting HLA-DR, -DQ and -DP (generated by Dr. D. Mason, Oxford and generously provided by Dr. M. Steel, Edinburgh) was tested on the BLCL and found negative. This can be taken as indicative that also HLA-DP-antigens are not expressed in these patients. Gladstone and Pious [3] have established mutant lymphoblastoid cell lines deficient in HLA-DR, -DQ and -DP. They found that these cells contain the structural genes for class-II-antigens but fail to express them [8]. Since we have observed a small number of class-II-antigen-positive cells in the skin biopsies of patients SM (Fig. 3b) and AH, we assume that the structural genes for class-II-antigens must be present.

Thus we are left with the hypothesis that our patients manifest an experiment of nature whereby a regulatory gene for the HLA-class-II-complex is affected similar to the mutants produced by Gladstone and Pious [3, 8]. Most interestingly, the clinical outcome is not combined ID as might be expected, but AG with a peculiar association of diarrhea and malabsorption.

References

1. Barnstable CJ, Bodmer WF, Brown G, Galfre G, Milstein C, Williams AF, Ziegler A (1978) Production of monoclonal antibodies to group A erythrocytes, HLA and other human cell surface antigens – new tools for genetic analysis. Cell 14:9–20
2. Durandy A, Virelizier JL, Griscelli C (1983) Enhancement by interferon of membrane HLA antigens in patients with combined immunodeficiency with defective HLA expression. Clin exp Immunol 52:173–178
3. Gladstone P, Pious D (1978) Stable variants affecting B cell alloantigens in human lymphoid cells. Nature 271: 459–461
4. Griscelli C, Durandy A, Virelizier JL (1980) Impaired cell to cell interaction in partial combined immunodeficiency with variable expression of HLA antigens. In: Seligmann M, Hitzig WH (eds) Primary Immunodeficiencies: INSERM Symposium No. 16. Elsevier/North-Holland, Amsterdam, pp 499–503
5. Hadam MR, Dopfer R, Peter HH, Niethammer D (1984) Congenital agammaglobulinaemia associated with lack of expression of HLA-D-region antigens. In: Griscelli C, Vossen J (eds) Progress in immunodeficiency research and therapy I. Elsevier, Amsterdam pp 43–50
6. Hadam MR, Dopfer R, Dammer G, Blum W, Peter HH, Schlesier M, Müller C, Niethammer D (1984) Lack of HLA-D-region antigens in congenital agammaglobulinaemia with malabsorption. (submitted)
7. Kuis W, Roord J, Zegers BJM, Schuurman RKB, Heijnen CJ, Baldwin WM, Goulmy E, Claas F, van de Griend RJ, Rijkers GT, van Rood JJ, Vossen JM, Ballieux RE, Stoop JW (1981) Clinical and immunological studies in a patient with the 'Bare-Lymphocyte' Syndrome. In: Touraine JL, Gluckman E, Griscelli C (eds) Bone marrow transplantation in Europe, Volume II. Excerpta Medica, Amsterdam, pp 201–208
8. Levine F, Pious D (1984) Revertants from the HLA class II regulatory mutant 6.1.6: implications for the regulation of Ia gene expression. J Immunol 132:959–962
9. Lohmeyer J, Rieber P, Feucht H, Johnson J, Hadam M, Riethmüller G (1981) A subset of human natural killer cells isolated and characterized by monoclonal antibodies. Eur J Immunol 11:997–1101
10. Müller C, Schüch K, Pawelec G, Wilms K, Wernet P (1982) Immunohistology of graft-versus-host disease mediated skin lesions and its correlation to a large granular lymphocyte surface phenotype and function. Blut 44: 89–94
11. Pawelec G, Shaw S, Ziegler A, Müller C, Wernet P (1982) Differential inhibition of HLA-D or SB directed secondary lymphoproliferative responses with monoclonal antibodies detecting human Ia-like determinants. J Immunol 129:1070–1075
12. Payne R, Brodsky FM, Peterlin BM, Young LM (1983) Bare lymphocytes without immunodeficiency. Human Immunol 6:219–227
13. Peter HH, Friedrich W, Dopfer R, Müller W, Kortmann C, Pichler WJ, Heinz F, Rieger ChHL (1983) NK cell function in severe combined immunodeficiency (SCID): Evidence of a common T and NK cell defect in some but not all SCID patients. J Immunol 131:2332–2339

14. Schuurman RKB, van Rood JJ, Vossen JM, Schellekens PThA, Feltkamp-Vroom ThM, Doyer E, Gmelig-Meyling F, Visser HKA (1979) Failure of lymphocyte-membrane HLA-A and -B expression in two siblings with combined immunodeficiency. Clin Immunol Immunopathol 14:418–434
15. Snyder DS, Beller DI, Unanue ER (1982) Prostaglandins modulate macrophage Ia expression. Nature 299:163–165
16. Touraine JL (1981) The Bare-Lymphocyte Syndrome: Report on the registry. Lancet I:319–321
17. Touraine JL, Bétuel H, Souillet G, Jeune M (1978) Combined immunodeficiency disease associated with absence of cell-surface HLA-A and -B antigens. J Pediatr 93:47–51
18. Zegers BJM, Heijnen CJ, Roord JJ, Kuis W, Schuurman RKB, Stoop JW, Ballieux RE (1983) Defective Expression of mononuclear cell membrane HLA antigens associated with combined immunodeficiency: Impaired cellular interactions. In: Wedgwood RJ, Rosen FS, Paul NW (eds) Primary immunodeficiency diseases. Birth Defects: Original Article Series. Alan Liss, New York, pp 93–96

Defect of Expression of MHC Genes Responsible for an Abnormal HLA Class I Phenotype and the Class II Negative Phenotype of Lymphocytes from Patients with Combined Immunodeficiency

B. Lisowska-Grospierre[1], D.J. Charron[2], C. de Préval[3], A. Durandy[1], P. Turmel[2], C. Griscelli[1], and B. Mach[3]

1 INSERM U132, Hopital des Enfants Malades, 75015 Paris, France
2 Laboratoire d'Immunogenétique, CHU Pitié-Salpetrière, 75013 Paris, France
3 Department de Microbiologie, Université de Geneve, 1205 Genève, Suisse

Introduction

An autosomal recessive combined immunodeficiency syndrome associated with a defective cell membrane expression of the HLA antigens has been described [9, 21, 22]. In the early observations, an absence of class II antigens was reported [21, 22]. We have also described patients in whom an absence of class II antigens was observed together with a decreased expression of class I antigens [7, 9, 12]. These latter patients have a profound defect of antibody production and of cell mediated immunity to thymus-dependent antigens. They suffered from repeated and severe bacterial and viral infections, which were the cause of death for most of them. The defect of class I and class II expression may contribute to the observed immunodeficiency, but the cellular mechanisms underlying this defect have not yet been elucidated. In this study we investigated the expression of class I and class II antigens both at protein and mRNA levels.

Material and Methods

Antibodies. The MAb anti-HLA class I clone W6/32 (Sera Lab) [2] and a rabbit anti-β_2 microglobulin (β_2m) (Dr. C. Vincent, Lyon), were used to detect class I antigens. The MAbs to native class II antigens were: MAb 2/06 [4], VI.15c, 147 (anti-αDR), 171 (anti-βDR) [10], MAb 8/12 (N. Rebai and B. Malissen, manuscript in preparation), MAb LB 14/16 (Dr. J Brochier, Lyon). Rabbit antisera to separated class II α and β chains, obtained by injecting DR subunits into rabbits, were a kind gift from Dr. J. P. Mach (Lausanne).

Cells and Cell Population Studies. Patients and control peripheral blood lymphocytes (PBLs) were isolated by Ficoll-Hypaque gradient centrifugation and, for biosynthetic studies, cultured in RPMI-1640 medium containing 10% human AB serum and an optimal dose of PHA (10 µg/ml) for 5 days. For immunofluorescence studies, cells were preincubated in RPMI-1640 serum-free medium for 30 min at 37 °, washed prior to the addition of antibodies, and the membrane antigens expression was assessed by the direct or indirect fluorescence test [7].

Cell Labeling and Immunoprecipitation. The nonadhering cells from patients and control PHA-stimulated cultures were collected at day 5, the percentage of blasts was determined, and the cells were preincubated in methionine-free MEM for 60 min. Then, $5 \cdot 10^6$ cells were incubated in 500 µl methionine-free MEM containing 100 µCi/ml [^{35}S]-meth-

Histocompatibility Testing 1984
Edited by E. D. Albert et al.

ionine (Amersham, 500 Ci/mmol) and 10% dialysed SVF at 37 ° for 3 h. Labeled cells were lysed in 50 m*M* Tris-HCl (pH 7.4), 150 m*M* NaCl, 2 m*M* EDTA, 2 m*M* PMSF, and 1% NP-40 for 30 min and centrifuged at 100 000 *g* for 30 min. Patients' and control lysates were adjusted to contain the same amount of radioactivity and were immunoprecipitated with antibodies listed above, using as immunoabsorbant *Staphylococcus aureus.* Washed precipitates were analyzed by SDS-polyacrylamide gel (12.5%) electrophoresis (1-D gel) [11]. In the two-dimensional gel analysis (2-D gel), the first dimension was a nonequilibrium pH gradient electrophoresis (NEPHGE), and the second a 10% polyacrylamide slab [5, 19]. Gels were fluorographed, dried, and exposed to Kodak AR film for 5–20 days. 1-D autoradiograms were scanned on a Vernon scanner.

RNA Preparation and Analysis. RNA preparation and Northern blot analysis were performed according to de Preval and Mach [20]. In brief, total RNA was prepared as described by Chirgwin et al. [6], denatured in glyoxal [18], electrophoresed in a 1.8% agarose gel, transferred to diazobensyloxymethyl paper, and hybridized with nick-translated ^{32}P-cDNA probes. Following hybridization with pHLA 44/2 HLA class I heavy chain probe [15], α DR [23], β DR [13], and Ii chain [14] cDNA probes, the filter was washed (final washes 0.1 × SSC at 68 °) and submitted to autoradiography. Dehybridization of the filter was performed in 99% formamide, 10 m*M* phosphate buffer pH 7.0, 5 m*M* EDTA at 68 °.

Results

Cell Population Studies

Study of PBLs in patients revealed normal or subnormal percentages of B cells, as assessed by sIg and Fc γ R phenotyping [7]. Membrane expression of class I and class II antigens on patients' PBLs and PHA-induced blasts is shown in Table 1. For class I, the percentages of the HLA-A, B, C and of β_2m positive cells varied from patient to patient and also varied with time. For class II, several monomorphic anti-DR antibodies failed to detect any positive cells in PBLs or in PHA blasts in eight patients. In a resting lymphocyte population of patient OT, a half of sIg+ B cells were DR positive, but his PHA blasts were not expressing the class II antigens.

Lymphoproliferative responses of patients' PBLs to PHA or PWM were normal when assessed by ^{3}H-thymidine incorporation (data not shown), but the percentage of blasts in the patient's mitogen-stimulated culture was in some experiments decreased as compared to the controls (10%–40% instead of 30%–70%). The HLA antigen expression of these blasts was abnormal as compared to the controls (Table 1).

HLA Class I Detection

In all nine patients the biosynthesis of class I antigens was quantitatively abnormal as judged from several experiments for each of them. Typical re-

Table 1. Membrane expression of class I and II antigens on resting and cultured lymphocytes

Controls / Patients	Resting lymphocytes			PHA-induced blasts		
	Class I	β_2 m	Class II	Class I	β_2m	Class II
	100	100	10	99	97	89[a]
AC	40	5	1	20	10	0[b]
JB	45	2	0	NT	NT	NT
RA	7	7	1	37	13	0[b]
DA	53	6	0	23	16	0[b]
NH	67	58	1	96	78	0[a]
OT	62	51	17[c]	98	84	0[a]
PA	80	75	0	NT	NT	NT
LS	30	45	2	NT	NT	NT
BA	51	98	0	NT	NT	NT

Detection was by immunofluorescence with MAb anti-class I W6/32 (SeraLab), MAb anti-β_2 m (MAb-018-SeraLab) and MAb anti-class II (Ortho-Pharm). Results are expressed as the percentage of immunofluorescent cells

[a] T cell lines; [b] PHA-induced T blasts

[c] Patient OT had an abnormally high level (32%) of sIg-bearing B cells

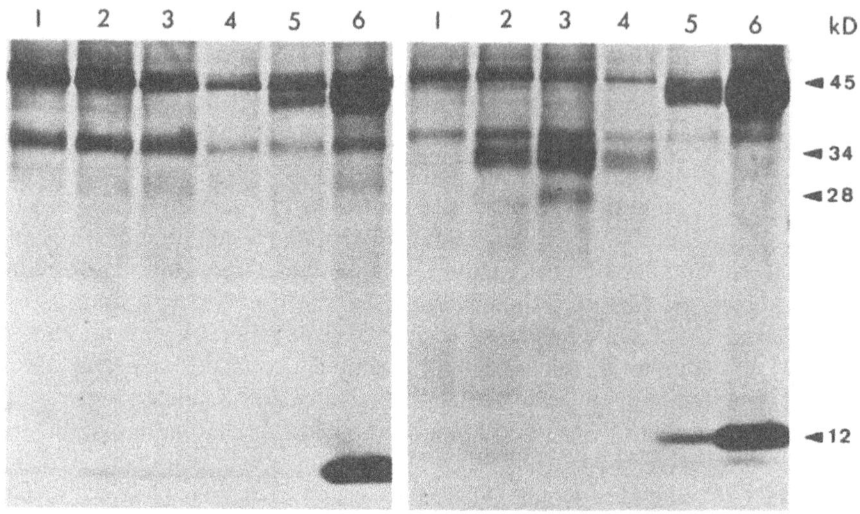

Fig. 1. 1-D gel electrophoretic analysis of immunoprecipitates of cell lysates of PHA blasts from a typical patient (RA, *left*) and control (*right*). [^{35}S]methionine-labeled cell lysates were precipitated with the following antibodies: 2 µl NMS (*1*), 3 µl each of Rb anti α and β chains (*2*), 20 µl of MAb anti-class II: 2/06 (*3*) and 8/12 (*4*), 3 µl of MAb W6/32 anti-class I (*5*), and 3 µl of rabbit anti-β_2-microglobulin (*6*)

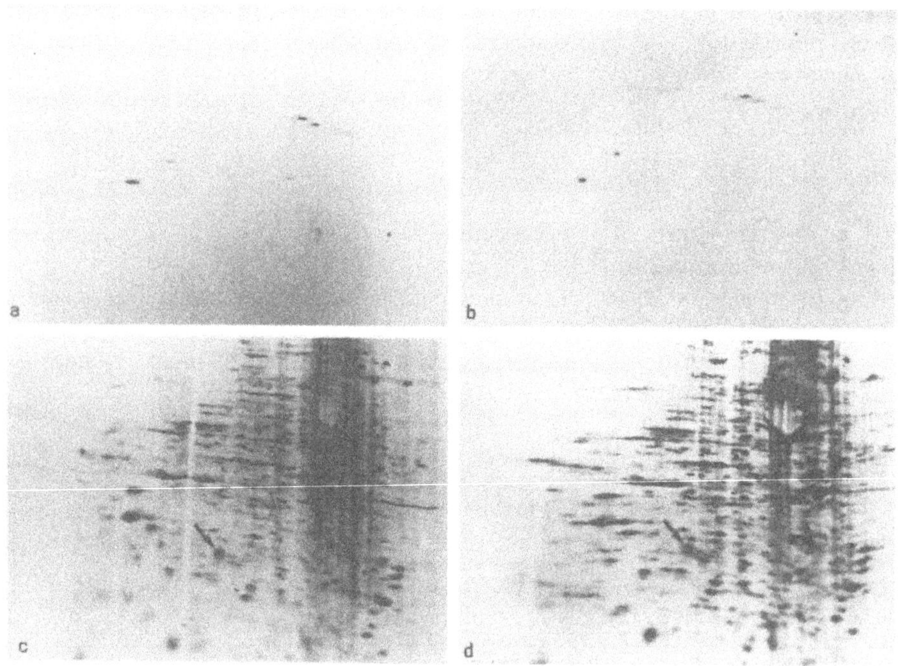

Fig. 2. 2-D gel electrophoretic analysis of patients' immunoprecipitates or total lysates of patients' PHA blasts. Precipitates were obtained with 5 µl of MAb 171 (*a*) or MAb 147 (*b*) from patient RA's [^{35}S]methionine-labeled cell lysate. For total lysates, 5 µl of patient RA (*c*) or patient AC (*d*) cell lysates were diluted with 45 µl IEF buffer. Arrows indicate the Ii chain.

sults are presented in Fig. 1. The heavy chain of class I antigen was found in decreased amounts as compared to the controls (lane 5), contrasting with a normal amount of the β_2 microglobulin (lane 6).
A quantitative estimation of the amount of the class I heavy chain in precipitates from patients' cells was obtained by scanning of the autoradiographs. When the density of the control heavy chain band was normalized to 1.0, the relative density of the patients' HLA 45K band varied from 0.16 to 0.77, with an average of 0.408 (the average density of the β_2m band was 0.90).
This quantitative defect of HLA class I expression was confirmed in the case of patient RA by Northern blot analysis of the HLA heavy chain mRNA. In the PBLs of this patient, containing at the time

of examination 7% of HLA class I-bearing cells, the amount of mRNA was decreased by a factor of 10 to 15 as compared to normal PBL controls (data not shown). The genomic DNA probe which was used [15] does not distinguish between the HLA-A, B, and C mRNAs and is able to detect these mRNA species in all subjects.

HLA Class II Detection

In all patients, the different monoclonal or rabbit antibodies used to isolate the HLA class II antigens repeatedly failed to precipitate any of the α and β chains, either from the cell lysates (Fig. 1 left lanes 2, 3, 4 as compared to right lanes 2, 3, 4) or from the culture supernatants (data not shown). 2-D gel electrophoresis of both immune precipitates and of total cell lysates was performed in four patients. Immunoprecipitates of class II antigens obtained using two antibodies able to detect the unassembled as well as assembled DR α or DR β chains failed to reveal any DR species (Fig. 2 panels a and b). Similar data were obtained with rabbit antisera to isolated α and β chains (data not shown). In contrast, the invariant (Ii) chain was readily detected when total lysates were analyzed in the case of four patients (Fig. 2 panels c and d).
The RNA studies were performed using PBLs of patient RA, containing 18% of sIg-bearing cells. Patient and control RNAs were analyzed for the presence of mRNA specific for HLA-DR α chain HLA-DR β chain, and for mRNA of DR-associated Ii chain utilizing previously isolated cDNA probes [13, 14, 23]. In the patient cells, no mRNA for HLA-DR α or β chain could be detected, whereas the mRNA for the Ii chain was present in amounts comparable to controls. Even after prolonged exposure of the same filters, no class II mRNA could be detected in the lane corresponding to the patient's RNA.

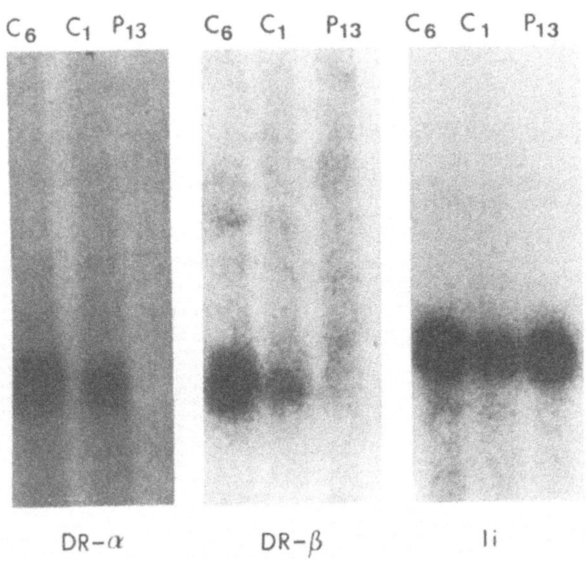

Fig. 3. Presence of Ii chain mRNA and absence of DR α and β chain mRNA in the patients' lymphocytes. Total RNA was electrophoresed, transferred to diazobensyloxymethyl paper, and hybridized with nick-translated ^{32}P-cDNA probes for α DR, β DR and Ii chain cDNA. *C6, C1,* 6 and 1 μg total RNA from cells of a healthy donor. *RA 13,* 13 μg total RNA from patient RA

Discussion

Molecular expression of MHC class I and II antigens varies in different cell populations and is clearly important in intercellular events leading to an immune response [3, 17]. In this respect, it is essential to assess the quantitative and qualitative defects of class I and class II MHC gene expression in immune deficiency, as these defects are likely to be responsible for the immunological manifestations of this disease. Qualitative deficiency in the expression of class II antigens has been shown in mice to result in a corresponding defect in the function of antigen-presenting cells [16].
In man, several types of immunodeficiency are described and are not always associated with an abnormal expression of HLA antigens. For example, the lymphocytes of patients with Severe Combined Immune Deficiency (SCID) express the MHC products normally. In the immunodeficiency that we have studied in which both T and B populations are present, the immune defect was thought to be associated with an even more profound defect of class II expression. The consistent reduction in the biosynthesis of class I polypeptides was confirmed by a low transcription level of the HLA class I heavy chain gene. However, the HLA class I expression can be enhanced to almost normal levels by incubation of patients' lymphocytes in the presence of α and β interferons [7]. The DR-negative phenotype of these cells was found to reflect not the deficient membrane insertion of class II antigens, but their abnormal synthesis. Several monomorphic anti-class II MAbs repeatedly failed to detect any of the α and β chains from the patient's cell lysates or from the culture supernatants. MAbs able to precipitate the nonassembled native DR subunits and the rabbit antisera to the isolated DR α and β chains did not reveal any DR specificities in patients cells. Because of the absence of protein synthesis, the level of activity of the HLA-DR genes on the RNAs was explored. The absence of HLA-DR α and β chains mRNA indicates that this disease involves a defect in gene expression and is not the result of a block of translation or assembly

as observed for instance, for class I antigens in the case of Daudi cells [20].

Because some of these DR-negative lymphocytes were seen to revert to a DR-positive phenotype following 3 weeks of culture in vitro (data not shown), the class II non-expression is not due to a massive deletion of both alleles of DR genes. It is very likely that we are dealing with a regulatory defect affecting the transcription of DR genes on both chromosomes. The situation in these patients resembles, therefore, the cases of DR-negative variants obtained experimentally [1, 8], in which we have also observed an absence of HLA DR mRNA with the presence of Ii chain mRNA (E.O. Long et al., manuscript in preparation; Levine et al., manuscript in preparation). This uncoupling of the expression of HLA-DR and Ii chain genes contrasts with the coordinate induction of both polypeptides in mitogen-stimulated PBL [5].

The total block of DR gene expression and a low transcription level of the HLA class I gene indicate a transactive, pleiotropic defect involving the major histocompatibility complex. Studies of HLA-DR expression in cells belonging to other cell lineages, such as epidermal cells, should be informative in these patients in distinguishing somatic mutation affecting the lymphocytes' lineage from a more general phenomenon, possibly a germline defect.

Summary

An autosomal recessive combined immunodeficiency syndrome associated with defective cell membrane expression of HLA antigens has been described. In several patients unable to mount the normal humoral and cellular immune responses and in whom a decreased expression of class I was found, we observed an absence of class II antigens. We studied the biosynthesis of HLA class I and class II molecules using the lymphocytes of these patients. A decreased amount of HLA-A, B, and C heavy chains but normal synthesis of β_2 microglobulin was observed. For class II antigens no biosynthesis of HLA-DR α and DR β chains could be detected at the protein level using monoclonal antibodies specific for either the HLA-DR α-β complex or its nonassociated α and β subunits. In contrast, the 31K Ii chain was readily detected when total lysates were analyzed by two-dimensional gel electrophoresis. In order to explore directly the level of activity of the HLA-DR genes, the RNAs were analyzed by Northern blot hybridization for the presence of mRNA specific for HLA- DR α chain and β chain and for mRNA of the DR- associated invariant chain Ii utilizing specific cDNA probes previously isolated. In the patients' cells no mRNA for HLA-DR α or β chain could be found, whereas mRNA for the Ii chain was present in amounts comparable to those in the controls. The hybridization results indicate that the absence of HLA-DR expression in the disease results from a block of class II gene expression and that this block occurs independently of a normal expression of the Ii chain gene and its product. This, therefore, strongly suggests a regulatory defect affecting the transcription of DR genes on both chromosomes.

References

1. Acolla RS (1983) Human B cell variants immunoselected against a single Ia antigen subset have lost expression of several Ia antigen subsets. J Exp Med 157:1053–1058
2. Barnstable CJ, Bodmer WF, Brown G, Galfre G, Milstein C, Williams AF, Ziegler A (1978) Production of monoclonal antibodies to group A erythrocytes, HLA and other human cell surface antigens: new tools for genetic analysis. Cell 14:9–20
3. Benaceraff B (1981) In: Dorf ME (ed) The role of the major histocompatibility complex in immunobiology. Garland, New York, p 255
4. Charron DJ, McDevitt HO (1979) Analysis of HLA-D region associated molecules with monoclonal antibody. Proc Natl Acad Sci USA, 76:6567–6571
5. Charron DJ, McDevitt HO (1980) Characterization of HLA-D region antigens by two-dimensional gel electrophoresis. J Exp Med 152:185–365
6. Chirgwin JM, Przybyla AE, MacDonald RJ, Rutter WJ (1979) Isolation of biologically active ribonucleic acid from sources enriched in ribonuclease. Biochemistry 18: 5294–5299
7. Durandy A, Virelizier JL, Griscelli C (1983) Enhancement by interferon of membrane HLA antigens in patients with combined immunodeficiency with defective HLA expression. Clin Exp Immunol 52:173–178
8. Gladstone P, Pious D (1978) Stable variants affecting B cell alloantigens in human lymphoid cells. Nature 271: 459–461
9. Griscelli C, Durandy A, Virelizier JL, Hors J, Lepage V, Colombani J (1980) In: Seligmann M, Hitzig WH (eds) Primary immunodeficiences. Elsevier/North Holland, pp 499–504
10. Goyert SM, Silver J (1981) Isolation of I-A subregion-like molecules from subhuman primates and man. Nature 294:266–268
11. Laemmli UK (1970) Cleavage of structural proteins during the assembly of the head of bacteriophage 4. Nature 227:680–685
12. Lisowska-Grospierre B, Durandy A, Virelizier JL, Fischer A, Griscelli C (1983) Combined immunodeficiency with defective expression of HLA: modulation of an abnormal HLA synthesis and functional studies. In: Wedgwood RJ, Rosen FS, Paul NW (eds) Primary immunodeficiency diseases. Riss, New York, Birth defect original article series no. 19 [3] pp 87–91
13. Long ED, Wake CT, Strubin M, Gross N, Accolla RS, Carrel S, Mach B (1982) Isolation of distinct cDNA clones encoding HLA-DR β chains by use of an expression assay. Proc Natl Acad Sci USA 79:7465–7469
14. Long EO, Strubin M, Wake CT, Gross N, Carrel S, Goodfellow P, Accolla RS, Mach B (1983) Isolation of cDNA clones for the p33 invariant chain associated with

HLA-DR antigens. Proc Natl Acad Sci USA 80:5714–5718
15. Malissen M, Damotte M, Birnbaum D, Trucy J, Jordan BR (1982) HLA cosmid clones show complete, widely spaced human class I genes with occasional clusters. Gene 20:485–489
16. Matis LA, Jones PP, Murphy DB, Hedrick SM, Lerner EA, Janeway CA, McNicholson JM, Schwartz RM (1982) Immune response gene function correlates with the expression of an Ia antigen. J Exp Med 155:500–523
17. McDevitt HO (1976) In: Katz DH, Benaceraff B (eds) The role of the products of the histocompatibility gene complex in immune response. Academic, New York, pp 257–275
18. McMaster GK, Carmichael GG (1977) Analysis of single and double-stranded nucleic acid on polyacrylamide and agarose gels by using glyoxal and acridine orange. Proc Natl Acad Sci USA 74:4835–4838
19. O'Farrell PH (1982) High resolution two dimensional electrophoresis of proteins. J Biol Chem 250:4007–4021
20. De Preval C, Mach B (1983) The absence of β_2 microglobulin in Daudi cells: active gene but inactive messenger RNA. Immunogenetics 17:133–140
21. Schuurman RKB, Van Rood JJ, Vossen JM, Schellekens PA, Felkampvroom TM, Doyer E, Gmelig-Meyling F, Visser HKA (1979) Failure of lymphocyte membrane expression in two siblings with combined immunodeficiency. Clin Immunol Immunopathol 14:418–421
22. Touraine JL, Betuel H, Souillet G, Jeune MJ (1978) Combined immunodeficiency disease associated with absence of cell surface HLA A and B antigens. J Pediatr 93:47–50
23. Wake CT, Long EO, Strubin M, Gross N, Accolla RS, Mach B (1982) Isolation of cDNA clones encoding HLA-DR α chains. Proc Natl Acad Sci USA 79:6979–6983

Inheritance and Possible Coinheritance of HLA-Linked Susceptibilities to Insulin-Dependent Diabetes Mellitus, Autoimmune Thyroid Diseases, and Rheumatoid Arthritis*

C. Torfs, B. Huey, H. Payami, J. Malmgren, G. Thomson, and M.-C. King

Epidemiology Program, School of Public Health, University of California, 140 Warren Hall, CA 94720, USA

To understand the clustering of autoimmune diseases in individuals and families, we examined the possible coinheritance of haplotypes predisposing to one or more of these diseases in 70 families with at least two sibs affected with one or more HLA-DR3 and/or HLA-DR4 associated diseases, namely insulin-dependent diabetes mellitus (IDDM), the autoimmune thyroid diseases (ATD) [Graves' disease (GD), Hashimoto's thyroiditis (HT)], and rheumatoid arthritis (RA). Affected sibs were typed for HLA-A, -B, -C, Bf, and GLO (antisera provided by Dr. C. Grumet, Stanford). We applied the classical sib pair method to the distributions of haplotypes identical by descent (IBD) in concordant sib pair data pooled from our study and from the literature. The estimated modes of inheritance are close to dominant for ATD and RA and close to recessive for IDDM. A strict single allele recessive model, however, can be ruled out for IDDM by other methods. Next we investigated the distribution of haplotypes IBD in sib pairs with two of these diseases. Results for pairs with various combinations of IDDM and ATD (IDDM + ATD-ATD; IDDM + ATD-IDDM; IDDM-ATD; IDDM + ATD-IDDM + ATD) and for pedigree analysis suggest that susceptibilities to IDDM and ATD cosegregate in families in which the IDDM proband also has ATD. The haplotypes which are presumably carrying both these susceptibilities are usually expressed as ATD in sibs and parents in whom they segregate. Comparison of cumulative risks of ATD to first-degree relatives of probands with ATD versus IDDM + ATD shows an increased risk to relatives of IDDM + ATD probands, suggesting an increased risk load of susceptibility to ATD in these probands. For pairs discordant for RA and ATD (RA-ATD; RA + ATD-ATD; RA + ATD-RA), results from sib pair distributions and from pedigree analysis suggest that the same haplotype does not predispose to both diseases. Next, we selected 17 families whose probands had either IDDM + ATD or IDDM only but had a sib with ATD, and typed or retyped them, including parents, for HLA-A, -B, -C, and DR (antisera provided by the Histocompatibility Workshop). Results show that haplotypes shared by IDDM + ATD probands and their ATD relatives carry mostly DR3 ($n = 7$) or DR4 (8) antigens, also DRw6 and DR blank (1 each) with HT; haplotypes not shared with ATD relatives carry DR1 (2), DR2 (1), DR3 (2), DR4 (4), DR5 (2), DRw6 (2), DR7 (3).

* All typing done in Dr. M.-C. King's lab, U. of California Berkeley, CA, with funds from NIH grant CA 27632. Research by H. Payami and G. Thomson supported by NIH grant HD 12731

Histocompatibility Testing 1984
Edited by E. D. Albert et al.

Genetic Polymorphism of the Fourth Component of Complement (C4)- and Type I Insulin-Dependent Diabetes

A. Marcelli-Barge[1], J.C. Poirier[1], M. Schmid[1], I. Deschamps[2], P. Prevost[1], and J. Hors[1]

1 INSERM U.93, Hôpital Saint Louis, 2, Place du Docteur Fournier, 75010 Paris, France
2 U.83 Hôpital Hérold, Paris, France

The C4 complement factors are controlled by genes located within the HLA region. We tested the structural C4 polymorphism by high-voltage electrophoresis and immunofixation of neuraminidase-treated samples, using the method of Awdeh and Alper [1], from IDDM patients, their first-degree relatives, genotyped for HLA-A, B, C, DR, Bf, and 97 healthy individuals. When gene frequencies in IDDM patients and controls are compared, it appears that the C4 silent allele (C4 BQ0) is significantly more frequent in the IDDM patients (32% versus 12%; $P < 10^{-5}$). It can also be noted that the frequency of C4 AQ0 is almost the same in patients as in controls (11% versus 10%, respectively). The genotype combinations of the silent allele BQ0 are shown in Table 1. The frequencies of the seven possible genotypes are compared in the IDDM patients and in controls. A significant excess of C4 BQ0 is observed in the patient group at a single gene dose only.

Table 1. C4 BQ0 Silent allele distribution and frequencies among diabetic patients (IDDM) and healthy controls

C4 silent allele pattern locus	IDDM patients (n = 45)		Normal controls (n = 97)		P value
	N	%	N	%	
A B					
[ ][0] / [ ][ ]	17	38	17	17	0.01
[ ][0] / [ ][0]	4	9	2	2	N.S.
[ ][ ] / [ ][ ]	16	36	59	61	0.005

C4 AQ0 allele distribution is normal among IDDM and controls. C4 BQ0 heterozygotes are more frequent in IDDM ($P<0.001$). C4 BQ0 homozygotes have normal frequency (N.S., not significant). Expressed alleles at C4 locus A and B are less frequent in IDDM ($P < 0.005$)

An increased incidence of C4 BQ0 is observed when the haplotypes bear either DR3 or DR4 (58% and 21% in IDDM patients and normal individuals, respectively; $P < 0.003$). Conversely, no significant increase of C4 BQ 0 was noted in relation to haplotypes bearing neither DR3 nor DR4. A significant increase in frequency for B18, BfF1, C4 A3 BQ0, DR3 was observed in IDDM (20% versus 5% in controls). The increased frequency of two other haplotypes, B12, BfS, C4 A3 B1, DR4 and B12, BfS, C4 A3 BQ0, DR4 was not significant. Our data suggest an effect induced by a single gene dose, since no excess of homozygous BQ0 was observed in our study. In addition, these findings are of particular interest since a decrease in the C4 level and/or hemolytic activity has been correlated with an impaired antiviral response.

Reference

1. Awdeh ZL, Alper CA (1980) Inherited structural polymorphism of the fourth component of human complement. Proc Natl Acad Sci USA 77:3576–3580

Histocompatibility Testing 1984
Edited by E. D. Albert et al.

Presence of Thyroid-Stimulating Immunoglobulins (TSI) in DR3 Positive Normal Individuals

J. Charreire[1], G. Karsenty[1], V. Lepage[2], and L. Degos[2]

1 INSERM U25, Hôpital Necker Enfants Malades, Paris, France
2 INSERM U90, Hôpital Saint-Louis, 75475 Paris, France

With the method of thyroid epithelial cell culture (TEC) that we developed in mice [1], monolayers of human TEC (HTEC) were used to detect thyroid-stimulating immunoglobulins (TSI) in a functional assay of cyclic AMP (cAMP) production. Under these experimental conditions, we previously demonstrated the presence of TSI in 92% of untreated Graves disease (GD) patients and their disappearance 6 months after neomercazole treatment in 55% of the GD patients [2]. In this study, TSI positivity was evaluated as the percentage of response when DEAE-trisacryl-purified IgGs from normal subjects were deposited onto HTEC for cAMP production. Among the 32 samples provided by the blood bank and used as controls, we found four TSI-positive subjects with euthyroid status. Since it has been clearly established that among Caucasians GD is associated with HLA-B8 and HLA-DR3 antigens [3], we investigated whether the presence of TSI in normal subjects could be related to these HLA antigens. For that purpose, IgGs were purified from the sera of 22 normal subjects with known HLA-A, B, C, DR, and DQ type (10B8 − DR3 −; 8B8 + DR3 +, 4B8 − DR3 +), and cAMP production was measured on three different HTECs. It was found that the mean cAMP levels (amount above the basal level) were:

4.0 ± 2.0 for B8− DR3−	positivity 0/10
17.0 ± 8.0 for B8+ DR3+	positivity 3/8
21.0 ± 8.0 for DR3+ B8−	positivity 2/4

It must be noted that the basal level of cAMP production by HTEC and medium without IgGs was 58.0 ± 3.0. Because of the small number of subjects in each group, no statistical differences were noted. In contrast, if we divided normal subjects into two groups as a function of their DR antigen expression, DR3− and DR3+ (10 and 12 subjects, respectively) cAMP production was 62.2 ± 2.0 for DR3− and 77.0 ± 6.9 for DR3+. This difference is highly significant ($0.02 < P < 0.01$).

These results clearly indicate that the expression of DR3, an HLA antigen significantly associated with GD, greatly favors the appearance of TSI in the sera of normal subjects. It also raises the issue that factors other than the presence of anti-receptor antibodies may be necessary for thyroid reactivity to be observed.

References

1. Salamero J, Michel-Béchet M, Charreire J (1983) Expression of H-2 antigens and thyroglobulin (Tg) on freshly dissociation and in vitro cultured monolayers of mouse thyroid epithelial cells (TEC). Tissue Antigens 22:231 − 238
2. Charreire J, Karsenty G, Bouchard P, Schaison B (1984) Effect of Neomercazole (NMZ) treatment in patients with Graves diseases (GD). Clin Exp Immunol 57:633
3. Briones-Urbina R, Bear JC, Farid NR (1982) Association of hypergammaglobulinemia G with HLA-DR3 in Graves' disease. Tissue Antigens 19:20 − 24

Histocompatibility Testing 1984
Edited by E. D. Albert et al.

Three Different HLA Associations in the Three Types of 21-Hydroxylase Congenital Adrenal Hyperplasia

S. Scholz[1], W. Höller[2], D. Knorr[2], F. Bidlingmaier[2], H. Zander[1], and E.D. Albert[1]

1 Labor für Immungenetik, Kinderpoliklinik der Universität München, Pettenkoferstraße 8 a, 8000 München 2, Federal Republic of Germany
2 Abteilung für pädiatrische Endokrinologie, Haunersche Kinderklinik der Universität München, 8000 München, Federal Republic of Germany

Introduction

Congenital adrenal hyperplasia (CAH) is a disorder of cortisol and aldosterone biosynthesis that mostly results from a 21-hydroxylase enzyme deficiency [1]. There is an incidence of about 1 : 7000 to 1 : 10 000 in central Europe [2–4]. It is characterized by increased plasma levels of 17-hydroxyprogesterone and elevated adrenal androgens, causing virilization.
The patients can be subdivided in three clinically accepted types: the salt-wasting (SW) form, the simple virilizing (SV) form (the two classical forms), and the recently described nonclassical (NC) late-onset or cryptic variant of the disease [5–7]. The three different syndromes are inherited in the same autosomal-recessive way [8]. The genetic base of the classical CAH was placed in the HLA region on chromosome 6 by Dupont in 1977 [9] and confirmed by associations with the HLA antigens B5 [10] and Bw47 [11].

Results

A total of 372 German CAH carriers were genotyped for HLA-A, B, C and in some cases for HLA-DR antigens. This group contained 240 healthy parents heterozygous for the CAH disease gene and 132 homozygous CAH patients. The patients were subdivided into 59 with SW, 60 with SV, and 15 with NC disease. The 264 affected haplotypes were designated as "pathological" and compared with the noninherited 240 unaffected "healthy" haplotypes of the parents. (Table 1). The 240 healthy haplotypes displayed HLA antigen distributions nearly identical to those of a normal control group. The pathological haplotypes, when compared all together with the healthy haplotypes, show the well known positive associations with HLA-B5, Bw47, and B14 and a slight negative association with B8. If we compare only the 59 SW patients and their 118 haplotypes with the healthy groups, we see only one association with Bw47. In contrast,

Table 1. Gene frequency distributions in controls, parents, and patients

HLA-B alleles	Control population $n = 400$	Unaffected haplotypes $n = 240$	SW+SV +NC $n = 264$	SW $n = 118$	SV $n = 120$	NC $n = 30$
5 (51/w52)	0.089	0.06	0.17	0.09	0.28*	0.03
7	0.134	0.14	0.11	0.18	0.07	0.03
8	0.075	0.10	0.04	0.03	0.04	0.07
12 (44/45)	0.125	0.12	0.09	0.06	0.11	0.10
13	0.041	0.03	0.02	0.02	0.03	0.0
14	0.013	0.0	0.08	0.03	0.01	0.47*
15 (w62/w63)	0.065	0.08	0.08	0.09	0.08	0.02
16 (38/39)	0.041	0.03	0.06	0.04	0.08	0.0
17 (w57/w58)	0.025	0.05	0.01	0.01	0.01	0.03
18	0.051	0.03	0.01	0.01	0.02	0.0
21 (49/w50)	0.038	0.03	0.01	0.01	0.01	0.0
w22 (w55/w56)	0.008	0.01	0.03	0.03	0.02	0.07
27	0.059	0.05	0.05	0.04	0.07	0.03
35	0.049	0.09	0.06	0.09	0.04	0.05
37	0.02	0.02	0.02	0.02	0.02	0.0
40 (w60/w61)	0.095	0.07	0.05	0.05	0.05	0.03
w41	0.005	0.02	0.02	0.01	0.03	0.0
w47	0.003	0.0	0.11	0.20*	0.05	0.07
Blank	0.063	0.05	0.01	0.00	0.02	0.00

* = $p \leqq 0.00001$

Histocompatibility Testing 1984
Edited by E. D. Albert et al.

Table 2. Unaffected and affected haplotype frequencies

HLA haplotype	Control $n = 240$ %	SW+SV+NC $n = 254$ %	SW $n = 118$ %	SV $n = 110$ %	NC $n = 30$ %
Aw33, B14, DR1	0.0	4.3	0.8	0.9	30.0
A2, B5	1.7	6.7	3.4	10.9*	3.3
A3, B5	1.3	6.3	2.5	11.8*	0.0
A3, Cw6, Bw47, DR7	0.0	8.7	15.3**	2.7	3.3
A1, B8	7.9	1.6	1.7	1.8	0.0

* $= p \leqq 0.010$; ** $= p \leqq 0.00001$

comparing the 60 SV patients and their 120 haplotypes with the healthy haplotypes we find only an association to B5. Finally, the NC group shows a nearly 100% association to B14. All these associations are statistically significant ($P \leq 0.00001$). Remarkable in this study is the fact that we could not find one single HLA-Bw47 or B14 antigen in the healthy haplotypes of the parents. If we further compare the antigens of the subsets with one another, we notice an additional positive association for B7 with the SW group and a negative association with the SV group. Looking at the haplotypes we find an excess of Aw33, B14, DR1 in the NC group, and no single Aw33, B14, DR1 haplotype in the unaffected family members. Furthermore, as shown in Table 2, there is a very high percentage of the haplotype A3, Cw6, Bw47, DR7 in the SW patients and the A2, B5 and A3, B5 haplotypes are increased significantly only in the SV group.

Discussion

The results of this study confirms the autosomal-recessive inheritance and the close genetic linkage of the 21-hydroxylase deficiency to the HLA system. It shows three distinct associations of certain HLA antigens to the three clinically accepted subtypes of the disease. These different associations to the disease variants indicate three genetically determined enzyme defect genes. In the single associated antigens we find an additional linkage to special so-called "superhaplotypes", which occur in the control population only very rarely. This, together with the fact that we do not see any Bw47 and B14 in the unaffected haplotypes of the parents, leads us to ask the following question: Are the defect genes old mutants in haplotypes which are for this reason now very rare, or are they relatively young mutants in particular haplotypes which have not been able to loose the gene by recombination in such a short time?

References

1. Bongiovanni AM, Eberlein W, Goldmann A, New M (1967) Disorders of adrenal steroid biogenesis. Recent Prog Horm Res 23:375
2. Prader A (1958) Die Häufigkeit des kongenitalen adrenogenitalen Syndroms. Helv Paedriatr Acta 13:426
3. Mauthe I, Laspe H, Knorr D (1977) Zur Häufigkeit des kongenitalen adrenogenitalen Syndroms (AGS): München 63–77. Klin Paedr 189:1727
4. Wallace AM, Beastall GH, Ross AM, Girdwood RWA, Kennedy R, Ferguson-Smith MA (1984) Management of congenital adrenal hyperplasia. Lancet I:1121
5. Newmark S, Dluhly R, Williams G, Pochi P, Rosel (1977) Partial 11- and 21-hydroxylase deficiency in hirsute women. Am J Obstet Gynecol 126:597
6. Zachmann M, Prader A (1978) Unusual heterozygotes of congenital adrenal hyperplasia due to 21-hydroxylase deficiency. Acta Endocrinol 87:557
7. Levine LS, Dupont B, Lorenzen F, Pang S, Pollack MS, Oberfield SE, Kohn D, Lerner A, Cacciari E, Mantero F, Scaroni C, Chimello G, Rondanini GE, Gargantini L, Giovanelli G, Virdis R, Bartolotta L, Migliori C, Pintor C, Tato L, Barboni F, New MI (1980) Cryptic 21-hydroxylase deficiency in families of patients with classical congenital adrenal hyperplasia. J Clin Endocrinol Metab 51:1193
8. Laron Z, Pollack MS, Zamir R, Roitman A, Dickerman Z, Levine LS, Lorenzen F, O'Neill GJ, Pang S, New MI, Dupont B (1980) Late-onset 21-hydroxylase deficiency and HLA in the Ashkenazi population: a new allele at the 21-hydroxylase locus. Hum Immunol 1:55
9. Dupont B, Oberfield SE, Smithwick EM, Lee TD, Levine LS (1977) Close genetic linkage between HLA and congenital adrenal hyperplasia (21-hydroxylase deficiency). Lancet II:1309
10. Grosse-Wilde H, Weil J, Albert ED, Scholz S, Bidlingmaier F, Sippel WG, Knorr D (1979) Genetic linkage studies between congenital adrenal hyperplasia and the HLA blood group system. Immunogenetics 8:41
11. Klouda PT, Harris R, Price DA (1978) HLA and congenital adrenal hyperplasia. Lancet II:1046

Distinct HLA-B Antigen Associations for the Salt-Wasting and Simple Virilizing Forms of Congenital Adrenal Hyperplasia Due to 21-Hydroxylase Deficiency*

B. Dupont[1], R. Virdis[2], A.J. Lerner[2], C. Nelson[2], M.S. Pollack[1], and M.I. New[2]

1 Human Immunogenetics Section, Memorial Sloan-Kettering Institute for Cancer Research, 1275 York Ave., New York, NY 10021 USA
2 Department of Pediatrics, Cornell University, Medical College New York, NY 10021 USA

The salt-wasting (SW) and simple virilizing (SV) forms of congenital adrenal hyperplasia (CAH) due to 21-hydroxylase deficiency (21-OH DEF) are both autosomal recessive defects of gene(s) closely linked to the HLA-B locus [1]. HLA-antigen associations with CAH have been described, in which an increase in Bw47, Bw60(40) and B51(5) and a decrease in B8 have been confirmed in several studies [2].

In this paper, we describe that the two classical forms of 21-hydroxylase deficiency display marked genetic linkage disequilibrium with distinct HLA-B determinants. HLA-B51(5) and HLA-B14 are selectively increased among patients with SV disease. In contrast, HLA-Bw60(40) and B27 (in Italy) are increased among patients with SW disease. The unique CAH 21-OH-DEF HLA-B antigen Bw47 is increased in both groups of patients, while HLA-B8 is significantly decreased in both groups.

The complete HLA genotypes were determined in 150 families of Caucasian patients with CAH: 83 North American families, 40 Italian, 11 Yugoslavian, and 16 Swiss. A total of 76 patients with SV disease and 74 with SW disease were studied. The HLA antigens of the patients were compared with the HLA antigens on the non-affected parental HLA haplotypes.

As demonstrated in Table 1, the HLA-B gene frequencies for HLA-B51(5) and B14 are significantly increased among patients with SV. In contrast, HLA-Bw60(40) is increased among the patients with SW.

As shown in Table 2, the B27 antigen is selectively increased among Italian patients with SW. In contrast, the unique CAH HLA-B antigen Bw47 is found in both SW and SV patients.

Table 1. Gene frequencies for HLA-B antigens with significant deviations among the patients

HLA-B antigen	Gene frequencies			
	Total CAH	SV	SW	Control
B51(5)	0.122	<u>0.183</u>	0.062	0.072
B14	0.038	<u>0.070</u>	0.007	0.028
Bw60 (40)	0.090	0.028	<u>0.151</u>	0.052
Bw47	0.045	<u>0.028</u>	<u>0.062</u>	0.004
B8	0.024	<u>0.014</u>	<u>0.034</u>	0.064

The statistically significant deviations are underlined

Table 2. Chi square test and *P* values for comparison between SV and SW

HLA antigen	SV+	SW+	SV−	SW−	χ^2	*P*
B51(5)	<u>26</u>	9	116	137	8.84	<0.005
B14	<u>10</u>	1	132	145	6.28	<0.025
B27(Italy)	0	<u>5</u>	52	25	6.55	<0.025
Bw60(40)	4	<u>22</u>	138	124	11.71	<0.001
Bw47	4	9	138	137	1.18	NS
B8	2	5	140	141	0.53	NS

The significant deviations are underlined

Conclusions

The data strongly suggest that the SV and SW forms of CAH are due to different mutational defects in the HLA-linked 21-hydroxylase locus. Recent data (P. White, M. I. New, B. Dupont, manuscript in preparation) have demonstrated that these diseases are due to a structural defect in the HLA-linked gene coding for adrenal 21-hydroxylase cytochrome P450.

References

1. Dupont B, Oberfield SE, Smithwick EM, Lee TD, Levine LS (1977) Close genetic linkage between HLA and congenital adrenal hyperplasia (21-hydroxylase deficiency). Lancet 2:1309–1311
2. Dupont B, Pollack MS, Levine LS, O'Neill GJ, Hawkins B, New MI (1980) Congenital adrenal hyperplasia and HLA: joint report from the Eighth International Histocompatibility Workshop. In: Terasaki PI (ed) Histocompatibility Testing 1980. UCLA, Los Angeles, pp 693–706

* Supported by USPHS NIH grants CA 22507, CA 08748, and HD 00072

Histocompatibility Testing 1984
Edited by E. D. Albert et al.

Defect of Ferritin Secretion in HLA-A3 Subjects and in Idiopathic Hemochromatosis

B. Martins da Silva[1], R. Fauchet[2], B. Genetet[2], L. Le Mignon[2], M. Simon[2], and M. de Sousa[1]

1 Abel Salazar Institute for the Biomedical Sciences, Largo da Escola Médica, 4000 Oporto, Portugal
2 Laboratoire Régional de Transfusion Sanguine, Rue Pierre Jean Gineste, F-35000 Rennes, France

We previously described an impairment of ferritin secretion in peripheral blood mononuclear cells from normal HLA-A3 subjects following stimulation in vitro with phytohemagglutinin (PHA) and concanavalin A (Con A) with or without addition of ferric citrate [1–3]. We now re-examine the association of ferritin secretion with HLA-A phenotype in a population of controls and idiopathic hemochromatosis (IH) patients in Brittany, the region where family studies first documented a linkage disequilibrium of the HLA-A3 antigen in IH [4].

Summary and Results

IH patients were identified according to clinical criteria defined by Simon et al. [5]. Peripheral blood samples from HLA-typed unrelated normal donors (24 males and 20 females), conjugal donors (3 husbands and 13 wives of IH patients), and IH patients (18 males and 7 females) were studied for ferritin release by a reverse hemolytic plaque assay described earlier [1–3]. The impairment of ferritin secretion following PHA activation in the presence of iron in the control HLA-A3 population was confirmed and extended to stimulation by ConA. Low levels of plaque-forming cells were found in the IH patients regardless of phenotype (Table 1).

References

1. Martins da Silva B, Pollack MS, Dupont B, de Sousa M (1982) A study of ferritin secretion by human peripheral blood mononuclear cells from HLA typed donors. In: Saltman P, Hegenauer J (eds) The biochemistry and physiology of iron. Elsevier/North Holland, Amsterdam, pp 733–737
2. De Sousa M, Martins da Silva B, Dörner MH, Munn G, Nishiya K, Grady R, Silverstone AE (1982) Iron as a target of immune surveillance. In: Saltman P, Hegenauer J (eds) The biochemistry and physiology of iron. Elsevier/North Holland, Amsterdam
3. Pollack MS, Martins da Silva B, Moshief DR, Groshen S, Bognacki J, Dupont B, de Sousa M (1983) Ferritin secretion by human mononuclear cells: Association with HLA phenotype. Clin Immunol Immunopathol 27:124–134
4. Simon M, Bourel M, Fauchet R, Genetet B (1976) Association of HLA-A3 and HLA-B14 antigens with idiopathic haemochromatosis. Gut 17:332–334
5. Simon M, Haspel P, Brissot P, Fauchet R, Edan G, Le Reun M, Le Mignon L, Genetet B, Bourel M (1981) Les hémochromatoses. Ann Med Interne (Paris) 132:413–433

Table 1. Statistical analysis of differences in number of PFC between A3+ and A3– subjects

	PHA			PHA + Fe			Con A			Con A + Fe		
	n A3+	A3–	*P*	*n* A3+	A3–	*P*	*n* A3+	A3–	*P*	*n* A3+	A3–	*P*
Unrelated donors	25	18	NS	23	20	0.002	17	15	0.04	18	14	0.04
IH	17	7	NS	18	7	NS	18	7	0.13	18	7	NS

[a] *P* value calculated by median test; and *n* represents number of individuals in each group

Immunogenetic Analysis of Leprosy in Japan

I. Kikuchi [1]*, T. Ozawa [2], and T. Sasazuki [1]*

1 Department of Human Genetics, Medical Research Institute, Tokyo Medical and Dental University, Tokyo 113, Japan
2 National Institute for Leprosy Research, Tokyo 189, Japan

Genetic control of the clinical manifestation of leprosy was investigated using 66 unrelated patients with leprosy and 192 members of 28 multiplex families. In the 66 unrelated patients with leprosy, HLA-DR2 and DQw1 were significantly increased (R.R. = 3.76, $\chi^2 = 16.60$, R.R. = 4.09, $\chi^2 = 11.10$, respectively) compared to healthy controls. In 34 tuberculoid patients, HLA-DR2 and -DQw1 were significantly increased (R.R. = 3.95, $\chi^2 = 11.10$, R.R. = 18.62, $\chi^2 = 12.64$, respectively). In 32 lepromatous patients, HLA-DR2 was significantly increased (R.R. = 3.57, $\chi^2 = 8.97$). Multiplex families with leprosy were analyzed by the affected sib pairs method [1]. Of 19 sib pairs affected with lepromatous leprosy, 8 shared two HLA haplotypes and 11 shared one HLA haplotype. This haplotype distribution differed from the random distribution ($\chi^2 = 7.20$, D.F. = 2, $P < 0.03$), suggesting the existence of the HLA-linked major gene for lepromatous leprosy. This method, however, could not distinguish between the recessive model with gene frequency of 0.48 and the dominant model with gene frequency of 0.19 for the HLA-linked disease susceptibility gene for lepromatous leprosy.

* Present address: Dept of Genetics, Medical Institute of Bioregulation, Kyushu University, 3-1-1 Maidashi, Higashi-Ku, Fukuoka 812, Japan

Tuberculoid patients showed vigorous immune response to *Mycobacterium leprae* antigen in vitro, whereas lepromatous patients did not show any response to this antigen. The non-responsiveness of lepromatous patients was antigen specific. The antigen-specific nonresponsiveness to *M. leprae* antigen was controlled by T cells but not by monocytes; T cells from tuberculoid patients showed a strong response to *M. leprae* antigen in the presence of monocytes from HLA-DR-identical or haplo-identical lepromatous patients, whereas T cells from lepromatous patients failed to respond to this antigen even in the presence of monocytes from HLA-DR-identical or haploidentical tuberculoid patients. Furthermore, it was demonstrated that antigen-specific suppressor T cell (Leu $2^{+}3^{-}$) was present in relapsed lepromatous patients. All these observations suggested that an HLA-linked gene controlled the clinical manifestation of leprosy through immune regulation by T cells.

Reference

1. Thomson G, Bodmer WF (1977) The genetics of HLA and disease associations. In: Christiansen TB, Fenchel TM (eds) Measuring selection in natural populations. Springer, Berlin Heidelberg New York, p 545

Affected Sib Methods*

E.J. Louis, G. Thomson, and H. Payami

Genetics Department, University of California, Berkeley, CA 94720, USA

The affected sib pair method is used extensively to distinguish between simple modes of inheritance of HLA associated diseases. Certain diseases, such as insulin dependent diabetes mellitus (IDDM), appear more complex than simple recessive or dominant traits. This finding has led to the development of several tests and extensions of the affected sib pair method to more complex models.

Numerical procedures for estimating mode of inheritance parameters, including the "disease" allele frequency and the relative penetrances of susceptible genotypes, have been derived, based on the expected haplotype sharing distributions of affected sib trios and pairs from sib trios as well as from affected sib pairs.

* Research supported by NIH grant HD 12731 and an NSF graduate fellowship to EJL

Histocompatibility Testing 1984
Edited by E. D. Albert et al.

Statistical tests of mode of inheritance hypotheses based on the affected sib sampling distribution have been derived (pairs from families with three or more affected sibs must be weighted appropriately according to the ascertainment method). These tests alleviate the normality assumption problems that invalidate many tests, including the likelihood ratio criteria.

Selection, recombination, admixture, nonrandom mating, and an environmental sib correlation can have a major effect on parameter estimates.

The DR3- and DR4-associated heterogeneity of IDDM, and the possible linkage of IDDM to Gm and Km types as well as to the insulin gene, have been impetus for the development of more complex sib pair and sib trio methods than single-locus, two-allele models. These methods include three-allele models in which two alleles exhibit negative complementation, and two-locus models, with epistatic interactions.

Haplotype sharing of affected sib pairs for a negative complementation model is bound by single-locus, two-allele expectations, while affected sib trio haplotype sharing is not. Affected sib pairs move towards recessive expectations, while affected sib trios move to a specific region outside of the single- locus, two-allele expectations.

Haplotype sharing from both affected sib pairs and sib trios for two-locus models is bound by single-locus expectations, unlike the negative complementation models.

Affected sib data for IDDM (pooled from the literature) follows the pattern of negative complementation. The sib pair data point falls near recessive expectations ($x_2^2 = 0.0002$ n.s.) while the sib trio point falls outside (but not significantly) the two-allele expectations and into the negative complementation region. This does not exclude the involvement of other loci, but it is supporting evidence of the hypothesis that negative complementation is a major component of the genetic predisposition to IDDM. The combined effects of multiple loci and negative complementation are currently being studied.

Genetic Interrelationship Amongst HLA-Associated Diseases*

H. Payami and G. Thomson

Genetics Department, University of California, Berkeley, CA 94720, USA

A number of diseases are associated with the same HLA antigen, and some of these diseases also exhibit clinical clustering. We have developed sib pair methods to aid in the understanding of the basis of the disease clustering. The expected HLA haplotype-sharing distributions of sib pairs with more than one disease have been calculated under two models as follows: model I, common allele predisposing to two diseases A and B; model II, different alleles at the same locus predisposing to diseases A and B. The expected haplotype-sharing distributions were derived for the three possible affectional status combinations of sib pairs: (1) AB-A (one sib is affected with two diseases, the other with only one); (2) AB-AB (both sibs affected with two diseases); and (3) A-B (each sib is affected with only one disease).

In many cases the expected distributions under the two hypotheses are quite distinct and allow discrimination between the alternate genetic models. The most informative haplotype-sharing distributions are for sib pairs with disease combinations AB-A and A-B rather than AB-AB. Some examples of cases where the two models can be easily distinguished by AB-A or A-B distributions are: (1) both diseases recessive; (2) one disease recessive and the other additive (A-B distribution requires a low penetrance for the recessive disease, or a low frequency for the common susceptibility allele); and (3) both diseases dominant (AB-A distribution requires a high penetrance for the unshared disease, and A-B distribution requires a low "disease" allele frequency).

Available data on insulin-dependent diabetes mellitus (IDDM) and autoimmune thyroid disease (ATD), and those on ATD and rheumatoid arthritis (RA), have been analyzed.

The associations of IDDM and ATD with DR3 suggest a common susceptibility allele for the two diseases. The observed haplotype sharing values for AB-A and AB-AB sib pairs do not allow discrimination between model I and model II. The ob-

*Research supported by NIH Grant HD 12731

served values for A-B sib pairs, however, are probably incompatible with both models, but due to the small sample size neither model can be rejected. The association of IDDM with DR4 and the excess of DR3/4 heterozygotes among patients suggests negative complementation of two susceptibility alleles in predisposing to IDDM. Preliminary results indicate that the observed values are more compatible with a model which assumes one allele predisposes to two diseases, and another predisposes to one, allowing for negative complementation for IDDM.

ATD (DR3 associated) and RA (DR4 associated) may be predisposed to by different alleles. The data favor the different allele hypothesis and are in agreement with the suggested near-dominant with high penetrance model for ATD and near-dominant with low penetrance model for RA. Model I can be ruled out if RA or ATD is recessive, additive, dominant, or close to any of them.

Is the Lod Score Method Reliable in HLA-Associated Diseases?

F. Clerget-Darpoux, C. Bonaïti-Pellie, and N. Feingold

INSERM U.155, Château de Longchamp, Bois de Boulogne, 75016 Paris, France

The lod score method is usually employed assuming (1) monogenic inheritance for the disease, (2) gametic equilibrium between the disease gene and the marker gene, and (3) known parameters at the disease locus. It is used to test the linkage and to estimate the recombination fraction θ between a putative susceptibility gene and a marker. However, the above assumptions may not be fulfilled in HLA-associated diseases and we show here that this may lead to erroneous conclusions.

1. *The disease may be determined by more than one locus.* Indeed, segregation analysis is most often inconclusive in HLA-associated diseases. In such a case the method may be inefficient. We have shown that in a two-locus model, if one of the loci is closely linked to the marker, one may conclude that linkage is loose [1] or even be unable to give evidence for linkage [2].

2. *Association between the disease gene and the marker.* We found that ignoring in the analysis the gametic disequilibrium due to such an association leads to a large underestimation of the lod score and to a slight underestimation of θ [3].

3. *Errors on parameters (gene frequency and penetrance) do not markedly affect the maximum lod score but induce a wrong θ estimate.* Indeed, we show that an underestimation of the gene frequency (q) and an overestimation of the penetrance (f) both lead to an overestimated recombination fraction θ. Most linkage analyses between HLA and specific diseases found in the literature were performed with a low gene frequency and concluded that the recombination fraction was large. For instance, in multiple sclerosis, assuming a dominant mode, $q = 0.005$, and $f = 0.05$, the estimate of θ was 0.12. Reanalyzing the same data with $q = 0.18$ and $f = 0.02$, we found a recombination fraction of zero. Similar results were obtained for insulin-dependent diabetes [4].

Thus the interpretation of familial data in HLA-associated diseases must be very cautious. The estimation of θ is much more sensitive to the use of wrong parameters than to the ignoring of association. In contrast, the power of the linkage test is sensitive to association between the disease and HLA but is almost unchanged by errors on parameters. When the assumption of monogenic inheritance is false, both the power of the test and the θ estimate may be affected.

Considering these results, the lod score method appears to be unreliable in estimating θ in HLA-associated diseases. Moreover, it seems illogical to look for a value for θ, since only a negligible recombination fraction can explain the population associations.

An alternative way of using the lod score function is, using a monogenic inheritance model, to seek the gene frequency and penetrance values consistent with a recombination fraction of zero.

References

1. Clerget-Darpoux F, Bonaïti-Pellie C (1980) Epistasis effect: an alternative to the hypothesis of linkage disequilibrium in HLA-associated diseases. Ann Hum Genet 44:195–204
2. Clerget-Darpoux F, Babron MC, Bonaïti-Pellie C (1984) HLA-associated diseases: a new method for performing linkage analysis with other markers than HLA. Am J Hum Genet 36:1075–1081

Histocompatibility Testing 1984
Edited by E. D. Albert et al.

3. Clerget-Darpoux F (1982) Bias of the estimated recombination fraction and lod score due to an association between a disease gene and a marker gene. Ann Hum Genet 46:363–372
4. Clerget-Darpoux F, Bonaïti-Pellie C, Hochez J (1984) Effects of misspecifying gene frequency and penetrance in lod score analysis (submitted)

HLA-DR, Gm Allotypes and Sex as Risk Factors for Celiac Disease

M. DeMarchi [1], A.O. Carbonara [1], W.R. Mayr [2], E. van Loghem [3], G.G. de Lange [3], N. Ansaldi [4], and E.S. Curtoni [1]

1 Istituto di Genetica Medica, Via Santena 19, 10126 Torino, Italy
2 Institut f. Blutgruppenserologie der Universität Wien, Spitalgasse 4, Wien, Austria
3 Central Blood Laboratory Blood Transfusion, Netherlands Red Cross, Amsterdam, The Netherlands
4 Istituto di Clinica Pediatrica, Universita di Torino, Torino, Italy

The susceptibility to celiac disease (CD) conferred by three independent genetic factors, i.e., HLA-DR, immunoglobulin allotypes, and sex, has been analyzed in a group of 140 Italian children (Table 1).

HLA-DR. Positive associations were found for DR3 and DR7, while DR1 and DR2 were negatively associated. Analysis of DR genotype associations showed higher risks for DR3/3 (15.0) and 3/7 (13.2) and lower risks for DR3/X (2.7), 7/X and 7/7 (1.6), in agreement with our previous study [2], except that RR values were computed versus the expected control genotype frequencies in this study [5]. This resulted in smaller 95% confidence limits, and highlighted the distinction between high- and low-risk genotypes better. As discussed elsewhere (Ninth Workshop Disease Studies), all the patients negative for DR3 and DR7 shared DR4 as a common antigen. This suggests that even this group in fact possesses an HLA gene predisposing to CD. Its RR value < 1 obtained by the usual Woolf's method does not indicate a negative association, but simply that its weight is lower than that of DR3 and DR7; indeed, comparison of DR4-positive genotypes with the X/X category (X = all alleles except DR3, 7, *and* 4) showed an RR as high as 46.

Sex. A sex ratio close to 1 was found in the high-risk genotypes, while there was a significant excess of girls in the low-risk genotypes (M/F = 0.44), indicating that their penetrance is increased in the context of the susceptible female "background", which entirely accounts for the higher prevalence of female patients.

Ig Allotypes. In the overall patient group no significant difference from controls was found for any Gm, A(2)m, and Km phenotypes. In agreement with our previous study [1], most (93%), and in the low-risk DR genotypes all but one (96%), of the male patients possessed the *fnb* haplotype. This sex-restricted association of Gm markers suggests that V_H genes might be involved in the humoral component of CD, as shown for anti-gliadin antibody response in experimental studies in mice [3] as well as in CD patients [4, 6].

References

1. Carbonara AO, DeMarchi M, van Loghem E, Ansaldi N (1983) Gm markers in celiac disease. Hum Immunol 6:91–95
2. DeMarchi M, Carbonara AO, Ansaldi N, Santini B, Barbera C, Borelli I, Rossino P, Rendine S (1983) HLA-DR3 and DR7 in coeliac disease: immunogenetic and clinical aspects. Gut 24:706–712
3. Kagnoff MF (1982) Two genetic loci control the murine immune response to A-gliadin, a wheat protein that activates coeliac sprue. Nature 296:158–160
4. Kagnoff MF, Weiss JB, Brown RJ, Lee T, Schanfield MS (1983) Immunoglobulin allotype markers in gluten-sensitive enteropathy. Lancet I:952–953
5. Lathrop M (1983) Estimating genotype relative risks. Tissue Antigens 22:160–166
6. Weiss JB, Austin RK, Schanfield MS, Kagnoff MF (1983) Gluten sensitive enteropathy: IgG heavy-chain (Gm) allotypes and the immune response to wheat gliadin. J Clin Invest 72:96–98

Table 1. Interaction of HLA-DR, sex, and Gm allotypes in CD

DR genotype	Male patients		Female patients		Sex	fnb
	n	% fnb	n	% fnb	χ^2	χ^2
3/3+3/7	25	88.0%	23	70.0%	ns	ns
3/X+7/X+7/7	27	96.3%	61	68.9%	6.6	8.0
4/4+4/X	2		2			

Histocompatibility Testing 1984
Edited by E. D. Albert et al.

The Relative Importance of MLC and HLA-DR Compatibility in Cadaver Kidney Transplantation

E. Langhoff, B.K. Jakobsen, P. Platz, L.P. Ryder, A. Svejgaard, and The Copenhagen Study Group of Kidney Transplantation

Tissue Typing Laboratory and Dept. of Nephrology, State University Hospital (Rigshospitalet), Tagenvej 20, 2200 Copenhagen O, Denmark

Analysis of the influence of DR compatibility on cadaver kidney graft survival (GS) has not given uniform results. However, there is now quite a number of mostly single-center studies favoring an association between DR compatibility and good GS. There have been fewer studies of the influence of MLC on cadaver kidney GS, and again the results are contradictory. To our knowledge, adequate attempts have not been made to answer the question as to which parameter, MLC or DR compatibility, has the most important influence – if any – on GS. Accordingly, we undertook such a study.

A series of 42 consecutive cadaver kidney donor-recipient pairs from whom frozen cells were available from before the transplantation were HLA-ABC- and DR-typed at least twice without knowledge of the fate of the graft. Leukocytes from each of these pairs were included in one of two large MLC experiments, in which responder cells from each recipient were tested against cells from the specific donor and about half of all the other donors. This allowed determination of the donor-specific MLC stabilized relative response (SSR) for 38 of the pairs, while 4 pairs had to be excluded because the recipient cells failed to respond or the donor cells to stimulate. Otherwise, no exclusions were made. All recipients were given conventional immunosuppressive therapy with azathioprine and prednisone. The observation time was at least 12 months after transplantation. Analysis of the kidneys rejected within this period revealed that the SSRs were significantly higher in patients rejecting than in those keeping their grafts ($P = 0.02$; Mann- Whitney rank sum test). Life-table analyses by the log rank method showed a significantly ($p = 0.006$) better GS (83% at 1 year) when the donor-specific SSR was < 51 than when it was higher (40%). This cut-off level is the one we use in HLA-D typing. There was a significant ($p = 0.004$) correlation between low MLC (SSR < 51) and compatibility for two DR antigens. DR-compatible kidneys fared better (70% at 1 year) than DR-incompatible ones (50%), but this difference was not significant ($P = 0.20$) and did not become significant when stratified for MLC reactivity. In contrast, the effect of SSR remained significant ($P = 0.05$) when stratified for DR match grade, indicating that MLC compatibility is more important than DR compatibility.

The above results were confirmed in a subsequent series of 19 transplants which showed a rate of 89% for 6-month GS when the donor-specific SSR was < 51, versus 40% for the remaining grafts.

In conclusion, low donor-specific MLC reactivity (expressed as SSR < 51) is an extremely reliable predictor of good GS in cadaver kidney transplantation, which seems biologically meaningful. Low MLC reactivity is significantly more frequent when there is DR compatibility, but the effect of MLC on GS is stronger than that of DR compatibility. Nevertheless, DR matching ensures low MLC reactivity (i.e., good GS) in the majority of cases, but the correlation is not absolute, mainly because there are still "blank" DR alleles and because some DR antigens (e.g., DR4) may be split. Consequently, larger numbers of transplants are needed to demonstrate the "secondary" effect of DR matching. It remains to be seen whether MLC compatibility has a similar effect in recipients treated with cyclosporin A.

Histocompatibility Testing 1984
Edited by E. D. Albert et al.

Long-Term Follow-Up of London Transplant Group (LTG) Renal Transplant Patients

H. Festenstein, P. Doyle, and J. Holmes *

Dept. of Immunology and Hill Centre *, London Hospital Medical College, Turner Street, London E1 2AD, UK

Since 1969, a total of 1284 cadaveric renal transplants have been performed within the LTG. Actuarial graft survival (GS: Peto program) for first grafts is 60% at 1 year, 46% at 5 years, and 36% at 10 years. Retransplants survive significantly less well: 48% at 1 year, 34% at 5 years, and 29% at 10 years ($P = 0.004$). To date 531 transplants have been done since 1978 and their 5-year GS is considerably higher (64% for first transplants, 44% for retransplants). The data show a consistent and highly significant effect of HLA-A and B antigen matching (broad groups) on GS ($P < 0.00001$) (see Fig. 1). Matching for HLA-B antigens alone produces as significant an effect as matching for both HLA-A and B antigens ($P < 0.00001$). HLA-A and B matching using cross-reacting groups (CREGs) does not demonstrate a significant influence on GS over and above that produced by HLA-A and B matching for broad groups inherent in the sample. An interesting finding is that first transplants in the medium-matched category (3B + 2, broad groups) show improved GS when they are also matched for two Bw4/6 antigens ($n = 318$) rather than one ($n = 257$) ($P = 0.025$). More stringent matching for HLA-A and B antigens using subtypic groups (splits) demonstrate a significant influence on GS ($P = 0.034$). For all transplants since 1978, GS is significantly improved by HLA-DR match (1 year GS 80% for zero DR mismatch, 73% for 1 DR mismatch and 64% for 2 DR mismatch, $P = 0.02$). Matching for both HLA-B and DR antigens produced an effect on graft survival that was greater than that for HLA-B or DR matching separately (1 year GS: 84% for zero B plus zero DR mismatch compared to 80% for all zero DR mismatched grafts and 74% for all zero B mismatched grafts).
GS is higher within DRw6-negative recipients than in DRw6-positive recipients, but the differences are not statistically significant. Multivariate analyses (Cox regression) on the whole data set, using the

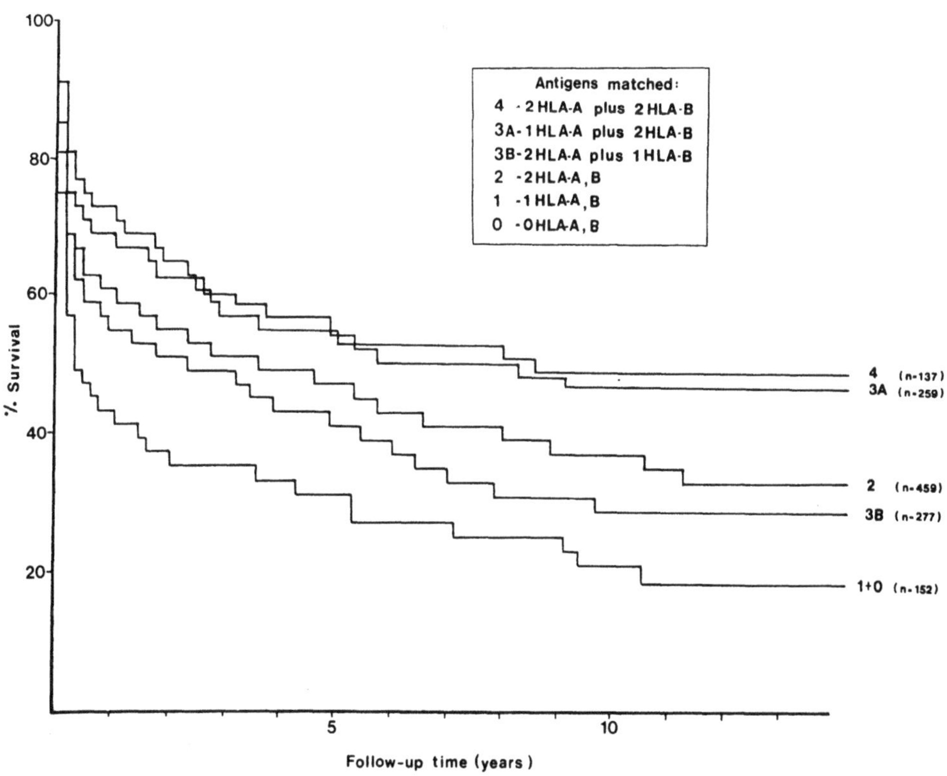

Fig. 1. Actuarial graft survival of all grafts by HLA-A, B match (broad groups); $n = 1284$; $P < 0.00001$

Histocompatibility Testing 1984
Edited by E. D. Albert et al.

parameters HLA-AB match (broad groups), donor sex, recipient sex, previous transplant, transfusions, sex compatibility, and centre, show significant beneficial effects (in order of significance) of HLA-A and B match grade, primary grafting, transfusions, and centre. The beneficial effects of transfusions are most marked in HLA-A, B match grades 3A, 2, 1, and 0. Using transplants from 1978 onwards, which probably represent the most uniform clinical experience, significant effects can only be found for transfusions and HLA-A, and -B and DR match grade. When female recipients are analysed separately, additional significant factors are pregnancy and donor sex: nulliparous females and female recipients of male kidneys show significantly higher GS than parous women and female recipients of female kidneys. Donor sex is not important in male graft survival. GS in men with poor HLA-A, B match (1 + 0) is significantly lower than in women with poor HLA-A, B poor match ($P < 0.001$).

The Influence of HLA-A, B Compatibility on Cadaver Donor Renal Transplantation in SEOPF

F. Sanfilippo[1], W. Vaughn[2], E. Spees[3], E. Heise[4], W. LeFor[5]

1 Duke University and Durham VA Medical Centers, Box 3712, Durham, NC 27710 USA
2 Vanderbilt University, Nashville, TN, USA
3 Johns Hopkins Medical School, Baltimore, MD, USA
4 Bowman Gray School of Medicine, Winston-Salem, NC, USA
5 University of South Florida, Tampa, FL, USA

Data collected prospectively on all 3811 transplants performed between June 1977 and July 1982 by the 42 member institutions of the South-Eastern Organ Procurement Foundation (SEOPF) were analyzed to determine the influence of donor-recipient HLA-A, B matching on patient and graft outcome. Patients receiving well-matched grafts used more shared organs, had a higher level of pretransplant sensitization, included fewer blacks and more retransplants. Multivariate analysis (Cox regression) including these four covariates (sharing, sensitization, race, transplant number) and five others (pretransplant transfusions, ATN, native nephrectomy, splenectomy, diabetes) revealed that poor HLA-A, B matching provided the greatest risk of graft loss due to irreversible rejection ($P < 10^{-5}$) for all variables examined.

The benefit of good HLA matching was found to increase with time post transplant, and the benefit of good matching on overall graft survival was significant in first transplant recipients as well as regrafted patients (Table 1). The most striking findings were the very poor long-term survival in all 0-matched recipients and the excellent results seen in four antigen-matched regrafted patients. The benefit of good HLA matching was additive to that of pretransplant transfusions, and recipients of well-matched shared kidneys had better graft sur-

Table 1. Influence of HLA-A, B match on graft survival

TXP	Match	N	Percent actuarial survival				
			6 mos	1 yr	2 yr	3 yr	4 yr
1	0	424	56±3	49±3	41±3	33±4	20±5
	1	882	60±2	53±2	46±2	41±2	39±3
	2	995	64±2	56±2	49±2	41±2	37±3
	3	443	66±2	61±2	54±3	48±3	39±4
	4	92	65±5	58±5	50±6	50±6	43±8
>1	0	101	49±5	38±5	27±6	23±6	12±7
	1	207	54±4	47±4	38±4	31±5	
	2	265	54±3	48±3	42±4	35±4	35±4
	3	148	54±4	50±4	40±5	37±6	37±6
	4	46	67±7	67±7	67±7	67±7	48±17

Histocompatibility Testing 1984
Edited by E. D. Albert et al.

vival than recipients of poorly matched locally obtained kidneys. Among patients who maintained graft function at least 1 year, well-matched recipients had lower serum creatinine levels and received significantly less immunosuppressive therapy. Matching by serologic cross-reactive group (CREG) specificities provided a better means of stratifying graft outcome by match number than matching strictly by typic and sub-typic specificities. In addition, the association between matching and outcome using CREGs was as significant ($P < 10^{-5}$) as by any other method.
We find that good HLA-A, B matching is associated with a significant decrease in graft loss from rejection and the need for less immunosuppression post transplant, and suggest that 0-matched transplants should be avoided.

Donor-Specific Blood Transfusion and Renal Graft Survival: A 3-Year Experience in Pediatrics

C. Kaplan[1], P. Niaudet[2], M.F. Gagnadoux[2], M.F. Reznikoff[1], J.Y. Muller[1], M. Broyer[2]

1 Unité d'immunologie leucoplaquettaire, CNTS-CHP, 6 rue Alexandre Cabanel, 75015 Paris, France
2 Hôpital Necker Enfants-Malades, Paris, France

The increased graft survival with donor-specific transfusion (DST) reported by Salvatierra and coworkers [1] encouraged us to carry out a similar trial for parental renal transplantation in children.
To date 20 patients have entered the study. The transfusion protocol consists in two or three transfusions at 4-week intervals before grafting. Serum samples obtained 10 and 20 days after each transfusion were tested for cytotoxic antibodies against the donor's isolated T and B cells at 4 °C, 22 °C, and 37 °C. The tests were also performed against a random panel of isolated T (37 °C) and B cells (22 °C).
Before the first transfusion, three patients who rejected a first cadaver kidney had positive cross-matches (B cells at 37 °C) and were no longer subject to the protocol. The remaining 17 patients have received donor-specific transfusions: 16 have negative cross-matches (T and B cells at all temperatures) and 15 have received transplants.
None has developed broad antibodies against the random panel. After grafting, six patients devel-

Table 1. DST: Humoral response to donor, random panel and renal function

Patients	RT/DST	DST Ab/panel		After graft		Renal function
		J0	After	Ab/panel	CM	
1	24/2	22% B	11% B	(+) B	(+) B	+
2	9/2	38% B	11% B	(+) B	–	CR
3	6/3	44% B	–	(+) B	–	CR
4	3/2	–	–	(+) B	(+) B	+
5	15/2	33% B	50% B	(+) B	–	+(RR)
6	>20/2	33% T	41% T	+T, B	–	CR
7	?/3	–	–	(+) B	(+) B	CR
8	>20/3	5% B	–	(+) B	(+) T, B	+(RR)
9	16/2	5% B	–B, 5% T	(+) T, B	–	+
10	2/3	83% T	–	(+) T, +B	–	CR
11	>20/3	50% B	27% B	+ B	–	+
12	6/3	–	–	–	(+) B	+
13	1/3	8% T	–	–	(+) B	CR
14	>20/2	–	–	(+) B	–	+
15	>20/2	–	–	–	–	+

CR, chronic rejection; RR, reversible rejection; ( ), transitory; RT, random transfusion; DST, donor-specific transfusion

Histocompatibility Testing 1984
Edited by E. D. Albert et al.

oped transient B-positive cross-match (predominantly at 22 °C).

All kidneys are presently functioning, with follow-up ranging from 2 months to 3.5 years. Nine patients have normal renal function, two of them experienced reversible acute rejection, and six patients have chronic rejection (Table 1).

The nature of the various immunologic mechanisms remains unclear, but the benefits derived from pretransplant DST in parental renal transplantation appear substantial.

Reference

1. Salvatierra O Jr, Amend W, Vincenti F, Potter D, Iwaki Y, Olpez G, Terasaki P, Duca R, Hanes D, Cochrum KC, Hopper S, Feduska NJ (1981) Pretreatment with donor-specific blood transfusions in related recipients with high MLC. Transplant Proc 13:142–149

Marrow Transplantation from Donors Other Than HLA Genotypically Identical Siblings: The Immunogenetics of Acute Graft Versus Host Disease

P.G. Beatty, R.A. Clift, J.A. Hansen, E.M. Mickelson, B. Nisperos, N. Fluornoy, and E.D. Thomas

Medical Oncology, Fred Hutchinson Cancer Research Center; Puget Sound Blood Center; and the Department of Medicine, University of Washington, 1124 Columbia Street, Seattle, WA 98104, USA

Abbreviations

AGVHD acute graft-versus-host disease, ALL acute lymphocytic leukemia, ANL acute non-lymphocytic leukemia, CML chronic myelogenous leukemia.

Bone marrow transplantation has become an accepted form of treatment for several hematologic malignancies [1]. However, only 40% of patients who are otherwise eligible for transplantation will have an HLA genotypically identical sibling. In 1975, the Seattle Marrow Transplant Team began using related donors other than HLA genotypically identical siblings in hopes of expanding the acceptable limits of disparity and thereby increasing the chance of a patient having an acceptable donor. This study analyzes how immunogenetic differences between patient and donor have an impact upon the incidence and day of onset of acute graft-versus-host disease (AGVHD), a major complication of marrow transplantation.

As of December 1, 1983, 101 patients in Seattle have received marrow grafts from donors other than HLA genotypically identical siblings for the treatment of an hematological malignancy. Forty-two had ALL, 44 ANL, and 15 CML. Forty-eight were in remission and 53 in relapse at the time of transplant. In all cases the donor and recipient were related and were genotypically identical for one haplotype ("haploidentical"). Twelve of 101 received marrow from a haploidentical donor who in addition was phenotypically identical for the A, B, and D/DR antigens of the nonshared haplotype, 60 received marrow from a donor who was incompatible for one antigen (A, B, or D/DR) of the nonshared haplotype, 23 received marrow from a

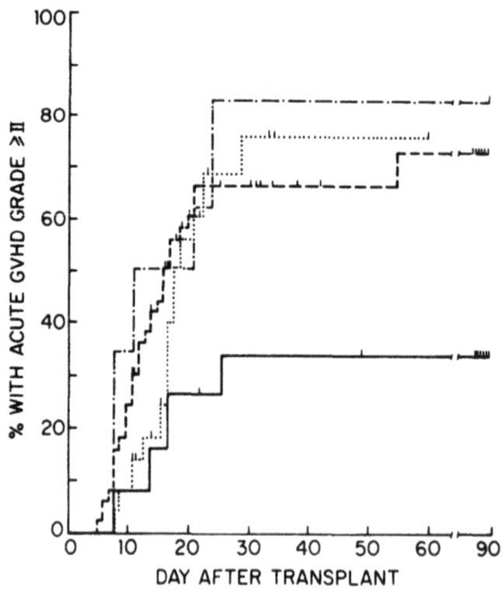

Fig. 1. Kaplan-Meir plots representing the cumulative percentage of patients who have developed grade II or greater AGVHD at the indicated day after transplant. Marks indicate censored patients who died on the indicated day, not having yet developed AGVHD ≥ II. Marks at day 90 indicate patients alive and felt to be past the time of risk for AGVHD. Increasing Degrees of Mismatch. —— Phenotypically identical (n = 12); – – – One antigen mismatched (n = 60); ··· Two antigen mismatched (n = 23); – · – Three antigen mismatched (n = 6)

Histocompatibility Testing 1984
Edited by E. D. Albert et al.

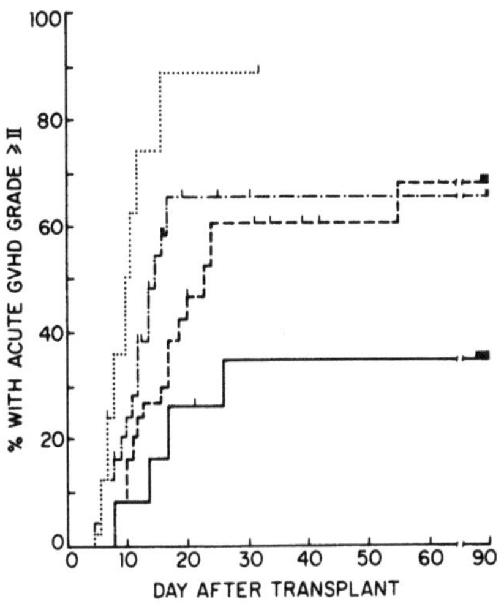

Fig. 2. One Antigen Mismatched. —— Phenotypically identical (n = 12); – – – A locus mismatch (n = 26); · · · B locus mismatch (n = 9); – · – D/DR locus mismatch (n = 25);

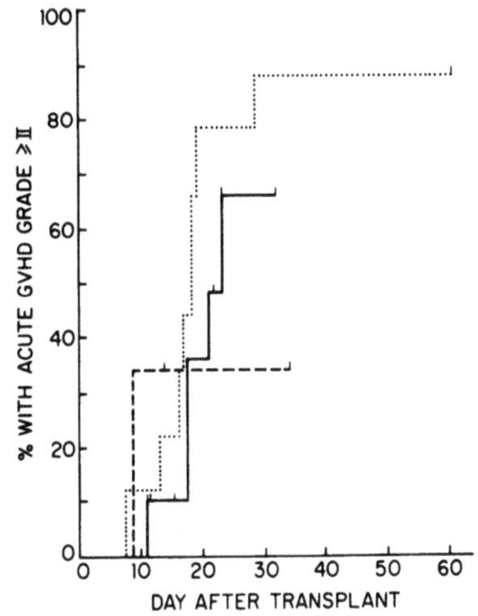

Fig. 3. Two Antigens Mismatched. —— A and B mismatched (n = 11); – – – A and D/DR mismatched (n = 3); · · · B and D/DR mismatched (n = 9)

haploidentical donor who was incompatible for two antigens (A, B; A, D/DR or B, D/DR), and six received marrow from a haploidentical donor who was incompatible for three antigens (A, B, and D/DR).

When the 48 mismatched patients transplanted while in remission are compared to a comparable group of matched patients, no difference is seen in survival. The 53 mismatched patients transplanted in relapse appeared to have a slightly poorer survival than matched relapse controls.

Actuarial analysis of the incidence and day of onset of significant AGVHD revealed a higher incidence in patients incompatible for one, two, or three antigens (65%–83%) compared to either the 12 patients phenotypically matched (35%) (Fig. 1) or the 578 control patients genotypically identical for both haplotypes (45%). Furthermore, patients mismatched for the antigens of one or more loci (A, B, or D/DR) developed AGVHD more rapidly (median = 14 days) than patients receiving grafts from HLA genotypically identical siblings (median = 25 days). Among the 60 patients grafted with marrow from a donor mismatched for one antigen, no significant difference was noted for A locus, versus B locus versus D/DR locus incompatibility (Fig. 2). Among the 23 patients incompatible for two antigens, there appeared to be no difference between a mismatch for two class I antigens (A, B) or a class I and a class II antigen (A, D/DR or B, D/DR) (Fig. 3). Thus incompatibility for either class I or class II antigens clearly influences the incidence and rate of onset of AGVHD, but does not have a clear impact upon survival of patients transplanted in remission.

Reference

1. Thomas ED (1983) Marrow transplantation for malignant diseases. J Clin Oncol 1:517–531

Immunological Investigation of Patients Treated for Leukaemia by Bone Marrow Transplantation (BMT)

E.H. Jones, S.M. Jackson and S.D. Lawler

Section of Human Genetics, Institute of Cancer Research, and The Royal Marsden Hospital, Fulham Road, London SW3 6JJ, UK

Studies in Patients Following a One-Haplotype Matched Graft. The chimaeric lymphocyte population of 24 leukaemic patients following an HLA one-haplotype matched BMT [1] was studied by HLA markers. After successful engraftment, the host was repopulated with B and T cells of donor HLA-ABC type and B lymphocytes of donor DR type, usually within 2 weeks after transplant. Lymphocytes of host HLA type were seen in varying proportions until successful engraftment occurred, and this was confirmed cytogenetically.

The use of sex chromosomes shows that, in leukaemic relapse, host cells reappear in bone marrow and dividing lymphoid cells of donor type may remain [2].

In leukaemic relapse following a one-haplotype matched BMT, peripheral blood lymphocytes may be exclusively of host or donor HLA type, or chimaeric. In one chimaeric case studied, peripheral blood T cells were of donor origin and B cells were of host origin. In the bone marrow, both the cells that formed rosettes with sheep red blood cells and the non-rosetting cells were of host HLA type.

T Cell Subpopulations. T cell subpopulations in 34 patients after an HLA-identical bone marrow graft were analysed by flow cytometry. The T helper subset ($OKT4^+$) was decreased and the T cytotoxic/suppressor subset ($OKT8^+$) increased after transplant, resulting in an inverted OKT4/OKT8 ratio (from 0.2 to 0.5) in BMT patients compared with normal controls (1.8).

HLA Antibody Studies. A sequential study of sera from 42 patients showed that 38% had lymphocytotoxic antibodies before, and 62% had antibodies at some time after BMT. HLA specificity could be defined in half the cases after BMT. In two cases, where the donor was matched for one haplotype, antibodies formed by recipient cells were specific for donor HLA antigens.

Summary. After a one-haplotype matched BMT for leukaemia, the patient was repopulated by donor lymphocytes by two weeks. After an HLA matched transplant the T helper subset decreased and the T cytotoxic/suppressor subset increased. 62% of patients had lymphocytotoxic antibodies after BMT.

References

1. Powles RL, Morganstern GR, Crofts M, Evans B, Lawler SD (1983) Mismatched family bone marrow transplantation. In: Gale RP (ed) Recent advances in bone marrow transplantation. Liss, New York, pp 757–767
2. Lawler SD, Baker MC, Harris H, Morganstern GR (1984) Cytogenetic studies on recipients of allogeneic bone marrow using the sex chromosomes as markers of cellular origin. Br J Haematol 56:431–443

Histocompatibility Testing 1984
Edited by E. D. Albert et al.

Chimerism Following Fetal Liver and Thymus Transplantation

H. Bétuel[1], J.L. Touraine[2], L. Gebuhrer[1], J. Lambert[1], M.G. Roncarolo[2]

1 Blood Transfusion Center, 69007 Lyon, France
2 Transplantation and Immunology Unit, Hôpital E. Herriot, 69007 Lyon, France

In severe combined immunodeficiency disease (SCID), fetal liver and thymus transplantation (FLTT) presents an alternative to bone marrow transplantation if no HLA-identical sib is available [1, 2]. Three infants afflicted with SCID were nurtured in sterile isolation before and long after transplantation. They received IP injections of fresh liver and thymus tissues from 8- to 13-week-old fetuses. The mean number of cells was 8.2×10^8. The procedure was repeated with different donors. Immunological reconstitution evolved slowly over 2 years. The numbers of T cells and of T subsets and the proliferative and cytotoxic responses gradually reached normal values. Immunoglobulin levels and antibody response developed after 3 years. Separation of T cells, B cells, and monocytes of the patient followed by iterative HLA typing documented the existence of a dual population, one from the host and the other from the donor(s). This was particularly evident in patient 1 (Ser S.), who received two transplants. He is now 86 months old and in good condition. The T cells are of donor origin, the B cells and monocytes are from the host; the monocytes of donor origin that were present at 60 months are now no longer detectable (Table 1).

Patient 2 (Aur C.) received five transplants. She is now 84 months old and in perfect health. The B cells are from the host and from the donor, while the monocytes are mainly from the host, with a small population of donor origin (Table 2).

Patient 3 (Jul. M) received two transplants, the last one 5 months ago. He is now 47 months old, and in good health. Most T and B cells are from the host; the T cells from the donor are still weakly represented.

In these three patients, despite complete HLA mismatch between host and donor(s), cooperation between T and B cells took place, giving rise to antibody production and resistance to infection [2]. These observations suggest that allogeneic restriction [3] may be less stringent in vivo in man than in experimental conditions in inbred animals. “Allo and X” recognition structures may exist on T cells, which could be driven to proliferate after proper elicitation [1].

References

1. Touraine JL, Betuel H (1981) Immunodeficiency diseases and expression of HLA antigens. Hum Immunol 2:147–153
2. Touraine JL, Griscelli C, Betuel H, Betend B, Souillet G (1983) Chimerism following liver transplantation: cell cooperation despite HLA mismatch. In: Primary immunodeficiency diseases. Birth Defects (Liss, New York, The National Foundation–March of Dimes) 19:143–145
3. Zinkernagel RM (1978) The thymus, its influence on recognition of “self-major histocompatibility Antigens” by T cells and consequences for reconstitution of immunodeficiency. Springer Semin Immunopathol 1:405–428

Table 1. Cell populations in patient 1

Patient 1	Origin	HLA-A	B	Bw	Cw	DR
T cells	Donor	1, 2	8, 18	6	7	Absent
B cells	Host	3, w33	14, w47	4, 6		4, 5, w52, w53
Monocytes	Host	3, w33	14, w47	4, 6		4, 5, w52, w53

Table 2. Cell populations in patient 2

Patient 2	HLA-A	B	Bw	Cw	DR	DQw
Host	2, 11	35, w62	6	3, 7	5, w6, w52	1
Donor	1	8	4	4	4	

Histocompatibility Testing 1984
Edited by E. D. Albert et al.

Annex

Reference Tables of Two-Locus Haplotype Frequencies for All MHC Marker Loci *

M.P. Baur [1], M. Neugebauer [1], and E.D. Albert [2]

1 Biometrical Department, Diabetes Research Institute, Auf'm Hennekamp 65, 4000 Düsseldorf, Federal Republic of Germany
2 Laboratory of Immungenetics, Pettenkoferstraße 8 a, 8000 Munich 2, Federal Republic of Germany

The following frequency tables were the basis for the population analysis of the Ninth International Histocompatibility Workshop (M. P. Baur et al., Population Analysis on the Basis of Deduced Haplotypes from Random Families, this volume), where the definition of the represented three major ethnic groups – CAU, ORI, NEG –, the computational procedure, and the description of the resulting parameter estimates are given). Due to the small amount of data available from healthy non-selected Negroid families, we included for this population the haplotypes of unrelated healthy individuals from disease families. We are aware that this introduces a bias in case of strong HLA-disease associations. Some of this distortion will cancel out due to the multiplicity of the various diseases included. On the other hand, we are confident that the information on race-specific distribution of haplotypes and disequilibria gained by this – admittedly unusual – measure is not influenced to a significant degree by this bias.

We refrained from printing complete three-way tables as had been done previously [1] due to the extremely high percentage of zero entries for frequencies as well as linkage parameters in tables like these. A selection of the most frequent three locus haplotype frequencies in the populations NEG, ORI and CAU is given in M. P. Baur et al., Reference tables of three locus haplotype frequencies and delta values in Negroids, Orientals and Caucasians, this volume. The total availability of all combinations of two-way frequencies and two-way disequilibria provides the means to approximate multilocus haplotype frequencies by ignoring higher order (≥ 3) linkage disequilibria. M. Neugebauer et al. (Analyses of Multilocus Pedigree Data by Computer, this volume) gave a procedure which recursively defines, for example, a four-locus haplotype frequency

$$\begin{aligned} f(a,b,c,d) = \; & f(d) * f(a,b,c) \\ & + f(a,b) * \text{delta}(c,d) \\ & + f(a,c) * \text{delta}(b,d) \\ & + f(b,c) * \text{delta}(a,d) \end{aligned}$$

as a function of the available gene frequencies, two-way haplotype frequencies, and two-way deltas. The additionally included term f (a, b, c) is (recursively) approximated by

$$\begin{aligned} f(a,b,c) = \; & f(c) * f(a,b) \\ & + f(a) * \text{delta}(b,c) \\ & + f(b) * \text{delta}(a,c) \end{aligned}$$

ignoring again the higher order interaction term delta (a, b, c). The general recursive approximation for an n-locus haplotype is given by

$$f(a_1,\ldots,a_i,\ldots,a_n) = f(a_1,\ldots,a_i,\ldots,a_{n-1}) * f(a_n) + \sum_{j=1}^{n-1} f(a_1,\ldots,\underset{\substack{i\neq j\\ i\neq n}}{a_i},\ldots,a_{n-2}) * \text{delta}(a_j,a_n)$$

which, implemented in FAP (M. Neugebauer et al., this volume), allowed the analysis of up to 11-locus haplotypes in the 2300 families of the Workshop Masterfile. For a similar approximation procedure see Morton et al. [2].

The layout of the two-locus tables is identical to the one used previously [1]. The specificities of the first locus are listed horizontally across the top of the table and those of the second locus vertically down the left margin. Broad specificities are not included; their frequencies are easily calculated as the sum of the corresponding split specificities. For each possible haplotype the table contains a block of four figures as follows:

1. Haplotype frequency per 10000;
2. Delta per 10000;
3. Relative delta;
4. Chi-square.

Symbols following the chi-square value indicate the nominal level of significance:

$* = P \leq 0.05 \quad \# = P \leq 0.01 \quad \$ = P \leq 0.001.$

Three dots printed instead of a figure for the chi-square indicate that due to the small sample size, the expected number for this haplotype is too small to calculate a meaningful test statistic.

	A1		Bf F1
B8	672	B18	60
	532		55
	0.64		0.48
	552.4 $		...

Figure 1. Layout of reference tables

* Supported by Deutsche Forschungsgemeinschaft Ba 660/5-1 Al 92/13-2.

Figure 1 shows two examples from population CAU, the first of which represents the results for the (A1, B8) haplotype, which has a frequency of 672/10 000; its delta equals 532/10 000, corresponding to a relative delta of 0.64. The chi-square statistic of 552.4 is significant at least at the level $P < 0.001$, as indicated by the $ sign.

The second example, haplotype (B18, BfF1), gives estimates for the frequency of 60/10 000. The delta is 55/10 000, the relative delta is 0.48; the three dots indicate that the sample size was too small to give a meaningful chi-square test statistic. The strong positive association between B18 and Bf F1 is not questioned, though, and would definitely yield a significant result in a larger sample.

Marginal frequencies on the right side and at the bottom of a table are the respective gene frequencies of the alleles represented in this row or column of the table. Differences in frequency estimates for the same allele in different tables are caused by the different sample sizes available for the estimation.

The following table of contents lists the reference tables with the corresponding sample sizes in the ethnic groups CAU, ORI, NEG, for which enough information was available in the Workshop Masterfile.

References

1. Baur MP, Danilovs J (1980) Reference tables of two and three-locus haplotype frequencies for HLA-A, B, C, DR, Bf and GLO. In: Terasaki PI (ed) Histocompatibility testing 1980. UCLA Tissue Typing Laboratory, Los Angeles
2. Morton NE, Simpson SP, Lew R, Yee S (1983) Estimation of haplotype frequencies. Tissue Antigens 22:257–262

Table 1. Table of contents for haplotype frequencies

Haplotype frequencies for population CAU
A-B (N=2106)

	A1	A2	A3	A11	A23	A24	A25	A26
B7	74 -89 -0.55 13.8$	260 -65 -0.20 4.5*	477 324 0.33 189.3$	30 -41 -0.58 6.2*	0 -15 -1.00 3.9*	142 25 0.03 1.4	5 -22 -0.82 4.6*	9 -28 -0.76 5.4*
B8	672 532 0.64 552.4$	110 -166 -0.60 32.9$	19 -110 -0.85 25.4$	19 -41 -0.69 7.3#	0 -13 -1.00 3.3	42 -57 -0.58 8.7#	9 -14 -0.62 2.2	14 -17 -0.56 2.5
B13	19 -22 -0.54 3.1	78 -4 -0.05 0.1	14 -24 -0.64 3.9*	0 -17 -1.00 4.2*	0 -3 -1.00 0.9	33 3 0.01 0.1	5 -1 -0.29 0.1	9 0 -0.06 0.0
B18	19 -59 -0.76 11.0$	162 4 0.01 0.0	13 -60 -0.82 12.9$	24 -10 -0.31 0.8	5 -2 -0.36 0.2	95 38 0.08 6.4*	138 125 0.54 263.1$	19 1 0.00 0.0
B27	16 -32 -0.68 5.7*	130 32 0.13 3.2	57 11 0.04 0.7	14 -7 -0.35 0.6	5 0 0.00 0.0	26 -8 -0.26 0.6	5 -2 -0.40 0.3	19 8 0.02 1.2
B35	29 -121 -0.81 27.2$	178 -121 -0.41 16.4$	257 117 0.13 26.3$	204 138 0.24 71.7$	14 0 -0.06 0.0	153 45 0.05 4.9*	5 -20 -0.81 4.0*	28 -6 -0.19 0.3
B37	76 53 0.40 31.6$	38 -6 -0.15 0.3	14 -6 -0.33 0.6	0 -9 -1.00 2.3	0 -1 -1.00 ...	5 -10 -0.69 1.8	0 -3 -1.00 0.8	5 0 -0.03 0.0
B38	31 -3 -0.11 0.1	33 -35 -0.52 5.7*	22 -9 -0.32 0.8	15 0 -0.02 0.0	0 -2 -1.00 0.8	35 10 0.05 0.0	0 -5 -1.00 1.3	87 79 0.34 174.5$
B39	19 -9 -0.35 0.9	69 11 0.08 0.7	7 -19 -0.74 3.7	9 -3 -0.29 0.3	0 -2 -1.00 0.6	33 12 0.07 1.7	18 13 0.07 7.6#	9 2 0.01 0.2
BW41	0 -12 -1.00 3.3	28 2 0.03 0.0	7 -4 -0.42 0.5	0 -5 -1.00 1.3	0 0 -1.00 ...	5 -3 -0.47 0.5	0 -1 -1.00 ...	27 24 0.27 42.1$
BW42	5 2 0.08 0.2	5 -1 -0.27 0.1	9 6 0.28 2.6	5 3 0.16 ...	0 0 -1.00 ...	0 -1 -1.00 0.6	0 0 -1.00 ...	0 0 -1.00 ...
B44	89 -89 -0.50 12.7$	503 148 0.17 20.9$	68 -97 -0.59 16.0$	14 -63 -0.82 13.6$	52 34 0.28 16.3$	88 -39 -0.31 3.3	20 -9 -0.34 0.9	17 -23 -0.59 3.5
B45	0 -5 -1.00 1.5	9 -2 -0.23 0.2	0 -4 -1.00 1.3	0 -2 -1.00 0.6	9 8 0.21 ...	9 5 0.13 1.3	0 0 -1.00 ...	5 4 0.09 ...
BW46	0 0 -1.00 ...	5 4 1.00 ...	0 0 -1.00 ...	0 0 -1.00 ...	0 0 -1.00 ...	0 0 -1.00 ...	0 0 -1.00 ...	0 0 -1.00 ...
BW47	0 -2 -1.00 0.9	0 -6 -1.00 2.0	14 11 0.52 8.9#	0 -1 -1.00 ...	0 0 -1.00 ...	0 -1 -1.00 0.6	0 0 -1.00 ...	0 0 -1.00 ...

	A28	A29	A30	A31	A32	AW33	AW34	AW36	AW43	AW66	AX	SUM
B7	38 -14 -0.29 1.1	33 0 -0.02 0.0	9 -30 -0.77 5.8*	24 -9 -0.29 0.7	24 -19 -0.45 2.2	0 -16 -1.00 4.1*	0 0 -1.00 ...	0 0 -1.00 ...	0 0 0.00 ...	6 4 0.35 ...	12 8 0.26 3.8	1143
B8	15 -29 -0.67 4.9*	14 -14 -0.51 1.8	14 -19 -0.58 2.8	9 -19 -0.68 3.2	19 -17 -0.49 2.1	5 -8 -0.65 1.5	0 0 -1.00 ...	5 5 1.00 ...	0 0 0.00 ...	0 0 -1.00 ...	5 2 0.05 0.2	971
B13	0 -12 -1.00 3.1	0 -7 -1.00 1.9	126 116 0.42 302.3$	0 -7 -1.00 1.9	5 -5 -0.55 0.7	0 -3 -1.00 0.9	0 0 -1.00 ...	0 0 -1.00 ...	0 0 0.00 ...	0 0 -1.00 ...	0 0 -1.00 ...	289
B18	14 -11 -0.46 1.2	0 -15 -1.00 3.7	43 24 0.07 6.9#	9 -6 -0.45 0.7	6 -14 -0.71 2.5	5 -2 -0.39 0.3	0 0 -1.00 ...	0 0 -1.00 ...	0 0 0.00 ...	0 0 -1.00 ...	0 -1 -1.00 ...	552
B27	14 -1 -0.12 0.1	2 -7 -0.80 1.5	12 0 0.00 0.0	19 9 0.03 1.8	19 6 0.02 0.6	5 0 -0.02 0.0	0 0 -1.00 ...	0 0 -1.00 ...	0 0 0.00 ...	0 0 -1.00 ...	0 0 -1.00 ...	343
B35	70 21 0.05 2.2	17 -13 -0.45 1.5	26 -9 -0.29 0.7	28 -2 -0.09 0.1	33 -6 -0.18 0.3	5 -10 -0.68 1.7	0 0 -1.00 ...	0 0 -1.00 ...	0 0 0.00 ...	0 0 -1.00 ...	5 1 0.04 0.1	1052
B37	0 -6 -1.00 1.6	9 4 0.03 0.9	0 -4 -1.00 1.2	5 0 0.00 0.0	5 0 -0.16 0.0	0 -1 -1.00 ...	0 0 -1.00 ...	0 0 -1.00 ...	0 0 0.00 ...	0 0 -1.00 ...	0 0 -1.00 ...	157
B38	0 -10 -1.00 2.6	5 -1 -0.30 0.1	0 -7 -1.00 1.9	5 -1 -0.30 0.1	9 0 -0.02 0.0	0 -3 -1.00 0.8	0 0 -1.00 ...	0 0 -1.00 ...	0 0 0.00 ...	0 0 -1.00 ...	0 0 -1.00 ...	242
B39	9 0 -0.04 0.0	0 -5 -1.00 1.3	0 -6 -1.00 1.6	19 13 0.07 6.4*	5 -2 -0.35 0.2	0 -2 -1.00 0.7	0 0 -1.00 ...	0 0 -1.00 ...	0 0 0.00 ...	5 5 0.34 ...	0 0 -1.00 ...	202
BW41	0 -3 -1.00 0.9	0 -2 -1.00 0.6	19 16 0.18 17.6$	0 -2 -1.00 0.6	5 2 0.02 0.1	0 0 -1.00 ...	0 0 -1.00 ...	0 0 -1.00 ...	0 0 0.00 ...	0 0 -1.00 ...	0 0 -1.00 ...	91
BW42	0 0 -1.00 ...	0 0 -1.00 ...	0 0 -1.00 ...	0 0 -1.00 ...	0 0 -1.00 ...	0 0 -1.00 ...	0 0 -1.00 ...	0 0 -1.00 ...	0 0 0.00 ...	0 0 -1.00 ...	0 0 -1.00 ...	24
B44	100 42 0.10 7.7#	180 143 0.56 139.7$	16 -26 -0.63 4.2*	24 -12 -0.34 1.1	52 5 0.01 0.1	19 0 0.00 0.0	0 0 -1.00 ...	0 0 -1.00 ...	0 0 0.00 ...	0 -1 -1.00 ...	0 -3 -1.00 1.0	1242
B45	0 -1 -1.00 ...	9 8 0.20 ...	0 0 -1.00 ...	0 0 -1.00 ...	0 -1 -1.00 ...	0 0 -1.00 ...	0 0 -1.00 ...	0 0 -1.00 ...	0 0 0.00 ...	0 0 -1.00 ...	0 0 -1.00 ...	41
BW46	0 0 -1.00 ...	0 0 -1.00 ...	0 0 -1.00 ...	0 0 -1.00 ...	0 0 -1.00 ...	0 0 -1.00 ...	0 0 -1.00 ...	0 0 -1.00 ...	0 0 0.00 ...	0 0 -1.00 ...	0 0 -1.00 ...	5
BW47	5 4 0.17 ...	0 0 -1.00 ...	0 0 -1.00 ...	0 0 -1.00 ...	0 0 -1.00 ...	5 5 0.20 ...	0 0 -1.00 ...	0 0 -1.00 ...	0 0 0.00 ...	0 0 -1.00 ...	0 0 -1.00 ...	24

Haplotype frequencies for population CAU
A-B (N=2106)

	A1	A2	A3	A11	A23	A24	A25	A26	A28	A29	A30	A31	A32	AW33	AW34	AW36	AW43	AW66	AX	SUM
BW48	0 0 0.00 ...	0 0 0.00 ...	0 0 0.00 ...	0 0 0.00 ...	0 0 0.00 ...	0 0 0.00 ...	0 0 0.00 ...	0 0 0.00 ...	0 0 0.00 ...	0 0 0.00 ...	0 0 0.00 ...	0 0 0.00 ...	0 0 0.00 ...	0 0 0.00 ...	0 0 0.00 ...	0 0 0.00 ...	0 0 0.00 ...	0 0 0.00 ...	0 0 0.00 ...	0
B49	9 -16 -0.65 2.8	43 -7 -0.16 0.4	14 -9 -0.42 1.0	5 -5 -0.56 0.8	24 21 0.15 39.1$	28 9 0.06 1.2	0 -3 -1.00 0.0	19 13 0.08 6.4*	0 -7 -1.00 1.9	0 -4 -1.00 1.2	24 18 0.10 11.3$	14 9 0.05 3.2	0 -6 -1.00 1.5	0 -2 -1.00 0.6	0 0 -1.00 ...	0 0 -1.00 ...	0 0 0.00 ...	0 0 -1.00 ...	0 0 -1.00 ...	180
BW50	9 -6 -0.45 0.8	62 30 0.37 8.2#	0 -14 -1.00 3.7	5 -1 -0.30 0.1	9 7 0.07 ...	9 -2 -0.23 0.1	0 -2 -1.00 0.6	0 -3 -1.00 0.8	0 -4 -1.00 1.2	5 2 0.02 0.2	9 5 0.05 1.5	0 -2 -1.00 0.7	0 -3 -1.00 0.0	5 3 0.03 ...	0 0 -1.00 ...	0 0 -1.00 ...	0 0 0.00 ...	0 0 -1.00 ...	0 0 -1.00 ...	113
B51	28 -61 -0.69 11.1$	233 55 0.12 5.4*	71 -11 -0.14 0.5	62 23 0.04 3.2	5 -3 -0.43 0.4	43 -20 -0.33 1.7	14 0 -0.08 0.0	9 -11 -0.56 1.5	38 9 0.02 0.7	5 -12 -0.73 2.2	5 -16 -0.77 2.0	62 44 0.16 24.2$	47 23 0.07 5.3*	0 -8 -1.00 2.1	0 0 -1.00 ...	0 0 -1.00 ...	0 0 0.00 ...	0 0 -1.00 ...	0 -1 -1.00 ...	622
BW52	22 -5 -0.22 0.3	47 -8 -0.16 0.4	14 -11 -0.46 1.4	76 64 0.35 75.6$	0 -2 -1.00 0.6	24 4 0.02 0.2	0 -4 -1.00 1.0	2 -3 -0.69 0.7	5 -3 -0.45 0.4	0 -5 -1.00 1.3	0 -6 -1.00 1.5	5 0 -0.13 0.0	0 -6 -1.00 1.7	0 -2 -1.00 0.6	0 0 -1.00 ...	0 0 -1.00 ...	0 0 0.00 ...	0 0 -1.00 ...	0 0 -1.00 ...	195
BW53	0 -6 -1.00 1.9	19 4 0.11 0.3	0 -6 -1.00 1.7	3 0 -0.09 0.0	0 0 -1.00 ...	0 -4 -1.00 1.3	0 0 -1.00 ...	0 -1 -1.00 ...	19 17 0.33 25.2$	0 -1 -1.00 ...	9 7 0.14 ...	0 -1 -1.00 ...	0 -1 -1.00 ...	0 0 -1.00 ...	0 0 -1.00 ...	0 0 -1.00 ...	0 0 0.00 ...	0 0 -1.00 ...	2 2 0.05 ...	52
BW54	5 4 1.00 ...	0 0 -1.00 ...	0 0 -1.00 ...	0 0 -1.00 ...	0 0 -1.00 ...	0 0 -1.00 ...	0 0 -1.00 ...	0 0 -1.00 ...	0 0 -1.00 ...	0 0 -1.00 ...	0 0 -1.00 ...	0 0 -1.00 ...	0 0 -1.00 ...	0 0 -1.00 ...	0 0 -1.00 ...	0 0 -1.00 ...	0 0 0.00 ...	0 0 -1.00 ...	0 0 -1.00 ...	5
BW55	28 5 0.04 0.3	24 -21 -0.47 3.1	9 -11 -0.58 1.8	62 52 0.35 60.0$	0 -1 -1.00 ...	9 -6 -0.45 0.8	0 -3 -1.00 0.9	9 4 0.02 0.6	9 2 0.01 0.1	0 -4 -1.00 1.0	5 0 -0.10 0.0	0 -4 -1.00 1.0	0 -5 -1.00 1.4	5 3 0.02 0.6	0 0 -1.00 ...	0 0 -1.00 ...	0 0 0.00 ...	0 0 -1.00 ...	0 0 -1.00 ...	160
BW56	5 -9 -0.67 1.7	33 3 0.04 0.1	26 12 0.13 2.4	12 5 0.05 0.0	0 -1 -1.00 ...	5 -5 -0.54 0.8	5 2 0.02 0.5	0 -2 -1.00 0.8	5 0 0.00 0.0	0 -2 -1.00 0.7	0 -3 -1.00 0.8	5 2 0.02 0.2	5 1 0.01 0.1	0 -1 -1.00 ...	5 5 0.49 ...	0 0 -1.00 ...	0 0 0.00 ...	0 0 -1.00 ...	0 0 -1.00 ...	106
BW57	166 124 0.50 93.6$	60 -22 -0.28 1.9	14 -24 -0.64 3.9*	0 -17 -1.00 4.2*	0 -3 -1.00 0.9	16 -13 -0.46 1.5	5 -1 -0.29 0.1	0 -9 -1.00 2.1	0 -13 -1.00 3.1	0 -8 -1.00 1.9	5 -4 -0.50 0.6	0 -8 -1.00 1.9	24 13 0.05 3.4	0 -3 -1.00 0.0	0 0 -1.00 ...	0 0 -1.00 ...	0 0 0.00 ...	0 0 -1.00 ...	0 0 -1.00 ...	290
BW58	0 -24 -1.00 6.2*	85 36 0.29 7.7#	14 -8 -0.39 0.9	9 -1 -0.18 0.1	5 3 0.02 0.6	0 -17 -1.00 4.2*	5 1 0.00 0.0	0 -5 -1.00 1.3	5 -2 -0.38 0.3	5 0 -0.02 0.0	5 0 -0.16 0.0	5 0 -0.02 0.0	7 0 0.00 0.0	28 25 0.17 54.5$	0 0 -1.00 ...	0 0 -1.00 ...	0 0 0.00 ...	0 0 -1.00 ...	0 0 -1.00 ...	173
BW59	0 0 0.00 ...	0 0 0.00 ...	0 0 0.00 ...	0 0 0.00 ...	0 0 0.00 ...	0 0 0.00 ...	0 0 0.00 ...	0 0 0.00 ...	0 0 0.00 ...	0 0 0.00 ...	0 0 0.00 ...	0 0 0.00 ...	0 0 0.00 ...	0 0 0.00 ...	0 0 0.00 ...	0 0 0.00 ...	0 0 0.00 ...	0 0 0.00 ...	0 0 0.00 ...	0
BW60	24 -29 -0.56 4.3*	196 88 0.33 22.0$	25 -24 -0.50 3.2	14 -9 -0.41 0.0	9 4 0.03 0.5	22 -16 -0.43 1.8	5 -3 -0.46 0.4	9 -2 -0.28 0.2	24 6 0.02 0.5	0 -10 -1.00 2.5	0 -12 -1.00 2.0	33 22 0.08 9.7#	14 0 -0.03 0.0	0 -5 -1.00 1.3	0 0 -1.00 ...	0 0 -1.00 ...	0 0 0.00 ...	3 2 0.18 ...	0 0 -1.00 ...	378
BW61	14 -14 -0.53 2.0	37 -21 -0.37 2.4	31 4 0.02 0.1	29 16 0.08 4.6*	0 -2 -1.00 0.6	37 16 0.09 2.9	5 0 -0.00 0.0	5 -1 -0.26 0.1	0 -9 -1.00 2.2	0 -5 -1.00 1.3	0 -6 -1.00 1.6	0 -5 -1.00 1.3	32 24 0.12 16.7$	0 -2 -1.00 0.7	5 5 0.49 ...	0 0 -1.00 ...	0 0 0.00 ...	0 0 -1.00 ...	10 9 0.27 ...	205
BW62	47 -40 -0.47 5.1*	279 104 0.24 19.3$	52 -29 -0.37 2.8	5 -33 -0.87 7.0#	5 -3 -0.43 0.4	125 62 0.11 15.2$	0 -14 -1.00 3.4	5 -14 -0.75 2.7	43 14 0.03 1.7	0 -17 -1.00 4.2*	0 -20 -1.00 4.9*	9 -8 -0.50 1.0	38 15 0.04 2.1	5 -3 -0.45 0.4	0 0 -1.00 ...	0 0 -1.00 ...	0 0 0.00 ...	0 0 -1.00 ...	1 0 -0.53 ...	614

Haplotype frequencies for population CAU
A-B ($N = 2106$)

	A1	A2	A3	A11	A23	A24	A25	A26	A28
BW63	9 0 -0.05 0.0	28 9 0.19 1.3	5 -3 -0.43 0.4	0 -3 -1.00 0.9	0 0 -1.00 ...	14 7 0.12 1.8	0 -1 -1.00 ...	0 -1 -1.00 ...	0 -2 -1.00 0.7
BW64	5 -10 -0.69 1.9	24 -7 -0.26 0.6	21 6 0.06 0.6	5 -1 -0.30 0.1	0 -1 -1.00 ...	2 -9 -0.83 1.9	0 -2 -1.00 0.6	14 10 0.09 6.2*	0 -4 -1.00 1.2
BW65	19 -18 -0.50 2.3	43 -31 -0.43 4.1*	59 24 0.11 4.1*	5 -11 -0.70 1.9	0 -3 -1.00 0.8	16 -10 -0.41 1.1	0 -5 -1.00 1.4	5 -3 -0.42 0.3	38 26 0.10 12.4$
BW67	0 0 0.00 ...	0 0 0.00 ...	0 0 0.00 ...	0 0 0.00 ...	0 0 0.00 ...	0 0 0.00 ...	0 0 0.00 ...	0 0 0.00 ...	0 0 0.00 ...
BW71	0 0 -1.00 ...	0 0 -1.00 ...	0 0 -1.00 ...	0 0 -1.00 ...	0 0 -1.00 ...	0 0 -1.00 ...	0 0 -1.00 ...	0 0 -1.00 ...	5 5 1.00 ...
BW72	0 -3 -1.00 1.0	5 -2 -0.40 0.4	0 -3 -1.00 0.9	0 -1 -1.00 ...	0 0 -1.00 ...	9 6 0.23 2.9	0 0 -1.00 ...	5 4 0.14 ...	5 4 0.13 ...
BW73	0 -1 -1.00 ...	14 10 1.00 7.4#	0 -1 -1.00 ...	0 0 -1.00 ...	0 0 -1.00 ...	0 0 -1.00 ...	0 0 -1.00 ...	0 0 -1.00 ...	0 0 -1.00 ...
BX	0 -4 -1.00 1.4	15 4 0.15 0.5	2 -2 -0.61 0.5	5 3 0.07 0.6	0 0 -1.00 ...	3 0 -0.23 0.0	0 0 -1.00 ...	0 0 -1.00 ...	5 3 0.09 ...
SUM	1439	2855	1335	631	142	1028	244	330	466

	A29	A30	A31	A32	AW33	AW34	AW36	AW43	AW66	AX	SUM
BW63	0 -1 -1.00 ...	0 -1 -1.00 ...	5 3 0.05 ...	5 2 0.04 0.5	0 0 -1.00 ...	0 0 -1.00 ...	0 0 -1.00 ...	0 0 0.00 ...	0 0 -1.00 ...	0 0 -1.00 ...	66
BW64	0 -2 -1.00 0.7	9 5 0.05 1.5	9 6 0.05 2.1	19 15 0.14 11.1$	5 3 0.03 ...	0 0 -1.00 ...	0 0 -1.00 ...	0 0 0.00 ...	0 0 -1.00 ...	0 0 -1.00 ...	113
BW65	5 -2 -0.35 0.2	5 -3 -0.45 0.4	5 -2 -0.35 0.2	5 -4 -0.50 0.6	57 53 0.37 158.5$	0 0 -1.00 ...	0 0 -1.00 ...	0 0 0.00 ...	0 0 -1.00 ...	0 0 -1.00 ...	262
BW67	0 0 0.00 ...	0 0 0.00 ...	0 0 0.00 ...	0 0 0.00 ...	0 0 0.00 ...	0 0 0.00 ...	0 0 0.00 ...	0 0 0.00 ...	0 0 0.00 ...	0 0 0.00 ...	0
BW71	0 0 -1.00 ...	0 0 -1.00 ...	0 0 -1.00 ...	0 0 -1.00 ...	0 0 -1.00 ...	0 0 -1.00 ...	0 0 -1.00 ...	0 0 0.00 ...	0 0 -1.00 ...	0 0 -1.00 ...	5
BW72	0 0 -1.00 ...	5 4 0.14 ...	0 0 -1.00 ...	0 0 -1.00 ...	0 0 -1.00 ...	0 0 -1.00 ...	0 0 -1.00 ...	0 0 0.00 ...	0 0 -1.00 ...	0 0 -1.00 ...	29
BW73	0 0 -1.00 ...	0 0 -1.00 ...	0 0 -1.00 ...	0 0 -1.00 ...	0 0 -1.00 ...	0 0 -1.00 ...	0 0 -1.00 ...	0 0 0.00 ...	0 0 -1.00 ...	0 0 -1.00 ...	14
BX	5 4 0.11 ...	0 0 -1.00 ...	0 0 -1.00 ...	3 2 0.04 ...	0 0 -1.00 ...	0 0 -1.00 ...	0 0 -1.00 ...	0 0 0.00 ...	0 0 -1.00 ...	0 0 -1.00 ...	38
SUM	294	346	294	381	149	10	5	0	14	35	

Haplotype frequencies for population CAU

A-C ($N = 2130$)

	A1	A2	A3	A11	A23	A24	A25	A26	A28	A29	A30	A31	A32	AW33	AW34	AW36	AW43	AW66	AX	SUM
CW1	23 -24 -0.52 3.3	115 18 0.08 1.1	41 -2 -0.07 0.1	26 5 0.01 0.2	0 -4 -1.00 1.1	22 -11 -0.35 1.0	24 16 0.07 6.0#	33 22 0.07 10.9$	15 0 -0.06 0.0	2 -7 -0.80 1.5	5 -6 -0.57 0.9	14 4 0.02 0.5	5 -7 -0.61 1.1	0 -4 -1.00 1.0	0 0 -1.00 ...	0 0 -1.00 ...	0 0 0.00 ...	0 0 -1.00 ...	10 8 0.20 ...	335
CW2	25 -33 -0.58 5.2*	125 5 0.02 0.1	61 6 0.02 0.2	23 -2 -0.13 0.1	0 -5 -1.00 1.4	58 16 0.04 1.4	0 -9 -1.00 2.3	5 -7 -0.62 1.1	19 0 -0.04 0.0	0 -11 -1.00 2.9	17 3 0.01 0.1	14 2 0.01 0.1	60 44 0.12 27.9$	9 3 0.03 0.5	0 0 -1.00 ...	0 0 -1.00 ...	0 0 0.00 ...	0 0 -1.00 ...	0 -1 -1.00 ...	416
CW3	89 -90 -0.51 13.2$	523 158 0.18 23.6$	129 -37 -0.23 2.4	91 10 0.02 0.4	14 -4 -0.27 0.3	164 35 0.04 2.7	9 -21 -0.71 3.8	35 -4 -0.12 0.1	84 24 0.06 2.5	5 -32 -0.87 7.2#	9 -34 -0.79 6.0#	38 2 0.01 0.0	42 -6 -0.14 0.2	28 11 0.09 1.7	0 0 -1.00 ...	0 0 -1.00 ...	0 0 0.00 ...	3 1 0.05 ...	1 -4 -0.82 0.9	1264
CW4	35 -131 -0.79 29.3$	236 -100 -0.30 10.3#	244 90 0.09 14.5$	204 130 0.23 58.0$	63 45 0.34 28.5$	141 22 0.02 1.1	5 -22 -0.82 4.8*	19 -17 -0.48 2.1	67 12 0.03 0.6	21 -13 -0.40 1.4	48 7 0.02 0.3	33 0 -0.01 0.0	42 -2 -0.07 0.1	5 -10 -0.68 1.8	0 0 -1.00 ...	0 0 -1.00 ...	0 0 0.00 ...	0 -1 -1.00 ...	6 1 0.02 0.0	1169
CW5	42 -57 -0.58 9.0#	373 171 0.34 46.4$	50 -42 -0.46 5.2*	14 -30 -0.69 5.1*	5 -5 -0.53 0.7	42 -28 -0.41 3.1	15 -1 -0.12 0.1	9 -12 -0.59 1.8	28 -4 -0.16 0.2	9 -11 -0.57 1.6	44 20 0.06 3.8	19 0 -0.05 0.0	43 16 0.04 2.3	8 0 -0.15 0.1	0 0 -1.00 ...	0 0 -1.00 ...	0 0 0.00 ...	0 0 -1.00 ...	0 -2 -1.00 0.7	701
CW6	266 145 0.20 46.9$	247 2 0.00 0.0	47 -64 -0.58 10.1#	14 -39 -0.74 7.4#	19 6 0.04 0.7	65 -20 -0.25 1.4	10 -10 -0.52 1.3	9 -17 -0.66 2.8	2 -37 -0.95 8.9#	14 -10 -0.45 1.2	114 85 0.27 58.5$	0 -23 -1.00 5.8*	33 0 0.00 0.0	9 -1 -0.21 0.1	0 0 -1.00 ...	0 0 -1.00 ...	0 0 0.00 ...	0 -1 -1.00 ...	0 -3 -1.00 0.9	849
CW7	625 275 0.26 71.1$	639 -67 -0.10 2.6	445 121 0.12 14.8$	66 -89 -0.58 15.7$	23 -13 -0.38 1.5	245 -3 -0.02 0.0	37 -22 -0.38 2.5	61 -15 -0.21 0.0	92 -23 -0.21 1.5	38 -35 -0.48 4.0*	36 -46 -0.58 8.3#	42 -27 -0.40 3.3	69 -24 -0.27 2.0	10 -22 -0.70 4.6*	0 -1 -1.00 ...	5 4 1.00 ...	0 0 0.00 ...	8 4 0.26 0.8	10 0 -0.09 0.0	2451
CW8	23 -28 -0.56 4.2*	66 -39 -0.37 4.6*	79 31 0.10 4.0*	10 -12 -0.57 1.8	0 -5 -1.00 1.2	19 -17 -0.49 2.2	0 -8 -1.00 2.0	14 3 0.01 0.1	38 21 0.06 5.7*	5 -5 -0.54 0.7	14 1 0.00 0.0	14 4 0.01 0.3	23 9 0.03 1.3	61 56 0.43 142.5$	0 0 -1.00 ...	0 0 -1.00 ...	0 0 0.00 ...	0 0 -1.00 ...	0 -1 -1.00 ...	366
CX	300 -49 -0.14 2.3	561 -144 -0.21 11.8$	224 -98 -0.31 9.9#	189 33 0.07 2.1	27 -9 -0.27 0.8	261 12 0.02 0.2	143 84 0.46 33.9$	129 52 0.22 10.3#	129 13 0.04 0.4	206 133 0.59 69.6$	60 -24 -0.29 2.1	112 42 0.19 7.3#	68 -25 -0.28 2.1	5 -27 -0.85 6.8#	9 7 1.00 ...	0 0 -1.00 ...	0 0 0.00 ...	7 3 0.19 0.4	18 7 0.21 1.3	2448
SUM	1428	2885	1320	637	151	1017	243	314	474	300	347	286	385	135	9	5	0	18	45	

A-DQ ($N = 2012$)

	A1	A2	A3	A11	A23	A24	A25	A26	A28	A29	A30	A31	A32	AW33	AW34	AW36	AW43	AW66	AX	SUM
DQW1	330 -121 -0.27 11.4$	891 -35 -0.04 0.6	650 218 0.24 37.9$	268 66 0.16 6.9#	29 -17 -0.38 2.0	333 -4 -0.02 0.0	92 20 0.14 1.8	112 14 0.07 0.6	119 -39 -0.25 3.1	44 -47 -0.52 7.6#	82 -33 -0.29 3.1	75 -20 -0.22 1.4	118 -8 -0.07 0.2	54 9 0.09 0.5	5 2 0.26 0.3	0 -1 -1.00 ...	0 0 0.00 ...	8 2 0.11 0.1	18 1 0.03 0.0	3228
DQW2	424 171 0.15 32.8$	391 -128 -0.25 11.0$	127 -114 -0.48 15.5$	77 -35 -0.32 3.0	40 14 0.12 1.8	165 -24 -0.13 0.9	20 -19 -0.50 2.5	51 -3 -0.08 0.1	70 -18 -0.21 1.1	141 90 0.39 39.5$	175 110 0.37 47.5$	30 -23 -0.44 2.7	59 -11 -0.17 0.5	35 10 0.08 0.9	5 3 0.39 ...	0 0 -1.00 ...	0 0 0.00 ...	0 -3 -1.00 0.9	0 -8 -1.00 2.3	1810
DQW3	240 -69 -0.27 7.5#	826 149 0.09 12.1$	273 -41 -0.13 1.7	120 -26 -0.19 1.4	47 13 0.12 1.3	254 7 0.01 0.1	74 22 0.13 2.4	59 -12 -0.18 0.6	185 69 0.18 11.4$	27 -39 -0.60 6.5*	48 -36 -0.43 4.3*	97 27 0.12 2.8	75 -17 -0.19 0.9	18 -14 -0.45 1.8	0 -1 -1.00 ...	5 4 1.00 ...	0 0 0.00 ...	2 -2 -0.58 0.4	8 -3 -0.35 0.4	2358
DQX	406 40 0.04 1.4	764 14 0.01 0.1	287 -61 -0.18 3.5	160 -2 -0.02 0.0	29 -8 -0.23 0.6	296 22 0.03 0.6	36 -21 -0.38 2.3	83 3 0.01 0.0	118 -9 -0.08 0.2	72 -1 -0.03 0.0	54 -39 -0.42 4.8*	96 18 0.08 1.2	141 38 0.13 4.1*	33 -3 -0.10 0.1	0 -2 -1.00 0.7	0 0 -1.00 ...	0 0 0.00 ...	10 5 0.32 1.2	26 12 0.32 3.1	2611
SUM	1400	2872	1337	625	145	1048	222	305	492	284	359	298	393	140	10	5	0	20	52	

Haplotype frequencies for population CAU
A-DR ($N = 1930$)

	A1	A2	A3	A11	A23	A24	A25	A26	A28	A29	A30	A31	A32	AW33	AW34	AW36	AW43	AW66	AX	SUM
DR1	64 -70 -0.53 9.2#	217 -50 -0.19 2.9	224 94 0.11 16.6$	102 42 0.07 6.6*	5 -8 -0.65 1.3	126 25 0.03 1.5	26 3 0.01 0.1	40 10 0.04 0.8	10 -34 -0.78 6.1*	10 -16 -0.62 2.3	32 -3 -0.10 0.1	26 -2 -0.11 0.1	28 -10 -0.28 0.7	41 28 0.23 13.2$	0 0 -1.00 ...	0 0 -1.00 ...	0 0 0.00 ...	0 0 -1.00 ...	6 1 0.03 0.1	957
DR2	156 -65 -0.30 5.2*	419 -21 -0.05 0.4	381 167 0.15 34.6$	92 -6 -0.07 0.1	15 -8 -0.36 0.7	186 20 0.02 0.6	72 34 0.16 6.0#	46 -2 -0.06 0.0	47 -26 -0.37 2.4	23 -20 -0.47 2.3	21 -37 -0.64 5.8*	33 -14 -0.31 1.1	60 -3 -0.06 0.1	5 -15 -0.76 2.9	0 -1 -1.00 ...	0 0 -1.00 ...	0 0 0.00 ...	10 8 1.00 ...	8 0 0.01 0.0	1574
DR3	497 326 0.31 159.8$	219 -120 -0.36 13.1$	92 -72 -0.44 8.1#	52 -23 -0.32 1.8	1 -16 -0.94 3.6	98 -29 -0.23 1.7	26 -2 -0.12 0.1	26 -11 -0.31 0.8	24 -32 -0.58 4.4*	31 -2 -0.08 0.0	64 19 0.06 1.8	16 -20 -0.57 2.7	31 -17 -0.37 1.5	26 10 0.08 1.3	0 0 -1.00 ...	0 0 -1.00 ...	0 0 0.00 ...	0 0 -1.00 ...	8 2 0.05 0.2	1211
DR4	132 -47 -0.27 3.3	457 99 0.11 8.4#	179 5 0.00 0.0	73 -6 -0.09 0.2	26 7 0.05 0.5	106 -28 -0.21 1.5	36 5 0.02 0.2	30 -9 -0.24 0.5	84 24 0.06 2.2	5 -30 -0.86 5.0*	12 -35 -0.75 6.1*	88 49 0.18 13.0$	35 -16 -0.32 1.3	9 -7 -0.48 0.9	0 0 -1.00 ...	0 0 -1.00 ...	0 0 0.00 ...	0 0 -1.00 ...	5 0 -0.18 0.0	1277
DR7	200 33 0.03 1.6	295 -37 -0.11 1.3	71 -89 -0.56 12.8$	40 -34 -0.46 3.8	31 13 0.10 2.2	87 -37 -0.31 2.9	16 -12 -0.45 1.3	41 4 0.02 0.1	51 -4 -0.09 0.1	124 91 0.37 56.5$	129 85 0.26 36.9$	31 -4 -0.15 0.2	45 -2 -0.07 0.0	21 5 0.04 0.3	5 4 0.43 ...	0 0 -1.00 ...	0 0 0.00 ...	0 0 -1.00 ...	0 -5 -1.00 1.3	1187
DRW8	31 -10 -0.26 0.6	108 25 0.12 2.1	16 -23 -0.60 3.4	26 7 0.03 0.6	0 -3 -1.00 0.9	41 10 0.04 0.7	0 -6 -1.00 1.5	5 -3 -0.46 0.4	19 5 0.02 0.4	14 6 0.02 0.8	0 -10 -1.00 2.3	10 1 0.00 0.0	21 9 0.03 1.4	0 -3 -1.00 0.8	0 0 -1.00 ...	0 0 -1.00 ...	0 0 0.00 ...	0 0 -1.00 ...	5 4 0.08 ...	296
DRW9	5 -5 -0.54 0.7	10 -11 -0.54 1.7	10 0 -0.04 0.0	5 0 0.00 0.0	0 0 -1.00 ...	0 -7 -1.00 1.8	0 -1 -1.00 ...	5 3 0.04 ...	16 12 0.17 8.6#	5 3 0.04 ...	0 -2 -1.00 0.6	5 3 0.04 ...	16 13 0.17 10.7#	0 0 -1.00 ...	0 0 -1.00 ...	0 0 -1.00 ...	0 0 0.00 ...	0 0 -1.00 ...	0 0 -1.00 ...	77
DRW10	25 13 0.19 3.6	22 0 -0.04 0.0	10 0 -0.10 0.0	0 -4 -1.00 1.1	5 4 0.05 ...	5 -3 -0.42 0.3	0 -1 -1.00 ...	0 -2 -1.00 ...	5 1 0.01 0.1	0 -1 -1.00 ...	0 -2 -1.00 0.6	5 2 0.03 ...	5 2 0.02 0.2	0 0 -1.00 ...	0 0 -1.00 ...	0 0 -1.00 ...	0 0 0.00 ...	0 0 -1.00 ...	0 0 -1.00 ...	82
DRW11	106 -67 -0.39 6.9#	419 72 0.08 4.5*	109 -58 -0.35 5.3*	54 -23 -0.31 1.7	21 2 0.02 0.1	207 76 0.08 10.0$	43 13 0.06 1.2	25 -12 -0.35 1.1	90 32 0.08 3.9*	17 -16 -0.51 2.0	41 -4 -0.11 0.1	31 -6 -0.18 0.3	54 4 0.01 0.1	16 0 -0.04 0.0	0 0 -1.00 ...	5 4 1.00 ...	0 0 0.00 ...	0 0 -1.00 ...	1 -4 -0.83 0.9	1239
DRW12	21 -8 -0.30 0.6	59 0 -0.02 0.0	36 7 0.04 0.4	10 -2 -0.26 0.2	5 2 0.01 0.2	16 -6 -0.29 0.4	14 9 0.04 3.0	5 -1 -0.25 0.1	31 21 0.10 8.0#	0 -5 -1.00 1.2	0 -7 -1.00 1.6	0 -6 -1.00 1.3	17 8 0.04 1.6	0 -2 -1.00 0.6	0 0 -1.00 ...	0 0 -1.00 ...	0 0 0.00 ...	0 0 -1.00 ...	0 0 -1.00 ...	214
DRW13	43 -33 -0.44 3.5	172 19 0.05 0.7	62 -11 -0.16 0.5	26 -7 -0.24 0.4	0 -7 -1.00 1.7	82 25 0.05 2.4	0 -12 -1.00 2.8	22 5 0.02 0.3	36 10 0.02 0.9	11 -3 -0.27 0.2	25 5 0.01 0.2	24 7 0.03 0.7	36 14 0.04 1.9	5 -1 -0.32 0.2	0 0 -1.00 ...	0 0 -1.00 ...	0 0 0.00 ...	0 0 -1.00 ...	0 -2 -1.00 0.5	544
DRW14	57 -23 -0.30 1.7	166 5 0.01 0.0	79 1 0.00 0.0	60 24 0.04 3.4	15 6 0.05 0.0	43 -17 -0.29 1.2	0 -13 -1.00 2.9	31 13 0.05 2.1	31 4 0.01 0.1	20 4 0.02 0.2	20 0 -0.07 0.0	18 0 0.00 0.0	20 -2 -0.14 0.1	5 -2 -0.36 0.2	5 4 0.47 ...	0 0 -1.00 ...	0 0 0.00 ...	0 0 -1.00 ...	5 2 0.05 0.4	575
DRX	71 -36 -0.34 3.1	241 26 0.05 0.9	90 -13 -0.14 0.5	69 41 0.07 7.6#	26 14 0.10 3.9*	58 -22 -0.28 1.5	10 -8 -0.46 0.9	34 10 0.04 0.9	28 -7 -0.23 0.4	18 -2 -0.16 0.1	29 0 0.00 0.0	19 -4 -0.19 0.2	38 7 0.02 0.3	7 -2 -0.32 0.2	0 0 -1.00 ...	0 0 -1.00 ...	0 0 0.00 ...	0 0 -1.00 ...	10 6 0.14 2.3	768
SUM	1408	2804	1359	629	150	1055	243	310	472	278	373	306	406	135	10	5	0	10	48	

Haplotype frequencies for population CAU

A-Bf ($N=675$)

	A1	A2	A3	A11	A23	A24	A25	A26	A28	A29	A30	A31	A32	AW33	AW34	AW36	AW43	AW66	AX	SUM
BF S	1459	2182	1017	611	59	637	208	237	358	89	237	228	252	74	15	15	0	15	30	7723
	77	55	-6	73	-20	-26	24	20	-30	-139	-37	-11	23	5	3	3	0	3	-16	
	0.19	0.09	-0.01	0.46	-0.26	-0.04	0.45	0.31	-0.08	-0.61	-0.14	-0.05	0.35	0.26	1.00	1.00	0.00	1.00	-0.36	
	1.6	0.6	0.0	3.2	1.6	0.4	0.0	0.6	0.8	26.2‡	1.6	0.2	0.7	0.1	0.3	0.3	...	0.3	1.9	
BF F	300	468	309	70	44	178	30	44	146	193	89	83	44	15	0	0	0	0	31	2044
	-65	-94	38	-71	23	2	-18	-12	43	132	16	19	-16	-2	-2	-2	0	-2	19	
	-0.18	-0.17	0.04	-0.51	0.28	0.00	-0.38	-0.23	0.11	0.56	0.06	0.08	-0.27	-0.18	-1.00	-1.00	0.00	-1.00	0.38	
	1.2	1.9	0.5	3.3	2.1	0.0	0.6	0.3	1.6	25.2‡	0.3	0.5	0.4	0.0	...	...	...	...	2.4	
BFF1	15	30	0	15	0	15	0	0	0	15	30	0	0	0	0	0	0	0	0	120
	-5	-2	-15	7	0	5	-2	-2	-5	11	26	-3	-3	0	0	0	0	0	0	
	-0.30	-0.09	-1.00	0.06	-1.00	0.04	-1.00	-1.00	-1.00	0.10	0.22	-1.00	-1.00	-1.00	-1.00	-1.00	0.00	-1.00	-1.00	
	0.2	0.0	1.3	0.4	...	0.2	...	...	...	...	...	...	...	...	...	...	...	...	...	
BFS07	15	59	0	0	0	30	0	0	0	0	0	0	0	0	0	0	0	0	0	104
	-3	30	-13	-6	0	21	-1	-2	-4	-2	-3	-2	-2	0	0	0	0	0	0	
	-0.19	0.40	-1.00	-1.00	-1.00	0.22	-1.00	-1.00	-1.00	-1.00	-1.00	-1.00	-1.00	-1.00	-1.00	-1.00	0.00	-1.00	-1.00	
	0.1	3.0	1.1	...	...	3.7	...	...	...	...	...	...	...	...	...	...	...	...	...	
BF V	0	15	0	0	0	0	0	0	0	0	0	0	0	0	0	0	0	0	0	15
	-2	11	-1	0	0	0	0	0	0	0	0	0	0	0	0	0	0	0	0	
	-1.00	1.00	-1.00	-1.00	-1.00	-1.00	-1.00	-1.00	-1.00	-1.00	-1.00	-1.00	-1.00	-1.00	-1.00	-1.00	0.00	-1.00	-1.00	
	...	...	...	...	...	...	...	...	...	...	...	...	...	...	...	...	...	...	...	
SUM	1789	2754	1326	696	103	860	238	281	504	297	356	311	296	89	15	15	0	15	61	

A-C2 ($N=344$)

	A1	A2	A3	A11	A23	A24	A25	A26	A28	A29	A30	A31	A32	AW33	AW34	AW36	AW43	AW66	AX	SUM
C2 1	1570	2558	1336	698	145	754	233	349	552	320	378	204	233	58	29	0	0	0	33	9450
	32	-103	-35	11	8	12	-14	19	3	18	21	11	13	3	2	0	0	0	2	
	0.35	-0.26	-0.08	0.27	1.00	0.28	-0.06	1.00	0.09	1.00	1.00	1.00	1.00	1.00	1.00	0.00	0.00	0.00	1.00	
	0.5	3.5	0.7	0.1	0.3	0.1	0.6	0.7	0.0	0.7	0.8	0.4	0.5	0.1	0.1	...	...	...	0.1	
C2 2	58	259	116	29	0	31	0	0	29	0	0	0	0	0	0	0	0	0	0	522
	-26	112	40	-8	-7	-9	-13	-17	0	-16	-19	-10	-11	-2	-1	0	0	0	-1	
	-0.32	0.30	0.09	-0.24	-1.00	-0.24	-1.00	-1.00	-0.04	-1.00	-1.00	-1.00	-1.00	-1.00	-1.00	0.00	0.00	0.00	-1.00	
	0.4	4.3*	0.9	0.1	...	0.1	...	0.7	0.0	0.6	0.7	...	...	...	...	...	...	...	...	
C2 3	0	0	0	0	0	0	0	0	0	0	0	0	0	0	0	0	0	0	0	0
	0	0	0	0	0	0	0	0	0	0	0	0	0	0	0	0	0	0	0	
	0.00	0.00	0.00	0.00	0.00	0.00	0.00	0.00	0.00	0.00	0.00	0.00	0.00	0.00	0.00	0.00	0.00	0.00	0.00	
	...	...	...	...	...	...	...	...	...	...	...	...	...	...	...	...	...	...	...	
C2 V	0	0	0	0	0	0	29	0	0	0	0	0	0	0	0	0	0	0	0	29
	-4	-7	-3	-1	0	-1	28	0	-1	0	0	0	0	0	0	0	0	0	0	
	-1.00	-1.00	-1.00	-1.00	-1.00	-1.00	1.00	-1.00	-1.00	-1.00	-1.00	-1.00	-1.00	-1.00	-1.00	0.00	0.00	0.00	-1.00	
	...	...	...	...	...	...	...	...	...	...	...	...	...	...	...	...	...	...	...	
SUM	1628	2817	1452	727	145	785	262	349	581	320	378	204	233	58	29	0	0	0	33	

Haplotype frequencies for population CAU
A-DP ($N = 117$)

	DPW1	DPW2	DPW3	DPW4	DPW5	DPW6	DPX	SUM
A1	237	159	81	690	61	0	291	1539
	171	-39	13	64	14	0	-221	
	0.47	-0.20	0.03	0.07	0.04	0.00	-0.43	
	6.4*	0.1	0.0	0.2	0.0	...	1.0	
A2	43	588	93	1261	218	0	1172	3375
	-100	152	-55	-111	70	0	46	
	-0.70	0.18	-0.38	-0.08	0.24	0.00	0.02	
	1.3	1.1	0.4	0.3	0.6	...	0.1	
A3	0	45	43	525	44	0	541	1198
	-50	-109	-9	38	-7	0	141	
	-1.00	-0.71	-0.19	0.05	-0.16	0.00	0.18	
	0.7	1.2	0.0	0.1	0.0	...	0.0	
A11	0	43	132	103	0	0	150	428
	-17	-11	113	-70	-18	0	7	
	-1.00	-0.22	0.28	-0.41	-1.00	0.00	0.03	
	...	0.0	...	0.6	...	...	0.0	
A23	43	0	0	114	0	0	14	171
	36	-21	-7	44	-6	0	-42	
	0.22	-1.00	-1.00	0.44	-1.00	0.00	-0.75	
	...	...	...	0.6	...	...	0.6	
A24	19	166	47	419	0	0	290	941
	-20	45	5	36	-40	0	-23	
	-0.53	0.05	0.01	0.06	-1.00	0.00	-0.08	
	...	0.2	...	0.1	...	...	0.0	
A25	0	85	46	43	85	0	82	341
	-14	41	31	-95	70	0	-31	
	-1.00	0.14	0.09	-0.69	0.21	0.00	-0.28	
	...	0.5	...	1.3	...	...	0.2	
A26	85	0	0	105	0	0	23	213
	76	-26	-8	18	-6	0	-47	
	0.37	-1.00	-1.00	0.15	-1.00	0.00	-0.68	
	...	...	...	0.1	...	...	0.6	
A28	0	70	0	304	0	0	139	513
	-21	4	-22	95	-21	0	-31	
	-1.00	0.01	-1.00	0.31	-1.00	0.00	-0.19	
	...	0.0	...	0.9	...	...	0.1	
A29	0	0	0	103	0	0	239	342
	-14	-43	-14	-35	-14	0	125	
	-1.00	-1.00	-1.00	-0.26	-1.00	0.00	0.55	
	...	0.6	...	0.2	...	...	2.5	
A30	0	50	0	0	0	0	35	85
	-3	39	-3	-34	-3	0	7	
	-1.00	0.53	-1.00	-1.00	-1.00	0.00	0.12	
	...	...	...	...	...	...	...	
A31	0	85	0	110	9	0	223	427
	-17	30	-18	-63	-9	0	81	
	-1.00	0.08	-1.00	-0.37	-0.52	0.00	0.28	
	...	0.2	...	0.5	...	...	0.8	
A32	0	0	0	145	0	0	25	170
	-6	-21	-7	76	-6	0	-31	
	-1.00	-1.00	-1.00	0.75	-1.00	0.00	-0.56	
	...	...	...	1.7	...	...	0.3	
AW33	0	0	0	146	0	0	25	171
	-6	-21	-7	76	-6	0	-31	
	-1.00	-1.00	-1.00	0.75	-1.00	0.00	-0.56	
	...	...	...	1.7	...	...	0.3	
AW34	0	0	0	0	0	0	85	85
	-3	-10	-3	-34	-3	0	57	
	-1.00	-1.00	-1.00	-1.00	-1.00	0.00	1.00	
	...	...	...	...	...	...	...	
AW36	0	0	0	0	0	0	0	0
	0	0	0	0	0	0	0	
	0.00	0.00	0.00	0.00	0.00	0.00	0.00	
	...	...	...	...	...	...	...	
AW43	0	0	0	0	0	0	0	0
	0	0	0	0	0	0	0	
	0.00	0.00	0.00	0.00	0.00	0.00	0.00	
	...	...	...	...	...	...	...	
AW66	0	0	0	0	0	0	0	0
	0	0	0	0	0	0	0	
	0.00	0.00	0.00	0.00	0.00	0.00	0.00	
	...	...	...	...	...	...	...	
AX	0	0	0	0	1	0	1	2
	0	0	0	0	1	0	0	
	-1.00	-1.00	-1.00	-1.00	0.48	0.00	0.25	
	...	...	...	...	...	...	...	
SUM	427	1291	442	4068	438	0	3335	

Haplotype frequencies for population CAU; A-C4A ($N = 541$)

	C4 A1	C4A12	C4A13	C4 A2	C4 A3	C4 A4	C4A51	C4 A6	C4AQ0	SUM
A1	0 -5 -1.00 ...	0 0 0.00 ...	18 9 0.20 ...	55 -49 -0.47 1.6	858 -284 -0.25 15.3¢	74 -25 -0.26 0.5	0 -2 -1.00 ...	150 87 0.27 8.1#	483 275 0.26 27.0¢	1638
A2	16 9 0.32 0.6	0 0 0.00 ...	16 4 0.09 0.1	142 -26 -0.16 0.3	1869 27 0.03 0.1	183 22 0.05 0.2	18 13 1.00 ...	122 20 0.07 0.3	268 -65 -0.20 1.1	2638
A3	0 -4 -1.00 ...	0 0 0.00 ...	0 -7 -1.00 ...	148 52 0.10 1.9	1157 104 0.23 2.2	92 0 0.00 0.0	0 -2 -1.00 ...	0 -57 -1.00 3.8*	111 -79 -0.42 2.5	1508
A11	0 -2 -1.00 ...	0 0 0.00 ...	0 -3 -1.00 ...	74 28 0.05 1.1	452 -50 -0.10 0.0	74 30 0.05 1.3	0 0 -1.00 ...	16 -11 -0.42 0.3	104 13 0.02 0.1	720
A23	0 0 -1.00 ...	0 0 0.00 ...	0 0 -1.00 ...	0 -7 -1.00 ...	129 39 1.00 3.1	0 -7 -1.00 ...	0 0 -1.00 ...	0 -4 -1.00 ...	0 -15 -1.00 1.0	129
A24	0 -2 -1.00 ...	0 0 0.00 ...	0 -3 -1.00 ...	37 -13 -0.27 0.2	597 43 0.18 0.6	94 46 0.08 2.7	0 0 -1.00 ...	25 -5 -0.16 0.1	41 -59 -0.59 2.4	794
A25	0 0 -1.00 ...	0 0 0.00 ...	0 -1 -1.00 ...	0 -18 -1.00 1.1	203 -3 -0.02 0.0	56 38 0.14 4.7*	0 0 -1.00 ...	18 7 0.02 0.2	19 -18 -0.49 0.6	296
A26	0 0 -1.00 ...	0 0 0.00 ...	0 0 -1.00 ...	18 0 0.00 0.0	217 24 0.29 0.6	18 1 0.00 0.0	0 0 -1.00 ...	0 -10 -1.00 0.6	23 -11 -0.34 0.3	276
A28	18 16 0.47 ...	0 0 0.00 ...	0 -2 -1.00 ...	55 24 0.05 1.2	327 -6 -0.02 0.0	18 -10 -0.38 0.3	0 0 -1.00 ...	0 -17 -1.00 1.1	61 0 0.00 0.0	479
A29	0 0 -1.00 ...	0 0 0.00 ...	0 -1 -1.00 ...	18 -6 -0.27 0.1	294 24 0.20 0.4	0 -23 -1.00 1.4	0 0 -1.00 ...	0 -14 -1.00 0.9	75 26 0.08 0.9	387
A30	0 0 -1.00 ...	0 0 0.00 ...	0 -1 -1.00 ...	18 -2 -0.15 0.0	264 53 0.53 2.2	0 -19 -1.00 1.2	0 0 -1.00 ...	18 5 0.02 0.1	11 -30 -0.74 1.5	331
A31	0 0 -1.00 ...	0 0 0.00 ...	18 16 0.31 ...	18 -2 -0.15 0.0	257 26 0.26 0.5	0 -19 -1.00 1.2	0 0 -1.00 ...	18 5 0.02 0.1	20 -21 -0.52 0.7	331
A32	0 0 -1.00 ...	0 0 0.00 ...	0 -1 -1.00 ...	0 -18 -1.00 1.1	258 52 0.58 2.4	0 -17 -1.00 1.1	0 0 -1.00 ...	18 7 0.02 0.2	19 -17 -0.49 0.6	295
AW33	0 0 -1.00 ...	0 0 0.00 ...	0 0 -1.00 ...	37 32 0.47 ...	36 -15 -0.30 0.9	0 -4 -1.00 ...	0 0 -1.00 ...	0 -2 -1.00 ...	1 -7 -0.89 0.5	74
AW34	0 0 -1.00 ...	0 0 0.00 ...	0 0 -1.00 ...	0 0 -1.00 ...	9 -3 -0.26 0.2	0 0 -1.00 ...	0 0 -1.00 ...	0 0 -1.00 ...	9 7 0.43 ...	18
AW36	0 0 -1.00 ...	0 0 0.00 ...	0 0 -1.00 ...	0 0 -1.00 ...	0 -12 -1.00 2.3	0 0 -1.00 ...	0 0 -1.00 ...	0 0 -1.00 ...	18 16 1.00 ...	18
AW43	0 0 0.00 ...	0 0 0.00 ...	0 0 0.00 ...	0 0 0.00 ...	0 0 0.00 ...	0 0 0.00 ...	0 0 0.00 ...	0 0 0.00 ...	0 0 0.00 ...	0
AW66	0 0 0.00 ...	0 0 0.00 ...	0 0 0.00 ...	0 0 0.00 ...	0 0 0.00 ...	0 0 0.00 ...	0 0 0.00 ...	0 0 0.00 ...	0 0 0.00 ...	0
AX	0 0 -1.00 ...	0 0 0.00 ...	0 0 -1.00 ...	19 13 0.28 ...	34 -5 -0.16 0.2	0 -3 -1.00 ...	0 0 -1.00 ...	0 -1 -1.00 ...	5 -1 -0.32 ...	58
SUM	36	0	54	639	6981	609	18	385	1268	

Haplotype frequencies for population CAU
A-C4B ($N=540$)

	C4 B1	C4B11	C4B12	C4 B2	C4 B3	C4 B4	C4 B5	C4B51	C4 B6	C4 B7	C4BQ0	SUM
A1	1344 149 0.32 4.3*	0 -2 -1.00 ...	0 -2 -1.00 ...	93 -60 -0.40 1.7	74 25 0.10 0.8	0 -5 -1.00 ...	19 7 0.10 0.2	0 -2 -1.00 ...	19 13 0.42 ...	19 16 1.00 ...	96 -132 -0.58 5.8*	1664
A2	1755 -143 -0.08 2.9	0 -4 -1.00 ...	19 14 1.00 ...	276 31 0.05 0.3	74 -4 -0.06 0.0	0 -9 -1.00 0.7	18 -1 -0.09 0.0	0 -4 -1.00 ...	18 8 0.30 0.5	0 -4 -1.00 ...	484 120 0.12 3.4	2644
A3	1079 -17 -0.02 0.1	0 -2 -1.00 ...	0 -2 -1.00 ...	148 7 0.01 0.0	19 -25 -0.58 1.0	19 13 0.41 ...	0 -10 -1.00 0.7	0 -2 -1.00 ...	0 -5 -1.00 ...	0 -2 -1.00 ...	262 52 0.04 0.9	1527
A11	390 -115 -0.23 5.5*	0 0 -1.00 ...	0 0 -1.00 ...	115 50 0.08 2.4	0 -20 -1.00 1.3	0 -2 -1.00 ...	19 14 0.20 ...	0 0 -1.00 ...	0 -2 -1.00 ...	0 0 -1.00 ...	180 83 0.14 4.8*	704
A23	103 10 0.26 0.2	0 0 -1.00 ...	0 0 -1.00 ...	0 -11 -1.00 0.7	0 -3 -1.00 ...	0 0 -1.00 ...	0 0 -1.00 ...	0 0 -1.00 ...	0 0 -1.00 ...	0 0 -1.00 ...	27 9 0.08 0.3	130
A24	624 52 0.23 0.0	0 -1 -1.00 ...	0 -1 -1.00 ...	94 20 0.03 0.4	37 13 0.05 0.5	0 -2 -1.00 ...	0 -5 -1.00 ...	0 0 -1.00 ...	0 -2 -1.00 ...	0 -1 -1.00 ...	41 -68 -0.63 2.9	796
A25	238 51 0.70 2.8	0 0 -1.00 ...	0 0 -1.00 ...	19 -4 -0.21 0.1	0 -7 -1.00 ...	0 0 -1.00 ...	0 -1 -1.00 ...	0 0 -1.00 ...	0 0 -1.00 ...	0 0 -1.00 ...	3 -32 -0.92 1.9	260
A26	239 26 0.31 0.6	0 0 -1.00 ...	0 0 -1.00 ...	19 -7 -0.31 0.2	0 -8 -1.00 ...	0 0 -1.00 ...	19 17 0.23 ...	0 0 -1.00 ...	0 0 -1.00 ...	0 0 -1.00 ...	20 -20 -0.51 0.7	297
A28	331 -26 -0.08 0.4	0 0 -1.00 ...	0 0 -1.00 ...	83 37 0.08 1.8	0 -14 -1.00 0.9	0 -1 -1.00 ...	0 -3 -1.00 ...	18 17 1.00 ...	0 -1 -1.00 ...	0 0 -1.00 ...	67 -1 -0.02 0.0	499
A29	296 30 0.28 0.7	19 18 1.00 ...	0 0 -1.00 ...	19 -14 -0.45 0.4	18 7 0.02 0.3	0 0 -1.00 ...	0 -2 -1.00 ...	0 0 -1.00 ...	0 0 -1.00 ...	0 0 -1.00 ...	19 -31 -0.63 1.3	371
A30	276 49 0.55 2.1	0 0 -1.00 ...	0 0 -1.00 ...	9 -19 -0.69 0.9	19 10 0.03 0.6	0 0 -1.00 ...	0 -1 -1.00 ...	0 0 -1.00 ...	0 0 -1.00 ...	0 0 -1.00 ...	12 -31 -0.72 1.5	316
A31	214 -24 -0.11 0.5	0 0 -1.00 ...	0 0 -1.00 ...	19 -11 -0.38 0.3	37 27 0.09 4.3*	0 0 -1.00 ...	0 -1 -1.00 ...	0 0 -1.00 ...	0 0 -1.00 ...	0 0 -1.00 ...	63 17 0.06 0.4	333
A32	201 -11 -0.05 0.1	0 0 -1.00 ...	0 0 -1.00 ...	12 -14 -0.56 0.5	0 -8 -1.00 ...	0 0 -1.00 ...	0 -1 -1.00 ...	0 0 -1.00 ...	0 0 -1.00 ...	0 0 -1.00 ...	83 42 0.17 2.8	296
AW33	37 -16 -0.31 1.0	0 0 -1.00 ...	0 0 -1.00 ...	19 12 0.18 ...	0 -1 -1.00 ...	19 19 0.50 ...	0 0 -1.00 ...	0 0 -1.00 ...	0 0 -1.00 ...	0 0 -1.00 ...	0 -9 -1.00 0.7	75
AW34	12 0 -0.07 0.0	0 0 -1.00 ...	0 0 -1.00 ...	0 -1 -1.00 ...	0 0 -1.00 ...	0 0 -1.00 ...	0 0 -1.00 ...	0 0 -1.00 ...	0 0 -1.00 ...	0 0 -1.00 ...	6 4 0.23 ...	18

Haplotype frequencies for population CAU
A-C4B ($N = 540$)

	C4 B1	C4B11	C4B12	C4 B2	C4 B3	C4 B4	C4 B5	C4B51	C4 B6	C4 B7	C4BQ0	SUM
AW36	0 -13 -1.00 2.6	0 0 -1.00 ...	0 0 -1.00 ...	0 -1 -1.00 ...	19 18 1.00 ...	0 0 -1.00 ...	0 0 -1.00 ...	0 0 -1.00 ...	0 0 -1.00 ...	0 0 -1.00 ...	0 -2 -1.00 ...	19
AW43	0 0 0.00 ...	0 0 0.00 ...	0 0 0.00 ...	0 0 0.00 ...	0 0 0.00 ...	0 0 0.00 ...	0 0 0.00 ...	0 0 0.00 ...	0 0 0.00 ...	0 0 0.00 ...	0 0 0.00 ...	0
AW66	0 0 0.00 ...	0 0 0.00 ...	0 0 0.00 ...	0 0 0.00 ...	0 0 0.00 ...	0 0 0.00 ...	0 0 0.00 ...	0 0 0.00 ...	0 0 0.00 ...	0 0 0.00 ...	0 0 0.00 ...	0
AX	44 2 0.14 0.0	0 0 -1.00 ...	0 0 -1.00 ...	0 -4 -1.00 ...	0 -1 -1.00 ...	0 0 -1.00 ...	0 0 -1.00 ...	0 0 -1.00 ...	0 0 -1.00 ...	0 0 -1.00 ...	14 6 0.12 ...	58
SUM	7183	19	19	925	297	38	75	18	37	19	1377	

Haplotype frequencies for population CAU; B-C ($N = 2080$)

	CW1	CW2	CW3	CW4	CW5	CW6	CW7	CW8	CX	SUM
B7	0 -36 -1.00 9.1#	0 -46 -1.00 11.5$	24 -118 -0.83 26.7$	4 -128 -0.97 33.3$	14 -67 -0.83 14.1$	13 -84 -0.87 18.8$	958 677 0.78 507.4$	0 -42 -1.00 10.5#	135 -150 -0.53 24.9$	1148
B8	0 -30 -1.00 7.4#	0 -38 -1.00 9.4#	5 -114 -0.96 28.9$	0 -110 -1.00 29.0$	5 -62 -0.93 14.5$	0 -81 -1.00 20.5$	738 503 0.69 328.0$	0 -35 -1.00 8.6#	212 -26 -0.11 0.9	960
B13	0 -9 -1.00 2.1	0 -11 -1.00 2.7	0 -36 -1.00 9.1#	0 -33 -1.00 8.4#	0 -20 -1.00 4.9*	262 237 0.87 520.2$	19 -53 -0.74 11.3$	0 -10 -1.00 2.5	16 -57 -0.78 12.0$	297
B18	1 -16 -0.94 3.7	5 -17 -0.78 3.2	1 -68 -0.99 17.0$	0 -64 -1.00 16.1$	92 52 0.10 16.4$	6 -40 -0.87 8.7#	166 29 0.07 1.8	0 -20 -1.00 4.8*	287 148 0.35 46.3$	558
B27	101 90 0.29 155.7$	213 199 0.59 613.9$	34 -9 -0.23 0.6	0 -40 -1.00 9.0#	5 -19 -0.80 3.7	0 -29 -1.00 7.1#	0 -85 -1.00 24.7$	0 -12 -1.00 2.0	0 -87 -1.00 25.2$	353
B35	19 -15 -0.45 1.7	10 -32 -0.77 6.3*	47 -85 -0.65 14.7$	890 767 0.82 999.9$	5 -69 -0.93 16.5$	10 -79 -0.89 18.2$	6 -253 -0.98 76.5$	0 -39 -1.00 9.6#	76 -188 -0.71 41.7$	1063
B37	5 0 -0.03 0.0	0 -6 -1.00 1.4	0 -19 -1.00 4.8*	0 -17 -1.00 4.4*	5 -5 -0.56 0.8	130 116 0.80 231.9$	0 -38 -1.00 10.9$	0 -5 -1.00 1.3	19 -20 -0.52 3.0	159
B38	0 -7 -1.00 1.8	0 -9 -1.00 2.3	2 -28 -0.94 6.6*	5 -23 -0.83 4.6*	0 -17 -1.00 4.1*	0 -20 -1.00 4.9*	13 -47 -0.79 10.7#	0 -8 -1.00 2.1	229 167 0.89 127.8$	249
B39	5 -1 -0.24 0.1	0 -7 -1.00 1.8	1 -23 -0.96 5.6*	5 -17 -0.79 3.5	5 -8 -0.65 1.4	0 -16 -1.00 3.0*	69 20 0.13 2.2	0 -7 -1.00 1.7	117 67 0.44 25.0$	202
BW41	0 -2 -1.00 0.6	0 -3 -1.00 0.8	0 -10 -1.00 2.6	10 0 -0.01 0.0	0 -5 -1.00 1.4	0 -6 -1.00 1.7	12 -8 -0.44 1.1	0 -2 -1.00 0.7	65 43 0.66 24.2$	87
BW42	0 0 -1.00 ...	5 4 0.17 ...	5 2 0.10 0.3	0 -2 -1.00 0.7	0 -1 -1.00 ...	0 -1 -1.00 ...	7 1 0.06 0.1	0 0 -1.00 ...	7 1 0.06 0.0	24
B44	1 -38 -0.98 9.4#	34 -16 -0.33 1.4	39 -115 -0.75 23.5$	106 -37 -0.26 2.7	535 447 0.72 579.4$	4 -100 -0.96 25.3$	135 -168 -0.56 29.5$	0 -45 -1.00 11.4$	387 78 0.08 6.2*	1241
B45	0 0 -1.00 ...	0 -1 -1.00 ...	0 -4 -1.00 1.3	5 0 -0.02 0.0	0 -2 -1.00 0.7	29 25 0.63 38.0$	5 -5 -0.54 0.9	0 -1 -1.00 ...	5 -5 -0.54 0.9	44
BW46	0 0 -1.00 ...	0 0 -1.00 ...	3 2 0.54 ...	0 0 -1.00 ...	0 0 -1.00 ...	0 0 -1.00 ...	0 0 -1.00 ...	0 0 -1.00 ...	2 1 0.20 ...	5
BW47	0 0 -1.00 ...	0 0 -1.00 ...	0 -1 -1.00 0.6	0 -1 -1.00 ...	0 0 -1.00 ...	10 8 0.45 ...	0 -4 -1.00 1.4	0 0 -1.00 ...	10 5 0.33 1.4	20

	CW1	CW2	CW3	CW4	CW5	CW6	CW7	CW8	CX	SUM
BW48	0 0 0.00 ...	0 0 0.00 ...	0 0 0.00 ...	0 0 0.00 ...	0 0 0.00 ...	0 0 0.00 ...	0 0 0.00 ...	0 0 0.00 ...	0 0 0.00 ...	0
B49	0 -5 -1.00 1.3	0 -6 -1.00 1.6	0 -21 -1.00 5.3*	5 -15 -0.76 2.8	0 -12 -1.00 2.9	0 -14 -1.00 3.5	123 80 0.60 41.1$	0 -6 -1.00 1.5	49 5 0.04 0.2	177
BW50	0 -3 -1.00 0.8	0 -4 -1.00 1.0	0 -13 -1.00 3.5	10 -2 -0.26 0.2	5 -2 -0.39 0.3	91 81 0.76 153.6$	0 -27 -1.00 7.9#	0 -3 -1.00 0.9	10 -18 -0.65 3.5	116
B51	67 47 0.15 25.3$	39 14 0.04 1.7	10 -66 -0.87 14.7$	27 -44 -0.62 6.9#	19 -24 -0.57 3.3	6 -45 -0.89 9.9#	28 -122 -0.81 29.3$	0 -22 -1.00 5.3*	420 267 0.58 136.8$	616
BW52	0 -5 -1.00 1.4	0 -7 -1.00 1.7	2 -21 -0.92 4.9*	11 -10 -0.51 1.4	0 -13 -1.00 3.1	0 -15 -1.00 3.8	23 -23 -0.51 3.5	0 -6 -1.00 1.6	157 109 0.75 69.7$	193
BW53	5 3 0.07 ...	0 -1 -1.00 ...	0 -5 -1.00 1.5	29 23 0.54 22.6$	0 -2 -1.00 0.8	5 1 0.02 0.0	0 -11 -1.00 3.3	0 -1 -1.00 ...	10 -1 -0.18 0.1	49
BW54	0 0 -1.00 ...	0 0 -1.00 ...	0 0 -1.00 ...	0 0 -1.00 ...	0 0 -1.00 ...	0 0 -1.00 ...	0 0 -1.00 ...	0 0 -1.00 ...	5 4 1.00 ...	5
BW55	24 19 0.13 15.7$	0 -5 -1.00 1.4	128 109 0.81 148.6$	0 -17 -1.00 4.3*	0 -10 -1.00 2.5	0 -12 -1.00 3.0	0 -37 -1.00 10.5#	0 -5 -1.00 1.3	2 -35 -0.95 9.7#	154
BW56	82 79 0.76 385.3$	0 -3 -1.00 0.0	5 -7 -0.63 1.3	0 -11 -1.00 2.0	0 -7 -1.00 1.7	0 -8 -1.00 2.1	15 -10 -0.43 1.3	0 -3 -1.00 0.9	5 -21 -0.81 4.9*	107
BW57	0 -9 -1.00 2.1	0 -11 -1.00 2.7	0 -36 -1.00 8.0#	5 -28 -0.85 6.0*	0 -20 -1.00 4.6*	264 239 0.89 535.4$	16 -55 -0.78 12.4$	0 -10 -1.00 2.4	9 -63 -0.88 16.1$	294
BW58	0 -5 -1.00 1.2	0 -6 -1.00 1.5	48 27 0.18 8.2#	0 -19 -1.00 4.7*	10 -1 -0.17 0.1	10 -3 -0.31 0.3	39 -2 -0.06 0.0	0 -5 -1.00 1.4	63 21 0.16 2.8	170
BW59	0 0 0.00 ...	0 0 0.00 ...	0 0 0.00 ...	0 0 0.00 ...	0 0 0.00 ...	0 0 0.00 ...	0 0 0.00 ...	0 0 0.00 ...	0 0 0.00 ...	0
BW60	0 -11 -1.00 2.7	0 -14 -1.00 3.5	338 291 0.88 445.9$	0 -43 -1.00 10.7#	5 -21 -0.81 4.1*	0 -31 -1.00 7.5#	5 -86 -0.95 23.6$	0 -13 -1.00 3.2	28 -65 -0.70 13.2$	376
BW61	5 -1 -0.24 0.1	98 90 0.46 215.7$	14 -10 -0.44 1.2	6 -16 -0.74 3.1	5 -8 -0.65 1.4	0 -16 -1.00 3.0*	5 -43 -0.90 11.2$	0 -7 -1.00 1.7	69 19 0.12 1.0	202
BW62	10 -9 -0.50 1.2	5 -19 -0.80 3.8	527 449 0.83 660.6$	43 -28 -0.40 2.9	0 -43 -1.00 10.5#	0 -52 -1.00 12.8$	10 -141 -0.93 38.0$	0 -22 -1.00 5.4*	26 -128 -0.83 31.6$	621

Halotype frequencies for population CAU; B-C ($N = 2080$)

	CW1	CW2	CW3	CW4	CW5	CW6	CW7	CW8	CX	SUM
BW63	0 -1 -1.00 ...	0 -2 -1.00 0.6	5 -2 -0.36 0.2	0 -6 -1.00 1.7	0 -3 -1.00 1.0	5 0 -0.07 0.0	27 12 0.24 2.4	0 -1 -1.00 ...	26 10 0.22 1.9	63
BW64	0 -3 -1.00 0.8	0 -4 -1.00 0.0	0 -13 -1.00 3.3	0 -12 -1.00 3.1	0 -7 -1.00 1.8	0 -8 -1.00 2.2	0 -26 -1.00 7.6#	110 106 0.99 589.7$	1 -26 -0.96 7.2#	111
BW65	0 -8 -1.00 1.9	0 -10 -1.00 2.4	0 -32 -1.00 8.0#	0 -30 -1.00 7.4#	0 -18 -1.00 4.3*	0 -21 -1.00 5.2*	0 -64 -1.00 18.3$	264 254 1.00 999.9$	0 -65 -1.00 18.7$	264
BW67	0 0 0.00 ...	0 0 0.00 ...	0 0 0.00 ...	0 0 0.00 ...	0 0 0.00 ...	0 0 0.00 ...	0 0 0.00 ...	0 0 0.00 ...	0 0 0.00 ...	0
BW71	0 0 -1.00 ...	0 0 -1.00 ...	0 0 -1.00 ...	0 0 -1.00 ...	0 0 -1.00 ...	0 0 -1.00 ...	5 4 1.00 ...	0 0 -1.00 ...	0 0 -1.00 ...	5
BW72	0 0 -1.00 ...	0 0 -1.00 ...	5 1 0.05 0.1	0 -2 -1.00 0.8	0 -1 -1.00 ...	0 -1 -1.00 0.6	14 7 0.32 1.9	0 0 -1.00 ...	10 3 0.13 0.3	29
BW73	0 0 -1.00 ...	0 0 -1.00 ...	5 3 0.24 ...	0 -1 -1.00 ...	0 0 -1.00 ...	0 0 -1.00 ...	10 6 0.56 3.0	0 0 -1.00 ...	0 -3 -1.00 1.0	15
BX	0 0 -1.00 ...	0 -1 -1.00 ...	0 -4 -1.00 1.1	0 -3 -1.00 1.0	0 -2 -1.00 0.6	5 2 0.05 0.2	0 -8 -1.00 2.6	0 0 -1.00 ...	33 24 0.82 16.3$	38
SUM	325	409	1248	1161	710	850	2448	374	2490	

Haplotype frequencies for population CAU
B-DR (N= 1900)

	DR1	DR2	DR3	DR4	DR7	DRW8	DRW9	DRW10	DRW11	DRW12	DRW13	DRW14	DRX	SUM
B7	72 -35 -0.34 2.9	544 368 0.39 194.9$	31 -104 -0.77 19.7$	138 -5 -0.04 0.1	42 -89 -0.68 14.9$	37 3 0.01 0.1	0 -7 -1.00 1.8	0 -8 -1.00 1.0	79 -61 -0.44 6.6*	15 -8 -0.39 0.8	26 -34 -0.57 4.5*	63 0 -0.02 0.0	72 -9 -0.13 0.3	1119
B8	19 -74 -0.80 13.9$	48 -103 -0.69 17.9$	731 613 0.72 766.0$	42 -82 -0.66 13.2$	16 -97 -0.86 20.1$	21 -7 -0.28 0.5	5 -1 -0.30 0.1	0 -7 -1.00 1.7	12 -109 -0.90 23.8$	0 -20 -1.00 4.5*	11 -40 -0.79 7.3#	28 -26 -0.50 3.0	35 -35 -0.51 4.2*	968
B13	8 -20 -0.72 3.2	11 -34 -0.76 6.3*	10 -25 -0.72 4.2*	7 -30 -0.82 5.7*	195 160 0.62 163.6$	0 -8 -1.00 1.8	0 -1 -1.00 ...	5 3 0.03 ...	16 -20 -0.57 2.7	0 -5 -1.00 1.3	5 -10 -0.69 1.6	18 1 0.00 0.0	20 -1 -0.08 0.0	295
B18	28 -28 -0.51 3.3	121 28 0.06 2.1	125 53 0.10 9.2#	42 -33 -0.45 3.5	25 -44 -0.64 6.5*	5 -12 -0.72 1.9	5 1 0.01 0.0	0 -4 -1.00 0.0	162 88 0.17 24.1$	11 -1 -0.14 0.1	14 -17 -0.56 2.1	15 -16 -0.56 2.2	36 -6 -0.17 0.3	589
B27	60 25 0.08 3.0*	52 -4 -0.08 0.1	22 -21 -0.50 2.4	65 19 0.06 1.7	5 -36 -0.88 7.4#	10 0 -0.07 0.0	11 8 0.12 5.2*	0 -2 -1.00 0.6	47 2 0.01 0.0	16 8 0.04 1.7	31 12 0.03 1.4	2 -18 -0.90 3.5	38 12 0.03 1.1	359
B35	292 191 0.22 84.7$	100 -63 -0.39 6.3*	59 -67 -0.53 8.7#	106 -27 -0.21 1.4	42 -80 -0.66 12.8$	42 11 0.04 0.8	5 -2 -0.35 0.2	5 -3 -0.42 0.3	150 19 0.02 0.7	26 3 0.02 0.1	57 1 0.00 0.0	50 -9 -0.16 0.4	109 32 0.05 3.1	1043
B37	6 -9 -0.62 1.3	21 -4 -0.19 0.2	5 -14 -0.75 2.5	16 -4 -0.24 0.3	5 -13 -0.74 2.3	16 11 0.07 4.9*	0 0 -1.00 ...	51 50 0.62 ...	16 -4 -0.22 0.2	0 -3 -1.00 0.7	27 18 0.12 7.6#	0 -8 -1.00 1.9	1 -10 -0.92 2.1	164
B38	32 7 0.03 0.4	13 -27 -0.68 4.4*	13 -17 -0.59 2.4	45 12 0.05 0.9	6 -23 -0.80 4.3*	9 1 0.00 0.0	0 -1 -1.00 ...	0 -1 -1.00 ...	18 -13 -0.44 1.4	5 0 -0.11 0.0	42 28 0.11 11.6$	53 38 0.16 20.4$	22 3 0.01 0.1	258
B39	23 3 0.02 0.1	55 23 0.13 3.7	5 -19 -0.80 3.5	14 -11 -0.47 1.3	11 -12 -0.54 1.6	26 20 0.10 12.8$	0 -1 -1.00 ...	0 -1 -1.00 ...	29 3 0.02 0.1	3 0 -0.33 0.1	5 -5 -0.55 0.7	5 -6 -0.57 0.8	28 13 0.07 2.4	204
BW41	0 -9 -1.00 2.1	11 -4 -0.30 0.3	11 0 -0.09 0.0	20 7 0.08 0.9	5 -6 -0.58 0.9	0 -2 -1.00 0.6	0 0 -1.00 ...	0 0 -1.00 ...	26 13 0.15 3.1	0 -1 -1.00 ...	5 0 -0.08 0.0	5 0 -0.13 0.0	17 10 0.10 2.6	100
BW42	0 -2 -1.00 ...	15 11 0.50 6.6*	5 2 0.08 0.2	0 -2 -1.00 0.7	0 -2 -1.00 0.7	0 0 -1.00 ...	0 0 -1.00 ...	0 0 -1.00 ...	0 -2 -1.00 0.7	0 0 -1.00 ...	5 4 0.15 ...	0 0 -1.00 ...	1 0 -0.48 ...	26
B44	67 -51 -0.44 5.5*	111 -82 -0.43 9.1#	41 -107 -0.73 19.4$	280 122 0.11 23.3$	287 142 0.14 34.1$	18 -18 -0.51 2.2	16 7 0.11 1.1	5 -4 -0.50 0.6	187 33 0.03 1.7	41 14 0.07 1.7	52 -13 -0.22 0.7	52 -17 -0.26 1.1	72 -17 -0.20 0.9	1229
B45	0 -3 -1.00 0.9	10 3 0.10 0.4	5 0 -0.02 0.0	5 0 -0.07 0.0	11 6 0.16 1.6	0 0 -1.00 ...	0 0 -1.00 ...	0 0 -1.00 ...	0 -4 -1.00 1.2	0 0 -1.00 ...	0 -1 -1.00 ...	5 3 0.07 ...	6 3 0.07 0.6	42
BW46	0 0 -1.00 ...	0 0 -1.00 ...	0 0 -1.00 ...	0 0 -1.00 ...	0 0 -1.00 ...	0 0 -1.00 ...	0 0 -1.00 ...	0 0 -1.00 ...	0 0 -1.00 ...	0 0 -1.00 ...	5 5 1.00 ...	0 0 -1.00 ...	0 0 -1.00 ...	5
BW47	0 -2 -1.00 ...	0 -3 -1.00 0.9	0 -2 -1.00 0.7	11 8 0.34 3.8	0 -2 -1.00 0.7	0 0 -1.00 ...	0 0 -1.00 ...	0 0 -1.00 ...	5 2 0.08 0.2	0 0 -1.00 ...	5 4 0.15 ...	5 4 0.14 ...	0 -1 -1.00 ...	26

Haplotype frequencies for population CAU
B-DR ($N = 1900$)

	DR1	DR2	DR3	DR4	DR7	DRW8	DRW9	DRW10	DRW11	DRW12	DRW13	DRW14	DRX	SUM
BW48	0 0 0.00 ...	0 0 0.00 ...	0 0 0.00 ...	0 0 0.00 ...	0 0 0.00 ...	0 0 0.00 ...	0 0 0.00 ...	0 0 0.00 ...	0 0 0.00 ...	0 0 0.00 ...	0 0 0.00 ...	0 0 0.00 ...	0 0 0.00 ...	0
B49	29 11 0.07 1.5	16 -12 -0.45 1.4	9 -12 -0.60 1.8	42 18 0.11 3.1	16 -5 -0.27 0.3	5 0 -0.10 0.0	0 0 -1.00 ...	0 -1 -1.00 ...	37 14 0.08 1.8	5 1 0.01 0.0	7 -2 -0.30 0.2	12 1 0.01 0.0	7 -6 -0.49 0.7	165
BW50	11 1 0.01 0.0	0 -16 -1.00 3.8	21 6 0.09 1.2	5 -8 -0.63 1.2	42 30 0.32 15.4$	5 2 0.02 0.2	0 0 -1.00 ...	0 0 -1.00 ...	5 -7 -0.62 1.1	5 3 0.03 ...	0 -5 -1.00 1.2	0 -5 -1.00 1.2	11 3 0.03 0.3	105
B51	37 -23 -0.39 2.1	51 -47 -0.48 5.6*	34 -41 -0.55 5.4*	89 8 0.01 0.2	64 -9 -0.14 0.3	32 13 0.05 1.9	11 6 0.09 1.8	0 -4 -1.00 1.1	168 89 0.16 23.3$	17 3 0.02 0.2	61 27 0.05 4.6*	28 -7 -0.22 0.4	36 -9 -0.22 0.5	628
BW52	21 3 0.02 0.1	82 53 0.34 22.0$	3 -18 -0.87 3.7	5 -18 -0.79 3.3	5 -16 -0.77 2.8	11 5 0.03 1.1	0 0 -1.00 ...	0 -1 -1.00 ...	11 -11 -0.53 1.4	5 1 0.01 0.0	11 1 0.01 0.0	5 -5 -0.53 0.6	26 12 0.07 2.4	185
BW53	0 -4 -1.00 1.1	2 -5 -0.76 1.1	0 -5 -1.00 1.4	5 -1 -0.25 0.1	5 0 -0.19 0.0	0 -1 -1.00 ...	0 0 -1.00 ...	0 0 -1.00 ...	10 3 0.08 0.4	0 0 -1.00 ...	14 11 0.23 8.0#	7 4 0.08 1.1	9 5 0.11 1.4	52
BW54	0 0 -1.00 ...	0 0 -1.00 ...	0 0 -1.00 ...	0 0 -1.00 ...	0 0 -1.00 ...	0 0 -1.00 ...	0 0 -1.00 ...	0 0 -1.00 ...	1 0 0.08 ...	0 0 -1.00 ...	0 0 -1.00 ...	0 0 -1.00 ...	4 4 0.78 ...	5
BW55	21 6 0.04 0.4	26 1 0.01 0.0	11 -7 -0.43 0.8	11 -8 -0.46 0.0	9 -9 -0.52 1.1	0 -4 -1.00 0.0	5 4 0.05 ...	0 0 -1.00 ...	16 -3 -0.20 0.2	0 -2 -1.00 0.7	16 7 0.05 1.3	32 23 0.15 11.8$	12 0 0.00 0.0	159
BW56	25 16 0.18 5.8*	20 5 0.06 0.4	5 -6 -0.57 0.8	16 4 0.05 0.3	0 -10 -1.00 2.4	11 8 0.09 4.6*	0 0 -1.00 ...	0 0 -1.00 ...	11 0 -0.08 0.0	0 -1 -1.00 ...	0 -4 -1.00 1.0	5 0 -0.08 0.0	2 -4 -0.71 0.7	95
BW57	16 -11 -0.43 1.1	25 -20 -0.45 2.2	1 -33 -0.97 7.4#	11 -25 -0.71 4.2*	189 155 0.60 154.6$	11 2 0.01 0.1	0 -1 -1.00 ...	0 -1 -1.00 ...	12 -24 -0.67 3.7	11 5 0.02 0.7	0 -15 -1.00 3.3	5 -11 -0.70 1.7	10 -10 -0.53 1.3	291
BW58	5 -11 -0.71 1.8	44 16 0.11 2.3	19 -1 -0.11 0.1	6 -16 -0.73 2.7	26 5 0.03 0.3	5 0 -0.05 0.0	0 0 -1.00 ...	5 4 0.04 ...	11 -10 -0.50 1.2	16 12 0.07 7.7#	5 -3 -0.47 0.4	5 -4 -0.50 0.5	28 15 0.09 3.7	175
BW59	0 0 0.00 ...	0 0 0.00 ...	0 0 0.00 ...	0 0 0.00 ...	0 0 0.00 ...	0 0 0.00 ...	0 0 0.00 ...	0 0 0.00 ...	0 0 0.00 ...	0 0 0.00 ...	0 0 0.00 ...	0 0 0.00 ...	0 0 0.00 ...	0
BW60	12 -22 -0.66 3.3	31 -25 -0.46 2.8	16 -27 -0.64 4.0*	92 45 0.14 9.9#	26 -16 -0.39 1.5	18 7 0.02 0.9	0 -2 -1.00 0.5	1 -1 -0.66 0.3	44 -1 -0.04 0.0	0 -7 -1.00 1.6	43 23 0.07 5.8*	40 19 0.06 3.7	40 13 0.04 1.4	363
BW61	11 -8 -0.46 0.9	32 0 -0.04 0.0	0 -25 -1.00 5.7*	23 -3 -0.15 0.1	16 -8 -0.36 0.7	11 5 0.02 0.7	0 -1 -1.00 ...	0 -1 -1.00 ...	75 48 0.26 19.7$	5 0 0.00 0.0	5 -5 -0.56 0.7	16 4 0.02 0.3	17 1 0.01 0.0	211
BW62	58 1 0.00 0.0	61 -30 -0.34 2.5	12 -38 -0.83 11.3$	156 61 0.16 20.0$	16 -52 -0.77 9.3#	0 -17 -1.00 3.7	16 12 0.17 6.4*	5 0 0.00 0.0	98 24 0.05 1.9	11 -1 -0.14 0.0	37 5 0.01 0.2	63 29 0.05 5.5*	52 9 0.02 0.4	585

Haplotype frequencies for population CAU
B-DR (N= 1900)

	DR1	DR2	DR3	DR4	DR7	DRW8	DRW9	DRW10	DRW11	DRW12	DRW13	DRW14	DRX	SUM
BW63	0 -5 -1.00 1.3	16 6 0.11 0.8	0 -7 -1.00 1.7	5 -2 -0.39 0.3	11 3 0.06 0.3	0 -1 -1.00 ...	0 0 -1.00 ...	0 0 -1.00 ...	0 -7 -1.00 1.8	0 0 -1.00 ...	21 18 0.29 17.0¢	11 7 0.12 2.0	0 -4 -1.00 0.0	64
BW64	5 -5 -0.56 0.7	5 -12 -0.73 2.2	11 -2 -0.22 0.1	14 0 -0.06 0.0	63 49 0.48 38.7¢	0 -2 -1.00 0.7	0 0 -1.00 ...	0 0 -1.00 ...	0 -14 -1.00 3.2	0 -2 -1.00 ...	5 0 -0.20 0.1	11 4 0.04 0.6	2 -6 -0.77 1.0	116
BW65	95 69 0.29 39.7¢	25 -16 -0.41 1.6	0 -32 -1.00 7.2#	11 -22 -0.68 3.6	42 10 0.04 0.8	0 -7 -1.00 1.6	0 -1 -1.00 ...	5 3 0.04 ...	5 -28 -0.85 5.5*	26 20 0.10 13.9¢	26 12 0.05 1.9	21 6 0.02 0.4	12 -7 -0.39 0.6	268
BW67	0 0 0.00 ...	0 0 0.00 ...	0 0 0.00 ...	0 0 0.00 ...	0 0 0.00 ...	0 0 0.00 ...	0 0 0.00 ...	0 0 0.00 ...	0 0 0.00 ...	0 0 0.00 ...	0 0 0.00 ...	0 0 0.00 ...	0 0 0.00 ...	0
BW71	0 0 -1.00 ...	0 0 -1.00 ...	0 0 -1.00 ...	5 4 1.00 ...	0 0 -1.00 ...	0 0 -1.00 ...	0 0 -1.00 ...	0 0 -1.00 ...	0 0 -1.00 ...	0 0 -1.00 ...	0 0 -1.00 ...	0 0 -1.00 ...	0 0 -1.00 ...	5
BW72	11 8 0.27 4.2*	5 0 -0.01 0.0	5 1 0.04 0.1	0 -3 -1.00 0.9	0 -3 -1.00 0.8	0 0 -1.00 ...	0 0 -1.00 ...	0 0 -1.00 ...	0 -3 -1.00 0.9	0 0 -1.00 ...	0 -1 -1.00 ...	11 9 0.30 ...	0 -1 -1.00 ...	32
BW73	0 -1 -1.00 ...	13 10 0.78 ...	0 -1 -1.00 ...	0 -1 -1.00 ...	0 -1 -1.00 ...	3 3 0.16 ...	0 0 -1.00 ...	0 0 -1.00 ...	0 -1 -1.00 ...	0 0 -1.00 ...	0 0 -1.00 ...	0 0 -1.00 ...	0 0 -1.00 ...	16
BX	5 1 0.03 0.1	9 3 0.07 0.2	5 0 0.00 0.0	0 -4 -1.00 1.2	0 -4 -1.00 1.0	5 4 0.09 ...	0 0 -1.00 ...	0 0 -1.00 ...	6 1 0.02 0.0	0 0 -1.00 ...	0 -1 -1.00 ...	0 -1 -1.00 ...	11 8 0.21 4.3*	41
SUM	969	1575	1215	1287	1180	301	74	82	1257	218	541	573	736	

Haplotype frequencies for population CAU; B-DQ ($N = 1964$)

	DQW1	DQW2	DQW3	DQX	SUM
B7	662 306 0.39 81.7$	58 -151 -0.72 29.8$	236 -40 -0.15 1.8	165 -112 -0.38 12.8$	1161
B8	114 -169 -0.63 38.2$	391 221 0.29 76.3$	75 -148 -0.67 28.2$	359 118 0.17 16.9$	939
B13	31 -64 -0.68 13.2$	214 160 0.66 118.9$	16 -54 -0.77 11.2$	35 -40 -0.54 6.0*	296
B18	170 -7 -0.04 0.1	84 -14 -0.15 0.6	147 16 0.04 0.5	148 7 0.02 0.1	549
B27	92 -18 -0.17 0.0	6 -53 -0.90 12.5$	97 15 0.06 0.8	147 59 0.23 10.9$	342
B35	401 64 0.09 3.9*	69 -118 -0.63 20.2$	265 17 0.02 0.3	306 39 0.05 1.7	1041
B37	55 9 0.09 0.5	5 -20 -0.81 4.0*	31 -2 -0.08 0.1	51 15 0.14 1.6	142
B38	134 53 0.32 10.5#	18 -26 -0.60 3.0*	68 9 0.05 0.3	29 -34 -0.55 5.2*	249
B39	74 8 0.06 0.3	17 -19 -0.54 2.6	45 -2 -0.07 0.1	67 15 0.10 1.2	203
BW41	22 -8 -0.29 0.8	10 -6 -0.42 0.8	42 19 0.26 4.2*	22 -2 -0.11 0.1	96
BW42	8 0 -0.01 0.0	0 -4 -1.00 1.1	0 -5 -1.00 1.5	17 11 0.57 4.6*	25
B44	231 -185 -0.45 27.7$	322 89 0.08 9.4#	507 200 0.20 38.6$	227 -102 -0.31 9.8#	1287
B45	5 -5 -0.56 1.0	10 4 0.13 0.5	5 -2 -0.40 0.3	15 6 0.23 1.1	35
BW46	3 1 0.26 ...	0 0 -1.00 ...	0 0 -1.00 ...	3 1 0.33 ...	6
BW47	10 2 0.11 0.1	0 -4 -1.00 1.1	10 4 0.21 0.7	5 0 -0.22 0.1	25
BW48	0 0 0.00 ...	0 0 0.00 ...	0 0 0.00 ...	0 0 0.00 ...	0
B49	64 7 0.06 0.3	22 -9 -0.30 0.7	65 23 0.17 3.4	24 -20 -0.47 2.6	175
BW50	15 -24 -0.62 4.5*	56 34 0.34 12.7$	4 -24 -0.86 5.7*	47 16 0.17 2.1	122
B51	157 -37 -0.20 2.3	79 -29 -0.28 2.1	189 45 0.10 3.9*	178 23 0.05 0.0	603
BW52	113 56 0.47 15.0$	10 -21 -0.69 3.7	18 -23 -0.57 3.6	36 -8 -0.21 0.5	177
BW53	15 0 0.01 0.0	5 -2 -0.39 0.3	10 0 -0.07 0.0	15 3 0.10 0.3	45
BW54	0 -1 -1.00 ...	0 0 -1.00 ...	5 4 1.00 ...	0 0 -1.00 ...	5
BW55	88 34 0.30 6.1*	16 -13 -0.47 1.7	20 -19 -0.50 2.6	44 1 0.01 0.0	168
BW56	49 13 0.17 1.3	5 -14 -0.75 2.8	15 -11 -0.44 1.3	43 14 0.17 1.9	112
BW57	48 -45 -0.49 6.7#	187 135 0.57 85.3$	19 -49 -0.73 9.7#	36 -37 -0.52 5.4*	290
BW58	70 10 0.08 0.5	41 7 0.05 0.4	23 -20 -0.48 2.7	52 4 0.03 0.1	186
BW59	0 0 0.00 ...	0 0 0.00 ...	0 0 0.00 ...	0 0 0.00 ...	0
BW60	119 0 0.00 0.0	25 -40 -0.62 6.4*	102 14 0.05 0.6	121 27 0.10 2.1	367
BW61	57 -11 -0.18 0.7	15 -23 -0.61 3.6	87 36 0.22 6.7#	55 0 0.00 0.0	214
BW62	181 -18 -0.09 0.5	21 -69 -0.61 18.7$	224 77 0.16 11.1$	190 32 0.07 1.8	616
BW63	44 24 0.59 8.7#	5 -5 -0.55 0.8	5 -9 -0.66 1.6	7 -8 -0.55 1.3	61
BW64	25 -10 -0.31 1.0	69 49 0.53 28.5$	14 -12 -0.48 1.6	4 -24 -0.86 5.7*	112
BW65	117 29 0.16 2.0	43 -5 -0.12 0.2	36 -27 -0.44 3.3	74 5 0.02 0.1	270
BW67	0 0 0.00 ...	0 0 0.00 ...	0 0 0.00 ...	0 0 0.00 ...	0
BW71	0 -1 -1.00 ...	0 0 -1.00 ...	5 4 1.00 ...	0 0 -1.00 ...	5
BW72	19 11 0.60 3.9*	5 0 0.01 0.0	0 -5 -1.00 1.6	2 -4 -0.70 0.9	26
BW73	15 10 1.00 6.2*	0 -2 -1.00 0.7	0 -3 -1.00 0.9	0 -3 -1.00 1.0	15
BX	13 2 0.07 0.1	0 -5 -1.00 1.5	0 -7 -1.00 2.2	22 13 0.50 5.0*	35
SUM	3241	1808	2385	2566	

Haplotype frequencies for population CAU; B-Bf (N=667)

	BF S	BF F	BFF1	BFS07	BF V	SUM
B7	1184 163 0.55 8.8#	135 -131 -0.49 6.3*	0 -15 -1.00 1.2	0 -13 -1.00 1.1	0 -1 -1.00 ...	1319
B8	1059 203 0.81 15.0$	17 -206 -0.92 17.0$	15 2 0.02 0.0	15 3 0.04 0.1	0 -1 -1.00 ...	1106
B13	270 61 1.00 5.4*	0 -54 -1.00 4.7*	0 -2 -1.00 ...	0 -2 -1.00 ...	0 0 -1.00 ...	270
B18	330 28 0.32 0.8	0 -78 -1.00 6.9#	60 55 0.48 ...	0 -3 -1.00 ...	0 0 -1.00 ...	390
B27	348 79 1.00 7.0#	0 -69 -1.00 6.1*	0 -3 -1.00 ...	0 -3 -1.00 ...	0 0 -1.00 ...	348
B35	524 -66 -0.11 2.5	240 85 0.14 4.3*	0 -8 -1.00 0.7	0 -7 -1.00 0.6	0 0 -1.00 ...	764
B37	15 -89 -0.86 22.9$	120 93 0.86 26.6$	0 -1 -1.00 ...	0 0 -1.00 ...	0 0 -1.00 ...	135
B38	209 36 0.70 2.2	15 -29 -0.67 1.7	0 -2 -1.00 ...	0 -1 -1.00 ...	0 0 -1.00 ...	224
B39	165 26 0.63 1.4	15 -20 -0.59 1.1	0 -1 -1.00 ...	0 -1 -1.00 ...	0 0 -1.00 ...	180
BW41	64 -16 -0.21 1.1	41 20 0.24 1.5	0 0 -1.00 ...	0 0 -1.00 ...	0 0 -1.00 ...	105
BW42	0 0 0.00 ...	0 0 0.00 ...	0 0 0.00 ...	0 0 0.00 ...	0 0 0.00 ...	0
B44	839 -265 -0.25 25.1$	599 305 0.26 30.9$	15 -1 -0.14 0.0	0 -14 -1.00 1.2	0 -1 -1.00 ...	1453
B45	60 -9 -0.14 0.4	15 -2 -0.18 0.0	0 0 -1.00 ...	15 14 0.16 ...	0 0 -1.00 ...	90
BW46	15 3 1.00 0.3	0 -2 -1.00 ...	0 0 -1.00 ...	0 0 -1.00 ...	0 0 -1.00 ...	15
BW47	15 -7 -0.35 0.9	15 9 0.37 ...	0 0 -1.00 ...	0 0 -1.00 ...	0 0 -1.00 ...	30
BW48	0 0 0.00 ...	0 0 0.00 ...	0 0 0.00 ...	0 0 0.00 ...	0 0 0.00 ...	0
B49	146 -4 -0.03 0.0	49 10 0.06 0.2	0 -1 -1.00 ...	0 -1 -1.00 ...	0 0 -1.00 ...	195
BW50	15 -65 -0.82 16.1$	0 -20 -1.00 1.8	0 0 -1.00 ...	75 74 0.71 ...	15 15 1.00 ...	105
B51	321 -50 -0.14 2.1	159 62 0.16 3.5	0 -5 -1.00 ...	0 -4 -1.00 ...	0 0 -1.00 ...	480
BW52	150 34 1.00 2.0	0 -29 -1.00 2.6	0 -1 -1.00 ...	0 -1 -1.00 ...	0 0 -1.00 ...	150
BW53	0 0 0.00 ...	0 0 0.00 ...	0 0 0.00 ...	0 0 0.00 ...	0 0 0.00 ...	0
BW54	0 0 0.00 ...	0 0 0.00 ...	0 0 0.00 ...	0 0 0.00 ...	0 0 0.00 ...	0
BW55	124 -3 -0.03 0.0	41 8 0.06 0.1	0 -1 -1.00 ...	0 -1 -1.00 ...	0 0 -1.00 ...	165
BW56	120 15 0.51 0.7	15 -11 -0.45 0.5	0 -1 -1.00 ...	0 0 -1.00 ...	0 0 -1.00 ...	135
BW57	360 70 0.82 5.1*	15 -60 -0.80 4.2*	0 -3 -1.00 ...	0 -3 -1.00 ...	0 0 -1.00 ...	375
BW58	45 -70 -0.61 13.1$	105 75 0.62 15.6$	0 -1 -1.00 ...	0 -1 -1.00 ...	0 0 -1.00 ...	150
BW59	0 0 0.00 ...	0 0 0.00 ...	0 0 0.00 ...	0 0 0.00 ...	0 0 0.00 ...	0
BW60	410 73 0.75 4.9*	10 -77 -0.89 6.1*	15 10 0.09 ...	0 -4 -1.00 ...	0 0 -1.00 ...	435
BW61	135 19 0.56 0.9	15 -14 -0.51 0.7	0 -1 -1.00 ...	0 -1 -1.00 ...	0 0 -1.00 ...	150
BW62	487 -85 -0.15 4.1*	253 103 0.17 6.4*	0 -8 -1.00 0.6	0 -7 -1.00 0.6	0 0 -1.00 ...	740
BW63	15 -19 -0.57 3.3	30 21 0.53 4.0*	0 0 -1.00 ...	0 0 -1.00 ...	0 0 -1.00 ...	45
BW64	105 12 0.45 0.5	15 -8 -0.38 0.3	0 0 -1.00 ...	0 0 -1.00 ...	0 0 -1.00 ...	120
BW65	180 -28 -0.14 1.2	90 35 0.16 1.0	0 -2 -1.00 ...	0 -2 -1.00 ...	0 0 -1.00 ...	270
BW67	0 0 0.00 ...	0 0 0.00 ...	0 0 0.00 ...	0 0 0.00 ...	0 0 0.00 ...	0
BW71	0 0 0.00 ...	0 0 0.00 ...	0 0 0.00 ...	0 0 0.00 ...	0 0 0.00 ...	0
BW72	0 -11 -1.00 3.4	15 12 1.00 ...	0 0 -1.00 ...	0 0 -1.00 ...	0 0 -1.00 ...	15
BW73	30 7 1.00 0.6	0 -5 -1.00 ...	0 0 -1.00 ...	0 0 -1.00 ...	0 0 -1.00 ...	30
BX	1 -11 -0.92 3.3	1 -1 -0.71 ...	15 15 0.88 ...	0 0 -1.00 ...	0 0 -1.00 ...	17
SUM	7741	2025	120	105	15	

Haplotype frequencies for population CAU; B-C2 ($N = 332$)

	C2 1	C2 2	C2 3	C2 V	SUM
B7	1302 17 0.22 0.2	59 -13 -0.19 0.1	0 0 0.00 ...	0 -3 -1.00 ...	1361
B8	1036 2 0.04 0.0	59 1 0.00 0.0	0 0 0.00 ...	0 -2 -1.00 ...	1095
B13	178 -17 -0.09 1.1	30 19 0.10 ...	0 0 0.00 ...	0 0 -1.00 ...	208
B18	473 -1 -0.00 0.0	0 -26 -1.00 1.0	0 0 0.00 ...	30 28 1.00 ...	503
B27	385 22 1.00 0.8	0 -20 -1.00 0.8	0 0 0.00 ...	0 0 -1.00 ...	385
B35	799 16 0.35 0.2	30 -13 -0.32 0.2	0 0 0.00 ...	0 -1 -1.00 ...	829
B37	59 3 1.00 0.1	0 -2 -1.00 ...	0 0 0.00 ...	0 0 -1.00 ...	59
B38	206 12 1.00 0.4	0 -10 -1.00 ...	0 0 0.00 ...	0 0 -1.00 ...	206
B39	118 7 1.00 0.2	0 -5 -1.00 ...	0 0 0.00 ...	0 0 -1.00 ...	118
BW41	148 8 1.00 0.3	0 -7 -1.00 ...	0 0 0.00 ...	0 0 -1.00 ...	148
BW42	0 0 0.00 ...	0 0 0.00 ...	0 0 0.00 ...	0 0 0.00 ...	0
B44	1450 25 0.30 0.3	59 -21 -0.27 0.2	0 0 0.00 ...	0 -4 -1.00 ...	1509
B45	118 7 1.00 0.2	0 -5 -1.00 ...	0 0 0.00 ...	0 0 -1.00 ...	118
BW46	30 2 1.00 0.1	0 -1 -1.00 ...	0 0 0.00 ...	0 0 -1.00 ...	30
BW47	30 2 1.00 0.1	0 -1 -1.00 ...	0 0 0.00 ...	0 0 -1.00 ...	30
BW48	0 0 0.00 ...	0 0 0.00 ...	0 0 0.00 ...	0 0 0.00 ...	0
B49	89 5 1.00 0.2	0 -4 -1.00 ...	0 0 0.00 ...	0 0 -1.00 ...	89
BW50	0 -27 -1.00 17.2$	30 28 1.00 ...	0 0 0.00 ...	0 0 -1.00 ...	30
B51	533 30 1.00 1.1	0 -27 -1.00 1.1	0 0 0.00 ...	0 -1 -1.00 ...	533
BW52	148 8 1.00 0.3	0 -7 -1.00 ...	0 0 0.00 ...	0 0 -1.00 ...	148
BW53	0 0 0.00 ...	0 0 0.00 ...	0 0 0.00 ...	0 0 0.00 ...	0
BW54	0 0 0.00 ...	0 0 0.00 ...	0 0 0.00 ...	0 0 0.00 ...	0
BW55	59 -51 -0.47 15.1$	59 53 0.47 ...	0 0 0.00 ...	0 0 -1.00 ...	118
BW56	118 -21 -0.16 2.1	30 22 0.16 ...	0 0 0.00 ...	0 0 -1.00 ...	148
BW57	444 25 1.00 0.9	0 -23 -1.00 0.9	0 0 0.00 ...	0 0 -1.00 ...	444
BW58	118 7 1.00 0.2	0 -5 -1.00 ...	0 0 0.00 ...	0 0 -1.00 ...	118
BW59	0 0 0.00 ...	0 0 0.00 ...	0 0 0.00 ...	0 0 0.00 ...	0
BW60	444 25 1.00 0.9	0 -23 -1.00 0.9	0 0 0.00 ...	0 0 -1.00 ...	444
BW61	89 -22 -0.21 2.0	30 24 0.21 ...	0 0 0.00 ...	0 0 -1.00 ...	119
BW62	503 -111 -0.21 13.1$	148 113 0.23 14.1$	0 0 0.00 ...	0 -1 -1.00 ...	651
BW63	59 3 1.00 0.1	0 -2 -1.00 ...	0 0 0.00 ...	0 0 -1.00 ...	59
BW64	178 10 1.00 0.4	0 -9 -1.00 ...	0 0 0.00 ...	0 0 -1.00 ...	178
BW65	237 13 1.00 0.5	0 -12 -1.00 ...	0 0 0.00 ...	0 0 -1.00 ...	237
BW67	0 0 0.00 ...	0 0 0.00 ...	0 0 0.00 ...	0 0 0.00 ...	0
BW71	0 0 0.00 ...	0 0 0.00 ...	0 0 0.00 ...	0 0 0.00 ...	0
BW72	0 0 0.00 ...	0 0 0.00 ...	0 0 0.00 ...	0 0 0.00 ...	0
BW73	59 3 1.00 0.1	0 -2 -1.00 ...	0 0 0.00 ...	0 0 -1.00 ...	59
BX	31 2 1.00 0.1	0 -1 -1.00 ...	0 0 0.00 ...	0 0 -1.00 ...	31
SUM	9441	534	0	30	

Haplotype frequencies for population CAU

B-C4A ($N=333$)

	C4 A1	C4A12	C4A13	C4 A2	C4 A3	C4 A4	C4A51	C4 A6	C4AQ0	SUM
B7	0 -4 -1.00 ...	0 0 0.00 ...	0 -7 -1.00 ...	75 -17 -0.19 0.2	1163 167 0.39 5.6*	56 -31 -0.37 0.8	0 -2 -1.00 ...	34 -19 -0.37 0.5	97 -62 -0.46 2.7	1425
B8	0 -3 -1.00 ...	0 0 0.00 ...	0 -5 -1.00 ...	19 -48 -0.72 2.3	415 -315 -0.43 26.0‡	0 -64 -1.00 4.1*	0 -1 -1.00 ...	0 -36 -1.00 2.4	612 460 0.53 118.9‡	1046
B13	0 0 -1.00 ...	0 0 0.00 ...	0 0 -1.00 ...	0 -11 -1.00 0.7	186 55 0.98 4.2*	0 -11 -1.00 0.7	0 0 -1.00 ...	0 -6 -1.00 ...	1 -22 -0.96 1.3	187
B18	0 -1 -1.00 ...	0 0 0.00 ...	0 -2 -1.00 ...	0 -31 -1.00 1.9	447 106 0.72 6.1*	38 8 0.02 0.1	0 0 -1.00 ...	0 -17 -1.00 1.1	3 -58 -0.95 3.6	488
B27	0 -1 -1.00 ...	0 0 0.00 ...	0 -1 -1.00 ...	0 -27 -1.00 1.7	300 -4 -0.02 0.0	75 48 0.12 5.1*	19 18 1.00 ...	0 -15 -1.00 0.9	42 -12 -0.24 0.2	436
B35	0 -2 -1.00 ...	0 0 0.00 ...	0 -4 -1.00 ...	131 77 0.13 6.9#	487 -68 -0.15 2.6	131 60 0.14 7.7#	0 -1 -1.00 ...	19 -11 -0.39 0.3	56 -47 -0.46 1.5	824
B37	0 0 -1.00 ...	0 0 0.00 ...	0 0 -1.00 ...	0 -6 -1.00 ...	112 34 1.00 2.6	0 -6 -1.00 ...	0 0 -1.00 ...	0 -3 -1.00 ...	0 -13 -1.00 0.9	112
B38	0 0 -1.00 ...	0 0 0.00 ...	19 18 0.32 ...	69 57 0.32 15.3‡	74 -56 -0.43 4.4*	0 -11 -1.00 0.7	0 0 -1.00 ...	0 -6 -1.00 ...	25 1 0.01 0.0	187
B39	0 0 -1.00 ...	0 0 0.00 ...	0 0 -1.00 ...	0 -5 -1.00 ...	75 9 0.33 0.2	0 -5 -1.00 ...	0 0 -1.00 ...	0 -3 -1.00 ...	19 7 0.09 0.3	94
BW41	0 0 -1.00 ...	0 0 0.00 ...	0 0 -1.00 ...	0 -6 -1.00 ...	92 14 0.41 0.4	0 -6 -1.00 ...	0 0 -1.00 ...	0 -3 -1.00 ...	20 6 0.06 0.2	112
BW42	0 0 0.00 ...	0 0 0.00 ...	0 0 0.00 ...	0 0 0.00 ...	0 0 0.00 ...	0 0 0.00 ...	0 0 0.00 ...	0 0 0.00 ...	0 0 0.00 ...	0
B44	19 14 0.42 ...	0 0 0.00 ...	0 -7 -1.00 ...	0 -87 -1.00 5.8*	1237 293 0.72 18.6‡	0 -83 -1.00 5.5*	0 -2 -1.00 ...	0 -50 -1.00 3.3	95 -74 -0.44 2.4	1351
B45	0 0 -1.00 ...	0 0 0.00 ...	0 0 -1.00 ...	19 12 0.11 ...	75 -3 -0.05 0.0	0 -6 -1.00 ...	0 0 -1.00 ...	0 -3 -1.00 ...	19 5 0.05 0.1	113
BW46	0 0 -1.00 ...	0 0 0.00 ...	0 0 -1.00 ...	0 0 -1.00 ...	0 -12 -1.00 2.4	0 0 -1.00 ...	0 0 -1.00 ...	0 0 -1.00 ...	19 17 1.00 ...	19
BW47	0 0 -1.00 ...	0 0 0.00 ...	0 0 -1.00 ...	0 0 -1.00 ...	19 6 1.00 0.4	0 0 -1.00 ...	0 0 -1.00 ...	0 0 -1.00 ...	0 -1 -1.00 ...	19
BW48	0 0 0.00 ...	0 0 0.00 ...	0 0 0.00 ...	0 0 0.00 ...	0 0 0.00 ...	0 0 0.00 ...	0 0 0.00 ...	0 0 0.00 ...	0 0 0.00 ...	0
B49	0 0 -1.00 ...	0 0 0.00 ...	0 0 -1.00 ...	0 -10 -1.00 0.6	130 12 0.23 0.2	19 9 0.05 0.4	0 0 -1.00 ...	0 -5 -1.00 ...	20 0 -0.06 0.0	169
BW50	0 0 -1.00 ...	0 0 0.00 ...	0 0 -1.00 ...	75 69 0.78 ...	0 -65 -1.00 11.7‡	0 -5 -1.00 ...	0 0 -1.00 ...	0 -3 -1.00 ...	19 7 0.09 0.3	94
B51	0 -1 -1.00 ...	0 0 0.00 ...	19 16 0.29 ...	75 39 0.08 2.6	418 38 0.23 0.7	0 -33 -1.00 2.0	0 0 -1.00 ...	0 -19 -1.00 1.2	32 -36 -0.53 1.3	544
BW52	0 0 -1.00 ...	0 0 0.00 ...	0 0 -1.00 ...	0 -8 -1.00 ...	131 39 1.00 3.1	0 -7 -1.00 ...	0 0 -1.00 ...	0 -4 -1.00 ...	0 -16 -1.00 1.0	131
BW53	0 0 0.00 ...	0 0 0.00 ...	0 0 0.00 ...	0 0 0.00 ...	0 0 0.00 ...	0 0 0.00 ...	0 0 0.00 ...	0 0 0.00 ...	0 0 0.00 ...	0
BW54	0 0 0.00 ...	0 0 0.00 ...	0 0 0.00 ...	0 0 0.00 ...	0 0 0.00 ...	0 0 0.00 ...	0 0 0.00 ...	0 0 0.00 ...	0 0 0.00 ...	0
BW55	0 0 -1.00 ...	0 0 0.00 ...	0 0 -1.00 ...	19 10 0.08 ...	38 -53 -0.59 5.7*	75 67 0.54 ...	0 0 -1.00 ...	0 -4 -1.00 ...	0 -16 -1.00 1.0	132
BW56	0 0 -1.00 ...	0 0 0.00 ...	0 0 -1.00 ...	0 -9 -1.00 0.6	103 -1 -0.02 0.0	19 10 0.07 ...	0 0 -1.00 ...	0 -5 -1.00 ...	28 9 0.07 0.3	150
BW57	0 0 -1.00 ...	0 0 0.00 ...	0 -1 -1.00 ...	0 -20 -1.00 1.2	34 -188 -0.85 29.2‡	0 -19 -1.00 1.2	0 0 -1.00 ...	285 273 0.69 355.5‡	0 -39 -1.00 2.5	319
BW58	19 18 0.49 ...	0 0 0.00 ...	0 0 -1.00 ...	0 -10 -1.00 0.6	112 -6 -0.06 0.1	19 8 0.05 0.4	0 0 -1.00 ...	19 13 0.08 ...	1 -19 -0.95 1.2	170
BW59	0 0 0.00 ...	0 0 0.00 ...	0 0 0.00 ...	0 0 0.00 ...	0 0 0.00 ...	0 0 0.00 ...	0 0 0.00 ...	0 0 0.00 ...	0 0 0.00 ...	0
BW60	0 -1 -1.00 ...	0 0 0.00 ...	0 -1 -1.00 ...	0 -26 -1.00 1.6	326 37 0.30 0.9	19 -6 -0.26 0.1	0 0 -1.00 ...	0 -15 -1.00 0.9	68 16 0.04 0.3	413
BW61	0 0 -1.00 ...	0 0 0.00 ...	0 0 -1.00 ...	19 7 0.04 0.2	144 13 0.22 0.2	19 7 0.04 0.3	0 0 -1.00 ...	0 -6 -1.00 ...	6 -17 -0.75 0.8	188
BW62	0 -2 -1.00 ...	0 0 0.00 ...	19 15 0.28 ...	19 -30 -0.62 1.2	551 21 0.09 0.2	112 65 0.11 5.5*	0 0 -1.00 ...	19 -9 -0.33 0.2	39 -56 -0.59 2.2	759

Haplotype frequencies for population CAU
B-C4A ($N = 333$)

	C4 A1	C4A12	C4A13	C4 A2	C4 A3	C4 A4	C4A51	C4 A6	C4AQ0	SUM
BW63	0 0 -1.00 ...	0 0 0.00 ...	0 0 -1.00 ...	0 -1 -1.00 ...	38 11 1.00 0.9	0 -1 -1.00 ...	0 0 -1.00 ...	0 0 -1.00 ...	0 -4 -1.00 ...	38
BW64	0 0 -1.00 ...	0 0 0.00 ...	0 0 -1.00 ...	19 10 0.08 ...	92 0 -0.00 0.0	0 -7 -1.00 ...	0 0 -1.00 ...	0 -4 -1.00 ...	21 4 0.04 0.1	132
BW65	0 0 -1.00 ...	0 0 0.00 ...	0 -1 -1.00 ...	94 74 0.26 16.5‡	149 -60 -0.29 3.3	38 19 0.07 1.2	0 0 -1.00 ...	0 -10 -1.00 0.6	20 -17 -0.47 0.5	301
BW67	0 0 0.00 ...	0 0 0.00 ...	0 0 0.00 ...	0 0 0.00 ...	0 0 0.00 ...	0 0 0.00 ...	0 0 0.00 ...	0 0 0.00 ...	0 0 0.00 ...	0
BW71	0 0 0.00 ...	0 0 0.00 ...	0 0 0.00 ...	0 0 0.00 ...	0 0 0.00 ...	0 0 0.00 ...	0 0 0.00 ...	0 0 0.00 ...	0 0 0.00 ...	0
BW72	0 0 0.00 ...	0 0 0.00 ...	0 0 0.00 ...	0 0 0.00 ...	0 0 0.00 ...	0 0 0.00 ...	0 0 0.00 ...	0 0 0.00 ...	0 0 0.00 ...	0
BW73	0 0 -1.00 ...	0 0 0.00 ...	0 0 -1.00 ...	19 17 0.47 ...	19 -7 -0.28 0.4	0 -1 -1.00 ...	0 0 -1.00 ...	0 0 -1.00 ...	0 -4 -1.00 ...	38
BX	0 0 -1.00 ...	0 0 0.00 ...	0 0 -1.00 ...	1 0 -0.27 ...	20 5 0.84 0.3	0 0 -1.00 ...	0 0 -1.00 ...	0 0 -1.00 ...	0 -2 -1.00 ...	21
SUM	38	0	57	653	6987	620	19	376	1262	

Haplotype frequencies for population CAU
B-C4B ($N = 334$)

	C4 B1	C4B11	C4B12	C4 B2	C4 B3	C4 B4	C4 B5	C4B51	C4 B6	C4 B7	C4BQ0	SUM
B7	1179 147 0.36 4.6*	0 -2 -1.00 ...	0 -2 -1.00 ...	112 -22 -0.17 0.3	56 13 0.05 0.2	0 -4 -1.00 ...	0 -10 -1.00 0.7	0 -2 -1.00 ...	0 -4 -1.00 ...	0 -2 -1.00 ...	93 -104 -0.53 4.1*	1440
B8	942 167 0.54 7.6#	0 -1 -1.00 ...	0 -1 -1.00 ...	19 -61 -0.81 4.4*	75 42 0.16 3.4	0 -3 -1.00 ...	0 -7 -1.00 ...	0 -1 -1.00 ...	0 -3 -1.00 ...	0 -1 -1.00 ...	46 -102 -0.69 4.0*	1082
B13	187 53 1.00 4.0*	0 0 -1.00 ...	0 0 -1.00 ...	0 -16 -1.00 1.0	0 -5 -1.00 ...	0 0 -1.00 ...	0 0 -1.00 ...	0 0 -1.00 ...	0 0 -1.00 ...	0 0 -1.00 ...	0 -25 -1.00 1.6	187
B18	410 75 0.56 3.3	0 0 -1.00 ...	0 0 -1.00 ...	19 -24 -0.57 0.9	19 5 0.02 0.1	0 -1 -1.00 ...	0 -3 -1.00 ...	0 0 -1.00 ...	0 -1 -1.00 ...	0 0 -1.00 ...	20 -43 -0.69 1.0	468
B27	337 25 0.21 0.4	0 0 -1.00 ...	0 0 -1.00 ...	56 15 0.04 0.4	0 -12 -1.00 0.8	0 -1 -1.00 ...	0 -2 -1.00 ...	0 0 -1.00 ...	0 -1 -1.00 ...	0 0 -1.00 ...	42 -17 -0.30 0.3	435
B35	333 -269 -0.45 24.9$	0 -1 -1.00 ...	0 -1 -1.00 ...	229 150 0.20 18.5$	0 -24 -1.00 1.5	0 -2 -1.00 ...	0 -5 -1.00 ...	0 -1 -1.00 ...	0 -2 -1.00 ...	0 -1 -1.00 ...	280 164 0.23 15.7$	842
B37	86 6 0.18 0.1	0 0 -1.00 ...	0 0 -1.00 ...	0 -9 -1.00 0.6	0 -2 -1.00 ...	0 0 -1.00 ...	0 0 -1.00 ...	0 0 -1.00 ...	0 0 -1.00 ...	0 0 -1.00 ...	26 11 0.11 0.5	112
B38	159 25 0.47 0.9	0 0 -1.00 ...	0 0 -1.00 ...	0 -16 -1.00 1.0	19 13 0.07 ...	0 0 -1.00 ...	0 0 -1.00 ...	0 0 -1.00 ...	0 0 -1.00 ...	0 0 -1.00 ...	9 -16 -0.65 0.7	187
B39	72 5 0.20 0.1	0 0 -1.00 ...	0 0 -1.00 ...	0 -8 -1.00 ...	0 -2 -1.00 ...	0 0 -1.00 ...	0 0 -1.00 ...	0 0 -1.00 ...	0 0 -1.00 ...	0 0 -1.00 ...	21 8 0.10 0.3	93
BW41	97 17 0.53 0.7	0 0 -1.00 ...	0 0 -1.00 ...	0 -9 -1.00 0.6	0 -2 -1.00 ...	0 0 -1.00 ...	0 0 -1.00 ...	0 0 -1.00 ...	0 0 -1.00 ...	0 0 -1.00 ...	15 0 -0.03 0.0	112
BW42	0 0 0.00 ...	0 0 0.00 ...	0 0 0.00 ...	0 0 0.00 ...	0 0 0.00 ...	0 0 0.00 ...	0 0 0.00 ...	0 0 0.00 ...	0 0 0.00 ...	0 0 0.00 ...	0 0 0.00 ...	0
B44	859 -79 -0.09 1.5	0 -1 -1.00 ...	0 -1 -1.00 ...	0 -122 -1.00 8.3#	19 -19 -0.52 0.7	0 -4 -1.00 ...	0 -9 -1.00 0.6	0 -1 -1.00 ...	0 -4 -1.00 ...	0 -1 -1.00 ...	433 252 0.22 25.1$	1311
B45	59 -20 -0.26 1.1	0 0 -1.00 ...	0 0 -1.00 ...	37 27 0.26 4.0*	0 -2 -1.00 ...	0 0 -1.00 ...	0 0 -1.00 ...	0 0 -1.00 ...	0 0 -1.00 ...	0 0 -1.00 ...	16 1 0.01 0.0	112
BW46	0 -13 -1.00 2.6	0 0 -1.00 ...	0 0 -1.00 ...	19 17 1.00 ...	0 0 -1.00 ...	0 0 -1.00 ...	0 0 -1.00 ...	0 0 -1.00 ...	0 0 -1.00 ...	0 0 -1.00 ...	0 -2 -1.00 ...	19
BW47	19 -7 -0.30 0.5	0 0 -1.00 ...	0 0 -1.00 ...	0 -3 -1.00 ...	0 0 -1.00 ...	0 0 -1.00 ...	0 0 -1.00 ...	0 0 -1.00 ...	0 0 -1.00 ...	0 0 -1.00 ...	19 14 0.42 ...	38

Haplotype frequencies for population CAU
B-C4B ($N = 334$)

	C4 B1	C4B11	C4B12	C4 B2	C4 B3	C4 B4	C4 B5	C4B51	C4 B6	C4 B7	C4BQ0	SUM
BW48	0 0 0.00 ...	0 0 0.00 ...	0 0 0.00 ...	0 0 0.00 ...	0 0 0.00 ...	0 0 0.00 ...	0 0 0.00 ...	0 0 0.00 ...	0 0 0.00 ...	0 0 0.00 ...	0 0 0.00 ...	0
B49	68 -53 -0.44 4.6*	0 0 -1.00 ...	19 19 1.00 ...	28 12 0.08 0.6	19 14 0.08 ...	19 18 0.49 ...	0 0 -1.00 ...	0 0 -1.00 ...	0 0 -1.00 ...	0 0 -1.00 ...	17 -5 -0.27 0.1	170
BW50	93 13 0.40 0.4	19 19 1.00 ...	0 0 -1.00 ...	0 -9 -1.00 0.6	0 -2 -1.00 ...	0 0 -1.00 ...	0 0 -1.00 ...	0 0 -1.00 ...	0 0 -1.00 ...	0 0 -1.00 ...	0 -14 -1.00 0.0	112
B51	411 21 0.14 0.2	0 0 -1.00 ...	0 0 -1.00 ...	19 -31 -0.63 1.2	19 3 0.01 0.0	0 -1 -1.00 ...	0 -3 -1.00 ...	0 0 -1.00 ...	0 -1 -1.00 ...	0 0 -1.00 ...	95 20 0.04 0.4	544
BW52	111 17 0.46 0.6	0 0 -1.00 ...	0 0 -1.00 ...	0 -11 -1.00 0.7	19 15 0.12 ...	0 0 -1.00 ...	0 0 -1.00 ...	0 0 -1.00 ...	0 0 -1.00 ...	0 0 -1.00 ...	1 -16 -0.94 1.0	131
BW53	0 0 0.00 ...	0 0 0.00 ...	0 0 0.00 ...	0 0 0.00 ...	0 0 0.00 ...	0 0 0.00 ...	0 0 0.00 ...	0 0 0.00 ...	0 0 0.00 ...	0 0 0.00 ...	0 0 0.00 ...	0
BW54	0 0 0.00 ...	0 0 0.00 ...	0 0 0.00 ...	0 0 0.00 ...	0 0 0.00 ...	0 0 0.00 ...	0 0 0.00 ...	0 0 0.00 ...	0 0 0.00 ...	0 0 0.00 ...	0 0 0.00 ...	0
BW55	19 -75 -0.80 11.5‡	0 0 -1.00 ...	0 0 -1.00 ...	0 -11 -1.00 0.7	0 -3 -1.00 ...	0 0 -1.00 ...	56 55 0.74 ...	0 0 -1.00 ...	19 18 0.49 ...	19 19 1.00 ...	19 1 0.01 0.0	132
BW56	106 0 -0.01 0.0	0 0 -1.00 ...	0 0 -1.00 ...	19 5 0.04 0.1	0 -4 -1.00 ...	0 0 -1.00 ...	19 18 0.24 ...	0 0 -1.00 ...	0 0 -1.00 ...	0 0 -1.00 ...	6 -14 -0.71 0.7	150
BW57	295 66 0.73 3.8	0 0 -1.00 ...	0 0 -1.00 ...	0 -29 -1.00 1.8	19 9 0.03 0.5	0 0 -1.00 ...	0 -1 -1.00 ...	0 0 -1.00 ...	0 0 -1.00 ...	0 0 -1.00 ...	5 -38 -0.69 2.2	319
BW58	140 33 0.76 1.9	0 0 -1.00 ...	0 0 -1.00 ...	0 -13 -1.00 0.8	0 -4 -1.00 ...	0 0 -1.00 ...	0 0 -1.00 ...	0 0 -1.00 ...	0 0 -1.00 ...	0 0 -1.00 ...	10 -10 -0.52 0.3	150
BW59	0 0 0.00 ...	0 0 0.00 ...	0 0 0.00 ...	0 0 0.00 ...	0 0 0.00 ...	0 0 0.00 ...	0 0 0.00 ...	0 0 0.00 ...	0 0 0.00 ...	0 0 0.00 ...	0 0 0.00 ...	0
BW60	200 -94 -0.32 6.0*	0 0 -1.00 ...	0 0 -1.00 ...	144 105 0.28 17.7‡	0 -11 -1.00 0.7	0 -1 -1.00 ...	0 -2 -1.00 ...	0 0 -1.00 ...	0 -1 -1.00 ...	0 0 -1.00 ...	68 11 0.03 0.1	412
BW61	136 1 0.02 0.0	0 0 -1.00 ...	0 0 -1.00 ...	19 1 0.01 0.0	0 -5 -1.00 ...	0 0 -1.00 ...	0 0 -1.00 ...	0 0 -1.00 ...	19 18 0.49 ...	0 0 -1.00 ...	14 -11 -0.46 0.3	188
BW62	507 -32 -0.06 0.4	0 0 -1.00 ...	0 0 -1.00 ...	112 42 0.06 1.6	37 14 0.05 0.5	0 -2 -1.00 ...	0 -5 -1.00 ...	0 0 -1.00 ...	0 -2 -1.00 ...	0 0 -1.00 ...	97 -6 -0.07 0.0	753

Haplotype frequencies for population CAU
B-C4B ($N = 334$)

	C4 B1	C4B11	C4B12	C4 B2	C4 B3	C4 B4	C4 B5	C4B51	C4 B6	C4 B7	C4BQ0	SUM
BW63	37 10 1.00 0.8	0 0 -1.00 ...	0 0 -1.00 ...	0 -2 -1.00 ...	0 0 -1.00 ...	0 0 -1.00 ...	0 0 -1.00 ...	0 0 -1.00 ...	0 0 -1.00 ...	0 0 -1.00 ...	0 -4 -1.00 ...	37
BW64	107 13 0.35 0.4	0 0 -1.00 ...	0 0 -1.00 ...	0 -11 -1.00 0.7	0 -3 -1.00 ...	0 0 -1.00 ...	0 0 -1.00 ...	0 0 -1.00 ...	0 0 -1.00 ...	0 0 -1.00 ...	24 6 0.05 0.1	131
BW65	158 -56 -0.26 2.9	0 0 -1.00 ...	0 0 -1.00 ...	103 75 0.28 12.2$	0 -8 -1.00 ...	19 18 0.48 ...	0 -1 -1.00 ...	19 18 1.00 ...	0 0 -1.00 ...	0 0 -1.00 ...	1 -39 -0.98 2.5	300
BW67	0 0 0.00 ...	0 0 0.00 ...	0 0 0.00 ...	0 0 0.00 ...	0 0 0.00 ...	0 0 0.00 ...	0 0 0.00 ...	0 0 0.00 ...	0 0 0.00 ...	0 0 0.00 ...	0 0 0.00 ...	0
BW71	0 0 0.00 ...	0 0 0.00 ...	0 0 0.00 ...	0 0 0.00 ...	0 0 0.00 ...	0 0 0.00 ...	0 0 0.00 ...	0 0 0.00 ...	0 0 0.00 ...	0 0 0.00 ...	0 0 0.00 ...	0
BW72	0 0 0.00 ...	0 0 0.00 ...	0 0 0.00 ...	0 0 0.00 ...	0 0 0.00 ...	0 0 0.00 ...	0 0 0.00 ...	0 0 0.00 ...	0 0 0.00 ...	0 0 0.00 ...	0 0 0.00 ...	0
BW73	37 10 1.00 0.8	0 0 -1.00 ...	0 0 -1.00 ...	0 -2 -1.00 ...	0 0 -1.00 ...	0 0 -1.00 ...	0 0 -1.00 ...	0 0 -1.00 ...	0 0 -1.00 ...	0 0 -1.00 ...	0 -4 -1.00 ...	37
BX	1 0 -0.30 ...	0 0 -1.00 ...	0 0 -1.00 ...	0 0 -1.00 ...	0 0 -1.00 ...	0 0 -1.00 ...	0 0 -1.00 ...	0 0 -1.00 ...	0 0 -1.00 ...	0 0 -1.00 ...	1 1 0.42 ...	2
SUM	7165	19	19	935	301	38	75	19	38	19	1378	

Haplotype frequencies for population CAU
B-DP ($N = 117$)

	DPW1	DPW2	DPW3	DPW4	DPW5	DPW6	DPX	SUM
B7	0 -36 -1.00 ...	151 41 0.05 0.2	47 9 0.02 ...	299 -47 -0.14 0.1	53 15 0.04 ...	0 0 0.00 ...	305 20 0.03 0.0	855
B8	256 216 0.56 ...	48 -72 -0.60 0.7	46 4 0.01 ...	386 4 0.01 0.0	44 3 0.01 ...	0 0 0.00 ...	160 -152 -0.49 1.5	940
B13	0 -21 -1.00 ...	79 13 0.03 0.0	0 -22 -1.00 ...	257 49 0.16 0.2	0 -22 -1.00 ...	0 0 0.00 ...	177 6 0.02 0.0	513
B18	0 -28 -1.00 ...	167 79 0.13 1.0	46 16 0.04 ...	157 -120 -0.43 1.1	65 55 0.13 ...	0 0 0.00 ...	228 0 0.00 0.0	683
B27	43 25 0.06 ...	71 16 0.04 0.1	43 24 0.06 ...	145 -28 -0.16 0.1	0 -18 -1.00 ...	0 0 0.00 ...	125 -16 -0.12 0.0	427
B35	0 -39 -1.00 ...	0 -120 -1.00 1.8	43 1 0.00 ...	463 81 0.15 0.4	0 -40 -1.00 ...	0 0 0.00 ...	434 121 0.19 0.9	940
B37	0 -14 -1.00 ...	64 20 0.07 0.1	43 28 0.09 ...	60 -78 -0.57 0.9	44 29 0.09 ...	0 0 0.00 ...	131 17 0.07 0.0	342
B38	19 12 0.07 ...	0 -21 -1.00 ...	0 -7 -1.00 ...	67 -1 -0.04 0.0	0 -7 -1.00 ...	0 0 0.00 ...	85 28 0.25 0.2	171
B39	0 -6 -1.00 ...	0 -21 -1.00 ...	0 -7 -1.00 ...	134 65 0.64 1.2	0 -7 -1.00 ...	0 0 0.00 ...	37 -19 -0.35 0.1	171
BW41	0 -1 -1.00 ...	0 -5 -1.00 ...	0 -1 -1.00 ...	43 26 1.00 ...	0 -1 -1.00 ...	0 0 0.00 ...	0 -13 -1.00 ...	43
BW42	0 0 0.00 ...	0 0 0.00 ...	0 0 0.00 ...	0 0 0.00 ...	0 0 0.00 ...	0 0 0.00 ...	0 0 0.00 ...	0
B44	0 -54 -1.00 0.8	217 52 0.05 0.3	38 -17 -0.33 0.1	506 -12 -0.03 0.0	44 -11 -0.22 0.0	0 0 0.00 ...	473 47 0.05 0.1	1278
B45	0 0 0.00 ...	0 0 0.00 ...	0 0 0.00 ...	0 0 0.00 ...	0 0 0.00 ...	0 0 0.00 ...	0 0 0.00 ...	0
BW46	0 0 0.00 ...	0 0 0.00 ...	0 0 0.00 ...	0 0 0.00 ...	0 0 0.00 ...	0 0 0.00 ...	0 0 0.00 ...	0
BW47	0 0 0.00 ...	0 0 0.00 ...	0 0 0.00 ...	0 0 0.00 ...	0 0 0.00 ...	0 0 0.00 ...	0 0 0.00 ...	0

	DPW1	DPW2	DPW3	DPW4	DPW5	DPW6	DPX	SUM
BW48	0 0 0.00 ...	0 0 0.00 ...	0 0 0.00 ...	0 0 0.00 ...	0 0 0.00 ...	0 0 0.00 ...	0 0 0.00 ...	0
B49	0 -6 -1.00 ...	85 63 0.43 ...	0 -7 -1.00 ...	71 2 0.02 0.0	0 -6 -1.00 ...	0 0 0.00 ...	14 -42 -0.75 0.6	170
BW50	0 0 0.00 ...	0 0 0.00 ...	0 0 0.00 ...	0 0 0.00 ...	0 0 0.00 ...	0 0 0.00 ...	0 0 0.00 ...	0
B51	43 21 0.05 ...	85 19 0.04 0.1	93 70 0.17 ...	103 -104 -0.51 1.1	0 -22 -1.00 ...	0 0 0.00 ...	189 18 0.05 0.0	513
BW52	0 -10 -1.00 ...	43 10 0.04 ...	43 32 0.13 ...	114 10 0.06 0.0	0 -10 -1.00 ...	0 0 0.00 ...	57 -28 -0.33 0.2	257
BW53	0 0 0.00 ...	0 0 0.00 ...	0 0 0.00 ...	0 0 0.00 ...	0 0 0.00 ...	0 0 0.00 ...	0 0 0.00 ...	0
BW54	0 0 0.00 ...	0 0 0.00 ...	0 0 0.00 ...	0 0 0.00 ...	0 0 0.00 ...	0 0 0.00 ...	0 0 0.00 ...	0
BW55	0 -10 -1.00 ...	73 40 0.18 ...	0 -10 -1.00 ...	118 14 0.09 0.0	0 -10 -1.00 ...	0 0 0.00 ...	65 -19 -0.24 0.1	256
BW56	0 -3 -1.00 ...	0 -10 -1.00 ...	0 -3 -1.00 ...	85 50 1.00 ...	0 -3 -1.00 ...	0 0 0.00 ...	0 -27 -1.00 ...	85
BW57	67 63 0.77 ...	0 -10 -1.00 ...	0 -3 -1.00 ...	19 -15 -0.46 ...	0 -3 -1.00 ...	0 0 0.00 ...	0 -28 -1.00 ...	86
BW58	0 0 0.00 ...	0 0 0.00 ...	0 0 0.00 ...	0 0 0.00 ...	0 0 0.00 ...	0 0 0.00 ...	0 0 0.00 ...	0
BW59	0 0 0.00 ...	0 0 0.00 ...	0 0 0.00 ...	0 0 0.00 ...	0 0 0.00 ...	0 0 0.00 ...	0 0 0.00 ...	0
BW60	0 -23 -1.00 ...	133 61 0.13 0.7	0 -24 -1.00 ...	186 -39 -0.18 0.1	125 101 0.24 ...	0 0 0.00 ...	112 -72 -0.40 0.5	556
BW61	0 -6 -1.00 ...	0 -21 -1.00 ...	0 -7 -1.00 ...	85 16 0.16 0.1	0 -6 -1.00 ...	0 0 0.00 ...	85 28 0.25 0.3	170
BW62	0 -43 -1.00 0.6	45 -86 -0.66 0.9	0 -44 -1.00 0.6	509 92 0.15 0.4	44 0 -0.02 0.0	0 0 0.00 ...	428 86 0.13 0.4	1026

Haplotype frequencies for population CAU; C-DR ($N = 1918$)

	CW1	CW2	CW3	CW4	CW5	CW6	CW7	CW8	CX	SUM
DR1	81 50 0.17 17.1$	51 9 0.02 0.5	91 -23 -0.21 1.2	293 182 0.21 71.1$	47 -20 -0.31 1.5	25 -57 -0.70 9.4#	117 -118 -0.50 16.7$	99 63 0.19 24.3$	159 -81 -0.34 7.9#	963
DR2	36 -15 -0.31 1.1	70 1 0.00 0.0	140 -48 -0.26 3.3	98 -65 -0.47 10.3#	73 -38 -0.35 3.4	66 -71 -0.52 9.3#	667 277 0.23 59.4$	30 -28 -0.50 3.4	413 14 0.01 0.1	1593
DR3	16 -22 -0.59 3.0	17 -34 -0.67 5.3*	49 -92 -0.66 15.1$	57 -80 -0.59 11.7$	108 24 0.04 1.5	27 -75 -0.74 13.4$	610 317 0.35 99.0$	10 -34 -0.78 6.1*	302 2 0.00 0.0	1196
DR4	35 -5 -0.15 0.2	62 8 0.02 0.2	279 129 0.12 27.7$	100 -44 -0.31 3.5	202 113 0.18 33.9$	49 -59 -0.55 7.9#	287 -20 -0.07 0.4	24 -22 -0.49 2.6	221 -94 -0.30 8.3#	1259
DR7	14 -24 -0.64 3.5	10 -40 -0.80 7.5#	53 -87 -0.62 13.5$	117 -19 -0.15 0.7	37 -46 -0.56 6.1*	435 333 0.44 256.2$	118 -171 -0.59 29.3$	99 55 0.17 15.3$	303 6 0.01 0.0	1186
DRW8	16 7 0.02 0.9	10 -1 -0.20 0.1	28 -5 -0.18 0.3	31 -1 -0.07 0.0	13 -6 -0.36 0.6	31 6 0.02 0.3	100 30 0.14 3.2	0 -10 -1.00 2.2	59 -12 -0.18 0.6	288
DRW9	5 2 0.03 ...	10 7 0.09 2.7	16 7 0.10 1.1	10 1 0.02 0.0	10 5 0.06 0.8	0 -6 -1.00 1.4	5 -13 -0.73 2.6	0 -2 -1.00 0.6	21 2 0.03 0.0	77
DRW10	5 2 0.03 ...	0 -2 -1.00 0.7	6 -2 -0.34 0.2	5 -3 -0.44 0.4	0 -4 -1.00 1.1	40 33 0.47 35.3$	0 -18 -1.00 4.8*	5 2 0.03 0.3	16 -2 -0.17 0.1	77
DRW11	52 12 0.04 0.8	98 45 0.12 8.6#	171 25 0.02 1.0	135 -6 -0.05 0.1	80 -6 -0.08 0.1	57 -48 -0.46 5.5*	235 -65 -0.22 4.2*	5 -40 -0.89 8.3#	399 90 0.10 7.7#	1232
DRW12	0 -6 -1.00 1.5	16 6 0.03 0.9	5 -20 -0.81 3.8*	27 1 0.01 0.0	32 16 0.08 3.6	16 -2 -0.17 0.1	33 -20 -0.39 2.2	26 18 0.08 7.7#	67 11 0.07 0.6	222
DRW13	10 -7 -0.43 0.7	37 14 0.03 1.7	109 45 0.09 7.2#	56 -5 -0.10 0.1	28 -9 -0.27 0.6	37 -9 -0.21 0.4	67 -64 -0.49 8.6#	32 12 0.03 1.5	164 29 0.07 1.6	540
DRW14	13 -5 -0.30 0.3	21 -3 -0.15 0.1	128 60 0.12 12.4$	71 5 0.01 0.1	31 -8 -0.23 0.5	23 -25 -0.53 3.1	99 -39 -0.29 3.1	30 9 0.02 0.8	153 10 0.02 0.2	569
DRX	43 17 0.06 2.4	30 -3 -0.13 0.1	114 19 0.03 0.9	155 63 0.09 10.2#	45 -10 -0.20 0.5	58 -10 -0.16 0.4	108 -85 -0.44 10.6#	13 -16 -0.56 2.0	229 30 0.05 1.2	795
SUM	326	432	1189	1155	706	864	2446	373	2506	

Haplotype frequencies for population CAU; C-DQ ($N = 1925$) ▶

	CW1	CW2	CW3	CW4	CW5	CW6	CW7	CW8	CX	SUM
DQW1	108 -1 -0.01 0.0	130 -6 -0.05 0.1	414 10 0.01 0.1	424 46 0.06 1.9	162 -70 -0.30 6.8#	137 -138 -0.50 22.5$	896 121 0.07 7.2#	140 19 0.06 0.0	831 22 0.01 0.2	3242
DQW2	16 -45 -0.74 8.5#	18 -58 -0.77 11.5$	75 -151 -0.67 28.3$	153 -58 -0.28 4.6*	109 -21 -0.17 0.0	455 300 0.43 153.4$	441 5 0.00 0.0	106 38 0.13 5.4*	450 -4 -0.01 0.0	1823
DQW3	68 -10 -0.14 0.4	138 39 0.12 4.2*	357 66 0.07 4.5*	266 -5 -0.02 0.0	302 135 0.24 30.2$	91 -107 -0.54 16.5$	515 -42 -0.08 1.1	49 -37 -0.44 4.4*	546 -35 -0.06 0.8	2332
DQX	146 58 0.23 10.6#	138 28 0.09 1.9	401 76 0.08 5.5*	322 18 0.02 0.3	145 -41 -0.23 2.7	169 -52 -0.24 3.7	540 -82 -0.13 3.9*	77 -19 -0.21 1.1	668 18 0.01 0.2	2606
SUM	338	424	1247	1165	718	852	2392	372	2495	

▼ B-DP ($N = 117$)

	DPW1	DPW2	DPW3	DPW4	DPW5	DPW6	DPX	SUM
BW63	0 -3 -1.00 ...	0 -10 -1.00 ...	0 -3 -1.00 ...	50 15 0.31 ...	0 -3 -1.00 ...	0 0 0.00 ...	35 7 0.12 ...	85
BW64	0 -3 -1.00 ...	0 -10 -1.00 ...	0 -3 -1.00 ...	85 50 1.00 ...	0 -3 -1.00 ...	0 0 0.00 ...	0 -27 -1.00 ...	85
BW65	0 -14 -1.00 ...	27 -16 -0.39 0.1	0 -14 -1.00 ...	120 -18 -0.14 0.1	0 -14 -1.00 ...	0 0 0.00 ...	195 81 0.36 1.0	342
BW67	0 0 0.00 ...	0 0 0.00 ...	0 0 0.00 ...	0 0 0.00 ...	0 0 0.00 ...	0 0 0.00 ...	0 0 0.00 ...	0
BW71	0 0 0.00 ...	0 0 0.00 ...	0 0 0.00 ...	0 0 0.00 ...	0 0 0.00 ...	0 0 0.00 ...	0 0 0.00 ...	0
BW72	0 0 0.00 ...	0 0 0.00 ...	0 0 0.00 ...	0 0 0.00 ...	0 0 0.00 ...	0 0 0.00 ...	0 0 0.00 ...	0
BW73	0 0 0.00 ...	0 0 0.00 ...	0 0 0.00 ...	0 0 0.00 ...	0 0 0.00 ...	0 0 0.00 ...	0 0 0.00 ...	0
BX	0 0 -1.00 ...	1 1 0.23 ...	0 0 -1.00 ...	2 1 0.44 ...	0 0 -1.00 ...	0 0 0.00 ...	0 0 -1.00 ...	3
SUM	428	1289	442	4064	439	0	3335	

Haplotype frequencies for population CAU; C-DP ($N=117$) ▼
◄ C-C2 ($N=340$)

	CW1	CW2	CW3	CW4	CW5	CW6	CW7	CW8	CX	SUM
C2 1	239 13 1.00 0.5	385 -5 -0.01 0.1	1138 -130 -0.27 9.5#	1060 32 0.52 0.7	853 -7 -0.02 0.0	735 -14 -0.03 0.2	2419 24 0.17 0.2	412 23 1.00 0.9	2200 68 0.54 1.7	9441
C2 2	0 -12 -1.00 ...	29 7 0.02 0.1	206 135 0.29 10.6#	29 -28 -0.50 0.6	59 11 0.02 0.1	59 17 0.03 0.3	118 -15 -0.12 0.1	0 -21 -1.00 0.8	29 -89 -0.76 3.2	529
C2 3	0 0 0.00 ...	0 0 0.00 ...	0 0 0.00 ...	0 0 0.00 ...	0 0 0.00 ...	0 0 0.00 ...	0 0 0.00 ...	0 0 0.00 ...	0 0 0.00 ...	0
C2 V	0 0 -1.00 ...	0 0 -1.00 ...	0 -3 -1.00 ...	0 -2 -1.00 ...	0 -2 -1.00 ...	0 -1 -1.00 ...	0 -6 -1.00 ...	0 0 -1.00 ...	29 22 1.00 ...	29
SUM	239	414	1344	1089	912	794	2537	412	2258	

	DPW1	DPW2	DPW3	DPW4	DPW5	DPW6	DPX	SUM
CW1	0 -6 -1.00 ...	0 -21 -1.00 ...	43 35 0.22 ...	128 58 0.58 0.0	0 -7 -1.00 ...	0 0 0.00 ...	0 -56 -1.00 1.0	171
CW2	0 -14 -1.00 ...	71 27 0.09 0.2	0 -14 -1.00 ...	145 6 0.03 0.0	44 29 0.09 ...	0 0 0.00 ...	82 -31 -0.28 0.2	342
CW3	43 -46 -0.52 0.4	207 -62 -0.23 0.3	0 -92 -1.00 1.4	974 122 0.10 0.4	169 77 0.22 0.0	0 0 0.00 ...	702 3 0.00 0.0	2095
CW4	0 -36 -1.00 ...	0 -111 -1.00 1.6	43 5 0.01 ...	409 56 0.11 0.2	0 -37 -1.00 ...	0 0 0.00 ...	416 126 0.22 1.1	868
CW5	0 -25 -1.00 ...	90 13 0.02 0.0	38 12 0.03 ...	277 34 0.10 0.1	0 -25 -1.00 ...	0 0 0.00 ...	193 -6 -0.03 0.0	598
CW6	67 30 0.08 ...	143 32 0.04 0.1	43 5 0.01 ...	275 -72 -0.21 0.3	44 6 0.02 ...	0 0 0.00 ...	284 -1 -0.01 0.0	856
CW7	256 156 0.48 3.9*	398 97 0.10 0.6	93 -9 -0.10 0.0	922 -24 -0.03 0.0	88 -13 -0.14 0.0	0 0 0.00 ...	572 -204 -0.26 1.2	2329
CW8	0 -17 -1.00 ...	27 -27 -0.51 0.2	0 -18 -1.00 ...	206 32 0.13 0.1	0 -18 -1.00 ...	0 0 0.00 ...	195 52 0.18 0.3	428
CX	62 -36 -0.37 0.2	355 56 0.06 0.2	182 60 0.23 0.0	731 -210 -0.22 1.2	94 -7 -0.08 0.0	0 0 0.00 ...	893 120 0.08 0.4	2317
SUM	428	1291	442	4067	439	0	3337	

Haplotype frequencies for population CAU
▼ C-C2 ($N=340$)

	C4 A1	C4A12	C4A13	C4 A2	C4 A3	C4 A4	C4A51	C4 A6	C4AQ0	SUM
CW1	0 0 -1.00 ...	0 0 0.00 ...	0 -1 -1.00 ...	0 -17 -1.00 1.1	218 21 0.24 0.4	56 39 0.15 5.1*	0 0 -1.00 ...	0 -10 -1.00 0.6	8 -26 -0.77 1.3	282
CW2	0 -1 -1.00 ...	0 0 0.00 ...	0 -2 -1.00 ...	0 -29 -1.00 1.8	372 42 0.29 0.0	37 8 0.02 0.1	19 18 1.00 ...	19 0 0.00 0.0	25 -33 -0.57 1.2	472
CW3	19 14 0.42 ...	0 0 0.00 ...	0 -7 -1.00 ...	56 -32 -0.37 0.8	973 7 0.02 0.0	223 138 0.26 14.0‡	0 -2 -1.00 ...	0 -53 -1.00 3.5	109 -61 -0.36 1.6	1380
CW4	0 -3 -1.00 ...	0 0 0.00 ...	19 13 0.26 ...	144 77 0.13 5.6*	643 -86 -0.12 2.1	130 66 0.12 4.3*	0 -1 -1.00 ...	19 -21 -0.54 0.7	88 -40 -0.32 0.9	1043
CW5	19 16 0.46 ...	0 0 0.00 ...	0 -3 -1.00 ...	0 -44 -1.00 2.7	615 133 0.64 7.0#	0 -41 -1.00 2.6	0 0 -1.00 ...	0 -26 -1.00 1.6	55 -29 -0.36 0.7	689
CW6	0 -2 -1.00 ...	0 0 0.00 ...	0 -3 -1.00 ...	74 25 0.04 0.8	362 -171 -0.32 10.7#	0 -46 -1.00 2.9	0 0 -1.00 ...	298 268 0.74 145.4‡	29 -65 -0.69 3.0	763
CW7	0 -9 -1.00 0.7	0 0 0.00 ...	0 -14 -1.00 1.1	93 -73 -0.44 2.6	1792 -20 -0.01 0.1	65 -93 -0.59 4.3*	0 -4 -1.00 ...	56 -45 -0.45 1.5	585 264 0.29 17.9‡	2591
CW8	0 -1 -1.00 ...	0 0 0.00 ...	0 -1 -1.00 ...	112 84 0.21 15.4‡	239 -60 -0.20 2.3	37 11 0.03 0.3	0 0 -1.00 ...	0 -16 -1.00 0.0	40 -12 -0.25 0.2	428
CX	0 -8 -1.00 ...	0 0 0.00 ...	37 24 0.56 3.0	167 15 0.03 0.1	1785 136 0.19 2.6	66 -78 -0.54 3.2	0 -3 -1.00 ...	0 -91 -1.00 6.8#	301 9 0.01 0.0	2356
SUM	38	0	56	646	6999	614	19	392	1240	

C-Bf ($N=671$)▼

	CW1	CW2	CW3	CW4	CW5	CW6	CW7	CW8	CX	SUM
BF S	240 32 0.52 1.5	318 38 0.46 1.6	1052 -37 -0.03 0.4	565 -146 -0.21 9.8#	596 -6 -0.01 0.0	702 -11 -0.02 0.1	2208 254 0.44 12.9‡	283 -14 -0.05 0.2	1743 -107 -0.06 2.4	7707
BF F	30 -25 -0.46 1.0	45 -29 -0.40 1.0	347 56 0.05 1.1	359 169 0.23 13.0‡	111 -49 -0.31 1.4	149 -40 -0.22 0.8	313 -208 -0.40 9.4#	104 24 0.08 0.7	599 105 0.07 2.5	2057
BFF1	0 -2 -1.00 ...	0 -3 -1.00 ...	15 -1 -0.12 0.0	0 -10 -1.00 0.8	60 51 0.46 20.1‡	0 -10 -1.00 0.8	15 -14 -0.51 0.7	0 -4 -1.00 ...	30 1 0.01 0.0	120
BFS07	0 -2 -1.00 ...	0 -3 -1.00 ...	0 -14 -1.00 1.2	0 -9 -1.00 0.7	15 7 0.07 0.4	60 50 0.53 19.4‡	0 -26 -1.00 2.4	0 -3 -1.00 ...	30 5 0.06 0.1	105
BF V	0 0 -1.00 ...	0 0 -1.00 ...	0 -1 -1.00 ...	0 0 -1.00 ...	0 0 -1.00 ...	15 14 1.00 ...	0 -3 -1.00 ...	0 0 -1.00 ...	0 -3 -1.00 ...	15
SUM	270	363	1414	924	762	926	2536	387	2402	

Haplotype frequencies for population CAU

C-C4B ($N=536$)

	C4 B1	C4B11	C4B12	C4 B2	C4 B3	C4 B4	C4 B5	C4B51	C4 B6	C4 B7	C4BQ0	SUM
CW1	224	0	0	56	0	0	0	0	0	0	2	282
	22	0	0	30	-7	0	-1	0	0	0	-36	
	0.28	-1.00	-1.00	0.12	-1.00	-1.00	-1.00	-1.00	-1.00	-1.00	-0.95	
	0.5	...	...	2.0	...	...	...	...	...	...	2.3	
CW2	374	0	0	37	0	0	0	0	0	0	42	453
	50	0	0	-4	-13	-1	-2	0	-1	0	-20	
	0.39	-1.00	-1.00	-0.12	-1.00	-1.00	-1.00	-1.00	-1.00	-1.00	-0.33	
	1.5	...	...	0.0	0.8	...	...	...	...	...	0.4	
CW3	794	0	0	265	19	0	75	0	19	19	171	1362
	-181	-2	-2	138	-21	-4	65	-2	14	16	-17	
	-0.19	-1.00	-1.00	0.17	-0.53	-1.00	1.00	-1.00	0.42	1.00	-0.09	
	7.4#	...	...	10.3#	0.7	...	25.7$	...	...	...	0.1	
CW4	414	0	0	247	19	0	0	0	0	0	385	1065
	-348	-1	-1	148	-12	-3	-7	-1	-3	-1	237	
	-0.46	-1.00	-1.00	0.18	-0.40	-1.00	-1.00	-1.00	-1.00	-1.00	0.26	
	33.7$	...	...	14.6$	0.3	...	...	...	...	...	26.6$	
CW5	353	0	0	0	0	0	0	0	0	0	337	690
	-140	0	0	-63	-20	-2	-4	0	-2	0	241	
	-0.29	-1.00	-1.00	-1.00	-1.00	-1.00	-1.00	-1.00	-1.00	-1.00	0.41	
	8.2#	...	...	4.1*	1.2	...	...	...	...	...	40.8$	
CW6	668	19	0	37	19	0	0	0	0	0	40	783
	107	18	0	-35	-3	-2	-5	0	-2	0	-67	
	0.48	1.00	-1.00	-0.49	-0.19	-1.00	-1.00	-1.00	-1.00	-1.00	-0.63	
	4.2*	...	...	1.1	0.0	...	...	...	...	...	2.9	
CW7	2174	0	0	112	179	0	0	0	0	0	160	2625
	294	-4	-4	-131	101	-9	-19	-4	-9	-4	-203	
	0.39	-1.00	-1.00	-0.54	0.46	-1.00	-1.00	-1.00	-1.00	-1.00	-0.56	
	11.8$	...	...	5.7*	9.6#	0.7	1.4	...	0.7	...	9.6#	
CW8	264	0	0	103	0	19	0	19	0	0	25	430
	-43	0	0	63	-12	17	-2	18	-1	0	-34	
	-0.14	-1.00	-1.00	0.16	-1.00	0.48	-1.00	1.00	-1.00	-1.00	-0.58	
	1.2	...	...	6.1*	0.7	...	...	...	...	...	1.3	
CX	1898	0	19	74	63	19	0	0	19	0	223	2315
	240	-3	15	-141	-5	10	-16	-3	10	-3	-97	
	0.37	-1.00	1.00	-0.66	-0.09	0.35	-1.00	-1.00	0.35	-1.00	-0.30	
	8.5#	...	...	7.1#	0.0	...	1.2	...	...	...	2.4	
SUM	7163	19	19	931	299	38	75	19	38	19	1385	

DR-C2 ($N=320$)

	DR1	DR2	DR3	DR4	DR7	DRW8	DRW9	DRW10	DRW11	DRW12	DRW13	DRW14	DRX	SUM
C2 1	652	1465	1330	1482	1469	250	63	63	1063	250	443	531	327	9408
	-20	59	50	-117	28	15	4	4	4	15	26	-56	-9	
	-0.04	0.65	0.62	-0.24	0.31	1.00	1.00	1.00	0.05	1.00	1.00	-0.10	-0.03	
	0.4	1.5	1.2	5.7*	0.3	0.5	0.1	0.1	0.0	0.5	0.9	3.2	0.2	
C2 2	63	31	31	219	63	0	0	0	63	0	0	94	0	564
	23	-54	-45	123	-22	-13	-3	-3	0	-13	-24	59	-19	
	0.04	-0.64	-0.60	0.26	-0.27	-1.00	-1.00	-1.00	-0.01	-1.00	-1.00	0.11	-1.00	
	0.5	1.4	1.1	6.5*	0.3	...	...	...	0.0	...	0.9	3.5	0.7	
C2 3	0	0	0	0	0	0	0	0	0	0	0	0	0	0
	0	0	0	0	0	0	0	0	0	0	0	0	0	
	0.00	0.00	0.00	0.00	0.00	0.00	0.00	0.00	0.00	0.00	0.00	0.00	0.00	
	...	...	...	...	...	...	...	...	...	...	...	...	...	
C2 V	0	0	0	0	0	0	0	0	0	0	0	0	31	31
	-1	-4	-3	-4	-4	0	0	0	-2	0	0	-1	30	
	-1.00	-1.00	-1.00	-1.00	-1.00	-1.00	-1.00	-1.00	-1.00	-1.00	-1.00	-1.00	1.00	
	...	...	...	...	...	...	...	...	...	...	...	...	...	
SUM	715	1516	1361	1701	1532	250	63	63	1126	250	443	625	358	

	DR1	DR2	DR3	DR4	DR7	DRW8	DRW9	DRW10	DRW11	DRW12	DRW13	DRW14	DRX	SUM
DQW1	732	1466	28	13	0	25	7	52	20	9	322	547	61	3282
	423	936	-344	-424	-402	-70	-17	27	-365	-65	146	348	-166	
	0.67	0.86	-0.92	-0.97	-1.00	-0.74	-0.72	0.54	-0.95	-0.88	0.41	0.86	-0.73	
	176.1$	541.5$	98.0$	130.8$	126.5$	15.0$	3.6	8.4#	115.1$	16.3$	35.5$	178.4$	36.2$	
DQW2	9	6	585	5	1195	7	5	0	1	0	5	6	31	1855
	-165	-293	374	-241	967	-47	-8	-13	-227	-41	-93	-105	-97	
	-0.95	-0.98	0.40	-0.98	0.97	-0.87	-0.65	-1.00	-1.00	-1.00	-0.95	-0.95	-0.76	
	39.3$	77.9$	170.2$	62.2$	999.9$	9.7#	1.3	3.2	58.8$	9.8#	21.5$	24.3$	18.1$	
DQW3	8	11	45	1201	3	29	19	0	891	172	1	0	64	2444
	-221	-383	-232	675	-296	-42	0	-17	589	116	-129	-147	-105	
	-0.97	-0.97	-0.84	0.87	-0.99	-0.60	0.01	-1.00	0.63	0.67	-0.99	-1.00	-0.62	
	57.8$	108.9$	53.8$	662.7$	82.1$	6.4*	0.0	4.5*	320.4$	60.7$	33.3$	38.6$	17.3$	
DQX	192	133	478	115	31	233	45	23	324	47	207	53	539	2420
	-35	-257	203	-207	-265	162	27	5	25	-7	78	-93	371	
	-0.16	-0.66	0.24	-0.64	-0.90	0.73	0.46	0.09	0.03	-0.15	0.19	-0.64	0.70	
	1.5	49.5$	41.3$	37.6$	66.3$	92.5$	9.5#	0.3	0.6	0.3	11.0$	15.5$	214.2$	
SUM	941	1616	1136	1334	1229	294	76	75	1236	228	535	606	695	

Haplotype frequencies for population CAU
DR-DQ (N=1848)▲
DR-Bf (N=526)▼

	DR1	DR2	DR3	DR4	DR7	DRW8	DRW9	DRW10	DRW11	DRW12	DRW13	DRW14	DRX	SUM
BF S	458	1408	1089	1201	830	215	51	21	1008	154	378	300	551	7664
	-127	258	60	84	-295	33	0	-57	197	10	-147	-70	58	
	-0.22	0.73	0.19	0.25	-0.26	0.59	-0.02	-0.73	0.80	0.23	-0.28	-0.19	0.39	
	7.6#	17.0$	1.0	1.9	22.9$	1.5	0.0	10.8#	13.4$	0.2	11.2$	3.6	1.8	
BF F	290	93	82	256	588	23	17	82	50	34	308	184	92	2099
	129	-221	-199	-49	280	-26	3	60	-171	-4	164	82	-42	
	0.21	-0.70	-0.71	-0.16	0.24	-0.54	0.05	0.74	-0.77	-0.14	0.30	0.22	-0.32	
	8.4#	13.7$	12.1$	0.7	22.1$	1.1	0.0	12.6$	11.1$	0.1	14.9$	5.2*	1.1	
BFF1	0	0	137	0	0	0	0	0	0	0	0	0	0	137
	-9	-20	119	-19	-19	-2	0	0	-13	-2	-8	-6	-8	
	-1.00	-1.00	1.00	-1.00	-1.00	-1.00	-1.00	-1.00	-1.00	-1.00	-1.00	-1.00	-1.00	
	0.7	1.4	52.5$	1.4	1.4	...	...	...	0.0	...	0.6	...	0.6	
BFS07	17	0	34	0	34	0	0	0	0	0	0	0	0	85
	10	-12	23	-11	22	-1	0	0	-8	-1	-5	-3	-4	
	0.13	-1.00	0.31	-1.00	0.30	-1.00	-1.00	-1.00	-1.00	-1.00	-1.00	-1.00	-1.00	
	...	0.9	3.1	0.9	2.6	...	...	...	0.6	...	...	...	...	
BF V	0	0	0	0	17	0	0	0	0	0	0	0	0	17
	0	-2	-1	-1	15	0	0	0	-1	0	0	0	0	
	-1.00	-1.00	-1.00	-1.00	1.00	-1.00	-1.00	-1.00	-1.00	-1.00	-1.00	-1.00	-1.00	
	...	...	...	...	...	...	...	...	...	...	...	...	...	
SUM	765	1501	1342	1457	1469	238	68	103	1058	188	686	484	643	

	BF S	BF F	BFF1	BFS07	BF V	SUM
C2 1	7326	1846	220	55	0	9449
	-38	75	12	-22	-25	
	-0.33	0.73	1.00	-0.30	-1.00	
	0.6	2.6	0.5	4.6*	17.5$	
C2 2	441	28	0	28	28	525
	32	-69	-11	24	27	
	0.27	-0.72	-1.00	0.30	1.00	
	0.4	2.4	...	...	...	
C2 3	0	0	0	0	0	0
	0	0	0	0	0	
	0.00	0.00	0.00	0.00	0.00	
	...	...	...	...	...	
C2 V	28	0	0	0	0	28
	6	-4	0	0	0	
	1.00	-1.00	-1.00	-1.00	-1.00	
	0.3	...	...	...	...	
SUM	7795	1876	220	83	28	

Haplotype frequencies for population CAU
C2-Bf (N=362)▲
Bf-DQ (N=632)▼

	BF S	BF F	BFF1	BFS07	BF V	SUM
DQW1	2181	650	0	16	0	2847
	-8	60	-35	-10	-4	
	-0.01	0.04	-1.00	-0.41	-1.00	
	0.0	0.7	3.2	0.4	...	
DQW2	1440	621	63	63	16	2203
	-254	165	35	42	12	
	-0.15	0.10	0.35	0.57	1.00	
	13.5$	6.1*	3.6	6.9#	...	
DQW3	2034	289	1	0	0	2324
	246	-191	-28	-21	-3	
	0.46	-0.40	-0.97	-1.00	-1.00	
	12.1$	7.0#	2.3	1.8	...	
DQX	2038	511	63	16	0	2628
	16	-32	30	-8	-3	
	0.03	-0.06	0.32	-0.36	-1.00	
	0.0	0.2	2.3	0.3	...	
SUM	7693	2071	127	95	16	

Haplotype frequencies for population CAU

C4A-DQ (N=526)▼

	C4 A1	C4A12	C4A13	C4 A2	C4 A3	C4 A4	C4A51	C4 A6	C4AQ0	SUM
DQW1	18 6 0.23 0.2	0 0 0.00 ...	38 20 0.52 1.8	251 63 0.15 1.7	2268 77 0.08 0.7	303 107 0.25 4.7*	0 -5 -1.00 ...	20 -98 -0.83 6.5*	227 -169 -0.43 6.4*	3125
DQW2	0 -7 -1.00 ...	0 0 0.00 ...	0 -12 -1.00 0.9	95 -37 -0.28 0.8	1267 -277 -0.18 11.3‡	19 -118 -0.86 7.4#	0 -3 -1.00 ...	264 180 0.61 27.2‡	559 279 0.28 21.6‡	2204
DQW3	19 9 0.33 0.6	0 0 0.00 ...	19 4 0.10 0.1	152 -3 -0.02 0.0	1940 127 0.16 2.1	204 42 0.09 0.8	19 14 1.00 ...	56 -41 -0.43 1.3	178 -149 -0.46 5.6*	2587
DQX	1 -6 -0.87 ...	0 0 0.00 ...	0 -11 -1.00 0.8	104 -21 -0.17 0.3	1535 72 0.12 0.8	102 -28 -0.22 0.5	0 -3 -1.00 ...	40 -36 -0.50 1.3	305 40 0.04 0.5	2087
SUM	36	0	57	602	7010	628	19	380	1269	

C2-DQ (N=327)▼

	C2 1	C2 2	C2 3	C2 V	SUM
DQW1	2993 4 0.02 0.0	180 5 0.01 0.0	0 0 0.00 ...	0 -9 -1.00 ...	3173
DQW2	2375 51 0.36 0.8	92 -43 -0.32 0.6	0 0 0.00 ...	0 -7 -1.00 ...	2467
DQW3	2670 -100 -0.25 2.0	272 110 0.28 3.7	0 0 0.00 ...	0 -8 -1.00 ...	2942
DQX	1382 45 0.55 1.0	6 -71 -0.92 2.7	0 0 0.00 ...	31 27 1.00 ...	1419
SUM	9420	550	0	31	

DR-C4A (N=502)▼

	C4 A1	C4A12	C4A13	C4 A2	C4 A3	C4 A4	C4A51	C4 A6	C4AQ0	SUM
DR1	0 -2 -1.00 ...	0 0 0.00 ...	20 15 0.28 ...	177 128 0.22 19.7‡	448 -106 -0.19 3.9*	79 29 0.05 1.0	0 -1 -1.00 ...	20 -7 -0.28 0.1	42 -52 -0.56 1.9	786
DR2	20 14 0.41 ...	0 0 0.00 ...	0 -9 -1.00 ...	59 -39 -0.41 1.1	1363 236 0.50 10.1#	112 11 0.02 0.1	0 -2 -1.00 ...	0 -55 -1.00 3.5	42 -151 -0.78 8.2#	1596
DR3	0 -4 -1.00 ...	0 0 0.00 ...	0 -7 -1.00 ...	39 -38 -0.50 1.2	633 -250 -0.28 14.1‡	0 -78 -1.00 4.9*	0 -2 -1.00 ...	0 -43 -1.00 2.7	580 428 0.40 79.8‡	1252
DR4	0 -5 -1.00 ...	0 0 0.00 ...	20 11 0.21 ...	98 1 0.00 0.0	1179 81 0.18 1.2	157 59 0.11 2.3	0 -2 -1.00 ...	20 -34 -0.64 1.4	81 -107 -0.57 4.2*	1555
DR7	0 -5 -1.00 ...	0 0 0.00 ...	0 -7 -1.00 ...	79 -8 -0.10 0.1	695 -101 -0.10 2.1	20 -68 -0.78 3.4	0 -2 -1.00 ...	275 225 0.74 62.1‡	143 -27 -0.17 0.3	1412
DRW8	0 0 -1.00 ...	0 0 0.00 ...	0 0 -1.00 ...	20 5 0.02 0.1	158 -8 -0.06 0.1	20 5 0.02 0.1	0 0 -1.00 ...	0 -7 -1.00 ...	39 10 0.05 0.2	237
DRW9	0 0 -1.00 ...	0 0 0.00 ...	0 0 -1.00 ...	0 -4 -1.00 ...	79 23 1.00 1.7	0 -4 -1.00 ...	0 0 -1.00 ...	0 -2 -1.00 ...	0 -9 -1.00 ...	79
DRW10	0 0 -1.00 ...	0 0 0.00 ...	0 0 -1.00 ...	0 -4 -1.00 ...	59 4 0.17 0.0	0 -4 -1.00 ...	0 0 -1.00 ...	0 -2 -1.00 ...	19 10 0.14 ...	78
DRW11	20 15 0.43 ...	0 0 0.00 ...	0 -6 -1.00 ...	20 -51 -0.72 2.3	1011 191 0.56 8.7#	39 -33 -0.47 0.0	0 -1 -1.00 ...	39 -1 -0.05 0.0	32 -108 -0.77 5.5*	1161
DRW12	0 0 -1.00 ...	0 0 0.00 ...	0 0 -1.00 ...	39 27 0.14 3.2	118 -20 -0.15 0.6	20 8 0.04 0.3	20 20 1.00 ...	0 -6 -1.00 ...	0 -23 -1.00 1.4	197
DRW13	0 -1 -1.00 ...	0 0 0.00 ...	0 -3 -1.00 ...	36 0 -0.03 0.0	385 -33 -0.08 0.5	59 22 0.04 0.7	0 0 -1.00 ...	0 -20 -1.00 1.2	113 41 0.08 1.4	593
DRW14	0 -1 -1.00 ...	0 0 0.00 ...	20 17 0.30 ...	17 -13 -0.46 0.4	346 -7 -0.02 0.0	39 7 0.02 0.1	0 0 -1.00 ...	0 -17 -1.00 0.0	79 18 0.04 0.3	501
DRX	0 -1 -1.00 ...	0 0 0.00 ...	0 -2 -1.00 ...	39 4 0.01 0.0	390 -2 -0.01 0.0	85 50 0.10 4.1*	0 0 -1.00 ...	0 -19 -1.00 1.1	43 -24 -0.36 0.5	557
SUM	40	0	60	623	7064	630	20	354	1213	

Haplotype frequencies for population CAU; DR-C4B ($N = 507$)▼ ▼
DR-DP ($N = 116$)▼

	C4 B1	C4B11	C4B12	C4 B2	C4 B3	C4 B4	C4 B5	C4B51	C4 B6	C4 B7	C4BQ0	SUM
DR1	370 -200 -0.35 13.4‡	0 -1 -1.00 ...	0 -1 -1.00 ...	121 48 0.07 1.9	25 0 -0.01 0.0	20 17 0.46 ...	0 -5 -1.00 ...	0 -1 -1.00 ...	0 -2 -1.00 ...	0 -1 -1.00 ...	270 152 0.22 12.8‡	806
DR2	1254 120 0.26 2.6	0 -2 -1.00 ...	0 -2 -1.00 ...	112 -32 -0.23 0.5	118 68 0.26 5.7*	0 -5 -1.00 ...	20 7 0.11 0.3	0 -2 -1.00 ...	0 -5 -1.00 ...	0 -2 -1.00 ...	96 -136 -0.59 5.7*	1600
DR3	1068 193 0.54 8.4#	0 -1 -1.00 ...	0 -1 -1.00 ...	0 -111 -1.00 7.1#	39 0 0.00 0.0	0 -4 -1.00 ...	0 -9 -1.00 ...	0 -1 -1.00 ...	0 -4 -1.00 ...	0 -1 -1.00 ...	128 -51 -0.29 1.0	1235
DR4	947 -156 -0.14 4.7*	0 -2 -1.00 ...	0 -2 -1.00 ...	136 -2 -0.02 0.0	79 30 0.11 1.1	20 14 0.41 ...	0 -11 -1.00 0.7	0 -2 -1.00 ...	0 -5 -1.00 ...	20 17 1.00 ...	356 128 0.10 5.1*	1560
DR7	1298 281 0.67 15.8‡	0 -2 -1.00 ...	0 -2 -1.00 ...	79 -50 -0.39 1.3	0 -44 -1.00 2.8	0 -5 -1.00 ...	0 -10 -1.00 0.7	0 -2 -1.00 ...	0 -5 -1.00 ...	0 -2 -1.00 ...	58 -150 -0.72 7.6#	1435
DRW8	123 -44 -0.27 2.1	20 20 1.00 ...	0 0 -1.00 ...	39 18 0.08 0.8	0 -6 -1.00 ...	0 0 -1.00 ...	0 -1 -1.00 ...	0 0 -1.00 ...	0 0 -1.00 ...	0 0 -1.00 ...	55 20 0.10 0.7	237
DRW9	39 -2 -0.07 0.0	0 0 -1.00 ...	0 0 -1.00 ...	0 -4 -1.00 ...	0 -1 -1.00 ...	0 0 -1.00 ...	0 0 -1.00 ...	0 0 -1.00 ...	0 0 -1.00 ...	0 0 -1.00 ...	20 11 0.23 ...	59
DRW10	39 -15 -0.29 0.8	0 0 -1.00 ...	0 0 -1.00 ...	0 -6 -1.00 ...	0 -1 -1.00 ...	0 0 -1.00 ...	0 0 -1.00 ...	19 19 1.00 ...	0 0 -1.00 ...	0 0 -1.00 ...	20 9 0.13 0.4	78
DRW11	988 163 0.46 6.3*	0 -1 -1.00 ...	0 -1 -1.00 ...	20 -84 -0.81 4.4*	39 2 0.01 0.0	0 -4 -1.00 ...	0 -8 -1.00 ...	0 -1 -1.00 ...	20 15 0.43 ...	0 -1 -1.00 ...	97 -72 -0.43 2.1	1164
DRW12	112 -13 -0.11 0.3	0 0 -1.00 ...	0 0 -1.00 ...	30 14 0.09 0.7	0 -5 -1.00 ...	0 0 -1.00 ...	0 0 -1.00 ...	0 0 -1.00 ...	0 0 -1.00 ...	0 0 -1.00 ...	36 10 0.07 0.2	178
DRW13	309 -112 -0.27 5.6*	0 0 -1.00 ...	20 19 1.00 ...	101 47 0.09 2.4	14 -4 -0.25 0.1	0 -1 -1.00 ...	20 15 0.21 ...	0 0 -1.00 ...	0 -1 -1.00 ...	0 0 -1.00 ...	132 45 0.09 1.5	596
DRW14	261 -104 -0.29 5.6*	0 0 -1.00 ...	0 0 -1.00 ...	128 81 0.17 8.3#	0 -15 -1.00 0.9	0 -1 -1.00 ...	39 35 0.47 ...	0 0 -1.00 ...	0 -1 -1.00 ...	0 0 -1.00 ...	89 14 0.03 0.2	517
DRX	280 -101 -0.27 5.0*	0 0 -1.00 ...	0 0 -1.00 ...	137 88 0.18 9.4#	0 -16 -1.00 0.9	0 -1 -1.00 ...	0 -3 -1.00 ...	0 0 -1.00 ...	20 18 0.47 ...	0 0 -1.00 ...	102 23 0.05 0.4	539
SUM	7088	20	20	905	314	40	79	19	40	20	1459	

	DPW1	DPW2	DPW3	DPW4	DPW5	DPW6	DPX	SUM
DR1	43 -4 -0.10 0.0	117 -26 -0.19 0.1	43 -5 -0.13 0.0	534 89 0.13 0.4	0 -48 -1.00 0.7	0 0 0.00 ...	372 0 -0.00 0.0	1109
DR2	0 -67 -1.00 0.0	114 -90 -0.44 0.6	0 -69 -1.00 1.0	837 204 0.22 1.5	133 63 0.17 0.8	0 0 0.00 ...	493 -37 -0.07 0.1	1577
DR3	278 241 0.61 ...	48 -63 -0.57 0.5	47 9 0.02 ...	355 8 0.02 0.0	0 -37 -1.00 ...	0 0 0.00 ...	135 -154 -0.54 1.6	863
DR4	0 -76 -1.00 1.1	302 70 0.07 0.3	172 92 0.25 1.6	505 -211 -0.30 1.5	142 63 0.17 0.7	0 0 0.00 ...	665 64 0.05 0.1	1786
DR7	67 15 0.04 0.1	93 -63 -0.41 0.4	0 -53 -1.00 0.7	442 -41 -0.09 0.1	0 -52 -1.00 0.7	0 0 0.00 ...	604 198 0.25 1.9	1206
DRW8	0 -14 -1.00 ...	0 -44 -1.00 0.6	0 -14 -1.00 ...	265 127 0.62 2.3	0 -14 -1.00 ...	0 0 0.00 ...	79 -36 -0.32 0.2	344
DRW9	0 -6 -1.00 ...	0 -21 -1.00 ...	47 39 0.24 ...	61 -7 -0.12 0.0	0 -7 -1.00 ...	0 0 0.00 ...	65 7 0.06 0.0	173
DRW10	0 -6 -1.00 ...	18 -3 -0.20 ...	0 -7 -1.00 ...	63 -5 -0.09 0.0	0 -7 -1.00 ...	0 0 0.00 ...	92 34 0.29 0.3	173
DRW11	43 -15 -0.27 0.1	320 143 0.13 1.8	90 29 0.08 0.2	507 -39 -0.07 0.1	86 26 0.07 0.2	0 0 0.00 ...	316 -141 -0.31 0.9	1362
DRW12	0 -6 -1.00 ...	27 5 0.03 ...	47 39 0.24 ...	0 -68 -1.00 1.4	0 -7 -1.00 ...	0 0 0.00 ...	96 40 0.35 0.5	172
DRW13	0 -25 -1.00 ...	71 -6 -0.09 0.0	0 -26 -1.00 ...	315 73 0.20 0.5	82 55 0.13 ...	0 0 0.00 ...	135 -67 -0.33 0.4	603
DRW14	0 -6 -1.00 ...	46 26 0.17 ...	0 -7 -1.00 ...	0 -68 -1.00 1.4	0 -7 -1.00 ...	0 0 0.00 ...	124 66 0.58 1.3	172
DRX	0 -19 -1.00 ...	142 82 0.20 1.6	0 -20 -1.00 ...	132 -52 -0.29 0.3	0 -19 -1.00 ...	0 0 0.00 ...	187 32 0.10 0.1	461
SUM	431	1300	446	4016	443	0	3365	

	C4 A1	C4A12	C4A13	C4 A2	C4 A3	C4 A4	C4A51	C4 A6	C4AQ0	SUM
C4 B1	10 -15 -0.61 1.9	0 0 0.00 ...	18 -20 -0.53 2.1	354 -108 -0.23 5.3*	5468 433 0.22 24.4$	34 -379 -0.92 71.8$	2 -10 -0.84 1.8	339 80 0.78 4.0*	927 24 0.07 0.1	7152
C4B11	0 0 -1.00 ...	0 0 0.00 ...	0 0 -1.00 ...	18 17 1.00 ...	0 -12 -1.00 2.4	0 0 -1.00 ...	0 0 -1.00 ...	0 0 -1.00 ...	0 -1 -1.00 ...	18
C4B12	0 0 -1.00 ...	0 0 0.00 ...	0 0 -1.00 ...	0 0 -1.00 ...	0 -12 -1.00 2.4	18 17 1.00 ...	0 0 -1.00 ...	0 0 -1.00 ...	0 -1 -1.00 ...	18
C4 B2	0 -2 -1.00 ...	0 0 0.00 ...	0 -4 -1.00 ...	82 25 0.04 0.7	240 -363 -0.62 48.3$	435 384 0.73 184.5$	0 -1 -1.00 ...	0 -31 -1.00 2.0	129 17 0.02 0.2	886
C4 B3	0 0 -1.00 ...	0 0 0.00 ...	0 -1 -1.00 ...	0 -20 -1.00 1.3	272 42 0.44 1.5	0 -18 -1.00 1.1	0 0 -1.00 ...	18 6 0.02 0.2	36 -4 -0.13 0.0	326
C4 B4	0 0 -1.00 ...	0 0 0.00 ...	0 0 -1.00 ...	16 13 0.20 ...	54 3 0.16 0.0	0 -3 -1.00 ...	0 0 -1.00 ...	0 -2 -1.00 ...	0 -8 -1.00 0.6	72
C4 B5	0 0 -1.00 ...	0 0 0.00 ...	0 0 -1.00 ...	0 -4 -1.00 ...	0 -50 -1.00 9.5#	72 68 1.00 ...	0 0 -1.00 ...	0 -2 -1.00 ...	0 -8 -1.00 0.6	72
C4B51	0 0 -1.00 ...	0 0 0.00 ...	0 0 -1.00 ...	0 0 -1.00 ...	0 -12 -1.00 2.4	0 0 -1.00 ...	0 0 -1.00 ...	0 0 -1.00 ...	18 16 1.00 ...	18
C4 B6	0 0 -1.00 ...	0 0 0.00 ...	0 0 -1.00 ...	0 -1 -1.00 ...	18 -6 -0.29 0.4	18 16 0.47 ...	0 0 -1.00 ...	0 0 -1.00 ...	0 -4 -1.00 ...	36
C4 B7	0 0 -1.00 ...	0 0 0.00 ...	0 0 -1.00 ...	0 0 -1.00 ...	18 5 1.00 0.4	0 0 -1.00 ...	0 0 -1.00 ...	0 0 -1.00 ...	0 -1 -1.00 ...	18
C4BQ0	26 21 0.68 ...	0 0 0.00 ...	36 29 0.61 ...	175 86 0.15 5.6*	970 -3 -0.00 0.0	2 -77 -0.98 5.2*	16 14 0.87 ...	5 -44 -0.90 2.7	153 -21 -0.12 0.2	1383
SUM	36	0	54	647	7040	579	18	362	1263	

Haplotype frequencies for population CAU
C4A-CB4 ($N=552$) ▲

	C4 A1	C4A12	C4A13	C4 A2	C4 A3	C4 A4	C4A51	C4 A6	C4AQ0	SUM
BF S	20 -10 -0.35 0.8	0 0 0.00 ...	20 -10 -0.35 0.8	275 -219 -0.44 22.8$	5243 -76 -0.11 0.8	552 83 0.58 3.4	20 5 1.00 0.3	394 76 0.79 4.2*	1155 151 0.50 5.7*	7679
BF F	20 12 0.37 ...	0 0 0.00 ...	20 12 0.37 ...	270 138 0.27 9.9#	1550 130 0.21 2.5	59 -65 -0.53 2.4	0 -3 -1.00 ...	20 -64 -0.76 3.3	110 -157 -0.59 6.6#	2049
BFF1	0 0 -1.00 ...	0 0 0.00 ...	0 0 -1.00 ...	0 -9 -1.00 0.6	135 26 0.54 1.1	0 -9 -1.00 ...	0 0 -1.00 ...	0 -5 -1.00 ...	22 1 0.01 0.0	157
BFS07	0 0 -1.00 ...	0 0 0.00 ...	0 0 -1.00 ...	79 73 0.78 ...	0 -68 -1.00 11.5$	0 -5 -1.00 ...	0 0 -1.00 ...	0 -3 -1.00 ...	20 7 0.08 0.2	99
BF V	0 0 -1.00 ...	0 0 0.00 ...	0 0 -1.00 ...	20 19 1.00 ...	0 -13 -1.00 2.3	0 0 -1.00 ...	0 0 -1.00 ...	0 0 -1.00 ...	0 -2 -1.00 ...	20
SUM	40	0	40	644	6928	611	20	414	1307	

Haplotype frequencies for population CAU; Bf-C4A ($N=508$) ▲
C2-C4A ($N=350$)▼

	C4 A1	C4A12	C4A13	C4 A2	C4 A3	C4 A4	C4A51	C4 A6	C4AQ0	SUM
C2 1	57 3 1.00 0.1	0 0 0.00 ...	0 0 0.00 ...	620 4 0.13 0.0	6606 231 0.67 17.4$	371 -279 -0.59 88.1$	29 1 1.00 0.1	486 -2 -0.01 0.0	1318 40 0.58 0.0	9487
C2 2	0 -2 -1.00 ...	0 0 0.00 ...	0 0 0.00 ...	29 -2 -0.08 0.0	114 -212 -0.65 15.6$	286 253 0.56 75.4$	0 0 -1.00 ...	29 4 0.01 0.0	29 -36 -0.56 0.9	487
C2 3	0 0 0.00 ...	0 0 0.00 ...	0 0 0.00 ...	0 0 0.00 ...	0 0 0.00 ...	0 0 0.00 ...	0 0 0.00 ...	0 0 0.00 ...	0 0 0.00 ...	0
C2 V	0 0 -1.00 ...	0 0 0.00 ...	0 0 0.00 ...	0 -1 -1.00 ...	0 -18 -1.00 2.1	29 27 1.00 ...	0 0 -1.00 ...	0 0 -1.00 ...	0 -3 -1.00 ...	29
SUM	57	0	0	649	6720	686	29	515	1347	

	C4 B1	C4B11	C4B12	C4 B2	C4 B3	C4 B4	C4 B5	C4B51	C4 B6	C4 B7	C4BQ0	SUM
BF S	5524 4 0.00 0.0	0 0 0.00 ...	0 -14 -1.00 3.3	866 172 0.81 10.2#	256 60 1.00 4.0*	39 -5 -0.14 0.2	79 18 1.00 1.2	0 0 0.00 ...	39 9 1.00 0.6	0 -14 -1.00 3.3	869 -226 -0.21 11.9‡	7672
BF F	1460 -2 -0.00 0.0	0 0 0.00 ...	20 16 1.00 ...	39 -144 -0.79 7.0#	0 -51 -1.00 3.4	20 8 0.17 0.3	0 -15 -1.00 1.0	0 0 0.00 ...	0 -7 -1.00 ...	20 16 1.00 ...	474 184 0.16 8.6#	2033
BFF1	54 -44 -0.46 3.8	0 0 0.00 ...	0 0 -1.00 ...	0 -11 -1.00 0.7	0 -3 -1.00 ...	0 0 -1.00 ...	0 0 -1.00 ...	0 0 0.00 ...	0 0 -1.00 ...	0 0 -1.00 ...	84 64 0.54 12.6‡	138
BFS07	137 38 0.97 2.6	0 0 0.00 ...	0 0 -1.00 ...	0 -11 -1.00 0.7	0 -3 -1.00 ...	0 0 -1.00 ...	0 0 -1.00 ...	0 0 0.00 ...	0 0 -1.00 ...	0 0 -1.00 ...	1 -18 -0.95 1.1	138
BF V	20 6 1.00 0.4	0 0 0.00 ...	0 0 -1.00 ...	0 -1 -1.00 ...	0 0 -1.00 ...	0 0 -1.00 ...	0 0 -1.00 ...	0 0 0.00 ...	0 0 -1.00 ...	0 0 -1.00 ...	0 -2 -1.00 ...	20
SUM	7195	0	20	905	256	59	79	0	39	20	1428	

Haplotype frequencies for population CAU; Bf-C4B ($N = 507$) ▲
C4B-DQ ($N = 523$)▼

	C4 B1	C4B11	C4B12	C4 B2	C4 B3	C4 B4	C4 B5	C4B51	C4 B6	C4 B7	C4BQ0	SUM
DQW1	2033 -249 -0.13 7.4#	0 -5 -1.00 ...	19 13 1.00 ...	417 130 0.21 4.9*	134 36 0.17 1.1	0 -11 -1.00 0.9	57 33 0.63 3.4	19 13 1.00 ...	19 7 0.27 0.3	0 -5 -1.00 ...	483 41 0.04 0.3	3181
DQW2	1983 391 0.62 22.9‡	0 -3 -1.00 ...	0 -3 -1.00 ...	76 -123 -0.62 5.7*	29 -38 -0.57 1.6	0 -7 -1.00 ...	0 -16 -1.00 1.1	0 -3 -1.00 ...	0 -7 -1.00 ...	0 -3 -1.00 ...	130 -177 -0.58 8.0#	2218
DQW3	1828 -27 -0.02 0.1	0 -4 -1.00 ...	0 -4 -1.00 ...	198 -35 -0.15 0.4	94 15 0.06 0.2	19 9 0.33 0.6	0 -19 -1.00 1.4	0 -4 -1.00 ...	0 -9 -1.00 0.7	17 12 0.86 ...	431 72 0.07 1.2	2587
DQX	1332 -114 -0.08 2.1	19 15 1.00 ...	0 -3 -1.00 ...	212 30 0.04 0.4	50 -11 -0.19 0.2	19 11 0.37 ...	19 4 0.06 0.1	0 -3 -1.00 ...	19 11 0.37 ...	2 -1 -0.48 ...	344 64 0.06 1.1	2016
SUM	7176	19	19	903	307	38	76	19	38	19	1388	

	DPW1	DPW2	DPW3	DPW4	DPW5	DPW6	DPX	SUM
DQW1	0 -114 -1.00 2.0	393 -41 -0.10 0.1	44 -104 -0.70 1.3	1448 143 0.07 0.4	220 72 0.24 0.6	0 0 0.00 ...	1156 48 0.02 0.1	3261
DQW2	43 -12 -0.24 0.0	194 -18 -0.09 0.0	88 15 0.04 0.0	542 -95 -0.15 0.3	0 -71 -1.00 1.0	0 0 0.00 ...	727 185 0.16 1.3	1594
DQW3	134 45 0.17 0.3	422 65 0.08 0.4	281 166 0.48 3.8	692 -316 -0.32 2.5	142 27 0.08 0.1	0 0 0.00 ...	856 -2 -0.00 0.0	2527
DQX	177 84 0.32 1.2	326 -23 -0.07 0.0	44 -75 -0.63 0.8	1320 272 0.17 1.8	92 -26 -0.23 0.1	0 0 0.00 ...	659 -230 -0.26 1.4	2618
SUM	354	1335	457	4002	454	0	3398	

DP-DQ ($N = 113$)▲

Haplotype frequencies for population CAU; DW-DQ ($N=91$)▼
C2-C4B ($N=348$)▼

	C4 B1	C4B11	C4B12	C4 B2	C4 B3	C4 B4	C4 B5	C4B51	C4 B6	C4 B7	C4BQ0	SUM
C2 1	6827 209 0.55 14.1¢	0 0 0.00 ...	29 2 1.00 0.1	830 -171 -0.35 21.1¢	201 -15 -0.08 0.8	57 3 1.00 0.1	0 -80 -1.00 52.4¢	0 0 0.00 ...	0 0 0.00 ...	29 2 1.00 0.1	1482 53 0.65 1.5	9455
C2 2	172 -209 -0.55 14.2¢	0 0 0.00 ...	0 -1 -1.00 ...	230 172 0.35 21.1¢	29 16 0.08 ...	0 -2 -1.00 ...	86 81 1.00 ...	0 0 0.00 ...	0 0 0.00 ...	0 -1 -1.00 ...	29 -53 -0.65 1.5	546
C2 3	0 0 0.00 ...	0 0 0.00 ...	0 0 0.00 ...	0 0 0.00 ...	0 0 0.00 ...	0 0 0.00 ...	0 0 0.00 ...	0 0 0.00 ...	0 0 0.00 ...	0 0 0.00 ...	0 0 0.00 ...	0
C2 V	0 0 0.00 ...	0 0 0.00 ...	0 0 0.00 ...	0 0 0.00 ...	0 0 0.00 ...	0 0 0.00 ...	0 0 0.00 ...	0 0 0.00 ...	0 0 0.00 ...	0 0 0.00 ...	0 0 0.00 ...	0
SUM	6999	0	29	1060	230	57	86	0	0	29	1511	

	DW1	DW2	DW3	DW4	DW5	DW6	DW7	DW8	DW9	DW10	DW11	DW12	DW13	DW14	DW15	DW16	DW17	DW18	DW19	DWX	SUM
DQW1	954 520 0.61 9.8#	656 434 0.99 12.5¢	0 -299 -1.00 4.5*	113 -113 -0.50 0.8	0 -451 -1.00 7.2#	107 70 0.97 ...	0 -221 -1.00 3.3	59 -68 -0.60 0.8	467 273 0.71 5.6*	0 -73 -1.00 1.0	0 -36 -1.00 ...	110 73 1.00 ...	59 22 0.30 ...	0 -73 -1.00 1.0	0 0 0.00 ...	0 0 0.00 ...	0 -73 -1.00 1.0	0 -36 -1.00 ...	432 264 0.98 7.9#	406 -203 -0.33 1.1	3363
DQW2	110 -162 -0.60 1.3	0 -138 -1.00 1.7	774 586 0.83 23.1¢	0 -142 -1.00 1.8	110 -173 -0.61 1.4	0 -22 -1.00 ...	628 489 0.94 21.2¢	0 -92 -1.00 1.1	0 -121 -1.00 1.5	0 -45 -1.00 ...	110 87 1.00 ...	0 -22 -1.00 ...	0 -22 -1.00 ...	0 -45 -1.00 ...	0 0 0.00 ...	0 0 0.00 ...	220 174 1.00 ...	0 -22 -1.00 ...	0 -92 -1.00 1.1	159 -223 -0.59 1.8	2111
DQW3	57 -334 -0.85 4.3*	0 -199 -1.00 2.8	0 -269 -1.00 3.9*	449 244 0.52 4.1*	978 571 0.61 12.1¢	0 -32 -1.00 ...	0 -199 -1.00 2.8	160 27 0.09 0.1	70 -104 -0.60 0.9	220 153 1.00 4.7*	0 -32 -1.00 ...	0 -32 -1.00 ...	0 -32 -1.00 ...	220 153 1.00 4.7*	0 0 0.00 ...	0 0 0.00 ...	0 -66 -1.00 0.9	0 -32 -1.00 ...	0 -132 -1.00 1.8	877 327 0.26 3.1	3031
DQX	171 -21 -0.12 0.0	3 -95 -0.97 1.1	117 -15 -0.12 0.0	114 13 0.02 0.0	256 55 0.05 0.2	2 -13 -0.88 ...	32 -66 -0.68 0.5	220 154 0.41 4.1*	40 -45 -0.54 0.3	0 -32 -1.00 ...	0 -15 -1.00 ...	0 -15 -1.00 ...	51 35 0.37 ...	0 -32 -1.00 ...	0 0 0.00 ...	0 0 0.00 ...	0 -32 -1.00 ...	110 94 1.00 ...	7 -58 -0.89 0.6	373 101 0.08 0.5	1496
SUM	1292	659	891	676	1344	109	660	439	577	220	110	110	110	220	0	0	220	110	439	1815	

Haplotype frequencies for population CAU
DW-DR ($N=89$)

	DW1	DW2	DW3	DW4	DW5	DW6	DW7	DW8	DW9	DW10	DW11	DW12	DW13	DW14	DW15	DW16	DW17	DW18	DW19	DWX	SUM
DR1	1101 938 0.67 63.1$	0 -82 -1.00 0.9	0 -112 -1.00 1.3	0 -84 -1.00 0.9	0 -183 -1.00 2.2	0 -13 -1.00 ...	0 -68 -1.00 0.7	0 -41 -1.00 ...	55 -17 -0.25 0.0	0 -27 -1.00 ...	0 -13 -1.00 ...	0 -13 -1.00 ...	0 -13 -1.00 ...	0 -27 -1.00 ...	0 0 0.00 ...	0 0 0.00 ...	0 -27 -1.00 ...	0 -13 -1.00 ...	0 -54 -1.00 ...	80 -134 -0.63 1.0	1236
DR2	0 -132 -1.00 1.5	674 606 1.00 57.3$	0 -91 -1.00 1.0	0 -69 -1.00 0.7	0 -149 -1.00 1.7	0 -10 -1.00 ...	0 -56 -1.00 0.6	0 -33 -1.00 ...	0 -59 -1.00 0.6	0 -22 -1.00 ...	0 -10 -1.00 ...	112 101 1.00 ...	0 -10 -1.00 ...	0 -22 -1.00 ...	0 0 0.00 ...	0 0 0.00 ...	0 -22 -1.00 ...	0 -10 -1.00 ...	0 -44 -1.00 ...	224 48 0.06 0.2	1010
DR3	0 -132 -1.00 1.5	0 -67 -1.00 0.7	849 757 0.92 67.8$	0 -69 -1.00 0.7	0 -149 -1.00 1.7	0 -10 -1.00 ...	0 -56 -1.00 0.6	0 -33 -1.00 ...	0 -59 -1.00 0.6	0 -22 -1.00 ...	0 -10 -1.00 ...	0 -10 -1.00 ...	0 -10 -1.00 ...	0 -22 -1.00 ...	0 0 0.00 ...	0 0 0.00 ...	0 -22 -1.00 ...	0 -10 -1.00 ...	0 -44 -1.00 ...	162 -13 -0.08 0.0	1011
DR4	0 -168 -1.00 2.3	0 -95 -1.00 1.1	0 -129 -1.00 1.5	643 544 0.92 33.5$	117 -94 -0.45 0.5	0 -15 -1.00 ...	0 -79 -1.00 0.9	0 -47 -1.00 ...	80 -3 -0.05 0.0	225 193 1.00 ...	0 -15 -1.00 ...	0 -15 -1.00 ...	0 -15 -1.00 ...	225 193 1.00 ...	0 0 0.00 ...	0 0 0.00 ...	0 -31 -1.00 ...	0 -15 -1.00 ...	0 -63 -1.00 0.7	139 -109 -0.44 0.6	1429
DR7	0 -162 -1.00 1.9	0 -62 -1.00 0.9	0 -112 -1.00 1.3	0 -84 -1.00 0.9	112 -71 -0.39 0.3	0 -13 -1.00 ...	562 493 1.00 37.6$	0 -41 -1.00 ...	0 -72 -1.00 0.8	0 -27 -1.00 ...	112 98 1.00 ...	0 -13 -1.00 ...	0 -13 -1.00 ...	0 -27 -1.00 ...	0 0 0.00 ...	0 0 0.00 ...	225 197 1.00 ...	0 -13 -1.00 ...	0 -54 -1.00 ...	225 10 0.01 0.0	1236
DRW8	0 -43 -1.00 ...	0 -22 -1.00 ...	0 -30 -1.00 ...	0 -22 -1.00 ...	0 -49 -1.00 ...	0 -3 -1.00 ...	0 -18 -1.00 ...	337 326 1.00 ...	0 -19 -1.00 ...	0 -7 -1.00 ...	0 -3 -1.00 ...	0 -3 -1.00 ...	0 -3 -1.00 ...	0 -7 -1.00 ...	0 0 0.00 ...	0 0 0.00 ...	0 -7 -1.00 ...	0 -3 -1.00 ...	0 -14 -1.00 ...	0 -58 -1.00 0.7	337
DRW9	0 -58 -1.00 0.6	0 -29 -1.00 ...	62 21 0.05 ...	0 -30 -1.00 ...	0 -66 -1.00 0.7	0 -4 -1.00 ...	0 -24 -1.00 ...	0 -14 -1.00 ...	0 -26 -1.00 ...	0 -9 -1.00 ...	0 -4 -1.00 ...	0 -4 -1.00 ...	0 -4 -1.00 ...	0 -9 -1.00 ...	0 0 0.00 ...	0 0 0.00 ...	0 -9 -1.00 ...	0 -4 -1.00 ...	0 -19 -1.00 ...	387 309 0.83 13.8$	449
DRW10	80 65 0.67 ...	0 -7 -1.00 ...	0 -9 -1.00 ...	0 -7 -1.00 ...	0 -16 -1.00 ...	0 0 -1.00 ...	0 -5 -1.00 ...	0 -3 -1.00 ...	0 -6 -1.00 ...	0 -2 -1.00 ...	0 0 -1.00 ...	0 0 -1.00 ...	0 0 -1.00 ...	0 -2 -1.00 ...	0 0 0.00 ...	0 0 0.00 ...	0 -2 -1.00 ...	0 0 -1.00 ...	0 -4 -1.00 ...	32 13 0.14 ...	112
DRW11	0 -177 -1.00 2.1	0 -90 -1.00 1.0	0 -122 -1.00 1.4	48 -44 -0.48 0.2	1257 1057 0.92 67.3$	0 -14 -1.00 ...	0 -75 -1.00 0.8	0 -44 -1.00 ...	0 -79 -1.00 0.9	0 -29 -1.00 ...	0 -14 -1.00 ...	0 -14 -1.00 ...	0 -14 -1.00 ...	0 -29 -1.00 ...	0 0 0.00 ...	0 0 0.00 ...	0 -29 -1.00 ...	0 -14 -1.00 ...	0 -60 -1.00 0.7	43 -191 -0.82 1.0	1348
DRW12	0 -58 -1.00 0.6	0 -29 -1.00 ...	0 -40 -1.00 ...	0 -30 -1.00 ...	0 -66 -1.00 0.7	0 -4 -1.00 ...	0 -24 -1.00 ...	0 -14 -1.00 ...	0 -26 -1.00 ...	0 -9 -1.00 ...	0 -4 -1.00 ...	0 -4 -1.00 ...	112 107 1.00 ...	0 -9 -1.00 ...	0 0 0.00 ...	0 0 0.00 ...	0 -9 -1.00 ...	0 -4 -1.00 ...	0 -19 -1.00 ...	337 259 0.70 9.7#	449
DRW13	0 -58 -1.00 0.6	0 -29 -1.00 ...	0 -40 -1.00 ...	0 -30 -1.00 ...	0 -66 -1.00 0.7	0 -4 -1.00 ...	0 -24 -1.00 ...	0 -14 -1.00 ...	0 -26 -1.00 ...	0 -9 -1.00 ...	0 -4 -1.00 ...	0 -4 -1.00 ...	0 -4 -1.00 ...	0 -9 -1.00 ...	0 0 0.00 ...	0 0 0.00 ...	0 -9 -1.00 ...	112 107 1.00 ...	337 317 0.74 ...	0 -77 -1.00 0.9	449
DRW14	139 35 0.05 0.1	0 -52 -1.00 ...	0 -71 -1.00 0.8	0 -53 -1.00 ...	0 -116 -1.00 1.3	112 103 1.00 ...	0 -43 -1.00 ...	0 -25 -1.00 ...	423 377 0.69 ...	0 -17 -1.00 ...	0 -8 -1.00 ...	0 -8 -1.00 ...	0 -8 -1.00 ...	0 -17 -1.00 ...	0 0 0.00 ...	0 0 0.00 ...	0 -17 -1.00 ...	0 -8 -1.00 ...	112 77 0.19 ...	0 -136 -1.00 1.6	786
DRX	0 -18 -1.00 ...	0 -9 -1.00 ...	0 -12 -1.00 ...	0 -9 -1.00 ...	0 -21 -1.00 ...	0 -1 -1.00 ...	0 -7 -1.00 ...	0 -4 -1.00 ...	33 24 0.18 ...	0 -2 -1.00 ...	0 -1 -1.00 ...	0 -1 -1.00 ...	0 -1 -1.00 ...	0 -2 -1.00 ...	0 0 0.00 ...	0 0 0.00 ...	0 -2 -1.00 ...	0 -1 -1.00 ...	0 -6 -1.00 ...	112 87 0.72 ...	145
SUM	1320	674	911	691	1486	112	562	337	591	225	112	112	112	225	0	0	225	112	449	1741	

Haplotype frequencies for population ORI
A-B ($N=956$)

	A1	A2	A3	A11	A23	A24	A25	A26	A28	A29	A30	A31	A32	AW33	AW34	AW36	AW43	AW66	AX	SUM
B7	0 -4 -1.00 ...	83 -47 -0.37 2.5	42 35 0.24 17.2¢	23 -32 -0.59 2.2	10 10 1.00 ...	259 112 0.35 12.5¢	0 0 0.00 ...	21 -12 -0.38 0.5	0 -9 -1.00 0.0	10 8 0.21 ...	0 -10 -1.00 1.1	10 -14 -0.59 0.9	0 -1 -1.00 ...	0 -28 -1.00 3.0	0 0 -1.00 ...	0 0 -1.00 ...	0 0 0.00 ...	0 -1 -1.00 ...	12 4 0.03 0.3	470
B8	10 10 0.49 ...	0 -5 -1.00 0.7	10 10 0.49 ...	0 -1 -1.00 ...	0 0 -1.00 ...	0 -5 -1.00 0.9	0 0 0.00 ...	0 0 -1.00 ...	0 0 -1.00 ...	0 0 -1.00 ...	0 0 -1.00 ...	0 0 -1.00 ...	0 0 -1.00 ...	0 0 -1.00 ...	0 0 -1.00 ...	0 0 -1.00 ...	0 0 0.00 ...	0 0 -1.00 ...	0 0 -1.00 ...	20
B13	0 -3 -1.00 ...	98 -6 -0.07 0.1	0 -5 -1.00 0.6	42 -1 -0.05 0.0	0 0 -1.00 ...	10 -106 -0.91 14.2¢	0 0 0.00 ...	21 -5 -0.22 0.1	0 -7 -1.00 0.8	0 -1 -1.00 ...	192 183 0.80 382.7¢	0 -19 -1.00 2.1	0 -1 -1.00 ...	0 -22 -1.00 2.4	0 0 -1.00 ...	0 0 -1.00 ...	0 0 0.00 ...	0 -1 -1.00 ...	13 7 0.04 0.8	376
B18	0 0 -1.00 ...	0 -8 -1.00 1.2	0 0 -1.00 ...	0 -3 -1.00 ...	0 0 -1.00 ...	20 10 0.48 1.5	0 0 0.00 ...	0 -1 -1.00 ...	0 0 -1.00 ...	10 10 0.32 ...	0 0 -1.00 ...	0 -1 -1.00 ...	0 0 -1.00 ...	0 -1 -1.00 ...	0 0 -1.00 ...	0 0 -1.00 ...	0 0 0.00 ...	0 0 -1.00 ...	1 0 0.02 ...	31
B27	10 8 0.08 ...	52 8 0.07 0.2	10 8 0.05 ...	21 3 0.02 0.0	0 0 -1.00 ...	39 -9 -0.20 0.3	0 0 0.00 ...	3 -7 -0.73 0.6	0 -2 -1.00 ...	0 0 -1.00 ...	0 -3 -1.00 ...	21 13 0.09 2.1	0 0 -1.00 ...	0 -6 -1.00 0.0	0 0 -1.00 ...	0 0 -1.00 ...	0 0 0.00 ...	0 0 -1.00 ...	0 -2 -1.00 ...	156
B35	10 0 -0.04 0.0	395 109 0.15 6.2*	10 -5 -0.36 0.2	94 -26 -0.22 0.7	0 0 -1.00 ...	329 10 0.01 0.1	0 0 0.00 ...	78 5 0.01 0.0	19 -1 -0.10 0.0	0 -3 -1.00 ...	0 -23 -1.00 2.6	83 30 0.06 1.9	0 -3 -1.00 ...	0 -61 -1.00 7.0#	0 -2 -1.00 ...	0 0 -1.00 ...	0 0 0.00 ...	0 -3 -1.00 ...	3 -13 -0.82 1.2	1021
B37	21 20 0.34 ...	1 -15 -0.94 2.0	0 0 -1.00 ...	10 3 0.05 0.1	0 0 -1.00 ...	10 -8 -0.47 0.6	0 0 0.00 ...	9 5 0.08 ...	10 9 0.15 ...	0 0 -1.00 ...	0 0 -1.00 ...	0 -2 -1.00 ...	0 0 -1.00 ...	0 -3 -1.00 ...	0 0 -1.00 ...	0 0 -1.00 ...	0 0 0.00 ...	0 0 -1.00 ...	0 0 -1.00 ...	61
B38	0 0 -1.00 ...	42 22 0.42 3.2	0 0 -1.00 ...	10 1 0.02 0.0	0 0 -1.00 ...	0 -21 -1.00 3.1	0 0 0.00 ...	10 5 0.07 ...	0 0 -1.00 ...	0 0 -1.00 ...	10 8 0.12 ...	0 -3 -1.00 ...	0 0 -1.00 ...	0 -3 -1.00 ...	0 0 -1.00 ...	0 0 -1.00 ...	0 0 0.00 ...	0 0 -1.00 ...	0 0 -1.00 ...	72
B39	0 -3 -1.00 ...	178 64 0.22 5.0*	0 -5 -1.00 0.6	73 25 0.07 1.5	0 0 -1.00 ...	93 -33 -0.27 1.3	0 0 0.00 ...	1 -27 -0.97 2.9	10 2 0.01 0.0	0 -1 -1.00 ...	0 -9 -1.00 0.0	52 31 0.08 4.7*	0 -1 -1.00 ...	0 -24 -1.00 2.6	0 0 -1.00 ...	0 0 -1.00 ...	0 0 0.00 ...	0 -1 -1.00 ...	0 -6 -1.00 0.7	407
BW41	0 0 -1.00 ...	0 -2 -1.00 ...	0 0 -1.00 ...	10 9 1.00 ...	0 0 -1.00 ...	0 -2 -1.00 ...	0 0 0.00 ...	0 0 -1.00 ...	0 0 -1.00 ...	0 0 -1.00 ...	0 0 -1.00 ...	0 0 -1.00 ...	0 0 -1.00 ...	0 0 -1.00 ...	0 0 -1.00 ...	0 0 -1.00 ...	0 0 0.00 ...	0 0 -1.00 ...	0 0 -1.00 ...	10
BW42	0 0 -1.00 ...	31 16 0.44 2.5	0 0 -1.00 ...	21 15 0.32 3.9*	0 0 -1.00 ...	0 -15 -1.00 2.3	0 0 0.00 ...	0 -3 -1.00 ...	0 0 -1.00 ...	0 0 -1.00 ...	0 0 -1.00 ...	0 -2 -1.00 ...	0 0 -1.00 ...	0 -2 -1.00 ...	0 0 -1.00 ...	0 0 -1.00 ...	0 0 0.00 ...	0 0 -1.00 ...	0 0 -1.00 ...	52
B44	0 -5 -1.00 0.6	24 -138 -0.85 16.7¢	41 32 0.22 11.9¢	20 -48 -0.71 3.0*	0 0 -1.00 ...	42 -139 -0.77 15.9¢	0 0 0.00 ...	10 -31 -0.76 2.6	0 -11 -1.00 1.2	0 -1 -1.00 ...	0 -13 -1.00 1.4	20 -9 -0.34 0.4	10 8 0.20 ...	414 379 0.69 437.8¢	0 -1 -1.00 ...	0 0 -1.00 ...	0 0 0.00 ...	0 -1 -1.00 ...	2 -6 -0.79 0.6	583
B45	0 0 -1.00 ...	0 -2 -1.00 ...	0 0 -1.00 ...	0 0 -1.00 ...	0 0 -1.00 ...	10 7 1.00 ...	0 0 0.00 ...	0 0 -1.00 ...	0 0 -1.00 ...	0 0 -1.00 ...	0 0 -1.00 ...	0 0 -1.00 ...	0 0 -1.00 ...	0 0 -1.00 ...	0 0 -1.00 ...	0 0 -1.00 ...	0 0 0.00 ...	0 0 -1.00 ...	0 0 -1.00 ...	10
BW46	0 -3 -1.00 ...	292 190 0.72 48.4¢	0 -5 -1.00 0.6	30 -12 -0.31 0.5	0 0 -1.00 ...	40 -73 -0.65 6.0#	0 0 0.00 ...	0 -25 -1.00 2.8	0 -7 -1.00 0.8	0 0 -1.00 ...	0 -8 -1.00 0.9	0 -18 -1.00 2.0	0 -1 -1.00 ...	4 -17 -0.82 1.6	0 0 -1.00 ...	0 0 -1.00 ...	0 0 0.00 ...	0 -1 -1.00 ...	0 -5 -1.00 0.6	366
BW47	0 0 -1.00 ...	4 -7 -0.67 0.7	0 0 -1.00 ...	0 -4 -1.00 ...	0 0 -1.00 ...	5 -7 -0.63 0.7	0 0 0.00 ...	8 5 0.12 ...	0 0 -1.00 ...	0 0 -1.00 ...	15 14 0.33 ...	0 -1 -1.00 ...	0 0 -1.00 ...	0 -2 -1.00 ...	0 0 -1.00 ...	0 0 -1.00 ...	0 0 0.00 ...	0 0 -1.00 ...	11 10 0.24 ...	43

Haplotype frequencies for population ORI
A-B ($N = 956$)

	A1	A2	A3	A11	A23	A24	A25	A26	A28	A29	A30	A31	A32	AW33	AW34	AW36	AW43	AW66	AX	SUM
BW48	0 -1 -1.00 ...	21 -25 -0.55 1.9	0 -2 -1.00 ...	0 -19 -1.00 2.2	0 0 -1.00 ...	73 21 0.18 1.2	0 0 0.00 ...	42 30 0.19 7.9#	0 -2 -1.00 ...	0 0 -1.00 ...	0 -3 -1.00 ...	31 22 0.14 5.8*	0 0 -1.00 ...	0 -9 -1.00 1.0	0 0 -1.00 ...	0 0 -1.00 ...	0 0 0.00 ...	0 0 -1.00 ...	0 -2 -1.00 ...	167
B49	0 0 -1.00 ...	5 -3 -0.44 0.2	0 0 -1.00 ...	0 -3 -1.00 ...	0 0 -1.00 ...	6 -3 -0.40 0.2	0 0 0.00 ...	0 -1 -1.00 ...	21 20 0.65 ...	0 0 -1.00 ...	0 0 -1.00 ...	0 -1 -1.00 ...	0 0 -1.00 ...	0 -1 -1.00 ...	0 0 -1.00 ...	0 0 -1.00 ...	0 0 0.00 ...	0 0 -1.00 ...	0 0 -1.00 ...	32
BW50	0 0 -1.00 ...	21 12 0.55 2.3	0 0 -1.00 ...	0 -3 -1.00 ...	0 0 -1.00 ...	0 -9 -1.00 1.3	0 0 0.00 ...	0 -1 -1.00 ...	10 9 0.31 ...	0 0 -1.00 ...	0 0 -1.00 ...	0 -1 -1.00 ...	0 0 -1.00 ...	0 -1 -1.00 ...	0 0 -1.00 ...	0 0 -1.00 ...	0 0 0.00 ...	0 0 -1.00 ...	0 0 -1.00 ...	31
B51	10 2 0.02 0.1	195 -17 -0.09 0.2	0 -11 -1.00 1.2	52 -37 -0.42 1.9	0 0 -1.00 ...	279 41 0.08 1.1	0 0 0.00 ...	64 10 0.01 0.2	10 -5 -0.36 0.2	0 -2 -1.00 ...	0 -17 -1.00 1.9	130 90 0.19 22.3$	0 -2 -1.00 ...	21 -24 -0.55 1.5	0 -1 -1.00 ...	0 0 -1.00 ...	0 0 0.00 ...	0 -2 -1.00 ...	1 -10 -0.92 1.1	762
BW52	10 3 0.03 0.1	78 -126 -0.62 11.2$	10 0 -0.11 0.0	52 -34 -0.40 1.6	0 0 -1.00 ...	505 276 0.55 50.2$	0 0 0.00 ...	12 -39 -0.77 3.5	21 6 0.03 0.2	0 -2 -1.00 ...	0 -16 -1.00 1.8	21 -16 -0.45 0.8	21 18 0.47 ...	0 -43 -1.00 4.9*	0 -1 -1.00 ...	0 0 -1.00 ...	0 0 0.00 ...	0 -2 -1.00 ...	2 -9 -0.83 0.9	732
BW53	0 0 -1.00 ...	10 2 0.07 0.0	0 0 -1.00 ...	0 -3 -1.00 ...	0 0 -1.00 ...	4 -4 -0.57 0.4	0 0 0.00 ...	0 -1 -1.00 ...	0 0 -1.00 ...	0 0 -1.00 ...	10 9 0.32 ...	0 -1 -1.00 ...	0 0 -1.00 ...	0 -1 -1.00 ...	0 0 -1.00 ...	0 0 -1.00 ...	0 0 0.00 ...	0 0 -1.00 ...	6 6 0.19 ...	30
BW54	10 3 0.03 0.1	167 -22 -0.12 0.4	0 -9 -1.00 1.1	105 25 0.04 0.9	0 0 -1.00 ...	344 132 0.28 12.3$	0 0 0.00 ...	31 -16 -0.36 0.7	10 -3 -0.28 0.1	0 -2 -1.00 ...	0 -15 -1.00 1.7	10 -24 -0.72 1.0	0 -2 -1.00 ...	0 -40 -1.00 4.5*	0 -1 -1.00 ...	0 0 -1.00 ...	0 0 0.00 ...	0 -2 -1.00 ...	1 -9 -0.91 0.9	678
BW55	0 -1 -1.00 ...	42 -15 -0.28 0.6	0 -2 -1.00 ...	104 79 0.43 28.4$	0 0 -1.00 ...	48 -16 -0.26 0.6	0 0 0.00 ...	0 -14 -1.00 1.6	10 6 0.03 ...	0 0 -1.00 ...	0 -4 -1.00 ...	0 -10 -1.00 1.1	0 0 -1.00 ...	0 -12 -1.00 1.3	0 0 -1.00 ...	0 0 -1.00 ...	0 0 0.00 ...	0 0 -1.00 ...	4 1 0.00 ...	208
BW56	0 0 -1.00 ...	32 -7 -0.21 0.2	0 -1 -1.00 ...	6 -10 -0.65 0.8	0 0 -1.00 ...	41 -3 -0.09 0.0	0 0 0.00 ...	31 21 0.15 4.3*	0 -2 -1.00 ...	10 9 0.24 ...	0 -2 -1.00 ...	0 -7 -1.00 0.8	0 0 -1.00 ...	0 -8 -1.00 0.9	10 10 0.32 ...	0 0 -1.00 ...	0 0 0.00 ...	10 9 0.23 ...	4 2 0.01 ...	144
BW57	21 20 0.28 ...	37 17 0.32 1.8	10 9 0.12 ...	0 -8 -1.00 0.9	0 0 -1.00 ...	5 -17 -0.78 1.9	0 0 0.00 ...	0 -4 -1.00 ...	0 -1 -1.00 ...	0 0 -1.00 ...	0 -1 -1.00 ...	0 -3 -1.00 ...	0 0 -1.00 ...	0 -3 -1.00 ...	0 0 -1.00 ...	0 0 -1.00 ...	0 0 0.00 ...	0 0 -1.00 ...	0 0 -1.00 ...	73
BW58	0 -2 -1.00 ...	31 -38 -0.56 2.9	0 -3 -1.00 ...	21 -8 -0.29 0.3	0 0 -1.00 ...	11 -66 -0.86 8.2#	0 0 0.00 ...	10 -7 -0.44 0.4	0 -4 -1.00 ...	0 0 -1.00 ...	0 -5 -1.00 0.6	0 -12 -1.00 1.4	10 9 0.22 ...	167 152 0.65 158.6$	0 0 -1.00 ...	0 0 -1.00 ...	0 0 0.00 ...	0 0 -1.00 ...	0 -3 -1.00 ...	250
BW59	0 0 -1.00 ...	63 31 0.38 4.1*	0 -1 -1.00 ...	0 -12 -1.00 1.5	0 0 -1.00 ...	41 5 0.07 0.1	0 0 0.00 ...	10 2 0.02 0.0	0 -1 -1.00 ...	0 0 -1.00 ...	0 -2 -1.00 ...	0 -5 -1.00 0.6	0 0 -1.00 ...	0 -6 -1.00 0.7	0 0 -1.00 ...	0 0 -1.00 ...	0 0 0.00 ...	0 0 -1.00 ...	0 -1 -1.00 ...	114
BW60	0 -6 -1.00 0.7	218 31 0.06 0.7	0 -9 -1.00 1.1	78 0 -0.01 0.0	0 0 -1.00 ...	219 10 0.02 0.1	0 0 0.00 ...	56 6 0.01 0.2	31 17 0.09 2.3	10 7 0.20 ...	0 -15 -1.00 1.7	23 -11 -0.34 0.4	0 -2 -1.00 ...	0 -40 -1.00 4.4*	10 8 0.29 ...	10 9 1.00 ...	0 0 0.00 ...	0 -2 -1.00 ...	13 2 0.01 0.0	668
BW61	0 -11 -1.00 1.3	376 52 0.06 1.2	0 -17 -1.00 1.9	119 -17 -0.13 0.3	0 0 -1.00 ...	346 -15 -0.04 0.1	0 0 0.00 ...	164 81 0.13 9.2#	52 28 0.15 3.6	0 -4 -1.00 ...	0 -26 -1.00 3.0	63 2 0.01 0.0	0 -4 -1.00 ...	0 -69 -1.00 8.1#	0 -2 -1.00 ...	0 0 -1.00 ...	0 0 0.00 ...	21 16 0.45 ...	19 0 0.00 0.0	1160
BW62	0 -9 -1.00 1.0	217 -46 -0.18 1.2	10 -3 -0.31 0.1	271 159 0.19 27.2$	0 0 -1.00 ...	228 -66 -0.23 2.3	0 0 0.00 ...	128 60 0.09 6.1*	0 -18 -1.00 2.1	0 -3 -1.00 ...	0 -21 -1.00 2.4	47 -1 -0.05 0.0	0 -3 -1.00 ...	0 -56 -1.00 6.4*	5 2 0.08 ...	0 0 -1.00 ...	0 0 0.00 ...	10 6 0.16 ...	29 14 0.09 1.3	945

Haplotype frequencies for population ORI
A-B (N=956)

	A1	A2	A3	A11	A23	A24	A25	A26	A28	A29	A30	A31	A32	AW33	AW34	AW36	AW43	AW66	AX	SUM
BW63	0 0 0.00 ...	0 0 0.00 ...	0 0 0.00 ...	0 0 0.00 ...	0 0 0.00 ...	0 0 0.00 ...	0 0 0.00 ...	0 0 0.00 ...	0 0 0.00 ...	0 0 0.00 ...	0 0 0.00 ...	0 0 0.00 ...	0 0 0.00 ...	0 0 0.00 ...	0 0 0.00 ...	0 0 0.00 ...	0 0 0.00 ...	0 0 0.00 ...	0 0 0.00 ...	0
BW64	0 0 0.00 ...	0 0 0.00 ...	0 0 0.00 ...	0 0 0.00 ...	0 0 0.00 ...	0 0 0.00 ...	0 0 0.00 ...	0 0 0.00 ...	0 0 0.00 ...	0 0 0.00 ...	0 0 0.00 ...	0 0 0.00 ...	0 0 0.00 ...	0 0 0.00 ...	0 0 0.00 ...	0 0 0.00 ...	0 0 0.00 ...	0 0 0.00 ...	0 0 0.00 ...	0
BW65	0 0 -1.00 ...	0 -5 -1.00 0.7	10 10 0.49 ...	0 -1 -1.00 ...	0 0 -1.00 ...	0 -5 -1.00 0.9	0 0 0.00 ...	0 0 -1.00 ...	0 0 -1.00 ...	0 0 -1.00 ...	10 10 0.49 ...	0 0 -1.00 ...	0 0 -1.00 ...	0 0 -1.00 ...	0 0 -1.00 ...	0 0 -1.00 ...	0 0 0.00 ...	0 0 -1.00 ...	0 0 -1.00 ...	20
BW67	0 0 -1.00 ...	0 -2 -1.00 ...	0 0 -1.00 ...	10 9 1.00 ...	0 0 -1.00 ...	0 -2 -1.00 ...	0 0 0.00 ...	0 0 -1.00 ...	0 0 -1.00 ...	0 0 -1.00 ...	0 0 -1.00 ...	0 0 -1.00 ...	0 0 -1.00 ...	0 0 -1.00 ...	0 0 -1.00 ...	0 0 -1.00 ...	0 0 0.00 ...	0 0 -1.00 ...	0 0 -1.00 ...	10
BW71	0 0 -1.00 ...	21 9 0.31 0.0	0 0 -1.00 ...	0 -4 -1.00 ...	0 0 -1.00 ...	18 5 0.17 0.3	0 0 0.00 ...	3 0 -0.00 ...	0 0 -1.00 ...	0 0 -1.00 ...	0 0 -1.00 ...	0 -1 -1.00 ...	0 0 -1.00 ...	0 -2 -1.00 ...	0 0 -1.00 ...	0 0 -1.00 ...	0 0 0.00 ...	0 0 -1.00 ...	0 0 -1.00 ...	42
BW72	0 0 -1.00 ...	0 -13 -1.00 1.9	0 0 -1.00 ...	10 4 0.09 0.3	0 0 -1.00 ...	28 12 0.34 1.3	0 0 0.00 ...	3 0 -0.18 ...	0 0 -1.00 ...	0 0 -1.00 ...	0 0 -1.00 ...	10 7 0.15 ...	0 0 -1.00 ...	0 -2 -1.00 ...	0 0 -1.00 ...	0 0 -1.00 ...	0 0 0.00 ...	0 0 -1.00 ...	0 0 -1.00 ...	51
BW73	0 0 -1.00 ...	0 -5 -1.00 0.8	0 0 -1.00 ...	0 -1 -1.00 ...	0 0 -1.00 ...	14 7 0.52 1.2	0 0 0.00 ...	0 -1 -1.00 ...	0 0 -1.00 ...	0 0 -1.00 ...	0 0 -1.00 ...	0 0 -1.00 ...	0 0 -1.00 ...	0 0 -1.00 ...	0 0 -1.00 ...	0 0 -1.00 ...	0 0 0.00 ...	0 0 -1.00 ...	7 7 0.32 ...	21
BX	0 -1 -1.00 ...	63 18 0.15 0.0	0 -1 -1.00 ...	0 -18 -1.00 2.1	0 0 -1.00 ...	55 5 0.04 0.1	0 0 0.00 ...	0 -11 -1.00 1.2	2 0 -0.40 ...	0 0 -1.00 ...	0 -3 -1.00 ...	1 -6 -0.88 0.7	0 0 -1.00 ...	1 -8 -0.90 0.8	5 5 0.15 ...	0 0 -1.00 ...	0 0 0.00 ...	0 0 -1.00 ...	34 31 0.20 ...	161
SUM	102	2797	153	1182	10	3122	0	715	206	40	237	522	41	607	30	10	0	41	162	

Haplotype frequencies for population ORI
A-C ($N = 969$)

	A1	A2	A3	A11	A23	A24	A25	A26	A28	A29	A30	A31	A32	AW33	AW34	AW36	AW43	AW66	AX	SUM
CW1	10 -6 -0.40 0.3	654 192 0.16 12.9¢	10 -12 -0.57 0.9	217 25 0.03 0.4	0 -1 -1.00 ...	578 66 0.06 1.4	0 0 0.00 ...	83 -34 -0.30 1.3	10 -23 -0.70 1.0	10 3 0.10 0.2	0 -38 -1.00 4.6*	30 -55 -0.65 4.5*	0 -6 -1.00 0.8	7 -92 -0.93 10.6#	10 5 0.19 ...	0 -1 -1.00 ...	0 0 0.00 ...	0 -7 -1.00 0.0	22 -5 -0.22 0.2	1641
CW2	10 9 0.09 ...	31 2 0.03 0.0	10 9 0.08 ...	0 -11 -1.00 1.3	0 0 -1.00 ...	21 -10 -0.35 0.6	0 0 0.00 ...	21 14 0.14 2.6	0 -1 -1.00 ...	0 0 -1.00 ...	0 -1 -1.00 ...	10 5 0.05 0.4	0 0 -1.00 ...	0 -5 -1.00 0.7	0 0 -1.00 ...	0 0 -1.00 ...	0 0 0.00 ...	0 0 -1.00 ...	0 -1 -1.00 ...	103
CW3	2 -25 -0.93 3.2	850 79 0.04 1.5	0 -38 -1.00 5.3*	224 -95 -0.30 4.3*	0 -2 -1.00 ...	622 -32 -0.04 0.3	0 0 0.00 ...	353 156 0.30 17.8¢	75 19 0.12 0.8	0 -10 -1.00 1.5	0 -63 -1.00 8.8#	191 47 0.12 2.1	0 -10 -1.00 1.5	179 12 0.03 0.1	0 -7 -1.00 1.1	0 -2 -1.00 ...	0 0 0.00 ...	10 -3 -0.28 0.2	33 -13 -0.30 0.6	2739
CW4	10 5 0.05 0.4	110 -38 -0.26 1.4	1 -6 -0.87 0.6	136 74 0.16 10.4#	0 0 -1.00 ...	125 -39 -0.24 1.4	0 0 0.00 ...	31 -6 -0.18 0.1	10 0 -0.08 0.0	0 -1 -1.00 ...	10 -1 -0.19 0.0	52 24 0.05 2.3	10 8 0.20 ...	10 -21 -0.69 1.7	0 -1 -1.00 ...	10 9 1.00 ...	0 0 0.00 ...	0 -2 -1.00 ...	13 4 0.02 0.2	528
CW5	0 0 -1.00 ...	21 4 0.08 0.1	31 30 0.49 ...	0 -6 -1.00 0.8	0 0 -1.00 ...	10 -8 -0.48 0.6	0 0 0.00 ...	0 -3 -1.00 ...	0 0 -1.00 ...	0 0 -1.00 ...	0 0 -1.00 ...	0 -2 -1.00 ...	0 0 -1.00 ...	0 -3 -1.00 ...	0 0 -1.00 ...	0 0 -1.00 ...	0 0 0.00 ...	0 0 -1.00 ...	0 0 -1.00 ...	62
CW6	41 37 0.38 ...	57 -48 -0.46 3.2	10 5 0.03 0.4	10 -33 -0.77 3.0	0 0 -1.00 ...	18 -99 -0.85 12.4¢	0 0 0.00 ...	10 -16 -0.63 1.2	21 13 0.07 2.3	0 -1 -1.00 ...	190 181 0.80 380.8¢	0 -19 -1.00 2.1	10 8 0.21 ...	0 -22 -1.00 2.5	0 0 -1.00 ...	0 0 -1.00 ...	0 0 0.00 ...	0 -1 -1.00 ...	11 5 0.03 0.3	378
CW7	10 -1 -0.17 0.0	328 -6 -0.02 0.0	41 24 0.19 3.8	196 57 0.06 2.9	10 9 1.00 ...	390 18 0.02 0.1	0 0 0.00 ...	60 -25 -0.30 0.9	31 6 0.04 0.2	0 -4 -1.00 ...	10 -17 -0.64 1.3	52 -10 -0.17 0.2	0 -4 -1.00 ...	31 -40 -0.57 2.8	0 -3 -1.00 ...	0 0 -1.00 ...	0 0 0.00 ...	10 4 0.09 0.3	21 1 0.00 0.0	1190
CW8	0 0 -1.00 ...	0 -7 -1.00 1.1	10 10 0.32 ...	0 -3 -1.00 ...	0 0 -1.00 ...	0 -8 -1.00 1.3	0 0 0.00 ...	0 -1 -1.00 ...	10 9 0.32 ...	0 0 -1.00 ...	10 9 0.32 ...	0 -1 -1.00 ...	0 0 -1.00 ...	0 -1 -1.00 ...	0 0 -1.00 ...	0 0 -1.00 ...	0 0 0.00 ...	0 0 -1.00 ...	0 0 -1.00 ...	30
CX	18 -15 -0.46 1.1	763 -172 -0.19 6.5*	30 -17 -0.37 0.0	384 -3 -0.01 0.0	0 -2 -1.00 ...	1159 120 0.06 2.9	0 0 0.00 ...	161 -77 -0.33 4.0*	49 -19 -0.29 0.8	31 17 0.63 3.2	15 -62 -0.81 7.6#	192 17 0.05 0.2	21 7 0.27 0.6	381 179 0.44 24.4¢	21 11 0.52 1.6	0 -2 -1.00 ...	0 0 0.00 ...	31 14 0.41 1.7	71 14 0.12 0.5	3327
SUM	101	2814	143	1167	10	3123	0	719	206	41	235	527	41	608	31	10	0	51	171	

Haplotype frequencies for population ORI
A-DR ($N = 756$)

	A1	A2	A3	A11	A23	A24	A25	A26	A28	A29	A30	A31	A32	AW33	AW34	AW36	AW43	AW66	AX	SUM
DR1	0 -3 -1.00 ...	119 -19 -0.14 0.3	0 -5 -1.00 ...	30 -27 -0.48 1.2	0 0 -1.00 ...	285 127 0.37 11.8‡	0 0 0.00 ...	26 -12 -0.34 0.4	0 -7 -1.00 0.6	0 -1 -1.00 ...	13 3 0.02 0.1	26 -1 -0.06 0.0	0 0 -1.00 ...	0 -31 -1.00 2.7	0 -1 -1.00 ...	0 0 -1.00 ...	0 0 0.00 ...	0 -2 -1.00 ...	0 -7 -1.00 0.7	499
DR2	0 -11 -1.00 1.1	362 -63 -0.15 1.2	14 -3 -0.22 0.1	181 5 0.00 0.0	0 -1 -1.00 ...	696 211 0.20 11.0‡	0 0 0.00 ...	92 -28 -0.24 0.7	13 -10 -0.47 0.5	0 -5 -1.00 ...	0 -29 -1.00 2.7	50 -34 -0.41 1.4	13 9 0.41 ...	0 -98 -1.00 9.4#	20 14 0.42 ...	0 -1 -1.00 ...	0 0 0.00 ...	13 5 0.11 0.3	76 50 0.35 8.7#	1530
DR3	13 12 0.15 ...	55 2 0.01 0.0	13 11 0.09 ...	0 -21 -1.00 1.9	0 0 -1.00 ...	12 -46 -0.80 4.4*	0 0 0.00 ...	0 -14 -1.00 1.3	12 9 0.06 ...	13 12 0.32 ...	0 -3 -1.00 ...	1 -9 -0.91 0.7	0 0 -1.00 ...	71 59 0.33 22.9‡	0 0 -1.00 ...	0 0 -1.00 ...	0 0 0.00 ...	0 0 -1.00 ...	1 -1 -0.69 ...	191
DR4	13 -3 -0.23 0.1	622 16 0.01 0.1	13 -12 -0.49 0.6	330 79 0.09 2.7	0 -2 -1.00 ...	774 84 0.06 1.4	0 0 0.00 ...	159 -12 -0.07 0.1	40 5 0.04 0.1	13 5 0.15 0.2	13 -28 -0.69 2.0	140 19 0.04 0.3	0 -5 -1.00 ...	13 -127 -0.91 11.0‡	0 -7 -1.00 0.8	13 10 1.00 ...	0 0 0.00 ...	0 -11 -1.00 1.1	35 -1 -0.05 0.0	2178
DR7	26 24 0.31 ...	41 -37 -0.48 1.0	26 23 0.20 ...	0 -32 -1.00 2.9	0 0 -1.00 ...	13 -76 -0.86 7.5#	0 0 0.00 ...	13 -8 -0.42 0.3	0 -4 -1.00 ...	0 0 -1.00 ...	138 132 0.70 ...	0 -15 -1.00 1.3	0 0 -1.00 ...	26 8 0.03 0.3	0 0 -1.00 ...	0 0 -1.00 ...	0 0 0.00 ...	0 -1 -1.00 ...	2 -2 -0.59 ...	285
DRW8	0 -5 -1.00 ...	232 35 0.07 0.7	0 -7 -1.00 0.7	57 -24 -0.30 0.7	0 0 -1.00 ...	217 -6 -0.03 0.0	0 0 0.00 ...	77 21 0.03 0.7	0 -10 -1.00 0.9	13 10 0.28 ...	0 -13 -1.00 1.1	92 53 0.10 6.1*	0 -1 -1.00 ...	17 -28 -0.63 1.6	0 -2 -1.00 ...	0 0 -1.00 ...	0 0 0.00 ...	0 -3 -1.00 ...	3 -8 -0.75 0.6	708
DRW9	0 -8 -1.00 0.8	451 125 0.15 5.7*	0 -13 -1.00 1.2	94 -40 -0.30 1.2	0 -1 -1.00 ...	279 -91 -0.25 2.9	0 0 0.00 ...	195 103 0.15 10.7#	13 -5 -0.30 0.1	0 -4 -1.00 ...	0 -22 -1.00 1.0	60 -4 -0.08 0.0	0 -2 -1.00 ...	13 -62 -0.83 4.8*	0 -4 -1.00 ...	0 -1 -1.00 ...	0 0 0.00 ...	40 34 0.72 ...	25 5 0.03 0.1	1170
DRW10	0 0 -1.00 ...	40 25 0.66 4.6*	0 0 -1.00 ...	0 -5 -1.00 ...	0 0 -1.00 ...	13 -3 -0.23 0.1	0 0 0.00 ...	0 -3 -1.00 ...	0 0 -1.00 ...	0 0 -1.00 ...	0 0 -1.00 ...	0 -2 -1.00 ...	0 0 -1.00 ...	0 -2 -1.00 ...	0 0 -1.00 ...	0 0 -1.00 ...	0 0 0.00 ...	0 0 -1.00 ...	0 0 -1.00 ...	53
DRW11	13 10 0.13 ...	111 1 0.00 0.0	0 -4 -1.00 ...	39 -6 -0.15 0.1	0 0 -1.00 ...	152 26 0.10 0.6	0 0 0.00 ...	0 -30 -1.00 2.7	13 7 0.04 ...	0 -1 -1.00 ...	26 18 0.10 3.5	41 19 0.05 1.4	0 0 -1.00 ...	0 -25 -1.00 2.2	0 -1 -1.00 ...	0 0 -1.00 ...	0 0 0.00 ...	0 -1 -1.00 ...	1 -5 -0.85 0.4	396
DRW12	0 -5 -1.00 ...	249 53 0.10 1.6	0 -7 -1.00 0.7	79 -1 -0.03 0.0	0 0 -1.00 ...	201 -22 -0.10 0.3	0 0 0.00 ...	60 4 0.01 0.0	15 4 0.03 0.1	0 -2 -1.00 ...	2 -11 -0.85 0.8	40 1 0.00 0.0	0 -1 -1.00 ...	40 -5 -0.12 0.1	0 -2 -1.00 ...	0 0 -1.00 ...	0 0 0.00 ...	0 -3 -1.00 ...	20 8 0.05 0.4	706
DRW13	0 -1 -1.00 ...	10 -70 -0.88 6.7#	13 10 0.08 ...	33 0 -0.01 0.0	0 0 -1.00 ...	54 -37 -0.41 1.8	0 0 0.00 ...	0 -22 -1.00 1.9	0 -4 -1.00 ...	0 0 -1.00 ...	0 -5 -1.00 ...	13 -2 -0.19 0.0	0 0 -1.00 ...	165 146 0.54 94.9‡	0 0 -1.00 ...	0 0 -1.00 ...	0 0 0.00 ...	0 -1 -1.00 ...	2 -2 -0.59 ...	290
DRW14	0 -4 -1.00 ...	88 -101 -0.54 6.1*	29 21 0.19 4.5*	81 2 0.00 0.0	0 0 -1.00 ...	116 -99 -0.46 5.5*	0 0 0.00 ...	90 36 0.06 2.2	0 -10 -1.00 0.9	0 -2 -1.00 ...	0 -12 -1.00 1.1	53 15 0.03 0.5	13 11 0.46 ...	197 153 0.25 46.0‡	13 10 0.28 ...	0 0 -1.00 ...	0 0 0.00 ...	0 -3 -1.00 ...	1 -10 -0.91 0.8	681
DRX	13 3 0.04 0.1	403 38 0.04 0.5	10 -4 -0.35 0.2	229 78 0.08 3.9*	13 11 1.00 ...	358 -57 -0.14 1.0	0 0 0.00 ...	76 -26 -0.26 0.7	53 32 0.23 4.4*	0 -4 -1.00 ...	3 -22 -0.88 1.8	39 -33 -0.46 1.4	0 -2 -1.00 ...	105 20 0.04 0.4	6 1 0.03 ...	0 -1 -1.00 ...	0 0 0.00 ...	0 -6 -1.00 0.6	4 -17 -0.82 1.3	1312
SUM	78	2783	118	1153	13	3170	0	788	159	39	195	555	26	647	39	13	0	53	170	

Haplotype frequencies for population ORI

A-Bf ($N=174$)

	A1	A2	A3	A11	A23	A24	A25	A26	A28	A29	A30	A31	A32	AW33	AW34	AW36	AW43	AW66	AX	SUM
BF S	172 22 1.00 0.4	2456 110 0.32 0.0	57 -92 -0.62 8.1#	2010 255 1.00 6.4*	0 0 0.00 ...	1605 -77 -0.08 0.6	0 0 0.00 ...	287 36 1.00 0.7	172 -27 -0.14 0.6	0 -49 -1.00 6.9#	734 -6 -0.01 0.0	345 44 1.00 0.9	115 15 1.00 0.3	460 -191 -0.29 8.4#	172 22 1.00 0.4	57 7 1.00 0.1	0 0 0.00 ...	0 0 0.00 ...	91 -57 -0.39 3.2	8733
BF F	0 -21 -1.00 ...	230 -108 -0.32 0.0	115 93 0.62 ...	0 -253 -1.00 6.3*	0 0 0.00 ...	322 79 0.08 0.6	0 0 0.00 ...	0 -35 -1.00 0.7	57 28 0.14 0.6	57 50 1.00 ...	115 8 0.01 0.0	0 -43 -1.00 0.9	0 -14 -1.00 ...	287 193 0.30 8.5#	0 -21 -1.00 ...	0 -6 -1.00 ...	0 0 0.00 ...	0 0 0.00 ...	80 58 0.39 ...	1263
BFF1	0 0 0.00 ...	0 0 0.00 ...	0 0 0.00 ...	0 0 0.00 ...	0 0 0.00 ...	0 0 0.00 ...	0 0 0.00 ...	0 0 0.00 ...	0 0 0.00 ...	0 0 0.00 ...	0 0 0.00 ...	0 0 0.00 ...	0 0 0.00 ...	0 0 0.00 ...	0 0 0.00 ...	0 0 0.00 ...	0 0 0.00 ...	0 0 0.00 ...	0 0 0.00 ...	0
BFS07	0 0 0.00 ...	0 0 0.00 ...	0 0 0.00 ...	0 0 0.00 ...	0 0 0.00 ...	0 0 0.00 ...	0 0 0.00 ...	0 0 0.00 ...	0 0 0.00 ...	0 0 0.00 ...	0 0 0.00 ...	0 0 0.00 ...	0 0 0.00 ...	0 0 0.00 ...	0 0 0.00 ...	0 0 0.00 ...	0 0 0.00 ...	0 0 0.00 ...	0 0 0.00 ...	0
BF V	0 0 0.00 ...	0 0 0.00 ...	0 0 0.00 ...	0 0 0.00 ...	0 0 0.00 ...	0 0 0.00 ...	0 0 0.00 ...	0 0 0.00 ...	0 0 0.00 ...	0 0 0.00 ...	0 0 0.00 ...	0 0 0.00 ...	0 0 0.00 ...	0 0 0.00 ...	0 0 0.00 ...	0 0 0.00 ...	0 0 0.00 ...	0 0 0.00 ...	0 0 0.00 ...	0
SUM	172	2686	172	2010	0	1927	0	287	229	57	849	345	115	747	172	57	0	0	171	

A-DQ ($N=779$)▼

	A1	A2	A3	A11	A23	A24	A25	A26	A28	A29	A30	A31	A32	AW33	AW34	AW36	AW43	AW66	AX	SUM
DQW1	17 -5 -0.27 0.2	706 -143 -0.17 3.8	42 3 0.03 0.0	366 11 0.01 0.0	0 -3 -1.00 ...	1018 60 0.03 0.6	0 0 0.00 ...	261 29 0.05 0.4	16 -34 -0.68 2.7	0 -11 -1.00 1.3	0 -65 -1.00 7.5#	143 -28 -0.17 0.6	26 16 1.00 4.7*	335 148 0.34 13.9$	31 19 0.71 3.5	0 -3 -1.00 ...	0 0 0.00 ...	13 1 0.04 0.0	63 9 0.07 0.2	3037
DQW2	26 22 0.30 ...	100 -39 -0.29 1.3	41 35 0.26 15.4$	31 -26 -0.47 1.2	0 0 -1.00 ...	57 -100 -0.64 7.7#	0 0 0.00 ...	17 -20 -0.56 1.0	0 -7 -1.00 0.7	13 11 0.31 ...	159 146 0.72 170.4$	13 -14 -0.54 0.7	0 0 -1.00 ...	41 10 0.02 0.3	0 -1 -1.00 ...	0 0 -1.00 ...	0 0 0.00 ...	0 -1 -1.00 ...	2 -6 -0.78 0.5	500
DQW3	26 1 0.01 0.0	1030 113 0.06 2.2	13 -28 -0.69 2.4	381 -1 -0.01 0.0	0 -3 -1.00 ...	1115 81 0.04 1.1	0 0 0.00 ...	260 9 0.02 0.0	68 13 0.12 0.4	1 -10 -0.92 1.2	40 -30 -0.43 1.6	176 -6 -0.04 0.0	0 -8 -1.00 0.0	77 -124 -0.62 9.5#	1 -11 -0.92 1.3	8 4 0.43 ...	0 0 0.00 ...	13 0 0.01 0.0	66 7 0.06 0.1	3277
DQX	8 -16 -0.67 1.3	963 70 0.04 0.9	33 -7 -0.20 0.2	391 18 0.02 0.1	13 9 1.00 ...	964 -41 -0.04 0.3	0 0 0.00 ...	227 -16 -0.07 0.1	83 30 0.26 1.9	24 12 0.46 1.3	17 -51 -0.75 4.6*	231 51 0.13 1.7	0 -7 -1.00 0.0	163 -33 -0.17 0.7	7 -4 -0.44 0.3	5 1 0.10 ...	0 0 0.00 ...	13 1 0.02 0.0	48 -8 -0.16 0.2	3190
SUM	77	2799	129	1169	13	3154	0	765	167	38	216	565	26	616	39	13	0	39	179	

Haplotype frequencies for population ORI
A-C4A ($N = 157$)

	C4 A1	C4A12	C4A13	C4 A2	C4 A3	C4 A4	C4A51	C4 A6	C4AQ0	SUM
A1	0 0 0.00 ...	0 -15 -1.00 ...	0 0 0.00 ...	0 -1 -1.00 ...	0 -65 -1.00 4.1*	0 -9 -1.00 ...	0 0 0.00 ...	128 126 1.00 ...	0 -12 -1.00 ...	128
A2	0 0 0.00 ...	319 4 0.00 0.0	0 0 0.00 ...	0 -49 -1.00 1.1	1831 87 0.10 0.3	255 56 0.10 0.4	0 0 0.00 ...	0 -32 -1.00 0.7	195 -63 -0.25 0.4	2600
A3	0 0 0.00 ...	0 -22 -1.00 ...	0 0 0.00 ...	64 60 0.32 ...	128 0 -0.01 0.0	0 -14 -1.00 ...	0 0 0.00 ...	0 -1 -1.00 ...	0 -18 -1.00 ...	192
A11	0 0 0.00 ...	255 -7 -0.03 0.0	0 0 0.00 ...	64 22 0.15 0.2	1366 -68 -0.06 0.3	126 -39 -0.24 0.2	0 0 0.00 ...	0 -27 -1.00 ...	358 142 0.18 2.1	2169
A23	0 0 0.00 ...	0 0 0.00 ...	0 0 0.00 ...	0 0 0.00 ...	0 0 0.00 ...	0 0 0.00 ...	0 0 0.00 ...	0 0 0.00 ...	0 0 0.00 ...	0
A24	0 0 0.00 ...	383 154 0.16 2.3	0 0 0.00 ...	0 -35 -1.00 0.7	1212 -52 -0.04 0.1	187 43 0.07 0.3	0 0 0.00 ...	0 -23 -1.00 ...	103 -84 -0.45 0.8	1885
A25	0 0 0.00 ...	0 0 0.00 ...	0 0 0.00 ...	0 0 0.00 ...	0 0 0.00 ...	0 0 0.00 ...	0 0 0.00 ...	0 0 0.00 ...	0 0 0.00 ...	0
A26	0 0 0.00 ...	64 25 0.09 0.3	0 0 0.00 ...	0 -5 -1.00 ...	252 37 0.35 0.3	0 -24 -1.00 ...	0 0 0.00 ...	0 -3 -1.00 ...	4 -27 -0.87 ...	320
A28	0 0 0.00 ...	0 -38 -1.00 0.7	0 0 0.00 ...	0 -5 -1.00 ...	192 -22 -0.11 0.1	128 103 0.35 ...	0 0 0.00 ...	0 -3 -1.00 ...	0 -31 -1.00 ...	320
A29	0 0 0.00 ...	0 -7 -1.00 ...	0 0 0.00 ...	0 0 -1.00 ...	59 16 0.76 0.3	0 -4 -1.00 ...	0 0 0.00 ...	0 0 -1.00 ...	5 0 -0.21 ...	64
A30	0 0 0.00 ...	0 -90 -1.00 1.8	0 0 0.00 ...	64 50 0.28 ...	688 183 0.74 3.4	0 -57 -1.00 1.1	0 0 0.00 ...	0 -9 -1.00 ...	0 -74 -1.00 1.4	752
A31	0 0 0.00 ...	0 -22 -1.00 ...	0 0 0.00 ...	0 -3 -1.00 ...	128 0 -0.01 0.0	64 49 0.28 ...	0 0 0.00 ...	0 -1 -1.00 ...	0 -18 -1.00 ...	192
A32	0 0 0.00 ...	0 -15 -1.00 ...	0 0 0.00 ...	0 -1 -1.00 ...	128 42 1.00 0.0	0 -9 -1.00 ...	0 0 0.00 ...	0 -1 -1.00 ...	0 -12 -1.00 ...	128
AW33	0 0 0.00 ...	128 27 0.04 0.1	0 0 0.00 ...	0 -15 -1.00 ...	551 -5 -0.01 0.0	0 -63 -1.00 1.2	0 0 0.00 ...	0 -10 -1.00 ...	151 68 0.09 1.1	830
AW34	0 0 0.00 ...	0 -20 -1.00 ...	0 0 0.00 ...	0 -2 -1.00 ...	71 -42 -0.38 0.8	0 -12 -1.00 ...	0 0 0.00 ...	0 -1 -1.00 ...	99 82 0.54 ...	170
AW36	0 0 0.00 ...	0 -7 -1.00 ...	0 0 0.00 ...	0 0 -1.00 ...	62 20 0.95 0.4	0 -4 -1.00 ...	0 0 0.00 ...	0 0 -1.00 ...	1 -4 -0.84 ...	63
AW43	0 0 0.00 ...	0 0 0.00 ...	0 0 0.00 ...	0 0 0.00 ...	0 0 0.00 ...	0 0 0.00 ...	0 0 0.00 ...	0 0 0.00 ...	0 0 0.00 ...	0
AW66	0 0 0.00 ...	0 0 0.00 ...	0 0 0.00 ...	0 0 0.00 ...	0 0 0.00 ...	0 0 0.00 ...	0 0 0.00 ...	0 0 0.00 ...	0 0 0.00 ...	0
AX	0 0 0.00 ...	64 41 0.25 ...	0 0 0.00 ...	0 -3 -1.00 ...	41 -85 -0.68 2.9	6 -8 -0.59 ...	0 0 0.00 ...	0 -1 -1.00 ...	79 60 0.35 ...	190
SUM	0	1213	0	192	6709	766	0	128	995	

Haplotype frequencies for population ORI
A-C4B ($N = 155$)

	C4 B1	C4B11	C4B12	C4 B2	C4 B3	C4 B4	C4 B5	C4B51	C4 B6	C4 B7	C4BQ0	SUM
A1	129 44 1.00 1.1	0 0 0.00 ...	0 0 -1.00 ...	0 -27 -1.00 ...	0 0 -1.00 ...	0 0 0.00 ...	0 0 0.00 ...	0 0 0.00 ...	0 0 0.00 ...	0 0 0.00 ...	0 -13 -1.00 ...	129
A2	1612 -113 -0.07 0.5	0 0 0.00 ...	0 -16 -1.00 ...	767 190 0.12 1.7	0 -16 -1.00 ...	0 0 0.00 ...	0 0 0.00 ...	0 0 0.00 ...	0 0 0.00 ...	0 0 0.00 ...	250 -41 -0.14 0.1	2629
A3	191 64 0.97 1.5	0 0 0.00 ...	0 0 -1.00 ...	0 -41 -1.00 0.9	0 0 -1.00 ...	0 0 0.00 ...	0 0 0.00 ...	0 0 0.00 ...	0 0 0.00 ...	0 0 0.00 ...	2 -18 -0.91 ...	193
A11	1161 -277 -0.19 3.1	0 0 0.00 ...	0 -13 -1.00 ...	837 356 0.21 6.7#	0 -13 -1.00 ...	0 0 0.00 ...	0 0 0.00 ...	0 0 0.00 ...	0 0 0.00 ...	0 0 0.00 ...	194 -49 -0.20 0.2	2192
A23	0 0 0.00 ...	0 0 0.00 ...	0 0 0.00 ...	0 0 0.00 ...	0 0 0.00 ...	0 0 0.00 ...	0 0 0.00 ...	0 0 0.00 ...	0 0 0.00 ...	0 0 0.00 ...	0 0 0.00 ...	0
A24	1394 227 0.37 2.4	0 0 0.00 ...	65 53 1.00 ...	318 -71 -0.18 0.3	0 -11 -1.00 ...	0 0 0.00 ...	0 0 0.00 ...	0 0 0.00 ...	0 0 0.00 ...	0 0 0.00 ...	0 -197 -1.00 4.2*	1777
A25	0 0 0.00 ...	0 0 0.00 ...	0 0 0.00 ...	0 0 0.00 ...	0 0 0.00 ...	0 0 0.00 ...	0 0 0.00 ...	0 0 0.00 ...	0 0 0.00 ...	0 0 0.00 ...	0 0 0.00 ...	0
A26	258 46 0.41 0.5	0 0 0.00 ...	0 -1 -1.00 ...	65 -5 -0.08 0.0	0 -1 -1.00 ...	0 0 0.00 ...	0 0 0.00 ...	0 0 0.00 ...	0 0 0.00 ...	0 0 0.00 ...	0 -35 -1.00 0.6	323
A28	194 -17 -0.09 0.1	0 0 0.00 ...	0 -1 -1.00 ...	129 58 0.23 0.0	0 -1 -1.00 ...	0 0 0.00 ...	0 0 0.00 ...	0 0 0.00 ...	0 0 0.00 ...	0 0 0.00 ...	0 -35 -1.00 0.6	323
A29	37 -4 -0.12 0.0	0 0 0.00 ...	0 0 -1.00 ...	0 -13 -1.00 ...	0 0 -1.00 ...	0 0 0.00 ...	0 0 0.00 ...	0 0 0.00 ...	0 0 0.00 ...	0 0 0.00 ...	27 20 0.35 ...	64
A30	617 119 0.46 1.4	0 0 0.00 ...	0 -4 -1.00 ...	7 -159 -0.96 3.3	0 -4 -1.00 ...	0 0 0.00 ...	0 0 0.00 ...	0 0 0.00 ...	0 0 0.00 ...	0 0 0.00 ...	135 51 0.08 0.6	759
A31	110 -16 -0.14 0.1	0 0 0.00 ...	0 0 -1.00 ...	0 -42 -1.00 0.9	0 0 -1.00 ...	0 0 0.00 ...	0 0 0.00 ...	0 0 0.00 ...	0 0 0.00 ...	0 0 0.00 ...	84 62 0.36 ...	194
A32	0 -84 -1.00 3.9*	0 0 0.00 ...	0 0 -1.00 ...	65 36 0.36 ...	0 0 -1.00 ...	0 0 0.00 ...	0 0 0.00 ...	0 0 0.00 ...	0 0 0.00 ...	0 0 0.00 ...	65 51 0.44 ...	130
AW33	516 -34 -0.06 0.1	0 0 0.00 ...	0 -4 -1.00 ...	0 -183 -1.00 3.0*	65 60 1.00 ...	0 0 0.00 ...	0 0 0.00 ...	0 0 0.00 ...	0 0 0.00 ...	0 0 0.00 ...	258 165 0.22 5.5*	839
AW34	97 -29 -0.24 0.3	0 0 0.00 ...	0 0 -1.00 ...	0 -42 -1.00 0.9	0 0 -1.00 ...	0 0 0.00 ...	0 0 0.00 ...	0 0 0.00 ...	0 0 0.00 ...	0 0 0.00 ...	97 75 0.44 ...	194

Haplotype frequencies for population ORI

A-C4B ($N = 155$)▼

	C4 B1	C4B11	C4B12	C4 B2	C4 B3	C4 B4	C4 B5	C4B51	C4 B6	C4 B7	C4BQ0	SUM
AW36	65 22 1.00 0.5	0 0 0.00 ...	0 0 -1.00 ...	0 -13 -1.00 ...	0 0 -1.00 ...	0 0 0.00 ...	0 0 0.00 ...	0 0 0.00 ...	0 0 0.00 ...	0 0 0.00 ...	0 -6 -1.00 ...	65
AW43	0 0 0.00 ...	0 0 0.00 ...	0 0 0.00 ...	0 0 0.00 ...	0 0 0.00 ...	0 0 0.00 ...	0 0 0.00 ...	0 0 0.00 ...	0 0 0.00 ...	0 0 0.00 ...	0 0 0.00 ...	0
AW66	0 0 0.00 ...	0 0 0.00 ...	0 0 0.00 ...	0 0 0.00 ...	0 0 0.00 ...	0 0 0.00 ...	0 0 0.00 ...	0 0 0.00 ...	0 0 0.00 ...	0 0 0.00 ...	0 0 0.00 ...	0
AX	186 60 0.91 1.3	0 0 0.00 ...	0 0 -1.00 ...	6 -35 -0.86 0.6	0 0 -1.00 ...	0 0 0.00 ...	0 0 0.00 ...	0 0 0.00 ...	0 0 0.00 ...	0 0 0.00 ...	0 -20 -1.00 ...	192
SUM	6567	0	65	2194	65	0	0	0	0	0	1112	

B-C ($N = 947$)▼

	CW1	CW2	CW3	CW4	CW5	CW6	CW7	CW8	CX	SUM
B7	2 -73 -0.97 8.5#	0 -4 -1.00 ...	8 -121 -0.94 15.7$	1 -24 -0.96 2.5	0 -2 -1.00 ...	0 -17 -1.00 1.9	387 330 0.79 216.4$	0 -1 -1.00 ...	76 -81 -0.52 6.3*	474
B8	0 -2 -1.00 ...	0 0 -1.00 ...	0 -5 -1.00 0.8	0 0 -1.00 ...	0 0 -1.00 ...	0 0 -1.00 ...	21 18 1.00 ...	0 0 -1.00 ...	0 -6 -1.00 0.0	21
B13	7 -53 -0.88 5.6*	0 -3 -1.00 ...	137 33 0.12 1.4	0 -20 -1.00 2.1	0 -1 -1.00 ...	215 200 0.55 277.8$	10 -35 -0.78 3.1	0 0 -1.00 ...	11 -114 -0.91 15.5$	380
B18	0 -4 -1.00 ...	0 0 -1.00 ...	0 -8 -1.00 1.1	0 -1 -1.00 ...	0 0 -1.00 ...	0 0 -1.00 ...	20 16 0.60 ...	0 0 -1.00 ...	11 1 0.03 0.0	31
B27	21 -3 -0.17 0.1	63 61 0.58 ...	21 -21 -0.52 1.5	11 2 0.02 0.1	0 0 -1.00 ...	0 -5 -1.00 0.6	0 -18 -1.00 2.1	0 0 -1.00 ...	42 -10 -0.20 0.3	158
B35	0 -160 -1.00 20.2$	11 0 0.00 0.0	564 286 0.39 42.7$	207 152 0.31 47.2$	0 -5 -1.00 0.7	0 -38 -1.00 4.3*	32 -88 -0.74 7.9#	0 -2 -1.00 ...	197 -138 -0.41 9.1#	1011
B37	0 -9 -1.00 1.1	0 0 -1.00 ...	9 -7 -0.48 0.5	0 -2 -1.00 ...	0 0 -1.00 ...	46 44 0.72 ...	0 -7 -1.00 0.8	0 0 -1.00 ...	8 -12 -0.62 1.1	63
B38	0 -11 -1.00 1.3	0 0 -1.00 ...	0 -19 -1.00 2.7	0 -3 -1.00 ...	0 0 -1.00 ...	0 -2 -1.00 ...	63 54 0.83 35.6$	0 0 -1.00 ...	11 -13 -0.55 1.1	74
B39	1 -62 -0.98 7.3#	0 -3 -1.00 ...	21 -89 -0.81 9.9#	0 -21 -1.00 2.3	0 -2 -1.00 ...	0 -15 -1.00 1.6	230 182 0.51 76.8$	0 0 -1.00 ...	150 16 0.06 0.3	402

Haplotype frequencies for population ORI; B-C ($N = 947$)

	CW1	CW2	CW3	CW4	CW5	CW6	CW7	CW8	CX	SUM
BW41	0 -1 -1.00 ...	0 0 -1.00 ...	0 -2 -1.00 ...	0 0 -1.00 ...	0 0 -1.00 ...	0 0 -1.00 ...	6 5 0.48 ...	0 0 -1.00 ...	5 1 0.18 ...	11
BW42	0 -7 -1.00 0.0	0 0 -1.00 ...	0 -14 -1.00 1.9	0 -2 -1.00 ...	0 0 -1.00 ...	0 -1 -1.00 ...	53 47 1.00 37.0$	0 0 -1.00 ...	0 -17 -1.00 2.5	53
B44	4 -91 -0.96 10.5#	0 -5 -1.00 0.7	22 -142 -0.87 17.2$	33 1 0.00 0.0	53 49 0.82 ...	0 -22 -1.00 2.4	32 -39 -0.56 2.5	0 -1 -1.00 ...	456 256 0.64 49.7$	600
B45	0 -1 -1.00 ...	0 0 -1.00 ...	0 -2 -1.00 ...	0 0 -1.00 ...	0 0 -1.00 ...	0 0 -1.00 ...	0 0 -1.00 ...	0 0 -1.00 ...	11 7 1.00 ...	11
BW46	304 247 0.82 124.7$	0 -3 -1.00 ...	32 -65 -0.67 6.1*	0 -18 -1.00 2.0	0 -1 -1.00 ...	0 -13 -1.00 1.4	0 -42 -1.00 4.6*	0 0 -1.00 ...	22 -96 -0.82 11.7$	358
BW47	4 -2 -0.42 0.1	11 11 0.25 ...	0 -11 -1.00 1.6	0 -1 -1.00 ...	0 0 -1.00 ...	12 10 0.25 ...	0 -4 -1.00 ...	0 0 -1.00 ...	16 2 0.06 0.0	43
BW48	21 -3 -0.17 0.1	0 -1 -1.00 ...	36 -7 -0.18 0.2	0 -8 -1.00 0.9	0 0 -1.00 ...	0 -5 -1.00 0.6	11 -7 -0.42 0.4	0 0 -1.00 ...	91 38 0.36 3.0*	159
B49	0 -4 -1.00 ...	0 0 -1.00 ...	11 2 0.08 0.1	0 -1 -1.00 ...	0 0 -1.00 ...	11 10 0.31 ...	0 -3 -1.00 ...	0 0 -1.00 ...	11 0 0.00 0.0	33
BW50	0 -4 -1.00 ...	0 0 -1.00 ...	21 12 0.53 2.2	11 9 0.31 ...	0 0 -1.00 ...	0 0 -1.00 ...	0 -3 -1.00 ...	0 0 -1.00 ...	0 -10 -1.00 1.5	32
B51	16 -106 -0.87 11.4$	0 -7 -1.00 0.9	115 -96 -0.46 6.3*	3 -38 -0.93 3.9*	0 -4 -1.00 ...	10 -19 -0.67 1.4	9 -83 -0.90 6.8#	0 -1 -1.00 ...	618 361 0.70 78.3$	771
BW52	22 -90 -0.80 8.9#	0 -7 -1.00 0.8	106 -87 -0.45 5.7*	0 -37 -1.00 4.1*	0 -4 -1.00 ...	0 -27 -1.00 2.9	26 -58 -0.69 4.7*	0 -1 -1.00 ...	553 318 0.67 65.6$	707
BW53	0 -4 -1.00 ...	0 0 -1.00 ...	0 -8 -1.00 1.2	13 11 0.37 ...	0 0 -1.00 ...	11 10 0.32 ...	0 -3 -1.00 ...	0 0 -1.00 ...	8 -2 -0.25 0.1	32
BW54	660 550 0.95 334.5$	0 -6 -1.00 0.8	0 -188 -1.00 26.5$	0 -36 -1.00 3.0*	0 -3 -1.00 ...	0 -26 -1.00 2.8	11 -70 -0.67 7.2#	0 -1 -1.00 ...	16 -212 -0.93 30.1$	687
BW55	139 105 0.59 37.0$	0 -1 -1.00 ...	24 -33 -0.59 2.7	0 -10 -1.00 1.2	0 0 -1.00 ...	0 -7 -1.00 0.8	15 -9 -0.41 0.5	0 0 -1.00 ...	33 -36 -0.53 2.9	211
BW56	89 66 0.53 20.0$	0 -1 -1.00 ...	4 -35 -0.90 4.4*	25 17 0.12 3.7	0 0 -1.00 ...	0 -5 -1.00 0.6	27 9 0.07 0.5	0 0 -1.00 ...	2 -46 -0.96 6.5*	147

	CW1	CW2	CW3	CW4	CW5	CW6	CW7	CW8	CX	SUM
BW57	0 -11 -1.00 1.3	0 0 -1.00 ...	9 -10 -0.56 0.8	0 -3 -1.00 ...	0 0 -1.00 ...	63 60 0.85 ...	0 -8 -1.00 0.0	0 0 -1.00 ...	2 -22 -0.92 2.0	74
BW58	11 -29 -0.73 2.5	0 -2 -1.00 ...	205 135 0.73 35.0$	0 -13 -1.00 1.4	0 -1 -1.00 ...	21 11 0.05 1.3	11 -18 -0.64 1.4	0 0 -1.00 ...	6 -76 -0.93 10.6#	254
BW59	95 76 0.76 36.1$	0 0 -1.00 ...	21 -10 -0.34 0.5	0 -5 -1.00 0.6	0 0 -1.00 ...	0 -4 -1.00 ...	0 -13 -1.00 1.5	0 0 -1.00 ...	0 -36 -1.00 5.5*	116
BW60	21 -66 -0.81 8.5#	11 4 0.04 0.2	307 121 0.25 10.0$	36 0 -0.02 0.0	0 -3 -1.00 ...	0 -25 -1.00 2.6	104 23 0.04 0.7	11 9 0.30 ...	187 -37 -0.17 0.0	677
BW61	25 -160 -0.87 17.8$	0 -11 -1.00 1.4	615 294 0.35 39.7$	21 -41 -0.67 3.2	0 -6 -1.00 0.8	0 -44 -1.00 5.1*	27 -112 -0.81 11.1$	0 -3 -1.00 ...	480 91 0.12 3.5	1168
BW62	76 -72 -0.49 4.4*	11 1 0.01 0.0	439 182 0.27 18.6$	180 129 0.26 36.6$	0 -5 -1.00 0.6	0 -35 -1.00 3.9*	31 -80 -0.72 6.0#	0 -2 -1.00 ...	197 -113 -0.37 6.5*	934
BW63	0 0 0.00 ...	0 0 0.00 ...	0 0 0.00 ...	0 0 0.00 ...	0 0 0.00 ...	0 0 0.00 ...	0 0 0.00 ...	0 0 0.00 ...	0 0 0.00 ...	0
BW64	0 0 0.00 ...	0 0 0.00 ...	0 0 0.00 ...	0 0 0.00 ...	0 0 0.00 ...	0 0 0.00 ...	0 0 0.00 ...	0 0 0.00 ...	0 0 0.00 ...	0
BW65	0 -2 -1.00 ...	0 0 -1.00 ...	0 -5 -1.00 0.8	0 0 -1.00 ...	0 0 -1.00 ...	0 0 -1.00 ...	0 -2 -1.00 ...	21 21 1.00 ...	0 -6 -1.00 0.0	21
BW67	0 -1 -1.00 ...	0 0 -1.00 ...	0 -2 -1.00 ...	0 0 -1.00 ...	0 0 -1.00 ...	0 0 -1.00 ...	11 10 1.00 ...	0 0 -1.00 ...	0 -3 -1.00 ...	11
BW71	11 4 0.11 0.3	0 0 -1.00 ...	0 -11 -1.00 1.6	0 -1 -1.00 ...	11 11 0.25 ...	0 -1 -1.00 ...	21 16 0.42 ...	0 0 -1.00 ...	0 -13 -1.00 2.0	43
BW72	0 -7 -1.00 0.0	0 0 -1.00 ...	11 -3 -0.25 0.1	0 -2 -1.00 ...	0 0 -1.00 ...	0 -1 -1.00 ...	21 15 0.31 3.6	0 0 -1.00 ...	21 3 0.10 0.1	53
BW73	0 -2 -1.00 ...	0 0 -1.00 ...	5 0 -0.13 0.0	0 0 -1.00 ...	0 0 -1.00 ...	0 0 -1.00 ...	10 7 0.40 ...	0 0 -1.00 ...	6 0 -0.14 0.0	21
BX	66 40 0.29 6.0#	0 -1 -1.00 ...	7 -37 -0.84 4.3*	0 -8 -1.00 0.9	0 0 -1.00 ...	0 -5 -1.00 0.6	11 -8 -0.44 0.4	0 0 -1.00 ...	80 25 0.23 1.7	164
SUM	1595	107	2750	541	64	389	1200	32	3327	

Haplotype frequencies for population ORI
B-DR (N=740)

	DR1	DR2	DR3	DR4	DR7	DRW8	DRW9	DRW10	DRW11	DRW12	DRW13	DRW14	DRX	SUM
B7	360 334 0.68 346.4$	28 -47 -0.63 2.8	0 -9 -1.00 0.8	22 -90 -0.81 7.4#	14 0 -0.08 0.0	14 -21 -0.61 1.1	0 -58 -1.00 5.2*	0 -2 -1.00 ...	27 6 0.02 0.1	14 -24 -0.64 1.3	0 -14 -1.00 1.2	0 -35 -1.00 2.0	35 -30 -0.47 1.3	514
B8	0 0 -1.00 ...	0 -3 -1.00 ...	27 26 1.00 ...	0 -5 -1.00 ...	0 0 -1.00 ...	0 -1 -1.00 ...	0 -2 -1.00 ...	0 0 -1.00 ...	0 0 -1.00 ...	0 -1 -1.00 ...	0 0 -1.00 ...	0 -1 -1.00 ...	0 -2 -1.00 ...	27
B13	0 -15 -1.00 1.3	27 -18 -0.42 0.7	0 -5 -1.00 ...	0 -68 -1.00 6.7#	125 116 0.41 114.7$	0 -21 -1.00 1.8	33 -2 -0.08 0.0	0 -1 -1.00 ...	14 1 0.00 0.0	64 41 0.14 5.8*	0 -8 -1.00 0.7	14 -7 -0.35 0.2	35 -4 -0.12 0.1	312
B18	0 -1 -1.00 ...	14 8 0.23 ...	14 13 0.33 ...	0 -8 -1.00 0.9	12 11 0.27 ...	0 -2 -1.00 ...	0 -4 -1.00 ...	0 0 -1.00 ...	0 -1 -1.00 ...	0 -2 -1.00 ...	0 0 -1.00 ...	0 -2 -1.00 ...	1 -3 -0.81 ...	41
B27	14 7 0.05 0.5	27 7 0.06 0.2	0 -2 -1.00 ...	14 -15 -0.54 0.8	14 10 0.07 ...	14 4 0.03 0.2	0 -15 -1.00 1.3	0 0 -1.00 ...	0 -5 -1.00 ...	54 44 0.35 15.1$	0 -3 -1.00 ...	0 -9 -1.00 0.8	0 -16 -1.00 1.5	137
B35	0 -53 -1.00 4.7*	149 -6 -0.04 0.0	0 -20 -1.00 1.7	390 159 0.19 11.6$	0 -30 -1.00 2.6	61 -11 -0.17 0.2	105 -15 -0.13 0.2	0 -5 -1.00 ...	54 11 0.03 0.3	95 16 0.02 0.3	0 -30 -1.00 2.7	17 -55 -0.77 3.8	178 44 0.05 1.4	1049
B37	0 -1 -1.00 ...	0 -5 -1.00 ...	0 0 -1.00 ...	20 11 0.34 1.3	0 0 -1.00 ...	0 -2 -1.00 ...	0 -4 -1.00 ...	14 14 0.34 ...	0 -1 -1.00 ...	0 -2 -1.00 ...	0 0 -1.00 ...	0 -2 -1.00 ...	7 2 0.05 ...	41
B38	14 10 0.13 ...	47 35 0.51 8.9#	0 -1 -1.00 ...	0 -17 -1.00 1.7	0 -1 -1.00 ...	0 -5 -1.00 ...	0 -8 -1.00 0.8	0 0 -1.00 ...	0 -2 -1.00 ...	0 -5 -1.00 ...	0 -1 -1.00 ...	0 -5 -1.00 ...	20 10 0.14 0.8	81
B39	0 -23 -1.00 1.9	27 -40 -0.60 2.3	0 -8 -1.00 0.7	104 3 0.01 0.0	0 -13 -1.00 1.1	85 53 0.12 7.3#	27 -25 -0.49 1.1	0 -2 -1.00 ...	0 -18 -1.00 1.5	68 34 0.08 2.7	11 -2 -0.20 0.0	52 20 0.05 1.1	85 26 0.07 1.1	459
BW41	0 0 0.00 ...	0 0 0.00 ...	0 0 0.00 ...	0 0 0.00 ...	0 0 0.00 ...	0 0 0.00 ...	0 0 0.00 ...	0 0 0.00 ...	0 0 0.00 ...	0 0 0.00 ...	0 0 0.00 ...	0 0 0.00 ...	0 0 0.00 ...	0
BW42	0 -1 -1.00 ...	27 21 0.60 ...	0 0 -1.00 ...	0 -8 -1.00 0.9	0 0 -1.00 ...	0 -2 -1.00 ...	0 -4 -1.00 ...	0 0 -1.00 ...	0 -1 -1.00 ...	14 11 0.29 ...	0 0 -1.00 ...	0 -2 -1.00 ...	0 -4 -1.00 ...	41
B44	14 -21 -0.61 1.1	14 -89 -0.86 7.2#	14 0 0.00 0.0	17 -136 -0.89 12.4$	27 6 0.02 0.2	18 -30 -0.63 1.7	17 -63 -0.79 4.5*	14 10 0.19 ...	0 -27 -1.00 2.4	27 -24 -0.48 1.1	203 182 0.66 130.9$	258 210 0.32 77.5$	75 -13 -0.16 0.2	698
B45	0 0 -1.00 ...	0 -1 -1.00 ...	0 0 -1.00 ...	0 -2 -1.00 ...	0 0 -1.00 ...	0 0 -1.00 ...	0 -1 -1.00 ...	0 0 -1.00 ...	14 13 1.00 ...	0 0 -1.00 ...	0 0 -1.00 ...	0 0 -1.00 ...	0 -1 -1.00 ...	14
BW46	13 -3 -0.22 0.1	18 -29 -0.63 1.7	0 -5 -1.00 ...	23 -47 -0.68 3.2	0 -9 -1.00 0.8	92 69 0.23 17.5$	105 68 0.24 10.6#	0 -1 -1.00 ...	0 -12 -1.00 1.1	4 -19 -0.84 1.4	9 0 -0.07 0.0	10 -11 -0.56 0.6	50 9 0.03 0.2	324
BW47	0 -2 -1.00 ...	0 -7 -1.00 0.7	0 0 -1.00 ...	14 2 0.04 0.0	19 17 0.33 ...	0 -3 -1.00 ...	0 -5 -1.00 ...	0 0 -1.00 ...	0 -1 -1.00 ...	17 13 0.25 ...	0 -1 -1.00 ...	0 -3 -1.00 ...	5 -1 -0.29 0.0	55

Haplotype frequencies for population ORI
B-DR ($N = 740$)

	DR1	DR2	DR3	DR4	DR7	DRW8	DRW9	DRW10	DRW11	DRW12	DRW13	DRW14	DRX	SUM
BW48	14	37	0	27	0	13	0	0	14	0	0	37	7	149
	6	15	-2	-5	-3	3	-16	0	8	-10	-3	27	-11	
	0.04	0.12	-1.00	-0.18	-1.00	0.02	-1.00	-1.00	0.06	-1.00	-1.00	0.19	-0.63	
	0.4	0.9	...	0.1	...	0.1	1.5	...	...	0.9	...	5.5*	0.7	
B49	0	0	0	0	0	0	0	0	27	0	0	0	0	27
	0	-3	0	-5	0	-1	-2	0	26	-1	0	-1	-2	
	-1.00	-1.00	-1.00	-1.00	-1.00	-1.00	-1.00	-1.00	1.00	-1.00	-1.00	-1.00	-1.00	
	...	...	...	...	...	...	...	...	...	...	...	...	...	
BW50	0	0	12	13	0	0	0	0	0	15	0	0	0	40
	-1	-5	11	4	0	-2	-4	0	-1	12	0	-2	-4	
	-1.00	-1.00	0.29	0.13	-1.00	-1.00	-1.00	-1.00	-1.00	0.32	-1.00	-1.00	-1.00	
	...	...	...	0.2	...	...	...	...	...	...	...	...	...	
B51	0	89	2	164	0	141	112	0	14	120	0	12	102	756
	-38	-22	-12	-2	-21	88	25	-3	-16	63	-22	-39	6	
	-1.00	-0.21	-0.87	-0.02	-1.00	0.14	0.04	-1.00	-0.55	0.09	-1.00	-0.77	0.01	
	3.3	0.5	0.9	0.0	1.8	12.7$	0.6	...	0.8	6.1*	1.9	2.7	0.0	
BW52	1	501	0	82	0	6	24	0	14	14	14	15	60	731
	-36	393	-13	-78	-21	-44	-59	-3	-15	-40	-7	-35	-32	
	-0.97	0.63	-1.00	-0.49	-1.00	-0.86	-0.72	-1.00	-0.53	-0.74	-0.36	-0.70	-0.36	
	2.0	133.1$	1.2	3.0*	1.8	3.4	3.9*	...	0.7	2.6	0.2	2.2	1.1	
BW53	0	0	0	7	0	6	0	14	14	0	0	0	0	41
	-1	-5	0	-1	0	3	-4	14	12	-2	0	-2	-4	
	-1.00	-1.00	-1.00	-0.23	-1.00	0.08	-1.00	0.34	0.31	-1.00	-1.00	-1.00	-1.00	
	...	...	...	0.0	...	...	...	...	...	...	...	...	...	
BW54	27	68	0	460	0	17	18	0	1	0	0	67	127	785
	-12	-47	-14	287	-22	-37	-72	-3	-30	-58	-22	13	27	
	-0.33	-0.42	-1.00	0.47	-1.00	-0.69	-0.80	-1.00	-0.97	-1.00	-1.00	0.02	0.04	
	0.4	1.9	1.3	49.1$	1.9	2.2	5.3*	...	2.5	5.1*	1.9	0.2	0.7	
BW55	0	6	0	54	0	27	77	0	43	27	0	0	9	243
	-11	-29	-4	0	-6	10	49	0	33	9	-6	-16	-21	
	-1.00	-0.83	-1.00	0.00	-1.00	0.04	0.23	-1.00	0.14	0.04	-1.00	-1.00	-0.71	
	0.0	2.2	...	0.0	0.6	0.5	7.3#	...	8.7#	0.3	0.6	1.4	1.4	
BW56	0	48	0	14	0	0	46	0	27	0	0	41	0	176
	-8	22	-2	-24	-4	-11	26	0	20	-12	-4	29	-21	
	-1.00	0.15	-1.00	-0.64	-1.00	-1.00	0.16	-1.00	0.12	-1.00	-1.00	0.18	-1.00	
	0.7	1.6	...	1.5	...	0.0	2.8	...	4.3*	1.1	...	5.5*	1.9	
BW57	0	0	0	0	41	0	0	0	27	0	0	0	14	82
	-3	-11	-1	-17	39	-5	-8	0	24	-5	-1	-5	4	
	-1.00	-1.00	-1.00	-1.00	0.48	-1.00	-1.00	-1.00	0.30	-1.00	-1.00	-1.00	0.05	
	...	1.1	...	1.7	...	...	0.8	...	...	...	...	...	0.1	
BW58	14	0	86	0	0	0	0	0	0	41	14	14	22	191
	4	-27	82	-41	-5	-12	-21	0	-7	27	8	1	-1	
	0.02	-1.00	0.44	-1.00	-1.00	-1.00	-1.00	-1.00	-1.00	0.15	0.04	0.00	-0.10	
	0.1	2.5	...	4.1*	...	1.1	1.9	...	0.6	4.1*	...	0.0	0.0	
BW59	0	0	0	108	0	0	0	0	0	0	0	0	0	108
	-5	-15	-1	84	-2	-7	-11	0	-3	-7	-2	-6	-13	
	-1.00	-1.00	-1.00	1.00	-1.00	-1.00	-1.00	-1.00	-1.00	-1.00	-1.00	-1.00	-1.00	
	...	1.4	...	28.6$	...	0.6	1.1	...	...	0.7	...	0.6	1.2	
BW60	0	92	42	149	15	0	48	0	14	64	18	63	185	690
	-34	-9	28	-2	-4	-47	-31	-3	-13	12	-2	15	97	
	-1.00	-0.10	0.15	-0.02	-0.26	-1.00	-0.40	-1.00	-0.50	0.02	-0.12	0.02	0.16	
	2.0	0.1	4.8*	0.0	0.1	4.1*	1.1	...	0.6	0.2	0.0	0.4	9.7#	
BW61	14	48	0	225	14	131	342	0	81	58	3	68	132	1116
	-42	-117	-21	-20	-18	53	213	-5	35	-25	-29	-8	-9	
	-0.76	-0.71	-1.00	-0.08	-0.57	0.09	0.22	-1.00	0.10	-0.31	-0.91	-0.12	-0.07	
	2.9	8.2#	1.9	0.2	0.9	3.3	33.2$	...	2.4	0.7	2.4	0.1	0.1	
BW62	29	145	0	224	14	14	192	0	23	54	25	14	75	809
	-12	25	-15	46	-9	-41	99	-4	-9	-6	1	-41	-27	
	-0.30	0.04	-1.00	0.07	-0.41	-0.75	0.14	-1.00	-0.30	-0.11	0.00	-0.75	-0.27	
	0.3	0.5	1.3	1.2	0.3	2.8	9.5#	...	0.3	0.1	0.0	2.7	0.7	

Haplotype frequencies for population ORI
B-DR ($N = 740$)

	DR1	DR2	DR3	DR4	DR7	DRW8	DRW9	DRW10	DRW11	DRW12	DRW13	DRW14	DRX	SUM
BW63	0 0 0.00 ...	0 0 0.00 ...	0 0 0.00 ...	0 0 0.00 ...	0 0 0.00 ...	0 0 0.00 ...	0 0 0.00 ...	0 0 0.00 ...	0 0 0.00 ...	0 0 0.00 ...	0 0 0.00 ...	0 0 0.00 ...	0 0 0.00 ...	0
BW64	0 0 0.00 ...	0 0 0.00 ...	0 0 0.00 ...	0 0 0.00 ...	0 0 0.00 ...	0 0 0.00 ...	0 0 0.00 ...	0 0 0.00 ...	0 0 0.00 ...	0 0 0.00 ...	0 0 0.00 ...	0 0 0.00 ...	0 0 0.00 ...	0
BW65	0 0 -1.00 ...	0 -1 -1.00 ...	0 0 -1.00 ...	14 11 1.00 ...	0 0 -1.00 ...	0 0 -1.00 ...	0 -1 -1.00 ...	0 0 -1.00 ...	0 0 -1.00 ...	0 0 -1.00 ...	0 0 -1.00 ...	0 0 -1.00 ...	0 -1 -1.00 ...	14
BW67	0 0 -1.00 ...	14 12 1.00 ...	0 0 -1.00 ...	0 -2 -1.00 ...	0 0 -1.00 ...	0 0 -1.00 ...	0 -1 -1.00 ...	0 0 -1.00 ...	0 0 -1.00 ...	0 0 -1.00 ...	0 0 -1.00 ...	0 0 -1.00 ...	0 -1 -1.00 ...	14
BW71	0 -1 -1.00 ...	0 -5 -1.00 ...	0 0 -1.00 ...	14 5 0.14 0.2	0 0 -1.00 ...	14 11 0.28 ...	0 -4 -1.00 ...	0 0 -1.00 ...	0 -1 -1.00 ...	0 -2 -1.00 ...	0 0 -1.00 ...	0 -2 -1.00 ...	14 9 0.24 ...	42
BW72	0 -2 -1.00 ...	14 6 0.12 0.4	0 0 -1.00 ...	26 14 0.32 1.5	0 -1 -1.00 ...	14 10 0.20 ...	0 -5 -1.00 ...	0 0 -1.00 ...	0 -1 -1.00 ...	0 -3 -1.00 ...	0 -1 -1.00 ...	0 -3 -1.00 ...	1 -5 -0.86 0.4	55
BW73	0 0 0.00 ...	0 0 0.00 ...	0 0 0.00 ...	0 0 0.00 ...	0 0 0.00 ...	0 0 0.00 ...	0 0 0.00 ...	0 0 0.00 ...	0 0 0.00 ...	0 0 0.00 ...	0 0 0.00 ...	0 0 0.00 ...	0 0 0.00 ...	0
BX	0 -7 -1.00 0.7	44 20 0.14 1.4	0 -2 -1.00 ...	18 -17 -0.50 0.9	0 -4 -1.00 ...	30 19 0.12 2.4	9 -9 -0.52 0.4	14 13 0.24 ...	0 -6 -1.00 ...	0 -11 -1.00 1.0	1 -3 -0.80 ...	12 1 0.00 0.0	36 15 0.11 0.9	164
SUM	514	1484	197	2203	295	697	1155	56	408	750	298	694	1275	

Haplotype frequencies for population ORI; B-DQ (N=759)

	DQW1	DQW2	DQW3	DQX	SUM
B7	266	13	107	127	513
	111	-12	-64	-32	
	0.31	-0.51	-0.38	-0.21	
	9.2#	0.6	2.0	0.8	
B8	0	26	0	0	26
	-7	25	-8	-7	
	-1.00	1.00	-1.00	-1.00	
	0.9	...	0.0	0.9	
B13	40	144	114	31	329
	-58	127	4	-71	
	-0.60	0.41	0.02	-0.70	
	3.0*	79.2$	0.0	5.7*	
B18	13	13	0	13	39
	1	11	-12	1	
	0.05	0.30	-1.00	0.03	
	0.0	...	1.5	0.0	
B27	45	17	53	17	132
	5	10	9	-23	
	0.06	0.08	0.10	-0.59	
	0.1	1.3	0.2	1.6	
B35	172	13	472	406	1063
	-147	-41	115	75	
	-0.46	-0.76	0.16	0.10	
	8.4#	2.8	4.8*	2.1	
B37	0	3	19	18	40
	-11	1	6	6	
	-1.00	0.02	0.21	0.20	
	1.3	...	0.3	0.3	
B38	32	5	13	15	65
	12	2	-8	-4	
	0.27	0.03	-0.40	-0.26	
	0.9	...	0.4	0.2	
B39	96	13	151	227	487
	-50	-11	-11	75	
	-0.35	-0.48	-0.08	0.22	
	2.0	0.5	0.1	4.3*	
BW41	0	0	0	0	0
	0	0	0	0	
	0.00	0.00	0.00	0.00	
	...	...	...	...	
BW42	36	0	17	0	53
	20	-2	0	-16	
	0.54	-1.00	-0.04	-1.00	
	2.7	...	0.0	1.8	
B44	458	26	52	146	682
	252	-6	-176	-66	
	0.53	-0.26	-0.77	-0.31	
	36.1$	0.2	16.7$	2.5	
B45	0	0	0	13	13
	-3	0	-3	9	
	-1.00	-1.00	-1.00	1.00	
	...	...	...	...	
BW46	107	0	63	159	329
	8	-16	-46	56	
	0.03	-1.00	-0.43	0.25	
	0.1	1.4	2.4	3.5	
BW47	0	16	15	22	53
	-15	13	-2	5	
	-1.00	0.26	-0.16	0.15	
	1.7	...	0.0	0.2	

	DQW1	DQW2	DQW3	DQX	SUM
BW48	98	0	36	37	171
	46	-8	-20	-15	
	0.39	-1.00	-0.37	-0.31	
	4.6*	0.7	0.9	0.6	
B49	0	0	13	13	26
	-7	0	4	5	
	-1.00	-1.00	0.25	0.27	
	0.9	...	0.2	0.3	
BW50	0	0	32	7	39
	-11	-1	19	-4	
	-1.00	-1.00	0.73	-0.42	
	1.3	...	3.1	0.2	
B51	96	31	363	287	777
	-137	-8	102	45	
	-0.59	-0.22	0.20	0.08	
	9.6#	0.2	4.0*	0.0	
BW52	528	4	92	113	737
	306	-33	-154	-116	
	0.59	-0.89	-0.63	-0.51	
	49.4$	2.6	12.0$	7.1#	
BW53	13	0	23	3	39
	1	-1	10	-8	
	0.05	-1.00	0.38	-0.75	
	0.0	...	0.9	0.8	
BW54	192	4	373	155	724
	-25	-32	130	-70	
	-0.12	-0.89	0.27	-0.31	
	0.4	2.6	8.6#	2.6	
BW55	9	9	127	79	224
	-58	-1	52	9	
	-0.87	-0.22	0.35	0.06	
	5.6*	0.0	4.2*	0.1	
BW56	92	13	27	39	171
	40	4	-29	-13	
	0.34	0.03	-0.53	-0.27	
	3.5	0.2	1.9	0.4	
BW57	26	40	13	0	79
	2	36	-13	-24	
	0.04	0.48	-0.51	-1.00	
	0.0	...	0.8	2.7	
BW58	40	16	40	49	145
	-3	9	-8	4	
	-0.09	0.06	-0.18	0.04	
	0.0	0.8	0.2	0.0	
BW59	0	6	90	36	132
	-39	0	46	-4	
	-1.00	-0.11	0.52	-0.13	
	4.4*	0.0	5.5*	0.1	
BW60	150	40	234	262	686
	-56	5	4	48	
	-0.27	0.01	0.01	0.10	
	1.8	0.1	0.0	1.3	
BW61	165	32	469	463	1129
	-174	-25	90	111	
	-0.52	-0.45	0.12	0.14	
	11.1$	1.0	2.8	4.3*	
BW62	226	26	272	296	820
	-20	-15	-2	40	
	-0.09	-0.36	-0.01	0.07	
	0.2	0.5	0.0	0.8	

	DQW1	DQW2	DQW3	DQX	SUM
BW63	0	0	0	0	0
	0	0	0	0	
	0.00	0.00	0.00	0.00	
	...	...	...	...	
BW64	0	0	0	0	0
	0	0	0	0	
	0.00	0.00	0.00	0.00	
	...	...	...	...	
BW65	0	3	13	11	27
	-7	2	4	3	
	-1.00	0.06	0.22	0.14	
	0.9	...	0.2	0.1	
BW67	13	0	0	0	13
	9	0	-3	-3	
	1.00	-1.00	-1.00	-1.00	
	...	...	...	...	
BW71	0	0	13	26	39
	-11	-1	0	14	
	-1.00	-1.00	-0.01	0.52	
	1.3	...	0.0	1.7	
BW72	26	0	23	4	53
	10	-2	5	-12	
	0.27	-1.00	0.15	-0.76	
	0.7	...	0.2	1.1	
BW73	0	0	0	0	0
	0	0	0	0	
	0.00	0.00	0.00	0.00	
	...	...	...	...	
BX	76	0	26	44	146
	32	-6	-22	-1	
	0.31	-1.00	-0.47	-0.03	
	2.6	0.6	1.2	0.0	
SUM	3015	513	3355	3118	

Haplotype frequencies for population ORI; B-Bf ($N = 174$)

	BF S	BF F	BFF1	BFS07	BF V	SUM
B7	287 -113 -0.28 4.6*	172 114 0.28 4.7*	0 0 0.00 ...	0 0 0.00 ...	0 0 0.00 ...	459
B8	0 -49 -1.00 6.9#	57 50 1.00 ...	0 0 0.00 ...	0 0 0.00 ...	0 0 0.00 ...	57
B13	920 67 0.54 0.8	57 -65 -0.54 0.8	0 0 0.00 ...	0 0 0.00 ...	0 0 0.00 ...	977
B18	0 0 0.00 ...	0 0 0.00 ...	0 0 0.00 ...	0 0 0.00 ...	0 0 0.00 ...	0
B27	287 36 1.00 0.7	0 -35 -1.00 0.7	0 0 0.00 ...	0 0 0.00 ...	0 0 0.00 ...	287
B35	345 -56 -0.14 1.1	115 57 0.14 1.2	0 0 0.00 ...	0 0 0.00 ...	0 0 0.00 ...	460
B37	0 -49 -1.00 6.9#	57 50 1.00 ...	0 0 0.00 ...	0 0 0.00 ...	0 0 0.00 ...	57
B38	57 -42 -0.43 2.5	57 43 0.43 ...	0 0 0.00 ...	0 0 0.00 ...	0 0 0.00 ...	114
B39	517 66 1.00 1.4	0 -64 -1.00 1.4	0 0 0.00 ...	0 0 0.00 ...	0 0 0.00 ...	517
BW41	0 0 0.00 ...	0 0 0.00 ...	0 0 0.00 ...	0 0 0.00 ...	0 0 0.00 ...	0
BW42	57 7 1.00 0.1	0 -6 -1.00 ...	0 0 0.00 ...	0 0 0.00 ...	0 0 0.00 ...	57
B44	230 -220 -0.49 15.7‡	287 222 0.49 15.9‡	0 0 0.00 ...	0 0 0.00 ...	0 0 0.00 ...	517
B45	0 0 0.00 ...	0 0 0.00 ...	0 0 0.00 ...	0 0 0.00 ...	0 0 0.00 ...	0
BW46	402 51 1.00 1.1	0 -50 -1.00 1.0	0 0 0.00 ...	0 0 0.00 ...	0 0 0.00 ...	402
BW47	115 15 1.00 0.3	0 -13 -1.00 ...	0 0 0.00 ...	0 0 0.00 ...	0 0 0.00 ...	115
BW48	57 7 1.00 0.1	0 -6 -1.00 ...	0 0 0.00 ...	0 0 0.00 ...	0 0 0.00 ...	57
B49	57 7 1.00 0.1	0 -6 -1.00 ...	0 0 0.00 ...	0 0 0.00 ...	0 0 0.00 ...	57
BW50	0 0 0.00 ...	0 0 0.00 ...	0 0 0.00 ...	0 0 0.00 ...	0 0 0.00 ...	0
B51	287 -12 -0.04 0.1	57 14 0.05 0.1	0 0 0.00 ...	0 0 0.00 ...	0 0 0.00 ...	344
BW52	172 -27 -0.14 0.5	57 28 0.14 0.6	0 0 0.00 ...	0 0 0.00 ...	0 0 0.00 ...	229
BW53	0 -49 -1.00 6.9#	57 50 1.00 ...	0 0 0.00 ...	0 0 0.00 ...	0 0 0.00 ...	57
BW54	460 58 1.00 1.2	0 -57 -1.00 1.2	0 0 0.00 ...	0 0 0.00 ...	0 0 0.00 ...	460
BW55	287 -12 -0.04 0.1	57 14 0.05 0.1	0 0 0.00 ...	0 0 0.00 ...	0 0 0.00 ...	344
BW56	345 44 1.00 0.9	0 -42 -1.00 0.9	0 0 0.00 ...	0 0 0.00 ...	0 0 0.00 ...	345
BW57	172 22 1.00 0.4	0 -21 -1.00 ...	0 0 0.00 ...	0 0 0.00 ...	0 0 0.00 ...	172
BW58	401 1 0.02 0.0	57 0 -0.01 0.0	0 0 0.00 ...	0 0 0.00 ...	0 0 0.00 ...	458
BW59	115 15 1.00 0.3	0 -13 -1.00 ...	0 0 0.00 ...	0 0 0.00 ...	0 0 0.00 ...	115
BW60	1149 45 0.28 0.3	115 -43 -0.28 0.3	0 0 0.00 ...	0 0 0.00 ...	0 0 0.00 ...	1264
BW61	517 16 0.22 0.1	57 -14 -0.21 0.1	0 0 0.00 ...	0 0 0.00 ...	0 0 0.00 ...	574
BW62	1316 167 1.00 3.8	0 -165 -1.00 3.8	0 0 0.00 ...	0 0 0.00 ...	0 0 0.00 ...	1316
BW63	0 0 0.00 ...	0 0 0.00 ...	0 0 0.00 ...	0 0 0.00 ...	0 0 0.00 ...	0
BW64	0 0 0.00 ...	0 0 0.00 ...	0 0 0.00 ...	0 0 0.00 ...	0 0 0.00 ...	0
BW65	0 0 0.00 ...	0 0 0.00 ...	0 0 0.00 ...	0 0 0.00 ...	0 0 0.00 ...	0
BW67	0 0 0.00 ...	0 0 0.00 ...	0 0 0.00 ...	0 0 0.00 ...	0 0 0.00 ...	0
BW71	0 0 0.00 ...	0 0 0.00 ...	0 0 0.00 ...	0 0 0.00 ...	0 0 0.00 ...	0
BW72	115 15 1.00 0.3	0 -13 -1.00 ...	0 0 0.00 ...	0 0 0.00 ...	0 0 0.00 ...	115
BW73	0 0 0.00 ...	0 0 0.00 ...	0 0 0.00 ...	0 0 0.00 ...	0 0 0.00 ...	0
BX	64 8 1.00 0.2	0 -7 -1.00 ...	0 0 0.00 ...	0 0 0.00 ...	0 0 0.00 ...	64
SUM	8731	1259	0	0	0	

Haplotype frequencies for population ORI; B-C4A ($N = 157$)

	C4 A1	C4A12	C4A13	C4 A2	C4 A3	C4 A4	C4A51	C4 A6	C4AQ0	SUM
B7	0 0 0.00 ...	255 193 0.43 11.3$	0 0 0.00 ...	64 54 0.30 ...	122 -219 -0.64 7.1#	64 25 0.05 0.3	0 0 0.00 ...	0 -6 -1.00 ...	5 -45 -0.90 0.8	510
B8	0 0 0.00 ...	0 0 0.00 ...	0 0 0.00 ...	0 0 0.00 ...	0 0 0.00 ...	0 0 0.00 ...	0 0 0.00 ...	0 0 0.00 ...	0 0 0.00 ...	0
B13	0 0 0.00 ...	0 -115 -1.00 2.3	0 0 0.00 ...	0 -17 -1.00 ...	851 208 0.66 3.6	0 -72 -1.00 1.4	0 0 0.00 ...	0 -11 -1.00 ...	107 11 0.01 0.0	958
B18	0 0 0.00 ...	0 0 0.00 ...	0 0 0.00 ...	0 0 0.00 ...	0 0 0.00 ...	0 0 0.00 ...	0 0 0.00 ...	0 0 0.00 ...	0 0 0.00 ...	0
B27	0 0 0.00 ...	0 -38 -1.00 0.7	0 0 0.00 ...	0 -5 -1.00 ...	255 41 0.39 0.4	64 40 0.13 ...	0 0 0.00 ...	0 -3 -1.00 ...	0 -31 -1.00 ...	319
B35	0 0 0.00 ...	0 -44 -1.00 0.8	0 0 0.00 ...	0 -6 -1.00 ...	255 8 0.07 0.0	49 21 0.06 ...	0 0 0.00 ...	0 -4 -1.00 ...	64 27 0.08 0.4	368
B37	0 0 0.00 ...	0 -15 -1.00 ...	0 0 0.00 ...	0 -1 -1.00 ...	64 -21 -0.25 0.3	64 54 0.46 ...	0 0 0.00 ...	0 -1 -1.00 ...	0 -12 -1.00 ...	128
B38	0 0 0.00 ...	0 -15 -1.00 ...	0 0 0.00 ...	64 62 0.49 ...	64 -21 -0.25 0.3	0 -9 -1.00 ...	0 0 0.00 ...	0 -1 -1.00 ...	0 -12 -1.00 ...	128
B39	0 0 0.00 ...	64 10 0.02 0.0	0 0 0.00 ...	0 -8 -1.00 ...	234 -65 -0.22 0.7	0 -33 -1.00 0.6	0 0 0.00 ...	0 -5 -1.00 ...	149 104 0.26 4.5*	447
BW41	0 0 0.00 ...	0 0 0.00 ...	0 0 0.00 ...	0 0 0.00 ...	0 0 0.00 ...	0 0 0.00 ...	0 0 0.00 ...	0 0 0.00 ...	0 0 0.00 ...	0
BW42	0 0 0.00 ...	0 0 0.00 ...	0 0 0.00 ...	0 0 0.00 ...	0 0 0.00 ...	0 0 0.00 ...	0 0 0.00 ...	0 0 0.00 ...	0 0 0.00 ...	0
B44	0 0 0.00 ...	64 -13 -0.17 0.0	0 0 0.00 ...	0 -11 -1.00 ...	511 82 0.39 0.8	0 -48 -1.00 0.9	0 0 0.00 ...	0 -7 -1.00 ...	64 0 0.00 0.0	639
B45	0 0 0.00 ...	0 0 0.00 ...	0 0 0.00 ...	0 0 0.00 ...	0 0 0.00 ...	0 0 0.00 ...	0 0 0.00 ...	0 0 0.00 ...	0 0 0.00 ...	0
BW46	0 0 0.00 ...	0 -38 -1.00 0.7	0 0 0.00 ...	0 -5 -1.00 ...	255 41 0.39 0.4	64 40 0.13 ...	0 0 0.00 ...	0 -3 -1.00 ...	0 -31 -1.00 ...	319
BW47	0 0 0.00 ...	0 -15 -1.00 ...	0 0 0.00 ...	0 -1 -1.00 ...	128 42 1.00 0.0	0 -9 -1.00 ...	0 0 0.00 ...	0 -1 -1.00 ...	0 -12 -1.00 ...	128

	C4 A1	C4A12	C4A13	C4 A2	C4 A3	C4 A4	C4A51	C4 A6	C4AQ0	SUM
BW48	0 0 0.00 ...	0 0 0.00 ...	0 0 0.00 ...	0 0 0.00 ...	0 0 0.00 ...	0 0 0.00 ...	0 0 0.00 ...	0 0 0.00 ...	0 0 0.00 ...	0
B49	0 0 0.00 ...	0 -7 -1.00 ...	0 0 0.00 ...	0 0 -1.00 ...	64 21 1.00 0.5	0 -4 -1.00 ...	0 0 0.00 ...	0 0 -1.00 ...	0 -5 -1.00 ...	64
BW50	0 0 0.00 ...	0 0 0.00 ...	0 0 0.00 ...	0 0 0.00 ...	0 0 0.00 ...	0 0 0.00 ...	0 0 0.00 ...	0 0 0.00 ...	0 0 0.00 ...	0
B51	0 0 0.00 ...	64 17 0.05 0.1	0 0 0.00 ...	64 57 0.31 ...	248 -9 -0.04 0.0	0 -28 -1.00 ...	0 0 0.00 ...	0 -4 -1.00 ...	8 -29 -0.79 0.4	384
BW52	0 0 0.00 ...	0 -7 -1.00 ...	0 0 0.00 ...	0 0 -1.00 ...	64 21 1.00 0.5	0 -4 -1.00 ...	0 0 0.00 ...	0 0 -1.00 ...	0 -5 -1.00 ...	64
BW53	0 0 0.00 ...	0 0 0.00 ...	0 0 0.00 ...	0 0 0.00 ...	0 0 0.00 ...	0 0 0.00 ...	0 0 0.00 ...	0 0 0.00 ...	0 0 0.00 ...	0
BW54	0 0 0.00 ...	255 201 0.51 13.9$	0 0 0.00 ...	0 -8 -1.00 ...	64 -235 -0.79 9.3#	128 94 0.23 4.6*	0 0 0.00 ...	0 -5 -1.00 ...	0 -44 -1.00 0.8	447
BW55	0 0 0.00 ...	0 -38 -1.00 0.7	0 0 0.00 ...	0 -5 -1.00 ...	255 41 0.39 0.4	64 40 0.13 ...	0 0 0.00 ...	0 -3 -1.00 ...	0 -31 -1.00 ...	319
BW56	0 0 0.00 ...	0 -45 -1.00 0.9	0 0 0.00 ...	0 -6 -1.00 ...	194 -62 -0.24 0.8	128 99 0.28 ...	0 0 0.00 ...	0 -4 -1.00 ...	61 23 0.07 0.2	383
BW57	0 0 0.00 ...	0 -15 -1.00 ...	0 0 0.00 ...	0 -1 -1.00 ...	0 -85 -1.00 4.1*	0 -9 -1.00 ...	0 0 0.00 ...	128 126 1.00 ...	0 -12 -1.00 ...	128
BW58	0 0 0.00 ...	64 2 0.00 0.0	0 0 0.00 ...	0 -9 -1.00 ...	359 17 0.10 0.0	0 -38 -1.00 0.7	0 0 0.00 ...	0 -6 -1.00 ...	87 36 0.08 0.5	510
BW59	0 0 0.00 ...	64 48 0.43 ...	0 0 0.00 ...	0 -1 -1.00 ...	64 -21 -0.25 0.3	0 -9 -1.00 ...	0 0 0.00 ...	0 -1 -1.00 ...	0 -12 -1.00 ...	128
BW60	0 0 0.00 ...	128 -57 -0.31 0.4	0 0 0.00 ...	0 -28 -1.00 ...	1141 113 0.22 0.7	64 -53 -0.46 0.5	0 0 0.00 ...	0 -19 -1.00 ...	200 47 0.06 0.3	1533
BW61	0 0 0.00 ...	64 2 0.00 0.0	0 0 0.00 ...	0 -9 -1.00 ...	381 38 0.23 0.2	0 -38 -1.00 0.7	0 0 0.00 ...	0 -6 -1.00 ...	66 15 0.03 0.1	511
BW62	0 0 0.00 ...	192 23 0.02 0.1	0 0 0.00 ...	0 -26 -1.00 ...	957 26 0.06 0.0	64 -41 -0.40 0.3	0 0 0.00 ...	0 -17 -1.00 ...	175 37 0.04 0.2	1388

Haplotype frequencies for population ORI
B-C4A (N = 157)

	C4 A1	C4A12	C4A13	C4 A2	C4 A3	C4 A4	C4A51	C4 A6	C4AQ0	SUM
BW63	0 0 0.00 ...	0 0 0.00 ...	0 0 0.00 ...	0 0 0.00 ...	0 0 0.00 ...	0 0 0.00 ...	0 0 0.00 ...	0 0 0.00 ...	0 0 0.00 ...	0
BW64	0 0 0.00 ...	0 0 0.00 ...	0 0 0.00 ...	0 0 0.00 ...	0 0 0.00 ...	0 0 0.00 ...	0 0 0.00 ...	0 0 0.00 ...	0 0 0.00 ...	0
BW65	0 0 0.00 ...	0 0 0.00 ...	0 0 0.00 ...	0 0 0.00 ...	0 0 0.00 ...	0 0 0.00 ...	0 0 0.00 ...	0 0 0.00 ...	0 0 0.00 ...	0
BW67	0 0 0.00 ...	0 0 0.00 ...	0 0 0.00 ...	0 0 0.00 ...	0 0 0.00 ...	0 0 0.00 ...	0 0 0.00 ...	0 0 0.00 ...	0 0 0.00 ...	0
BW71	0 0 0.00 ...	0 0 0.00 ...	0 0 0.00 ...	0 0 0.00 ...	0 0 0.00 ...	0 0 0.00 ...	0 0 0.00 ...	0 0 0.00 ...	0 0 0.00 ...	0
BW72	0 0 0.00 ...	0 -15 -1.00 ...	0 0 0.00 ...	0 -1 -1.00 ...	128 42 1.00 0.0	0 -9 -1.00 ...	0 0 0.00 ...	0 -1 -1.00 ...	0 -12 -1.00 ...	128
BW73	0 0 0.00 ...	0 0 0.00 ...	0 0 0.00 ...	0 0 0.00 ...	0 0 0.00 ...	0 0 0.00 ...	0 0 0.00 ...	0 0 0.00 ...	0 0 0.00 ...	0
BX	0 0 0.00 ...	0 -6 -1.00 ...	0 0 0.00 ...	0 0 -1.00 ...	50 0 -0.01 0.0	14 8 0.12 ...	0 0 0.00 ...	0 0 -1.00 ...	11 4 0.05 ...	75
SUM	0	1214	0	192	6703	767	0	128	997	

Haplotype frequencies for population ORI
B-C4B ($N = 155$)

	C4 B1	C4B11	C4B12	C4 B2	C4 B3	C4 B4	C4 B5	C4B51	C4 B6	C4 B7	C4BQ0	SUM
B7	424 85 0.48 1.0	0 0 0.00 ...	0 -2 -1.00 ...	65 -47 -0.43 0.4	0 -2 -1.00 ...	0 0 0.00 ...	0 0 0.00 ...	0 0 0.00 ...	0 0 0.00 ...	0 0 0.00 ...	27 -29 -0.53 0.3	516
B8	0 0 0.00 ...	0 0 0.00 ...	0 0 0.00 ...	0 0 0.00 ...	0 0 0.00 ...	0 0 0.00 ...	0 0 0.00 ...	0 0 0.00 ...	0 0 0.00 ...	0 0 0.00 ...	0 0 0.00 ...	0
B13	718 63 0.25 0.5	0 0 0.00 ...	0 -5 -1.00 ...	114 -97 -0.46 1.0	0 -5 -1.00 ...	0 0 0.00 ...	0 0 0.00 ...	0 0 0.00 ...	0 0 0.00 ...	0 0 0.00 ...	135 28 0.03 0.1	967
B18	0 0 0.00 ...	0 0 0.00 ...	0 0 0.00 ...	0 0 0.00 ...	0 0 0.00 ...	0 0 0.00 ...	0 0 0.00 ...	0 0 0.00 ...	0 0 0.00 ...	0 0 0.00 ...	0 0 0.00 ...	0
B27	311 100 0.90 2.2	0 0 0.00 ...	0 -1 -1.00 ...	0 -70 -1.00 1.5	0 -1 -1.00 ...	0 0 0.00 ...	0 0 0.00 ...	0 0 0.00 ...	0 0 0.00 ...	0 0 0.00 ...	11 -24 -0.69 0.3	322
B35	64 -179 -0.74 6.2*	0 0 0.00 ...	0 -1 -1.00 ...	243 161 0.56 6.6*	0 -1 -1.00 ...	0 0 0.00 ...	0 0 0.00 ...	0 0 0.00 ...	0 0 0.00 ...	0 0 0.00 ...	65 24 0.07 0.2	372
B37	65 -19 -0.24 0.2	0 0 0.00 ...	0 0 -1.00 ...	65 36 0.36 ...	0 0 -1.00 ...	0 0 0.00 ...	0 0 0.00 ...	0 0 0.00 ...	0 0 0.00 ...	0 0 0.00 ...	0 -13 -1.00 ...	130
B38	65 -19 -0.24 0.2	0 0 0.00 ...	0 0 -1.00 ...	0 -28 -1.00 ...	0 0 -1.00 ...	0 0 0.00 ...	0 0 0.00 ...	0 0 0.00 ...	0 0 0.00 ...	0 0 0.00 ...	65 51 0.44 ...	130
B39	452 155 1.00 3.8	0 0 0.00 ...	0 -2 -1.00 ...	0 -98 -1.00 2.1	0 -2 -1.00 ...	0 0 0.00 ...	0 0 0.00 ...	0 0 0.00 ...	0 0 0.00 ...	0 0 0.00 ...	0 -49 -1.00 0.9	452
BW41	0 0 0.00 ...	0 0 0.00 ...	0 0 0.00 ...	0 0 0.00 ...	0 0 0.00 ...	0 0 0.00 ...	0 0 0.00 ...	0 0 0.00 ...	0 0 0.00 ...	0 0 0.00 ...	0 0 0.00 ...	0
BW42	0 0 0.00 ...	0 0 0.00 ...	0 0 0.00 ...	0 0 0.00 ...	0 0 0.00 ...	0 0 0.00 ...	0 0 0.00 ...	0 0 0.00 ...	0 0 0.00 ...	0 0 0.00 ...	0 0 0.00 ...	0
B44	579 155 0.70 2.7	0 0 0.00 ...	0 -3 -1.00 ...	0 -141 -1.00 3.0	65 61 1.00 ...	0 0 0.00 ...	0 0 0.00 ...	0 0 0.00 ...	0 0 0.00 ...	0 0 0.00 ...	2 -69 -0.97 1.3	646
B45	0 0 0.00 ...	0 0 0.00 ...	0 0 0.00 ...	0 0 0.00 ...	0 0 0.00 ...	0 0 0.00 ...	0 0 0.00 ...	0 0 0.00 ...	0 0 0.00 ...	0 0 0.00 ...	0 0 0.00 ...	0
BW46	0 -211 -1.00 9.9#	0 0 0.00 ...	0 -1 -1.00 ...	323 252 1.00 18.4$	0 -1 -1.00 ...	0 0 0.00 ...	0 0 0.00 ...	0 0 0.00 ...	0 0 0.00 ...	0 0 0.00 ...	0 -35 -1.00 0.6	323
BW47	114 29 0.66 0.5	0 0 0.00 ...	0 0 -1.00 ...	15 -12 -0.47 ...	0 0 -1.00 ...	0 0 0.00 ...	0 0 0.00 ...	0 0 0.00 ...	0 0 0.00 ...	0 0 0.00 ...	0 -13 -1.00 ...	129

Haplotype frequencies for population ORI
B-C4B ($N = 155$)

	C4 B1	C4B11	C4B12	C4 B2	C4 B3	C4 B4	C4 B5	C4B51	C4 B6	C4 B7	C4BQ0	SUM
BW48	0 0 0.00 ...	0 0 0.00 ...	0 0 0.00 ...	0 0 0.00 ...	0 0 0.00 ...	0 0 0.00 ...	0 0 0.00 ...	0 0 0.00 ...	0 0 0.00 ...	0 0 0.00 ...	0 0 0.00 ...	0
B49	65 22 1.00 0.5	0 0 0.00 ...	0 0 -1.00 ...	0 -13 -1.00 ...	0 0 -1.00 ...	0 0 0.00 ...	0 0 0.00 ...	0 0 0.00 ...	0 0 0.00 ...	0 0 0.00 ...	0 -6 -1.00 ...	65
BW50	0 0 0.00 ...	0 0 0.00 ...	0 0 0.00 ...	0 0 0.00 ...	0 0 0.00 ...	0 0 0.00 ...	0 0 0.00 ...	0 0 0.00 ...	0 0 0.00 ...	0 0 0.00 ...	0 0 0.00 ...	0
B51	323 69 0.52 0.9	0 0 0.00 ...	0 -2 -1.00 ...	64 -20 -0.25 0.1	0 -2 -1.00 ...	0 0 0.00 ...	0 0 0.00 ...	0 0 0.00 ...	0 0 0.00 ...	0 0 0.00 ...	0 -42 -1.00 0.8	387
BW52	0 -42 -1.00 1.9	0 0 0.00 ...	0 0 -1.00 ...	0 -13 -1.00 ...	0 0 -1.00 ...	0 0 0.00 ...	0 0 0.00 ...	0 0 0.00 ...	0 0 0.00 ...	0 0 0.00 ...	65 58 1.00 ...	65
BW53	0 0 0.00 ...	0 0 0.00 ...	0 0 0.00 ...	0 0 0.00 ...	0 0 0.00 ...	0 0 0.00 ...	0 0 0.00 ...	0 0 0.00 ...	0 0 0.00 ...	0 0 0.00 ...	0 0 0.00 ...	0
BW54	137 -116 -0.46 2.5	0 0 0.00 ...	0 -2 -1.00 ...	65 -19 -0.24 0.1	0 -2 -1.00 ...	0 0 0.00 ...	0 0 0.00 ...	0 0 0.00 ...	0 0 0.00 ...	0 0 0.00 ...	185 142 0.41 8.5#	387
BW55	194 -17 -0.09 0.1	0 0 0.00 ...	0 -1 -1.00 ...	109 38 0.15 0.4	0 -1 -1.00 ...	0 0 0.00 ...	0 0 0.00 ...	0 0 0.00 ...	0 0 0.00 ...	0 0 0.00 ...	20 -15 -0.44 0.1	323
BW56	258 4 0.03 0.0	0 0 0.00 ...	0 -2 -1.00 ...	129 44 0.15 0.5	0 -2 -1.00 ...	0 0 0.00 ...	0 0 0.00 ...	0 0 0.00 ...	0 0 0.00 ...	0 0 0.00 ...	0 -42 -1.00 0.8	387
BW57	194 67 1.00 1.6	0 0 0.00 ...	0 0 -1.00 ...	0 -42 -1.00 0.9	0 0 -1.00 ...	0 0 0.00 ...	0 0 0.00 ...	0 0 0.00 ...	0 0 0.00 ...	0 0 0.00 ...	0 -21 -1.00 ...	194
BW58	129 -208 -0.62 6.2*	0 0 0.00 ...	0 -2 -1.00 ...	65 -47 -0.43 0.4	0 -2 -1.00 ...	0 0 0.00 ...	0 0 0.00 ...	0 0 0.00 ...	0 0 0.00 ...	0 0 0.00 ...	321 264 0.58 22.4$	515
BW59	65 22 1.00 0.5	0 0 0.00 ...	0 0 -1.00 ...	0 -13 -1.00 ...	0 0 -1.00 ...	0 0 0.00 ...	0 0 0.00 ...	0 0 0.00 ...	0 0 0.00 ...	0 0 0.00 ...	0 -6 -1.00 ...	65
BW60	1258 283 0.56 4.4*	0 0 0.00 ...	0 -9 -1.00 ...	194 -131 -0.40 1.2	0 -9 -1.00 ...	0 0 0.00 ...	0 0 0.00 ...	0 0 0.00 ...	0 0 0.00 ...	0 0 0.00 ...	32 -132 -0.81 2.2	1484
BW61	452 112 0.63 1.8	0 0 0.00 ...	0 -2 -1.00 ...	65 -46 -0.43 0.4	0 -2 -1.00 ...	0 0 0.00 ...	0 0 0.00 ...	0 0 0.00 ...	0 0 0.00 ...	0 0 0.00 ...	0 -56 -1.00 1.1	517
BW62	568 -359 -0.39 7.3#	0 0 0.00 ...	65 56 1.00 ...	639 329 0.30 8.1#	0 -8 -1.00 ...	0 0 0.00 ...	0 0 0.00 ...	0 0 0.00 ...	0 0 0.00 ...	0 0 0.00 ...	141 -15 -0.10 0.0	1413

Haplotype frequencies for population ORI
B-C4B ($N = 155$)

	C4 B1	C4B11	C4B12	C4 B2	C4 B3	C4 B4	C4 B5	C4B51	C4 B6	C4 B7	C4BQ0	SUM
BW63	0 0 0.00 ...	0 0 0.00 ...	0 0 0.00 ...	0 0 0.00 ...	0 0 0.00 ...	0 0 0.00 ...	0 0 0.00 ...	0 0 0.00 ...	0 0 0.00 ...	0 0 0.00 ...	0 0 0.00 ...	0
BW64	0 0 0.00 ...	0 0 0.00 ...	0 0 0.00 ...	0 0 0.00 ...	0 0 0.00 ...	0 0 0.00 ...	0 0 0.00 ...	0 0 0.00 ...	0 0 0.00 ...	0 0 0.00 ...	0 0 0.00 ...	0
BW65	0 0 0.00 ...	0 0 0.00 ...	0 0 0.00 ...	0 0 0.00 ...	0 0 0.00 ...	0 0 0.00 ...	0 0 0.00 ...	0 0 0.00 ...	0 0 0.00 ...	0 0 0.00 ...	0 0 0.00 ...	0
BW67	0 0 0.00 ...	0 0 0.00 ...	0 0 0.00 ...	0 0 0.00 ...	0 0 0.00 ...	0 0 0.00 ...	0 0 0.00 ...	0 0 0.00 ...	0 0 0.00 ...	0 0 0.00 ...	0 0 0.00 ...	0
BW71	0 0 0.00 ...	0 0 0.00 ...	0 0 0.00 ...	0 0 0.00 ...	0 0 0.00 ...	0 0 0.00 ...	0 0 0.00 ...	0 0 0.00 ...	0 0 0.00 ...	0 0 0.00 ...	0 0 0.00 ...	0
BW72	121 36 0.82 0.7	0 0 0.00 ...	0 0 -1.00 ...	0 -27 -1.00 ...	0 0 -1.00 ...	0 0 0.00 ...	0 0 0.00 ...	0 0 0.00 ...	0 0 0.00 ...	0 0 0.00 ...	8 -5 -0.44 ...	129
BW73	0 0 0.00 ...	0 0 0.00 ...	0 0 0.00 ...	0 0 0.00 ...	0 0 0.00 ...	0 0 0.00 ...	0 0 0.00 ...	0 0 0.00 ...	0 0 0.00 ...	0 0 0.00 ...	0 0 0.00 ...	0
BX	12 -44 -0.79 1.6	0 0 0.00 ...	0 0 -1.00 ...	41 22 0.32 ...	0 0 -1.00 ...	0 0 0.00 ...	0 0 0.00 ...	0 0 0.00 ...	0 0 0.00 ...	0 0 0.00 ...	34 24 0.31 ...	87
SUM	6568	0	65	2196	65	0	0	0	0	0	1111	

Haplotype frequencies for population ORI

C-DQ ($N=772$)▼

	CW1	CW2	CW3	CW4	CW5	CW6	CW7	CW8	CX	SUM
DQW1	479 -30 -0.06 0.3	39 8 0.11 0.2	573 -203 -0.26 7.0#	34 -133 -0.80 12.5‡	47 27 0.60 4.3*	65 -35 -0.35 1.4	434 72 0.09 1.8	0 -10 -1.00 1.3	1341 309 0.16 15.6‡	3012
DQW2	31 -54 -0.64 3.4	26 21 0.21 ...	85 -44 -0.35 1.7	0 -27 -1.00 2.4	0 -2 -1.00 ...	193 176 0.56 154.7‡	65 4 0.01 0.0	2 0 0.00 ...	103 -69 -0.40 3.5	505
DQW3	687 128 0.11 4.1*	26 -7 -0.24 0.2	997 146 0.08 3.9*	325 141 0.36 13.1‡	0 -20 -1.00 2.5	66 -43 -0.40 2.1	318 -78 -0.20 2.0	13 0 0.02 0.0	866 -263 -0.23 10.8#	3298
DQX	497 -42 -0.08 0.5	13 -19 -0.61 1.4	925 102 0.06 1.0	200 22 0.06 0.3	18 -2 -0.13 0.0	10 -95 -0.91 10.2#	386 2 0.00 0.0	23 11 0.42 1.1	1116 24 0.01 0.1	3188
SUM	1694	104	2580	559	65	334	1203	38	3426	

C-C4A ($N=157$)▼

	C4 A1	C4A12	C4A13	C4 A2	C4 A3	C4 A4	C4A51	C4 A6	C4AQ0	SUM
CW1	0 0 0.00 ...	319 133 0.13 2.0	0 0 0.00 ...	0 -28 -1.00 ...	798 -228 -0.22 2.9	299 182 0.28 5.7*	0 0 0.00 ...	0 -19 -1.00 ...	115 -36 -0.25 0.2	1531
CW2	0 0 0.00 ...	64 33 0.15 ...	0 0 0.00 ...	0 -4 -1.00 ...	192 20 0.24 0.1	0 -19 -1.00 ...	0 0 0.00 ...	0 -2 -1.00 ...	0 -24 -1.00 ...	256
CW3	0 0 0.00 ...	255 -39 -0.14 0.1	0 0 0.00 ...	0 -46 -1.00 0.0	1776 144 0.18 0.8	255 69 0.12 0.6	0 0 0.00 ...	0 -30 -1.00 ...	148 -93 -0.39 0.8	2434
CW4	0 0 0.00 ...	64 2 0.00 0.0	0 0 0.00 ...	0 -9 -1.00 ...	426 63 0.49 1.0	0 -38 -1.00 0.7	0 0 0.00 ...	0 -6 -1.00 ...	21 -29 -0.59 0.3	511
CW5	0 0 0.00 ...	0 -7 -1.00 ...	0 0 0.00 ...	0 0 -1.00 ...	64 21 1.00 0.5	0 -4 -1.00 ...	0 0 0.00 ...	0 0 -1.00 ...	0 -5 -1.00 ...	64
CW6	0 0 0.00 ...	0 -137 -1.00 2.8	0 0 0.00 ...	0 -21 -1.00 ...	876 113 0.30 0.9	64 -22 -0.27 0.1	0 0 0.00 ...	128 113 1.00 ...	69 -43 -0.39 0.3	1137
CW7	0 0 0.00 ...	319 109 0.11 1.2	0 0 0.00 ...	64 31 0.19 0.6	1186 25 0.04 0.0	0 -132 -1.00 2.7	0 0 0.00 ...	0 -21 -1.00 ...	162 -9 -0.06 0.0	1731
CW8	0 0 0.00 ...	0 0 0.00 ...	0 0 0.00 ...	0 0 0.00 ...	0 0 0.00 ...	0 0 0.00 ...	0 0 0.00 ...	0 0 0.00 ...	0 0 0.00 ...	0
CX	0 0 0.00 ...	192 -90 -0.32 0.7	0 0 0.00 ...	128 83 0.57 3.2	1389 -177 -0.11 1.3	148 -30 -0.17 0.1	0 0 0.00 ...	0 -29 -1.00 ...	480 247 0.32 5.0*	2337
SUM	0	1213	0	192	6707	766	0	128	995	

	CW1	CW2	CW3	CW4	CW5	CW6	CW7	CW8	CX	SUM
DR1	31 -57 -0.65 3.6	13 8 0.08 ...	51 -76 -0.61 5.1*	13 -12 -0.51 0.6	0 -2 -1.00 ...	13 -2 -0.19 0.0	339 277 0.62 110.4‡	0 0 -1.00 ...	45 -125 -0.74 11.1‡	505
DR2	160 -106 -0.40 4.6*	13 -2 -0.19 0.1	326 -63 -0.16 1.3	1 -77 -0.99 7.2#	13 3 0.05 0.1	0 -47 -1.00 4.4*	174 -12 -0.07 0.1	0 -3 -1.00 ...	830 315 0.31 25.7‡	1517
DR3	0 -33 -1.00 3.1	0 -1 -1.00 ...	137 87 0.61 15.8‡	0 -9 -1.00 0.8	0 0 -1.00 ...	0 -5 -1.00 ...	27 3 0.02 0.0	0 0 -1.00 ...	29 -36 -0.56 2.4	193
DR4	684 297 0.22 26.5‡	27 4 0.04 0.1	569 3 0.00 0.0	276 161 0.40 22.9‡	0 -14 -1.00 1.4	13 -56 -0.81 4.6*	157 -114 -0.42 5.3*	27 21 1.00 ...	447 -299 -0.40 17.5‡	2200
DR7	2 -48 -0.96 4.4*	27 24 0.23 ...	20 -53 -0.73 4.1*	0 -14 -1.00 1.2	0 -1 -1.00 ...	176 167 0.60 242.8‡	40 4 0.02 0.0	0 0 -1.00 ...	24 -73 -0.76 6.5*	289
DRW8	203 77 0.13 4.6*	0 -7 -1.00 0.6	155 -28 -0.16 0.5	8 -28 -0.79 1.0	0 -4 -1.00 ...	0 -22 -1.00 1.9	76 -9 -0.12 0.1	0 -1 -1.00 ...	271 28 0.06 0.4	715
DRW9	196 -9 -0.05 0.0	13 1 0.01 0.0	421 120 0.14 5.5*	47 -13 -0.23 0.3	0 -7 -1.00 0.7	26 -10 -0.30 0.3	93 -50 -0.36 1.8	0 -2 -1.00 ...	372 -24 -0.06 0.2	1168
DRW10	0 -8 -1.00 0.9	0 0 -1.00 ...	0 -13 -1.00 1.4	0 -2 -1.00 ...	13 13 0.24 ...	18 16 0.32 ...	0 -6 -1.00 ...	0 0 -1.00 ...	22 4 0.11 0.1	53
DRW11	81 13 0.04 0.2	0 -3 -1.00 ...	101 1 0.00 0.0	40 20 0.05 1.6	0 -2 -1.00 ...	40 28 0.09 5.1*	14 -33 -0.71 2.1	0 0 -1.00 ...	111 -19 -0.16 0.4	387
DRW12	54 -75 -0.58 4.4*	13 5 0.05 0.3	290 100 0.18 5.7*	40 1 0.00 0.0	0 -4 -1.00 ...	2 -20 -0.91 1.6	90 0 -0.01 0.0	0 -1 -1.00 ...	249 -1 -0.01 0.0	738
DRW13	11 -37 -0.78 2.8	0 -2 -1.00 ...	48 -23 -0.33 0.8	2 -12 -0.86 0.9	0 -1 -1.00 ...	0 -8 -1.00 0.7	0 -34 -1.00 3.0	0 0 -1.00 ...	219 124 0.67 18.8‡	280
DRW14	134 16 0.03 0.2	0 -6 -1.00 0.6	137 -35 -0.21 0.8	13 -21 -0.63 1.2	27 23 0.37 ...	13 -7 -0.39 0.3	51 -31 -0.39 1.1	0 -1 -1.00 ...	298 69 0.16 2.6	673
DRX	204 -21 -0.10 0.2	0 -13 -1.00 1.2	318 -11 -0.04 0.1	82 15 0.03 0.3	13 5 0.08 0.2	15 -25 -0.63 1.4	172 14 0.01 0.1	0 -2 -1.00 ...	479 43 0.05 0.6	1283
SUM	1760	106	2573	522	66	316	1235	27	3396	

C-DR ($N=749$)

Haplotype frequencies for population ORI

C-C4B ($N = 155$)▼

	C4 B1	C4B11	C4B12	C4 B2	C4 B3	C4 B4	C4 B5	C4B51	C4 B6	C4 B7	C4BQ0	SUM
CW1	616 -315 -0.34 5.6*	0 0 0.00 ...	0 -8 -1.00 ...	598 287 0.26 6.1*	0 -8 -1.00 ...	0 0 0.00 ...	0 0 0.00 ...	0 0 0.00 ...	0 0 0.00 ...	0 0 0.00 ...	205 47 0.05 0.3	1419
CW2	247 78 0.88 1.6	0 0 0.00 ...	0 -1 -1.00 ...	0 -56 -1.00 1.2	0 -1 -1.00 ...	0 0 0.00 ...	0 0 0.00 ...	0 0 0.00 ...	0 0 0.00 ...	0 0 0.00 ...	11 -17 -0.62 ...	258
CW3	1260 -313 -0.20 3.7	0 0 0.00 ...	65 49 1.00 ...	665 139 0.08 0.0	0 -15 -1.00 ...	0 0 0.00 ...	0 0 0.00 ...	0 0 0.00 ...	0 0 0.00 ...	0 0 0.00 ...	407 141 0.17 1.7	2397
CW4	387 48 0.27 0.3	0 0 0.00 ...	0 -2 -1.00 ...	65 -47 -0.43 0.4	0 -2 -1.00 ...	0 0 0.00 ...	0 0 0.00 ...	0 0 0.00 ...	0 0 0.00 ...	0 0 0.00 ...	65 6 0.02 0.0	517
CW5	62 20 0.91 0.4	0 0 0.00 ...	0 0 -1.00 ...	0 -13 -1.00 ...	0 0 -1.00 ...	0 0 0.00 ...	0 0 0.00 ...	0 0 0.00 ...	0 0 0.00 ...	0 0 0.00 ...	2 -4 -0.72 ...	64
CW6	943 147 0.35 1.4	0 0 0.00 ...	0 -7 -1.00 ...	199 -66 -0.25 0.4	0 -7 -1.00 ...	0 0 0.00 ...	0 0 0.00 ...	0 0 0.00 ...	0 0 0.00 ...	0 0 0.00 ...	71 -63 -0.47 0.6	1213
CW7	1639 491 0.82 11.5‡	0 0 0.00 ...	0 -10 -1.00 ...	102 -281 -0.73 4.0*	0 -10 -1.00 ...	0 0 0.00 ...	0 0 0.00 ...	0 0 0.00 ...	0 0 0.00 ...	0 0 0.00 ...	8 -185 -0.96 3.8	1749
CW8	0 0 0.00 ...	0 0 0.00 ...	0 0 0.00 ...	0 0 0.00 ...	0 0 0.00 ...	0 0 0.00 ...	0 0 0.00 ...	0 0 0.00 ...	0 0 0.00 ...	0 0 0.00 ...	0 0 0.00 ...	0
CX	1411 -152 -0.10 0.9	0 0 0.00 ...	0 -14 -1.00 ...	565 42 0.03 0.1	65 50 1.00 ...	0 0 0.00 ...	0 0 0.00 ...	0 0 0.00 ...	0 0 0.00 ...	0 0 0.00 ...	342 77 0.09 0.5	2383
SUM	6565	0	65	2194	65	0	0	0	0	0	1111	

C-Bf ($N = 174$)▼

	CW1	CW2	CW3	CW4	CW5	CW6	CW7	CW8	CX	SUM
BF S	1419 114 0.60 1.6	230 29 1.00 0.6	2193 77 0.25 0.5	517 -39 -0.07 0.4	0 0 0.00 ...	1060 67 0.46 0.7	1490 -46 -0.05 0.2	0 0 0.00 ...	1826 -197 -0.20 3.5	8735
BF F	75 -113 -0.60 1.6	0 -28 -1.00 0.6	230 -75 -0.25 0.5	121 40 0.07 0.4	0 0 0.00 ...	77 -66 -0.46 0.7	270 48 0.05 0.2	0 0 0.00 ...	491 198 0.20 3.5	1264
BFF1	0 0 0.00 ...	0 0 0.00 ...	0 0 0.00 ...	0 0 0.00 ...	0 0 0.00 ...	0 0 0.00 ...	0 0 0.00 ...	0 0 0.00 ...	0 0 0.00 ...	0
BFS07	0 0 0.00 ...	0 0 0.00 ...	0 0 0.00 ...	0 0 0.00 ...	0 0 0.00 ...	0 0 0.00 ...	0 0 0.00 ...	0 0 0.00 ...	0 0 0.00 ...	0
BF V	0 0 0.00 ...	0 0 0.00 ...	0 0 0.00 ...	0 0 0.00 ...	0 0 0.00 ...	0 0 0.00 ...	0 0 0.00 ...	0 0 0.00 ...	0 0 0.00 ...	0
SUM	1494	230	2423	638	0	1137	1760	0	2317	

Haplotype frequencies for population ORI
DR-C4A ($N = 149$)

	C4 A1	C4A12	C4A13	C4 A2	C4 A3	C4 A4	C4A51	C4 A6	C4AQ0	SUM
DR1	0 0 0.00 ...	268 200 0.43 10.6#	0 0 0.00 ...	67 56 0.30 ...	134 -220 -0.62 6.4*	67 27 0.06 0.3	0 0 0.00 ...	0 -6 -1.00 ...	0 -55 -1.00 0.0	536
DR2	0 0 0.00 ...	0 -147 -1.00 2.9	0 0 0.00 ...	67 44 0.25 ...	874 106 0.27 0.7	0 -85 -1.00 1.6	0 0 0.00 ...	0 -15 -1.00 ...	220 99 0.11 1.5	1161
DR3	0 0 0.00 ...	0 -36 -1.00 0.7	0 0 0.00 ...	0 -5 -1.00 ...	267 75 0.76 1.3	0 -20 -1.00 ...	0 0 0.00 ...	0 -3 -1.00 ...	24 -5 -0.21 ...	291
DR4	0 0 0.00 ...	342 186 0.17 4.3*	0 0 0.00 ...	0 -24 -1.00 ...	711 -96 -0.12 0.6	67 -22 -0.26 0.1	0 0 0.00 ...	0 -15 -1.00 ...	102 -24 -0.20 0.1	1222
DR7	0 0 0.00 ...	0 -132 -1.00 2.5	0 0 0.00 ...	67 46 0.26 ...	913 220 0.62 3.4	0 -76 -1.00 1.4	0 0 0.00 ...	67 53 0.44 ...	0 -108 -1.00 2.0	1047
DRW8	0 0 0.00 ...	0 -33 -1.00 0.6	0 0 0.00 ...	0 -4 -1.00 ...	262 85 0.94 1.9	0 -19 -1.00 ...	0 0 0.00 ...	0 -3 -1.00 ...	5 -22 -0.82 ...	267
DRW9	0 0 0.00 ...	134 -46 -0.26 0.2	0 0 0.00 ...	0 -28 -1.00 ...	1145 204 0.42 2.3	67 -37 -0.36 0.3	0 0 0.00 ...	0 -16 -1.00 ...	76 -71 -0.49 0.7	1422
DRW10	0 0 0.00 ...	0 -8 -1.00 ...	0 0 0.00 ...	0 0 -1.00 ...	67 23 1.00 0.5	0 -4 -1.00 ...	0 0 0.00 ...	0 0 -1.00 ...	0 -6 -1.00 ...	67
DRW11	0 0 0.00 ...	67 -26 -0.29 0.1	0 0 0.00 ...	0 -14 -1.00 ...	402 -85 -0.18 0.7	138 64 0.12 2.2	0 0 0.00 ...	67 57 0.46 ...	63 -13 -0.18 0.0	737
DRW12	0 0 0.00 ...	67 -51 -0.44 0.4	0 0 0.00 ...	0 -18 -1.00 ...	454 -165 -0.27 2.2	134 65 0.10 1.1	0 0 0.00 ...	0 -12 -1.00 ...	282 184 0.22 6.4*	937
DRW13	0 0 0.00 ...	67 50 0.43 ...	0 0 0.00 ...	0 -2 -1.00 ...	0 -88 -1.00 3.0*	0 -9 -1.00 ...	0 0 0.00 ...	0 -1 -1.00 ...	67 53 0.44 ...	134
DRW14	0 0 0.00 ...	201 87 0.11 1.2	0 0 0.00 ...	0 -17 -1.00 ...	508 -85 -0.14 0.6	130 64 0.10 1.1	0 0 0.00 ...	0 -11 -1.00 ...	59 -34 -0.37 0.2	898
DRX	0 0 0.00 ...	127 -35 -0.22 0.2	0 0 0.00 ...	0 -25 -1.00 ...	878 29 0.07 0.1	134 39 0.06 0.3	0 0 0.00 ...	0 -16 -1.00 ...	144 10 0.01 0.0	1283
SUM	0	1273	0	201	6615	737	0	134	1042	

Haplotype frequencies for population ORI
DR-C4B ($N = 148$)

	C4 B1	C4B11	C4B12	C4 B2	C4 B3	C4 B4	C4 B5	C4B51	C4 B6	C4 B7	C4BQ0	SUM
DR1	394	0	0	68	0	0	0	0	0	0	79	541
	26	0	-3	-37	-3	0	0	0	0	0	20	
	0.15	0.00	-1.00	-0.36	-1.00	0.00	0.00	0.00	0.00	0.00	0.04	
	0.1	...	...	0.3	...	...	...	...	...	...	0.1	
DR2	609	0	0	338	0	0	0	0	0	0	239	1186
	-197	0	-7	105	-7	0	0	0	0	0	109	
	-0.25	0.00	-1.00	0.11	-1.00	0.00	0.00	0.00	0.00	0.00	0.11	
	2.6	...	...	0.0	...	...	...	...	...	...	1.7	
DR3	0	0	0	0	0	0	0	0	0	0	294	294
	-199	0	-1	-57	-1	0	0	0	0	0	262	
	-1.00	0.00	-1.00	-1.00	-1.00	0.00	0.00	0.00	0.00	0.00	1.00	
	9.5#	...	...	1.1	...	...	...	...	...	...	...	
DR4	952	0	0	135	0	0	0	0	0	0	80	1167
	158	0	-7	-93	-7	0	0	0	0	0	-47	
	0.42	0.00	-1.00	-0.41	-1.00	0.00	0.00	0.00	0.00	0.00	-0.36	
	1.6	...	...	0.8	...	...	...	...	...	...	0.3	
DR7	1052	0	0	0	0	0	0	0	0	0	74	1126
	286	0	-7	-220	-7	0	0	0	0	0	-49	
	0.79	0.00	-1.00	-1.00	-1.00	0.00	0.00	0.00	0.00	0.00	-0.40	
	5.6*	...	...	4.6*	...	...	...	...	...	...	0.4	
DRW8	242	0	0	0	0	0	0	0	0	0	29	271
	58	0	-1	-52	-1	0	0	0	0	0	0	
	0.67	0.00	-1.00	-1.00	-1.00	0.00	0.00	0.00	0.00	0.00	-0.03	
	0.9	...	...	1.0	...	...	...	...	...	...	...	
DRW9	897	0	68	397	0	0	0	0	0	0	9	1371
	-35	0	59	128	-8	0	0	0	0	0	-141	
	-0.04	0.00	1.00	0.12	-1.00	0.00	0.00	0.00	0.00	0.00	-0.94	
	0.1	...	...	1.3	...	...	...	...	...	...	2.6	
DRW10	68	0	0	0	0	0	0	0	0	0	0	68
	22	0	0	-12	0	0	0	0	0	0	-6	
	1.00	0.00	-1.00	-1.00	-1.00	0.00	0.00	0.00	0.00	0.00	-1.00	
	0.5	...	...	...	...	...	...	...	...	...	...	
DRW11	474	0	0	208	0	0	0	0	0	0	63	745
	-32	0	-4	62	-4	0	0	0	0	0	-18	
	-0.06	0.00	-1.00	0.10	-1.00	0.00	0.00	0.00	0.00	0.00	-0.23	
	0.1	...	...	0.5	...	...	...	...	...	...	0.1	
DRW12	609	0	0	271	0	0	0	0	0	0	0	880
	10	0	-5	98	-5	0	0	0	0	0	-96	
	0.04	0.00	-1.00	0.14	-1.00	0.00	0.00	0.00	0.00	0.00	-1.00	
	0.0	...	...	1.1	...	...	...	...	...	...	1.8	
DRW13	135	0	0	0	0	0	0	0	0	0	0	135
	43	0	0	-25	0	0	0	0	0	0	-14	
	1.00	0.00	-1.00	-1.00	-1.00	0.00	0.00	0.00	0.00	0.00	-1.00	
	0.0	...	...	...	...	...	...	...	...	...	...	
DRW14	669	0	0	139	0	0	0	0	0	0	100	908
	51	0	-5	-36	-5	0	0	0	0	0	0	
	0.18	0.00	-1.00	-0.22	-1.00	0.00	0.00	0.00	0.00	0.00	0.00	
	0.2	...	...	0.2	...	...	...	...	...	...	0.0	
DRX	703	0	0	406	68	0	0	0	0	0	131	1308
	-186	0	-8	149	59	0	0	0	0	0	-12	
	-0.21	0.00	-1.00	0.14	1.00	0.00	0.00	0.00	0.00	0.00	-0.09	
	2.1	...	...	1.8	...	...	...	...	...	...	0.0	
SUM	6804	0	68	1962	68	0	0	0	0	0	1098	

Haplotype frequencies for population ORI

DR-DQ ($N = 739$)▼

	DR1	DR2	DR3	DR4	DR7	DRW8	DRW9	DRW10	DRW11	DRW12	DRW13	DRW14	DRX	SUM
DQW1	349 191 0.54 25.9$	1426 952 0.89 241.1$	0 -46 -1.00 5.1*	55 -626 -0.92 79.1$	14 -75 -0.84 7.1#	202 -16 -0.08 0.1	47 -310 -0.87 32.6$	41 24 0.63 3.7	18 -103 -0.85 9.9#	0 -228 -1.00 26.4$	211 119 0.58 17.1$	631 417 0.86 92.8$	83 -292 -0.78 27.8$	3077
DQW2	6 -18 -0.76 1.2	14 -60 -0.81 4.6*	71 64 0.43 42.4$	31 -76 -0.71 5.5*	259 245 0.88 335.9$	0 -34 -1.00 2.9	59 2 0.01 0.0	3 0 0.01 ...	27 8 0.02 0.2	16 -19 -0.56 0.9	0 -14 -1.00 1.2	0 -33 -1.00 2.8	1 -58 -0.98 5.1*	487
DQW3	51 -120 -0.70 9.9#	0 -514 -1.00 67.5$	26 -24 -0.49 1.4	1847 1107 0.75 235.9$	0 -97 -1.00 11.2$	46 -190 -0.81 18.4$	387 0 -0.00 0.0	0 -17 -1.00 2.0	296 163 0.62 23.3$	593 345 0.70 57.3$	0 -99 -1.00 11.4$	3 -229 -0.99 27.0$	90 -317 -0.78 31.4$	3339
DQX	108 -51 -0.32 1.9	101 -376 -0.79 37.7$	57 9 0.09 0.2	284 -403 -0.59 32.7$	20 -70 -0.78 6.1*	463 242 0.49 30.7$	670 309 0.39 32.1$	11 -5 -0.36 0.2	56 -66 -0.55 4.1*	135 -95 -0.42 4.6*	87 -4 -0.06 0.0	63 -152 -0.71 12.5$	1049 669 0.79 144.1$	3104
SUM	514	1541	154	2217	293	711	1163	55	397	744	298	697	1223	

DR-Bf ($N = 167$)▼

	DR1	DR2	DR3	DR4	DR7	DRW8	DRW9	DRW10	DRW11	DRW12	DRW13	DRW14	DRX	SUM
BF S	360 -56 -0.14 1.0	991 -181 -0.16 4.1*	261 -17 -0.06 0.1	1214 160 1.00 3.5	1058 139 1.00 2.0	180 -27 -0.14 0.5	1309 68 0.36 0.6	0 -51 -1.00 6.6#	720 43 0.42 0.4	900 67 0.53 0.7	0 -103 -1.00 13.4$	600 5 0.06 0.0	1089 -42 -0.04 0.2	8682
BF F	120 57 0.14 1.0	360 182 0.16 4.1*	60 18 0.06 0.1	0 -159 -1.00 3.5	0 -139 -1.00 3.0	60 28 0.14 0.5	120 -68 -0.36 0.6	60 52 1.00 ...	60 -42 -0.42 0.4	60 -66 -0.53 0.7	120 104 1.00 ...	85 -4 -0.06 0.0	215 43 0.04 0.2	1320
BFF1	0 0 0.00 ...	0 0 0.00 ...	0 0 0.00 ...	0 0 0.00 ...	0 0 0.00 ...	0 0 0.00 ...	0 0 0.00 ...	0 0 0.00 ...	0 0 0.00 ...	0 0 0.00 ...	0 0 0.00 ...	0 0 0.00 ...	0 0 0.00 ...	0
BFS07	0 0 0.00 ...	0 0 0.00 ...	0 0 0.00 ...	0 0 0.00 ...	0 0 0.00 ...	0 0 0.00 ...	0 0 0.00 ...	0 0 0.00 ...	0 0 0.00 ...	0 0 0.00 ...	0 0 0.00 ...	0 0 0.00 ...	0 0 0.00 ...	0
BF V	0 0 0.00 ...	0 0 0.00 ...	0 0 0.00 ...	0 0 0.00 ...	0 0 0.00 ...	0 0 0.00 ...	0 0 0.00 ...	0 0 0.00 ...	0 0 0.00 ...	0 0 0.00 ...	0 0 0.00 ...	0 0 0.00 ...	0 0 0.00 ...	0
SUM	480	1351	321	1214	1058	240	1429	60	780	960	120	685	1304	

Haplotype frequencies for population ORI

DQ-Bf ($N = 172$) ▶

	BF S	BF F	BFF1	BFS07	BF V	SUM
DQW1	2150 -183 -0.20 2.7	525 184 0.20 2.7	0 0 0.00 ...	0 0 0.00 ...	0 0 0.00 ...	2675
DQW2	1337 89 0.49 0.0	94 -88 -0.49 0.0	0 0 0.00 ...	0 0 0.00 ...	0 0 0.00 ...	1431
DQW3	2473 111 0.32 0.0	235 -110 -0.32 0.0	0 0 0.00 ...	0 0 0.00 ...	0 0 0.00 ...	2708
DQX	2764 -14 -0.02 0.0	422 15 0.02 0.0	0 0 0.00 ...	0 0 0.00 ...	0 0 0.00 ...	3186
SUM	8724	1276	0	0	0	

DQ-C4B ($N = 153$) ▼

	C4 B1	C4B11	C4B12	C4 B2	C4 B3	C4 B4	C4 B5	C4B51	C4 B6	C4 B7	C4BQ0	SUM
DQW1	1796 -103 -0.05 0.4	0 0 0.00 ...	0 -6 -1.00 ...	732 116 0.08 0.6	0 -16 -1.00 ...	0 0 0.00 ...	0 0 0.00 ...	0 0 0.00 ...	0 0 0.00 ...	0 0 0.00 ...	335 13 0.02 0.0	2863
DQW2	1168 186 0.38 1.9	0 0 0.00 ...	0 -3 -1.00 ...	130 -187 -0.59 2.5	0 -9 -1.00 ...	0 0 0.00 ...	0 0 0.00 ...	0 0 0.00 ...	0 0 0.00 ...	0 0 0.00 ...	179 13 0.01 0.0	1477
DQW3	1901 198 0.23 1.4	0 0 0.00 ...	0 -5 -1.00 ...	641 89 0.06 0.4	0 -16 -1.00 ...	0 0 0.00 ...	0 0 0.00 ...	0 0 0.00 ...	0 0 0.00 ...	0 0 0.00 ...	24 -263 -0.92 5.6*	2566
DQX	1772 -281 -0.14 2.6	0 0 0.00 ...	24 17 1.00 ...	648 -17 -0.03 0.0	65 45 1.00 ...	0 0 0.00 ...	0 0 0.00 ...	0 0 0.00 ...	0 0 0.00 ...	0 0 0.00 ...	586 238 0.31 4.1*	3095
SUM	6637	0	24	2151	65	0	0	0	0	0	1124	

DQ-C4A ($N = 153$) ▼

	C4 A1	C4A12	C4A13	C4 A2	C4 A3	C4 A4	C4A51	C4 A6	C4AQ0	SUM
DQW1	0 0 0.00 ...	462 116 0.13 0.0	0 0 0.00 ...	0 -54 -1.00 1.2	1633 -249 -0.13 2.2	273 54 0.10 0.3	0 0 0.00 ...	65 28 0.30 0.5	389 105 0.15 0.9	2822
DQW2	0 0 0.00 ...	0 -170 -1.00 3.5	0 0 0.00 ...	155 128 0.77 ...	1131 198 0.43 2.3	82 -25 -0.24 0.1	0 0 0.00 ...	0 -17 -1.00 ...	30 -109 -0.79 1.7	1398
DQW3	0 0 0.00 ...	394 64 0.07 0.3	0 0 0.00 ...	0 -51 -1.00 1.1	1515 -279 -0.16 2.8	256 48 0.08 0.2	0 0 0.00 ...	65 30 0.32 0.6	460 190 0.26 3.1	2690
DQX	0 0 0.00 ...	370 -8 -0.02 0.0	0 0 0.00 ...	39 -20 -0.35 0.2	2394 330 0.32 3.6	164 -75 -0.32 0.6	0 0 0.00 ...	0 -39 -1.00 0.9	126 -184 -0.59 2.7	3093
SUM	0	1226	0	194	6673	775	0	130	1005	

Haplotype frequencies for population ORI

Bf-C4B ($N = 146$)▼

	C4 B1	C4B11	C4B12	C4 B2	C4 B3	C4 B4	C4 B5	C4B51	C4 B6	C4 B7	C4BQ0	SUM
BF S	5769 -88 -0.23 0.5	0 0 0.00 ...	68 8 1.00 0.1	1986 110 0.45 1.0	0 -60 -1.00 7.7#	0 0 0.00 ...	0 0 0.00 ...	0 0 0.00 ...	0 0 0.00 ...	0 0 0.00 ...	1012 31 0.24 0.1	8835
BF F	861 89 0.23 0.5	0 0 0.00 ...	0 -7 -1.00 ...	137 -109 -0.45 1.0	69 61 1.00 ...	0 0 0.00 ...	0 0 0.00 ...	0 0 0.00 ...	0 0 0.00 ...	0 0 0.00 ...	98 -30 -0.24 0.1	1165
BFF1	0 0 0.00 ...	0 0 0.00 ...	0 0 0.00 ...	0 0 0.00 ...	0 0 0.00 ...	0 0 0.00 ...	0 0 0.00 ...	0 0 0.00 ...	0 0 0.00 ...	0 0 0.00 ...	0 0 0.00 ...	0
BFS07	0 0 0.00 ...	0 0 0.00 ...	0 0 0.00 ...	0 0 0.00 ...	0 0 0.00 ...	0 0 0.00 ...	0 0 0.00 ...	0 0 0.00 ...	0 0 0.00 ...	0 0 0.00 ...	0 0 0.00 ...	0
BF V	0 0 0.00 ...	0 0 0.00 ...	0 0 0.00 ...	0 0 0.00 ...	0 0 0.00 ...	0 0 0.00 ...	0 0 0.00 ...	0 0 0.00 ...	0 0 0.00 ...	0 0 0.00 ...	0 0 0.00 ...	0
SUM	6630	0	68	2123	69	0	0	0	0	0	1110	

Bf-C4A ($N = 147$) ▼

	C4 A1	C4A12	C4A13	C4 A2	C4 A3	C4 A4	C4A51	C4 A6	C4AQ0	SUM
BF S	0 0 0.00 ...	1151 13 0.09 0.0	0 0 0.00 ...	68 -51 -0.43 2.0	6173 116 0.15 0.9	610 70 1.00 1.3	0 0 0.00 ...	135 16 1.00 0.3	712 -161 -0.19 4.3*	8849
BF F	0 0 0.00 ...	135 -12 -0.09 0.0	0 0 0.00 ...	68 52 0.43 ...	672 -115 -0.15 0.9	0 -69 -1.00 1.3	0 0 0.00 ...	0 -15 -1.00 ...	276 162 0.19 4.3*	1151
BFF1	0 0 0.00 ...	0 0 0.00 ...	0 0 0.00 ...	0 0 0.00 ...	0 0 0.00 ...	0 0 0.00 ...	0 0 0.00 ...	0 0 0.00 ...	0 0 0.00 ...	0
BFS07	0 0 0.00 ...	0 0 0.00 ...	0 0 0.00 ...	0 0 0.00 ...	0 0 0.00 ...	0 0 0.00 ...	0 0 0.00 ...	0 0 0.00 ...	0 0 0.00 ...	0
BF V	0 0 0.00 ...	0 0 0.00 ...	0 0 0.00 ...	0 0 0.00 ...	0 0 0.00 ...	0 0 0.00 ...	0 0 0.00 ...	0 0 0.00 ...	0 0 0.00 ...	0
SUM	0	1286	0	136	6845	610	0	135	988	

Haplotype frequencies for population ORI
C4A-C4B ($N = 154$)▼

	C4 A1	C4A12	C4A13	C4 A2	C4 A3	C4 A4	C4A51	C4 A6	C4AQ0	SUM
C4 B1	0	1050	0	130	4462	65	0	130	721	6558
	0	239	0	2	63	-446	0	45	98	
	0.00	0.56	0.00	0.03	0.03	-0.87	0.00	1.00	0.30	
	...	3.6	...	0.0	0.1	18.9‡	...	1.1	0.8	
C4B11	0	0	0	0	0	0	0	0	0	0
	0	0	0	0	0	0	0	0	0	
	0.00	0.00	0.00	0.00	0.00	0.00	0.00	0.00	0.00	
	...	...	...	...	...	...	...	...	...	
C4B12	0	0	0	0	65	0	0	0	0	65
	0	-7	0	0	21	-4	0	0	-5	
	0.00	-1.00	0.00	-1.00	1.00	-1.00	0.00	-1.00	-1.00	
	...	...	...	...	0.5	...	...	...	...	
C4 B2	0	65	0	0	1332	651	0	0	165	2213
	0	-208	0	-42	-151	478	0	-26	-44	
	0.00	-0.76	0.00	-1.00	-0.10	0.79	0.00	-1.00	-0.22	
	...	3.6	...	0.9	0.9	28.4‡	...	...	0.2	
C4 B3	0	0	0	0	65	0	0	0	0	65
	0	-7	0	0	21	-4	0	0	-5	
	0.00	-1.00	0.00	-1.00	1.00	-1.00	0.00	-1.00	-1.00	
	...	...	...	...	0.5	...	...	...	...	
C4 B4	0	0	0	0	0	0	0	0	0	0
	0	0	0	0	0	0	0	0	0	
	0.00	0.00	0.00	0.00	0.00	0.00	0.00	0.00	0.00	
	...	...	...	...	...	...	...	...	...	
C4 B5	0	0	0	0	0	0	0	0	0	0
	0	0	0	0	0	0	0	0	0	
	0.00	0.00	0.00	0.00	0.00	0.00	0.00	0.00	0.00	
	...	...	...	...	...	...	...	...	...	
C4B51	0	0	0	0	0	0	0	0	0	0
	0	0	0	0	0	0	0	0	0	
	0.00	0.00	0.00	0.00	0.00	0.00	0.00	0.00	0.00	
	...	...	...	...	...	...	...	...	...	
C4 B6	0	0	0	0	0	0	0	0	0	0
	0	0	0	0	0	0	0	0	0	
	0.00	0.00	0.00	0.00	0.00	0.00	0.00	0.00	0.00	
	...	...	...	...	...	...	...	...	...	
C4 B7	0	0	0	0	0	0	0	0	0	0
	0	0	0	0	0	0	0	0	0	
	0.00	0.00	0.00	0.00	0.00	0.00	0.00	0.00	0.00	
	...	...	...	...	...	...	...	...	...	
C4BQ0	0	122	0	65	784	65	0	0	64	1100
	0	-13	0	44	46	-20	0	-13	-39	
	0.00	-0.10	0.00	0.25	0.13	-0.24	0.00	-1.00	-0.39	
	...	0.0	...	...	0.2	0.1	...	...	0.3	
SUM	0	1237	0	195	6708	781	0	130	950	

Haplotype frequencies for population NEG
A-B ($N = 330$)

	A1	A2	A3	A11	A23	A24	A25	A26	A28	A29	A30	A31	A32	AW33	AW34	AW36	AW43	AW66	AX	SUM
B7	118 21 0.03 0.2	317 95 0.09 1.9	170 77 0.12 2.6	0 -25 -1.00 1.0	68 -40 -0.38 0.6	59 -4 -0.08 0.0	0 0 0.00 ...	59 7 0.02 0.0	115 -7 -0.07 0.0	89 28 0.07 0.5	118 -25 -0.18 0.2	0 -22 -1.00 0.9	59 33 0.18 1.6	30 -25 -0.47 0.5	0 -59 -1.00 2.4	30 -6 -0.20 0.1	0 -10 -1.00 ...	0 -3 -1.00 ...	34 -25 -0.43 0.4	1266
B8	325 284 0.58 74.1$	30 -63 -0.68 1.8	0 -38 -1.00 1.5	0 -10 -1.00 ...	85 39 0.08 1.3	0 -26 -1.00 0.0	0 0 0.00 ...	4 -17 -0.82 0.5	30 -21 -0.42 0.4	0 -25 -1.00 0.9	30 -30 -0.51 0.6	0 -9 -1.00 ...	0 -10 -1.00 ...	30 6 0.01 0.1	0 -24 -1.00 0.9	0 -15 -1.00 0.6	0 -4 -1.00 ...	0 -1 -1.00 ...	0 -24 -1.00 0.9	534
B13	0 -10 -1.00 ...	30 4 0.03 0.0	0 -10 -1.00 ...	0 -2 -1.00 ...	0 -12 -1.00 ...	0 -7 -1.00 ...	0 0 0.00 ...	0 -5 -1.00 ...	0 -13 -1.00 ...	30 23 0.16 ...	59 42 0.32 3.9*	0 -2 -1.00 ...	0 -2 -1.00 ...	0 -6 -1.00 ...	0 -6 -1.00 ...	0 -3 -1.00 ...	0 0 -1.00 ...	0 0 -1.00 ...	30 23 0.16 ...	149
B18	29 -2 -0.09 0.0	29 -42 -0.60 1.1	59 29 0.07 1.0	0 -8 -1.00 ...	59 23 0.06 0.6	59 38 0.10 2.5	0 0 0.00 ...	0 -16 -1.00 0.6	59 19 0.05 0.3	0 -19 -1.00 0.7	59 12 0.03 0.1	0 -6 -1.00 ...	0 -8 -1.00 ...	0 -17 -1.00 0.7	0 -18 -1.00 0.7	30 18 0.06 ...	0 -3 -1.00 ...	0 0 -1.00 ...	30 10 0.03 0.2	413
B27	0 -13 -1.00 ...	16 -14 -0.48 0.3	0 -12 -1.00 ...	30 26 0.15 ...	0 -14 -1.00 0.6	22 13 0.08 ...	0 0 0.00 ...	0 -6 -1.00 ...	0 -16 -1.00 0.6	0 -8 -1.00 ...	7 -12 -0.65 0.3	0 -2 -1.00 ...	89 85 0.49 ...	0 -7 -1.00 ...	0 -7 -1.00 ...	0 -4 -1.00 ...	0 -1 -1.00 ...	0 0 -1.00 ...	13 5 0.03 ...	177
B35	1 -59 -0.98 2.3	88 -51 -0.37 0.8	59 0 0.00 0.0	118 101 0.53 22.7$	57 -11 -0.17 0.1	118 78 0.17 5.7*	0 0 0.00 ...	30 -2 -0.09 0.0	61 -16 -0.21 0.1	30 -7 -0.22 0.1	37 -53 -0.59 1.3	51 37 0.22 ...	0 -16 -1.00 0.6	59 23 0.06 0.6	30 -7 -0.20 0.1	0 -23 -1.00 0.9	0 -6 -1.00 ...	0 -1 -1.00 ...	59 21 0.05 0.5	798
B37	59 45 0.28 ...	0 -30 -1.00 1.3	0 -12 -1.00 ...	0 -3 -1.00 ...	30 15 0.09 0.5	0 -8 -1.00 ...	0 0 0.00 ...	0 -6 -1.00 ...	0 -16 -1.00 0.6	0 -8 -1.00 ...	30 10 0.06 0.2	0 -2 -1.00 ...	0 -3 -1.00 ...	59 51 0.30 ...	0 -7 -1.00 ...	0 -4 -1.00 ...	0 -1 -1.00 ...	0 0 -1.00 ...	0 -7 -1.00 ...	178
B38	30 19 0.14 ...	0 -25 -1.00 1.1	30 19 0.14 ...	0 -2 -1.00 ...	0 -12 -1.00 ...	0 -6 -1.00 ...	0 0 0.00 ...	59 53 0.37 ...	0 -13 -1.00 ...	0 -6 -1.00 ...	0 -16 -1.00 0.6	0 -2 -1.00 ...	0 -2 -1.00 ...	0 -6 -1.00 ...	29 22 0.16 ...	0 -3 -1.00 ...	0 0 -1.00 ...	0 0 -1.00 ...	0 -6 -1.00 ...	148
B39	0 -1 -1.00 ...	0 -4 -1.00 ...	0 -1 -1.00 ...	0 0 -1.00 ...	0 -2 -1.00 ...	0 -1 -1.00 ...	0 0 0.00 ...	0 0 -1.00 ...	0 -2 -1.00 ...	30 29 1.00 ...	0 -2 -1.00 ...	0 0 -1.00 ...	0 0 -1.00 ...	0 0 -1.00 ...	0 0 -1.00 ...	0 0 -1.00 ...	0 0 -1.00 ...	0 0 -1.00 ...	0 0 -1.00 ...	30
BW41	0 -13 -1.00 ...	0 -30 -1.00 1.3	0 -12 -1.00 ...	0 -3 -1.00 ...	0 -14 -1.00 0.6	30 21 0.12 ...	0 0 0.00 ...	59 52 0.30 ...	89 72 0.45 11.0$	0 -8 -1.00 ...	0 -19 -1.00 0.8	0 -2 -1.00 ...	0 -3 -1.00 ...	0 -7 -1.00 ...	0 -7 -1.00 ...	0 -4 -1.00 ...	0 -1 -1.00 ...	0 0 -1.00 ...	0 -7 -1.00 ...	178
BW42	0 -42 -1.00 1.6	59 -39 -0.40 0.7	0 -40 -1.00 1.6	0 -11 -1.00 ...	0 -47 -1.00 1.8	0 -27 -1.00 1.0	0 0 0.00 ...	0 -22 -1.00 0.8	30 -24 -0.45 0.4	59 32 0.07 1.4	346 282 0.57 49.1$	8 -1 -0.20 ...	30 18 0.09 ...	30 5 0.01 0.0	0 -26 -1.00 0.0	0 -16 -1.00 0.6	0 -4 -1.00 ...	0 -1 -1.00 ...	0 -26 -1.00 0.0	562
B44	30 -24 -0.45 0.4	151 26 0.04 0.2	30 -21 -0.43 0.4	0 -14 -1.00 ...	30 -30 -0.51 0.6	40 4 0.01 0.0	0 0 0.00 ...	0 -28 -1.00 1.1	32 -36 -0.54 0.8	92 58 0.13 3.6	45 -35 -0.44 0.6	0 -12 -1.00 ...	30 15 0.08 ...	30 -1 -0.06 0.0	89 55 0.13 3.4	0 -20 -1.00 0.8	59 53 0.64 ...	30 28 1.00 ...	24 -9 -0.29 0.1	712
B45	0 -20 -1.00 0.8	148 101 0.46 8.0#	53 33 0.13 2.1	0 -5 -1.00 ...	0 -22 -1.00 0.9	30 17 0.07 ...	0 0 0.00 ...	30 19 0.07 ...	0 -25 -1.00 0.0	0 -12 -1.00 ...	0 -29 -1.00 1.2	0 -4 -1.00 ...	0 -5 -1.00 ...	0 -11 -1.00 ...	6 -6 -0.52 ...	0 -7 -1.00 ...	0 -1 -1.00 ...	0 0 -1.00 ...	0 -12 -1.00 ...	267
BW46	0 0 0.00 ...	0 0 0.00 ...	0 0 0.00 ...	0 0 0.00 ...	0 0 0.00 ...	0 0 0.00 ...	0 0 0.00 ...	0 0 0.00 ...	0 0 0.00 ...	0 0 0.00 ...	0 0 0.00 ...	0 0 0.00 ...	0 0 0.00 ...	0 0 0.00 ...	0 0 0.00 ...	0 0 0.00 ...	0 0 0.00 ...	0 0 0.00 ...	0 0 0.00 ...	0
BW47	0 0 0.00 ...	0 0 0.00 ...	0 0 0.00 ...	0 0 0.00 ...	0 0 0.00 ...	0 0 0.00 ...	0 0 0.00 ...	0 0 0.00 ...	0 0 0.00 ...	0 0 0.00 ...	0 0 0.00 ...	0 0 0.00 ...	0 0 0.00 ...	0 0 0.00 ...	0 0 0.00 ...	0 0 0.00 ...	0 0 0.00 ...	0 0 0.00 ...	0 0 0.00 ...	0

Haplotype frequencies for population NEG
A-B (N = 330)

	A1	A2	A3	A11	A23	A24	A25	A26	A28	A29	A30	A31	A32	AW33	AW34	AW36	AW43	AW66	AX	SUM
BW48	0 -1 -1.00 ...	0 -4 -1.00 ...	0 -1 -1.00 ...	0 0 -1.00 ...	30 27 1.00 ...	0 -1 -1.00 ...	0 0 0.00 ...	0 0 -1.00 ...	0 -2 -1.00 ...	0 0 -1.00 ...	0 -2 -1.00 ...	0 0 -1.00 ...	0 0 -1.00 ...	0 0 -1.00 ...	0 0 -1.00 ...	0 0 -1.00 ...	0 0 -1.00 ...	0 0 -1.00 ...	0 0 -1.00 ...	30
B49	29 13 0.07 0.4	30 -5 -0.18 0.0	30 15 0.08 0.5	0 -3 -1.00 ...	0 -17 -1.00 0.7	0 -9 -1.00 ...	0 0 0.00 ...	0 -8 -1.00 ...	30 10 0.05 0.2	56 46 0.23 ...	0 -23 -1.00 0.9	0 -3 -1.00 ...	0 -3 -1.00 ...	0 -8 -1.00 ...	0 -9 -1.00 ...	0 -5 -1.00 ...	30 28 0.32 ...	0 0 -1.00 ...	3 -6 -0.70 ...	208
BW50	0 -4 -1.00 ...	29 19 0.38 ...	0 -3 -1.00 ...	0 0 -1.00 ...	0 -4 -1.00 ...	0 -2 -1.00 ...	0 0 0.00 ...	0 -1 -1.00 ...	0 -5 -1.00 ...	0 -2 -1.00 ...	0 -6 -1.00 ...	0 0 -1.00 ...	0 0 -1.00 ...	30 27 0.49 ...	0 -2 -1.00 ...	0 -1 -1.00 ...	0 0 -1.00 ...	0 0 -1.00 ...	0 -2 -1.00 ...	59
B51	1 -14 -0.94 0.5	58 22 0.13 0.5	59 44 0.23 4.6*	0 -3 -1.00 ...	30 12 0.06 0.3	0 -9 -1.00 ...	0 0 0.00 ...	0 -8 -1.00 ...	0 -19 -1.00 0.8	0 -9 -1.00 ...	0 -23 -1.00 0.9	59 55 0.32 ...	0 -3 -1.00 ...	0 -8 -1.00 ...	0 -9 -1.00 ...	0 -5 -1.00 ...	0 -1 -1.00 ...	0 0 -1.00 ...	0 -9 -1.00 ...	207
BW52	0 -4 -1.00 ...	0 -10 -1.00 ...	0 -3 -1.00 ...	0 0 -1.00 ...	30 25 0.45 ...	0 -2 -1.00 ...	0 0 0.00 ...	0 -1 -1.00 ...	0 -5 -1.00 ...	0 -2 -1.00 ...	0 -6 -1.00 ...	30 29 0.49 ...	0 0 -1.00 ...	0 -2 -1.00 ...	0 -2 -1.00 ...	0 -1 -1.00 ...	0 0 -1.00 ...	0 0 -1.00 ...	0 -2 -1.00 ...	60
BW53	15 -33 -0.70 0.9	44 -68 -0.61 1.8	0 -46 -1.00 1.8	0 -12 -1.00 ...	63 8 0.01 0.0	7 -24 -0.78 0.7	0 0 0.00 ...	50 23 0.06 0.8	0 -61 -1.00 2.4	11 -19 -0.64 0.5	104 31 0.05 0.5	0 -10 -1.00 ...	0 -12 -1.00 ...	89 60 0.14 4.7*	34 4 0.01 0.0	207 188 0.68 67.6‡	0 -5 -1.00 ...	0 -1 -1.00 ...	18 -11 -0.41 0.2	642
BW54	0 0 0.00 ...	0 0 0.00 ...	0 0 0.00 ...	0 0 0.00 ...	0 0 0.00 ...	0 0 0.00 ...	0 0 0.00 ...	0 0 0.00 ...	0 0 0.00 ...	0 0 0.00 ...	0 0 0.00 ...	0 0 0.00 ...	0 0 0.00 ...	0 0 0.00 ...	0 0 0.00 ...	0 0 0.00 ...	0 0 0.00 ...	0 0 0.00 ...	0 0 0.00 ...	0
BW55	0 -4 -1.00 ...	30 19 0.39 ...	0 -3 -1.00 ...	30 29 0.49 ...	0 -4 -1.00 ...	0 -2 -1.00 ...	0 0 0.00 ...	0 -1 -1.00 ...	0 -5 -1.00 ...	0 -2 -1.00 ...	0 -6 -1.00 ...	0 0 -1.00 ...	0 0 -1.00 ...	0 -2 -1.00 ...	0 -2 -1.00 ...	0 -1 -1.00 ...	0 0 -1.00 ...	0 0 -1.00 ...	0 -2 -1.00 ...	60
BW56	0 -1 -1.00 ...	0 -4 -1.00 ...	0 -1 -1.00 ...	0 0 -1.00 ...	0 -2 -1.00 ...	0 -1 -1.00 ...	0 0 0.00 ...	0 0 -1.00 ...	30 27 1.00 ...	0 0 -1.00 ...	0 -2 -1.00 ...	0 0 -1.00 ...	0 0 -1.00 ...	0 0 -1.00 ...	0 0 -1.00 ...	0 0 -1.00 ...	0 0 -1.00 ...	0 0 -1.00 ...	0 0 -1.00 ...	30
BW57	30 7 0.03 0.1	118 66 0.27 3.4	27 5 0.02 0.0	0 -5 -1.00 ...	30 4 0.02 0.0	19 4 0.01 ...	0 0 0.00 ...	0 -11 -1.00 ...	30 1 0.00 0.0	0 -13 -1.00 ...	43 9 0.03 0.1	0 -4 -1.00 ...	0 -5 -1.00 ...	0 -12 -1.00 ...	0 -13 -1.00 ...	0 -8 -1.00 ...	0 -2 -1.00 ...	0 0 -1.00 ...	0 -13 -1.00 ...	297
BW58	45 -34 -0.44 0.6	122 -59 -0.33 0.9	121 45 0.07 1.0	0 -21 -1.00 0.8	0 -88 -1.00 3.6	30 -21 -0.43 0.4	0 0 0.00 ...	93 50 0.14 2.2	161 60 0.07 1.5	0 -49 -1.00 1.9	145 27 0.03 0.3	0 -17 -1.00 0.7	0 -21 -1.00 0.8	59 13 0.03 0.1	113 64 0.15 3.2	0 -30 -1.00 1.2	0 -8 -1.00 ...	0 -2 -1.00 ...	147 98 0.23 7.6#	1036
BW59	0 0 0.00 ...	0 0 0.00 ...	0 0 0.00 ...	0 0 0.00 ...	0 0 0.00 ...	0 0 0.00 ...	0 0 0.00 ...	0 0 0.00 ...	0 0 0.00 ...	0 0 0.00 ...	0 0 0.00 ...	0 0 0.00 ...	0 0 0.00 ...	0 0 0.00 ...	0 0 0.00 ...	0 0 0.00 ...	0 0 0.00 ...	0 0 0.00 ...	0 0 0.00 ...	0
BW60	0 -15 -1.00 0.6	89 52 0.30 3.1	30 15 0.08 0.5	0 -3 -1.00 ...	0 -17 -1.00 0.7	30 19 0.10 ...	0 0 0.00 ...	30 21 0.11 ...	0 -19 -1.00 0.8	0 -9 -1.00 ...	0 -23 -1.00 0.9	30 26 0.15 ...	0 -3 -1.00 ...	0 -8 -1.00 ...	0 -9 -1.00 ...	0 -5 -1.00 ...	0 -1 -1.00 ...	0 0 -1.00 ...	0 -9 -1.00 ...	209
BW61	28 20 0.20 ...	31 12 0.14 0.3	18 10 0.10 ...	0 -1 -1.00 ...	0 -8 -1.00 ...	30 25 0.24 ...	0 0 0.00 ...	0 -3 -1.00 ...	0 -9 -1.00 ...	0 -4 -1.00 ...	0 -11 -1.00 ...	0 -1 -1.00 ...	0 -1 -1.00 ...	0 -4 -1.00 ...	0 -4 -1.00 ...	0 -2 -1.00 ...	0 0 -1.00 ...	0 0 -1.00 ...	0 -4 -1.00 ...	107
BW62	0 -20 -1.00 0.8	89 42 0.19 1.5	30 10 0.04 0.2	30 24 0.12 ...	0 -22 -1.00 0.9	30 16 0.06 ...	0 0 0.00 ...	0 -10 -1.00 ...	30 4 0.02 0.0	0 -12 -1.00 ...	0 -29 -1.00 1.2	0 -4 -1.00 ...	0 -5 -1.00 ...	0 -11 -1.00 ...	59 46 0.18 ...	0 -7 -1.00 ...	0 -1 -1.00 ...	0 0 -1.00 ...	0 -12 -1.00 ...	268

Haplotype frequencies for population NEG

A-B ($N=330$)▼

	A1	A2	A3	A11	A23	A24	A25	A26	A28	A29	A30	A31	A32	AW33	AW34	AW36	AW43	AW66	AX	SUM
BW63	0 -13 -1.00 ...	58 27 0.18 0.9	0 -12 -1.00 ...	0 -3 -1.00 ...	59 44 0.27 4.6*	0 -8 -1.00 ...	0 0 0.00 ...	0 -6 -1.00 ...	30 13 0.08 0.3	0 -8 -1.00 ...	30 10 0.06 0.2	0 -2 -1.00 ...	0 -3 -1.00 ...	0 -7 -1.00 ...	0 -7 -1.00 ...	0 -4 -1.00 ...	0 -1 -1.00 ...	0 0 -1.00 ...	1 -6 -0.88 ...	178
BW64	0 -10 -1.00 ...	0 -25 -1.00 1.1	0 -10 -1.00 ...	0 -2 -1.00 ...	0 -12 -1.00 ...	0 -7 -1.00 ...	0 0 0.00 ...	0 -5 -1.00 ...	89 75 0.55 ...	0 -6 -1.00 ...	15 -1 -0.12 0.0	0 -2 -1.00 ...	0 -2 -1.00 ...	30 23 0.16 ...	0 -6 -1.00 ...	0 -3 -1.00 ...	0 0 -1.00 ...	0 0 -1.00 ...	15 8 0.06 ...	149
BW65	29 15 0.09 ...	30 0 -0.04 0.0	0 -12 -1.00 ...	0 -3 -1.00 ...	59 44 0.27 4.6*	0 -8 -1.00 ...	0 0 0.00 ...	0 -6 -1.00 ...	30 13 0.08 0.3	30 21 0.13 ...	0 -19 -1.00 0.8	0 -2 -1.00 ...	0 -3 -1.00 ...	0 -7 -1.00 ...	0 -7 -1.00 ...	0 -4 -1.00 ...	0 -1 -1.00 ...	0 0 -1.00 ...	0 -7 -1.00 ...	178
BW67	0 0 0.00 ...	0 0 0.00 ...	0 0 0.00 ...	0 0 0.00 ...	0 0 0.00 ...	0 0 0.00 ...	0 0 0.00 ...	0 0 0.00 ...	0 0 0.00 ...	0 0 0.00 ...	0 0 0.00 ...	0 0 0.00 ...	0 0 0.00 ...	0 0 0.00 ...	0 0 0.00 ...	0 0 0.00 ...	0 0 0.00 ...	0 0 0.00 ...	0 0 0.00 ...	0
BW71	0 -5 -1.00 ...	0 -12 -1.00 ...	0 -5 -1.00 ...	0 -1 -1.00 ...	30 24 0.34 ...	0 -3 -1.00 ...	0 0 0.00 ...	0 -2 -1.00 ...	15 8 0.11 ...	0 -3 -1.00 ...	30 21 0.32 ...	0 0 -1.00 ...	0 -1 -1.00 ...	0 -2 -1.00 ...	0 -3 -1.00 ...	0 -1 -1.00 ...	0 0 -1.00 ...	0 0 -1.00 ...	0 -3 -1.00 ...	75
BW72	0 -51 -1.00 1.0	144 25 0.05 0.2	6 -43 -0.88 1.5	0 -13 -1.00 ...	170 112 0.18 8.3#	0 -33 -1.00 1.3	0 0 0.00 ...	0 -27 -1.00 1.0	89 23 0.04 0.3	55 22 0.05 0.6	33 -43 -0.57 1.0	0 -11 -1.00 ...	0 -13 -1.00 ...	0 -29 -1.00 1.1	82 50 0.11 2.9	29 9 0.03 0.1	0 -5 -1.00 ...	0 -1 -1.00 ...	69 37 0.08 1.6	677
BW73	0 0 0.00 ...	0 0 0.00 ...	0 0 0.00 ...	0 0 0.00 ...	0 0 0.00 ...	0 0 0.00 ...	0 0 0.00 ...	0 0 0.00 ...	0 0 0.00 ...	0 0 0.00 ...	0 0 0.00 ...	0 0 0.00 ...	0 0 0.00 ...	0 0 0.00 ...	0 0 0.00 ...	0 0 0.00 ...	0 0 0.00 ...	0 0 0.00 ...	0 0 0.00 ...	0
BX	0 -10 -1.00 ...	13 -12 -0.50 0.3	14 3 0.02 ...	0 -2 -1.00 ...	30 17 0.13 ...	0 -6 -1.00 ...	0 0 0.00 ...	0 -5 -1.00 ...	23 9 0.07 ...	0 -6 -1.00 ...	7 -9 -0.58 0.2	0 -2 -1.00 ...	0 -2 -1.00 ...	0 -6 -1.00 ...	30 23 0.16 ...	0 -3 -1.00 ...	0 0 -1.00 ...	0 0 -1.00 ...	30 23 0.16 ...	147
SUM	769	1753	736	208	860	504	0	414	973	482	1138	178	208	446	472	296	89	30	473	

A-DQ ($N=284$)▼

	A1	A2	A3	A11	A23	A24	A25	A26	A28	A29	A30	A31	A32	AW33	AW34	AW36	AW43	AW66	AX	SUM
DQW1	139 -197 -0.59 5.0*	795 139 0.14 1.7	451 131 0.27 2.8	92 8 0.06 0.0	297 16 0.04 0.0	154 -27 -0.15 0.2	0 0 0.00 ...	135 -32 -0.20 0.3	426 -18 -0.04 0.0	280 51 0.15 0.6	361 -108 -0.23 1.4	35 -20 -0.37 0.4	137 67 0.63 3.1	114 -67 -0.37 1.3	177 -3 -0.02 0.0	101 17 0.13 0.2	70 14 0.17 0.2	0 0 0.00 ...	216 39 0.15 0.4	3980
DQW2	377 190 0.29 7.6#	148 -216 -0.59 5.6*	155 -22 -0.13 0.1	0 -46 -1.00 1.7	194 38 0.07 0.4	50 -50 -0.51 0.0	0 0 0.00 ...	34 -59 -0.64 1.5	331 83 0.10 1.1	141 14 0.03 0.1	390 128 0.14 2.6	13 -17 -0.58 0.4	32 -6 -0.18 0.0	148 47 0.13 0.8	121 20 0.06 0.2	35 -11 -0.25 0.1	0 -30 -1.00 1.1	0 0 0.00 ...	47 -51 -0.52 1.0	2216
DQW3	290 80 0.13 1.2	543 133 0.11 1.0	74 -125 -0.63 3.3	69 17 0.10 0.2	176 1 0.00 0.0	164 50 0.15 0.9	0 0 0.00 ...	194 89 0.28 2.0	233 -44 -0.16 0.3	89 -53 -0.38 0.8	173 -120 -0.41 2.1	35 0 0.00 0.0	0 -43 -1.00 1.7	123 9 0.03 0.0	90 -22 -0.21 0.2	35 -16 -0.33 0.2	70 35 0.33 1.4	0 0 0.00 ...	129 18 0.05 0.1	2487
DQX	40 -70 -0.64 1.6	161 -54 -0.25 0.5	124 19 0.03 0.1	50 22 0.12 0.6	38 -53 -0.59 1.1	89 29 0.07 0.5	0 0 0.00 ...	60 5 0.01 0.0	129 -17 -0.12 0.1	65 -9 -0.14 0.0	257 102 0.10 2.5	57 39 0.32 2.7	7 -15 -0.70 0.4	73 13 0.03 0.1	68 8 0.02 0.0	40 12 0.07 0.2	0 -17 -1.00 0.6	0 0 0.00 ...	53 -4 -0.09 0.0	1311
SUM	846	1647	804	211	705	457	0	423	1119	575	1181	140	176	458	456	211	140	0	445	

Haplotype frequencies for population NEG
A-C ($N=345$)

	A1	A2	A3	A11	A23	A24	A25	A26	A28	A29	A30	A31	A32	AW33	AW34	AW36	AW43	AW66	AX	SUM
CW1	0 -6 -1.00 ...	0 -14 -1.00 0.6	29 23 0.28 ...	0 -1 -1.00 ...	0 -6 -1.00 ...	29 24 0.30 ...	0 0 0.00 ...	0 -3 -1.00 ...	0 -8 -1.00 ...	0 -3 -1.00 ...	0 -9 -1.00 ...	0 -1 -1.00 ...	29 27 0.32 ...	0 -3 -1.00 ...	0 -3 -1.00 ...	0 -2 -1.00 ...	0 0 -1.00 ...	0 0 -1.00 ...	0 -3 -1.00 ...	87
CW2	60 -34 -0.37 0.6	202 -6 -0.03 0.0	0 -83 -1.00 3.5	29 4 0.02 0.0	246 144 0.20 8.7#	15 -47 -0.76 1.5	0 0 0.00 ...	0 -48 -1.00 2.0	87 -31 -0.27 0.4	0 -60 -1.00 2.5	173 38 0.04 0.5	21 0 -0.00 0.0	58 33 0.19 1.8	47 -5 -0.11 0.0	87 27 0.06 0.5	29 -5 -0.17 0.0	0 -13 -1.00 ...	0 -3 -1.00 ...	157 97 0.22 6.5*	1211
CW3	0 -74 -1.00 3.1	175 10 0.01 0.0	87 21 0.03 0.3	16 -3 -0.18 0.0	41 -39 -0.49 0.8	87 37 0.08 1.1	0 0 0.00 ...	106 67 0.18 4.6*	202 108 0.12 5.2*	0 -47 -1.00 1.9	58 -48 -0.46 0.0	29 12 0.08 0.4	29 9 0.05 0.2	44 2 0.01 0.0	58 11 0.02 0.1	29 1 0.00 0.0	0 -10 -1.00 ...	0 -2 -1.00 ...	0 -46 -1.00 1.9	961
CW4	15 -93 -0.86 3.5	157 -82 -0.34 1.4	74 -21 -0.23 0.2	116 88 0.50 11.2$	58 -58 -0.50 1.3	163 90 0.20 4.8*	0 0 0.00 ...	24 -31 -0.58 0.8	2 -133 -0.99 5.9*	40 -29 -0.43 0.5	192 37 0.04 0.4	37 13 0.09 0.3	0 -27 -1.00 1.2	119 59 0.16 2.4	92 23 0.06 0.3	197 157 0.63 25.1$	0 -15 -1.00 0.7	29 25 1.00 ...	76 7 0.02 0.0	1391
CW5	0 -21 -1.00 0.8	63 15 0.07 0.2	0 -18 -1.00 0.7	0 -5 -1.00 ...	87 64 0.25 6.8#	0 -13 -1.00 ...	0 0 0.00 ...	0 -10 -1.00 ...	0 -26 -1.00 1.1	0 -13 -1.00 ...	44 13 0.05 0.2	0 -4 -1.00 ...	58 52 0.27 ...	0 -11 -1.00 ...	0 -13 -1.00 ...	0 -7 -1.00 ...	0 -2 -1.00 ...	0 0 -1.00 ...	24 10 0.04 ...	276
CW6	160 56 0.08 1.3	77 -151 -0.66 4.8*	150 58 0.10 1.6	0 -26 -1.00 1.1	90 -21 -0.19 0.2	59 -9 -0.15 0.1	0 0 0.00 ...	87 33 0.09 0.8	177 47 0.06 0.7	75 9 0.02 0.0	99 -48 -0.33 0.7	0 -22 -1.00 0.9	0 -26 -1.00 1.1	62 4 0.01 0.0	116 51 0.12 1.6	29 -8 -0.25 0.1	29 14 0.14 0.5	0 -3 -1.00 ...	117 51 0.12 1.7	1327
CW7	370 185 0.31 8.0#	547 140 0.11 2.6	109 -53 -0.33 0.9	0 -47 -1.00 2.2	123 -75 -0.38 1.4	129 6 0.01 0.0	0 0 0.00 ...	87 -8 -0.09 0.0	205 -26 -0.12 0.2	258 140 0.36 7.8#	158 -105 -0.40 2.2	0 -40 -1.00 1.9	0 -47 -1.00 2.2	124 21 0.06 0.2	131 15 0.04 0.1	0 -68 -1.00 3.2	29 2 0.02 0.0	0 -6 -1.00 ...	93 -23 -0.20 0.2	2363
CW8	29 0 -0.02 0.0	29 -35 -0.55 0.9	0 -25 -1.00 1.0	0 -7 -1.00 ...	77 45 0.13 2.5	0 -19 -1.00 0.7	0 0 0.00 ...	10 -4 -0.35 0.1	174 137 0.40 20.2$	29 10 0.03 0.2	14 -27 -0.67 0.8	0 -6 -1.00 ...	0 -7 -1.00 ...	0 -15 -1.00 0.6	0 -18 -1.00 0.7	0 -10 -1.00 ...	0 -3 -1.00 ...	0 0 -1.00 ...	15 -3 -0.19 0.0	377
CX	151 -6 -0.04 0.0	472 126 0.09 2.4	242 103 0.19 3.6	42 1 0.01 0.0	119 -49 -0.30 0.7	40 -64 -0.62 1.8	0 0 0.00 ...	92 10 0.03 0.1	134 -62 -0.32 0.0	99 -1 -0.02 0.0	379 155 0.17 5.2*	87 52 0.37 3.4	29 -11 -0.29 0.2	38 -48 -0.56 1.3	9 -89 -0.91 3.7	6 -51 -0.90 2.1	58 35 0.37 2.3	0 -5 -1.00 ...	12 -86 -0.88 3.5	2009
SUM	785	1722	691	203	841	522	0	406	981	501	1117	174	203	434	493	290	116	29	494	

Haplotype frequencies for population NEG
A-DR (N=290)

	A1	A2	A3	A11	A23	A24	A25	A26	A28	A29	A30	A31	A32	AW33	AW34	AW36	AW43	AW66	AX	SUM
DR1	20 -21 -0.52 0.4	152 67 0.15 1.9	35 -6 -0.16 0.0	86 75 0.39 ...	10 -27 -0.74 0.7	0 -25 -1.00 0.8	0 0 0.00 ...	69 47 0.12 3.2	35 -22 -0.40 0.3	0 -29 -1.00 0.0	69 6 0.01 0.0	0 -6 -1.00 ...	0 -8 -1.00 ...	17 -6 -0.29 0.1	0 -26 -1.00 0.9	35 22 0.10 ...	0 -6 -1.00 ...	0 0 0.00 ...	0 -24 -1.00 0.8	528
DR2	104 -12 -0.11 0.1	192 -45 -0.19 0.4	259 143 0.21 6.5*	0 -29 -1.00 1.1	77 -29 -0.28 0.3	118 47 0.11 1.1	0 0 0.00 ...	35 -25 -0.43 0.4	135 -25 -0.16 0.2	60 -22 -0.28 0.2	40 -134 -0.77 4.0*	0 -20 -1.00 0.7	69 43 0.29 2.5	29 -36 -0.56 0.7	103 27 0.06 0.3	0 -35 -1.00 1.2	69 49 0.41 3.0*	0 0 0.00 ...	182 113 0.28 6.5*	1472
DR3	276 155 0.23 7.4#	135 -109 -0.45 2.0	76 -43 -0.37 0.6	0 -30 -1.00 1.1	66 -43 -0.40 0.7	0 -73 -1.00 2.6	0 0 0.00 ...	1 -61 -0.98 2.2	140 -26 -0.16 0.2	117 31 0.07 0.4	452 271 0.27 15.8$	35 14 0.12 0.3	3 -22 -0.89 0.7	111 42 0.11 0.9	50 -28 -0.36 0.4	34 -2 -0.08 0.0	19 -1 -0.10 0.0	0 0 0.00 ...	5 -66 -0.93 2.2	1520
DR4	172 109 0.15 6.4*	214 86 0.13 2.1	0 -62 -1.00 2.1	69 53 0.28 ...	0 -57 -1.00 1.0	69 30 0.07 0.8	0 0 0.00 ...	69 36 0.09 1.3	104 17 0.02 0.1	0 -44 -1.00 1.5	0 -94 -1.00 3.4	35 24 0.19 ...	0 -13 -1.00 ...	0 -35 -1.00 1.2	0 -40 -1.00 1.4	0 -18 -1.00 0.6	0 -10 -1.00 ...	0 0 0.00 ...	63 25 0.06 0.6	795
DR7	69 -25 -0.27 0.3	104 -88 -0.46 1.6	73 -21 -0.23 0.2	0 -24 -1.00 0.8	145 58 0.09 1.4	0 -57 -1.00 2.0	0 0 0.00 ...	0 -49 -1.00 1.7	238 107 0.11 3.2	138 71 0.14 2.6	195 52 0.05 0.7	0 -16 -1.00 ...	35 14 0.09 0.3	35 -18 -0.35 0.2	119 57 0.12 1.8	0 -28 -1.00 0.0	0 -16 -1.00 ...	0 0 0.00 ...	47 -9 -0.17 0.1	1198
DRW8	0 -7 -1.00 ...	0 -16 -1.00 ...	0 -7 -1.00 ...	0 -1 -1.00 ...	35 27 0.28 ...	23 18 0.18 ...	0 0 0.00 ...	0 -3 -1.00 ...	0 -11 -1.00 ...	0 -5 -1.00 ...	12 0 -0.04 ...	0 0 -1.00 ...	35 33 0.32 ...	0 -4 -1.00 ...	0 -4 -1.00 ...	0 -2 -1.00 ...	0 0 -1.00 ...	0 0 0.00 ...	0 -4 -1.00 ...	105
DRW9	35 21 0.13 ...	0 -27 -1.00 0.0	3 -10 -0.78 ...	0 -3 -1.00 ...	0 -12 -1.00 ...	0 -7 -1.00 ...	0 0 0.00 ...	0 -6 -1.00 ...	0 -18 -1.00 0.6	0 -9 -1.00 ...	35 14 0.09 0.3	0 -1 -1.00 ...	0 -2 -1.00 ...	0 -7 -1.00 ...	66 57 0.35 ...	35 31 0.18 ...	0 -1 -1.00 ...	0 0 0.00 ...	0 -7 -1.00 ...	174
DRW10	0 -21 -1.00 0.7	64 19 0.08 0.3	35 13 0.05 0.3	34 28 0.14 ...	40 20 0.08 0.6	0 -12 -1.00 ...	0 0 0.00 ...	0 -10 -1.00 ...	0 -29 -1.00 1.0	35 19 0.07 ...	0 -32 -1.00 1.1	0 -3 -1.00 ...	0 -4 -1.00 ...	0 -11 -1.00 ...	34 20 0.07 ...	0 -6 -1.00 ...	0 -3 -1.00 ...	0 0 0.00 ...	35 22 0.08 ...	277
DRW11	49 -82 -0.63 1.0	366 97 0.07 1.5	100 -30 -0.24 0.3	0 -33 -1.00 1.2	150 29 0.05 0.3	67 -13 -0.17 0.1	0 0 0.00 ...	121 52 0.15 1.4	149 -33 -0.18 0.2	93 0 -0.01 0.0	208 10 0.01 0.0	35 12 0.10 0.2	0 -28 -1.00 1.0	103 28 0.07 0.4	49 -36 -0.43 0.6	104 64 0.31 3.6	35 12 0.10 0.2	0 0 0.00 ...	36 -42 -0.54 0.8	1665
DRW12	34 7 0.02 0.1	40 -15 -0.28 0.2	0 -26 -1.00 0.9	0 -6 -1.00 ...	29 4 0.01 0.0	69 52 0.16 ...	0 0 0.00 ...	0 -13 -1.00 ...	69 31 0.10 0.9	0 -18 -1.00 0.6	41 0 -0.00 0.0	0 -4 -1.00 ...	0 -5 -1.00 ...	28 12 0.04 ...	19 1 0.00 0.0	0 -7 -1.00 ...	16 11 0.08 ...	0 0 0.00 ...	0 -15 -1.00 ...	345
DRW13	17 -18 -0.53 0.3	69 -3 -0.05 0.0	96 60 0.15 3.4	17 8 0.04 ...	17 -15 -0.48 0.2	35 13 0.03 0.3	0 0 0.00 ...	35 16 0.04 0.4	0 -48 -1.00 1.7	0 -24 -1.00 0.8	35 -18 -0.35 0.2	0 -5 -1.00 ...	0 -7 -1.00 ...	60 40 0.09 2.5	35 12 0.03 0.2	0 -10 -1.00 ...	0 -5 -1.00 ...	0 0 0.00 ...	35 14 0.03 0.3	451
DRW14	18 -61 -0.78 1.7	244 81 0.10 1.5	61 -18 -0.23 0.2	0 -20 -1.00 0.7	104 31 0.05 0.4	0 -48 -1.00 1.7	0 0 0.00 ...	85 43 0.12 1.5	192 81 0.09 2.2	120 63 0.12 2.4	84 -35 -0.30 0.4	35 21 0.17 ...	32 14 0.09 0.4	1 -44 -0.98 1.5	0 -51 -1.00 1.8	0 -24 -1.00 0.8	0 -13 -1.00 ...	0 0 0.00 ...	34 -13 -0.29 0.1	1010
DRX	0 -37 -1.00 1.3	35 -41 -0.54 0.8	51 13 0.03 0.2	0 -9 -1.00 ...	52 17 0.04 0.3	104 81 0.18 9.1#	0 0 0.00 ...	0 -19 -1.00 0.6	35 -16 -0.33 0.2	0 -26 -1.00 0.9	19 -37 -0.66 0.9	0 -6 -1.00 ...	0 -7 -1.00 ...	67 46 0.11 3.1	43 18 0.04 0.4	35 23 0.10 ...	0 -6 -1.00 ...	0 0 0.00 ...	35 13 0.03 0.2	476
SUM	794	1615	789	206	725	485	0	415	1097	563	1190	140	174	451	518	243	139	0	472	

Haplotype frequencies for population NEG; B-C ($N = 334$)

	CW1	CW2	CW3	CW4	CW5	CW6	CW7	CW8	CX	SUM
B7	29 18 0.24 ...	56 -91 -0.62 2.5	116 -4 -0.04 0.0	80 -94 -0.54 2.3	0 -34 -1.00 1.4	146 -13 -0.09 0.1	699 413 0.43 29.4$	0 -50 -1.00 2.0	126 -137 -0.52 3.5	1252
B8	0 -4 -1.00 ...	29 -32 -0.53 0.7	43 -7 -0.15 0.0	0 -72 -1.00 3.0	0 -14 -1.00 ...	18 -48 -0.73 1.5	345 225 0.56 19.3$	15 -5 -0.30 0.1	75 -35 -0.32 0.5	525
B13	0 0 -1.00 ...	0 -16 -1.00 0.7	0 -13 -1.00 ...	10 -9 -0.51 0.2	0 -3 -1.00 ...	87 68 0.54 9.8#	0 -32 -1.00 1.5	0 -5 -1.00 ...	48 17 0.15 0.4	145
B18	0 -3 -1.00 ...	87 59 0.11 1.2	29 -9 -0.26 0.1	22 -34 -0.61 0.9	44 33 0.12 ...	0 -51 -1.00 2.1	112 19 0.06 0.2	29 12 0.03 0.3	84 -1 -0.02 0.0	407
B27	0 -1 -1.00 ...	138 114 0.64 20.9$	0 -19 -1.00 0.7	7 -20 -0.75 0.6	29 23 0.12 ...	0 -25 -1.00 1.0	0 -45 -1.00 2.1	0 -7 -1.00 ...	29 -13 -0.32 0.2	203
B35	0 -6 -1.00 ...	55 -41 -0.43 0.7	133 54 0.07 1.5	467 353 0.50 46.1$	0 -22 -1.00 0.8	32 -71 -0.69 2.1	29 -157 -0.84 6.3*	29 -3 -0.13 0.0	72 -99 -0.58 2.7	817
B37	0 -1 -1.00 ...	36 15 0.10 0.4	0 -16 -1.00 0.6	25 1 0.00 0.0	0 -4 -1.00 ...	55 33 0.22 1.9	0 -39 -1.00 1.8	0 -6 -1.00 ...	58 21 0.16 0.5	174
B38	0 0 -1.00 ...	0 -16 -1.00 0.7	0 -13 -1.00 ...	0 -19 -1.00 0.8	0 -3 -1.00 ...	0 -18 -1.00 0.7	29 -3 -0.13 0.0	0 -5 -1.00 ...	117 86 0.75 10.4#	146
B39	0 0 -1.00 ...	0 -2 -1.00 ...	0 -2 -1.00 ...	0 -3 -1.00 ...	0 0 -1.00 ...	17 13 0.53 ...	12 5 0.24 ...	0 0 -1.00 ...	0 -5 -1.00 ...	29
BW41	0 -1 -1.00 ...	29 5 0.03 0.0	0 -19 -1.00 0.7	0 -27 -1.00 1.1	0 -5 -1.00 ...	0 -25 -1.00 1.0	87 41 0.26 1.6	0 -7 -1.00 ...	87 44 0.28 1.0	203
BW42	0 -4 -1.00 ...	79 6 0.01 0.0	0 -58 -1.00 2.3	29 -55 -0.66 1.5	0 -16 -1.00 0.6	0 -77 -1.00 3.2	35 -104 -0.75 3.6	0 -24 -1.00 0.9	469 340 0.70 40.4$	612
B44	29 23 0.28 ...	26 -56 -0.69 1.6	29 -38 -0.57 0.9	175 77 0.13 2.5	117 98 0.38 18.1$	0 -89 -1.00 3.7	149 -10 -0.07 0.0	0 -28 -1.00 1.1	175 27 0.05 0.2	700
B45	0 -1 -1.00 ...	0 -27 -1.00 1.1	0 -22 -1.00 0.9	0 -32 -1.00 1.3	0 -5 -1.00 ...	12 -17 -0.60 0.4	17 -35 -0.68 1.1	0 -9 -1.00 ...	204 155 0.84 21.1$	233
BW46	0 0 0.00 ...	0 0 0.00 ...	0 0 0.00 ...	0 0 0.00 ...	0 0 0.00 ...	0 0 0.00 ...	0 0 0.00 ...	0 0 0.00 ...	0 0 0.00 ...	0
BW47	0 0 0.00 ...	0 0 0.00 ...	0 0 0.00 ...	0 0 0.00 ...	0 0 0.00 ...	0 0 0.00 ...	0 0 0.00 ...	0 0 0.00 ...	0 0 0.00 ...	0

	CW1	CW2	CW3	CW4	CW5	CW6	CW7	CW8	CX	SUM
BW48	0 0 -1.00 ...	29 26 1.00 ...	0 -2 -1.00 ...	0 -3 -1.00 ...	0 0 -1.00 ...	0 -3 -1.00 ...	0 -6 -1.00 ...	0 0 -1.00 ...	0 -5 -1.00 ...	29
B49	0 -1 -1.00 ...	0 -23 -1.00 0.9	0 -19 -1.00 0.7	0 -27 -1.00 1.1	0 -5 -1.00 ...	0 -25 -1.00 1.0	204 157 1.00 23.5$	0 -7 -1.00 ...	0 -42 -1.00 1.9	204
BW50	0 0 -1.00 ...	29 22 0.42 ...	0 -5 -1.00 ...	0 -7 -1.00 ...	0 -1 -1.00 ...	11 3 0.07 ...	19 6 0.12 ...	0 -1 -1.00 ...	0 -11 -1.00 ...	59
B51	29 27 0.32 ...	6 -17 -0.75 0.5	0 -19 -1.00 0.7	0 -27 -1.00 1.1	0 -5 -1.00 ...	0 -25 -1.00 1.0	0 -46 -1.00 2.1	0 -7 -1.00 ...	169 126 0.78 15.9$	204
BW52	0 0 -1.00 ...	0 -6 -1.00 ...	0 -5 -1.00 ...	0 -7 -1.00 ...	0 -1 -1.00 ...	0 -6 -1.00 ...	0 -12 -1.00 ...	0 -1 -1.00 ...	58 46 1.00 ...	58
BW53	0 -5 -1.00 ...	22 -56 -0.72 1.7	103 39 0.06 0.9	481 388 0.68 67.6$	0 -17 -1.00 0.7	0 -84 -1.00 3.5	7 -144 -0.95 6.4*	14 -12 -0.48 0.2	37 -102 -0.74 3.4	664
BW54	0 0 0.00 ...	0 0 0.00 ...	0 0 0.00 ...	0 0 0.00 ...	0 0 0.00 ...	0 0 0.00 ...	0 0 0.00 ...	0 0 0.00 ...	0 0 0.00 ...	0
BW55	0 0 -1.00 ...	0 -6 -1.00 ...	46 40 0.76 ...	0 -7 -1.00 ...	0 -1 -1.00 ...	0 -7 -1.00 ...	0 -12 -1.00 ...	0 -1 -1.00 ...	13 1 0.01 ...	59
BW56	0 0 -1.00 ...	0 -2 -1.00 ...	29 26 1.00 ...	0 -3 -1.00 ...	0 0 -1.00 ...	0 -3 -1.00 ...	0 -6 -1.00 ...	0 0 -1.00 ...	0 -5 -1.00 ...	29
BW57	0 -2 -1.00 ...	0 -34 -1.00 1.4	0 -27 -1.00 1.1	1 -39 -0.98 1.6	0 -7 -1.00 ...	203 166 0.65 28.0$	88 21 0.09 0.3	0 -11 -1.00 ...	0 -61 -1.00 2.7	292
BW58	0 -8 -1.00 ...	0 -121 -1.00 5.1*	29 -69 -0.71 2.0	64 -78 -0.55 1.9	0 -27 -1.00 1.1	638 507 0.57 83.4$	270 35 0.04 0.3	0 -41 -1.00 1.6	26 -190 -0.88 7.9#	1027
BW59	0 0 0.00 ...	0 0 0.00 ...	0 0 0.00 ...	0 0 0.00 ...	0 0 0.00 ...	0 0 0.00 ...	0 0 0.00 ...	0 0 0.00 ...	0 0 0.00 ...	0
BW60	0 -1 -1.00 ...	0 -23 -1.00 0.9	146 126 0.69 30.5$	0 -27 -1.00 1.1	0 -5 -1.00 ...	0 -25 -1.00 1.0	58 11 0.07 0.1	0 -7 -1.00 ...	0 -42 -1.00 1.9	204
BW61	0 0 -1.00 ...	29 17 0.18 ...	0 -9 -1.00 ...	0 -14 -1.00 ...	0 -2 -1.00 ...	0 -12 -1.00 ...	0 -23 -1.00 1.1	0 -3 -1.00 ...	76 54 0.65 5.6*	105
BW62	0 -1 -1.00 ...	0 -30 -1.00 1.2	175 150 0.63 33.6$	0 -36 -1.00 1.5	0 -6 -1.00 ...	58 24 0.11 0.7	0 -59 -1.00 2.7	0 -10 -1.00 ...	29 -25 -0.48 0.5	262

Haplotype frequencies for population NEG
B-C ($N = 334$)

	CW1	CW2	CW3	CW4	CW5	CW6	CW7	CW8	CX	SUM
BW63	0	0	1	0	87	0	0	0	87	175
	-1	-20	-15	-23	82	-21	-39	-6	50	
	-1.00	-1.00	-0.94	-1.00	0.48	-1.00	-1.00	-1.00	0.36	
	...	0.8	0.6	0.0	...	0.9	1.8	...	2.9	
BW64	0	29	0	0	0	0	0	117	0	146
	0	12	-13	-19	-3	-18	-32	111	-30	
	-1.00	0.09	-1.00	-1.00	-1.00	-1.00	-1.00	0.79	-1.00	
	...	0.3	...	0.8	...	0.7	1.5	...	1.3	
BW65	0	0	0	0	0	0	0	204	0	204
	-1	-23	-19	-27	-5	-25	-46	196	-42	
	-1.00	-1.00	-1.00	-1.00	-1.00	-1.00	-1.00	1.00	-1.00	
	...	0.9	0.7	1.1	...	1.0	2.1	...	1.9	
BW67	0	0	0	0	0	0	0	0	0	0
	0	0	0	0	0	0	0	0	0	
	0.00	0.00	0.00	0.00	0.00	0.00	0.00	0.00	0.00	
	...	...	...	...	...	...	...	...	...	
BW71	0	58	0	0	0	0	15	0	0	73
	0	49	-6	-9	-1	-8	-1	-2	-14	
	-1.00	0.77	-1.00	-1.00	-1.00	-1.00	-0.10	-1.00	-1.00	
	...	...	...	...	...	...	0.0	...	0.7	
BW72	0	420	87	0	0	0	66	0	39	612
	-4	347	28	-84	-16	-77	-73	-24	-89	
	-1.00	0.64	0.05	-1.00	-1.00	-1.00	-0.53	-1.00	-0.70	
	...	67.1¢	0.5	3.5	0.6	3.2	1.8	0.9	2.8	
BW73	0	0	0	0	0	0	0	0	0	0
	0	0	0	0	0	0	0	0	0	
	0.00	0.00	0.00	0.00	0.00	0.00	0.00	0.00	0.00	
	...	...	...	...	...	...	...	...	...	
BX	0	29	0	36	0	2	46	0	31	144
	0	12	-13	16	-3	-15	13	-5	1	
	-1.00	0.09	-1.00	0.13	-1.00	-0.89	0.12	-1.00	0.01	
	...	0.3	...	0.5	...	0.6	0.2	...	0.0	
SUM	87	1186	966	1397	277	1279	2287	408	2109	

Haplotype frequencies for population NEG B-Bf ($N=99$)

	BF S	BF F	BFF1	BFS07	BF V	SUM
B7	792 227 0.36 1.0	396 -203 -0.34 1.6	0 -11 -1.00 ...	0 -11 -1.00 ...	0 0 0.00 ...	1188
B8	495 166 0.46 1.7	198 -151 -0.43 1.4	0 -6 -1.00 ...	0 -6 -1.00 ...	0 0 0.00 ...	693
B13	0 -93 -1.00 1.8	198 98 1.00 1.0	0 -1 -1.00 ...	0 -1 -1.00 ...	0 0 0.00 ...	198
B18	99 -41 -0.30 0.2	198 48 0.33 0.3	0 -2 -1.00 ...	0 -2 -1.00 ...	0 0 0.00 ...	297
B27	0 0 0.00 ...	0 0 0.00 ...	0 0 0.00 ...	0 0 0.00 ...	0 0 0.00 ...	0
B35	891 374 0.65 5.7*	198 -351 -0.64 5.1*	0 -10 -1.00 ...	0 -10 -1.00 ...	0 0 0.00 ...	1089
B37	0 0 0.00 ...	0 0 0.00 ...	0 0 0.00 ...	0 0 0.00 ...	0 0 0.00 ...	0
B38	99 52 1.00 ...	0 -49 -1.00 ...	0 0 -1.00 ...	0 0 -1.00 ...	0 0 0.00 ...	99
B39	0 0 0.00 ...	0 0 0.00 ...	0 0 0.00 ...	0 0 0.00 ...	0 0 0.00 ...	0
BW41	0 -140 -1.00 2.7	297 147 1.00 2.0	0 -2 -1.00 ...	0 -2 -1.00 ...	0 0 0.00 ...	297
BW42	66 -215 -0.77 3.3	528 228 0.76 3.7	0 -5 -1.00 ...	0 -5 -1.00 ...	0 0 0.00 ...	594
B44	198 -83 -0.30 0.5	396 96 0.33 0.7	0 -5 -1.00 ...	0 -5 -1.00 ...	0 0 0.00 ...	594
B45	0 -140 -1.00 2.7	297 147 1.00 2.0	0 -2 -1.00 ...	0 -2 -1.00 ...	0 0 0.00 ...	297
BW46	0 0 0.00 ...	0 0 0.00 ...	0 0 0.00 ...	0 0 0.00 ...	0 0 0.00 ...	0
BW47	0 0 0.00 ...	0 0 0.00 ...	0 0 0.00 ...	0 0 0.00 ...	0 0 0.00 ...	0
BW48	0 0 0.00 ...	0 0 0.00 ...	0 0 0.00 ...	0 0 0.00 ...	0 0 0.00 ...	0
B49	198 104 1.00 2.2	0 -99 -1.00 2.0	0 -1 -1.00 ...	0 -1 -1.00 ...	0 0 0.00 ...	198
BW50	0 -46 -1.00 ...	99 49 1.00 ...	0 0 -1.00 ...	0 0 -1.00 ...	0 0 0.00 ...	99
B51	0 0 0.00 ...	0 0 0.00 ...	0 0 0.00 ...	0 0 0.00 ...	0 0 0.00 ...	0
BW52	99 52 1.00 ...	0 -49 -1.00 ...	0 0 -1.00 ...	0 0 -1.00 ...	0 0 0.00 ...	99
BW53	99 -124 -0.56 1.4	373 135 0.58 1.6	0 -4 -1.00 ...	0 -4 -1.00 ...	0 0 0.00 ...	472
BW54	0 0 0.00 ...	0 0 0.00 ...	0 0 0.00 ...	0 0 0.00 ...	0 0 0.00 ...	0
BW55	99 52 1.00 ...	0 -49 -1.00 ...	0 0 -1.00 ...	0 0 -1.00 ...	0 0 0.00 ...	99
BW56	0 0 0.00 ...	0 0 0.00 ...	0 0 0.00 ...	0 0 0.00 ...	0 0 0.00 ...	0
BW57	66 -74 -0.53 0.8	231 81 0.55 0.9	0 -2 -1.00 ...	0 -2 -1.00 ...	0 0 0.00 ...	297
BW58	627 -61 -0.09 0.1	723 -8 -0.01 0.0	0 -13 -1.00 ...	99 85 1.00 ...	0 0 0.00 ...	1449
BW59	0 0 0.00 ...	0 0 0.00 ...	0 0 0.00 ...	0 0 0.00 ...	0 0 0.00 ...	0
BW60	198 104 1.00 2.2	0 -99 -1.00 2.0	0 -1 -1.00 ...	0 -1 -1.00 ...	0 0 0.00 ...	198
BW61	0 -46 -1.00 ...	99 49 1.00 ...	0 0 -1.00 ...	0 0 -1.00 ...	0 0 0.00 ...	99
BW62	198 104 1.00 2.2	0 -99 -1.00 2.0	0 -1 -1.00 ...	0 -1 -1.00 ...	0 0 0.00 ...	198
BW63	198 104 1.00 2.2	0 -99 -1.00 2.0	0 -1 -1.00 ...	0 -1 -1.00 ...	0 0 0.00 ...	198
BW64	0 -93 -1.00 1.8	198 98 1.00 1.0	0 -1 -1.00 ...	0 -1 -1.00 ...	0 0 0.00 ...	198
BW65	198 57 0.36 0.4	99 -50 -0.34 0.4	0 -2 -1.00 ...	0 -2 -1.00 ...	0 0 0.00 ...	297
BW67	0 0 0.00 ...	0 0 0.00 ...	0 0 0.00 ...	0 0 0.00 ...	0 0 0.00 ...	0
BW71	0 0 0.00 ...	0 0 0.00 ...	0 0 0.00 ...	0 0 0.00 ...	0 0 0.00 ...	0
BW72	132 -196 -0.60 2.4	462 112 0.33 0.8	99 92 1.00 ...	0 -6 -1.00 ...	0 0 0.00 ...	693
BW73	0 0 0.00 ...	0 0 0.00 ...	0 0 0.00 ...	0 0 0.00 ...	0 0 0.00 ...	0
BX	0 -27 -1.00 ...	59 29 1.00 ...	0 0 -1.00 ...	0 0 -1.00 ...	0 0 0.00 ...	59
SUM	4752	5049	99	99	0	

Haplotype frequencies for population NEG; B-DQ ($N=276$)

	DQW1	DQW2	DQW3	DQX	SUM
B7	744	107	258	226	1335
	203	-188	-64	50	
	0.26	-0.64	-0.20	0.04	
	4.1*	4.9*	0.5	0.5	
B8	114	377	72	71	634
	-142	236	-80	-11	
	-0.56	0.48	-0.53	-0.15	
	3.9*	15.0‡	1.7	0.1	
B13	35	141	0	0	176
	-35	102	-42	-22	
	-0.51	0.74	-1.00	-1.00	
	0.9	9.6#	1.6	0.7	
B18	156	67	92	37	352
	13	-10	7	-8	
	0.06	-0.14	0.03	-0.20	
	0.1	0.1	0.0	0.1	
B27	92	13	24	12	141
	35	-17	-9	-6	
	0.42	-0.58	-0.30	-0.35	
	1.0	0.4	0.1	0.1	
B35	425	70	164	150	809
	97	-108	-31	44	
	0.20	-0.61	-0.16	0.06	
	1.5	2.6	0.2	0.6	
B37	92	0	35	14	141
	35	-30	1	-4	
	0.42	-1.00	0.01	-0.24	
	1.0	1.1	0.0	0.0	
B38	53	0	35	18	106
	10	-23	9	4	
	0.16	-1.00	0.12	0.04	
	0.1	0.8	0.1	...	
B39	28	0	0	7	35
	14	-7	-7	2	
	0.66	-1.00	-1.00	0.08	
	...	...	...	...	
BW41	48	122	35	7	212
	-37	75	-15	-20	
	-0.44	0.45	-0.32	-0.75	
	0.8	4.3*	0.2	0.5	
BW42	156	110	166	202	634
	-100	-30	13	119	
	-0.39	-0.22	0.03	0.22	
	1.0	0.3	0.0	5.7*	
B44	352	146	159	82	739
	53	-17	-19	-14	
	0.12	-0.11	-0.11	-0.16	
	0.5	0.1	0.1	0.1	
B45	151	54	70	7	282
	37	-8	2	-29	
	0.22	-0.14	0.01	-0.81	
	0.6	0.0	0.0	0.8	
BW46	0	0	0	0	0
	0	0	0	0	
	0.00	0.00	0.00	0.00	
	...	...	...	...	
BW47	0	0	0	0	0
	0	0	0	0	
	0.00	0.00	0.00	0.00	
	...	...	...	...	
BW48	18	0	18	0	36
	3	-7	9	-4	
	0.16	-1.00	0.34	-1.00	
	...	...	...	...	
B49	28	35	141	7	211
	-56	-11	90	-20	
	-0.67	-0.25	0.56	-0.75	
	1.8	0.1	5.9*	0.5	
BW50	35	25	0	10	70
	7	9	-16	1	
	0.16	0.17	-1.00	0.01	
	0.1	...	...	...	
B51	35	0	0	70	105
	-7	-22	-24	56	
	-0.18	-1.00	-1.00	0.62	
	0.1	0.8	0.9	...	
BW52	0	0	70	0	70
	-27	-15	53	-8	
	-1.00	-1.00	1.00	-1.00	
	1.3	...	...	...	
BW53	147	115	130	93	485
	-48	7	13	29	
	-0.25	0.02	0.03	0.07	
	0.6	0.0	0.1	0.4	
BW54	0	0	0	0	0
	0	0	0	0	
	0.00	0.00	0.00	0.00	
	...	...	...	...	
BW55	28	0	18	25	71
	0	-15	1	16	
	-0.03	-1.00	0.02	0.25	
	0.0	...	...	...	
BW56	35	0	0	0	35
	21	-7	-7	-4	
	1.00	-1.00	-1.00	-1.00	
	...	...	...	...	
BW57	152	48	57	25	282
	38	-14	-10	-11	
	0.23	-0.23	-0.16	-0.33	
	0.6	0.1	0.1	0.1	
BW58	421	167	297	145	1030
	4	-60	48	10	
	0.01	-0.27	0.06	0.01	
	0.0	0.7	0.4	0.0	
BW59	0	0	0	0	0
	0	0	0	0	
	0.00	0.00	0.00	0.00	
	...	...	...	...	
BW60	35	35	88	17	175
	-35	-3	46	-5	
	-0.51	-0.10	0.34	-0.26	
	0.9	0.0	1.8	0.1	
BW61	47	44	0	0	91
	10	24	-21	-11	
	0.19	0.34	-1.00	-1.00	
	0.1	1.0	0.8	...	
BW62	106	88	87	1	282
	-7	25	19	-35	
	-0.07	0.12	0.09	-0.97	
	0.0	0.4	0.2	1.1	
BW63	82	18	28	13	141
	25	-12	-5	-5	
	0.30	-0.42	-0.18	-0.30	
	0.5	0.2	0.0	0.1	
BW64	15	148	0	13	176
	-55	109	-42	-9	
	-0.79	0.80	-1.00	-0.44	
	2.1	10.0‡	1.6	0.1	
BW65	90	35	70	16	211
	5	-11	19	-11	
	0.04	-0.25	0.12	-0.42	
	0.0	0.1	0.3	0.2	
BW67	0	0	0	0	0
	0	0	0	0	
	0.00	0.00	0.00	0.00	
	...	...	...	...	
BW71	35	35	18	0	88
	0	15	-2	-11	
	-0.02	0.23	-0.15	-1.00	
	0.0	0.4	0.0	...	
BW72	219	193	219	39	670
	-51	44	57	-48	
	-0.19	0.09	0.11	-0.56	
	0.5	0.5	0.8	0.9	
BW73	0	0	0	0	0
	0	0	0	0	
	0.00	0.00	0.00	0.00	
	...	...	...	...	
BX	75	25	66	8	174
	5	-13	24	-14	
	0.04	-0.35	0.18	-0.65	
	0.0	0.2	0.5	0.3	
SUM	4049	2218	2417	1315	

Haplotype frequencies for population NEG
B-DR (N=285)

	DR1	DR2	DR3	DR4	DR7	DRW8	DRW9	DRW10	DRW11	DRW12	DRW13	DRW14	DRX	SUM
B7	137 66 0.15 2.1	461 249 0.22 11.4$	103 -101 -0.50 1.0	68 -38 -0.36 0.5	102 -58 -0.37 0.8	0 -13 -1.00 ...	0 -27 -1.00 0.9	21 -15 -0.43 0.2	142 -82 -0.37 1.2	13 -28 -0.69 0.7	137 77 0.20 3.4	68 -62 -0.48 1.1	111 43 0.10 0.9	1363
B8	0 -31 -1.00 1.0	68 -27 -0.29 0.3	341 249 0.48 23.0$	68 20 0.04 0.3	34 -38 -0.53 0.7	0 -5 -1.00 ...	0 -12 -1.00 ...	34 17 0.07 ...	17 -83 -0.83 2.5	0 -18 -1.00 0.6	0 -26 -1.00 0.9	18 -40 -0.70 0.0	34 3 0.01 0.0	614
B13	0 -8 -1.00 ...	34 7 0.05 0.1	0 -25 -1.00 0.9	0 -12 -1.00 ...	137 117 0.77 22.1$	0 -1 -1.00 ...	0 -2 -1.00 ...	0 -4 -1.00 ...	0 -27 -1.00 0.0	0 -4 -1.00 ...	0 -7 -1.00 ...	0 -15 -1.00 ...	0 -8 -1.00 ...	171
B18	0 -17 -1.00 0.6	41 -11 -0.23 0.1	34 -16 -0.34 0.2	0 -26 -1.00 0.9	34 -5 -0.16 0.0	0 -3 -1.00 ...	0 -6 -1.00 ...	0 -8 -1.00 ...	187 131 0.46 10.7#	0 -9 -1.00 ...	0 -14 -1.00 ...	45 12 0.04 0.1	0 -16 -1.00 ...	341
B27	0 -6 -1.00 ...	68 47 0.40 3.5	3 -17 -0.85 0.5	0 -10 -1.00 ...	0 -15 -1.00 ...	21 20 0.19 ...	0 -2 -1.00 ...	0 -3 -1.00 ...	14 -8 -0.38 0.1	0 -3 -1.00 ...	0 -5 -1.00 ...	31 16 0.14 ...	0 -6 -1.00 ...	137
B35	119 78 0.16 4.9*	69 -52 -0.43 0.8	75 -42 -0.36 0.6	102 41 0.06 0.9	0 -92 -1.00 3.3	0 -7 -1.00 ...	34 18 0.10 ...	68 47 0.19 3.2	34 -94 -0.74 2.6	96 72 0.25 6.9#	34 0 -0.02 0.0	153 78 0.11 2.7	0 -38 -1.00 1.3	784
B37	0 -6 -1.00 ...	28 7 0.06 0.1	6 -13 -0.71 0.3	0 -10 -1.00 ...	0 -15 -1.00 ...	0 0 -1.00 ...	0 -2 -1.00 ...	34 30 0.23 ...	0 -21 -1.00 0.8	0 -3 -1.00 ...	17 11 0.08 ...	17 4 0.03 ...	34 27 0.21 ...	136
B38	0 -4 -1.00 ...	68 52 0.61 ...	0 -14 -1.00 ...	34 26 0.28 ...	0 -11 -1.00 ...	0 0 -1.00 ...	0 -1 -1.00 ...	0 -2 -1.00 ...	0 -16 -1.00 ...	0 -2 -1.00 ...	0 -4 -1.00 ...	0 -9 -1.00 ...	0 -4 -1.00 ...	102
B39	0 -1 -1.00 ...	20 15 0.51 ...	0 -4 -1.00 ...	0 -2 -1.00 ...	0 -3 -1.00 ...	0 0 -1.00 ...	0 0 -1.00 ...	0 0 -1.00 ...	14 8 0.30 ...	0 0 -1.00 ...	0 -1 -1.00 ...	0 -2 -1.00 ...	0 -1 -1.00 ...	34
BW41	68 57 0.30 ...	0 -31 -1.00 1.1	34 3 0.02 0.0	34 18 0.10 ...	68 44 0.24 2.6	0 -1 -1.00 ...	0 -3 -1.00 ...	0 -5 -1.00 ...	0 -33 -1.00 1.2	0 -5 -1.00 ...	0 -8 -1.00 ...	0 -19 -1.00 0.6	0 -9 -1.00 ...	204
BW42	0 -33 -1.00 1.1	74 -26 -0.27 0.3	393 296 0.54 32.2$	34 -16 -0.33 0.2	11 -65 -0.86 1.9	0 -6 -1.00 ...	0 -12 -1.00 ...	34 16 0.06 0.5	34 -72 -0.68 1.8	34 14 0.05 0.3	34 5 0.01 0.0	0 -61 -1.00 2.1	0 -31 -1.00 1.0	648
B44	0 -36 -1.00 1.2	137 26 0.04 0.2	53 -53 -0.51 0.0	102 46 0.07 1.3	173 88 0.14 3.2	34 27 0.28 ...	0 -14 -1.00 ...	0 -18 -1.00 0.6	60 -57 -0.49 1.0	0 -21 -1.00 0.7	46 14 0.03 0.2	68 0 -0.01 0.0	42 6 0.01 0.0	715
B45	0 -13 -1.00 ...	48 6 0.02 0.0	34 -6 -0.17 0.0	0 -20 -1.00 0.7	34 2 0.01 0.0	0 -2 -1.00 ...	11 5 0.03 ...	0 -6 -1.00 ...	111 66 0.29 3.4	0 -7 -1.00 ...	34 22 0.08 ...	0 -25 -1.00 0.8	0 -13 -1.00 ...	272
BW46	0 0 0.00 ...	0 0 0.00 ...	0 0 0.00 ...	0 0 0.00 ...	0 0 0.00 ...	0 0 0.00 ...	0 0 0.00 ...	0 0 0.00 ...	0 0 0.00 ...	0 0 0.00 ...	0 0 0.00 ...	0 0 0.00 ...	0 0 0.00 ...	0
BW47	0 0 0.00 ...	0 0 0.00 ...	0 0 0.00 ...	0 0 0.00 ...	0 0 0.00 ...	0 0 0.00 ...	0 0 0.00 ...	0 0 0.00 ...	0 0 0.00 ...	0 0 0.00 ...	0 0 0.00 ...	0 0 0.00 ...	0 0 0.00 ...	0

Haplotype frequencies for population NEG
B-DR ($N=285$)

	DR1	DR2	DR3	DR4	DR7	DRW8	DRW9	DRW10	DRW11	DRW12	DRW13	DRW14	DRX	SUM
BW48	0 -1 -1.00 ...	5 0 -0.06 ...	0 -4 -1.00 ...	0 -2 -1.00 ...	0 -3 -1.00 ...	0 0 -1.00 ...	0 0 -1.00 ...	0 0 -1.00 ...	29 23 0.82 ...	0 0 -1.00 ...	0 -1 -1.00 ...	0 -2 -1.00 ...	0 -1 -1.00 ...	34
B49	0 -10 -1.00 ...	8 -23 -0.75 0.6	26 -4 -0.16 0.0	0 -15 -1.00 ...	0 -23 -1.00 0.8	0 -1 -1.00 ...	0 -3 -1.00 ...	0 -5 -1.00 ...	137 103 0.60 10.0$	34 28 0.14 ...	0 -8 -1.00 ...	0 -19 -1.00 0.6	0 -9 -1.00 ...	205
BW50	0 -3 -1.00 ...	0 -10 -1.00 ...	29 19 0.33 ...	0 -4 -1.00 ...	0 -7 -1.00 ...	0 0 -1.00 ...	0 0 -1.00 ...	0 -1 -1.00 ...	0 -10 -1.00 ...	0 -1 -1.00 ...	0 -2 -1.00 ...	34 27 0.45 ...	5 2 0.02 ...	68
B51	0 -4 -1.00 ...	34 18 0.21 ...	34 19 0.22 ...	0 -7 -1.00 ...	0 -11 -1.00 ...	0 0 -1.00 ...	0 -1 -1.00 ...	0 -2 -1.00 ...	34 17 0.20 ...	0 -2 -1.00 ...	0 -4 -1.00 ...	0 -9 -1.00 ...	0 -4 -1.00 ...	102
BW52	0 -3 -1.00 ...	0 -10 -1.00 ...	0 -9 -1.00 ...	34 29 0.46 ...	0 -7 -1.00 ...	0 0 -1.00 ...	0 0 -1.00 ...	0 -1 -1.00 ...	34 23 0.40 ...	0 -1 -1.00 ...	0 -2 -1.00 ...	0 -6 -1.00 ...	0 -2 -1.00 ...	68
BW53	53 25 0.05 0.7	26 -57 -0.69 1.4	69 -11 -0.15 0.1	0 -41 -1.00 1.4	34 -29 -0.47 0.5	14 8 0.09 ...	60 49 0.25 ...	0 -14 -1.00 ...	190 101 0.23 4.2*	7 -9 -0.58 ...	0 -23 -1.00 0.8	17 -34 -0.67 0.8	68 41 0.09 1.0	538
BW54	0 0 0.00 ...	0 0 0.00 ...	0 0 0.00 ...	0 0 0.00 ...	0 0 0.00 ...	0 0 0.00 ...	0 0 0.00 ...	0 0 0.00 ...	0 0 0.00 ...	0 0 0.00 ...	0 0 0.00 ...	0 0 0.00 ...	0 0 0.00 ...	0
BW55	17 13 0.21 ...	0 -10 -1.00 ...	0 -9 -1.00 ...	34 29 0.46 ...	0 -7 -1.00 ...	0 0 -1.00 ...	0 0 -1.00 ...	0 -1 -1.00 ...	0 -10 -1.00 ...	0 -1 -1.00 ...	17 14 0.22 ...	0 -6 -1.00 ...	0 -2 -1.00 ...	68
BW56	0 -1 -1.00 ...	34 29 1.00 ...	0 -4 -1.00 ...	0 -2 -1.00 ...	0 -3 -1.00 ...	0 0 -1.00 ...	0 0 -1.00 ...	0 0 -1.00 ...	0 -5 -1.00 ...	0 0 -1.00 ...	0 -1 -1.00 ...	0 -2 -1.00 ...	0 -1 -1.00 ...	34
BW57	34 20 0.08 ...	34 -7 -0.20 0.1	0 -40 -1.00 1.4	0 -20 -1.00 0.7	46 14 0.06 0.2	0 -2 -1.00 ...	34 28 0.14 ...	0 -6 -1.00 ...	34 -10 -0.24 0.1	0 -7 -1.00 ...	22 10 0.04 ...	68 42 0.17 2.2	0 -13 -1.00 ...	272
BW58	15 -40 -0.73 0.0	136 -29 -0.18 0.2	68 -91 -0.58 1.0	56 -26 -0.33 0.3	94 -31 -0.26 0.3	0 -10 -1.00 ...	0 -21 -1.00 0.7	0 -28 -1.00 0.0	257 81 0.09 1.4	0 -32 -1.00 1.1	68 21 0.05 0.3	253 150 0.18 7.8#	119 66 0.15 2.7	1066
BW59	0 0 0.00 ...	0 0 0.00 ...	0 0 0.00 ...	0 0 0.00 ...	0 0 0.00 ...	0 0 0.00 ...	0 0 0.00 ...	0 0 0.00 ...	0 0 0.00 ...	0 0 0.00 ...	0 0 0.00 ...	0 0 0.00 ...	0 0 0.00 ...	0
BW60	0 -8 -1.00 ...	0 -25 -1.00 0.9	34 8 0.06 0.1	34 21 0.13 ...	0 -19 -1.00 0.7	0 -1 -1.00 ...	0 -2 -1.00 ...	0 -4 -1.00 ...	34 6 0.04 0.0	34 29 0.17 ...	34 26 0.16 ...	0 -15 -1.00 ...	0 -8 -1.00 ...	170
BW61	0 -5 -1.00 ...	48 29 0.28 1.5	38 20 0.19 0.7	0 -9 -1.00 ...	0 -14 -1.00 ...	0 0 -1.00 ...	0 -2 -1.00 ...	0 -2 -1.00 ...	0 -19 -1.00 0.7	0 -3 -1.00 ...	0 -4 -1.00 ...	3 -8 -0.75 ...	34 28 0.24 ...	123
BW62	0 -13 -1.00 ...	0 -41 -1.00 1.5	34 -6 -0.17 0.0	68 47 0.19 3.3	34 2 0.01 0.0	0 -2 -1.00 ...	34 28 0.14 ...	34 27 0.10 ...	0 -44 -1.00 1.6	0 -7 -1.00 ...	0 -11 -1.00 ...	68 42 0.17 2.2	0 -13 -1.00 ...	272

Haplotype frequencies for population NEG

B-DR (N=285)▼

	DR1	DR2	DR3	DR4	DR7	DRW8	DRW9	DRW10	DRW11	DRW12	DRW13	DRW14	DRX	SUM
BW63	34 27 0.21 ...	34 13 0.11 0.3	0 -19 -1.00 0.7	34 23 0.19 ...	0 -15 -1.00 ...	0 0 -1.00 ...	0 -2 -1.00 ...	0 -3 -1.00 ...	34 12 0.10 0.2	0 -3 -1.00 ...	0 -5 -1.00 ...	0 -12 -1.00 ...	0 -6 -1.00 ...	136
BW64	0 -8 -1.00 ...	0 -26 -1.00 0.9	11 -14 -0.57 0.3	0 -12 -1.00 ...	160 140 0.93 31.7‡	0 -1 -1.00 ...	0 -2 -1.00 ...	0 -4 -1.00 ...	0 -27 -1.00 0.0	0 -4 -1.00 ...	0 -7 -1.00 ...	0 -15 -1.00 ...	0 -6 -1.00 ...	171
BW65	34 23 0.12 ...	34 2 0.01 0.0	0 -30 -1.00 1.0	34 18 0.10 ...	34 10 0.05 0.1	0 -1 -1.00 ...	0 -3 -1.00 ...	0 -5 -1.00 ...	0 -33 -1.00 1.2	34 28 0.14 ...	0 -8 -1.00 ...	34 14 0.08 0.3	0 -9 -1.00 ...	204
BW67	0 0 0.00 ...	0 0 0.00 ...	0 0 0.00 ...	0 0 0.00 ...	0 0 0.00 ...	0 0 0.00 ...	0 0 0.00 ...	0 0 0.00 ...	0 0 0.00 ...	0 0 0.00 ...	0 0 0.00 ...	0 0 0.00 ...	0 0 0.00 ...	0
BW71	0 -3 -1.00 ...	0 -12 -1.00 ...	0 -12 -1.00 ...	17 10 0.13 ...	34 24 0.32 ...	0 0 -1.00 ...	0 -1 -1.00 ...	0 -1 -1.00 ...	0 -13 -1.00 ...	0 -2 -1.00 ...	0 -3 -1.00 ...	34 26 0.34 ...	0 -3 -1.00 ...	85
BW72	10 -25 -0.72 0.6	0 -105 -1.00 3.8*	83 -18 -0.19 0.1	0 -52 -1.00 1.8	143 62 0.10 1.7	0 -6 -1.00 ...	23 9 0.05 ...	13 -5 -0.30 0.1	253 141 0.25 6.4*	55 34 0.12 1.7	0 -29 -1.00 0.0	51 -14 -0.22 0.1	51 17 0.04 0.3	682
BW73	0 0 0.00 ...	0 0 0.00 ...	0 0 0.00 ...	0 0 0.00 ...	0 0 0.00 ...	0 0 0.00 ...	0 0 0.00 ...	0 0 0.00 ...	0 0 0.00 ...	0 0 0.00 ...	0 0 0.00 ...	0 0 0.00 ...	0 0 0.00 ...	0
BX	0 -8 -1.00 ...	48 22 0.15 0.6	0 -24 -1.00 0.9	30 17 0.11 ...	12 -7 -0.40 0.1	34 32 0.32 ...	8 5 0.03 ...	34 29 0.16 ...	0 -27 -1.00 0.0	0 -4 -1.00 ...	0 -6 -1.00 ...	0 -15 -1.00 ...	3 -4 -0.65 ...	169
SUM	521	1557	1502	783	1184	103	204	272	1649	307	443	962	501	

C-DQ (N=287)▼

	CW1	CW2	CW3	CW4	CW5	CW6	CW7	CW8	CX	SUM
DQW1	51 9 0.14 0.1	422 -15 -0.04 0.0	434 38 0.06 0.2	555 48 0.06 0.3	114 6 0.05 0.0	551 30 0.04 0.1	1136 80 0.05 0.4	176 -6 -0.04 0.0	606 -189 -0.24 2.7	4045
DQW2	19 -3 -0.18 0.0	309 71 0.08 0.9	209 -5 -0.03 0.0	164 -110 -0.40 1.9	26 -30 -0.55 0.6	305 22 0.02 0.1	492 -80 -0.14 0.6	146 47 0.13 0.8	526 94 0.06 0.9	2196
DQW3	0 -24 -1.00 0.0	239 -23 -0.09 0.1	283 45 0.06 0.4	313 9 0.01 0.0	105 42 0.21 1.1	312 0 -0.00 0.0	563 -70 -0.11 0.4	87 -22 -0.21 0.2	525 47 0.03 0.2	2427
DQX	35 21 0.23 ...	114 -30 -0.21 0.2	54 -76 -0.59 1.7	221 54 0.05 0.7	16 -18 -0.54 0.3	119 -52 -0.31 0.6	420 71 0.07 0.7	44 -15 -0.27 0.2	312 49 0.05 0.4	1335
SUM	105	1084	960	1253	261	1287	2611	453	1969	

Haplotype frequencies for population NEG; C-DR ($N=293$)▼
C4A-C4B ($N=82$)▼

	CW1	CW2	CW3	CW4	CW5	CW6	CW7	CW8	CX	SUM
DR1	0 -4 -1.00 ...	10 -46 -0.83 1.4	10 -41 -0.81 1.2	151 85 0.19 3.9*	0 -12 -1.00 ...	0 -70 -1.00 2.5	217 85 0.22 2.3	34 11 0.03 0.2	100 -1 -0.02 0.0	522
DR2	34 18 0.21 ...	131 -38 -0.23 0.4	171 16 0.02 0.1	61 -134 -0.69 3.7	68 28 0.13 0.7	118 -93 -0.44 1.7	598 205 0.18 4.0*	34 -34 -0.51 0.6	342 37 0.03 0.2	1557
DR3	0 -15 -1.00 ...	106 -61 -0.37 0.9	178 25 0.03 0.2	103 -90 -0.47 1.7	17 -21 -0.57 0.4	118 -90 -0.44 1.6	498 111 0.10 1.5	11 -56 -0.84 1.7	505 204 0.16 5.9*	1536
DR4	0 -7 -1.00 ...	34 -51 -0.60 1.1	137 59 0.08 1.6	68 -30 -0.31 0.4	102 82 0.35 10.0#	56 -50 -0.48 0.9	102 -95 -0.48 1.0	34 0 -0.02 0.0	251 97 0.15 2.4	784
DR7	34 22 0.24 ...	280 150 0.16 6.5*	68 -49 -0.42 0.8	117 -32 -0.22 0.3	0 -29 -1.00 1.0	240 78 0.08 1.5	34 -264 -0.89 10.4#	160 107 0.27 7.6#	253 20 0.02 0.1	1186
DRW8	0 0 -1.00 ...	21 10 0.11 ...	0 -9 -1.00 ...	47 34 0.38 ...	34 31 0.32 ...	0 -13 -1.00 ...	0 -25 -1.00 1.0	0 -4 -1.00 ...	0 -19 -1.00 0.7	102
DRW9	0 -1 -1.00 ...	0 -18 -1.00 0.6	34 17 0.11 ...	50 28 0.19 1.3	0 -3 -1.00 ...	34 11 0.07 0.2	0 -42 -1.00 1.7	0 -7 -1.00 ...	53 19 0.14 0.4	171
DRW10	0 -2 -1.00 ...	40 10 0.04 0.1	34 7 0.03 0.1	34 0 -0.01 0.0	0 -6 -1.00 ...	68 31 0.13 0.9	82 13 0.06 0.1	0 -11 -1.00 ...	15 -38 -0.72 1.0	273
DRW11	0 -15 -1.00 ...	226 49 0.05 0.5	119 -40 -0.26 0.4	173 -30 -0.15 0.2	34 -6 -0.17 0.0	214 -5 -0.03 0.0	525 118 0.10 1.6	68 -3 -0.05 0.0	256 -60 -0.19 0.5	1615
DRW12	0 -2 -1.00 ...	28 -8 -0.25 0.1	62 28 0.09 0.8	75 32 0.11 0.8	0 -8 -1.00 ...	16 -30 -0.66 0.7	93 7 0.03 0.0	34 19 0.06 ...	34 -32 -0.49 0.6	342
DRW13	0 -4 -1.00 ...	17 -31 -0.65 0.7	62 18 0.04 0.2	106 50 0.13 1.6	0 -10 -1.00 ...	73 12 0.03 0.1	102 -9 -0.09 0.0	0 -19 -1.00 0.6	84 -2 -0.04 0.0	444
DRW14	0 -9 -1.00 ...	151 42 0.05 0.6	118 19 0.02 0.1	150 24 0.03 0.2	0 -24 -1.00 0.8	324 188 0.22 9.8#	121 -129 -0.52 2.9	69 25 0.06 0.5	64 -131 -0.67 3.6	997
DRX	34 29 0.30 ...	51 0 -0.00 0.0	0 -45 -1.00 1.6	126 67 0.16 2.7	0 -11 -1.00 ...	102 38 0.09 0.8	150 32 0.09 0.4	0 -20 -1.00 0.7	5 -86 -0.95 3.1	468
SUM	102	1095	993	1261	255	1363	2522	444	1962	

	C4 A1	C4A12	C4A13	C4 A2	C4 A3	C4 A4	C4A51	C4 A6	C4AQ0	SUM
C4 B1	366 -196 -0.35 1.8	0 0 0.00 ...	0 0 0.00 ...	443 41 0.20 0.1	4527 -1 -0.00 0.0	122 42 1.00 0.5	309 68 0.54 0.5	122 42 1.00 0.5	709 7 0.02 0.0	6598
C4B11	0 0 0.00 ...	0 0 0.00 ...	0 0 0.00 ...	0 0 0.00 ...	0 0 0.00 ...	0 0 0.00 ...	0 0 0.00 ...	0 0 0.00 ...	0 0 0.00 ...	0
C4B12	0 0 0.00 ...	0 0 0.00 ...	0 0 0.00 ...	0 0 0.00 ...	0 0 0.00 ...	0 0 0.00 ...	0 0 0.00 ...	0 0 0.00 ...	0 0 0.00 ...	0
C4 B2	122 39 0.05 0.2	0 0 0.00 ...	0 0 0.00 ...	122 62 0.11 ...	710 40 0.13 0.1	0 -11 -1.00 ...	0 -35 -1.00 ...	0 -11 -1.00 ...	22 -81 -0.79 0.7	976
C4 B3	122 80 0.18 ...	0 0 0.00 ...	0 0 0.00 ...	0 -29 -1.00 ...	362 27 0.18 0.1	0 -5 -1.00 ...	0 -17 -1.00 ...	0 -5 -1.00 ...	4 -47 -0.92 ...	488
C4 B4	0 0 0.00 ...	0 0 0.00 ...	0 0 0.00 ...	0 0 0.00 ...	0 0 0.00 ...	0 0 0.00 ...	0 0 0.00 ...	0 0 0.00 ...	0 0 0.00 ...	0
C4 B5	0 0 0.00 ...	0 0 0.00 ...	0 0 0.00 ...	0 0 0.00 ...	0 0 0.00 ...	0 0 0.00 ...	0 0 0.00 ...	0 0 0.00 ...	0 0 0.00 ...	0
C4B51	0 0 0.00 ...	0 0 0.00 ...	0 0 0.00 ...	0 0 0.00 ...	0 0 0.00 ...	0 0 0.00 ...	0 0 0.00 ...	0 0 0.00 ...	0 0 0.00 ...	0
C4 B6	0 0 0.00 ...	0 0 0.00 ...	0 0 0.00 ...	0 0 0.00 ...	0 0 0.00 ...	0 0 0.00 ...	0 0 0.00 ...	0 0 0.00 ...	0 0 0.00 ...	0
C4 B7	0 0 0.00 ...	0 0 0.00 ...	0 0 0.00 ...	0 0 0.00 ...	0 0 0.00 ...	0 0 0.00 ...	0 0 0.00 ...	0 0 0.00 ...	0 0 0.00 ...	0
C4BQ0	244 78 0.11 0.4	0 0 0.00 ...	0 0 0.00 ...	45 -72 -0.62 0.5	1265 -66 -0.05 0.1	0 -23 -1.00 ...	57 -13 -0.20 0.0	0 -23 -1.00 ...	329 123 0.14 0.8	1940
SUM	854	0	0	610	6864	122	366	122	1064	

Haplotype frequencies for population NEG

DR-DQ ($N = 288$)▼

	DR1	DR2	DR3	DR4	DR7	DRW8	DRW9	DRW10	DRW11	DRW12	DRW13	DRW14	DRX	SUM
DQW1	394 180 0.57 7.7#	1317 678 0.72 41.2$	234 -353 -0.60 12.0$	0 -321 -1.00 16.9$	104 -395 -0.79 17.3$	28 -13 -0.33 0.2	0 -83 -1.00 4.1*	236 124 0.75 6.9#	410 -265 -0.39 6.1*	17 -121 -0.88 5.4*	329 147 0.54 5.0*	922 514 0.85 34.7$	38 -83 -0.69 2.9	4029
DQW2	21 -96 -0.82 3.1	64 -288 -0.82 10.4#	732 407 0.36 22.2$	17 -159 -0.90 5.8*	1103 827 0.86 104.8$	0 -22 -1.00 0.9	102 56 0.34 2.5	0 -61 -1.00 2.3	95 -277 -0.75 9.2#	52 -24 -0.32 0.3	0 -99 -1.00 3.9*	23 -201 -0.90 7.5#	14 -52 -0.79 1.6	2223
DQW3	31 -96 -0.76 2.0	58 -324 -0.85 12.5$	170 -182 -0.52 4.2*	728 535 0.88 61.3$	12 -287 -0.96 11.0$	57 32 0.40 1.6	72 21 0.14 0.4	17 -49 -0.75 1.5	994 589 0.46 39.0$	225 141 0.54 9.4#	0 -108 -1.00 4.3*	18 -226 -0.93 8.9#	35 -37 -0.52 0.8	2417
DQX	85 14 0.03 0.1	147 -63 -0.30 0.8	324 130 0.11 3.4	53 -52 -0.50 0.0	22 -142 -0.87 4.7*	19 5 0.06 ...	35 7 0.04 0.1	24 -12 -0.35 0.2	178 -44 -0.20 0.4	52 6 0.02 0.0	123 63 0.16 2.3	50 -84 -0.63 1.0	216 176 0.67 26.3$	1328
SUM	531	1586	1460	798	1241	104	209	277	1677	346	452	1013	303	

DR-Bf ($N = 102$)▼

	DR1	DR2	DR3	DR4	DR7	DRW8	DRW9	DRW10	DRW11	DRW12	DRW13	DRW14	DRX	SUM
BF S	458 142 0.38 1.3	392 -13 -0.04 0.0	686 9 0.01 0.0	490 84 0.18 0.4	386 -137 -0.26 0.8	0 0 0.00 ...	98 8 0.07 0.0	196 15 0.07 0.0	588 -269 -0.31 1.0	294 113 0.54 1.4	262 -8 -0.03 0.0	621 16 0.02 0.0	136 46 0.44 0.5	4607
BF F	228 -127 -0.36 1.1	490 32 0.08 0.1	686 -77 -0.10 0.2	392 -65 -0.14 0.2	752 161 0.29 1.0	0 0 0.00 ...	98 -3 -0.04 0.0	196 -7 -0.04 0.0	1274 307 0.34 2.5	98 -105 -0.52 1.2	326 21 0.07 0.0	654 -27 -0.04 0.0	0 -100 -1.00 2.2	5194
BFF1	0 -6 -1.00 ...	0 -8 -1.00 ...	98 84 1.00 ...	0 -8 -1.00 ...	0 -10 -1.00 ...	0 0 0.00 ...	0 -1 -1.00 ...	0 -3 -1.00 ...	0 -17 -1.00 ...	0 -3 -1.00 ...	0 -5 -1.00 ...	0 -12 -1.00 ...	0 -1 -1.00 ...	98
BFS07	0 -6 -1.00 ...	0 -8 -1.00 ...	0 -13 -1.00 ...	0 -8 -1.00 ...	0 -10 -1.00 ...	0 0 0.00 ...	0 -1 -1.00 ...	0 -3 -1.00 ...	0 -17 -1.00 ...	0 -3 -1.00 ...	0 -5 -1.00 ...	39 26 0.31 ...	59 57 0.59 ...	98
BF V	0 0 0.00 ...	0 0 0.00 ...	0 0 0.00 ...	0 0 0.00 ...	0 0 0.00 ...	0 0 0.00 ...	0 0 0.00 ...	0 0 0.00 ...	0 0 0.00 ...	0 0 0.00 ...	0 0 0.00 ...	0 0 0.00 ...	0 0 0.00 ...	0
SUM	686	882	1470	882	1138	0	196	392	1862	392	588	1314	195	

Reference Tables of Three-Locus Haplotype Frequencies and Delta Values in Caucasians, Orientals, and Negroids*

M.P. Baur[1], M. Neugebauer[1], and E.D. Albert[2]

1 Biometrical Department, Diabetes Research Institute, Auf'm Hennekamp 65, 4000 Düsseldorf, Federal Republic of Germany
2 Laboratory of Immunogenetics, Pettenkoferstr. 8 a, 8000 München 2, Federal Republic of Germany

The frequencies given were determined by haplotype counting based on the results of the FAP [1]. The selection criteria were the same as those used for the production of the gene frequencies and the two-point haplotype frequencies [2].
We have listed the most common frequencies together with the delta values, which were calculated as described by Baur and Danilovs [3]. Significance testing by way of 2×2×2 chi squares is problematic with respect to the three-way delta. For a discussion of the problem of significance testing of higher-order interactions, see Baur et al. [4]. Only haplotypes which were found at least three times in the respective sample were included in the tables.

* Supported by Deutsche Forschungsgemeinschaft grant Al 92/13-2, and Ba 660/5-1

References

1. Neugebauer M, Willems J, Baur MP (1984) Analysis of multilocus pedigree data by computer (this volume)
2. Baur MP, Neugebauer M, Albert E (1984) Reference tables of two-locus haplotype frequencies for all NHC marker loci (this volume)
3. Baur MP, Danilovs JA (1980) Population analysis of HLA-A, B, C, DR and other genetic markers. In: Terasaki PI (ed) Histocompatibility testing 1980. UCLA Tissue Typing Laboratory, Los Angeles, pp 955–994
4. Baur MP, Neugebauer M, Deppe H, Sigmund M, Luton T, Mayr WR, Albert E (1984) Population analysis on the basis of deduced haplotypes from random families (this volume)

Three-locus haplotype frequencies (per 10 000) in Caucasians

HLA-A, C, B ($n = 2065$)

Haplotype HLA- A	C	B	Haplotype frequency	Delta value
2	w2	27	68	5
11	w3	w55	52	37
2	w3	w60	177	63
2	w3	w62	226	52
24	w3	w62	111	46
2	w4	35	151	78
3	w4	35	227	86
11	w4	35	189	101
24	w4	35	125	26
2	w5	44	332	145
2	w6	13	74	0
30	w6	13	112	90
1	w6	37	73	47
1	w6	w57	158	105
2	w6	w57	51	−22
1	w7	7	66	−82
2	w7	7	234	−16
3	w7	7	378	156
24	w7	7	127	24
1	w7	8	512	247
2	w7	8	92	−72
2	w7	18	100	56
2	w7	44	50	−14
3	w8	w65	61	24
w33	w8	w65	58	51

HLA-A, B, DR ($n = 1889$)

Haplotype HLA- A	B	DR	Haplotype frequency	Delta value
2	w62	4	86	25
2	13	7	55	2
30	13	7	83	59
2	44	7	57	−37
29	44	7	111	76
1	w57	7	101	59
2	18	w11	84	33
24	35	w11	53	23
24	35	w11	53	23
2	44	w11	61	19
3	35	1	133	72
11	35	1	79	43
2	7	2	127	− 9
3	7	2	260	115
24	7	2	69	3
25	18	2	69	44
2	44	2	62	9
1	8	3	477	280
2	8	3	74	−98
3	7	4	50	−12
2	51	w11	78	18
2	w62	w11	53	10

Histocompatibility Testing 1984
Edited by E. D. Albert et al.

Three-locus haplotype frequencies (per 10 000) in Caucasians

HLA-A, C, DR ($n = 1897$)

Haplotype HLA-			Haplotype frequency	Delta value
A	C	DR		
2	w3	2	60	3
2	w3	4	116	10
2	w3	w11	71	0
3	w4	1	116	57
11	w4	1	81	44
2	w5	4	130	46
1	w6	7	121	38
2	w6	7	134	15
30	w6	7	76	42
1	w7	2	66	-51
2	w7	2	202	30
3	w7	2	226	73
24	w7	2	72	- 6
1	w7	3	353	157
1	w7	4	51	-10
2	w7	4	99	3
2	w7	w11	88	13

HLA-C, B, DR ($n = 1869$)

Haplotype HLA-			Haplotype frequency	Delta value
C	B	DR		
w3	w60	4	82	30
w3	w62	2	55	-16
w3	w62	4	142	62
w3	w62	w11	89	22
w4	35	1	263	138
w4	35	2	83	-40
w4	35	4	70	-32
w4	35	w11	118	6
w4	35	w13	52	5
w4	35	w14	51	2
w4	44	7	66	39
w5	18	3	83	66
w5	44	4	196	108
w5	44	w11	60	- 7
w6	13	7	185	129
w6	w57	7	171	116
w7	7	1	55	15
w7	7	2	471	196
w7	7	4	129	12
w7	7	w11	66	-30
w7	7	w14	53	5
w7	8	3	544	280
w7	18	w11	70	31
w8	w64	7	59	43
w8	w65	1	96	65

HLA-DR, C4A, C4B ($n = 502$)

Haplotype HLA-			Haplotype frequency	Delta value
DR	C4A	C4B		
1	3	1	241	3
1	2	Q0	83	41
1	3	Q0	146	- 29
2	3	1	1210	50
2	4	2	94	32
2	3	3	120	23
3	3	1	477	-183
3	Q0	1	563	131
3	3	Q0	104	40
4	3	1	763	- 41
4	4	2	139	75
4	3	3	80	15
4	3	Q0	272	6
7	3	1	842	- 84
7	6	1	278	64
7	Q0	1	112	- 29
w8	3	1	104	6
w11	3	1	959	51
w12	3	1	101	14
w13	3	1	241	0
w13	3	Q0	111	21
w14	3	1	195	- 19
w14	3	Q0	80	16

Three-locus haplotype frequencies (per 10 000) in Orientals

HLA-A, C, B ($n=943$)

Haplotype HLA- A	C	B	Haplotype frequency	Delta value
2	w1	w46	236	114
2	w1	w54	169	−25
11	w1	w54	95	10
24	w1	w54	334	101
11	w1	w55	64	34
2	w3	13	61	21
2	w3	35	232	32
24	w3	35	169	− 2
w33	w3	w58	152	97
2	w3	w60	102	1
24	w3	w60	120	26
2	w3	w61	144	−49
24	w3	w61	201	21
26	w3	w61	119	33
w31	w3	w61	51	12
2	w3	w62	95	−20
24	w3	w62	157	47
26	w3	w62	99	35
2	w4	35	59	− 1
24	w4	35	74	13
11	w4	w62	106	69
30	w6	13	184	164
2	w7	7	64	−38
24	w7	7	218	82
2	w7	39	94	21
24	w7	39	61	7

HLA-A, B, DR ($n=736$)

Haplotype HLA- A	B	DR	Haplotype frequency	Delta value
24	7	1	251	123
2	7	1	54	−42
2	35	2	68	17
24	w52	2	428	202
w33	w58	3	59	50
2	35	4	160	24
11	35	4	77	26
24	35	4	80	−47
2	39	4	54	13
2	51	4	61	23
24	51	4	68	− 3
24	w52	4	58	−48
2	w54	4	92	−34
11	w54	4	68	− 1
24	w54	4	261	80
2	w59	4	54	18
2	w61	4	80	− 4
24	w61	4	91	25
11	w62	4	95	28
30	13	7	125	114
2	w46	w8	62	25
31	51	w8	68	48
2	w46	w9	83	31
2	w61	w9	117	0
24	w61	w9	59	−36
26	w61	w9	93	44
2	w62	w9	57	− 2
2	w61	w11	54	28
w33	w44	w13	152	115
w33	w44	w14	200	140

Three-locus haplotype frequencies (per 10 000) in Orientals

HLA-A, C, DR ($n = 745$)

Haplotype HLA- A	C	DR	Haplotype frequency	Delta value
2	w1	2	80	19
24	w1	2	66	−35
2	w1	4	178	−54
11	w1	4	97	− 7
24	w1	4	337	85
26	w1	4	54	9
2	w1	w8	113	40
2	w1	w9	82	−13
24	w1	w11	50	15
2	w3	2	95	− 3
11	w3	2	54	34
24	w3	2	94	−49
w33	w3	3	70	46
2	w3	4	178	−13
24	w3	4	191	14
26	w3	4	75	1
31	w3	4	53	3
24	w3	w8	56	17
2	w3	w9	171	6
24	w3	w9	77	−23
26	w3	w9	96	18
2	w3	w12	109	4
24	w3	w12	90	10
2	w4	4	80	3
11	w4	4	108	57
30	w6	7	136	124
2	w7	1	67	−24
24	w7	1	220	96
2	w7	2	71	28
24	w7	4	57	− 4

HLA-C, B, DR ($n = 731$)

Haplotype HLA- C	B	DR	Haplotype frequency	Delta value
w1	w46	w8	90	57
w1	w46	w9	76	33
w1	w54	2	68	−27
w1	w54	4	449	208
w1	w54	w14	68	12
w1	w55	w9	50	20
w1	w59	4	95	56
w3	13	w12	54	29
w3	35	2	107	20
w3	35	4	243	56
w3	35	w9	86	1
w3	35	w12	78	14
w3	w58	3	85	59
w3	w60	w12	59	25
w3	w60	w14	50	27
w3	w61	4	123	9
w3	w61	w8	99	50
w3	w61	w9	126	− 6
w3	w62	2	86	30
w3	w62	4	68	−24
w3	w62	w9	114	35
w4	35	4	87	20
w4	w62	4	136	81

Three-locus haplotype frequencies (per 10 000) in Negroids

HLA-A, C, B ($n=336$)

Haplotype HLA- A	C	B	Haplotype frequency	Delta value
2	w2	w72	131	51
23	w2	w72	105	50
11	w2	35	119	87
24	w4	35	119	76
w36	w4	w53	202	150
28	w6	w58	120	46
3	w6	w58	97	38
2	w7	7	214	47
1	w7	8	249	146
2	w7	w58	100	50

HLA-A, B, DR ($n=286$)

Haplotype HLA- A	B	DR	Haplotype frequency	Delta value
2	7	2	105	23
3	7	2	123	52
1	8	3	280	192
30	w42	3	254	143
28	w64	7	105	75
2	w58	w11	116	69
28	w58	w14	105	68

HLA-C, B, DR ($n=289$)

Haplotype HLA- C	B	DR	Haplotype frequency	Delta value
w2	w72	7	111	52
w2	w72	w11	174	89
w3	7	2	103	55
w4	35	1	104	65
w4	35	w14	103	50
w4	44	7	107	77
w4	w53	w11	130	59
w5	44	4	104	86
w6	w58	w11	129	11
w6	w58	w14	209	107
w7	7	1	104	33
w7	7	2	321	102
w7	7	w13	104	50
w7	8	3	270	138
w7	49	w11	138	75
w7	w58	w11	120	38
w8	w64	7	128	103

Index of Authors

The page numbers indicate the articles to which each author has contributed

www.ingramcontent.com/pod-product-compliance
Ingram Content Group UK Ltd.
Pitfield, Milton Keynes, MK11 3LW, UK
UKHW051840180926
475695UK00004B/125
9783642697722